Growth Disorders

Second Edition

Christopher J. H. Kelnar
Professor of Paediatric Endocrinology
University of Edinburgh, UK

Martin O. Savage
Professor of Paediatric Endocrinology
Barts and the London School of Medicine and Dentistry, UK

Paul Saenger
Professor of Pediatrics
Albert Einstein College of Medicine, USA

Chris T. Cowell
Clinical Associate Professor, Director of Clinical Research, and Head
Institute of Endocrinology and Diabetes
University of Sydney, Australia

Hodder Arnold
A MEMBER OF THE HODDER HEADLINE GROUP

First published in Great Britain in 1998 by Chapman & Hall
This second edition published in 2007 by
Hodder Arnold, an imprint of Hodder Education and a member of the
Hodder Headline Group, an Hachette Livre UK Company
338 Euston Road, London NW1 3BH

www.hoddereducation.com

Whilst the advice and information in this book are believed to be true and
accurate at the date of going to press, neither the author[s] nor the
publisher can accept any legal responsibility or liability for any errors or
omissions that may be made. In particular (but without limiting the
generality of the preceding disclaimer) every effort has been made to
check drug dosages; however it is still possible that errors have been
missed. Furthermore, dosage schedules are constantly being revised and
new side-effects recognized. For these reasons the reader is strongly
urged to consult the drug companies' printed instructions before
administering any of the drugs recommended in this book.

British Library Cataloguing in Publication Data
A catalogue record for this book is available from the British Library

Library of Congress Cataloging-in-Publication Data
A catalog record for this book is available from the Library of Congress

ISBN   978 0 340 81240 2

1 2 3 4 5 6 7 8 9 10

Commissioning Editor: Sarah Burrows
Project Editor: Francesca Naish
Production Controller: Joanna Walker
Cover Designer: Helen Townson
Indexer: Laurence Errington

Typeset in 10/12 Minion by Charon Tec Ltd (A Macmillan Company), Chennai, India
www.charontec.com
Printed and bound in Italy

What do you think about this book? Or any other Hodder Arnold
title? Please visit our website: www.hoddereducation.com

Contents

Contributors

M. Lynn Ahmed
Department of Paediatrics
University of Cambridge
Addenbrooke's Hospital
Cambridge
UK

S. Faisal Ahmed
Consultant Paediatric Endocrinologist
Honorary Senior Lecturer
Department of Child Health
Royal Hospital For Sick Children
Glasgow
UK

Jesús Argente
Professor and Chief of Pediatrics
Department of Endocrinology
Hospital Infantil Universitario Nino Jesus
Department of Paediatrics
University Autonoma of Madrid

Swati Banerjee MD
Pediatric Endocrinology
Children's Hospital Central California
Madera
USA

Jennifer A. Batch
Professor of Pediatrics and Child Health
University of Queensland
Royal Children's Hospital
Herston
Australia

Louise A. Baur MBBS BSc (Med) PhD FRACP
Professor of Paediatrics and Child Health
University of Sydney
Australia

R. Mark Beattie
Consultant Paediatric Gastroenterologist
Honorary Senior Lecturer
Paediatric Medical Unit
Southampton General Hospital
Southampton
UK

V. Beauloye MD PhD
Unit of Pediatric Endocrinology
School of Medicine
Catholic University of Louvain
Brussels
Belgium

Barry B. Bercu MD
Professor, Departments of Pediatrics, Molecular Pharmacology
and Physiology
University of South Florida College of Medicine
Tampa
and
ALL Children's Hospital
St Petersburg
Florida
USA

Fabio Broglio MD PhD
Division of Endocrinology
Department of Internal Medicine
University of Turin
Turin
Italy

Mark F. H. Brougham
Specialist Registrar in Paediatric Oncology
Department of Paediatric Haematology and Oncology
Royal Hospital for Sick Children
Edinburgh
UK

John M. H. Buckler DM DSc FRCP FRCPCH DCH
Honorary Senior Lecturer
Department of Paediatrics & Child Health
Leeds General Infirmary
Leeds
UK

Stef van Buuren
Professor of Applied Statistics in Prevention
TNO Quality of Life
Leiden
The Netherlands

Cecilia Camacho-Hübner
Department of Endocrinology
St Bartholomew's Hospital
London
UK

Noël Cameron MSc PhD Cbiol FIBiol
Professor of Human Biology
Department of Human Sciences
Loughborough University
Loughborough
UK

Julie A. Chowen PhD
Department of Endocrinology
Hospital Infantil Universitario Niño Jesús
Madrid
Spain

Melissa Colsman
Child Behavioral Health
Department of Pediatrics
University of Michigan
Ann Arbor
USA

Chris Cowell
Clinical Associate Professor,
University of Sydney
Director of Clinical Research
Head, Institute of Endocrinology and Diabetes
The Children's Hospital at Westmead
Westmead
Australia

Henriette A. Delemarre–van de Waal PhD
Professor in Pediatric Endocrinology
Department of Pediatrics
VU University Medical Center
Amsterdam
The Netherlands

Elizabeth Denney–Wilson
Post-Doctoral Fellow
New South Wales Centre for Overweight and Obesity
University of Sydney
Australia

Frank B. Diamond MD
Professor
University of South Florida College of Medicine
Tampa
USA

Malcolm D. C. Donaldson
Department of Child Health
Royal Hospital for Sick Children
Glasgow
UK

Amanda J. Drake
Senior Lecturer
Department of Child Life and Health
University of Edinburgh
Edinburgh
UK

Stenvert L. S. Drop MD PhD
Professor
Sophia Children's Hospital
Erasmus Medical Center
Rotterdam
The Netherlands

David B. Dunger MB BS DCH MRCP MD FRCP FRCPCH
Professor of Paediatrics
Department of Paediatrics
University of Cambridge
Addenbrooke's Hospital
Cambridge
UK

Leo Dunkel
Professor of Paediatrics
Kuopio University Hospital
and
University of Kuopio
Kuopio
Finland

Laura M. Frago
Contracted Professor
Department of Endocrinology
Hospital Infantil Universitario Nino Jesus
Department of Paediatrics
University Autonoma of Madrid

Oliver Fricke MD
Universitöts-Kinderklinik
Köln
Germany

Ezio Ghigo
Endocrine Division
Department of Medicine
University of Turin
Turin
Italy

Jane Gilmour
Behavioural Sciences Unit
Institute of Child Health
University College London
London
UK

John M. Graham, Jr. MD ScD
Professor of Pediatrics
David Geffen School of Medicine at UCLA
Director of Clinical Genetics and Dysmorphology
Director of Clinical Training in Medical Genetics
Cedars-Sinai Medical Center
Los Angeles
USA

Ristan M. Greer
Discipline of Paediatrics and Child Health
University of Queensland
Royal Children's Hospital
Herston
Australia

Melvin M. Grumbach MD DM Hon causa (University of Geneva)
D Hon Causa (University René Descartes, Paris)
Edward B. Shaw Professor of Pediatrics
Emeritus Chairman
Department of Pediatrics
University of California
San Francisco
USA

Annette Grüters
Zentrum für Kinder und Jugendmedizin
Der Humboldt-Universität
Berlin
Germany

Lars Hagenäs MD PhD
Pediatric Endocrine Unit
Pediatric Clinic
Karolinska Institute and University Hospital
Stockholm
Sweden

Katerina Harwood
Division of Pediatric Endocrinology
Montefiore Medical Center
New York
USA

Peter C. Hindmarsh
Professor of Paediatric Encrinology
Developmental Encrinology Research Group
Molecular Genetics Unit
Institute of Child Health
University College London
London
UK

Raymond L. Hintz MD
Professor Emeritus
Department of Pediatrics
Stanford University School of Medicine
Stanford
USA

Ze'ev Hochberg MD PhD
Professor of Pediatrics
Division of Endocrinology
Meyer Children's Hospital
Rambam Medical Center
Technicon–Israel Institute of Technology
Haifa
Israel

Jeff M. P. Holly
Professor of Clinical Sciences
Department of Clinical Science at North Bristol
University of Bristol
Southmead Hospital
Bristol
UK

Linda B. Johnston
Clinical Senior Lecturer in Paediatric Endocrinology
Centre for Endocrinology
Barts and the London Queen Mary School of Medicine
London
UK

Christopher J. H. Kelnar
Professor of Paediatric Endocrinology
University of Edinburgh
Edinburgh
UK

Professor J. M. Ketelslegers MD PhD
Unit of Diabetes and Nutrition
School of Medicine
Catholic University of Louvain
Brussels
Belgium

Ralph S. Lachman
County of Los Angeles Department of Health Services
Harbor-UCLA Medical Center
Torrance
USA

Ann Christin Lindgren
Pediatric Endocrinology Unit
Department of Woman and Child Health
Astrid Lindgrens Children's Hospital
Karolinska Hospital
Stockholm
Sweden

Malcolm F. MacNicol
Consultant Orthopaedic Surgeon
Royal Hospital for Sick Children
Edinburgh
UK

M. Maes MD PhD
Professor
Unit of Pediatric Endocrinology
School of Medicine
Catholic University of Louvain
Brussels
Belgium

D. Maiter MD PhD
Professor
Unit of Diabetes and Nutrition
School of Medicine
Catholic University of Louvain
Brussels
Belgium

Joan diMartino-Nardi MD
Department of Pediatrics
Division of Pediatric Encorinology
Albert Einstein College of Medicine
New York
USA

Geert R. Mortier MD PhD
Department of Medical Genetics
Ghent University Hospital
Ghent
Belgium

Sabine M. P. F. de Muinck Keizer Schönau
Assistant Professor
Sophia Children's Hospital
Erasmus Medical Center
Rotterdam
The Netherlands

Primus E. Mullis
Paediatric Encrinology/Diabetology and Metabolism
University Children's Hospital
University of Bern
Bern
Switzerland

Wendy Paterson MSC
Auxologist
Department of Child Health
Royal Hospital for Sick Children
Glasgow
UK

Michael A. Patton
Professor
Reader in Medical Genetics
St George's Hospital Medical School
London
UK

Michael A. Preece
Biochemistry, Endocrinology and Metabolism Unit
Institute of Child Health
University College London
London
UK

Palany Raghupathy MD DCH FRCP
Senior Consultant in Paediatric Endocrinology and
Director of Academic Studies
Sagar Apollo Hospital
Bangalore
India
and
Former Professor of Paediatrics and Head
Department of Child Health
Christian Medical College Hospital
Vellore
India

Nazneen Rahman MA BM BCh MRCP PhD
Professor of Human Genetics
Institute of Cancer Research
Sutton
UK

Michael B. Ranke MD, FRCP (Edin)
Section Paediatric Endocrinology
Universitats-Kinderklinik
Tubingen
Germany

David L. Rimoin MD PhD
Professor of Pediatrics, Medicine and Human Genetics
David Geffen School of Medicine at UCLA
Steven Spielberg Chair of Pediatrics
Director, Medical Genetics-Birth Defects Center
Cedars-Sinai Medical Center
Los Angeles
USA

Ron Rosenfeld
Senior Vice-President for Medical Affairs
Lucile Packard Foundation for Children's Health
Stanford University
and
Professor of Pediatrics
Professor of Cell and Developmental Biology
Oregon Health and Sciences University
Portland
USA

Paul Saenger
Professor of Pediatrics
Division of Pediatric Endocrinology
Albert Einstein College of Medicine
New York
USA

Vincenzo de Sanctis
Department of Reproduction and Growth
Ferrara
Italy

David E. Sandberg PhD
Director of Child Behavioural Health
Department of Pediatrics
University of Michigan
Ann Arbor
USA

Martin O. Savage
Professor of Paediatric Endocrinology
Department of Endocrinology
Barts and the London School of Medicine and Dentistry
London
UK

Franz Schaefer MD
Professor of Pediatrics
Head, Division of Pediatric Nephrology
Director, KfH Kidney Center for Children and Adolescents
Hospital for Pediatric and Adolescent Medicine
Heidelberg
Germany

Eckhard Schönau
Universitöts-Kinderklinik
Köln
Germany

David Skuse
Professor of Behavioural and Brain Sciences
Behavioural and Brain Sciences Unit
Institute of Child Health
University College London
UK
and
Honorary Consultant at Great Ormond Street Hospital for Sick Children
Head of Social Communication Disorders Clinic
Great Ormond Street Hospital for Sick Children
London
UK

Olle Söder MD PhD
Professor and Chairman
Department of Woman and Child Health
Pediatric Endocrinology Unit
Karolinska Institutet and University Hospital
Stockholm
Sweden

Helen L. Storr MD PhD
Department of Endocrinology
Barts and the London School of Medicine and Dentistry
London
UK

J. P. Thissen MD PhD
Professor
Unit of Diabetes and Nutrition
School of Medicine

Catholic University of Louvain
Brussels
Belgium

Dov Tiosano MD
Division of Endocrinology
Meyer Children's Hospital
Ramban Medical Center
Haifa
Israel

L. E. Underwood MD PhD
Professor
Division of Pediatric Endocrinology
School of Medicine
University of North Carolina
Chapel Hill
USA

Jerry K. H. Wales DM MA BM BCh MRCP FRCPCH (Hon) DCH (Hon)
Senior Lecturer in Paediatric Endocrinology
Child Health
Sheffield Children's Hospital
Sheffield
UK

W. Hamish B. Wallace
Consultant Paediatric Oncologist
Departments of Paediatric Haematology & Oncology
Royal Hospital for Sick Children
Edinburgh
UK

Jan-Maarten Wit
Professor of Pediatrics
Department of Paediatrics
Leiden University Medical Center
Leiden
The Netherlands

Beatrix Wonke
Former Consultant Haematologist
Thalassaemia Services
The Whittington Hospital
London

Katie Woods MBBS MRCP MD
Assistant Professor of Pediatric Endocrinology
Department of Pediatrics
Doernbechers Children's Hospital
Portland
USA

Elke Wühl
Consultant Pediatric Nephrologist
Division of Pediatric Nephrology
Hospital for Pediatric and Adolescent Medicine
Heidelberg
Germany

Foreword

The advances in knowledge of the hormonal and environmental influences on human growth and maturation are a landmark in human biology and medicine. About five decades ago growth hormone was purified from human pituitaries and the first growth hormone-deficient patient was treated with human growth hormone (hGH). Concurrently, the revolution in molecular biology and genetics began, introducing terms such as genomics, proteomics, transcriptomics, metabolomics, epigenetics, and systems analysis. The first mutation in the human 'growth hormone cascade' was detected over 25 years ago. The completion of the Human Genome Project, a monumental achievement, promises to facilitate identification of single gene mutations that affect growth, as well as to unravel the molecular interactions of multiple gene products that regulate diverse aspects of growth. These developments should lead to advances in the specificity of diagnosis and treatment of disordered growth.

Clinical studies and trials are exploring the potential role of hGH and IGF-1 in treatment of a variety of conditions associated with impaired growth. The prevalence of growth hormone deficiency is about 1 in 3,500 children, but about 3 percent of infants are born small for gestational age (SGA) and are at risk for the 'metabolic syndrome' in adolescence or adulthood. Human growth hormone treatment of SGA children is increasingly used to improve long-term growth.

This timely volume, 'Growth Disorders,' is to my mind the most balanced, comprehensive, insightful, and definitive treatment available on normal growth and the broad range of conditions, disorders, and diseases that may impair or increase linear growth in infancy, childhood, and adolescence. The study of human growth and puberty and their disorders and the hormonal, genetic, and environmental factors that affect growth is the mother's milk of pediatric endocrinology, and addresses fundamental biologic processs. The four distinguished Editors have enlisted authoritative, eminent contributors largely from the United Kingdom and Europe, representing a wide range of disciplines and expertise.

The book is divided into five sections as follows: 1) Physiology of Linear Growth; 2) Growth Assessment; 3) Chronic Pediatric Disorders and Management of the Associated Growth Disturbance; 4) Endocrine Causes of Abnormal Growth; and 5) Treatment of Growth Disorders. The chapters in each of these sections are current and provocative. The reader may find the "Key Learning Points" section highlighted at the end of each chapter a useful starting point. Symbols in the bibliography identify prismatic papers and key review articles.

Controversial issues in the diagnosis of growth disorders and their treatment are addressed in a lucid, balanced, readable, concise, and provocative manner. In discussing broad aspects the authors have presented the reader with their well-considered opinions and recommendations emanating from their experience and knowledge. Throughout the book, psychosocial issues of growth disorders are presented.

The advances in this field of the life sciences and of clinical pediatrics are legion, leading to an explosive advancement of knowledge in fundamental aspects of growth. These advances, including molecular, cellular and developmental biology, genetics and genomics, and new imaging techniques have advanced diagnosis and the assessment of therapies.

This book is an invaluable and compelling resource, a treasure trove of up-to-date knowledge and practical and useful clinical insight for physicians and other health professionals who care for infants, children, and adolescents.

Melvin M. Grumbach, M.D.
Department of Pediatrics
University of California San Francisco

Preface to the first edition

If you can look into the seeds of time,
And say which grain will grow and which will not...

William Shakespeare, Macbeth, Act 1 Scene 3.

Linear growth is a biological process which is of fundamental importance to the physical and psychological make up of a child and adolescent. It is a process that is, however, vulnerable to a wide range of insults. Patients with growth disorders, varying from the infant who fails to thrive to the emotionally stressed adolescent with delayed puberty, constitute a significant and fundamental part of the practice of clinical paediatrics.

On an individual basis, poor growth is the 'final common pathway' for many organic and emotional problems of childhood and growth monitoring is important in the early detection of childhood disease. In public health terms, growth assessment remains one of the most useful indices of health and economic well-being in both developing and socially heterogeneous developed countries.

In this book, we have sought to approach growth and growth disorders from physiological and pathophysiological standpoints respectively. Individual principal physiological mechanisms underlying normal growth are set out, as is their interrelationship which results in the complex and dynamic phenomenon of linear growth. The process of accurate growth assessment, fundamental for the detection and diagnosis of abnormal growth, is described in detail together with the often complex and multifaceted pathogenesis of growth disorders. Management of abnormal stature and growth is discussed in depth – a knowledge of what can and cannot be achieved by a particular treatment modality is crucial for a satisfactory outcome for the child or adolescent and his or her parents.

The book is divided into broad sections. First, historical and worldwide perspectives of human growth are described. This section provides the background to the descriptions of the physiological processes that modulate growth of the fetus, in infancy, childhood and adolescence. Contributors to this section include basic and molecular scientists, obstetricians and perinatologists, and paediatric and adult endocrinologists.

The section on growth assessment starts by defining abnormal growth and then covers the practical auxological, endocrinological, radiological and psychological aspects of patient assessment. The contributors are drawn from an appropriately wide range of disciplines including paediatric endocrinology, auxology, radiology and psychology.

The section on aetiology and management comprises approximately two-thirds of the book and continues to reflect a multidisciplinary approach across a wide range of medical subspecialties where there is wide experience of system-related growth disorders. All major physiological systems are covered, with an extended section concentrating on the endocrine basis of abnormal growth, seen principally by the paediatric endocrinologist.

A detailed account of management covers both short and tall stature and disorders of the timing of puberty. There are logical and evidence-based analyses of the various therapeutic options currently available. Both successes and disappointments are described objectively with contributions from oncologists, surgeons and endocrinologists.

Our aim has been to produce a wide-ranging, stimulating and balanced account of the challenging field of growth and growth disorders. We believe that the views of international specialists from a diverse background of scientific and clinical disciplines provide a challenging review of the major areas of concern and controversy in this field.

We hope that this book will enable a wide range of medical and paramedical practitioners to learn more about the subject of growth. Above all, we intend it to be a practical help and guide for the clinician to the diverse physical and emotional disorders in children which are associated with disturbances of linear growth, and to their appropriate investigation and management.

We are grateful to our many contributors and to Helen Heyes, Lara Wilson and Jane Sugarman of Chapman and Hall who have helped to guide the project to completion.

C.J.H. Kelnar, M.O. Savage, H.F. Stirling
and P. Saenger
Edinburgh, London, Coventry and New York
February 1998

Preface to the second edition

The questions are the same but the answers are different.

[allegedly said by Albert Einstein in response to a complaint from a student about why the examination questions were the same as those set the previous year]

Teach thy tongue to say 'I do not know' and thou shalt progress.

Maimonides 12thC AD

Since the first edition of this book there have been many developments in the understanding of growth disorders at the molecular, cellular and biochemical levels, and in their management. This extensively revised second edition reflects these advances and also the better evidence base for our treatments where this has become available over the last nine years. It is a pleasure to welcome a number of new authors for this edition and those retained have extensively revised their contributions to reflect this progress and the developing evidence base.

Understanding normal and abnormal growth remains as fundamental to the clinical practice of paediatrics and paediatric endocrinology as ever, despite or even because of such advances in the basic science underpinning growth and its perturbations, and the development of new treatment modalities. Once again, our aim has been to produce a wide-ranging, stimulating and balanced account of the challenging field of growth and growth disorders. Even now, managing growth disorders in children remains both a science and an art – many tests in paediatric endocrinology (not least tests of growth hormone secretory ability) give the least useful information when there is most uncertainty from a clinical assessment and vice versa. We still fall into the trap of thinking that because we can measure something (or think we can) it must be an important and relevant measurement: what we can measure easily is not necessarily more important than what we cannot.

Height is not a validated proxy for quality of life. We are still poor at measuring quality of life in children with chronic disorders or short stature or, conversely, at measuring the emotional cost of coping in psychological terms. Whilst non-compliance is the commonest reason for therapeutic failure, we are beginning to explore the underlying genetic differences between individuals that may affect outcome (pharmacogenomics).

We recognise that well designed randomised controlled trials in large enough cohorts of patients (requiring national and international cooperative research) are necessary to distinguish absence of effect from no effect and need to show potentially clinically (rather than just statistically) significant benefit. However, significant side effects and harm are not generally identifiable in such studies. Large scale long term surveillance is necessary and should be the responsibility of all clinicians involved in (for example) GH therapy in children whether or not such patients are being formally followed up and treated in adulthood.

Instead of 'knowing all the answers' we are now (perhaps) beginning to ask (some of) the right questions and admitting that a 'right' answer today may not be the right answer next year, let alone in another nine years from now.

We hope that this new edition will again prove a practical help and guide for the clinician to the diverse physical and emotional disorders in children that are associated with disturbances of linear growth, and to their appropriate investigation and management.

We are grateful to our many contributors, to Professor Melvin Grumbach for writing the Foreword to this edition and to Joanna Koster, Sarah Burrows, Naomi Wilkinson and Francesca Naish of Hodder Arnold who have helped to see this second edition through to completion.

C.J.H. Kelnar, M.O. Savage, P. Saenger and
C. Cowell

List of abbreviations used

aa	amino acid	CRH	corticotropin-releasing hormone
ACE	angiotensin-converting enzyme	CRI	chronic renal insufficiency
ACTH	adrenocorticotrophic hormone	CRP	c-reactive protein
ADHD	attention deficit hyperactivity disorder	CRSP	Collaborative Research Support Program
AGA	appropriate gestational age	CS	Cockayne syndrome
AGRP	Agouti-related peptide	CSF	cerebral spinal fluid
AHO	Albright hereditary osteodystrophy	CSH	chorionic somatomammotrophin pseudogene
AIS	androgen insensitive syndrome		
ALL	acute lymphoblastic leukemia	CT	computed tomography
ALP	alkaline phosphatase	CTS	constitutional tall stature
ALS	acid labile subunit		
ANP	atrial natriuretic peptide	DE	dopamine
AP	anteroposterior	DEB	diepoxybutane
APECED	autoimmune polyendocrinopathy– candidosis– ectodermal dystrophy	DEXA	dual X-ray absorptiometry
		DHEA	dihydroepiandrosterone
AUC	area under the curve		
AVV	arginine vasopressin	EDTA	European Dialysis and Transplant Association
BMI	body mass index	EGF	epidermal growth factor
BMP	bone morphogenic protein	EPO	erythropoietin
BMT	bone marrow transplantation	ESRD	end stage renal disease
BOCD	Blomstrand lethal osteochondrodysplasia		
BPD	bronchopulmonary dysplasia	FDA	Food and Drug Administration
		FFA	free fatty acid
CA	catecholamine	FGD	familial glucocorticoid deficiency
CAH	congenital adrenal hyperplasia	FGF	fibroblast growth factor
CART	cocaine-and-amphetamine-related transcript	FGFR	fibroblast growth factor receptor
		FISH	fluorescence *in situ* hybridization
CBCL	child behaviour checklist	FMPP	familial male precocious puberty
CCD	cleidocranial dysplasia	FSGS	focal segmental glomerulosclerosis
CDK	cyclin-dependent kinase	FSH	follicle-stimulating hormone
CDMP	cartilage-derived morphogenic protein	FSIVGTT	frequently sampled intravenous GTT (q.v.)
CFCS	cardiofaciocutaneous syndrome	FSS	familial short stature
CDGA	constitutional delay in adolescence		
CDGP	constitutional delay in puberty	GABA	gamma-amino butyric acid
CGD	constitutional delay in growth	GDF	growth and differentiation factor
CGH	comparative genomic hybridization	GFR	glomerular filtration rate
ChAT	choline acetyl transferase	GH	growth hormone
CHD	chromodomain helicase DNA-binding (gene)	GHD	growth hormone deficiency
		GHIF	growth hormone inhibiting factor
CHH	cartilage hair hypoplasia	GHIS	growth hormone insensitivity syndrome
CJD	Creutzfeld–Jacob disease	GHND	growth hormone neurosecretory dysfunction
CNS	central nervous system		
CNTF	ciliary neurotopic factor	GHRH	growth hormone releasing hormone
CPHD	combined pituitary hormone deficiency	GHRHR	growth hormone releasing hormone receptor
CPP	central precocious puberty		
CRF	chronic renal failure	GHRP-6	His-D-Trp-Ala-Trp-D-Phe -Lys-NH$_2$

GHS	growth hormone secretagogue		NAS	nonsense-mediated altered splicing
GIPP	gonadotropin-independent precocious puberty		NCDS	National Child Development Study
			NCGS	National Cooperative Growth Study
GLP	glucagen-like peptide		NCP	noncollagenous matrix protein
GLUT	glucose transporter		NE	norepinephrine
GnRH	gonadotropin-releasing hormone		NGF	nerve growth factor
GTT	glucose tolerance test		NHANES	National Health and Nutrition Examination Survey US
HCG	human chorionic gonadotropin		NIDDM	non-insulin-dependent diabetes mellitus
hGH	human growth hormone		NLSY	National Longitudinal Survey of Youth
HH	hypogonadotropic hypogonadism		NPY	neuropeptide Y
HPA	hypothalamic-pituitary-adrenal			
5-HT	5-hydroxytryptamine		OI	osteogenesis imperfecta
htSD	height standard deviation		OPPG	osteoporosis–pseudoglioma syndrome
IBD	inflammatory bowel disease		PA	premature adrenarche
ICP	infant–childhood–puberty (model)		PACAP	pituitary adenylate cyclase-activating peptide
IDDM	insulin-dependent diabetes mellitus		PAH	predicted adult height
IGFBP-3	insulin-like growth factor binding protein 3		PCOS	polycystic ovarian syndrome
IGF-I	insulin-like growth factor I		PCM	pre-cortical melanotroph
IGT	impaired glucose tolerance		PCR	polymerase chain reaction
IIH	idiopathic intracranial hypertension		PDGF	platelet-derived growth factor
IL-6	interleukin 6		PHM	peptide histidine–methionine
IMAGe syndrome	intrauterine growth restriction, metaphyseal dysplasia, adrenal hypoplasia congenita, genital abnormalities		PHP	pseudohypoparathyroidism
			POMC	pro-opiomelanocortin
			PNAH	primary nodular adrenal hyperplasia
INCAP	Institute of Nutrition of Central America and Panama		PP	pancreatic polypeptide
			PRA	plasma renin activity
IOTF	International Obesity Task Force		PRL	prolactin
ISS	idiopathic short stature		PSP	Psychosocial Screening Project
ITT	insulin tolerance test		PTH	parathyroid hormone
IUGR	intrauterine growth retardation		PTP	phosphotyrosin phosphatase
IVU	intravenous urography		PVN	paraventricular nucleus
			PWS	Prader–Willi syndrome
KIGS	Kabi International Growth Study			
			QOL	quality of life
LAP	latency-associated peptide			
LBM	lean body mass		rGH	recombinant growth hormone
LEPR	leptin receptor		RTA	renal tubule acidosis
LH	luteinizing hormone		RTS	Rubinstein–Taybi syndrome
LIFA	ligand-mediated immunofunctional assay			
LPS	lipopolysaccharide		SADDAN	severe achondroplasia with developmental delay and acanothis nigricans
LWPES	Lawson Wilkins Pediatric Endocrine Society			
			SCE	sister chromatid exchange
			SCFE	slipped capital femoral epiphysis
MAPK	mitogen-activated protein kinase			
MAS	McCune–Albright syndrome		SD	standard deviation
MCH	melanin-concentrating hormone		SDS	standard deviation score
MED	multiple epiphyseal dysplasia		SEDC	spondyloepiphyseal dysplasia congenita
MEPE	matrix extracellular phosphoglycoprotein		SEMD	spondylometa-epiphyseal dysplasia
MMC	mitomycin C		SES	socioeconomic status
MPS	mucopolysaccharidoses		SGA	small for gestational age
MRI	magnetic resonance imaging		SHBG	sex hormone binding globulin
			SHOX	short stature homeobox (gene)
NAFLD	non-alcoholic fatty liver disease		SLE	systemic lupus erythematosus
NAPRTCS	North Atlantic Pediatric Renal Transplant Registry		SOCS	suppressor of cytokine signaling
			SS	somatostatin

TBI	total-body irradiation	VEGF	vascular endothelial growth factor
TH	tyrosine hydroxylase	VHM	ventromedial nucleus
TmP	maximal tubular phosphate (transportation capacity)	VIP	vasoactive intestinal peptide
		VLBW	very low birth weight
TS	Turner syndrome		
TSH	thyroid-stimulating hormone	WHO	World Health Organization
		WRS	Wiedemann–Rautenstrauch syndrome
UC	ulcerative colitis		

1

Historical background and worldwide perspectives

MICHAEL A PREECE, NOËL CAMERON

UNDERSTANDING NORMAL GROWTH: THE AMERICAN AND EUROPEAN GROWTH STUDIES OF THE TWENTIETH CENTURY

By definition a growth disorder is a presentation of human growth that is outside the recognized limits of normality. Thus it could be argued that the ability to recognize a growth disorder depends completely on our ability to recognize the limits of normal growth. Modern research into human growth is generally accepted as being initiated by the encyclopedists of eighteenth century France, and in particular George Louis LeClerc, the Compte de Buffon.[1] Buffon's treatise on natural science (*Histoire Naturelle, Générale et Particulière*) contained a table of data (on page 77 of Supplement 14 published in 1778) recording the growth of the son of his friend and colleague Count Philibert Geuneau de Montbeillard. That record is thought to be the first serial study of human growth[2] and faithfully records a normal pattern of growth in height not dissimilar in any way from the growth of modern children (Fig. 1.1). However, it was not until the middle of the twentieth century that research on normal human growth and development had advanced to the degree that it was possible to identify and treat children who demonstrated abnormal growth.

To a large extent this timing was due to the initiation and development of a series of longitudinal growth studies in the USA. From 1904 to 1948, 17 such studies were started and 11 completed. Their complexity varied from the relatively simple elucidation of the development of height and weight to data yielding correlations between behavior, personality,

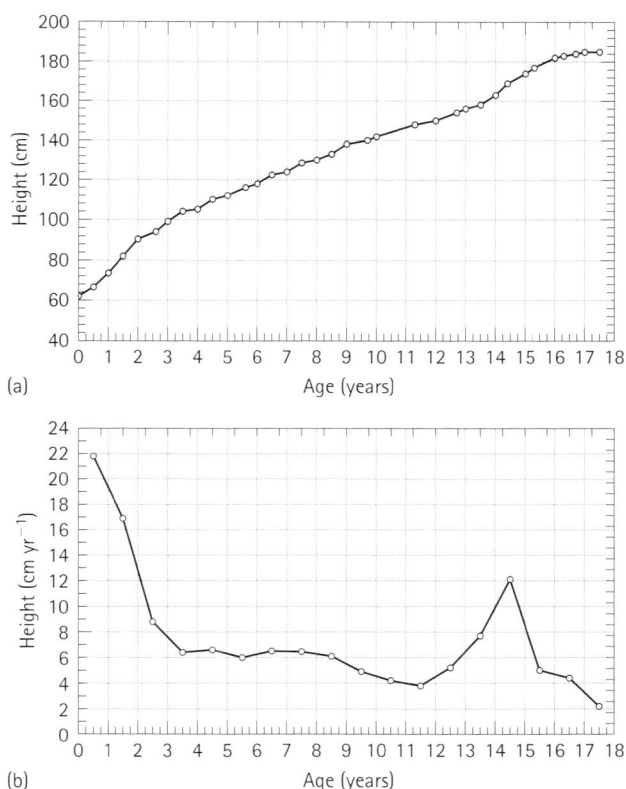

Figure 1.1 The growth of De Montbeillard's son 1759–1777. (a) Distance, (b) velocity. (Redrawn from Tanner JM. *Growth at Adolescence*, 2nd edn. Oxford: Blackwell Scientific Publications, 1962.)

social background, and physical development. By the 1950s these studies had reached a level of maturity sufficient for the data to be analyzed to demonstrate not simply the pattern of normal growth in a variety of physical dimensions but also the extent of normal variation. Thus, in 1959, it was possible for two American psychologists, Leona M. Bayer and Nancy Bayley, to publish a book entitled *Growth Diagnosis* in which they sought 'to convert selected segments of developmental data into simple techniques for appraising growth.'[3] We have no way of knowing how widely this information was disseminated but it seems reasonably certain that much of it stayed in the United States and was not widely recognized in Europe. After the Second World War, the European emergence of expertise on normal and thus abnormal human growth was linked to the rise of a group of scientists with backgrounds in clinical medicine, most commonly pediatrics, but research interests that encompassed biology and physiology and who possessed enough statistical knowledge to make sense of human variation. Such scientists, the natural academic offspring of the Encyclopedists of the Enlightenment, were, in the two decades following the Second World War, beginning to acquire positions of importance in Europe within the areas that would be critical to develop the diagnostic and treatment tools for abnormal growth and development.

In Europe, in particular, the appointment in 1945 of Professor (later Sir) Alan Moncrieff (1901–1971) to the directorship of the newly formed Institute of Child Health as the postgraduate medical school attached to the Hospital for Sick Children, Great Ormond Street, London, was critical in that he recognized the study of human growth as the basic science of pediatrics. Whilst Moncrieff's own interests were in respiratory diseases he encouraged a team of younger pediatricians who were developing expertise in child growth including James Tanner (1915–) and Frank Falkner (1918–2003). The former was invited to lead the newly formed Department of Growth and Development whilst the latter was assigned as Moncrieff's medical officer. Falkner's future was eventually to lie in the USA but between 1958 and 1962 he and Tanner were instrumental in coordinating a series of growth studies throughout western Europe.

In 1951 Tanner's Harpenden Growth Study had been running for 3 years and an expansion of interest in child growth was beginning to present possibilities for collaboration in continental Europe. Thus it was that a group of European pediatricians, that included Alan Moncrieff and James Tanner in London, Robert Debré (1883–1978) in Paris, Anders Wallgren (1889–1973) in Stockholm, and Guido Fanconi (1892–1979) and Andrea Prader (1919–2001) in Zurich created a coordinated series of child growth studies which eventually established the global importance of growth as a reflection of child health. In 1951 Frank Falkner was appointed to take charge of the London study and in 1953 he went to Paris to spend a year with Debré setting up the French study. During this time he played a leading role in creating the International Children's Centre (ICC) in Paris that coordinated the studies. The ICC started a series of coordination meetings under the care of

Dr Natalie Masse (1919–1975), which formed an important training ground for subsequent generations of pediatricians and non-clinical scientists. Every 2 or 3 years the members of the growth study teams would meet in Paris to exchange experiences and discuss results. In doing so they developed an expertise in the study of human growth that could not be bettered anywhere in the world. By the end of the twentieth century the names of the pediatricians and scientists involved were synonymous with various aspects of the clinical appraisal of normal and abnormal growth.

The fundamental problem in trying to describe human growth and development is that of variability. This variability is not only in the timing of the critical periods within the whole pattern of growth (e.g., puberty) but also in the magnitude and rate of change coincident with the period. In addition for a radical change in, say, height to occur there must also be changes in the anatomical parts that make up total height and these changes are themselves variable. Acceleration, for instance, in height velocity may be the result of different changes in the length of the spine, femur, and/or tibia each of which may contribute differently to the total process. In addition, not only may the process be variable within a single child it may also be variable between different children of the same or opposite sexes. The mathematical and statistical problems arising from the seemingly simple process of an increase in height are thus complex and their elucidation was reliant on the close collaboration of clinicians, biologists, and statistical mathematicians. Such collaboration does not seem to have been a characteristic of the earlier American studies.

Tanner[4] highlights the fact that the North American growth studies that pioneered our knowledge of normal growth had little or no influence on therapeutic pediatrics because the importance of growth as a reflection of health had not clearly been recognized and its implications for monitoring treatment remained unrealized in the middle of the twentieth century. 'Modern methods of auxology,' writes Tanner, 'came to be applied to the therapeutic field mostly after (Andrea) Prader had joined the International Children's Centre study of normal growth', and Tanner himself had returned (from physiology research) to clinical medicine to initiate the Growth Disorder Clinics at the Hospital for Sick Children, Great Ormond Street in 1963.

However, it would be wrong to dismiss the importance of the North American growth studies of the first half of the twentieth century to the development of therapeutic pediatrics. Although some significant studies were initiated by educational psychologists and developmental psychologists with philosophies relating to the 'whole child' (e.g., Iowa, Berkeley) many others (e.g., Denver, Harvard, Fels, Brush Foundation) were directed by pediatricians and/or anthropologists with a direct interest in the biology of normal growth and subsequently its disorders. Their contributions were numerous and sometimes fundamentally important. In 1923, for instance, the educational psychologist Bird T. Baldwin (1875–1928), Director of the Iowa Child Welfare Research and initiator of the Iowa longitudinal study, collaborated with Thomas D. Wood of the Life Extension Institute to develop growth reference charts based on representative samples of 130 000 American boys and girls. These 'Baldwin–Wood tables' were used as American growth standards for many years and superseded British or European charts by over 40 years (see below).[5] Prior to this Baldwin had created the first norms for pubertal changes based on the appearance of pubic hair in boys and a combination of breast development, menarche, and axillary hair in girls.[6] It would be over half a century before the Europeans would create norms for pubertal development[7] and these would be modifications and advances based on the work of the Americans Reynolds and Wines[8] and Nicholson and Hanley.[9] Baldwin was also responsible for the collection between 1918 and 1928 of hand–wrist radiographs on 1300 children aged from birth to 17 years that pioneered years of research into the development of accurate and sensitive methods to determine skeletal maturity. Later the psychologist Frank Shuttleworth (1899–1958) worked on data from the Harvard longitudinal growth study to develop an understanding of the importance of growth increment and particularly the concept of growth velocity that is fundamental to the diagnosis and treatment of growth disorders. Norms for growth 'velocity' would not appear in Europe for another 30 years. T. Wingate Todd's (1885–1938) studies of skeletal maturity in the Brush Foundation longitudinal study started in 1930, gave rise to the Greulich–Pyle Atlas methods for the assessment of skeletal maturity that are still in use almost 60 years after their conception.[10,11] It was not until the 1960s that bone-specific scoring methods for skeletal maturity assessment were developed in Europe.[12] The psychologist Nancy Bayley (1899–1994), who worked on the 1928 Berkeley Growth Study developed the widely used 'Bayley Scales of Infant Development' in addition to the Bayley–Pinneau technique for adult height prediction initially based on Todd's Atlas but later on the Greulich–Pyle Atlas of Skeletal Maturity.[13] Height prediction in Europe would not emerge until the late 1960s.

GROWTH DISORDER CLINICS

The North American studies before World War II did much to provide a basic understanding of the process of human growth and did much to influence the later development of the methods we now use to investigate the child with a suspected growth disorder. However, there is little doubt that the development of European experience in the diagnosis and treatment of children with growth disorders occurred essentially after the Second World War.

The classification of various abnormalities of growth has taken time. Now we recognize categories where growth is disordered secondary to endocrine disease, chronic inflammatory conditions, renal or gastrointestinal disease and a whole raft of dysmorphic syndromes. However, in the past there were only crude classifications – it is not that long since all-embracing terms such as dwarf or midget were common currency. Textbooks of the 1950s and 1960s still used these terms although there was certainly recognition of cretinism as a defined etiology with available treatment. By then also there was a beginning of understanding of dysmorphic syndromes which really started to develop with the publication of the first edition of Smith's classic *Recognisable Patterns of Human Malformation*.[14] Similarly, there have been advances in understanding the mechanisms underlying how non-endocrine chronic disease impacts on growth; this is developed more in Chapters 20–27.

The initiation of the international impetus to understand abnormalities of human growth is most accurately fixed in London University's Institute of Child Health in James Tanner's Department of Growth and Development during the 1960s and 1970s. In 1963 the first Growth Disorder Clinic was established at the Hospital for Sick Children, Great Ormond Street under the direction of Tanner who notes that 'a few years earlier M. Raben in Boston had for the first time successfully treated a child with growth hormone deficiency with human growth hormone.'[4] In fact, Maurice Raben's landmark publication in 1958[15] was to be the first of many American papers discussing human growth hormone treatment prior to the first research paper emanating from the London group in 1967. In 1962 Raben published a further two articles describing both the physiological aspects and clinical uses of growth hormone.[16,17] It was not a coincidence that the London growth clinics, in which so much excellent work was done in the advancement of treatment for children with growth disorders, was founded, at least in part, on the pioneering work of these American doctors. In 1967 the London team published the results on treating 26 children 'with short stature' with human growth hormone.[18] The growth hormone preparation was prepared by the Raben method.[19] Of the 26 children so treated only 16 were 'presumed hyposomatotrophic dwarfs', three had had craniopharyngiomas removed, two had rheumatoid arthritis and had been treated with large doses of steroids, and there was one case each of renal dwarfism, gonadal dysgenesis, and pinealoma. The remaining two children were probably normal short children. Tanner and Whitehouse reported catch-up growth in 10 of the 16 hyposomatotrophic dwarfs and the three craniopharyngioma patients with little or no real response, in terms of increased growth velocity, from the other categories. The London clinic was to spawn a series of 18 coordinated growth clinics throughout the UK within the next 15 years. No such national collaboration was apparent in the rest of Europe or the USA and thus by far the largest collection of children with growth disorders of various etiologies could be found by amalgamating the data from the UK growth disorder clinics.

The ability to diagnose and treat growth disorders depends on the availability of a variety of techniques that allow the accurate assessment of both the morphological and physiological status of the juvenile patient. Morphological techniques include appropriate growth charts, anthropometric methods, maturity assessment, and adult height prediction techniques. Physiological techniques include tests to stimulate the hypothalamic–pituitary axis and the ability to measure the subsequent release of a variety of pituitary hormones. We will consider each of these in what follows.

THE DEVELOPMENT OF GROWTH REFERENCE CHARTS

Henry Pickering Bowditch (1840–1911)[20] was the first to provide percentile charts for growth in height and weight of Boston children. He used the method described as 'Galton's percentile grades'. Francis Galton (1822–1911) was the first to demonstrate that the Laplace–Gauss distribution or the 'normal distribution' could be applied to human psychological attributes, including intelligence.[21] From this finding, he coined the use of percentile scores for measuring relative standing on various measurements in relation to the normal distribution.[22] This, of course, was ideal for illustrating growth in height because its adherence to a normal distribution from birth to adulthood. However, it was the Baldwin–Wood charts of 1925 (revised 1927) that were based on a representative sample of 74 000 boys and 55 000 girls from 12 schools in the eastern and central USA and could properly be described as the first American 'reference charts'.

The problem with many of the analyses of longitudinal data was that they were analyzed in a cross-sectional manner. The information on growth increments supplied by the longitudinality of the study design was ignored in favor of cross-sectionally calculated means of height or weight attained by age. Frank Shuttleworth (1899–1958), a psychologist from Iowa, was the first to develop growth charts that took account of the fact that children grew at individually different rates,[23] a phenomenon that Tanner[24] was later to call 'tempo of growth'. Shuttleworth's publications between 1934 and 1949 chronicle the first serious approach to understanding individual differences in the tempo of growth and how to illustrate for the purposes of assessing normality. Tanner[4] maintains that Shuttleworth 'never cast his data in a mould suitable for engendering practical standards' but the illustrations in these works clearly demonstrate how close Shuttleworth came to developing tempo-conditional references that were not going to be further developed for another 30 years.[25]

Nancy Bayley, using data from the Berkeley growth Study made the most significant advances of the next 20 years. In 1959, working with Leona M. Bayer, she published *Growth Diagnosis: Selected Methods for Interpreting and Predicting Physical Development From One Year to Maturity*.[3] This volume is divided into two parts. Part one deals with methodology and covers data collection, analysis and interpretation. Part two is a series of case histories of firstly normal children exhibiting different tempos of growth, and then a variety of disorders; giantism (*sic*), dwarfism, precocious menarche, obesity in boys, growth following castration in adolescent girls, growth in a hypogonadal boy, and female pseudohermaphrodism. The auxological techniques developed in the earlier American longitudinal studies are here organized for

the first time in a veritable workshop manual of the assessment and diagnosis of growth disorders. The anthropometric techniques (weight, height, sitting height, biacromial, and bi-iliac diameters) come from Stolz and Stolz's *Somatic Development of Adolescent Boys*.[26] They feature no measures of subcutaneous fat although Bayley later (p. 38) discusses normal fat distribution. Skeletal maturity uses the 'new' Greulich–Pyle Atlas technique for the hand and wrist only published earlier that year.[11] Nicholson and Hanley's[9] methods for assessing secondary sexual development (genitalia in boys, breasts and pubic hair in girls) are illustrated prior to an interesting and unusual series of illustrations of 'androgynic patterns of body form' (from hyper-feminine, through feminine, hypo-feminine, bisexual, hypo-masculine, masculine, and hyper-masculine). Height prediction using the recent Bayley–Pinneau tables[13] precedes the section on 'height and weight curves'.

These are not entitled as standards or references for growth because they are indeed a variety of different curves or patterns of growth (Fig. 1.2). Curves for 'accelerated' and 'retarded' children are above and below those of average rate

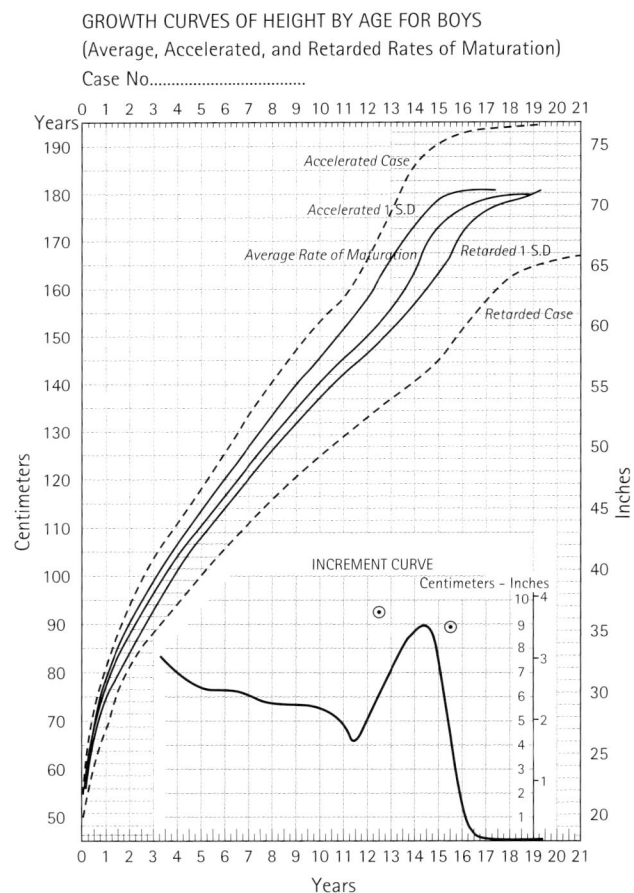

Figure 1.2 Bayley's growth curves of height by age for boys. (Reprinted from *Journal of Pediatrics*, vol. 48. Bayley N. Growth curves of height and weight by age for boys and girls, scaled according to physical maturity, pp. 187–94; copyright 1956, with permission from Elsevier.)

of maturation. On the same graphs an 'increment curve' or growth velocity curve is depicted. The only attempt to provide limits of normality are curves for plus and minus one standard deviation either side of the average distance curve. No percentiles are depicted and thus no outer limits of normality above or below which the pediatrician would be advised to take further action. However, here is a pioneering piece of work that for the first time seeks to combine the various techniques from anthropology, human biology, statistics, and clinical medicine into a comprehensive manual for the assessment of child growth on an individual basis.

Growth charts that were representative of the American population were not destined to be produced until the advent of the National Health Examination Surveys (NHES) of the 1960s and the later National Health and Nutrition Examination Survey (NHANES) which have continued to the present day. In each of the cross-sectional surveys, a national probability sample of the civilian, non-institutionalized population of the United States was examined. Survey-specific sample weights were applied to the national survey sample data to assure representation of the US population according to age, sex, and racial/ethnic composition at the time the surveys were conducted. Supplemental data sources provided data for birth to 2 months of age. The large sample size in these surveys and the pooling of older data added precision for calculation of the outlying percentile estimates, especially the 3rd and 97th percentiles, to better assess children who are growing at the extremes. Traditionally these references were published by the National Centre for Health Statistics (NCHS) but are now to be found on the websites of the Centers for Disease Control (CDC) in Atlanta, Georgia (http://www.cdc.gov/growthcharts/). These cross-sectional reference charts were the first, and remain the only, nationally representative growth references for the USA. Meanwhile in Europe the science of human growth was beginning to move forward rapidly.

J.M. Tanner and R.H. Whitehouse were the first to develop growth charts for British children, which they published in 1959.[27] Further modifications took place to produce their 1965 charts.[28,29] The sampling source for the 1965 charts was a combination of three datasets; the Child Study Centre, London longitudinal study (1948–1954), the cross-sectional London County Council survey (1959), and finally children from the Harpenden Longitudinal Growth Study (1948 onwards). Because of its wide dissemination and clarity of explanation this 1966 paper formed the technical basis for research teams through Europe to develop their own charts. Thus in other European countries auxologists and community health teams set up large scale cross-sectional studies involving the most appropriate stratified random sampling techniques to arrive at externally valid national growth charts. In the UK the 'Tanner–Whitehouse' chart, whilst not initially promoted as a universal 'standard of reference' became widely used as the national reference to assess the growth and development of both samples and individuals throughout the country. Thus whilst other countries were developing externally valid growth charts the UK was relying on a growth chart that had never claimed external validity.

In the course of time the original Tanner–Whitehouse chart was updated to become a 'clinical longitudinal chart'[7] but it was not until 1996, 30 years after the first appearance of the Tanner–Whitehouse chart that a team, primarily from the Institute of Child Health London under the statistical guidance of Professor Tim J. Cole from Cambridge, produced an alternative, and purportedly externally valid, national chart.[30] That chart went through a further modification in 1997 following a critical comparative analysis by Wright and colleagues at the University of Newcastle upon Tyne[31] to achieve its present form.[32] Almost at the same time Tanner was working with John Buckler from Leeds to update the 1976 reference and produce the latest 'Buckler–Tanner' chart.[33]

For a while there were a variety of charts circulating in the UK, often causing significant confusion. For this reason the Royal College of Paediatrics and Child Health commissioned a review of the existing charts and reference sets which resulted in a critical appraisal concluding that the UK90[32] and Buckler–Tanner[33] charts were the only ones that were appropriate for clinical use.[34]

ANTHROPOMETRY

The anthropometry peculiar to somatic growth that we use today had its recent development in the American longitudinal studies of the first half of this century. One common characteristic of the study designs was the desire to maintain accuracy of measurement. Administrative problems and staff changes meant that this was not always possible, but runs of ten years with the same measurement team are to be found in the Berkeley Growth Study of 1927,[35] and the Yale Study of the same year.[36]

Research workers were aware of the need for comparability of measurements and published precise accounts of their methods and techniques, with suitable adaptations for the measurement of growth. The three most important and informative accounts from this period are those of Frank Shuttleworth[37] for the Harvard Growth Study of 1922 (made in the School of Education), Harold Stuart[38] for the Center for Research in Child Health and Development Study of 1930, and Katherine Simmons in her reports of the Brush Foundation's Studies of 1931.[39] Stuart provides the most complete account of measurements used for auxology using the techniques that resulted from the International Congress of 1912, 'with diversions from these techniques at appropriate times'. H.V. Meredith (1936) is unique in his perception of the problems involved in the measurement of human growth at the time of the early US studies. The multitude of papers he published on the growth of children from Iowa City, Massachusetts, Alabama, Toronto (Canada) and Minnesota contain excellent examples of reliability control. He was convinced that long-term studies of physical growth would only be valid if preliminary detailed investigations were made into the accuracy with which body dimensions could be measured during growth. If the growth increment from one age to the next was less than the 90th centile of the differences between repeated measurements of a chosen dimension, he thought it unwise to take the measurement. Detailed descriptions of the measurements his team used are included in his reports.[40] He and his colleague Virginia Knott (1941) criticized the sparsity of modern techniques and the lack of information pertaining to their reliability. These American studies almost exclusively used accepted anthropological instrumentation such as Martin anthropometers which would be modified when they did not precisely meet the needs of the auxological situation. An anthropometer may, for instance, have been fixed to a board to facilitate the measurement of recumbent length. In addition, American studies promoted the development of instrumentation such as skinfold calipers. They did much to influence more recent researchers in the field of growth and development on both sides of the Atlantic.

The Harpenden Longitudinal Growth Study, set up by J.M. Tanner and R.H. Whitehouse in 1949, became the strongest influence in British studies of human growth and did much to advance auxological anthropometry in Europe. Whitehouse was dissatisfied with the instrumentation available and developed the Harpenden range of instruments that are recognized today as being among the best in the world. They are accepted internationally for their accuracy, consistency, and ease of use. Their principal advance was to eliminate graduated rules for measuring linear distances and instead to use counter mechanisms.

The International Children's Centre Coordinated Longitudinal Growth Studies had a major effect on standardizing anthropometric measurements and growth study design. But it was the International Biological Project (IBP) that brought together scientists from all over the world under the umbrella of research in 'human biology' during the years 1962–72 and gave rise to one of the standard texts for research into the human biological sciences. Weiner and Lourie's IBP handbook now revised and in its second edition[41] formed the source for many scientists who wish to use standard techniques. During the 1980s two further texts were to become established reference works for the measurement of human growth. The first was Cameron's *The Measurement of Human Growth*[42] and the second the text edited by Tim Lohman, Alex Roche and Reynaldo Martorell entitled *Anthropometric Standardization Reference Manual*.[43]

Noël Cameron (1948–) had worked with Tanner and Whitehouse from 1973 to 1983. He assessed the growth status of children attending Tanner's growth disorder clinics and measured children in a variety of research projects under way during that time. His volume, which detailed the techniques used in the growth disorder clinics, was the first to be devoted to anthropometric measurements on children, as opposed to adults, and included a variety of other growth assessment techniques, e.g., skeletal maturity.

Tim Lohman's *Anthropometric Standardization Reference Manual* sought to do two things: first, to provide a detailed account of how to undertake a variety of anthropometric measurements on children; and second, to establish these techniques as *the* standard techniques to be universally adopted. The volume resulted from a consultative conference held in the USA in 1984 at which various teams of experts (mostly American) were given groups of dimensions on which to make recommendations concerning their assessment and standardization.

Reliability

It seems almost absurd to emphasize the role of accurate measurement in the identification of growth disorders but it was not forever thus and it is a fact that the most successful centers for the study of human growth have placed particular emphasis on anthropometric measurement procedures. In a recurrent theme it was the elucidation of the fact that errors of measurement are normally distributed that allowed anthropometric methods to assume appropriate importance within the pediatric armamentarium.

The development of methods to assess reliability has been characterized by a diverse terminology. Thus whilst one group publish data on 'accuracy' another publishes similar data on 'precision' and a third on 'reproducibility'. One group use the statistics of 'standard deviation of differences' another 'standard errors of measurement', a third 'technical errors of measurement', and yet a fourth coefficients of 'reliability', 'reproducibility', 'objectivity' or 'stability'. Only in the last 40 years have we begun to see some degree of agreement over the fundamental statistics that describe reliability and thus allow for direct comparisons between different growth clinics.

All sources agree that the way in which one assesses reliability is through a test–retest study in which the same children are measured on two occasions with sufficient delay between occasions to prevent the magnitude of dimensions being remembered. It is now accepted that the results of such a study are analyzed to obtain a statistic called the 'technical error of measurement'[43] or 'standard error of measurement'.[42] The statistics are almost exactly the same save for the addition of a term in the standard error of measurement that corrects for bias. The technical error of measurement assumes no bias. When multiplied by 1.96 these statistics provide the 95% limits within which the 'true' magnitude of a dimension will lie for a particular observer.

SKELETAL MATURITY

Three techniques were developed in clinical situations to estimate skeletal maturity; the atlas technique of Greulich and Pyle[11], the Tanner–Whitehouse bone-specific scoring technique,[12,44–46] and the Fels hand–wrist method.[47,48] All use the left hand and wrist to estimate a skeletal age or bone age yet the latter two are different both in concept and in method from the former.

Atlas techniques

The Atlas technique had its origins in the pioneer work of T. Wingate Todd, who published an *Atlas of Skeletal Maturation* in 1937.[49] A *Skiagraphic Atlas* showing the development of the bones of the hand and wrist had, in fact, been published in London in 1898 by a surgeon called John Poland.[50] This contained anatomical descriptions of the development of each bone and a series of 'Roentgens' of children (mostly boys) from 12 months to 17 years of age. As a system of skeletal maturity assessment its appearance was an isolated event, until Todd's Atlas. This was based on the hand–wrist radiographs of 1000 children from the Brush Foundation Study of Human Growth and Development, which started in 1929 in Cleveland, Ohio. The children were only admitted to the study on the application of a pediatrician and were thus, in the Midwest of the 1930s, a socially advantaged group later described by Greulich and Pyle as 'above average in economic and educational status'.

From each chronological age group the films were arrayed, concentrating on one bone at a time, in order of increasing maturity. The film exhibiting the modal maturity for the age group was selected and the maturity indicators of that particular bone described. The appearance of these indicators was taken as typical for a healthy child of that age and sex. Having described these indicators for each bone and each age, the series was re-examined to identify radiographs showing, for every bone, the modal maturity for that age and sex. Each of these standards was assigned a 'skeletal age' determined by the age of the children on whom the standard was based and it is those standards that appeared in the Atlas. Continuing Todd's work, Drs William Walter Greulich, Idell Pyle, and Normand Hoerr published a variety of atlases between 1950 and 1969 to describe the skeletal maturation of the hand and wrist, knee, and foot and ankle.[10,11,51] That for the hand and wrist is the best known and is referred to universally as the 'Greulich–Pyle Atlas'.

Bone-specific techniques

Bone-specific techniques were developed in an attempt to overcome the two main disadvantages of the atlas techniques. These were the concept of the 'evenly maturing skeleton' and the difficulty of using 'age' in a system measuring maturity. Acceptance of the evenly maturing skeleton was compulsory if one used the atlas method of comparing the radiograph with standard plates. This acceptance decreased the significance of individual variation within the bones of the hand–wrist. Similarly, the acceptance of 'age' from the standards implied the acceptance of a chronological time series when, in fact, maturity advanced according to a developmental rather than a chronological clock.

THE OXFORD METHOD

R.M. Acheson, working on radiographs from about 500 pre-school children in Oxford, England, devised a scoring system for the hand and wrist and knee that 'permitted maturation to be rated on a scale that did not require direct consideration of the size of the bone and was independent of the age of the child'.[52] The system, like all subsequent bone-specific systems, depended upon assigning a number or score to each maturity indicator or combination of maturity indicators. However, Acheson's scores were arbitrary; they were not weighted in the statistical sense, because 'the decision as to what did, and what did not, constitute a maturity indicator was somewhat arbitrary in any case'. The problem of this technique, called the 'Oxford method' by Acheson, is that it does not deal with the problem of dysmaturity in that similar total scores from different individuals may be the result of the maturity of different bones. Even though the Oxford method fell some way short of an acceptable technique it did allow Acheson to investigate the nature of maturity indicators. The fundamental flaws in the 'Oxford method', however, led Tanner and his colleagues to develop their techniques a few years later.

THE TANNER–WHITEHOUSE METHOD

In 1959 and 1962 J.M. Tanner and R.H. Whitehouse, working in England, published their first attempt at a bone-specific scoring system. This was known as TW1 but was later revised and published as TW2[12,44] and most recently as TW3.[46] The basic rationale was that the development of each single bone reflected a single process that they defined as maturation. 'Scores' could be assigned to the presence of particular maturity indicators within the developing bones. Ideally each of the 'n' scores from each of the bones in a particular individual ought to be the same. This common score, with suitable standardization, would be the individual's maturity. To arrive at a practical technique a variety of modifications to this rationale had to be made. In addition Tanner and his colleagues were highly critical of the method and how it operated in practice – in how well it served the pediatric and research communities for whom it was intended. Their monitoring of the system promoted the various modifications that resulted in TW2 and most recently TW3.

The underlying rationale of the Tanner–Whitehouse techniques was based on dissatisfaction with a maturity system based on chronological age and thus the need to define a maturity scale that does not refer directly to age. Concentrating on the bones of the hand and wrist, they defined series of eight maturity indicators for each bone and nine for the radius. These maturity indicators were then evaluated, not in relation to chronological age, but in relation to their appearance within the full passage of each specific bone from immaturity to maturity. Thus, for example, it was possible to say that a particular indicator on the lunate first appeared at 13% maturity and that a process of fusion in the first metacarpal started at 85% maturity. In addition the metacarpals and phalanges, being greater in number than the carpal bones, would weight the final scores in favour of the 'long' bones and so rays 2 and 4 were omitted from the final calculations. The scores were weighted so that half of the mature score derived from the carpal bones and half from the long and short bones. The scores were so proportioned that the final mature score totalled 1000 points. Five thousand radiographs of normal British children were then rated, using this technique, to arrive at population 'standards' that related bone maturity scores to chronological ages. The resulting curve of bone maturity score against age was sigmoid demonstrating a non-linear relationship between skeletal maturity and chronological age.

However, the contribution of the carpus to 50% of total maturity presented a problem in terms of the repeatability of assessing maturity indicators (i.e., the carpus is less reliable) and because the carpus was known neither to play a major role in growth in height nor in epiphyseal fusion. Subsequently Tanner and his colleagues changed the scores assigned to the individual bones to allow the calculation of a bone maturity score based on the radius, ulna and short bones (RUS) only or the carpal bones (CARPAL) only in addition to the full 20-bone score (TW2(20)) and called this system TWII.

The Tanner–Whitehouse II skeletal maturity system thus addressed the disadvantages of both the Greulich–Pyle Atlas method and the Oxford method. It allowed an assessment of skeletal maturity that was age independent and, because of the three systems available from a single rating (TW2(20), RUS, CARPAL), allowed considerable flexibility both in the assessment and the monitoring of skeletal maturity.

TW3 uses a more recent standardizing sample to allow for secular trends in growth and maturity and the TW2(20) bone score has been abolished to leave two separate assessments via the radius, ulna and short bones or the carpal bones.

THE ROCHE–WAINER–THISSEN TECHNIQUE

In 1975 Roche, Wainer, and Thissen[53] published a technique to estimate the skeletal maturity of the knee.[54] Roche in particular was critical of the hand–wrist techniques because the bones of the hand and wrist exhibit few maturational changes over the age ranges of 11–15 in boys and 9–13.5 in girls.[55] In addition, the usefulness of the hand–wrist techniques was limited at early ages when few centers were visible and in later ages when some areas (e.g., the carpus) reach their adult maturity levels prior to others. He chose the knee as an area for assessment because he believed that the area investigated should be closely related to the reason for assessment; maturity of the knee relates closely to growth in height. Thus when one is dealing with growth disorders or height prediction the knee ought to give a more appropriate estimation of skeletal maturity but this may not actually be the case.

However, Roche was to change his opinion in the next decade and with his colleagues Cameron Chumlea and David Thissen he produced a hand–wrist scoring technique in 1988 known as the Fels hand–wrist method.[47,48]

THE FELS HAND–WRIST TECHNIQUE

The theoretical basis for the Fels hand–wrist method is little different from that of the earlier Tanner–Whitehouse methods. Roche and his colleagues went through the laborious process of identifying suitable maturity indicators from 13 823 serial radiographs of children from the Fels Longitudinal Growth study. The radiographs were taken between 1932 and 1972 and thus may appear to be rather dated and susceptible to the problems of secular change. From a possible 130 maturity indicators taken from the literature, 98 were finally selected that conformed to the criteria of universality, discriminative ability, reliability, validity, and completeness. In addition to graded indicators Roche and his colleagues also used metric ratios of lengths of radius, ulna, metacarpals and phalanges. They maintain that the Fels method differs from previous methods in terms of the observations made, the chronological ages when assessments are possible, the maturity indicators, the statistical methods, and scale of maturity. In order to translate the ratings of the bones into a skeletal 'age' specific computer software (FELShw) is required.[47] The data entry forms reflect the fact that the method can use ratings from the radius, ulna, all carpal bones and, like the TW systems, the phalanges of rays I, III, and V. The output is an 'estimated skeletal age' and an 'estimated standard error' to provide an idea of the confidence of the estimated age.

Height prediction

Early fascination with prediction focussed on the prediction of adult stature because of the clinical importance of being able to estimate, with low, or at least clinically insignificant errors, the adult height of an individual from data obtained at pubertal or prepubertal examinations and the information that the errors of prediction provide with regard to the relative importance of the variables thought to influence adult stature.

Orthopedic surgeons Gill and Abbott[56] were interested in the effect of leg lengthening operations on adult height. Such operations demanded accurate methods of estimating the future rate of growth, the ultimate length of the extremities, and final height. The technique developed then was based on the belief that canalization was a strong enough phenomenon to allow accurate prediction of adult height and that the accuracy would increase when an estimate of bone maturation was also considered. In addition, they determined that the relative proportions of the length of the femur and tibia to stature are maintained with only small age variations throughout the adolescent period. Further, Gill and Abbot took the age-adjusted proportions of the femur and tibia to stature and multiplied the final proportions by predicted final height. The method was validated by investigating the serial predictions of 33 girls and 12 boys using the percentile (canalization) method. A child's present height was entered on a growth chart, drawn up by Gill and Abbott from the Whitehouse Conference data of 1932, at either the appropriate chronological age or, if the skeletal age and chronological age differed by more than 6 months, at the skeletal age, and the centile followed to a final height estimation at 18.5 years for boys and 16.5 years for girls. This technique produced an average error of ±2.5 cm and 90 percent confidence limits of ±5.1 cm.

Frank Shuttleworth was the first to predict 'mature height' for biological interest rather than clinical necessity.[23] Data from the Harvard Longitudinal Growth Study were used to develop two types of tables presented separately for boys and girls and for northern Europeans and Italians. The first used the variables of initial height and chronological age and the second included, in addition to the previous variables, the annual height increment for ages 10.5 to 14.5 years in girls and 12.5 and 16.5 years in boys. Shuttleworth emphasized that these latter tables should be used with 'some discrimination if their value is to be realized. The interval on which the gain (annual increment) is based should be within two or three weeks of the exact one year period. The original measurements must be taken with care, by the same method, at the same time of day, and to the nearest quarter of an inch. Finally, these tables must not be used outside the specified age ranges'. Shuttleworth also included the probable error of estimate for each age specific column of his tables; ±4 cm at worse.

These two early methods highlight the original clinical and biological interest in prediction techniques and both relied on the phenomenon of canalization and the use of a maturity variable to infer the possibility of deviations from the genetically determined growth canal; Gill and Abbott[56] used skeletal maturity, and Shuttleworth[23] used height velocity as the refining variable.

Prediction techniques have been developed using three approaches. In the first and simplest case single cross-sectional variables have been used to predict adult height. The use of parental height is a prime example of this method. However, in all other methods for predicting a future event in the growth and development of a child the current age of the child (chronological age, CA), is a necessary variable. Any measured variable associated with a child during growth implicitly carries the information of chronological age. Thus height is actually height-for-age, and its use becomes an example of the second case in which combinations of cross-sectionally obtained variables have been used. Shuttleworth's technique is an example in which present height and age are the initial variables. The third case involves longitudinally obtained data. These data relate to the changing rate of somatic growth and/or maturation over a set period of time. Shuttleworth's second technique is such a situation in which height velocity from one age to the next is used in conjunction with cross-sectionally derived variables.

Almost without exception the more recent prediction techniques are multivariate techniques employing regression equations. This fact alone indicates that multivariate techniques reduce the errors of prediction. The problem involved in multivariable techniques is the variety of data required to accomplish a prediction. Some authors have tried to overcome this problem by allowing the substitution of population mean values for the missing data. Others[44,46,57] have provided a number of alternative equations depending on the available data.

PHYSIOLOGICAL ASSESSMENT

Before considering tests we should quickly review the history of our understanding of the physiological control of growth. Writing in the 1950s Lawson Wilkins summarized the understanding of growth regulation at that time.[58] In general the pattern of understanding was much as today with the recognition of extrinsic factors such as nutrition and acquired disease, interplaying with intrinsic factors such as genes and the endocrine system. However, there was a considerable absence of detail. The manner of the interaction between genes and phenotype was still largely unknown but certainly had moved away from the earlier ideas that all genetic influence on growth was mediated through the endocrine system.[59] There was also recognition of the importance of the central nervous system as a pathway particularly via the hypothalamic pathways.[60]

As a general picture little has changed, but there has been considerable progress in understanding of the mechanisms by which the environment and acquired disease, genes and the endocrine system interact. As an example we might consider the growth hormone axis where key events over a number of years have revolutionized our thinking. We now understand the interaction of growth hormone releasing hormone and somatostatin, both released from specific centres in the hypothalamus, which control the episodic synthesis and release of growth hormone (GH) from the anterior pituitary. We also understand much more about the embryology of the pituitary and are gradually unravelling the genetic regulation of this process and the differentiation of the various hormone producing cells within the gland.[61] For many years it was uncertain whether GH was directly involved in linear growth and even when this became clear it was originally thought that it acted directly on growing tissues. The next major clarification came with the discovery of sulphation factor[62] later renamed somatomedin[63] and yet later characterized as insulin-like growth factor I and II (IGF-I and IGF-II).[64] Subsequently a whole family of specific binding proteins for the IGFs has been defined[65] and we now have a much clearer understanding of the way in which they interact in health and disease.

Apart from their involvement in the embryology, development and function of the endocrine system genes may be directly involved in growth disorders. Many skeletal and other growth disorders have been clinically recognized for decades, but apart from the major chromosomal disorders (e.g., Down syndrome) it has only been in the last two decades that we have started to identify and characterize single gene or contiguous gene defects causing recognizable malformation syndromes.[66]

Biochemical investigation of growth disorders does not share such a distinguished history with auxology and anthropometry. In the 1950s it was not even clear that growth hormone was directly related to growth. Methods of measurement of GH were in their infancy and not really established until immunoassays were developed in the early 1960s.[67,68] Then it became clear that GH, as with many pituitary hormones was secreted in an episodic manner such that single basal samples were of little value. Then the concept of tests of GH 'reserve' was developed and to some extent these remain the mainstay of biochemical investigation of growth disorders. Reference to a typical text book of the era (e.g., Hubble's *Paediatric Endocrinology*, 1969) contain descriptions of tests many of which are still used today[69] of which the insulin tolerance test is probably the most venerable. This has had a rather tarnished reputation more recently because of concerns over safety[70] but it continues to be used especially in adults and older children.

It is salutary to look back at the endocrine measurements that were available in the middle of the twentieth century. In Lawson Wilkins classical textbook[58] he lists the methods available for measurement of the various hormones. Most depended on bioassays which were seldom sensitive enough for clinical use and a few steroids were measurable using chromatographic or fluorometric assays. The contrast with the armoury of hormonal measurements available to us only 50 years later is stark.

In the 1970s it was discovered that GH did not act directly on tissues stimulating growth, but rather worked through the intermediary IGF-I which circulates in blood bound to a specific binding protein. Understanding of this system has expanded exponentially over the last 30 years although it has still failed to find a better test of the GH axis.[71]

There has been a continued search for better tests with better safety profiles and more diagnostic reliability. However, there still remains a lack of the perfect test and diagnosis of growth disorders still depends on a combination of clinical auxology, clinical judgement and various biochemical investigations that will be discussed in appropriate chapters later in this volume.

Of course not all growth disorders are caused by disturbance of the GH axis and in many cases there are perfectly reliable tests that can quickly lead to a diagnosis; the measurement of thyroid hormone in blood would be a clear example. Other great successes are the fantastic advances in imaging that have occurred over the past few decades: computerized axial tomography, ultrasound and magnetic resonance imaging are striking examples of progress.

APPROACHES TO TREATMENT

In the pre-GH era treatment was very limited. Hypothyroidism was treatable originally with desiccated thyroid and then pure L-thyroxine. It has also been used empirically in other short stature conditions but without benefit. Similarly, androgens were occasionally used to treat short stature (particularly in the form of anabolic steroids) but apart from those conditions where androgen deficiency was a genuine part of the problem they were of little value. One major exception is in constitutional delay of growth and puberty which will be discussed in Chapter 41.

The advent of GH for therapeutic use has made a major difference. Raben's classical report of the first case of GH deficiency treated has already been mentioned[15] and in the years that followed much was achieved. In the first 25 years the GH was extracted from human pituitary glands removed at post-mortem. Because of the scarcity of the hormone supplies were always constrained and the dosing was crude, typically 5–10 IU per dose two or three times per week irrespective of body size.[72]

Then, in 1985, more or less contemporaneously in the USA and UK a number of cases of Creutzfeldt–Jakob disease (CJD) in unusually young patients were identified. The one thing they had in common was GH treatment and over subsequent years many more cases have appeared in several countries.[73] In 2004 the world total is about 170 cases. It is now inescapable that the CJD is caused by contamination of the pituitary-derived GH with the infectious prion protein co-purified from pituitaries taken from patients with preclinical disease.

Pituitary GH was discontinued in most countries in mid-1985. Fortunately, material prepared by recombinant DNA technology was already in clinical trial and by late 1986 most GH-deficient children were back on treatment and doing well. This will be discussed extensively in Chapter 35. Also, over the last 20 years, the use of GH to treat other causes of growth failure has been explored in many countries. Whilst by no means a panacea for short stature it has proved useful in a number of conditions where GH deficiency is not the cause of the poor growth; perhaps the best example is Turner syndrome. These options are all considered in following chapters.

REFERENCES

1 Cameron N. *Human Growth and Development*. New York: Academic Press; 2002.

2 Scammon RE. The first seriatim study of human growth. *Am J Phys Anthropol* 1927; **10**: 329–36.

3 Bayer LM, Bayley N. *Growth Diagnosis*. Chicago: University of Chicago Press; 1959.

4 Tanner JM. *A History of the Study of Human Growth*. Cambridge: Cambridge University Press; 1981.

5 Baldwin BT, Wood TD. *Weight-height-age Tables. Tables for Boys and Girls of School Age.* New York: American Child Health Association; 1923.

6 Baldwin BT. *A Measuring Scale for Physical Growth and Physiological Age. The Fifteenth Year Book of the National Society for the Study of Education.* Bloomington, Illinois: Public School Publishing Company, 1916: 11–23.

7 Tanner JM, Whitehouse RH. Clinical longitudinal standards for height, weight, height velocity, weight velocity, and the stages of puberty. *Arch Dis Child* 1976; **51**: 170–9.

8 Reynolds EL, Wines JV. Physical changes associated with adolescence in boys. *Am J Dis Child* 1948; **75**: 329–50.

9 Nicholson AB, Hanley C. Indices of physiological maturity. *Child Dev* 2005; **24**: 3–38.

10 Greulich WW, Pyle SI. *Radiographic Atlas of Skeletal Development of the Hand and Wrist.* Palo Alto: Stanford University Press, 1950.

11 Greulich WW, Pyle SI. *Radiographic Atlas of Skeletal Development of the Hand and Wrist.* Palo Alto: Stanford University Press, 1959.

12 Tanner JM, Whitehouse RH, Healy MJR. A new system for estimating skeletal maturity from the hand and wrist with standards derived from a study of 2,600 healthy British children. Paris: Centre International de l'Enfance, 1962.

13 Bayley N, Pinneau S. Tables for predicting adult height from skeletal age. *J Pediatr* 1952; **40**: 423–41.

14 Smith DW. *Recognizable Patterns of Human Malformation: Genetic, Embryologic and Clinical Aspects.* Philadelphia: Saunders, 1970.

15 Raben MS. Treatment of a pituitary dwarf with human growth hormone. *J Clin Endocrinol* 1958; **18**: 901–3.

16 Raben MS. Growth hormone. 1. Physiological aspects. *N Engl J Med* 1962; **266**: 71–114.

17 Raben MS. Growth hormone. 1. Clinical use of human growth hormone. *N Engl J Med* 1962; **266**: 82–86.

18 Tanner JM, Whitehouse RH. Growth response of 26 children with short stature given human growth hormone. *BMJ* 1967; **2**: 69–75.

19 Raben MS. Human growth hormone. *Recent Prog Horm Res* 1959; **15**: 71–114.

20 Bowditch Hp. *The Growth of Children Studied by Galton's Percentile Grades.* 22nd Annual Report of the State Board of Health of Massachusetts. Boston: Wright & Potter, 1891: 479–525.

21 Simonton DK. Francis Galton's hereditary genius: Its place in the history and psychology of science. In: Sternberg RJ, ed. *The Anatomy of Impact: What Makes the Great Works of Psychology Great.* Washington: American Psychological Association, 2003: 3–18.

22 Jensen A. Galton's legacy to research on intelligence. *J Biosoc Sci* 2002; **34**: 145–72.

23 Shuttleworth FK. The physical and mental growth of girls and boys aged six to sixteen in relation to age at maximum growth. *Monogr Soc Res Child Dev* 1939; **4**: 1–291.

24 Tanner JM. *Growth at Adolescence.* Oxford: Blackwell Scientific Publications, 1955.

25 Cameron N. Conditional standards for growth in height of British children from 5.0 to 15.99 years of age. *Ann Hum Biol* 1980; **7**: 331–7.

26 Stolz HR, Stolz LM. *Somatic Growth of Adolescent Boys.* New York: Macmillan, 1951.

27 Tanner JM, Whitehouse RH. Standards for height and weight of British children from birth to maturity. *Lancet* 1959; **2**: 1086–8.

28 Tanner JM, Whitehouse RH, Takaishi M. Standards from birth to maturity for height, weight, height velocity, and weight velocity: British children, 1965 - I. *Arch Dis Child* 1966; **41**: 454–71.

29 Tanner JM, Whitehouse RH, Takaishi M. Standards from birth to maturity for height, weight, height velocity, and weight velocity: British children, 1965 - II. *Arch Dis Child* 1966; **41**: 613–35.

30 Freeman JV, Cole TJ, Chinn S, *et al.* Cross-sectional stature and weight reference curves for the UK, 1990. *Arch Dis Child* 1995; **73**: 17–24.

31 Wright CM, Corbett SS, Drewett RF. Sex differences in weight in infancy and the British 1990 national growth standards. *BMJ* 1997; **313**: 513–14.

32 Cole TJ, Freeman JV, Preece MA. British 1990 growth reference centiles for weight, height, body mass index and head circumference fitted by maximum penalized likelihood. *Stat Med* 1998; **17**: 407–29.

33 Tanner JM, Buckler JM. Revision and update of Tanner-Whitehouse clinical longitudinal charts for height and weight. *Eur J Pediatr* 1997; **156**: 248–9.

34 Wright C, Booth I, Buckler JM, *et al.* Growth reference charts for use in the United Kingdom. *Arch Dis Child* 2002; **86**: 11–14.

35 Bayley N. *Studies in the Development of Young Children.* Berkeley: University of California Press; 1940.

36 Gessell A, Thompson H. *The Psychology of Early Growth.* New York: Macmillan; 1938.

37 Shuttleworth FK. Sexual maturation and the physical growth of girls aged six to sixteen. *Dev Monogr* 1937; **2**: 1.

38 Stuart HC. Studies from the Center for Research in Child Health and Development, School of Public Health, Harvard University. *Child Dev Monogr* 1939; **4**: 1.

39 Simmons K. The Brush Foundation study of child growth and development. *Child Dev Monogr* 1944; **9**: 1.

40 Meredith HV. The reliability of anthropometric measurements taken on eight- and nine-year old white males. *Child Dev* 1936; **7**: 262.

41 Weiner JS, Lourie JA. *Practical Human Biology.* London: Academic Press; 1981.

42 Cameron N. *The Measurement of Human Growth.* London: Croom Helm; 1984.

43 Lohman TG, Roche A, Martorell R. *Anthropometric Standardization Reference Manual.* Champagne, Illinois: Human Kinetrics Books; 1988.

44 Tanner JM, Whitehouse RH, Marshall WA, *et al. Assessment of Skeletal Maturity and Prediction of Adult Height (TW2 Method).* London: Academic Press; 1975.

45 Tanner JM, Landt KW, Cameron N, *et al.* Prediction of adult height from height and bone age in childhood: A new system

of equations (TW Mark II) based on a sample including very tall and very short children. *Arch Dis Child* 1983; **58**: 767–76.

46 Tanner JM, Healy MJR, Goldstein H, Cameron N. *Assessment of Skeletal Maturity and Prediction of Adult Height (TW3 Method)*. London: Academic Press; 2001.

47 Roche AF, Chumlea C, Thissen D. *Assessing the Skeletal Maturity of the Hand–Wrist: Fels Method*. Springfield, Illinois: CC Thomas; 1988.

48 Chumlea C, Roche A, Thissen D. The FELS method for assessing the skeletal maturity of the hand-wrist. *Am J Hum Biol* 1989; **1**: 175–83.

49 Todd TW. *Atlas of Skeletal Maturation (Hand)*. St. Louis: C.V. Mosby Co; 1937.

50 Poland JG. *Skiagraphic Atlas Showing the Development of the Bones of the Wrist and Hand, for the Use of Students and Others*. London: Smith, Elder; 1898.

51 Pyle SI, Hoerr NL. *Radiographic Atlas of Skeletal Development of the Knee*. Springfield, Illinois: Charles C. Thomas; 1955.

52 Acheson RM. Maturation of the skeleton. In: Falkner F, ed. *Human Development*. Philadelphia: Saunders; 1966: 465–502.

53 Roche AF, Wainer H, Thissen D. *Skeletal Maturity. The Knee Joint As A Biological Indicator*. New York: Plenum; 1975.

54 Roche AF, Wainer H. *Predicting Adult Stature for Individuals*. Basel: S Karger AG; 1975.

55 Roche AF. Associations between rates of maturation of the bones of the hand-wrist. *Am J Phys Anthropol* 1970; **33**: 341–8.

56 Gill GG, Abbott LC. Practical method of predicting the growth of the femur and tibia in the child. *Arch Surg* 1942; **45**: 286–315.

57 Tanner JM, Whitehouse RH, Cameron N, *et al*. *Assessment of Skeletal Maturity and Prediction of Adult Height (TW2 Method)*. London: Academic Press, 1983.

58 Wilkins L. *The Diagnosis and Treatment of Endocrine Disorders in Childhood and Adolescence*. Oxford: Blackwell Scientific Publications; 1957.

59 Stockard CR. *The Genetic and Endocrine Basis for Differences in Form and Behaviour*. Philadelphia: Wistar Institute; 1941.

60 Bauer J. *Constitution and Disease. Applied Constitutional Pathology*. New York: Grune & Stratton; 1945.

61 Dattani MT, Preece MA. Growth hormone deficiency and related disorders: Novel insights into aetiology, diagnosis and treatment. *Lancet* 2004; **363**: 1977–87.

62 Salmon WD, Daughaday WH. A hormonally controlled serum factor which stimulates sulfate incorporation by cartilage in vitro. *J Lab Clin Med* 1957; **49**: 825–36.

63 Van den Brande JL, Van Buul S. Somatomedins. *Isr J Med Sci* 1975; **11**: 693–8.

64 Rinderknecht E, Humbel RE. Amino-terminal sequences of two polypeptides from human serum with nonsuppressible insulin-like and cell-growth-promoting activities: Evidence for structural homology with insulin B chain. *Proc Natl Acad Sci USA* 1976; **73**: 4379–81.

65 Ballard J, Baxter R, Binoux M, *et al*. On the nomenclature of the IGF binding proteins. *Acta Endocrinol* 1989; **121**: 751–2.

66 Preece MA. Genetically determined growth disorders. In: Cameron N, ed. *Human Growth and Development*. Amsterdam: Academic Press; 2002: 237–51.

67 Glick SM, Roth J, Yalow RS, Berson SA. Immunoassay of human growth hormone in plasma. *Nature* 1963; **199**: 784–7.

68 Hunter WM, Greenwood FC. A radioimmunoelectrophoretic assay for human growth hormone. *Biochem J* 1964; **91**: 43–56.

69 Laron Z. The hypothalamus and the pituitary gland. In: Hubble D, ed. *Paediatric Endocrinology*. Oxford: Blackwell Scientific Publications; 1969: 35–111.

70 Shah A, Stanhope R, Matthew D. Hazards of pharmacological tests of growth hormone secretion in childhood. *BMJ* 1992; **304**: 173–4.

71 Mitchell H, Dattani MT, Nanduri V, *et al*. Failure of IGF-I and IGFBP-3 to diagnose growth hormone insufficiency. *Arch Dis Child* 1999; **80**: 443–7.

72 Milner RDG, Russell Fraser T, Brook CGD, *et al*. Experience with human growth hormone in Great Britain: The report of the M.R.C. Working Party. *Clin Endocrinol* 1979; **11**: 15–38.

73 Brown P, Preece MA, Brandel J-P, *et al*. Iatrogenic Creutzfeldt Jakob disease at the Millenium. *Neurology* 2000; **55**: 1075–81.

PHYSIOLOGY OF LINEAR GROWTH

2

Cellular growth

OLLE SÖDER

INTRODUCTION

Multicellular organisms such as the human being are dependent on intricate systems for control of global and tissue growth. The lack of such needs is one major advantage of unicellular organisms such as bacteria over complex multi-cellular and multi-tissue species. Thus, most prokaryotes are characterized by a relative simplicity of their control of cellular multiplication and show a continuous rapid proliferation under optimal environmental conditions including nutrient supply, temperature and osmotic balance. Similarly, under culture conditions *in vitro* eukaryotic immortalized single cell lines derived from transformed normal cells or malignancies may show much the same growth behavior. However, by definition this situation is very different from the socially well-controlled cellular growth patterns of intact cells in their tissue of origin *in vivo*. Precisely how tissue and organ growth is coordinated within the body of a single individual and how this is integrated into the control of global growth is still poorly understood.

Large adult mammals consist of about 5×10^{13} cells and 200 different cell types which together compose multiple tissues and organs. It is obvious that there is a need for well tuned processes controlling the proliferation of single cells within the tissues of such multi-cellular higher order species of animals, not only regulating cell numbers but also the timely appearance and spatial orientation in the tissue architecture. Further, as will be discussed later, the needs for such control may vary in different tissues and may also show

temporal differences. The general principle of the tissue and organ size control in higher animals is a social regulation executed by endocrine, paracrine, autocrine, and juxtacrine negative and positive signals delivered by hormones and growth factors as well as by mechanical forces.[1–3] Although our knowledge of the biological and biochemical mechanisms of this control has advanced during recent years it is still far from complete.

In single cells the control is exerted at the level of proliferation and anti-proliferation genes and by genes governing cellular decisions to live or die, the perturbation of which may lead to uncontrolled cellular growth as in cancer. However, growth control in malignant cells and the integrated control of growth at the secular level is beyond the scope of this chapter. The normal life cycle of specialized adult human cells includes birth, hypertrophy, proliferation, differentiation, and death. This introductory chapter discusses how such cellular events may contribute to the growth of human tissues and organs *in vivo*.

COMPARISON OF CELLULAR GROWTH PATTERNS *IN VIVO* AND *IN VITRO*

Most of our knowledge of cellular growth has been obtained from studies of cells maintained in cultures *in vitro*.[4] As intact cells usually grow poorly in culture, immortalized cell lines derived from normal diploid animals cells have frequently been used for such studies. The major disadvantage with transformed cells is that they are, by definition, perturbed with respect to their growth control, and it is always debatable whether results from such cells are relevant for the growth physiology of normal cells *in vivo*. Despite these limitations, primary cultures of intact cells may sometimes be useful and it seems that most differentiated cell types retain their growth patterns *in vitro*, at least for an initial limited period of time. Thus, lymphoid cells stimulated by antigen or polyclonal mitogens proliferate readily in a suspension culture, whereas anchorage-dependent cells such as epithelial cells grow well in monolayers and show density dependence and contact inhibition. However, it is rarely possible to create *in vitro* cell culture models that mimic fully the situation *in vivo*, and just by varying culture parameters such as bottom shape of culture wells, presence or not of an extracellular matrix surface stroma or composition of the culture medium very different growth patterns may follow.[4]

FACTORS CONTRIBUTING TO SIZE OF TISSUES AND ORGANS *IN VIVO*

In everyday medicine, routine auxology from clinical examinations of children produce robust data demonstrating growth (or lack of growth) at the level of the whole body or of an organ. Translating such data into growth at the cellular level of human beings is not a simple task and is hampered by lack of non-invasive ethically acceptable methodology. The most obvious factor contributing to tissue and organ size *in vivo* is the number of cells present. At the time of organogenesis and tissue expansion during embryonic and fetal development stimulation of cell proliferation (hyperplasia) is a prerequisite for growth. However, it is simplistic to regard hyperplasia resulting in an increased cell number as the most important factor contributing to tissue size. Other factors such as size of individual cells, rate of cell loss by programmed cell death (apoptosis)[5] and the volume of the intercellular space (extracellular matrix and fluids) also contribute and may be equally or more important (Fig. 2.1). Expansion of the extracellular matrix results in a dilution of the cell density and may thus seem paradoxical with respect to cell numbers. The relative contributions of these components to tissue growth vary in different tissues and organs and may also show temporal variation during pre- and postnatal development.

The epiphyseal growth plate as a model of tissue growth

The epiphyseal growth plate is an illustrative and pertinent example of a tissue in which all above mentioned mechanisms of tissue size control are operative and contributing to longitudinal bone growth (Fig. 2.1; see also Chapter 3 of this book). In the resting zone of the growth cartilage, mitotically quiescent cells are stimulated by endocrine and paracrine/autocrine signals (growth hormone (GH),

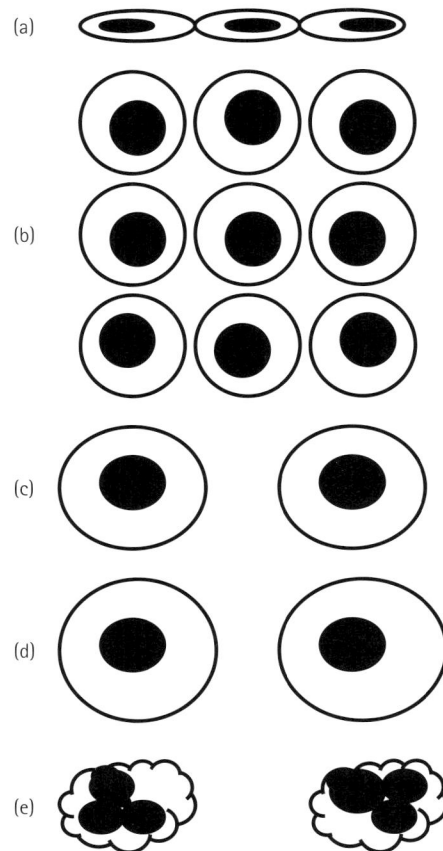

Figure 2.1 Factors contributing to tissue growth in the epiphyseal growth plate *in vivo*. See text for details. (a) Resting non-proliferating cells. (b) Active cell divisions (hyperplasia). (c) Increase of cellular size (hypertrophy). (d) Expansion of extracellular matrix volume. (e) Cell death by apoptosis.

insulin-like growth factor-I (IGF-I)) to start clonal proliferation (hyperplasia) which is morphologically reflected as columns of cells in the proliferation zone. Following this proliferative phase, the size of the individual chondrocytes then increases, defining the hypertrophy zone. In parallel the cell density is diluted by a stimulated secretory activity of the cells adding cartilage specific extracellular matrix factors to the expanding intercellular space. Finally, the hypertrophic growth plate chondrocytes undergo a well controlled programmed cell death (apoptotis) ending their contribution to the growth process. All these components (hyperplasia, hypertrophy, expansion of cartilage matrix, apoptosis) add to the volume of the tissue and thus to the longitudinal bone growth.

It is obvious that different classes of factors may be involved in the regulation of the above processes. Any substance stimulating clonal proliferation of epiphyseal growth plate chondrocytes *in vivo* may serve as a growth factor at the tissue level and would thus be regarded as a growth stimulator at the systemic level. However, from the present discussion it is also obvious that a differentiation factor halting proliferation and/or hypertrophy of the chondrocytes and instead stimulating their secretion of cartilage matrix components is also a growth stimulating factor from a clinical perspective (i.e., resulting in increased height) since the net outcome of such action is an increased tissue volume. *In vitro*, however, such differentiation factors are often seen as growth inhibitors as their effects may require mitotic quiescence. It is also obvious that pro- and anti-apoptotic factors may contribute to tissue growth and re-modelling by regulating cell survival. The balance of newly added cells following recruitment and clonal expansion of chondrocytes and their survival time in the tissue adds to the longitudinal growth rate and affects final stature.

It is concluded that growth at the tissue and organ level is the result of a complex regulation involving growth promoting factors that are not necessarily mitogenic. There are also examples of mitogenic factors *in vitro* that do not expand tissue volume as the size of the daughter cells progressively decreases during clonal expansion. In the following text some of the above components and their contribution to body growth are discussed in greater detail.

CELLULAR GROWTH *IN VITRO*

The cell cycle

Eukaryotic somatic cells reproduce by duplicating their contents, including their chromosomes, and increase in size before division into two genetically identical daughter cells. The cycle of cell division is the fundamental means by which all somatic cells are propagated.[6] It can be divided into several distinct phases (Fig. 2.2). The most distinct event is mitosis – the process of nuclear division – which is immediately followed by the physical cleavage of the mother cell into two daughter cells (cytokinesis). These two morphologically distinct parts of the cell cycle are both included in the mitosis (M) phase which has a very constant duration of about 1 h in most eukaryotic cells. In the period between two M phases – the interphase – cycling cells are preparing themselves for the next mitosis and cytokinesis. This preparation includes DNA replication that takes place during the S phase (S = synthesis) and other events occurring in the two gap (G) phases: before (G1) and after (G2) the S phase. The duration of the S phase is also usually very constant in eukaryotic cells. Thus, the S phase usually occupies 6–8 h of the cell cycle, which is the time required to replicate the total chromatin of a normal cell. In contrast to constantly dividing cells, most cells in adult tissues are not proliferating; instead they are in a resting state and perform their specialized functions while being reversibly or irreversibly retired from the division cycle. Such noncycling (quiescent) cells are referred to as being in a prolonged (sometimes indefinite) G1 phase called G0. In humans, the cell cycle time of cycling normal adult tissue cells varies from 9 to 10 h in, for example, rapidly cycling activated lymphocytes, to

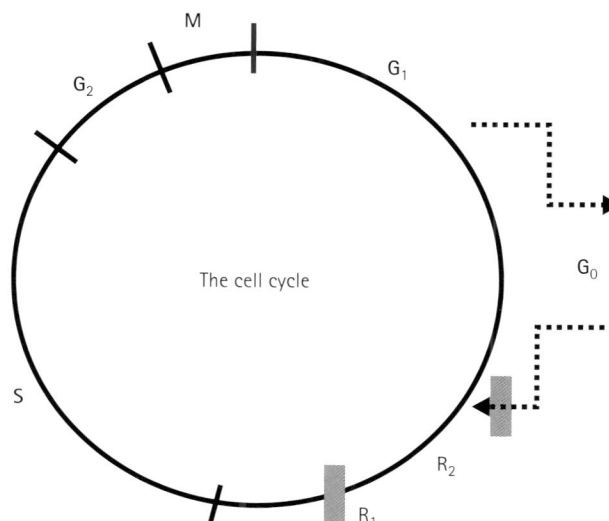

Figure 2.2 The mammalian cell cycle. See text for explanation. Cycling cells enter G_1 after mitosis (M) and are allowed to pass into S phase (DNA synthesis) and cell division provided progression growth factors are present to allow passage over the G_1 restriction point R_1. Quiescent cells are retired in a prolonged G_1 phase (G0) and may be recruited back into the active cell cycle by competence growth factors, allowing passage over the restriction point R_2.

25–30 h, which is typical of the surface epithelial cells of the small intestine. The time difference in cycle length of different cell types is a result of a variation in the duration of the G1 phase, whereas the S, G2 and M phases are of a more constant duration. In embryonic and fetal tissues, the cell cycle duration may be faster, such as in early embryonic stem cells, which display a very rapid cell cycle transition time. An exceptionally rapid eukaryotic cell cycle is found in fly embryos with duration of less than 10 min.[7]

Cell cycle regulation

Cell cycle control is complex and involves a series of intricate interactions between multiprotein enzymes that regulate the process.[2,8–10] The general principles of the regulatory system seem to be shared by most eukaryotic cells and have been best studied in yeast. The common, intracellular, cell cycle control system consists of a family of cyclically operating protein kinases and their associated regulatory protein complexes. The regulatory proteins are called cyclins and the kinases are referred to as cyclin dependent kinases (CDKs). Mitotic cyclins can be divided into several families which are characterized by accumulation and rapid degradation in a manner that triggers the different phases of the cell cycle at the right time and right order of sequence.[11] A number of regulatory proteins control the activity of the CDKs. Cyclins activate them and are important for their spatial orientation at their intracellular sites of action. Thus, the cyclin proteins activate CDKs to phosphorylate other proteins on threonine and serine residues at specific time points of the cell cycle. Several kinases and phosphatases regulate their activity. Inhibitors of CDKs suppress their binding and function. Ubiquitin-dependent proteases can degrade cyclins and other regulatory proteins at specific checkpoints of the cell cycle. One important target of cyclin/CDK complexes acting in the G1 phase is the retinoblastoma protein (Rb) that operates as an inhibitor of cell cycle progression.[12] If Rb is phosphorylated by the cyclin/CDK complex, its inhibitory effect is counteracted and the cells start to proliferate. Other critical targets for the cyclin/CDK complexes are p53, the centromeric and the lamin proteins. The CDKs are regulated by a network of inhibitors which include p15, p16, p27, and WAF1. Inactivation of phosphorylation of Rb by these inhibitors maintains Rb activity, thus keeping the growth of the cells arrested. The p53 tumor-suppressor gene product is a DNA-binding phosphoprotein made of 393 amino acids; it affects cell cycle progression at specific checkpoints in the G1 and G2 phases. Its effects in apoptosis are discussed below.

Growth factors regulate cell cycle events

The progression through the cell cycle involves decisions on the part of the cell about whether to proceed or not at specific checkpoints located at precise sites of the cycle.[8] In mammals, the most important checkpoint is found in the G1 phase, 1.5 h before the onset of the S phase and it is often referred to as the restriction point (R) or 'start' in yeast (Fig. 2.2). Without receiving the proper signals eukaryotic cells stop dividing and become blocked in G1 phase at R.[8,9,13] The transitions from G0 to G1 and that from G1 (through R) into the S phase are regulated by mitogenic peptide growth factors, possessing more or less target cell specificity.[14] For cells resting in G0 phase, one proposed model suggests that two separate factors are needed for activation and start of cell cycle progression. For T lymphocytes, the specific antigen exerts the first signal resulting in the transition from G0 to G1, cytologically referred to as blast transformation. The event is referred to as competence formation, which occurs without start of proliferation, and the factor(s) required for this process is thus named the competence factor. In this specific case competence formation triggers production of the lymphocyte growth factor interleukin 2 (IL-2), acting in an autocrine and paracrine manner to induce progression from G1 into S phase of the activated T cells. IL-2 is thus a progression growth factor that can exert its action only on competent cells. The described series of events initiates clonal proliferation of the T cells. Examples of growth factors with broader target cell specificity are platelet-derived growth factor (PDGF), insulin-like growth factor I (IGF-I) and transforming growth factor-α (TGF-α).[14] Thus, at the level of single cells, mitogenic growth factors exert their regulatory action by allowing passage through checkpoints in the cell cycle.

Many factors known to be effective as growth stimulators *in vivo* may be poor mitogens when tested on cells *in vitro* and their observed action in the cell cycle may seem paradoxical. Such factors may act as cell cycle inhibitors and exert their growth-promoting actions through stimulation of cell size and/or production of extracellular matrix components, or by serving as survival factors through inhibition of programmed cell death. One important family of differentiation factors that belongs to this category is the transforming growth factor-β (TGF-β) gene superfamily, which includes members such as TGF-β, anti-müllerian hormone and inhibin.[15] The physiological relevance of *in vitro* growth factors on growth regulation *in vivo* has been challenged by data accumulating from gene deletion experiments in mice. For some growth factors, gene disruption in knock-out mice has produced the expected growth disturbances, whereas elimination of other peptide growth factors has not shown any growth failure *in vivo*. For example, deletion of the genes encoding IGF-I or the IGF-I receptor results in severe growth failure of the offspring,[16] an effect that might be the result of a prolongation of the cell cycle time.[17] On the contrary, removal of TGF-α has failed to show any systemic growth reduction *in vivo*[18] and EGF, one of the archetypes of peptide growth factors, still awaits disclosure of its growth function *in vivo*. Interestingly, deletion of the T-lymphocyte factor IL-2 discussed above results in a much reduced proliferative responsiveness of the T cells to antigen and polyclonal activators *in vitro* but without apparent major effect on the immune function *in vivo*.[19]

It is not unlikely that the physiological role of several of the discovered *in vitro* growth factors may turn out to be unrelated to growth regulation. Accordingly, EGF has been found to potently suppress gastric acid secretion, a role that is relevant for its presence in breast milk and a putative function to protect important breast milk factors from being degraded in the stomach of the recipient infant.[20] It is thus fair to say that the physiological relevance *in vivo* of several growth factors with established effects *in vitro* still awaits confirmation.

Programmed cell death: apoptosis

Cell death occurs in tissues and organs as a natural process in the formation and maintenance of tissue architecture and homeostasis. Apoptosis and necrosis are the two main types of cell death. Necrosis is described as accidental cell death in the late stages of dying or injured tissues. It is characterized by swelling of cellular organelles and disruption of membranes. Necrosis is always accidental and results in activation of inflammatory cells. In contrast, apoptosis or programmed cell death is a highly regulated process of cell deletion and is composed of a constitutive suicide program expressed in most if not all cells. It may be triggered by a variety of extrinsic and intrinsic signals and is characterized by typical morphological criteria.[5,21,22] These include shrinkage of the cell, fragmentation and condensation of chromatin, blebbing of membranes, and, finally, compaction of cellular material into membrane-enclosed vesicles.

Apoptosis is a regulated and energy-dependent 'committed cell suicide' resulting in rapid phagocytosis of dying cells without any signs of an inflammatory cell response.

Our basic knowledge on apoptosis derives from studies in the nematode *Caenorhabditis elegans*.[23–25] Classical apoptosis, which is largely mediated by cysteine proteases known as caspases, is evolutionarily conserved and found in all animals. Caspases are cysteine proteases that cleave their substrate proteins specifically behind an aspartate residue, playing critical roles in initiation and execution of apoptosis.[26] Structurally, caspases are classified as initiator and effector caspases. Initiator caspases (caspases-2, -8, -9, and -10) activate themselves by dimerization, and effector caspases (caspases -3, -6, and -7) are cleaved into their active forms by initiator caspases and cleave cellular target proteins according to their substrate specificity.

Apoptosis occurs after activation via two different pathways: the death receptor pathway and mitochondrial pathway. The former pathway is initiated by binding of a ligand to a death receptor and the latter pathway may be activated by extracellular cues and internal insults such as DNA damage caused by irradiation or chemotherapy. The two apoptotic pathways are not independent but interact in several ways.

DEATH RECEPTOR PATHWAY

The death receptor pathway or extrinsic pathway of apoptosis is initiated by ligand-receptor binding at the cell surface. FAS (or APO-1/CD95) is the best-characterized member of the tumor necrosis factor (TNF) superfamily of receptors that activate the extrinsic apoptosis pathway. FAS carries a conserved 80 amino acid long intracellular region called a death domain (DD). FAS could be activated by a membrane FasL, being a 40 kDa type II transmembrane protein that is homologous to TNF. FasL could also be shed by proteolysis into the intercellular space as a soluble form that is less potent in inducing apoptosis than the membrane-bound form.[27] Binding of FasL to FAS leads to receptor trimerization and recruitment of adaptor proteins to the cytoplasmic death domain. This results in a series of steps activating procaspase-8 which cleaves its downstream effector caspases, including procaspase-3. This activates caspase-3 and the completion of the cell death program.[28–30]

MITOCHONDRIAL PATHWAY

DNA damage caused by most anticancer drugs and other cellular stresses could activate the mitochondrial pathway of apoptosis.[31,32] After activation, the permeability of the mitochondrial outer membrane is increased, and the structural organization of the cristae changed to make cytochrome *c* accessible for release.[33] After the release of cytochrome *c* into the cytosol this protein interacts with other proteins to form a heptameric complex which is known as an apoptosome. This is followed by activation of procaspase-9 which activates downstream effector caspases (caspase-3, -6, and -7), resulting in DNA fragmentation and apoptosis.[34–36] It is not yet known how cytochrome *c* manages to cross the mitochondrial outer membrane, but it is clear that the Bcl-2 family is intimately involved in the regulation of this process. Bcl-2 family proteins are divided into two groups, one that suppresses apoptosis including several identified members, and one that promotes apoptosis comprising more than ten known proteins. Most Bcl-2 family proteins can interact with each other and function as agonists or antagonists of each other, directly influencing the response to cellular stress.[37–41] The expression level of Bcl-2 family members can influence the response of cancer cells to chemotherapy, both negatively and positively.[36,42] This knowledge has formed the basis of novel therapeutic targets in cancer therapy.

A model for tissue size homeostasis which has recently attracted attention employs the view that cell maintenance in a tissue microenvironment is dependent on specific survival signals, which rescue the cells from activation of an intrinsic default pathway that leads to programmed cell death.[1] Compatible with this view, several factors that originally have been regarded as mitogenic growth factors seem instead to act as survival factors.[43] The basic idea behind this hypothesis is that a certain concentration of survival factor is needed at the tissue level to prevent activation of the apoptotic suicide program of the constituent cells. If the total cell mass of the tissue is increased, more survival factor is consumed. This lowers the concentration of the survival factor, thus forcing the cells into apoptosis. The cell loss leads to less consumption and an increased concentration of the survival factor, thus balancing cell death and survival to keep the tissue cell mass at the desired level.[1]

Cellular senescence

Cellular senescence is a loss of replicative capacity after a fixed number of population doublings in cell culture. This phenomenon is commonly termed the Hayflick limit[44] and states that human fibroblasts from young donors are allowed to pass about 50 doublings before the aging process slows the cycling capacity dramatically and finally stops the proliferation. Cellular senescence seems to reflect the chronological age of the individual animal serving as a cell donor to the cultures. Thus, cells taken from fetal tissues have the capacity to go through more division cycles than cells from adolescents or elderly subjects. From more recent quantitative studies it is clear that the cells decline in replicative capacity in a stochastic manner, with a half-life of approximately eight doublings, whereas the apparent 50-cell doubling limit reflects the propagation of the last surviving clone. The relevance of either figure to survival of cells in the body has been extensively discussed and the relationship between cellular senescence *in vitro* and normal aging of whole organisms *in vivo* is still obscure. Further, contrasting the well established *in vitro* findings it has been shown that stem cells in some renewing tissues undergo more than 1000 divisions in a lifetime with no morphological sign of senescence.[45] The molecular mechanism behind cellular senescence is an accumulating defect in chromosome telomere elongation which is a result of defective telomerase activity.[46] Telomerase and telomeres are involved in the control of cell proliferation as well as the unlimited proliferation capacity of malignant cells. Human telomeres are specialized chromosomal end structures composed of TTAGGG repeats and function by protecting chromosomes from degradation, fusion and recombination. Data derived from stem cell populations and different tissues with varying proliferative patterns indicate that telomerase is active *in vivo* where and when it is needed to maintain tissue integrity. However, data from the immune system indicate that replicative senescence may be an important factor behind immune exhaustion in human immunodeficiency virus disease.[47]

CELLULAR GROWTH PATTERNS OF TISSUES *IN VIVO*

At the systemic level homeostatic mechanisms must operate to control and adjust the rate of cell renewal and cell death in order to keep tissues and organs at their optimal size. The needs vary in different tissues. Mammalian tissues may be divided into three major categories with respect to their intrinsic proliferative activity *in vivo*. In permanent tissues, cells are permanently growth arrested and cannot be replaced by proliferation of their differentiated neighbor cells if they are lost. Many highly differentiated cell types such as nerve cells, skeletal muscle, and lens cells of the eye belong to this category. This group also includes a variety of terminally differentiated cells that have lost the intracellular machinery needed for cell division, such as erythrocytes and neutrophils. Cells of permanent tissues may renew their subcellular constituents and can alter in size and change structural features, but the fully differentiated cells of permanent tissues never divide under normal conditions. The clinical consequence is poor if any regenerative ability, which is obvious for nervous tissue. Another important clinical implication is that permanent cell types are rarely involved in malignant transformation. The major advances in stem cell biology during recent years (see below) may change the therapeutic scene in the future but the clinical applications of these techniques are yet of limited functional relevance for permanent tissues.

A second type of intrinsic growth pattern is found in so-called expanding tissues. Here, the tissue balances cell deaths and births to maintain the organ size. A good example of this is the liver which contains fully differentiated hepatocytes that may divide on demand to produce daughter cells of the same type. The normal turnover time of individual liver cells may well be several years, but this can be speeded up when needed. In experimental liver regeneration in rats, two-thirds of the liver is removed surgically and the remaining part studied for the regeneration pattern.[48] In such experiments, regenerating liver cells start to divide within 24 h of the injury and continue to proliferate until the loss of liver cell mass is repaired. Gene expression analyses and studies with parabiotic animals have revealed that the regenerative process is associated with activation of a number of growth factors and cytokines including hepatocyte growth factor, members of the epidermal growth factor superfamily and interleukin-6.[48,49] Interestingly, the active regulation of liver cell mass operates also to reduce liver size if too many cells are present. Thus, increased apoptosis of liver cells is observed during the regression phase after experimentally induced liver cell hyperplasia *in vivo*.[50] Another typical example of cells that rest outside the cell division cycle until there is a need for more cells is the immunocomponent lymphocytes which proliferate only if activated by the proper antigenic stimulus.

The third type of intrinsic growth pattern is found in renewing tissues with a continuous high rate of proliferation. This kind of pattern is typical of the intestinal epithelium, the epidermis and the bone marrow. In these tissues, stem cells (see below) produce daughter cells that either repopulate the stem cell compartment where they continue to proliferate, or become differentiated cells that undergo further maturation, ending up as terminally differentiated cells which are eventually eliminated through programmed cell death (see above). In certain tissues (e.g., the epiphyseal growth plate; Fig. 2.1), the number of stem cells are finite and not self-renewing; the growth process is therefore irreversibly terminated when all stem cells have been consumed. Most renewing tissues, however, have an indefinite number of stem cells as a result of the self-renewal process, so securing a continuous supply of differentiated progeny with a reproductive capacity greatly exceeding the full life expectancy of the host. Renewing tissues are often sites of malignant transformation.

STEM CELLS

Stem cells are undifferentiated cells capable of self-renewal and differentiation to cells of different lineages. Embryonic stem cells are pluripotent cells derived from the inner cell mass of blastocyst stage embryos, possessing long-lasting capacity to self-renew and differentiate into cell types of all three germ layers (endodermal, ectodermal, mesodermal).

Somatic stem cells are found in differentiated tissues and can renew themselves in addition to generating the specialized cell types of their tissue of origin.[51] Somatic stem cells have been discovered in tissues that were previously not thought to contain these kinds of cells, such as the brain. Some of these somatic stem cells appear to be capable of developing into cell types of other tissues, but have a reduced differentiation potential as compared to embryo-derived stem cells. Therefore, somatic stem cells are referred to as multipotent rather than pluripotent. In renewing tissues unipotent stem cells are responsible for producing only one type of daughter cell with regard to the differentiated function.

Accumulating evidence indicates that the adult bone marrow also harbors a population of stem cells, including a small population of cells seeded to peripheral blood, with multipotent if not pluripotent capacity, in addition to the clinically widely used hematopoietic stem cells. From such findings and other observations it is obvious that stem cell biology holds great promise for use with a therapeutic intention for regenerating damaged tissues. However, as discussed elsewhere, for permanent highly differentiated cell types such as neuronal cells, such therapy is not just a matter of stem cell transfer and subsequent proliferation of the donor cells. Stem cells introduced into the nervous system must acquire a physiological function dependent on integration of neurons into functional neuronal networks. Although promising results have been achieved after transplantation of neuronal cells into the injured brain (e.g., in Parkinson's disease) it is still unclear whether these results are due to cell replacement, trophic support, or induced paracrine changes supporting endogenous neuroprotection and/or regeneration. The clinical potential for pediatric patients of advances in stem cell biology has recently been reviewed.[52]

MODELS OF TISSUE AND ORGAN SIZE CONTROL IN MULTICELLULAR ORGANISMS

Our knowledge of the regulation of proliferation of single cells has increased dramatically over the last decades, particularly with respect to cell cycle control, peptide growth factors, malignant transformation and tumor-suppression factors. However, at the global level our understanding of the mechanisms behind integrative growth and size control is still incomplete as is our insight into how organ growth is coordinated within a single individual.

From examples such as experimental liver regeneration in rats described above it is obvious that there must be well tuned mechanisms operating as tissue-size sensors. Recent findings in insects challenge our current concepts of organ size regulation in mammals. In such models it seems that organs carry intrinsic information about their size and that changes in cell numbers may be compensated by regulation of cell size. Further, it seems that evolutionary well conserved mechanisms are operative to connect external nutrient supply to cell size.[53–55] Also, in reptiles, the number of cells does not seem to determine the size of an organ. In salamanders with a varying degree of ploidy ($n = 1–5$), the organ size is maintained at the same level despite the cell number of the tissue being inversely proportional to the level of chromosomal ploidy. This is achieved through an increase in the size of individual cells that is directly proportional to the degree of ploidy, pentaploid cells being five times larger than haploid cells. However, the question still remains; how does an organ know what is the correct cell mass? Experiments in *Drosophila* have verified the results from salamanders.[2,3,55–57] Environmental factors such as nutrient availability and functional load seem also to play an important role. The latter phenomenon is well known among clinicians in cases of unilateral nephrectomy where the remaining kidney shows rapid compensatory growth. The same compensatory phenomenon has also been implicated to occur in adipose tissue.[58]

For certain tissues such as the epidermis (stratified squamous epithelium), an old hypothesis suggests that growth control is exerted by soluble factors that act as growth inhibitors at high concentrations. The originally proposed model, referred to as the chalone hypothesis, implied that the growth inhibitors consisted of tissue-specific peptides (chalones) that are secreted in constant amounts by each individual cell, thus resulting in high tissue concentrations when the total cell mass became high. The cells then stop multiplying until the concentration of chalones was lowered as a result of a loss of cell mass; this then resulted in a relapse of proliferative activity.[59] More recently the chalone hypothesis has been revisited to include some well-characterized growth inhibitory factors that are non-tissue specific, such as members of the TGF-β superfamily.[60]

Other tissue growth control models have instead discussed the bioavailability of peptide growth factors as the crucial regulatory step. Many hormones, growth factors, and cytokines are bound to and transported by binding proteins or soluble receptors in plasma and tissue fluids, leaving only a minor fraction available for direct interaction at the target receptor level. The IGF-I system constitutes a well-characterized example, which includes the ligands IGF-I and IGF-II, and at least six distinct ligand-binding proteins (IGFBPs);[14,16] see also Chapter 7. In blood plasma, 99 percent of IGF-I is bound to IGFBPs, leaving only 1 percent free to exert biological function. Thus, an increase of the level of free IGF-I obtained by lowering IGFBP levels might produce an equally effective biological response as direct stimulation of IGF-I synthesis. Regulation of ligand bioavailability by tuning its binding to specific proteins, rather than controlling production of the ligand itself is thus a possible target for systemic growth regulation. As mentioned above, lack of IGF-I function may result in a prolongation of the cell cycle transit time.[17] Several studies have demonstrated that nutrient availability may be a key factor in tissue and body size control.[57] This concept is compatible with the important function of many growth factors to regulate nutrient transport at the cellular level.

Another factor that has recently been implicated as a regulator of body size is the proto-oncogene c-Myc. Mice made incrementally deficient in c-Myc show smaller organs due to a decreased number of cells.[61] This indicates that, if c-Myc represents a physiological regulator of body and organ size in mammals, the mechanisms of such control differ from those of lower species discussed above.

KEY LEARNING POINTS

- Growth of tissues and organs *in vivo* depends on the number of cells present, the size of individual cells and the volume of the intercellular space. Cell numbers in tissues are the net yield of cell multiplication and cell death by apoptosis.
- Factors increasing tissue and organ size *in vivo* may exert their action at the cellular level by stimulating proliferation (mitogenic factors), increasing cell volume, allowing cell survival (anti-apoptotic factors) and expanding the extracellular matrix (many differentiation factors). Thus, factors stimulating growth *in vivo* may not necessarily be mitogenic.
- Mitogenic growth factors exert their effects in the cell cycle. Cycling cells need progression growth factors allowing passage over a restriction point in G1 to enter S phase. Cells withdrawing from the cycle may die by apoptosis or become quiescent in G0. Recruitment back to cycle requires competence growth factors allowing passage over a G0–G1 restriction point.
- Differentiated cells of adult tissues show three different patterns of growth *in vivo*. Cells belonging to permanent tissues (e.g., neuronal cells) do not divide whereas cells of expanding tissues (e.g., liver) are not normally dividing but may regenerate by cell division if required. In renewing tissues (e.g., bone marrow) cells show continuous multiplication.
- Stem cells are undifferentiated cells found in almost all tissues, holding great therapeutic potentials for regenerative purposes. Multipotent or pluripotent stem cells have been found in bone marrow. Such cells do not seem to be restricted by the replicative senescence (Hayflick limit) demonstrated for different cell types *in vitro*.
- Apoptosis is a highly regulated process of physiological cell death of great importance for control of tissue architecture and size. Apoptosis occurs through two major pathways; an extrinsic death receptor pathway activated by exogenous ligands and an intrinsic mitochondrial pathway activated by cellular stressors and cytotoxic compounds.
- Tissues and organs carry intrinsic information about their optimal size *in vivo*. The size sensing mechanisms are unknown but availability of growth and survival factors, growth inhibitors, and nutrient supply as well as functional demands seem to be of importance.

REFERENCES

◆ = Key review paper
● = Seminal primary article

◆　1　Raff MC. Social control of cell survival and cell death. *Nature* 1992; **356**: 397–400.
◆　2　Conlon IJ, Raff MC. Size control in animal development. *Cell* 1999; **96**: 235–44.
◆　3　Ingber DE. Mechanical control of tissue growth: Function follows form. *Proc Natl Acad Sci USA* 2005; **102**: 11571–2.
◆　4　Abbot A. Cell culture: biology's new dimension. *Nature* 2003; **424**: 870–2.
◆　5　Schwartzman RA, Cidlowski JA. Apoptosis: The biochemistry and molecular biology of programmed cell death. *Endocrine Rev* 1993; **14**: 133–51.
　　6　Murray A, Hunt T, eds. *The Cell Cycle*. Oxford: Oxford University Press, 1993.
◆　7　O'Farrell PH, Stumpff J, Su TT. Embryonic cleavage cycles: how is a mouse like a fly? *Curr Biol* 2004; **14**: R35–45.
◆　8　Hartwell LH, Weinert TA. Checkpoints: controls that ensure the order of cell cycle events. *Science* 1989; **246**: 629–34.
◆　9　Pardee AB. G1 events and regulation of cell proliferation. *Science* 1989; **246**: 603–8.
◆　10　Zetterberg A. Control of mammalian cell proliferation. *Curr Opin Cell Biol* 1990; **2**: 296–300.
◆　11　Sherr CJ. Mammalian G1 cyclins. *Cell* 1993; **73**: 1059–65.
◆　12　Cobrink D, Dowdy SF, Hinds PW, *et al.* The retino-blastoma protein and the regulation of cell cycling. *Trends Biochem Sci* 1992; **17**: 312–5.
●　13　Pardee AB. A restriction point for control of normal animal cell proliferation. *Proc Natl Acad Sci USA* 1974; **71**: 1286–90.
　　14　Sporn MB, Roberts AB, eds. *Peptide Growth Factors and Their Receptors*. Berlin: Springer Verlag, 1990.
◆　15　Kingsley DM. The TGF-b superfamily: new members, new receptors and new genetic tests of function in different organisms. *Genes Dev* 1994; **8**: 133–46.
●　16　Liu JP, Baker J, Perkins AS, *et al.* Mice carrying null mutations of the genes encoding insulin-like growth factor-I (IGF-I) and type 1 IGF receptor (IGF1R). *Cell* 1993; **75**: 59–72.
●　17　Baserga R, Porcu P, Rubini M, Sell C. Cell cycle control by the IGF-I receptor and its ligands. *Adv Exp Med Biol* 1993; **343**: 105–12.
●　18　Luetteke NC, Qui TH, Pfeiffer RL, *et al.* TGF alpha deficiency results in hair follicle and eye abnormalities in targeted and waved-1 mice. *Cell* 1993; **73**: 263–78.
●　19　Schorle H, Holtschke T, Hunig T, *et al.* Development and function of T cells in mice rendered interleukin-2 deficient by gene targeting. *Nature* 1991; **352**: 621–4.
　　20　Kohut A, Mahelova O, Mojzis J, Mirossay L. Effect of sialoadenectomy on stomach lesions induced by indomethacin and ethanol in relation to gastric vascular

permeability, the gastrin level and HCl secretion in rats. *Physiol Res* 1992; **41**: 381–6.

● 21 Lockshin RA, Williams CM. Programmed cell death. V. Cytolytic enzymes in relation to the breakdown of the intersegmental muscles of silkmoths. *J Insect Physiol* 1965; **11**: 831–44.

◆ 22 Kerr JF, Wyllie AH, Currie AR. Apoptosis: a basic biological phenomenon with wide-ranging implications in tissue kinetics. *Br J Cancer* 1972; **26**: 239–57.

◆ 23 Brenner S. New directions in molecular biology. *Nature* 1974; **248**: 785–7.

● 24 Sulston JE. Post-embryonic development in the ventral cord of *Caenorhabditis elegans*. *Philos Trans R Soc Lond B Biol Sci* 1976; **275**: 287–97.

◆ 25 Ellis HM, Horvitz HR. Genetic control of programmed cell death in the nematode *C. elegans*. *Cell* 1986; **44**: 817–29.

◆ 26 Earnshaw WC, Martins LM, Kaufmann SH. Mammalian caspases: structure, activation, substrates, and functions during apoptosis. *Annu Rev Biochem* 1999; **68**: 383–424.

◆ 27 Nagata S. Apoptosis by death factor. *Cell* 1997; **88**: 355–65.

● 28 Chinnaiyan AM, Tepper CG, Seldin MF, *et al*. FADD/MORT1 is a common mediator of CD95 (Fas/APO-1) and tumor necrosis factor receptor-induced apoptosis. *J Biol Chem* 1996; **271**: 4961–5.

◆ 29 Kim R, Emi M, Tanabe K. Caspase-dependent and -independent cell death pathways after DNA damage [Review]. *Oncol Rep* 2005; **14**: 595–9.

30 Krueger A, Schmitz I, Baumann S, *et al*. Cellular FLICE-inhibitory protein splice variants inhibit different steps of caspase-8 activation at the CD95 death-inducing signaling complex. *J Biol Chem* 2001; **276**: 20633–40.

◆ 31 Kroemer G, Reed JC. Mitochondrial control of cell death. *Nature Med* 2000; **6**: 513–19.

◆ 32 Reed JC. Dysregulation of apoptosis in cancer. *J Clin Oncol* 1999; **17**: 2941–53.

◆ 33 Reed JC, Green DR. Remodeling for demolition: Changes in mitochondrial ultrastructure during apoptosis. *Mol Cell* 2002; **9**: 1–3.

● 34 Zou H, Henzel, WJ, Liu X, *et al*. Apaf-1, a human protein homologous to *C. elegans* CED-4, participates in cytochrome c-dependent activation of caspase-3. *Cell* 1997; **90**: 405–13.

● 35 Chereau D, Zou H, Spada AP, Wu JC. A nucleotide binding site in caspase-9 regulates apoptosome activation. *Biochemistry* 2005; **44**: 4971–6.

◆ 36 Zhang L, Yu J, Park BH, *et al*. Role of BAX in the apoptotic response to anticancer agents. *Science* 2000; **290**: 989–92.

◆ 37 Antonsson B, Martinou JC. The Bcl-2 protein family. *Exp Cell Res* 2000; **256**: 50–7.

● 38 Guo B, Godzik A, Reed JC. Bcl-G, a novel pro-apoptotic member of the Bcl-2 family. *J Biol Chem* 2001; **276**: 2780–5.

● 39 Ke N, Godzik A, Reed JC. Bcl-B, a novel Bcl-2 family member that differentially binds and regulates Bax and Bak. *J Biol Chem* 2001; **276**: 12481–4.

40 Oda E, Ohki R, Murasawa H, *et al*. Noxa, a BH3-only member of the Bcl-2 family and candidate mediator of p53-induced apoptosis. *Science* 2000; **288**: 1053–8.

◆ 41 Green DR, Reed JC. Mitochondria and apoptosis. *Science* 1998; **281**: 1309–12.

● 42 Campos L, Rouault, JP, Sabido O, *et al*. High expression of Bcl-2 protein in acute myeloid leukemia cells is associated with poor response to chemotherapy. *Blood* 1993; **81**: 3091–6.

● 43 Williams GT, Smith CA, Spooncer E, *et al*. Haematopoietic colony stimulating factors promote cell survival by suppressing apoptosis. *Nature* 1990; **343**: 76–9.

● 44 Hayflick L. The limited in vitro lifetime of human diploid cell strains. *Exp Cell Res* 1965; **37**: 614–36.

◆ 45 Rubin H. The disparity between human cell senescence in vitro and lifelong replication in vivo. *Nature Biotechnol* 2002; **20**: 675–81.

● 46 Lundblad V, Szostak JW. A mutant with a defect in telomere elongation leads to senescence in yeast. *Cell* 1989; **57**: 633–43.

47 Effros R, Pawelec G. Replicative senescence of T cells: does the Hayflick limit lead to immune exhaustion? *Immunol Today* 1997; **18**: 450–4.

◆ 48 Michalopoulos GK, DeFrances MC. Liver regeneration. *Science* 1997; **276**: 60–6.

49 Furlong RA. The biology of the hepatocyte growth factor/scatter factor. *Bioessays* 1992; **14**: 613–7.

● 50 Bursch W, Taper HS, Lauer B, Schulte-Hermann R. Quantitative histological and histochemical studies on the occurrence and stages of controlled cell death (apoptosis) during regression of rat liver hyperplasia. *Virchow's Arch B Cell Pathol Mol Pathol* 1985; **50**: 153–66.

◆ 51 Mayhall EA, Paffett-Lugassy N, Zon LI. The clinical potential of stem cells. *Curr Opin Cell Biol* 2004; **16**: 713–20.

◆ 52 Pediatric Research, Special Review Issue. *Clinical Potential of Stem Cells in Pediatric Medicine*. The Woodlands, Philadelphia: Lippincott Williams & Wilkins, 2006.

◆ 53 Stocker H, Hafen E. Genetic control of cell size. *Curr Opin Genet Dev* 2000; **10**: 529–35.

◆ 54 Potter CJ, Xu T. Mechanisms of size control. *Curr Opin Genet Dev* 2001; **11**: 279–86.

◆ 55 Johnston LA, Gallant P. Control of growth and organ size in Drosophila. *Bioessays* 2002; **24**: 54–64.

● 56 Brogiolo W, Stocker H, Ikeya T, *et al*. An evolutionary conserved function of the Drosophila insulin receptor and insulin-like peptides in growth control. *Curr Biol* 2001; **11**: 213–21.

● 57 Colombani J, Raisin S, Pantalacci S, *et al*. A nutrient sensor mechanism controls Drosophila growth. *Cell* 2003; **114**: 739–49.

58 Hausman DB, Lu J, Ryan DH, *et al.* Compensatory growth of adipose tissue after partial lipectomy: involvement of serum factors. *Exp Biol Med* 2004; **229**: 512–20.

59 Refsum SB, Haskjold E, Bjerknes R, Iversen OH. Circadian variation in cell proliferation and maturation. A hypothesis for the growth regulation of the rat corneal epithelium. *Virchow's Arch B Cell Pathol Mol Pathol* 1991; **60**: 225–30.

60 Strain AJ. Transforming growth factor-beta: the elusive hepatic chalone. *Hepatology* 1992; **16**: 269–70.

◆ 61 Trumpp A, Refaeli Y, Oskarsson,T, *et al.* C-Myc regulates mammalian body size by controlling cell number but not cell size. *Nature* 2001; **414**: 768–73.

3

Bone and cartilage growth and metabolism

DOV TIOSANO, ZE'EV HOCHBERG

LONGITUDINAL GROWTH AT THE GROWTH PLATE

The skeleton is made of two tissues, cartilage and bone, three cell types, chondrocyte, osteoblast and osteoclast, and more than 216 different skeletal elements throughout the body. After developing a given skeletal element, mesenchymal cells in this element differentiate in most cases into chondrocytes, the cell type specific for cartilage. The cartilaginous template is eventually replaced by bone containing osteoblasts and osteoclasts. This process of bone formation is called endochondral ossification. In some skeletal elements, mesenchymal cells differentiate directly into osteoblasts in a process called intramembranous ossification.[1]

Positioned between the epiphyseal bone crest and its metaphyseal boundary, the growth plate is a highly organized functional unit, commissioned to continuous delivery of new cartilage cells and matrix, to be succeeded by bone formation. Endochondral ossification at the growth plate can be divided for didactic purposes into two consecutive phases: (1) chondroplasia – the process of cartilage differentiation and growth; and (2) osteogenesis – the process of calcification and ossification of cartilage tissue.[2]

PRIMARY AND SECONDARY OSSIFICATION CENTERS

In early fetal life a rod of hyaline cartilage, condensed with mesenchymal cells, prefigures a long bone. Nutrient vessels deliver pluripotent stem cells, which give rise to the bone marrow, as a source of building blocks for the ossification centers (Fig. 3.1). The first step in the formation of a center of primary ossification takes place when chondrocytes deep in the center of the primitive shaft enlarge greatly. Their intervening glycoprotein matrix is then calcified and compressed into thin and often perforated septa. Chondrocyte cytoplasm becomes vacuolated and accumulates glycogen, and as they undergo further hypertrophy, they degenerate through a process of apoptosis. The lacunae formed in the calcified cartilage by cell death do not remain empty for long. The periosteal collar overlying the calcified cartilage wall invades chondrocyte lacunae by osteogenic buds from the deep periosteal layers. These are blind-ended capillaries that accompany embryonic medullary tissue, vascular mesenchymal osteoprogenitor cells, osteoclasts, osteoblasts, hematopoietic and marrow stromal cells.

As bones enlarge, secondary ossification centers are established in the bone epiphyses through a similar process. In long bones of the limbs, growth chondrocytes continue to proliferate between primary and secondary ossification centers. This cartilage then forms the growth plate, as a distinct plate of cells between bones of the secondary ossification centre and the primary spongiosa.

HISTOLOGICAL APPEARANCE OF THE GROWTH PLATE

An organized region of rapid growth develops as the future growth plate between epiphysis and diaphysis. Transverse

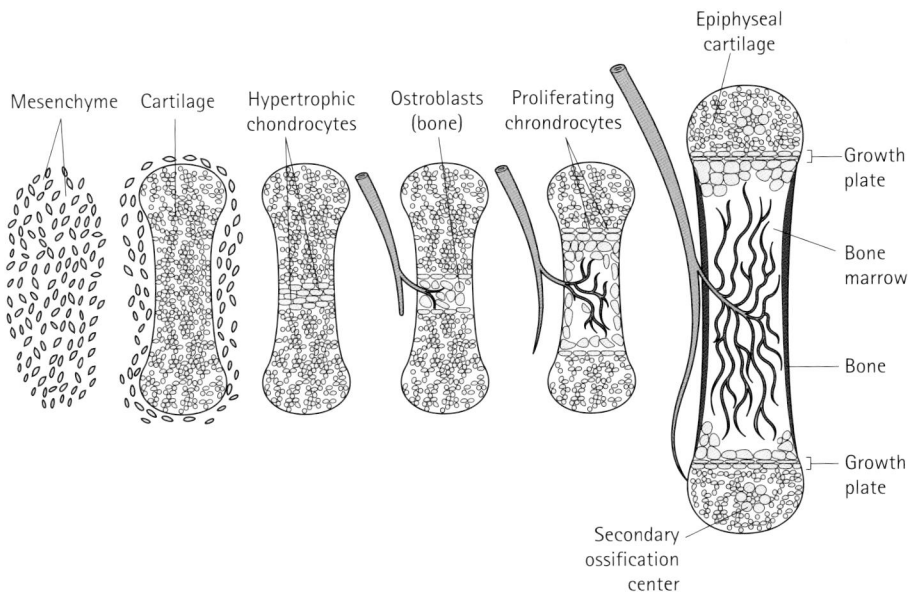

Figure 3.1 Bone development from its mesenchymal analage. Hyaline cartilage transforms into a primary then a secondary ossification center. Nutrient vessels deliver pluripotent stem cells as a source for building blocks. Between the primary and secondary ossification centers, a growth plate becomes the site of enchondral ossification.

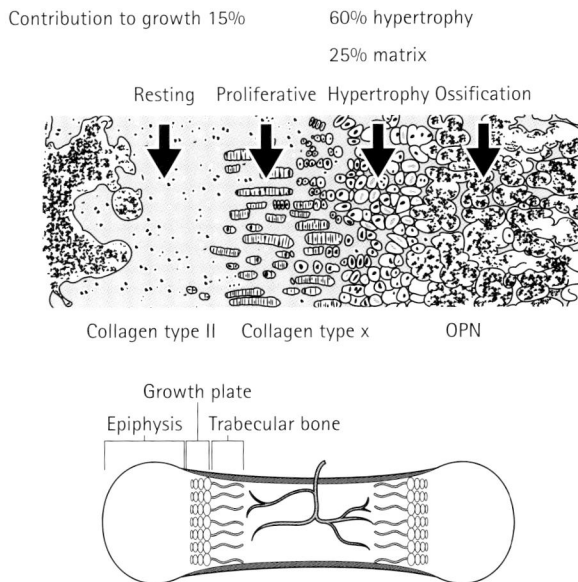

Figure 3.2 Photomicrograph of longitudinal cell columns of the growth plate. Adjoining the upper epiphysis, the first layer of reserve cells in the resting zone differentiate into collagen type II-producing proliferating chondrocytes, which will become collagen type X-producing hypertrophic chondrocytes, before they undergo apoptosis and die at the ossification front. OPN, osteopontin.

or latitudinal growth is due to transverse mitosis and appositional growth resulting from matrix deposition by cells from the perichondrial ring at this level. The future growth plate thus expands in concert with the shaft and adjacent future epiphysis (Fig. 3.2).

On the epiphyseal end of the plate, a zone of reserve chondroprogenitor cells makes the resting zone. Further towards the shaft of the bone is an actively mitotic zone – the proliferative zone. More frequent divisions in the long axis soon create longitudinal columns of flat chondrocytes, each in a flattened lacuna, surrounded by cartilage matrix. The cells become rounded, with prominent rotund or oval nuclei and a low cytoplasm/nucleus ratio with gap junctions between cells. Proliferating chondrocytes secrete a surrounding basophilic halo of matrix, composed of a delicate network of type II collagen filaments, type IX collagen, a high level of oxidative enzyme activity and cartilage proteoglycan core proteins that make the hallmark of differentiation into chondrocytes.

Traced centrally in the shaft, the cells cease to divide and show increasing maturity to make the hypertrophic zone. They increase in size, change orientation from transverse to longitudinal, accumulate glycogen and display surface projections into reciprocal recesses in the lacuna walls. The projections increase greatly as the cells hypertrophy, although the largest cells apparently lose their projections.

In the process of endochondral ossification, mineralization of the growth plate is closely associated with type X collagen production in the hypertrophic zone. There is a sharp redox change and energy metabolism is depressed. The chondrocytes enter an apoptotic process.

The calcified lacunae become the zone of bone formation, and are invaded by vascular elements of bone marrow, osteoblasts and osteoclasts. As the bone reaches maturity, epiphyseal and metaphyseal ossification processes gradually encroach upon the growth plate from either side, eventually meeting to make a bony fusion of the epiphysis and metaphysis as the longitudinal growth of bone ends. As growth ceases, the cartilaginous plate thins gradually; metaphyseal and epiphyseal vessels unite as a bony fusion is accomplished by ossification around these vessels.

ONTOGENESIS CARTILAGE

Reserve zone

In the first layer of cells, adjacent to the epiphysis, chondroprogenitor cells form the germinative 'reserve cells', also known as 'resting cells'. These are derived from a common mesenchymal progenitor cell for chondroblast, osteoblast, myotubes and adipocytes. The resting zone cartilage makes important contributions to endochondral bone formation at the growth plate: (1) it contains stem-like cells that give rise to clones of proliferative chondrocytes; (2) it produces a growth plate-orienting factor, a morphogen that directs the alignment of the proliferative clones into columns parallel to the long axis of the bone; and (3) it may also produce a morphogen that inhibits terminal differentiation of nearby proliferative zone chondrocytes. Thus, it may be partially responsible for organization of the growth plate into distinct zones of proliferation and hypertrophy. Numerous factors take part in these cascades of transforming events such as BMP, β-catenin, Pbx1, and Wnt proteins.

BONE MORPHOGENIC PROTEINS

The transforming growth factor-β (TGF-β) superfamily comprises a number of functionally diverse growth factors/signaling molecules that elicit their response upon binding to serine-threonine kinase receptors (Table 3.1). As members of the TGF-β superfamily, bone morphogenic proteins (BMPs) direct the transformation of the pluripotent mesenchymal stem cell to form chondrocytes and osteoblasts. Of the 15 members of the BMP family, BMP2 and BMP4 are specifically important for this differentiation process. Targeted disruption of either BMP2 or BMP4 leads to early embryonic lethality[3] whereas mutations in BMP5 and BMP6 display mild skeletal phenotypes, indicating a highly redundant role of BMPs in regulating bone development.[4]

The chordin-like protein (CHL2) behaves as a secreted BMP-binding inhibitor; its levels decrease during chondroblast differentiation.[5]

Cartilage-derived morphogenetic protein 1 and 2 (CDMP1 and CDMP2) are closely related to the BMPs. CDMP1 is predominantly expressed at sites of skeletal morphogenesis. Expression is normally restricted to the primordial cartilage of appendicular skeleton, with little expression in the axial skeleton such as vertebrae and ribs. Mutations in the CDMP1 gene have been reported in brachydactyly type C.[6]

Growth/differentiation factor 5 (GDF5) enhances cartilage formation by promoting chondroprogenitor cell aggregation, and amplifying the responses of cartilage differentiation markers.[7] Mutations in the human GDF5 gene cause chondrodysplasia Grebe type, acromesomelic chondrodysplasia Hunter–Thompson type, and brachydactyly type C, all of which are characterized by limb defects, with increasing severity toward the distal regions.[8,9]

The BMP antagonist Noggin binds with equal avidity to BMP2 and BMP4 and competitively inhibits their interaction with the BMP receptor. It specifically blocks chondrogenic differentiation, rather than osteogenic differentiation of the mesodermal stem cell.[10] Mutations in the noggin gene result in proximal symphalangism and multiple synostoses syndrome.[11]

β-Catenin regulates important biological processes in embryonic development and tumorigenesis. It is expressed in prechondrogenic mesenchymal cells, but significantly decreases in differentiated chondrocytes. Accumulation of β-catenin inhibits chondrogenesis by stabilizing cell–cell adhesion.[12]

Pre-B cell leukemia transcription factor (Pbx1) is a TALE (three amino acid loop extension) class homeodomain protein. Its role is in coordinating the extent and/or timing of proliferation until terminal differentiation. It is important for programming chondrocyte proliferation and differentiation.[13]

Important regulators of skeletal development are the Wnt family members. These are signaling molecules that regulate cell proliferation and differentiation during embryonic development and tumor formation. Wnt5a and Wnt5b coordinate chondrocyte proliferation and differentiation by differentially regulating cyclin D1, p130, and chondrocyte-specific Col2a1 expression, which are important cell cycle regulators.[14]

Proliferating zone

In this matrix-rich zone, the flattened chondrocytes undergo cell division in a longitudinal direction, and organize in typical columns ordination (Fig. 3.3, page 29). Proliferating chondrocytes synthesize substantial amounts of extracellular matrix proteins, which are essential for matrix structure. At a given moment, either by a finite numbers of cell divisions or by changes in exposure to local PTH-related peptide (PTHrP), proliferating chondrocytes lose their capacity to divide, and become hypertrophic chondrocytes, coinciding with an increase in size. This location is called the transition zone.

PTHrP, INDIAN HEDGEHOG, AND THE FIBROBLAST GROWTH FACTORS

Ihh is a key mitogen on the transition zone.[15] It belongs to a family of morphogen hedgehog proteins that play a crucial role in embryonic patterning and development. Hedgehogs bind to a patched receptor (Ptc), thereby releasing a membrane smoothened (Smo) protein with an intrinsic intracellular activity. Released Smo proteins result in a downstream signal to activate specific intracellular targets. Ihh and Smo regulate chondrocyte proliferation at least in part by modulating the transcription of cyclin D1.[16,17]

Table 3.1 Genetic defects in the ontogenesis and function of the growth plate

Area	Defect	Reference
Reserve cells		
BMP2 or BMP4	Early embryonic lethality	3,4
BMP5, BMP6	Mild skeletal phenotypes	5
Chordin-like protein (**CHL2**)	BMP-binding inhibitor	6
Cartilage-derived morphogenetic protein 1 and 2 (**CDMP1 and CDMP2**)	Brachydactyly type C	7
GDF5 gene		8–10
Growth factors/signaling molecules that are closely related to the subfamily of bone morphogenetic proteins	Chondrodysplasia Grebe type, acromesomelic chondrodysplasia Hunter–Thompson type, and brachydactyly type C, all of which are mainly characterized by defects of the limbs, with increasing severity toward the distal region	
Noggin	Proximal symphalangism and multiple synostoses syndrome	11,12
Pbx1	Aplasia of proximal limb axis structures	14
Wnt5a and Wnt5b	Coordinate chondrocyte proliferation	15
Proliferating zone		
Indian hedgehog	Mitogen in the endochondral skeleton	16
Patched receptor (Ptc)	Indian hedgehog receptor	17,18
TGF-β2	Relay between Ihh and PTHrP	20
Constitutively activated PTH/PTHrP receptor mutations	Jansen-type metaphyseal chondrodysplasia Abrogated chondrocyte differentiation	23
Homozygous inactivation PTH/PTHrP receptor mutations	Blomstrand lethal osteochondrodysplasia (BOCD) Type I and II	24,25
FGFR1, -2 and -3	Accelerated endochondral ossification Inhibiting Ihh expression	27
FGFR2	Crouzon	24
Activating mutations of the FGFR3	Achondroplasia (97% of mutations have a Gly to Arg mutation) SADDAN (severe achondroplasia with developmental delay and acanthosis nigricans), and thanatophoric dysplasia	29,30
SOX9	Col2A1 expression is directly regulated by SOX9 Campomelic dysplasia	31
Gene mutations in type II, IX, or X collagens	Spondyloepiphyseal dysplasia and hypochondriasis, multiple epiphyseal dysplasia and Schmid metaphyseal chondrodysplasia; all are associated with short stature	33
ECM molecules: aggrecan, biglycan, glypican, and chondroitin	Autosomal recessive chondrodysplasias, including diastrophic dysplasia, atelosteogenesis type II, and achondrogenesis type 1B	34
EXT 1 and 2(Exostosis) an endoplasmic reticulum (ER)-resident type II transmembrane glycoprotein whose expression in cells results in the alteration of the synthesis and display of cell surface heparan sulfate glycosaminoglycans (GAGs)	Absence of the proteoglycan heparan sulfate, which is an important signaling molecule involved in transport of growth factors in cartilage, including Ihh and FGFs Leading to disorganization of growth plate chondrocytes	26
Hypertrophic zone		
Runx2/Cbfa1	Decreased numbers of hypertrophic chondrocytes	34
Haploinsufficiency of RUNX2	Cleidocranial dysplasia	40

(Continued)

Table 3.1 (Continued)

Area	Defect	Reference
Vascular invasion		
Hypoxia-inducible factor-1α (HIF-1α)	Anaerobic glycolysis regulator	42
VEGF	Induces invasion of vessels into the cartilage	43
Apoptosis		
Hypophosphatemia	Rachitic expansion of the calcified hypertrophic zone	45–47
Osteoblasts		
Cbfa1 type II isoform	Regulates osteoblast differentiation	53
Twist proteins	Regulates Runx2 binding to DNA	56
	Saethre–Chotzen syndrome	
Osterix	Differentiation of preosteoblasts	57
Osteoprotegerin (OPG)	Inhibits the formation of osteoclast-like cells	58
	Juvenile Paget's disease	60
RANKL	Induces formation of OCLs	61
Osteopontin	Facilitates the attachment of osteoblasts and osteoclasts to the extracellular matrix	63
Osteocalcin	Mineralized matrix of bone	64
Osteonectin	Adhesive of cell and ECM-binding glycoprotein	67
LRP5	Osteoporosis-pseudoglioma syndrome (OPPG): reduced bone mass	70

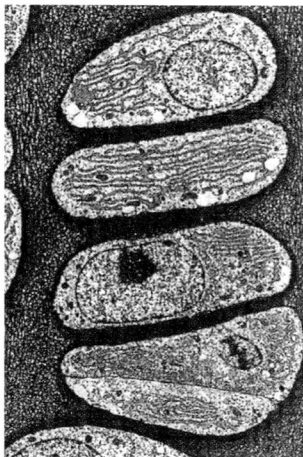

Figure 3.3 Electron micrograph of proliferating chondrocytes in rat growth plate (proximal tibia, 35 days, ×2550). The width of this cell is 7 μm, so that each division is associated with addition 7 μm in growth in a period of approx. 2 days. The cell will undergo about 4 such divisions. From Hunziker EB.[1]

Ihh is expressed by chondrocytes making the transition from a proliferating into a hypertrophic phenotype. Expression of Ihh at this stage is up-regulated by BMPs but inhibited by FGFs. Ihh activates adjacent chondrocytes and diffuses toward the lateral perichondrium, where it can bind to its receptor Ptc. BMP and Ihh signals regulate chondrocytes proliferation and the onset of hypertrophic differentiation. At the same time, BMP delays the maturation of terminally hypertrophic cells.[18] TGFβ2 acts as a signal relay between Ihh and PTHrP in the regulation of cartilage hypertrophic differentiation. TGFβ2 mediates the effect of Ihh on hypertrophic differentiation and PTHrP expression.[19]

PTHrP is generated from the periarticular perichondrium. It diffuses toward the early hypertrophic zone, which expresses high levels of PTH/PTHrP receptors, and inhibits differentiation of proliferating chondrocytes to cells capable of synthesizing Ihh. Because Ihh and PTHrP are not expressed in close proximity to each other, and the matrix surrounding chondrocytes allows only limited diffusion of growth factors, intermediates may play a role between Ihh and PTHrP signaling[20] (Fig. 3.4). In two human conditions the function of the PTH/PTHrP receptor in the transition zone is disturbed.[21] A constitutively activated PTH/PTHrP receptor causes Jansen-type metaphyseal chondrodysplasia, which is characterized by abrogated chondrocyte differentiation and severe dwarfism.[22] On the other hand, homozygous inactivation of this receptor causes Blomstrand lethal osteochondrodysplasia (BOCD) and dwarfism.[23] BOCD presents in two forms, a severe form (type I) and a milder form (type II). This disease is characterized by accelerated endochondral ossification, which is the mirror image of the Jansen-type metaphyseal chondrodysplasia that results from an activating mutation.[24]

Exostosis (EXT 1 and 2) is an endoplasmic reticulum (ER)-resident type II transmembrane glycoprotein whose expression in cells results in the alteration of the synthesis and display of cell surface heparan sulfate glycosaminoglycans (GAGs). In the absence of the proteoglycan heparan sulfate, which is an important signaling molecule involved in transport of growth factors in cartilage, Ihh and FGFs lead to disorganization of growth plate chondrocytes.[25]

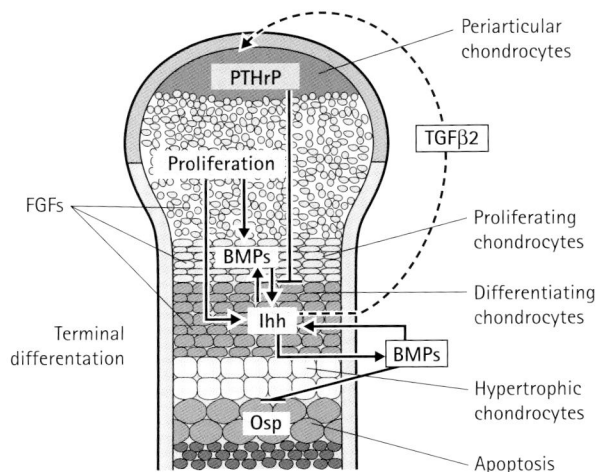

Figure 3.4 During endochondral ossification *Ihh* is expressed in the differentiating chondrocytes. Ihh induces the expression of *PTHrP* in periarticular chondrocytes; *TGF-β2* acts as a signal relay between Ihh and PTHrP in the regulation of cartilage hypertrophic differentiation. PTHrP signaling keeps chondrocytes in a proliferating state by blocking premature hypertrophic differentiation. Ihh in addition regulates the expression of BMP genes in the perichondrium/periosteum and in part of the proliferating chondrocytes. BMP and Ihh signaling together up-regulate chondrocyte proliferation, thereby pushing cells out of the range of PTHrP signaling. BMP signaling also negatively regulates the development of terminally differentiated hypertrophic chondrocytes.

Some of the FGFs are major regulators of embryonic bone development. At least 23 members were identified and they interact with at least four receptors (FGFR). They inhibit chondrocyte proliferation by inhibiting Ihh expression. Both FGF1 and -2 as well as FGFR1, -2, and -3 are expressed in chondrocytes.[26] The FGFR express in two splice variants IIIb and IIIc. FGFR2-IIIc is a positive regulator of ossification that affects mainly the osteoblast, while FGFR3-IIIc has a negative role on both chondrocytes and osteoblasts. FGF18, a ligand for FGFR2-IIIc and FGFR3-IIIc acts as a coordinator of osteogenesis via these two receptors.[27]

In humans, activating mutations of the FGFR3 cause achondroplasia; 97 percent of mutations are a Gly to Arg mutation in codon 380.[28] In addition, three other types of chrondrodysplasia due to mutations in FGFR3 gene have been described. One is a mild form of chrondrodysplasia, and two are severe types, severe achondroplasia with developmental delay and acanthosis nigricans (SADDAN), and thanatophoric dysplasia.[29]

FGF and PTHrP signals independently inhibit chondrocyte differentiation through two integrated parallel pathways that mediate both overlapping and distinct functions during longitudinal bone growth. The balance between BMP and FGF is crucial in regulating proliferation, Ihh expression and terminal differentiation of chondrocytes.

SOX9 is expressed during chondrocyte differentiation to become a target of PTHrP signaling in prehypertrophic chondrocytes in the growth plate. During chondrogenesis

in the mouse, Sox9 is co-expressed with type II collagen (Col2a1) to become the major cartilage matrix protein. Col2A1 expression is directly regulated by SOX9 and abnormal regulation of COL2A1 during chondrogenesis is implicated in skeletal abnormalities associated with campomelic dysplasia.[30] Sox9 is up-regulated by FGFs in chondrocytes and is mediated by the mitogen-activated protein kinase (MAPK) cascade, during chondrocyte differentiation.[31]

EXTRACELLULAR MATRIX PROTEINS

As the process of differentiation and cell commitment to the chondrocyte cascade of maturation progresses several protein are expressed and secreted to the ECM. The major group of matrix proteins consists of the collagens, of which type II is expressed predominantly in the proliferating zone, type IX in the pre-hypertrophic zone, and type X in the hypertrophic zone (Table 3.2). Gene mutations in type II, IX or X collagens causes spondylo-epiphyseal dysplasia and hypochondrogenesis, multiple epiphyseal dysplasia and Schmid metaphyseal chondrodysplasia.[32]

Aggrecan, biglycan, glypican, and chondroitin belong to another group of proteoglycans that require free sulfate groups for their activation and for cross-linking of the ECM. Several autosomal recessive chondrodysplasias, including diastrophic dysplasia, atelosteogenesis type II, and achondrogenesis type 1B[33] results from defective synthesis of sulfated proteoglycans.

The cell surface adhesion receptors integrins mediate the attachment of the chondrocytes to the surrounding ECM macromolecules.

The metalloproteinases (MMP) and their inhibitors are involved in maintaining the ECM and in initiating angiogenesis. MMP-13 (collagenase-3) is essential in the transition zone of the growth plate, and plays an important role in the degradation of collagen II and expression of collagen X.[34,35] Mice lacking MMP-9 display abnormal growth plate vascularization and bone formation, whereas disruption of tissue inhibitors of MMP-1 in mice increases basement membrane invasiveness of chondroprogenitor cells.

Hypertrophic zone

Hypertrophic chondrocytes have a longitudinal, round appearance and secrete large amounts of matrix proteins (Fig. 3.5). These proteins are located in small membrane-enclosed particles that are released from chondrocytes to the matrix, and contain large amounts of annexins and connective tissue growth factors (CTGF, CCN2). These matrix vesicles generate calcium-phosphate hydroxyapatite, which has a major role in the mineralization of the vesicles and their surroundings. CTGF is a key regulator in coupling ECM remodeling to angiogenesis at the growth plate. The mineralization process, in combination with low oxygen tension, attracts blood vessels from the underlying primary spongiosum.[36]

Table 3.2 Proteins involved in the regulation of bone formation and modulation

Protein	Role
Osteonectin (SPARC)	Calcium apatite and matrix protein binding
	Modulation of cell attachment
α-2-HS-glycoprotein	Chemotaxis for monocytes
	Mineralization via matrix vesicles
Osteocalcin (bone GLA protein)	Stabilization of hydroxyapatite
	Binding of calcium
	Chemotaxis for monocytes
	Regulation of bone formation
Matrix-GLA-protein	Inhibition of matrix mineralization
Osteopontin (bone sialoprotein I)	Cell attachment
	Calcium binding
Bone sialoprotein II	Cell attachment
	Calcium binding
24K Phosphoprotein (α-1procollagen N-propeptide)	Residue from collagen processing
Biglycan (proteoglycan I)	Regulation of collagen fiber growth
	Mineralization and bone formation
	Growth factor binding
Decorin (proteoglycan II)	Collagen fibrillogenesis
	Growth factor binding
Thrombospondin and fibronectin	Cell attachment
	Growth factor binding
	Hydroxyapatite formation

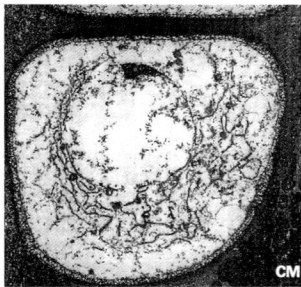

Figure 3.5 Electron micrograph of a hypertrophic chondrocyte in rat growth plate (proximal tibia, 35 days, ×2550). The cell has increased its longitudinal size within approx. 2 days five-fold to about 38 μm, as compared to the 7 μm of the proliferating cell in Fig. 3.3, so that the growth of each cell contributes 31 μm over that period. From Hunziker EB.[1]

RUNX2/Cbfa1 is an essential transcription factor for osteoblast and chondrocyte differentiation from early commitment step to final differentiation. It came to prominent attention because mice missing Runx2 have no osteoblasts and exhibit abnormalities of chondrocyte maturation. Their bones either lack or have decreased numbers of hypertrophic chondrocytes, and those hypertrophic chondrocytes already present, fail to mineralize their matrix and have decreased or absent expression of osteopontin and MMP13.[37,38] RUNX2 is expressed in the late condensation stage of chondrogenesis, mainly in the prehypertrophic and hypertrophic chondrocytes. It is highly expressed in perichondrial cells and in osteoblasts. Haploinsufficiency of RUNX2 causes cleidocranial dysplasia.[39] It also plays a role in the expression of vascular endothelial growth factor (VEGF) in growth plate chondrocytes to attract vasculature to lacunae of the terminal hypertrophic cells.[40]

VASCULAR INVASION AND VASCULAR ENDOTHELIAL GROWTH FACTOR

Epiphyseal cartilage remains largely avascular due to the production of angiogenic inhibitors. As a result, the center of the epiphysis is hypoxic, and survival of these chondrocytes is dependent on anaerobic glycolysis regulated by hypoxia-inducible factor-1 (HIF-1).[41] When the chondrocytes differentiate into mature hypertrophic cells they produce angiogenic stimulators and attract metaphyseal blood vessels. Metaphyseal vascular invasion is associated with apoptosis of terminal hypertrophic chondrocytes and recruitment of osteoblasts and osteoclasts, resulting in the replacement of mineralized cartilage with bone and marrow.

Vascular invasion is regulated by several factors including VEGF produced by hypertrophic chondrocytes. VEGF exists as three isoforms: a soluble $VEGF_{120}$, a matrix-bound $VEGF_{188}$, and $VEGF_{164}$. All isoforms bind the receptors Flt-1 (VEGF receptor-1) and Flk-1 (VEGF receptor-2), whereas only $VEGF_{164}$ binds neuropilin-1 (NRP-1). Progressive growth of normal avascular epiphyseal cartilage results in a state of increasing hypoxia, inducing VEGF expression. Soluble VEGF isoforms diffuse from the hypoxic center

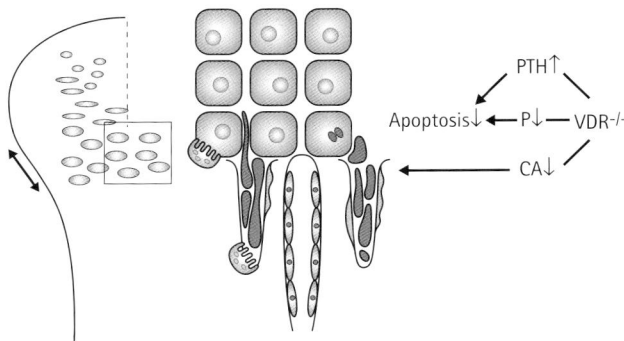

Figure 3.6 Apoptosis of the late hypertrophic chondrocyte is regulated by phosphorus in a dose and time dependent manner. Low phosphate is the major determinant of decreased chondrocyte apoptosis that leads to rachitic changes in the growth plate.

toward the periphery, thereby stimulating epiphyseal vessel outgrowth that reduces hypoxic stress. VEGF then induces invasion of vessels into the cartilage, initiating secondary ossification. Proteases mediating cartilage resorption, such as MMP-9, release bound VEGF that acts upon endothelial cells, osteoclasts, and osteoblasts, thereby coupling metaphyseal vascularization, cartilage resorption, and bone formation.[42]

APOPTOSIS OF THE TERMINAL CHONDROCYTE

The terminal chondrocyte of the hypertrophic zone undergoes programmed cell death, apoptosis, leaving a scaffold for new bone formation. Early in the process, phosphatidylserine is translocated from the inner surface of the plasma membrane to the outer surface; permitting binding of circulating annexin V. Annexin V forms the voltage-dependent Ca^{2+} channels in the phospholipid bilayer, thereby regulating the permeability of the channel pore to ions. Elevated intracellular calcium levels activate proteases, lipases, and nucleases.[43]

Apoptosis of the late hypertrophic chondrocyte is regulated by phosphorus. Inorganic phosphate induces chondrocyte apoptosis in a dose and time dependent manner.[42,44] Hypophosphatemia blocks the translocation of phosphatidyl-serine from the inner surface of the plasma membrane to its outer surface. Low phosphate is the major determinant of decreased chondrocyte apoptosis that leads to rachitic changes in the growth plate, as seen in humans with hypophosphatemic rickets in the absence of hyperparathyroidism. In hypocalcemic rickets with hyperparathyroidism, as in vitamin D receptor mutations,[45] rachitic bone changes are detected in the presence of phosphaturia before calcium levels decrease (Fig. 3.6).

Survival and maintenance of the differentiated phenotype of chondrocytes are regulated by growth factors and cytokines. Pro-inflammatory cytokines such as interleukin-1

exert catabolic effects during cartilage destruction that is mediated by nitric oxide (NO) production. Direct production of NO induces dedifferentiation and apoptosis by modulating various intracellular signaling processes such as activation of p38 kinase, extracellular signal-regulated kinase (ERK) and mitogen-activated proteins (MAP) kinases that are widely involved in signal transduction. IGF1 blocks this process, and thereby has an inhibitory effect on apoptosis of the terminal hypertrophic chondrocyte.[15]

Thus, rachitic hypophosphatemia is associated with a marked decrease in apoptosis, leading to the characteristic rachitic expansion of the calcified hypertrophic zone of the growth plate. Phosphorous has a major role in the growth plate maturation and apoptosis of hypertrophic chondrocytes (Fig. 3.6).

THE BONE AND ITS ONTOGENESIS

The osteoblasts

Osteoblasts originate from common progenitors, which are capable of differentiating into other mesenchymal cell lineages such as chondrocytes, myoblasts, bone marrow stromal cells, and adipocytes (Fig. 3.7). During this differentiation process various hormones and cytokines regulate osteoblast differentiation. Among these, BMPs are the most potent inducers: BMPs not only stimulate osteoprogenitor cells to differentiate into mature osteoblasts, but also induce non-osteogenic cells to differentiate into osteoblast lineage cells. The counter regulatory mechanism of BMP stimulation is noggin, a 60 kDa homodimeric protein that is expressed in mature osteoblasts, and inhibits osteoblast differentiation and bone formation.[46]

The common progenitor gives rise to both chondrocytes and osteoblasts, a division arguably dictated by Sox9 and Cbfa1/Runx2. Like chondrocytes, pre-osteoblasts are also self-renewing, and exit the cell cycle to form osteocytes. When subjected to compression, they undergo chondrogenesis in relation with up-regulation of Sox9. Sonic and Indian hedgehogs (Ihh) play important roles in regulation of osteoblast differentiation by interacting with BMPs to up-regulate the core binding factor a1 (Cbfa1) expression.

Cbfa1/Runx2 is essential but not sufficient for osteoblast differentiation and bone formation. Cbfa1-deficient mice completely lacked bone formation due to maturational arrest of osteoblasts, and osteoclastogenesis is markedly retarded. In humans, the cleidocranial dysplasia (CCD) phenotype reveals perturbation of the Cbfa1 gene structure.[47]

Several isoforms for each of the three Cbfa transcription factors have been identified. The Cbfa1 type I isoform is a 513 amino acid protein (designated p56/type I) that initiates in exon 2.[48] The second major isoform, til-1 (designated p57 or type II isoform), initiates in exon 1 and is only 15 amino acids longer than the p56/type I isoform.[49]

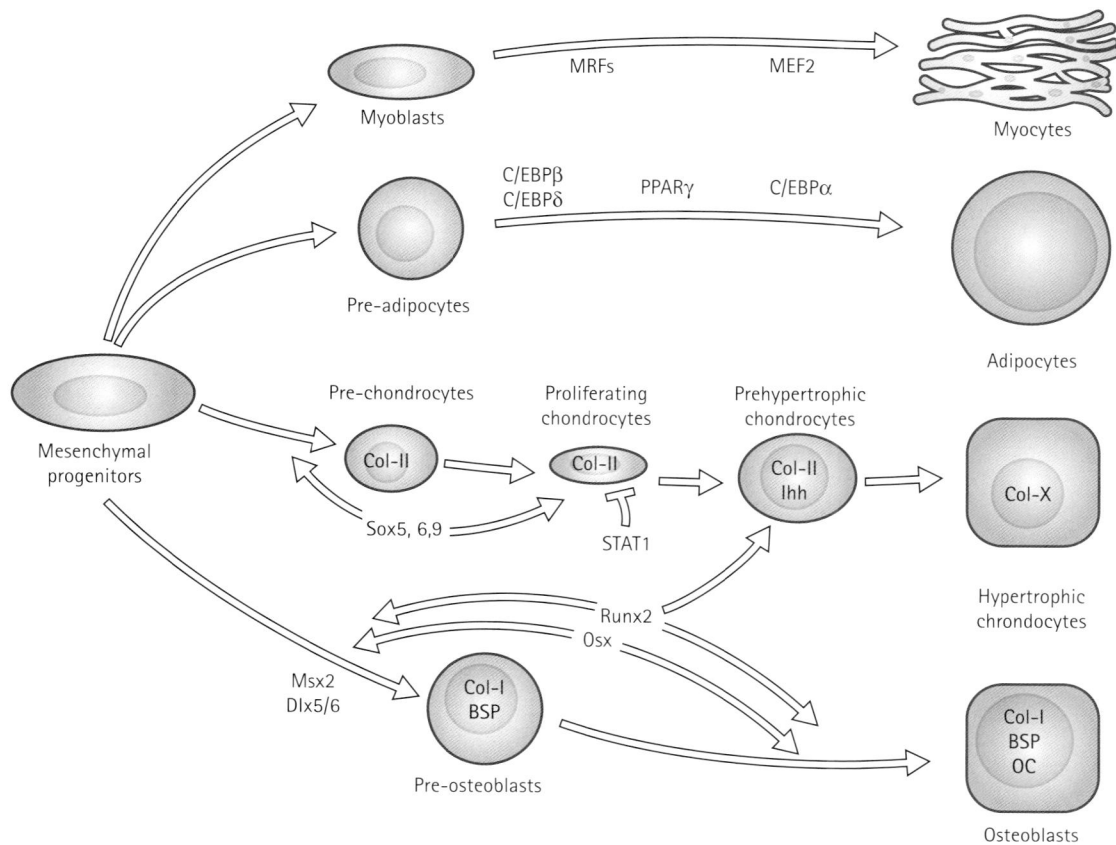

Figure 3.7 Transcriptional control stem cell differentiation. Osteoblasts differentiate from mesenchymal progenitor cells under the control of MRFs and MEF2 and to chondrocytes under the control of Sox5, -6, -9 and STAT1. Runx2 is essential for osteoblast differentiation and is also involved in chondrocyte maturation. Osterix (Osx) acts downstream of Runx2 to induce mature osteoblasts that express osteoblast markers, including osteocalcin. (Abbreviations: MRFs, myogenic regulatory factors (including MyoD, myogenin, myogenic factor 5 and myogenic regulatory factor 4); MEF2, myocyte-enhancer factor 2; C/EBP, CCAAT-enhancer-binding protein; PPARγ, peroxisome proliferator-activated receptor γ; STAT1, signal transducers and activators of transcription-1; Runx2, runt-related transcription factor 2; Col-I/II/X, type I/II/X collagen; Ihh, Indian hedgehog; BSP, bone sialoprotein; OC, osteocalcin.) Adapted from Harada S and Rodan GA. Control of osteoblast function and regulation of bone mass. *Nature* 2003; **423**: 349–355. With permission from Macmillan Publishers Ltd: Nature, copyright 2003.

Type I transcript is constitutively expressed in nonosseous mesenchymal tissues and during osteoblast differentiation. However, expression of the type II transcript is regulated during osteoblast differentiation and is induced by BMP2.[50]

TGF-β inhibits the expression of the cbfa1 and osteocalcin genes, whose expression is controlled by Runx2/Cbfa1 in osteoblast-like cell lines. This inhibition is mediated by Smad3, which interacts with Cbfa1 and represses its transcriptional activity at the Cbfa1-binding CBFA1 gene promoter sequence.[51] Tob, a member of the emerging family of anti-proliferative proteins, negatively regulates osteoblast proliferation and differentiation by suppressing the activity of the receptor-regulated Smad proteins.[52]

Twist proteins transiently inhibit Runx2 function during skeletogenesis. Twist 1 and 2 are expressed in Runx2-expressing cells throughout the skeleton early during development, and osteoblast-specific gene expression occurs only after their expression decreases. Twist1 and Twist2 bind directly to the DNA-binding domain of Runx2, therefore decreasing the ability of Runx2 to bind to DNA. Mutations in Twist 1 and 2 cause premature osteoblast differentiation as seen in the Saethre–Chotzen syndrome.[53]

Osterix (Osx) is a novel zinc finger-containing transcription factor that acts downstream of Runx2. It is required for the differentiation of preosteoblasts into fully functioning osteoblasts and is a negative regulator of Sox9 and of the chondrocyte phenotype.[54] Although, Osx null preosteoblasts express typical chondrocyte marker genes, they do not deposit bone matrix or differentiate into osteoblasts.

The osteoblast role in osteoclastogenesis

Two molecules produced by osteoblasts play important roles in osteoclastogenesis. These are osteoprotegerin (OPG) and RANKL (receptor activator of NFκB ligand) (Fig. 3.8).

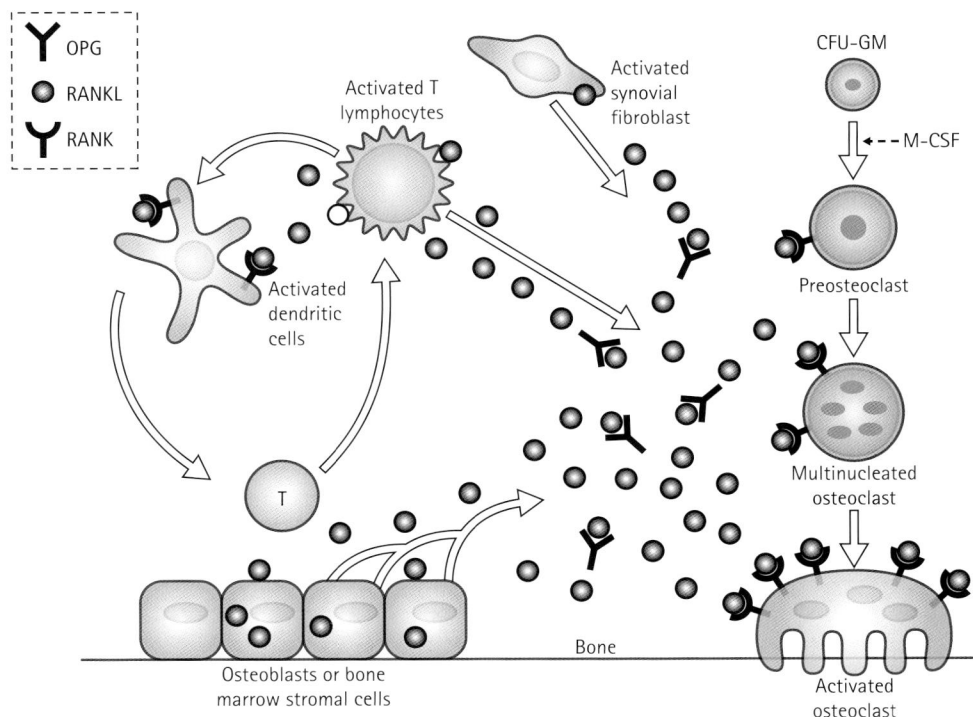

Figure 3.8   Hormonal control of bone resorption. RANKL expression is induced in osteoblasts, activated T cells, synovial fibroblasts and bone marrow stromal cells, and subsequently binds to its specific membrane-bound receptor RANK, thereby triggering a network of TRAF-mediated kinase cascades that promote osteoclast differentiation, activation and survival. Conversely, OPG expression is induced by factors that block bone catabolism and promote anabolic effects. OPG binds and neutralizes RANKL, leading to a block in osteoclastogenesis and decreased survival of pre-existing osteoclasts. RANKL induces the expression of the osteoclast-associated receptor (OSCAR). The interaction between osteoblasts and osteoclasts is regulated by many hormones and factors. PTH, PTHrP, PGE2, IL-2, IL-6, TNF, and corticosteroids are pro-resorptive, while estrogens, calcitonin, BMP2/4, and TGF-β are anabolic and anti-osteoclastic factors. Adapted from Boyle WJ, Simonet WS, Lacey DL.[69] With permission from Macmillan Publishers Ltd: Nature, copyright 2003.

OPG is a secretory protein of the TNF receptor family. It inhibits the formation of osteoclast-like cells (OCLs), as well as bone resorption by acting as a decoy receptor for RANKL. OPG knockout mice exhibit severe osteopenia due to accelerated bone resorption.[55,56] Mutations in the OPG gene are associated with idiopathic hyperphosphatasia (also known as juvenile Paget's disease) in humans. This is an autosomal recessive bone disease characterized by deformities of long bones and kyphosis.[57] Individuals with this disorder exhibit widening of the long-bone diaphyses with a propensity to fracture, accelerated bone turnover, and are typically of short stature.

RANKL belongs to the TNF ligand family and binds to OPG. RANKL appears on osteoclast lineage cells in either a soluble or the membrane-bound form, the latter requiring cell-to-cell contact. The soluble form of RANKL, together with macrophage colony-stimulating factor (CSF) induces formation of OCLs even in the absence of osteoblast lineage cells. RANKL-deficient mice exhibit severe osteopetrosis and complete lack of osteoclasts as a result of an inability of osteoblasts to support osteoclastogenesis. The formation of OCLs induced by soluble RANKL is abolished by the addition of OPG, indicating a specific interaction between RANKL and OPG in osteoclastogenesis.[58]

In the transition of pre-osteoblasts to mature osteoblasts during bone development and fracture healing, vascularization is enhanced by the production of osteoblast-derived VEGF-A. The latter is stimulated in the presence of anabolic factors such as IGF-I or BMPs.[59]

OSTEOBLASTS AND THE BONE MATRIX

Bone matrix is predominantly a mixture of tough fibers (type I collagen fibrils), which resist pulling forces, and solid particles (calcium phosphate as hydroxyapatite crystals), which resist compression. The volume occupied by the collagen is nearly equal to that occupied by the calcium phosphate. The collagen fibrils in adult bone are arranged in regular plywood-like layers, with the fibrils in each layer lying parallel to one another but at right angles to the fibrils in the layers on either side.

The organic matrix of collagen-based calcified tissues consists of a supporting collagen meshwork and various noncollagenous matrix proteins (NCP). The two major NCPs are bone sialoprotein and osteopontin, and generally co-distribute and accumulate in cement lines and in the spaces among the mineralized collagen fibrils. Genes expressed at or near the time of mineralization include osteopontin and osteocalcin.

Osteopontin

Osteopontin is a phosphorylated glycoprotein secreted to the mineralizing extracellular matrix by osteoblasts during bone development. It facilitates the attachment of osteoblasts and osteoclasts to the extracellular matrix, allowing them to perform their respective functions during osteogenesis.[60] Following PTH treatment, immediate changes in osteoblast gene expression involve induction of primary response genes. PTH regulates Nurr1 expression.[61] Along with vitamin D, Nurr1 activates the OPN promoter in a synergistic fashion whereas Nurr1-mediated transactivation of the OPN promoter is repressed by estrogen.[62]

Osteocalcin

Osteocalcin is a small bone γ-carboxyglutamic acid (Gla) protein that is associated with the mineralized matrix of bone. Its interaction with synthetic hydroxyapatite depends on its content of three residues of Gla, the amino acid formed post-translationally from glutamic acid by a vitamin K-dependent process.[63]

Osteonectin

Osteonectin (OSN) is an adhesive of cell and ECM-binding glycoprotein. It supports bone remodeling and the maintenance of bone mass.[64]

Low-density lipoprotein receptor-related protein 5

LRP5 (low-density lipoprotein receptor-related protein 5) is another signaling pathway that controls osteoblast proliferation. Mice with disruption of LRP5 develop a low bone mass phenotype secondary to decreased osteoblast proliferation. The phenotype of the Lrp5-deficient mice mirrored human osteoporosis-pseudoglioma syndrome. In autosomal recessive osteoporosis–pseudoglioma syndrome (OPPG) obligate carriers of mutant LRP5 genes had reduced bone mass when compared to age and gender matched controls. Interestingly, mutations at the N-terminal part of the gene, before the first EGF-like domain, resulted in an increased bone density, affecting mainly the cortices of the long bones and the skull by increasing Wnt signaling.[65]

THE PHOSPHORUS CONNECTION

The ability of cells to actively transport phosphate is a requirement for mineralization in bone and as a prerequisite for osteopontin expression. This signal is an integral part of a tightly coordinated program that ensures mineralization is not induced before osteoblasts cease proliferation. The phosphate signal ties osteopontin expression to alkaline phosphatase (ALP). In the differentiating cell, these signals ensure that induction of the early differentiation marker ALP does not begin until antiproliferation signals are enacted, and expression of osteopontin is not induced until ALP is active at the cell surface. ALP is localized to the plasma membrane and oriented such that its catalytic subunit is ectoplasmic. Within the extracellular environment, ALP cleaves a phosphate from β-glycerol phosphate to leave free glycerol. The free phosphate enters the cell through a

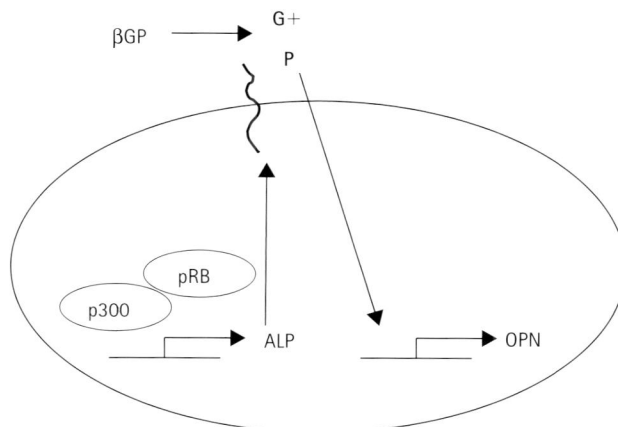

Figure 3.9 Alkaline phosphatase (ALP) is localized to the plasma membrane and oriented such that its catalytic subunit is ectoplasmic. Within the extracellular environment, ALP cleaves a phosphate (P) from β-glycerol phosphate (βGP) to leave free glycerol (G). Free phosphate enters the cell through a Na-dependent phosphate transporter, which is subject to inhibition by foscarnet. Transport of phosphate results in up-regulation of osteopontin (OPN). Induction of ALP does not begin until proliferation has shut down, and expression of osteopontin is not induced until ALP is active at the cell surface.

Na-dependent phosphate transporter, which results in the up-regulation of osteopontin RNA levels (Fig. 3.9).

The osteopontin promoter has functional response elements for the vitamin D receptor and the estrogen receptor. Osteopontin facilitates the attachment of osteoblasts and osteoclasts to the extracellular matrix. It acts as a cytokine, and exposure of cells to purified osteopontin leads to downstream events that include calcium mobilization and possible activation of the calcium ATPase pump. Osteopontin modulates hydroxyapatite crystal elongation during bone formation. The tight link between osteopontin expression and phosphate levels, combined with the ability of osteopontin to modulate calcium levels, suggests that the various biological activities attributed to osteopontin may be related to an overall role in regulating calcium localization or transport in conditions of high cellular phosphate levels.[66]

Serum calcium and phosphate concentrations are maintained in narrow ranges, and are primarily regulated by PTH and vitamin D. In the second level of tuning, phosphate homeostasis depends on FGF-23 and PHEX, both of which are from an osteoblast origin. FGF-23 is a 26 kDa circulating protein consisting of an N-terminal FGF homology domain and a novel 71 amino acid C-terminus of uncertain function.

PHEX is an osteoblast cell surface metalloprotease phosphate-regulating endopeptidase, mutations in PHEX are the cause for the X-linked dominant hypophosphatemic rickets (XLH). Phex expression is regulated by vitamin D3, glucocorticoids, IGF and GH (Fig. 3.10). PTHrP and PTH, through the common type-1 PTH/PTHrP receptor and via the cAMP pathway, down-regulate PHEX expression. Thus, bone-derived PTHrP acts in a paracrine/autocrine manner

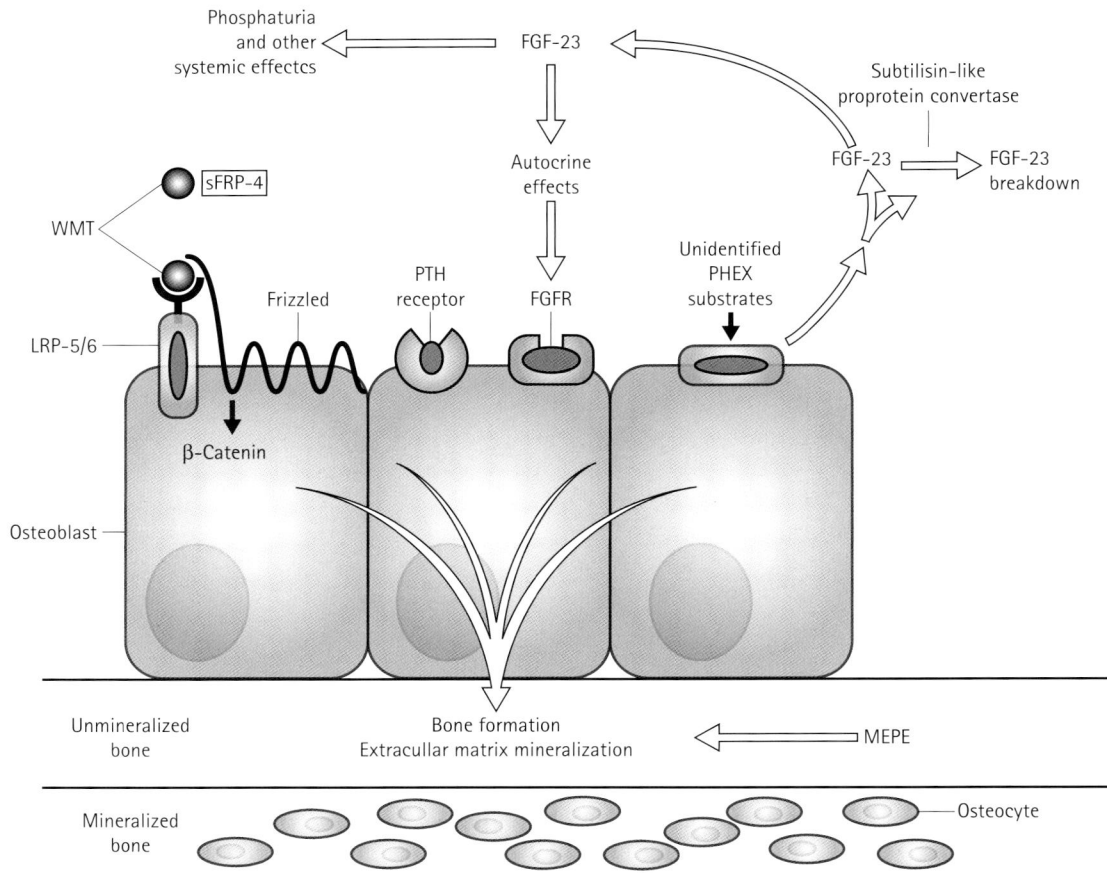

Figure 3.10   Osteoblasts express components necessary for coordinating mineralization of ECM and phosphate handling by the kidney. FGF-23, secreted from osteoblasts under the control of PHEX and possibly G_s-dependent pathways, regulates renal phosphate handling, as well as local osteoblast-mediated bone mineralization. The LRP-Wnt signaling pathway in osteoblasts regulates bone mass and, in conjunction with PHEX and FGF-23, participates in coordinating renal phosphate conservation to meet the needs of osteoblast-mediated mineralization. Adapted from Quarles LD. Evidence for a bone-kidney axis regulating phospate homeostasis. *J Clin Invest* 2003; **112**: 642–6.

to regulate phosphorus metabolism through the FGF23 pathway. The role of PTHrP may be important for the timing of PHEX expression in differentiating osteoprogenitor cells, in order to maintain adequate phosphorus level at the growth plate.[67] FGF23 suppresses the renal 25-hydroxyvitamin D-1α OHase expression cooperating or competing with several humoral factors such as PTH and $1,25(OH)_2D_3$ itself. Thus, FGF-23 secreted from osteoblasts under the control of PHEX and possibly G_sα-dependent pathways has systemic actions to regulate renal phosphate handling as well as potential autocrine effects to regulate osteoblast-mediated bone mineralization.

Wnt interact with a receptor complex containing a member of the frizzled-related protein (FRP) family of heptahelical receptors and LRP-5 and LRP-6. The binding and sequestration of Wnt by FRP prevents Wnt-dependent activation of the frizzled/LRP receptor complex. The inhibition of renal phosphate reabsorption is associated with FRP-4 antagonizing Wnt-dependent β-catenin pathways in the kidney.[68]

Osteoblasts express all of the implicated components of the bone–kidney axis to coordinate systemic phosphate homeostasis and mineralization. These include PHEX, FGF-23, matrix extracellular phosphoglycoprotein and LRP-5/Wnt, as well as FRP, FGF, and PTH receptors. In addition, autocrine effects of FGF23 on osteoblasts could regulate the production of ECM proteins that regulate mineralization.

Osteoclasts

Osteoclasts are multinucleated giant cells, of monocyte/macrophage origin, with the capacity to resorb mineralized tissues (Fig. 3.11). Osteoblasts/stromal cells are crucially involved in osteoclast development. Cell-to-cell contact between cells of the osteoblast and monocyte lineages is necessary for inducing differentiation of the osteoclasts.

Two hematopoietic factors are necessary for osteoclastogenesis and for the subsequent activation of RANK on

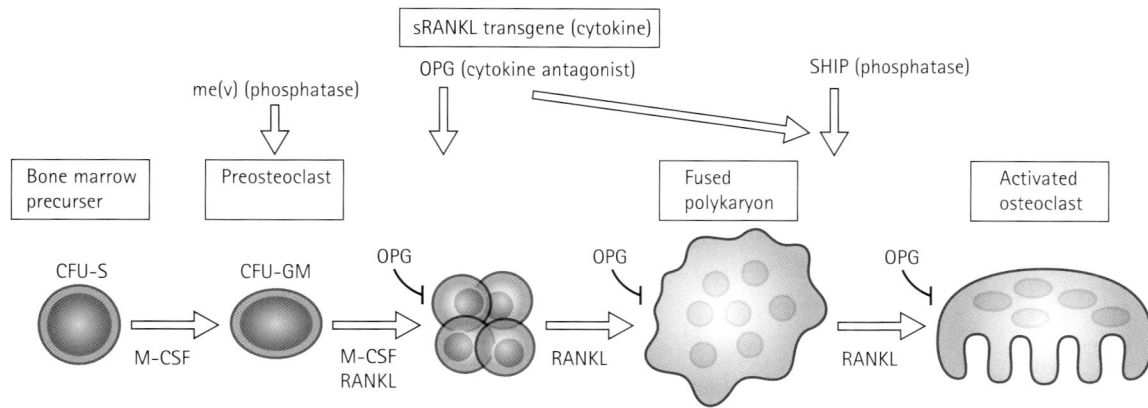

Figure 3.11 Development schema of hematopoietic precursor cell differentiation into mature osteoclasts, which are multinucleated cells fused from 10–20 individual preosteoclasts. M-CSF (CSF-1) and RANKL are essential for osteoclastogenesis, and their action during lineage allocation and maturation is shown. OPG can bind and neutralize RANKL, and can negatively regulate both osteoclastogenesis and activation of mature osteoclasts. RANKL stimulates osteoclast activation by inducing secretion of protons and lytic enzymes into a sealed resorption vacuole formed between the basal surface of the osteoclast and the bone surface. Adapted from Boyle WJ, Simonet WS, Lacey DL.[69] With permission from Macmillan Publishers Ltd: Nature, copyright 2003.

the surface of hematopoietic precursor cells. These are the TNF-related cytokine RANKL (receptor activator of NF-B ligand) and the polypeptide growth factor colony-stimulating factor-1 (CSF-1). Together, CSF-1 and RANKL are required to induce expression of genes that typify the osteoclast lineage, including those encoding tartrate-resistant acid phosphatase (TRAP), cathepsin K (CATK), calcitonin receptor and the β_3-integrin, leading to the development of mature osteoclasts.[69]

Osteoprotegerin (OPG) acts as a decoy receptor by blocking RANKL binding to its cellular receptor RANK. OPG is also produced by osteoblasts in response to anabolic agents such as estrogens and BMPs. Expression of RANKL and OPG is therefore coordinated to regulate bone resorption and density by controlling the activation state of RANK on the osteoclast.[70]

The osteoclast differentiation is severely blocked in mice lacking DNAX-activating protein (DAP12), a membrane adaptor molecule that contains immunoreceptor, a tyrosine-based activation motif (ITAM motif) which activates calcium signaling in immune cells.

RANKL induces another member of the immunoglobulin superfamily receptor, osteoclast associated receptor (OSCAR). The ligand for OSCAR is not known yet. OSCAR associates with an adaptor protein (Fc receptor) that like DAP12 contains an ITAM motif and is essential in immune responses indicating that there are two ITAM-mediated co-stimulatory pathways that seem to work together to promote osteoclast differentiation.

Phosphorylation of ITAM stimulated by immunoreceptors and RANKL–RANK interaction results in the recruitment of Syk family kinases, leading to the activation of PLC and calcium signalling, which is critical for NFATc1 induction. NFATc1 induction is also dependent on c-Fos and TRAF6, both of which are activated by RANKL.[71]

Signaling by RANKL is essential for the induction of osteoclast differentiation, and it must be strictly regulated to maintain bone homeostasis. RANKL induces the interferon-β (IFN-β) gene expression in osteoclast precursor cells, and the latter inhibits differentiation by interfering with RANKL-induced expression of c-Fos, an essential transcription factor for the formation of osteoclasts. IFN-β-gene induction mechanism is dependent on c-Fos itself. Thus an auto-regulatory mechanism operates, whereby RANKL induced c-Fos, which induces its own inhibitor. The importance of this regulatory mechanism for bone homeostasis is emphasized by the observation that mice deficient in IFN-β signaling exhibit severe osteopenia that is accompanied by enhanced osteoclastogenesis.[72]

Activating mutations of the RANK gene are associated with osteolytic and non-osteolytic forms of hyperphosphatasia as in expansile skeletal hyperphosphatasia and familial expansile osteolysis.[73]

Activation of osteoclast surface receptors for IL-1, c-Fms, TNF-α, PGE2 and TGF-β potentiate osteoclastogenesis *in vitro*, and can stimulate bone resorption *in vivo*. Thus, RANK-deficient mice are resistant to bone resorption induced by TNF-α, IL-1β, 1,25-dihydroxyvitamin D_3 and PTHrP, which, excluding PTH, are the major calciotropic factors that are known to induce increases in bone resorption and serum hypercalcemia.[74]

The mature, multinucleated osteoclast is activated by signals, which lead to initiation of bone remodeling. The osteoclast cell body is polarized, and in response to activation of RANK by its ligand, it undergoes internal structural changes that prepare it to resorb bone. Such structural changes include rearrangements of actin cytoskeleton and formation of a tight junction between the bone surface and basal membrane, which form a sealed compartment. This external compartment is then acidified by the export of hydrogen ions generated by the ATP6i complex. Secretion continues with the export of the lytic enzymes TRAP, and pro-cathepsin K (CATK) into a resorption pit (Howship's lacunae). Through this process the osteoclast erodes the underlying bone. Degradation products (collagen fragments, soluble calcium and phosphate) are processed within the osteoclast and released into the circulation.[75]

The RANKL–OPG axis may be further influenced by osteoclast inhibitory lectin (OCIL), a newly recognized inhibitor of osteoclast formation. In addition to its capacity to limit osteoclast formation, OCIL also inhibits bone resorption by mature, giant-cell tumor-derived osteoclasts.[76]

The mechanism for the regulation of osteoclast life span involves T-cell-mediated cytotoxicity. Cytotoxic T cells express ligand for Fas and Fas-mediated apoptosis. Fas is a death receptor of osteoclasts.[77]

ENDOCRINE CONTROL OF THE GROWTH PLATE AND BONE

The major systemic hormones that regulate longitudinal bone growth are growth hormone (GH) and insulin-like growth factor I (IGF-I), thyroid hormones, and glucocorticoids, whereas during puberty the sex steroids (androgens and estrogens) contribute a great deal to this process.

Thyroid hormones

The actions of thyroid hormones have a key role in normal skeletal development, linear growth, and the maintenance of adult bone mass. Thus, childhood hypothyroidism is characterized by growth arrest, epiphyseal dysgenesis, and delayed bone age (Fig. 3.12).

Thyroid hormone receptor, TRα1, α2 and β1 are expressed in reserve and proliferative chondrocytes but not in the hypertrophic zone. They are necessary for chondrocyte differentiation in combination with glucocorticoids and TGF-β.[78] Induction of hypothyroidism in experimental animals induces a drastic change in epiphyseal growth plate structure and its adjacent bone.[79] The width of the epiphyseal growth plate and that of the articular cartilage are markedly diminished, as are the volumes of both epiphyseal and metaphyseal bone trabecules. Reserve chondroprogenitor cells occupy a broader than normal segment of the growth plate. Cartilage cell columns lose their vertical organization and are jumbled. They show narrowing of the epiphyseal growth plate and disappearance of the subchondral metaphyseal trabecular bone. They contain an abnormal matrix rich in heparan sulfate, and hypertrophic chondrocyte differentiation fails to progress. But most importantly, the growth plate is totally disengaged from its neighboring bone. The hypertrophic zone is completely sealed off from the bone marrow, and thus, osteoclasts, osteoblasts and growth factors are prevented from their

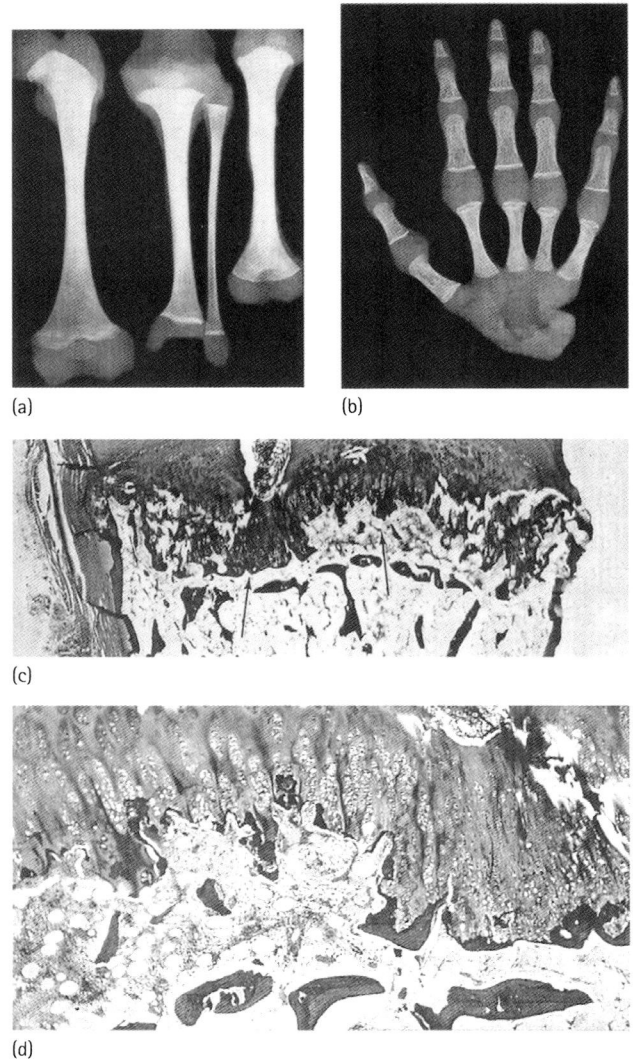

(a)   (b)

(c)

(d)

Figure 3.12 (a) and (b) Radiograms of a femur, tibia, and fibula, humerus and hand removed at autopsy from a 6-year-old child with cretinism. Ossification centers of the distal femur and proximal tibia are present but femur head, tibial distal epiphysis and capitulum of the humerus, which appear usually at age 4 months, are absent, indicating the onset of the disease between gestational 34 weeks and postnatal 4 months. (c) Photomicrograph of the fibula shows the complete disengagement of the cartilage from the underlying metaphysis, implying a complete arrest of osteogenesis. ($\times$12) (d) Though cartilage cells line up in columns, cores of calcified cartilage matrix do not extend into the metaphysis. Osseous tissue opposes directly the growth plate cartilage, indicating total impairment of osteogenesis. ($\times$35)

task of osteogenesis. Hypothyroid growth plates are grossly disorganized. The bone–cartilage interface is inactive, and these tissues are completely dissociated. These effects are associated with the absence of collagen X expression and increased PTHrP expression.[80]

Thyroid hormones modulate the Ihh–BMP–PTHrP signaling loop, to induce FGFR1 and to influence FGF signaling. They play a major role in the regulation of FGFs- and VEGF-induced angiogenesis during endochondral ossification.[81]

The mechanism underlying this drastic disarray in bone and cartilage is complex, as thyroid hormones affect such a wide range of tissues and genes.[82] One of these target tissues is the pituitary somatotroph. The growth hormone gene was among the first to be shown to possess a thyroid response element in its non-coding promoter,[83] and the secondary growth hormone deficiency that develop during hypothyroidism is dose dependent. Indeed, clinicians have known for many years that growth hormone response to pharmacological stimuli is low in hypothyroidism and recovers upon replacement therapy. In hypothyroidism there is also a profound decrease in growth hormone receptors.[84] But growth hormone deficiency is certainly not the only relevant component of hypothyroidism. Growth hormone replacement therapy, given to hypothyroid animals accelerated growth, increased to some extent the number of proliferating cells in the growth plate and broke down the sealing of the cartilage–bone interface, with no effect on cellular organization or on hypertrophic cell morphology. Yet, these effects are not as enormous as those seen after replacement therapy with thyroid hormones. Thyroid hormones exert direct effects on cartilage growth and maturation.[85]

Interestingly, TSH receptors are expressed in osteoblast and osteoclast precursors. TSH inhibits osteoclast formation and survival by attenuating JNK/c-jun and NFκB signaling, triggered in response to RANKL and TNFα. TSH also inhibits osteoblast differentiation and type 1 collagen expression by down-regulating Wnt and VEGF signaling.[86]

Growth hormone: The IGF–I axis

GROWTH HORMONE AND THE GROWTH PLATE (TABLE 3.3)

Growth hormone increases longitudinal bone growth directly by stimulating prechondrocyte differentiation in the resting zone, followed by a IGF-I-dependent clonal expansion in the proliferating zone. Cartilage-derived IGF-I moderates local action of GH by reducing GHR availability[87–89].

GH receptor (GHR) is expressed in the reserve cells, the hypertrophic layer, and in small amounts also in the proliferative layer of the growth plate.[90]

The transition from reserve cell zone to proliferating cartilage is associated with expression of high concentration of IGF-I, IGF-I receptors and the cell's responsiveness to IGF-I. GH stimulation of proliferation is, therefore, an indirect effect of reserve cells that were stimulated by GH to advance into their proliferating phase. Interestingly,

IGF-I null mice show a 30 percent decrease in linear dimension of the terminal hypertrophic chondrocytes.

In the cartilage–bone interface, GH stimulates mobilization of osteoclasts to the resorption front.[91] Similarly, IGF-I elicits a significant increase in osteoclastic acid phosphatase activity.[92]

GH and IGF-I markedly enhance DNA synthesis, expression of cartilage specific type II collagen, and proteoglycan. Both GH and IGF-I accelerate the maturational process of chondroplasia. Yet, GH also induces osteogenesis. It regulates the transformation of the cartilage into bone.[93]

The differences between GH and IGF-I are quite obvious in transgenic animals overexpressing either GH or IGF-I. Thus, GH-transgenic animals grow to approximately twice the size of their normal littermates whereas IGF-I transgenic mice do not grow more than their non-transgenic siblings. Local administration of GH, but not IGF-I, stimulates the transcription of the IGF-I gene and antibodies to IGF-I abolish the stimulatory effect of locally administered GH.[94]

Surrounding the growth plate, GH also influences bone itself, connective tissue, vasculature and the bone marrow. GH stimulates bone turnover and remodeling. Osteoclasts express IGF-I receptors,[95] and IGF-I is involved in osteoclast mobilization and in GH effects on bone resorption.

GROWTH HORMONE AND THE BONE

Growth hormone stimulates osteoblast proliferation and differentiated functions such as ALP, osteocalcin, and type I collagen expression. Whereas circulating levels of IGF-I are GH dependent, GH may not be the only determinant of bone IGF-I. Regulatory effects on IGF-I were demonstrated for estrogen, PTH, and glucocorticoids.[96]

GH stimulates osteoclast activity on bone resorption through an IGF-I-independent osteoclast differentiation and indirect activation of mature osteoclasts.[97]

Glucocorticoids

Glucocorticoid receptors (GRs) are expressed in bone cells,[98] and in all layers of the growth plate where glucocorticoids are potent negative regulators of enchondral ossification[99]. Most prominently, they increased apoptosis in terminal hypertrophic cells.[100]

Glucocorticoids in excess rapidly deplete the amount of functional Runx2 nuclear protein, with an accompanying inhibitory effect on Runx2-dependent gene expression.[101] They reduce IGF-I, GHR, and IGF-IR expression in the growth plate, and inhibit basal and IGF-I induced DNA synthesis. Differential regulation of IGFBPs could account in part for glucocorticoid-induced growth arrest.

Glucocorticoids contribute to the control of T_3 levels within the growth plate by regulating deiodinase activity. In the bone, glucocorticoids stimulate osteoclastogenesis

Table 3.3   Regulation of the growth plate and bone by the GH–IGF-I axis

Cells	Growth hormone (GH)	Insulin-type growth factor I (IGF-I)
Reserve cells		
Progenitor to chondrocytes	Expression of GH receptors	
	↑ Differentiation into chondrocytes	
Proliferating chondrocytes		
Longitudinal cell division		Expression of IGF-I and IGF-I receptors
		↑ Proliferation
Hypertrophic chondrocytes		
Cell hypertrophy	Expression of GH receptors	Expression of IGF-I
Longitudinal orientation	↑ Longitudinal orientation	↑ Longitudinal orientation
Apoptosis		↓ Apoptosis
Cartilage—bone interface		
Lacuna in the calcified matrix	GH binding and activity in osteoclasts	IGF immunoreactivity in osteoclasts
Bone marrow invasion	↑ Marrow invasion	↑ Marrow invasion
	↑ Mobilization of osteoclasts	↑ Mobilization of osteoclasts
Bone resorption	Differentiation of osteoclasts	
Extracellular matrix		
Cartilage matrix		IGF-I immunoreactivity in matrix elements
Calcification of matrix		
Bone matrix		^{35}S incorporation into cartilage proteoglycans
Bone marrow		
Differentiation of lineages	Expression of GH receptor in all lineages	Expression of IGF-I and IGF receptor in all lineages
Lineages maturation	↑ Maturation of erythro- and granulopoiesis	↑ Maturation of erythro- and granulopoiesis
Cell proliferation	↑ Proliferation of erythro- and granulopoiesis	↑ Proliferation of erythro- and granulopoiesis
Bone		
Resorption and formation	↑ Resorption and formation	IGF-I expression in osteoblasts
Bone turnover and remodeling	Shorten resorption and reversal time	Expression of IGF-I receptors in osteoclasts
Bone mineral density (BMD)	↓ BMD in GHD	↑ Bone matrix apposition
	↑ BMD with GH therapy	
Bone markers	↓ All markers in GHD	Support of osteoclast formation and activation
	↑ Markers with GH therapy	

and increase the expression of receptor activator of nuclear factor-κB ligand and CSF-1, and decrease the expression of osteoprotegerin. However, the most significant effect of glucocorticoids in bone is the inhibition of osteoblastogenesis by increasing osteoblast apoptosis.[102] This inhibition is caused by a decrease in the number of osteoblasts secondary to a shift in the differentiation of mesenchymal cells away from the osteoblastic lineage, and an increase in the death of mature osteoblasts.[103] Excess glucocorticoids directly affect bone-forming cells *in vivo*. Glucocorticoid-induced loss of bone strength results in part from increased death of osteocytes, independent of bone loss. They have effects on osteoblast gene expression, including down-regulation of type I collagen and osteocalcin, and up-regulation of interstitial collagenase. They suppress the expression of IGF-I and regulate IGF-binding proteins synthesis. A summary of the effects of glucocorticoids is given in Table 3.4.

Sex hormones

ESTROGENS

Estrogen receptors (ERs), ERα and ERβ are highly expressed in pre-hypertrophic and proliferative chondrocytes, and to a lesser degree in the late hypertrophic zone, indicating that estrogens have direct effects on chondrocytes in the growth plate.[104] Estrogens increase chondrocyte differentiation, ECM generation and the concentration of matrix growth factors.

ERβ is involved in abrogating the effects on longitudinal growth, growth plate width, radial skeletal growth and suppression of osteocalcin and IGF-I, which are mediated by ERs.[104]

The pubertal growth spurt is supported by low estrogen levels, whereas growth plate fusion is mediated by the

Table 3.4 Glucocorticoid effects on growth plate cartilage and bone

	Effect
Calcium metabolism	↓ Calcium intestinal absorption
	↓ Calcium renal reabsorption
	↑ Plasma PTH
	Normal vitamin D level and function
Cartilage	↓ IGF-I generation
	↓ Matrix collagen and mineralization
	↑ Matrix proteoglycans
Bone	↓ Osteoblast function
	↑ Osteoclast number and surface binding
	↓ IGF-I generation
	↓ Matrix collagen and mineralization
Catabolic effects	Myopathy
	↓ Fibroblast DNA, RNA and protein

exclusive action of high levels of estrogen, demonstrating the biphasic effects of estrogen on longitudinal growth. Indeed, patients with a loss of function mutation in the ER or aromatase gene loss of function demonstrate continued longitudinal growth into adulthood resulting in tall stature due to absence of growth plate fusion and severe osteoporosis, despite high levels of testosterone.[105,106]

During osteoblast differentiation, the androgen receptor (AR), ERα and ERβ expression profiles are different. ERβ expression is relatively constant throughout differentiation, exhibiting more constitutive expression. In contrast, AR levels are lowest during proliferation, and then increase throughout differentiation with highest levels in the most mature mineralizing cells.[107] Estrogen increases gene transcription of the TGF-β type I receptor, which contains several Runx binding sequences, and enhances Smad dependent gene expression by TGF-β in osteoblasts.[108]

Estrogen exerts its anti-resorptive effects on bone, at least in part, by stimulating ER and OPG expression in osteoblasts.[109]

ANDROGENS

Androgens are an important bone regulator in both women and men.[110] While some of the androgenic effects are induced through aromatization into estrogen, bone cells and epiphyseal chondrocytes express AR[111] and respond to androgen by proliferation, differentiation, mineralization and expression of genes consistent with bone formation.[112]

Expression and activity of aromatase and 5α-reductase in osteoblast-like cells, indicate that local metabolism of sex steroids may contribute to bone mass and bone remodeling.

The role of adrenal androgens is well established for its rapid maturational impact on bone development in children

with congenital adrenal hyperplasia. The effect is greatest on the short bones, intermediate on the cuboid bones and minimal on the long bones of the hand. These differences may relay to the differential expression of both ERα and ERβ in the growth plate and mineralized bone, with ER more highly expressed in cortical than in cancellous bone and ERβ most evident at cancellous than cortical sites.[113] For a reason not completely understood, this effect is not exerted before birth or within the first 6 months of life.

ADIPOSITY AND BONE MORPHOGENESIS

Bone-forming cells share a common mesenchymal precursor in the bone marrow with the adipocyte. Osteoblast development is controlled by several phenotype-specific transcription factors, among them Runx2/Cbfa1 and Dlx5, whereas formation of terminally differentiated adipocytes in the marrow requires the activity of PPAR-γ2. Rosiglitazone, a PPAR-γ2 agonist, inhibits the mineralization the ECM, and suppresses the expression of Runx2/ Cbfa1 and other osteoblast-specific genes such as collagen type-1, osteopontin, ALP and osteocalcin.[114]

On the other hand, Lovastatin, a lipid-lowering drug, enhances osteoblast differentiation by expression of Cbfa1/ Runx2 and by increasing osteocalcin expression. By enhancing osteoblast gene expression and by inhibiting adipogenesis, Lovastatin shunts uncommitted osteoprogenitor cells in marrow from the adipocytic to the osteoblastic differentiation pathway.[115]

Human marrow stromal cells express the leptin receptor. Leptin enhances chondrocyte proliferation and osteoblast differentiation and inhibits adipocyte differentiation.[116,117] Leptin also increases the abundance of the IGF-I receptor in chondrocytes and the progenitor cell population.[118]

Partly, leptin regulates bone formation indirectly via the sympathetic nervous system, β-adrenergic receptors of osteoblasts down-regulate their proliferation, and decreases bone mass.[119,120]

Weight, gravity, and bone

The capacity of bone tissue to alter its mass and structure in response to mechanical demands has long been recognized but the cellular mechanisms involved remained poorly understood (Fig. 3.13). Bone not only develops as a structure designed specifically for mechanical tasks, but it can adapt during life toward more efficient mechanical performance. Mechanical adaptation of bone is a cellular process and needs a biological system that senses the mechanical loading. The loading information must then be communicated to the effector cells that form new bone or destroy old bone.

Bone loss is observed after exposure to weightlessness in both astronauts and in-flight animals. This physiological

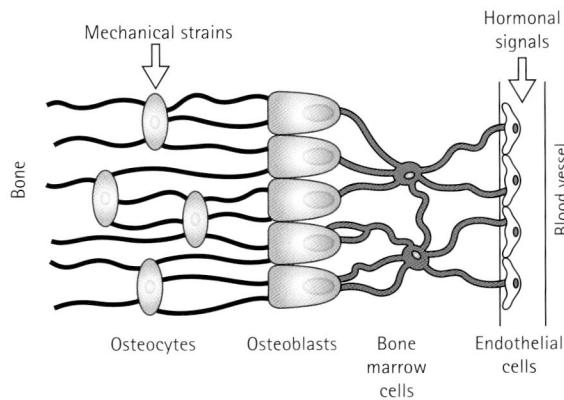

Figure 3.13 ECF flow through the canalicular network is altered during bone matrix compression and tension, whereas osteocyte cellular activity is increased after bone loading. Adapted from Marotti G. The osteocyte as a wiring transmission system. *J Musculoskelet Neuronal Interact* 2000 Dec; **1**(2): 133–6. With permission from Marotti.

consequence of microgravity is the rapid loss of weight-bearing bone that is associated with skeletal unloading. Whereas exercise (mechanical loading) has been shown to increase bone formation and stimulate osteoblast function, the mechanisms underlying signal transduction of mechano-perception is yet to be fully understood. Osteoblasts respond to mechanical stress such as fluid shear, bending, flexing, and compression. The type of stress and amount of stress determine the osteoblast response.

The *in vivo* operating cell stress derived from bone loading is likely the flow of interstitial fluid along the surface of osteocytes and lining cells. The response of bone cells to fluid flow includes prostaglandin synthesis and expression of prostaglandin synthase inducible cyclooxygenase (COX-2). Bone cells rapidly produce nitric oxide (NO) in response to fluid flow as a result of activation of endothelial nitric oxide synthase, which also mediates the adaptive response of bone tissue to mechanical loading. The possible regulatory sensors include mechano-sensitive calcium channels, autocrine responses to stress, response to FAK/integrin, alterations in the cytoskeleton as well as other known growth factor and cytokine receptors. The secondary signal may include growth factor related kinases such as ERK, p38 and JNK map kinase (MAPK) pathways. In fact, normal osteoblast response to stress and growth factors requires normal Earth gravity.

Under microgravity, marrow stromal differentiation into osteoblasts is suppressed and cells fail to express ALP, collagen I, Runx2 and osteonectin. On the other hand, PPARγ2 is highly expressed in response to microgravity. These changes did not correct after 35 days of re-adaptation to normal gravity.[121]

Mechanical loading of the skeleton causes interstitial fluid flow throughout the lacunar and canalicular spaces in bone. The osteoblasts and osteocytes lining these spaces respond to this mechano-stimulation provided by the fluid flow. The mechano-transduction of this response into alterations in biochemical markers determines bone development and remodeling in response to mechanical stressors. Increased shear forces (without significant changes in the chemotransport characteristics) result in enhanced mineralized extracellular matrix deposition (the hallmark of the complete osteoblastic differentiation). The combined effect of fluid shear forces on the mineralized extracellular matrix production and distribution emphasizes the importance of mechano-sensation on osteoblastic cell function.[122]

The bone structure

Three types of bones are found in the skeleton: flat, cuboid, and long bones. These are derived by distinct types of development: intramembranous, osteogenesis, and endochondral ossification, combining osteogenesis and chondroplasia.

During intramembranous ossification, a group of mesenchymal cells within a highly vascularized area of the embryonic connective tissue proliferates, forming early cell condensations within which cells differentiate directly into osteoblasts. These cells will synthesize a woven bone matrix, while at the periphery mesenchymal cells continue to differentiate into osteoblasts. Blood vessels are incorporated between the woven bone trabeculae and will form the hematopoietic bone marrow. Later this woven bone will be replaced by mature lamellar bone.

The development and growth of long bones involve both cellular processes. The main difference between intramembranous and endochondral bone formation is the presence of a growth plate in endochondral bone.

Long bones have either one or two wider extremities, the epiphyses, a cylindrical hollow portion in the middle, the midshaft or diaphysis, and a transition zone between them, the metaphysis. The external part of the bones is formed by a thick and dense layer of calcified tissue, the cortex (compact bone) that in the diaphysis encloses the bone medullary cavity. The cortex becomes progressively thinner toward the metaphysis and the epiphysis, and the internal space is filled with a network of thin, calcified trabeculae forming the cancellous or trabecular bone. The spaces enclosed by these thin trabeculae are also filled with hematopoietic bone marrow and are continuous with the diaphyseal medullary cavity. The outer cortical bone surfaces at the epiphyses are covered with a layer of articular cartilage that does not calcify.

THE OSTEON

The principal organizing feature of compact bone is the osteon, or the Haversian system (Fig. 3.14). The permanent bone formed by the periosteum when first laid down is cancellous in structure. Later the osteoblasts contained in its spaces become arranged in concentric layers characteristic of the Haversian systems, and are included as bone corpuscles.

The bone cells, the osteocytes, derive from osteoblasts, which have been trapped in the bone matrix that they produced, and which becomes calcified. Osteocytes have

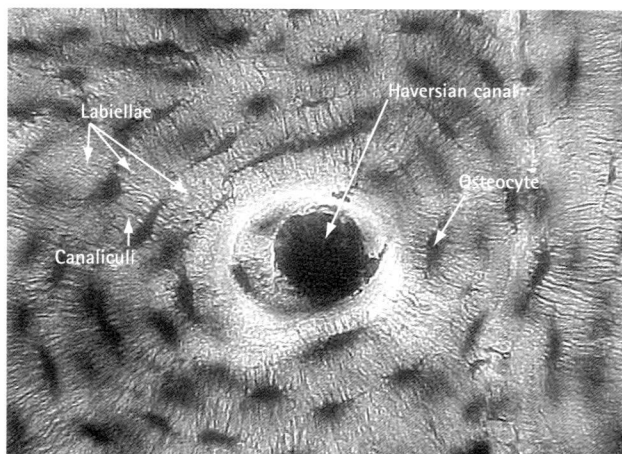

Figure 3.14 The osteon, or the Haversian system. A central haversian canal is surrounded by layers of lamellae and canaliculi. Please see Plate 1.

numerous long cell processes rich in microfilaments, which are in contact with cell processes from other osteocytes or with processes from the cells lining the bone surface (osteoblasts or flat lining cells). These processes are organized during the formation of the matrix and before its calcification; they form a network of thin canaliculi permeating the entire bone matrix. Osteocytic canaliculi are mainly directed toward the bone surface. Between the osteocyte plasma membrane and the bone matrix itself is the periosteocytic space. This space exists both in the lacunae and in the canaliculi, and it is filled with extracellular fluid (ECF), the only source of nutrients for the osteocyte. The lacunæ are connected with each other and with the central Haversian canal.

Each Haversian canal contains one or two blood vessels, with a small quantity of delicate connective tissue and some nerve filaments. In such larger canals there are also lymphatic vessels, and cells with branching processes that communicate through the canaliculi with the branched processes of certain bone cells in the substance of the bone. Thus, the whole of the bone is permeated by a system of blood vessels running through the bony canals in the centers of the Haversian systems. The Haversian system is supplied with nutrient fluids derived from the vessels in the Haversian canal and distributed through the canaliculi and lacunæ.

Osteoblasts undergo either apoptosis or they differentiate into osteocytes or bone-lining cells after termination of bone matrix synthesis. MT1-MMP-activated TGF-β maintains osteoblast survival during transdifferentiation into osteocytes, and maintains mature osteocyte viability.[122] During this transition from osteoblasts to osteocytes, the cells lose numerous osteoblastic phenotypes and acquire osteocytic morphology and high expression of osteocalcin.

The young osteocyte has most of the ultrastructural characteristics of the osteoblast from which it was derived. The older osteocyte, located deeper within the calcified bone, shows a further decrease in cell volume and organelles, and an accumulation of cytoplasmic glycogen. These cells synthesize small amounts of new bone matrix at the surface of the osteocytic lacunae, which subsequently calcifies. Osteocytes express low levels of a number of osteoblast markers, including osteocalcin, osteopontin, osteonectin, and the osteocyte markers. They are connected with each other in bone and with osteoblasts on the bone surface through canaliculi, forming cellular networks.[123]

Matrix extracellular phosphoglycoprotein (MEPE) is predominantly expressed by osteocytes, with significant expression within mineralized bone.[124] MEPE stimulates new bone formation by activating integrin signaling pathways in osteoblasts.[124]

Osteocytes regulate osteoblast differentiation by sclerostin. The latter is expressed exclusively by osteocytes and inhibits the differentiation and mineralization of pre-osteoblastic cells. Although sclerostin shares some of the actions of the BMP antagonist noggin, sclerostin does not inhibit alkaline phosphatase (ALP) activity, and does not antagonize BMP-stimulated ALP activity or Smad phosphorylation. Its unique localization and action on osteoblasts suggest that sclerostin may be the previously proposed osteocyte-derived factor that is transported to osteoblasts at the bone surface and inhibits bone formation. Sclerosteosis, a skeletal disorder characterized by high bone mass due to increased osteoblast activity, is caused by loss of the sclerostin gene product.[125]

REFERENCES

1   Hunziker EB. Mechanism of longitudinal bone growth and its regulation by growth plate chondrocytes. *Microsc Res Tech* 1994; **28**: 505–19.

2   Hochberg Z. *Endocrine Control of Bone Maturation*. Basel: Karger; 2002.

3   Winnier G, Blessing M, Labosky PA, Hogan BL. Bone morphogenetic protein-4 is required for mesoderm formation and patterning in the mouse. *Genes Dev* 1995; **9**: 2105–16.

4   Monsoro-Burq AH, Duprez D, Watanabe Y, *et al*. The role of bone morphogenetic proteins in vertebral development. *Development* 1996; **122**: 360–716.

5   Nakayama N, Han CY, Cam L, *et al*. A novel chordin-like BMP inhibitor, CHL2, expressed preferentially in chondrocytes of developing cartilage and osteoarthritic joint cartilage. *Development* 2004; **131**: 229–40.

6   Schwabe GC, Turkmen S, Leschik G, *et al*. Brachydactyly type C caused by a homozygous missense mutation in the prodomain of CDMP1. *Am J Med Genet* 2004; **124A**: 356–63.

7   Hatakeyama Y, Tuan RS, Shum L. Distinct functions of BMP4 and GDF5 in the regulation of chondrogenesis. *J Cell Biochem* 2004; **91**: 1204–17.

8   Buxton P, Edwards C, Archer CW, Francis-West P. Growth/differentiation factor-5 (GDF-5) and skeletal development. *J Bone Joint Surg Am* 2001; **83A(Suppl 1, Pt 1)**: S23–30.

9 Thomas JT, Lin K, Nandedkar M, *et al.* A human chondrodysplasia due to a mutation in a TGF-beta superfamily member. *Nat Genet* 1996; **12**: 315–17.

10 Nifuji A, Kellermann O, Noda M. Noggin inhibits chondrogenic but not osteogenic differentiation in mesodermal stem cell line C1 and skeletal cells. *Endocrinology* 2004; **145**: 3434–42.

11 Gong Y, Krakow D, Marcelino J, *et al.* Heterozygous mutations in the gene encoding noggin affect human joint morphogenesis. *Nat Genet* 1999; **21**: 302–4.

12 Ryu JH, Kim SJ, Kim SH, *et al.* Regulation of the chondrocyte phenotype by beta-catenin. *Development* 2002; **129**: 5541–50.

13 Selleri L, Depew MJ, Jacobs Y, *et al.* Requirement for Pbx1 in skeletal patterning and programming chondrocyte proliferation and differentiation. *Development* 2001; **128**: 3543–57.

14 Yang Y, Topol L, Lee H, Wu J. Wnt5a and Wnt5b exhibit distinct activities in coordinating chondrocyte proliferation and differentiation. *Development* 2003; **130**: 1003–15.

15 Chung UI, Schipani E, McMahon AP, Kronenberg HM. Indian hedgehog couples chondrogenesis to osteogenesis in endochondral bone development. *J Clin Invest* 2001; **107**: 295–304.

16 Karp SJ, Schipani E, St-Jacques B, *et al.* Indian hedgehog coordinates endochondral bone growth and morphogenesis via parathyroid hormone related-protein-dependent and -independent pathways. *Development* 2000; **127**: 543–8.

17 Long F, Zhang XM, Karp S, *et al.* Genetic manipulation of hedgehog signaling in the endochondral skeleton reveals a direct role in the regulation of chondrocyte proliferation. *Development* 2001; **128**: 5099–108.

18 Minina E, Wenzel HM, Kreschel C, *et al.* BMP and Ihh/PTHrP signaling interact to coordinate chondrocyte proliferation and differentiation. *Development* 2001; **128**: 4523–34.

19 Alvarez J, Sohn P, Zeng X, *et al.* TGFbeta2 mediates the effects of hedgehog on hypertrophic differentiation and PTHrP expression. Development 2002; **129**: 1913–24.

20 Lanske B, Karaplis AC, Lee K, *et al.* PTH/PTHrP receptor in early development and Indian hedgehog-regulated bone growth. *Science* 1996; **273**: 663–6.

21 Kobayashi T, Chung UI, Schipani E, *et al.* PTHrP and Indian hedgehog control differentiation of growth plate chondrocytes at multiple steps. *Development* 2002; **129**: 2977–86.

22 Schipani E, Kruse K, Juppner H. A constitutively active mutant PTH-PTHrP receptor in Jansen-type metaphyseal chondrodysplasia. *Science* 1995; **268**: 98–100.

23 Jobert AS, Zhang P, Couvineau A, *et al.* Absence of functional receptors for parathyroid hormone and parathyroid hormone-related peptide in Blomstrand chondrodysplasia. *J Clin Invest* 1998; **102**: 34–40.

24 Karaplis AC, Luz A, Glowacki J, *et al.* Lethal skeletal dysplasia from targeted disruption of the parathyroid hormone-related peptide gene. *Genes Dev* 1994; **8**: 277–89.

25 Duncan G, McCormick C, Tufaro F. The link between heparan sulfate and hereditary bone disease: finding a function for the EXT family of putative tumor suppressor proteins. *J Clin Invest* 2001; **108**: 511–16.

26 Peters KG, Werner S, Chen G, Williams LT. Two FGF receptor genes are differentially expressed in epithelial and mesenchymal tissues during limb formation and organogenesis in the mouse. *Development* 1992; **114**: 233–43.

27 Liu Z, Xu J, Colvin JS, Ornitz DM. Coordination of chondrogenesis and osteogenesis by fibroblast growth factor 18. *Genes Dev* 2002; **16**: 859–69.

28 Vajo Z, Francomano CA, Wilkin DJ. The molecular and genetic basis of fibroblast growth factor receptor 3 disorders: the achondroplasia family of skeletal dysplasias, Muenke craniosynostosis, and Crouzon syndrome with acanthosis nigricans. *Endocr Rev* 2000; **21**: 23–39.

29 Francomano CA, McIntosh I, Wilkin DJ. Bone dysplasias in man: molecular insights. *Curr Opin Genet Dev* 1996; **6**: 301–8.

30 Bell DM, Leung KK, Wheatley SC, *et al.* SOX9 directly regulates the type-II collagen gene. *Nat Genet* 1997; **16**: 174–8.

31 Murakami S, Kan M, McKeehan WL, de Crombrugghe B. Up-regulation of the chondrogenic Sox9 gene by fibroblast growth factors is mediated by the mitogen-activated protein kinase pathway. *Proc Natl Acad Sci USA* 2000; **97**: 1113–18.

32 Horton W. Morphology of connective tissue: cartilage. In: Royce PM, Steinmann B, eds. *Connective Tissue and its Heritable Disorders*. New York: Wiley-Liss Inc., 1993: 641–75.

33 Rossi A, Superti-Furga A. Mutations in the diastrophic dysplasia sulfate transporter (DTDST) gene (SLC26A2): 22 novel mutations, mutation review, associated skeletal phenotypes, and diagnostic relevance. *Hum Mutat* 2001; **17**: 159–71.

34 Ortega N, Behonick D, Stickens D, Werb Z. How proteases regulate bone morphogenesis. *Ann NY Acad Sci* 2003; **995**: 109–16.

35 Wu CW, Tchetina EV, Mwale F, *et al.* Proteolysis involving matrix metalloproteinase 13 (collagenase-3) is required for chondrocyte differentiation that is associated with matrix mineralization. *J Bone Miner Res* 2002; **17**: 639–51.

36 Kirsch T, Harrison G, Golub EE, Nah HD. The roles of annexins and types II and X collagen in matrix vesicle-mediated mineralization of growth plate cartilage. *J Biol Chem* 2000; **275**: 35577–83.

37 Komori T, Yagi H, Nomura S, *et al.* Targeted disruption of Cbfa1 results in a complete lack of bone formation owing to maturational arrest of osteoblasts. *Cell* 1997; **89**: 755–64.

38 Takeda S, Bonnamy JP, Owen MJ, *et al.* Continuous expression of Cbfa in nonhypertrophic chondrocytes uncovers its ability to induce hypertrophic chondrocyte differentiation and partially rescues Cbfa1-deficient mice. *Genes Dev* 2001; **15**: 467–81.

39 Bergwitz C, Prochnau A, Mayr B, *et al.* Identification of novel CBFA1/RUNX2 mutations causing cleidocranial dysplasia. *J Inherit Metab Dis* 2001; **24**: 648–56.

40 Zelzer E, Glotzer DJ, Hartmann C, *et al.* Tissue specific regulation of VEGF expression during bone development requires Cbfa1/Runx2. *Mech Dev* 2001; **106**: 97–106.

41 Semenza GL. HIF-1 and human disease: one highly involved factor. *Genes Dev* 2000; **14**: 1983–91.

42 Mansfield K, Rajpurohit R, Shapiro IM. Extracellular phosphate ions cause apoptosis of terminally differentiated epiphyseal chondrocytes. *J Cell Physiol* 1999; **179**: 276–86.

43 Wang W, Xu J, Kirsch T. Annexin-mediated Ca^{2+} influx regulates growth plate chondrocyte maturation and apoptosis. *J Biol Chem* 2003; **278**: 376–29.

44 Mansfield K, Teixeira CC, Adams CS, Shapiro IM. Phosphate ions mediate chondrocyte apoptosis through a plasma membrane transporter mechanism. *Bone* 2001; **28**: 1–8.

45 Donohue MM, Demay MB. Rickets in VDR null mice is secondary to decreased apoptosis of hypertrophic chondrocytes. *Endocrinology* 2002; **143**: 3691–4.

46 Wu XB, Li Y, Schneider A, *et al.* Impaired osteoblastic differentiation, reduced bone formation, and severe osteoporosis in noggin-overexpressing mice. *J Clin Invest* 2003; **112**: 924–34.

47 Mundlos S. Cleidocranial dysplasia: clinical and molecular genetics. *J Med Genet* 1999; **36**: 177–82.

48 Harada H, Tagashira S, Fujiwara M, *et al.* Cbfa1 isoforms exert functional differences in osteoblast differentiation. *J Biol Chem* 1999; **274**: 6972–8.

49 Stewart M, Terry A, Hu M, *et al.* Proviral insertions induce the expression of bone-specific isoforms of PEBP2alphaA (CBFA1): evidence for a new myc collaborating oncogene. *Proc Natl Acad Sci USA* 1997; **94**: 8646–51.

50 Banerjee C, Javed A, Choi JY, *et al.* Differential regulation of the two principal Runx2/Cbfa1 n-terminal isoforms in response to bone morphogenetic protein-2 during development of the osteoblast phenotype. *Endocrinology* 2001; **142**: 4026–39.

51 Derynck R, Zhang YE. Smad-dependent and Smad-independent pathways in TGF-beta family signalling. *Nature* 2003; **425**: 577–84.

52 Yoshida Y, Tanaka S, Umemori H, *et al.* Negative regulation of BMP/Smad signaling by Tob in osteoblasts. *Cell* 2000; **103**: 1085–97.

53 Bialek P, Kern B, Yang X, *et al.* A twist code determines the onset of osteoblast differentiation. *Dev Cell* 2004; **6**: 423–35.

54 Nakashima K, Zhou X, Kunkel G, *et al.* The novel zinc finger-containing transcription factor osterix is required for osteoblast differentiation and bone formation. *Cell* 2002; **108**: 17–29.

55 Simonet WS, Lacey DL, Dunstan CR, *et al.* Osteoprotegerin: a novel secreted protein involved in the regulation of bone density. *Cell* 1997; **89**: 309–19.

56 Bucay N, Sarosi I, Dunstan CR, *et al.* Osteoprotegerin-deficient mice develop early onset osteoporosis and arterial calcification. *Genes Dev* 1998; **12**: 1260–8.

57 Whyte MP, Obrecht SE, Finnegan PM, *et al.* Osteoprotegerin deficiency and juvenile Paget's disease. *N Engl J Med* 2002; **347**: 175–84.

58 Yasuda H, Shima N, Nakagawa N, *et al.* Identity of osteoclastogenesis inhibitory factor (OCIF) and osteoprotegerin (OPG): a mechanism by which OPG/OCIF inhibits osteoclastogenesis in vitro. *Endocrinology* 1998; **139**: 1329–37.

59 Deckers MM, Karperien M, van der Bent C, *et al.* Expression of vascular endothelial growth factors and their receptors during osteoblast differentiation. *Endocrinology* 2000; **141**: 1667–74.

60 Sodek J, Chen J, Nagata T, *et al.* Regulation of osteopontin expression in osteoblasts. *Ann NY Acad Sci* 1995; **760**: 223–41.

61 Tetradis S, Bezouglaia O, Tsingotjidou A. Parathyroid hormone induces expression of the nuclear orphan receptor Nurr1 in bone cells. *Endocrinology* 2001; **142**: 663–70.

62 Lammi J, Huppunen J, Aarnisalo P. Regulation of the osteopontin gene by the orphan nuclear receptor NURR1 in osteoblasts. *Mol Endocrinol* 2004; **18**: 1546–57.

63 Nishimoto SK, Araki N, Robinson FD, Waite JH. Discovery of bone gamma-carboxyglutamic acid protein in mineralized scales. The abundance and structure of Lepomis macrochirus bone gamma-carboxyglutamic acid protein. *J Biol Chem* 1992; **267**: 11600–5.

64 Delany AM, Amling M, Priemel M, *et al.* Osteopenia and decreased bone formation in osteonectin-deficient mice. *J Clin Invest* 2000; **105**: 915–23.

65 Gong Y, Slee RB, Fukai N, *et al.* LDL receptor-related protein 5 (LRP5) affects bone accrual and eye development. *Cell* 2001; **107**: 513–23.

66 Beck GR Jr, Zerler B, Moran E. Phosphate is a specific signal for induction of osteopontin gene expression. *Proc Natl Acad Sci USA* 2000; **97**: 8352–7.

67 Vargas MA, St-Louis M, Desgroseillers L, *et al.* Parathyroid hormone-related protein(1-34) regulates Phex expression in osteoblasts through the protein kinase A pathway. *Endocrinology* 2003; **144**: 4876–85.

68 Berndt T, Craig TA, Bowe AE, *et al.* Secreted frizzled-related protein 4 is a potent tumor-derived phosphaturic agent. *J Clin Invest* 2003; **112**: 785–94.

69 Boyle WJ, Simonet WS, Lacey DL. Osteoclast differentiation and activation. *Nature* 2003; **423**: 337–42.

70 Udagawa N, Takahashi N, Yasuda H, *et al.* Osteoprotegerin produced by osteoblasts is an important regulator in osteoclast development and function. *Endocrinology* 2000; **141**: 3478–84.

71 Koga T, Inui M, Inoue K, *et al.* Costimulatory signals mediated by the ITAM motif cooperate with RANKL for bone homeostasis. *Nature* 2004; **428**: 758–63.

72 Takayanagi H, Kim S, Matsuo K, *et al.* RANKL maintains bone homeostasis through c-Fos-dependent induction of interferon-beta. *Nature* 2002; **416**: 744–9.

73 Whyte MP, Hughes AE. Expansile skeletal hyperphosphatasia is caused by a 15-base pair tandem duplication in TNFRSF11A encoding RANK and is allelic to familial expansile osteolysis. *J Bone Miner Res* 2002; **17**: 26–9.

74 Li J, Sarosi I, Yan XQ, *et al.* RANK is the intrinsic hematopoietic cell surface receptor that controls osteoclastogenesis and regulation of bone mass and calcium metabolism. *Proc Natl Acad Sci USA* 2000; **97**: 1566–71.

75 Li YP, Chen W, Liang Y, *et al.* Atp6i-deficient mice exhibit severe osteopetrosis due to loss of osteoclast-mediated extracellular acidification. *Nat Genet* 1999; **23**: 447–51.

76 Zhou H, Kartsogiannis V, Quinn JM, *et al.* Osteoclast inhibitory lectin, a family of new osteoclast inhibitors. *J Biol Chem* 2002; **277**: 48808–15.

77 Kawakami A, Eguchi K, Matsuoka N, *et al.* Fas and Fas ligand interaction is necessary for human osteoblast apoptosis. *J Bone Miner Res* 1997; **12**: 1637–46.

78 Robson H, Siebler T, Stevens DA, *et al.* Thyroid hormone acts directly on growth plate chondrocytes to promote hypertrophic differentiation and inhibit clonal expansion and cell proliferation. *Endocrinology* 2000; **141**: 3887–97.

79 Lewinson D, Harel Z, Shenzer P, *et al.* Effect of thyroid hormone and growth hormone on recovery from hypothyroidism of epiphyseal growth plate cartilage and its adjacent bone. *Endocrinology* 1989; **124**: 937–45.

80 Bassett JH, Williams GR. The molecular actions of thyroid hormone in bone. *Trends Endocrinol Metab* 2003; **14**: 356–64.

81 Stevens DA, Harvey CB, Scott AJ, *et al.* Thyroid hormone activates fibroblast growth factor receptor-1 in bone. *Mol Endocrinol* 2003; **17**: 1751–66.

82 Williams GR, Robson H, Shalet SM. Thyroid hormone actions on cartilage and bone: interactions with other hormones at the epiphyseal plate and effects on linear growth. *J Endocrinol* 1998; **157**: 391–403.

83 Yaffe BM, Samuels HH. Hormonal regulation of the growth hormone gene. Relationship of the rate of transcription to the level of nuclear thyroid hormone-receptor complexes. *J Biol Chem* 1984; **259**: 6284–91.

84 Hochberg Z, Bick T, Harel Z. Alterations of human growth hormone binding by rat liver membranes during hypo- and hyperthyroidism. *Endocrinology* 1990; **126**: 325–9.

85 Burch WM, Van Wyk JJ. Triiodothyronine stimulates cartilage growth and maturation by different mechanisms. *Am J Physiol* 1987; **252(2, Pt 1)**: E176–82.

86 Abe E, Marians RC, Yu W, *et al.* TSH is a negative regulator of skeletal remodeling. *Cell* 2003; **115**: 151–62.

87 Hunziker EB, Wagner J, Zapf J. Differential effects of insulin-like growth factor I and growth hormone on developmental stages of rat growth plate chondrocytes in vivo. *J Clin Invest* 1994; **93**: 1078–86.

88 Mohan S, Bautista CM, Wergedal J, Baylink DJ. Isolation of an inhibitory insulin-like growth factor (IGF) binding protein from bone cell-conditioned medium: a potential local regulator of IGF action. *Proc Natl Acad Sci USA* 1989; **86**: 8338–42.

89 Leung K, Rajkovic IA, Peters E, *et al.* Insulin-like growth factor I and insulin down-regulate growth hormone (GH) receptors in rat osteoblasts: evidence for a peripheral feedback loop regulating GH action. *Endocrinology* 1996; **137**: 2694–702.

90 Barnard R, Haynes KM, Werther GA, Waters MJ. The ontogeny of growth hormone receptors in the rabbit tibia. *Endocrinology* 1988; **122**: 2562–9.

91 Lewinson D, Shenzer P, Hochberg Z. Growth hormone involvement in the regulation of tartrate-resistant acid phosphatase-positive cells that are active in cartilage and bone resorption. *Calcif Tissue Int* 1993; **52**: 216–21.

92 Trippel SB, Wroblewski J, Makower AM, *et al.* Regulation of growth-plate chondrocytes by insulin-like growth-factor I and basic fibroblast growth factor. *J Bone Joint Surg Am* 1993; **75**: 177–89.

93 Maor G, Hochberg Z, von der Mark K, *et al.* Human growth hormone enhances chondrogenesis and osteogenesis in a tissue culture system of chondroprogenitor cells. *Endocrinology* 1989; **125**: 1239–45.

94 Yakar S, Rosen CJ, Beamer WG, *et al.* Circulating levels of IGF-I directly regulate bone growth and density. *J Clin Invest* 2002; **110**: 771–81.

95 Hou P, Sato T, Hofstetter W, Foged NT. Identification and characterization of the insulin-like growth factor I receptor in mature rabbit osteoclasts. *J Bone Miner Res* 1997; **12**: 534–40.

96 McCarthy TL, Casinghino S, Centrella M, Canalis E. Complex pattern of insulin-like growth factor binding protein expression in primary rat osteoblast enriched cultures: regulation by prostaglandin E2, growth hormone, and the insulin-like growth factors. *J Cell Physiol* 1994; **160**: 163–75.

97 Hill PA, Reynolds JJ, Meikle MC. Osteoblasts mediate insulin-like growth factor-I and -II stimulation of osteoclast formation and function. *Endocrinology* 1995; **136**: 124–31.

98 Silvestrini G, Mocetti P, Ballanti P, *et al.* Cytochemical demonstration of the glucocorticoid receptor in skeletal cells of the rat. *Endocr Res* 1999; **25**: 117–28.

99 Annefeld M. Changes in rat epiphyseal cartilage after treatment with dexamethasone and glycosaminoglycan-peptide complex. *Pathol Res Pract* 1992; **188**: 649–52.

100 Chrysis D, Ritzen EM, Savendahl L. Growth retardation induced by dexamethasone is associated with increased apoptosis of the growth plate chondrocytes. *J Endocrinol* 2003; **176**: 331–7.

101 Chang DJ, Ji C, Kim KK, *et al.* Reduction in transforming growth factor beta receptor I expression and transcription factor CBFa1 on bone cells by glucocorticoid. *J Biol Chem* 1998; **273**: 4892–6.

102 Delany AM, Dong Y, Canalis E. Mechanisms of glucocorticoid action in bone cells. *J Cell Biochem* 1994; **56**: 295–302.

103 Hofbauer LC, Gori F, Riggs BL, *et al.* Stimulation of osteoprotegerin ligand and inhibition of osteoprotegerin production by glucocorticoids in human osteoblastic lineage cells: potential paracrine mechanisms of glucocorticoid-induced osteoporosis. *Endocrinology* 1999; **140**: 4382–9.

104 Nilsson O, Chrysis D, Pajulo O, *et al.* Localization of estrogen receptors-alpha and -beta and androgen receptor in the human growth plate at different pubertal stages. *J Endocrinol* 2003; **177**: 319–26.

105 Smith EP, Boyd J, Frank GR, *et al*. Estrogen resistance caused by a mutation in the estrogen-receptor gene in a man. *N Engl J Med* 1994; **331**: 1056–61.

106 Morishima A, Grumbach MM, Simpson ER, *et al*. Aromatase deficiency in male and female siblings caused by a novel mutation and the physiological role of estrogens. *J Clin Endocrinol Metab* 1995; **80**: 3689–98.

107 Arts J, Kuiper GG, Janssen JM, *et al*. Differential expression of estrogen receptors alpha and beta mRNA during differentiation of human osteoblast SV-HFO cells. *Endocrinology* 1997; **138**: 5067–70.

108 McCarthy TL, Chang WZ, Liu Y, Centrella M. Runx2 integrates estrogen activity in osteoblasts. *J Biol Chem* 2003; **278**: 4312–19.

109 Bord S, Ireland DC, Beavan SR, Compston JE. The effects of estrogen on osteoprotegerin, RANKL, and estrogen receptor expression in human osteoblasts. *Bone* 2003; **32**: 136–41.

110 Hofbauer LC, Khosla S. Androgen effects on bone metabolism: recent progress and controversies. *Eur J Endocrinol* 1999; **140**: 271–86.

111 Carrascosa A, Audi L, Ferrandez MA, Ballabriga A. Biological effects of androgens and identification of specific dihydrotestosterone-binding sites in cultured human fetal epiphyseal chondrocytes. *J Clin Endocrinol Metab* 1990; **70**: 134–40.

112 Somjen D, Weisman Y, Mor Z, *et al*. Regulation of proliferation of rat cartilage and bone by sex steroid hormones. *J Steroid Biochem Mol Biol* 1991; **40**: 717–23.

113 Bord S, Horner A, Beavan S, Compston J. Estrogen receptors alpha and beta are differentially expressed in developing human bone. *J Clin Endocrinol Metab* 2001; **86**: 2309–14.

114 Lecka-Czernik B, Gubrij I, Moerman EJ, *et al*. Inhibition of Osf2/Cbfa1 expression and terminal osteoblast differentiation by PPARgamma2. *J Cell Biochem* 1999; **74**: 357–71.

115 Li X, Cui Q, Kao C, *et al*. Lovastatin inhibits adipogenic and stimulates osteogenic differentiation by suppressing PPARgamma2 and increasing Cbfa1/Runx2 expression in bone marrow mesenchymal cell cultures. *Bone* 2003; **33**: 65–29.

116 Thomas T, Gori F, Khosla S, *et al*. Leptin acts on human marrow stromal cells to enhance differentiation to osteoblasts and to inhibit differentiation to adipocytes. *Endocrinology* 1999; **140**: 1630–8.

117 Nakajima R, Inada H, Koike T, Yamano T. Effects of leptin to cultured growth plate chondrocytes. *Horm Res* 2003; **60**: 91–8.

118 Maor G, Rochwerger M, Segev Y, Phillip M. Leptin acts as a growth factor on the chondrocytes of skeletal growth centers. *J Bone Miner Res* 2002; **17**: 1034–43.

119 Ducy P, Schinke T, Karsenty G. The osteoblast: a sophisticated fibroblast under central surveillance. *Science* 2000; **289**: 1501–4.

120 Takeda S, Elefteriou F, Levasseur R, *et al*. Leptin regulates bone formation via the sympathetic nervous system. *Cell* 2002; **111**: 305–17.

121 Noble BS, Peet N, Stevens HY, *et al*. Mechanical loading: biphasic osteocyte survival and targeting of osteoclasts for bone destruction in rat cortical bone. *Am J Physiol Cell Physiol* 2003; **284**: C934–43.

122 Wronski TJ, Morey ER. Skeletal abnormalities in rats induced by simulated weightlessness. *Metab Bone Dis Relat Res* 1982; **4**: 69–75.

123 Karsdal MA, Andersen TA, Bonewald L, Christiansen C. Matrix metalloproteinases (MMPs) safeguard osteoblasts from apoptosis during transdifferentiation into osteocytes: MT1-MMP maintains osteocyte viability. *DNA Cell Biol* 2004; **23**: 155–65.

124 Nampei A, Hashimoto J, Hayashida K, *et al*. Matrix extracellular phosphoglycoprotein (MEPE) is highly expressed in osteocytes in human bone. *J Bone Miner Metab* 2004; **22**: 176–84.

125 van Bezooijen RL, Roelen BA, Visser A, *et al*. Sclerotin is an osteocyte-expressed negative regulator of bone formation, but not a classical BMP antagonist. *J Exp Med* 2004; **199**: 805–14.

4

Genetic control of growth

PRIMUS E MULLIS

INTRODUCTION

Growth is an inherent property of life. Normal somatic growth requires the integrated function of many of the hormonal, metabolic, and other growth factors involved in the hypothalamo–pituitary–growth axis.

The application of the powerful tool molecular biology has made it possible to ask questions not only about hormone production and action but also to characterize many of the receptor molecules that initiate responses to the hormones. Therefore, significant progress has been made in unravelling the events that lead to the final cellular expression of hormonal stimulation. As more details of intracellular signaling emerge the complexities of parallel and intersecting pathways of transduction have become more evident. We are beginning to understand how cells may regulate the expression of genes and how hormones intervene in regulatory processes to adjust the expression of individual genes. In addition, great strides have been made in understanding how individual cells talk to each other through locally released factors to coordinate growth, differentiation, secretion, and other responses within a tissue. In this chapter we focus (1) on the different components of the growth hormone axis; (2) on some developmental aspects; and (3) we examine the different altered genes and their related growth factors and/or regulatory systems that play an important physiological and pathophysiological role in growth. Further, as we have already entered the 'postgenomic' area, in which not only a defect at the molecular but also its functional

impact at the cellular level becomes important, we are concentrating in the last part on some of the most important aspects of cell biology and secretion.

DIFFERENT COMPONENTS OF THE GROWTH HORMONE AXIS

The overall growth hormone (GH) axis is shown in Fig. 4.1. GH is regulated by two hypothalamic peptides, GH-releasing hormone (GHRH), which is stimulatory, and GH-inhibiting factor (GHIF) which is inhibitory. There are membrane receptors for both GHRH and GHIF (somatostatin) on anterior pituitary cells. These two peptides are in turn influenced by an array of neurotransmitters. Pituitary GH encoded by the *GH-1* gene is secreted in pulses and binds to GH receptors (GHR) in the liver and other target organs. Receptor occupancy increases production and release of insulin-like growth factor-I (IGF-I). This mediator of GH action binds to IGF-I receptors in target tissues such as growth plates at the end of the long bones. There is a tight feedback control of GH release, involving GH and IGF-I in regulation of GHIF and probably GHRH. Additional genes are of importance to the GH axis including pituitary transcription factors (e.g., Pit1; POU1F1). Further, classification of genetic defects in the development of the GH axis illustrates that, basically, the site of these defects, both reported and hypothetical, may be located at any level from the hypothalamus to the target receptors of skeletal tissues (Fig. 4.1, Table 4.1).

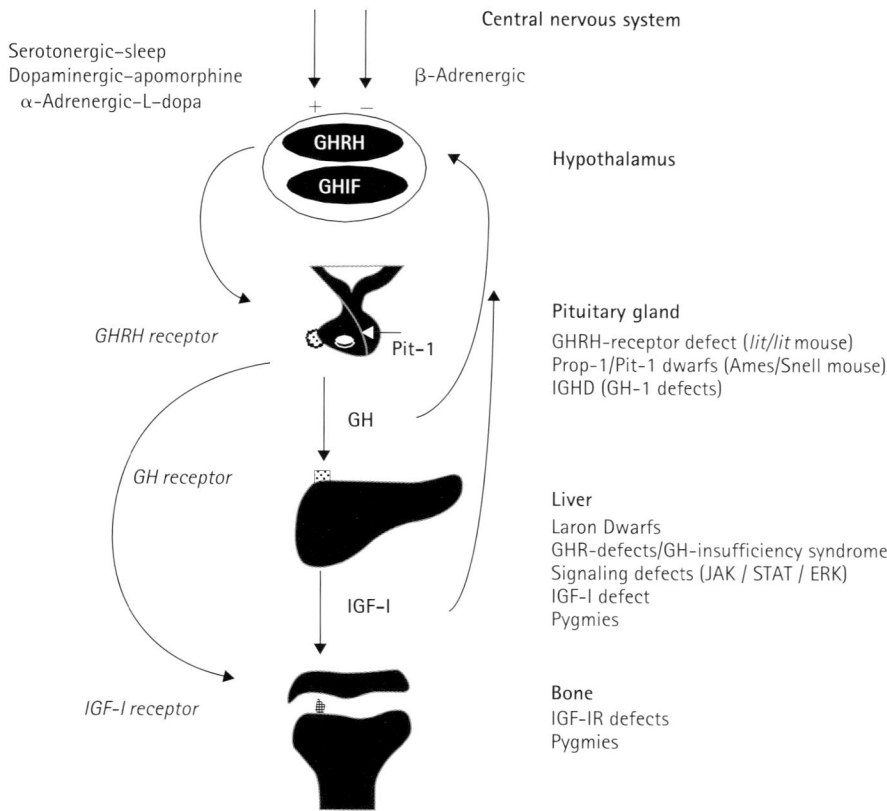

Figure 4.1   Regulation of growth hormone (GH) secretion/GHRH–GH axis. GH secretion is regulated by various factors. The sites of derangements responsible for various familial disorders of the GH axis are indicated on the right.

Table 4.1   Alteration of the GHRH–GH axis affecting growth in humans

Hypothalamus
  Transcription factors
  GHRH gene
Pituitary gland
  Transcription factors
    (i) TPIT
    (ii) SOX3
    (iii) HESX1
    (iv) LHX3
    (v) LHX4
    (vi) PROP1
    (vii) POU1F1
  GHRH receptor
  GH-gene cluster
    (i) GH-deficiency/bio-inactivity
GH target organs
  GH-receptor (primary: extracellular, transmembrane, intracellular)
    (i) GH insensitivity
    (ii) Signaling (JAK/STAT/ERK)
  GH insensitivity (secondary)
    (i) Malnutrition (e.g., anorexia)
    (ii) Liver disease (e.g., Byler's disease)
IGF-I defects
IGF-I transport/clearance
IGF-I resistance
  IGF-I receptor defect
  IGF-I signaling

DEVELOPMENT OF THE PITUITARY GLAND AND ITS IMPACT ON HORMONAL DEFICIENCIES

Overview

Discovery of transcription factors responsible for pituitary cell differentiation and organogenesis has had an immediate impact on understanding and diagnosis of pituitary hormone deficiencies. Importantly, combined pituitary hormone deficiencies have been associated with mutations in transcription factor coding genes that control organogenesis or multiple cell lineages, whereas isolated hormone deficiencies are often caused by transcription factors controlling late cell differentiation. However, as there may be a strong phenotypic variability in familial combined pituitary hormone deficiency caused by different transcription factors, e.g., PROP1 (Table 4.2), it is of high clinical importance to have some knowledge about the various steps in pituitary gland development (Fig. 4.2).[1–12]

As summarized in Fig. 4.2 the formation of the pituitary gland involves many factors that control various processes during development; these include factors for early patterning (Fig. 4.3; Rathke's pouch: dorsal: Pax-6; ventral: Isl-1, Brn-4; early pituitary gland: within anterior lobe: dorsal: Pax-6, Prop-1; ventral: Isl-1, Brn-4, Lhx-4, GATA-2; within intermediate lobe: Six-3, Pax-6) and organogenesis, for control of cell proliferation, and finally, for differentiation of individual lineages. Some of these transcription factors

Table 4.2   Comparison of phenotypes caused by a defect of various transcription factors of the pituitary gland

Factor	POU1F1	PROP1	LHX3	HESX1	LHX4
Hormonal deficiencies	GH, PRL, TSH	GH, PRL, TSH, – LH, FSH, (ACTH)	GH, PRL, TSH, LH, FSH, (ACTH)	GH, PRL, TSH, LH, FSH ACTH	GH, TSH, – ACTH
anterior pituitary posterior pituitary	n- > hypo normal	hypo > hyper normal	hypo- normal	hypo- ectopic	hypo- ectopic
Other manifestations	none	none	neck rotation no: 160° to 180° patients: 75° to 85°	eyes, brain septo-optic dysplasia	sella turcica skull defects

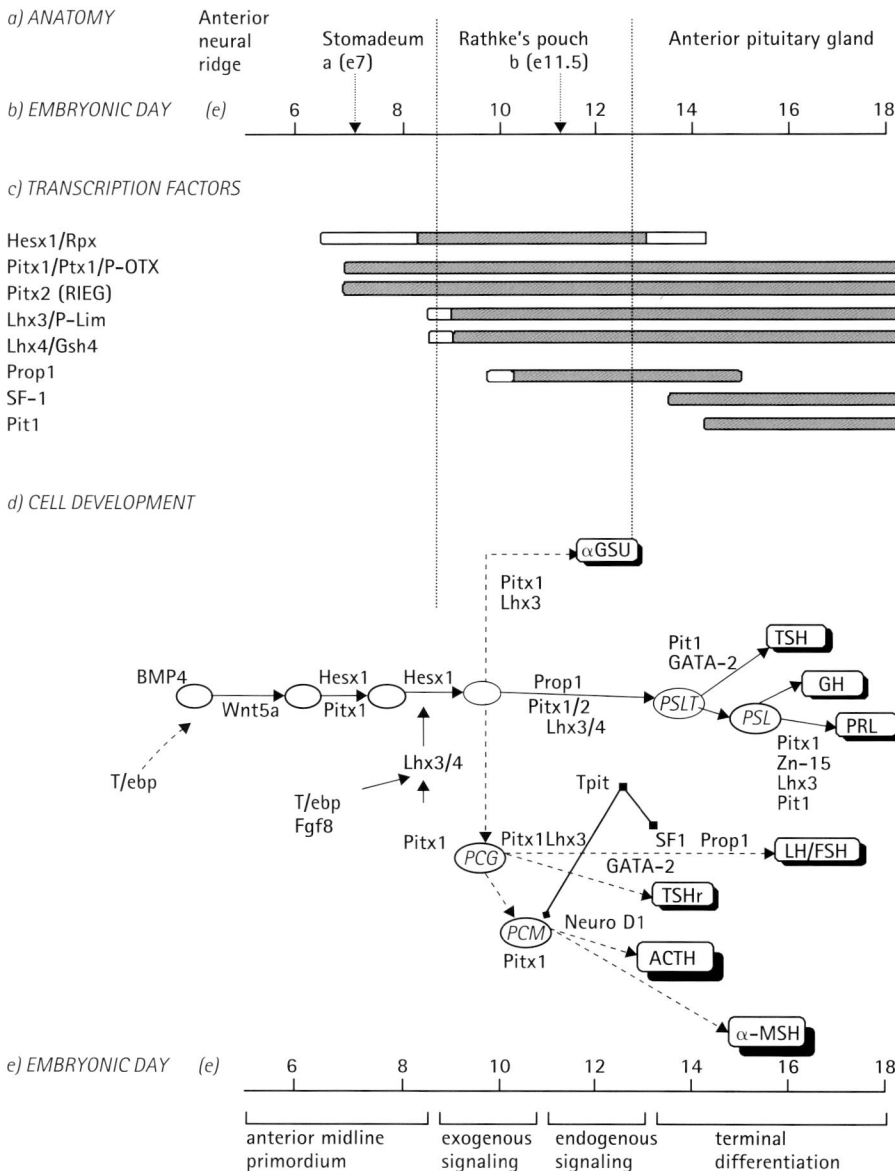

Figure 4.2   Pituitary gland development. In this figure a model of cell lineage determination in pituitary ontogeny is depicted.

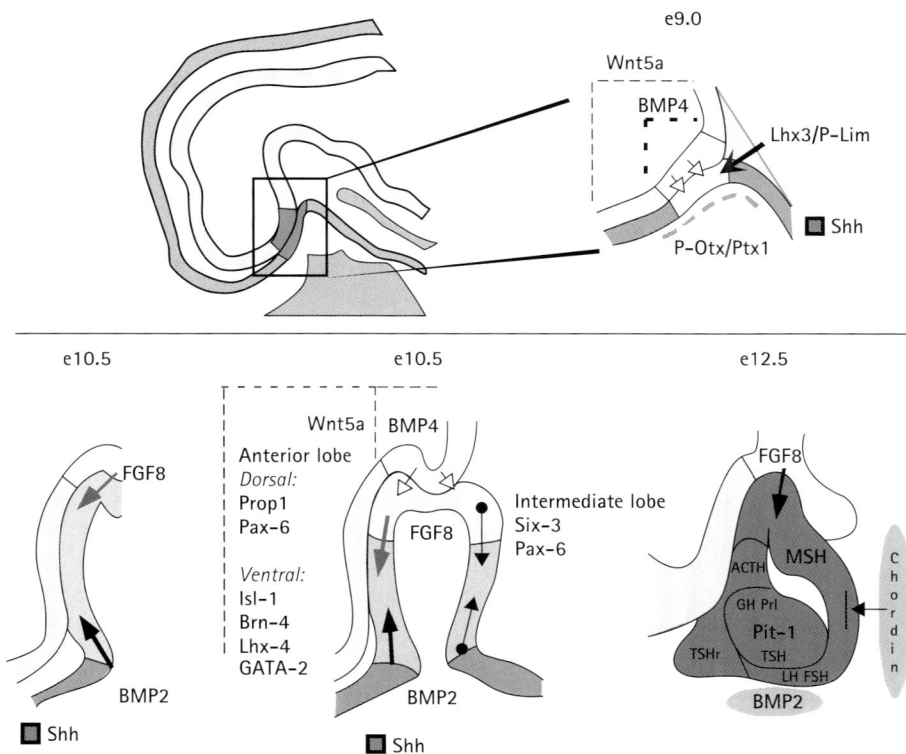

Figure 4.3 Signaling mechanism in pituitary morphogenesis. The pituitary primordium, Rathke's pouch, derives from the oral ectoderm. Signaling gradients generate overlapping patterns of transcription factor expression in pituitary development. At e9.0 Sonic hedgehog (Shh) and P-OTX/Pit1/2 are expressed throughout the oral ectoderm. BMP4 is originally present in the ventral diencephalon, whereas expression of FGF8 occurs at e10.5. In this early stage Shh expression is excluded from the Rathke's pouch creating a molecular compartment border between oral and pouch ectoderm. BMP2 expression is detected at this border region at e10.5. Expression of the BMP antagonist chordin in the caudal mesenchyme also potentially serves to maintain a ventrodorsal BMP2 gradient. These different gradients of transcription factors dorsally (Pax-6, Prop1), ventrally (Brn-4, Isl-1, Lhx-4, GATA-2) based on the variability of FGF8 and BMP2 transcription levels are important for pituitary commitment, and appearance of the cell lineages which in turn are necessary for later cell determination and differentiation.

contribute to more than one process at different times. For example, the Pitx-1 and Pitx-2 factor contribute to very early organogenesis, but they are also involved in late functions such as expansion of the gonadatotroph and thyro-throph lineages in Pitx[13] and the control of hormone-coding gene transcription (Fig. 4.2d).

Lineage commitment and differentiation

All lineages of the anterior and intermediate pituitary gland derive from the epithelial cells of the Rathke's pouch which projects as a diverticulum from the roof of the stomadeum – in humans – at the middle of the fourth week (Fig. 4.3). Molecular markers indicate that the pouch cells are not equivalent along the dorso-ventral axis, and this may be taken as an indication that the commitment to different pituitary lineages may be determined at an early developmental stage. In mice, at stage (e9.5–11.5), transcription factors such as Prop1 and Pax6 are preferentially expressed in the

dorsal pouch, whereas factors Isl-1, Brn-4, Lhx4 and GATA-2 are primarily expressed on the ventral side. Only one of these factors, Prop1, may be a commitment factor. Prop1 is initially expressed in the dorsal pouch and developing anterior pituitary where the somato-lactotrophs and definitive thyrotrophs will eventually appear.[14,15] Further Prop1 is required for expression of Pit1, which itself is necessary for differentiation of the same lineages.[16] Therefore, if data suggest that Prop1 may commit the dorsal pituitary to give rise to the somato-lactotroph and thyrotroph lineages, there is no evidence of a counterpart of Prop1 that may commit the ventral pituitary to give rise to gonadotroph or corticotroph lineages. Isl1 and GATA-2 may be candidate factors for this function.[12,17,18] Based on the description of gradients of signaling molecules and transcription factors in and around the development of the pituitary gland, a combinatorial model was proposed in which these regulatory molecules define territories within the developing gland. Only the unique combination of signals and/or factors would be responsible for differentiation toward one rather than the other lineages.[19] This model, however, reflects the fact that precise relations among all the lineages are not clear at all.[20] As it has been recently shown that the corticotroph and gonadotroph lineages (both arise ventrally) may have a common precursor[17,18,21] a simple binary model to account for all pituitary differentiation events starting from a common precursor has been proposed (Fig. 4.2d). This model would be consistent with the clearly commitment of the dorsal pituitary by Prop1 to form the pre-somato-lacto-thyrotroph precursors (PSLT), from which TSH, GH and PRL lineages will later arise through the action of Pit1, GATA-2, and other factors. Further, pre-corticol-gonadotrophs (PCG) are committed at a similar time, and these will later be driven to differentiate into corticotrophs via pre-cortico-melanotrophs (PCMs) under the influence of Tpit or NeuroD1, or even later into gonadotrophs under the influence of SF1 and GATA-2. However, for the time being it is not clear which factors may commit the ventral pituitary to the PCG fate. Signaling gradients are also likely to be involved and affect differentiation in this model, but these gradients may rather act in a stochastic fashion on a cell-by-cell basis rather than by defining specific territories within the developing gland.

Pituitary hormones and maintenance of normal cell function

In addition, it is not only important to get a certain function, but also to maintain it. Therefore, it has to be highlighted that a specific cell function (production of any hormone) might be lost over time because of a lack of cellular cross-talk as is has to be suggested in patients suffering from *PROP1* gene defects in terms of ACTH production.[14] Further, not only the different transcription factors but also the distinct and well-tuned hormonal feedback-loops [e.g., GH-releasing hormone (GHRH), GHRH receptor, GH, GH receptor, IGF-I] may play a major role at the level of maintenance of each hormonal cell activity. As an example, GHRH-receptor-mutant mice (*little*-mouse) present with a hypoplastic anterior gland and phenotypically with dwarfism lacking GH secretion.

Transcription factors of clinical importance

HESX1

The *paired-like* homeobox gene HESX1, a transcriptional repressor, has been implicated in patients suffering from septo-optic dysplasia (SOD) often referred as 'de Morsier syndrome' (OMIM 182230). It is characterized by the classical triad of optic nerve hypoplasia, midline defects mainly combined with neuro-radiological abnormalities, such as agenesis of the corpus callosum and the absence of the septum pellucidum and pituitary hypoplasia with consequent panhypopituitarism. Dattani *et al.* described the first HESX1 gene defect (R160C) in two siblings.[22] Importantly, the phenotype is highly variable, and may include any two of the

three classical features even within a family, suggesting incomplete penetrance.[22–28] In addition to the two homozygous missense mutations (R160C, I26T), three heterozygous mutations (S170L, T181A and Q6H) have been described in association with milder phenotypes characterized by isolated GHD with or without an ectopic posterior pituitary gland. Recently, a *de novo* heterozygous mutation (insertion: 306/307 ins AG) within exon 2 was reported in a family from Japan.[26] This patient, however, presented with severe combined pituitary hormone deficiency (CPHD) including ACTH deficiency.[26]

PROP1

Wu *et al.* described four families in which CPHD was associated with homozygosity or compound heterozygosity for inactivating mutations of the *PROP1* gene.[29] PROP1 (prophet of Pit1) is a paired-like homeodomain transcription factor and, originally, a mutation in this gene (Ser83Pro) was found causing the Ames dwarf (*df*) mouse phenotype.[30] In mice, *Prop1* gene mutation primarily cause GH, PRL and TSH deficiency, and in humans, *PROP1* gene defects also appear to be a major cause of CPHD. In agreement with the model of Prop1 playing a role in commitment of dorsal lineages (GH, PRL and TSH) Prop1 mutant mice exhibit a dorsal expansion of gonadotrophs that normally arise on the ventral side.

To date, many different missense, frameshift and splice site mutations, deletions, and insertions have been reported, and it has been realized that the clinical phenotype varied not only among the different gene mutations but also among the affected siblings with the same mutation.[1,2] In addition, although the occurrence of the hormonal deficiency varies from patient to patient,[1] the affected patients as adults were not only GH, PRL and TSH deficient, but also gonadotropin deficient (Table 4.2). The three tandem repeats of the dinucleotides GA at location 296–302 in the PROP1 gene represent a 'hot-spot' for CPHD.[1–3] Low levels of cortisol have also been described in some patients with *PROP1* gene mutations.[31,32] In addition, pituitary enlargement with subsequent involution has been reported in patients with PROP1 mutations.[31] The mechanism, however, underlying this phenomenon still remains unknown.

POU1F1 (PIT1)

The pituitary transcription factor PIT-1 is a member of the POU-family of homeo-proteins which regulates important differentiating steps during embryological development of the pituitary gland and regulates target gene function within the postnatal life.[33–38] Further, it is 291 amino acids in length, contains a transactivation domain as well as two conserved DNA-binding domains: the POU-homeo-domain and the POU-specific-domain.[33–38] As PIT1 is confined to the nuclei of somatotropes, lactotropes and thyrotropes in the anterior pituitary gland, the target genes of PIT1 include the *GH*, prolactin (PRL) and the *TSH* subunit, and the *POU1F1* gene itself.[39] Therefore, the defects in the human *POU1F1* gene known so far have all resulted in a total deficiency of GH and PRL, whereas a variable hypothyroidism due to an insufficient TSH secretion, at least during childhood, has been described.[40–42] Although it is important to stress that the clinical variability is due to other factors than the exact location of the mutation reported, the type of inheritance, however, seems to correlate well with the genotype.[35,37,38,42–48] Beside one exception, which is the C-terminal located mutation in the *POU1F1* gene (V272ter), the following rule was deduced: mutations lying within the DNA-binding domains, either POU-specific and/or POU homeodomain, cause autosomal recessively inherited CPHD, whereas CPHD caused by mutations outside these two specific regions may follow the autosomal–dominant pattern of inheritance.[49,50]

LHX3

LHX3 encodes a LIM-type homeodomain protein that contains two amino-terminal tandemly repeated LIM motifs and a carboxy terminal homeodomain with DNA-binding activity.[51,52] In Lhx3 −/− mice, the Rathke's pouch formed but failed to differentiate, except for the corticotroph lineage, which, however, failed to differentiate. Further, it is selectively expressed in both anterior and intermediate pituitary in the mature mice and is also transiently expressed in the developing ventral neural cord brainstem.[52] The Lhx3 protein acts synergistically with the Pit1 protein to transcriptionally activate genes that control pituitary differentiation. Two mutations in LHX3, a missense mutation changing a tyrosine to a cysteine (Y116C) and an intragenic deletion that results in a truncated protein lacking the DNA-binding homeodomain, have been identified in humans. These mutations were identified in patients with retarded growth and combined pituitary hormone deficiency, except for ACTH, and also abnormal neck (rigid cervical spine leading to limited head rotation) and cervical spine development (Table 4.2).[53] Further, in some of the affected subjects severe pituitary hypoplasia was diagnosed, whereas one patient presented at the age of 19 years with an enlarged anterior pituitary gland that was not documented ten years earlier.[53]

LHX4

Machinis *et al.* reported a family with an LHX4 germline splice-site mutation that resulted in a disease phenotype characterized by short stature due to GHD (as well as deficits of other anterior pituitary hormones associated with hypoplastic anterior hypophysis) and by pituitary and hindbrain defects (Chiari malformation type 1; OMIM 118420) in combination with abnormalities of the sella turcica of the central skull base (Table 4.2).[54] Most importantly, the affected subjects presented with a heterozygous intronic point mutation (G → C transversion) involving the invariant dinucleotide (AG) of the splice-acceptor site preceding exon 5.[54]

SOX3

Sox3 is a member of the Sox family (approx. 20 genes) that encode a group of proteins that carry a 79 amino acid DNA-binding domain (HMG box).[55] Recently, in both mice and humans, Sox3/SOX3, in humans a single exon gene on the X chromosome (Xq26-17), has been implicated in X-linked hypopituitarism.[55–57] In humans, in a single pedigree with X-linked GHD and mental retardation, a polyalanine expansion (26 alanine residues instead of 15) was identified in SOX3, C-terminal to the HMG box domain.[55] The phenotype consists of variable mental retardation, facial anomalies and IGHD. The final height of the untreated subjects ranged from 135 to 159 cm. Additionally, a deletion of nine alanine residues within the same polyalanine tract was found in two boys with mental retardation, short stature, microcephaly and abnormal facies.[58] This may be a gene of high clinical as well as scientific importance as interestingly, another group of patients with X-linked hypopituitarism harbors duplications of the region of the X chromosome that includes SOX3. The phenotype in these subjects is most likely due to the increased dosage of the gene.[59]

Different genes involved and their related defects

As summarized in Table 4.3, there are many potential as well as well established genetic defects affecting the growth axis. Because the strategy that led to the identification of many of these molecular defects was a candidate-gene approach based on a specific phenotype reported in genetically engineered mice, in this table, mice and human data are indicated and referenced. However, it is noteworthy that patients' phenotype may differ from that of mice carrying a targeted disruption of the corresponding gene as for instance patients with a LHX4 mutation do segregate as an autosomal dominant trait whereas, in mice, the Lhx4 +/− genotype is asymptomatic. From the clinical point of view some of the affected transcription factor gene defects can be suggested after the analysis of the magnetic resonance imaging data of hypothalamus and pituitary gland as well as of the concomitant anomalies (Table 4.2).

CLASSIFICATION OF ISOLATED GROWTH HORMONE DEFICIENCY

Structure and function of GH and CS genes

The *GH* gene cluster consists of five very similar genes in the order 5′[GH-1, CSHP (chorionic somatomammotropin pseudogene), CSH-1 (chorionic somatomammotropin gene), GH-2, CSH-2] 3′ encompassing a distance of about 65 000 bp (65 kb) on the long arm of chromosome 17 at bands q22–24 (Fig. 4.4a).[73] The *GH-2* gene encodes a protein (GH-V) that is expressed in the placenta rather than in the pituitary gland and differs from the primary sequence of

Table 4.3 Potential and well-established gene defects affecting the growth axis in mice and humans

Mutant gene/transgene	Rodent mutant/human disease	Phenotype	References
PRIMORDIA			
Bmp4 Bone morphogenetic protein	Knock-out (KO) and gene mutated animals	Initial invagination fails to occur, animals die at, or near the time of pituitary development	60, 61
Pitx1–Noggin	Transgenic mice	Noggin: Bmp antagonist using the regulatory sequences of the *Pitx1* gene, targets expression throughout the oral ectoderm and within Rathke's pouch. Pituitary development is arrested at e10	62
Fgf8 Fibroblast growth factor	KO	Lethal: dead during gastrulation	63
Titf1 (TITF, T/ebp) thyroid transcription factor 1	KO	Lethal at birth: thyroid, lung problems; no pituitary gland, all three lobes of pituitary gland are absent (importance of extrinsic signalling)	64
TTF–1 /TITF–1/ NKX2.1	Haploinsufficiency	Choreoathetosis, hypothyroidism, respiratory problems	65, 66
Rpx/Hesx1 Rathke's pouch homeobox; Homeobox gene expression in embryonic stem cells;	KO: expression in prospective forebrain, optic vesicles, Rathke's pouch	Hypoplastic nasal cavities, aplastic olfactory epithelium, micro- to anophthalmia, alterations of septum pellucidum, anterior commissures, corpus callosum; hypoplastic adenohypophysis	22
HESX1	Combined pituitary hormonal deficiencies, optic nerve hypoplasia, brain abnormalities	Septo-optic dysplasia variable forms	22
Pitx1 (P-OTX, Ptx1) Bicoid-related pituitary homeobox 1 factor	Knock-down: Loss of Lhx3 and αGSU-expression; KO: expression in midline stomadeum, anterior pituitary, branchial arch and hindlimb	pituitary cell differentiation may be normal, proliferation is altered (see *Lxh3*)	13, 67
PITX2 (RIEG)	Rieger syndrome Autosomal dominant disease	Cleft palate, tibia-, fibula-, patella-alterations, anterior chamber ocular abnormalities, dental hypoplasia, mild craniofacial dysmorphism, protuberant umbilicus, variable degrees of hypopituitarism	68
Lhx3 (P-Lim)	KO: expression in stomadeum, Rathke's pouch, pituitary gland, developing hindbrain, spinal cord, motoneural development, pineal gland	Lethal: Rathke's pouch is formed but does not invaginate normally, absence of thyro-, gonado-, somato- and lactotrope, hypoplastic adrenal gland	69
LHX3	Combined pituitary hormonal deficiencies, rigid cervical spine	Complete deficit in all anterior pituitary hormones except ACTH	53
Lhx4 (Gsh-1)	KO: expression not required for pouch induction, necessary for expansion of specialized cells	Mild hypopituitarism (reduced somatotrope and lactotropes); GHRH deficiency in nucleus arcuatus	70
LHX4	Combined pituitary hormonal deficiencies, abnormalities of skull base	Complete deficit GH, TSH, ACTH, normal PRL, LH/FSH	54
Lhx3, Lhx4 **double mutant**		Lethal: no definitive pouch ?	71

Multiple cell types

Prop1 Prophet of Pit1	Ames dwarf (df/df)	Nearly complete loss of somatotropes, lactotropes, thyrotropes, gonadotropes	30
PROP1 Human Prop1	Combined pituitary hormonal deficiencies	Variable loss of GH, PRL, TSH, LH, FSH function, later in life possibly loss of ACTH	1, 29
Pit1 (GHF1) Pituitary transcription factor 1	Snell dwarf (dw/dw)	Loss of somatotropes, lactotropes, and thyrotropes	34
POU1F1 POU domain, class1 transcription factor 1	Human hypopituitarism	Loss of GH and PRL, variable loss of TSH	37
Dat1 Dopamine transporter 1	KO: reduced number of somato-, lactotropes	Increased dopaminergic tone, anterior pituitary hypoplasia, dwarfism	72

Isolated GH deficiency

GHRH–receptor	Little mouse/IGHD	Short stature	117
GH	Short stature, hypoglycemia		see Table 5
	Bio-inactivity		101

IGF-I deficiency

GH–receptor	Extracellular	GH-insensitivity syndrome	158
	Transmembrane	GH-insensitivity syndrome	175
	Intracellular	GH-insensitivity syndrome	177
GH–receptor signalling	STAT5b	Intrauterine and postnatal growth retardation; GH-insensitivity syndrome; immunodeficiency; respiratory problems	151
IGF-I		Intrauterine and postnatal growth retardation; sensoneural deafness; mental retardation; hyeractivity	152

IGF-I resistance

IGF-I receptor		Intrauterine and postnatal growth retardation; variable phenotype, distinct from IGF-I synthesis defect, gene dosage (I)	195, 198

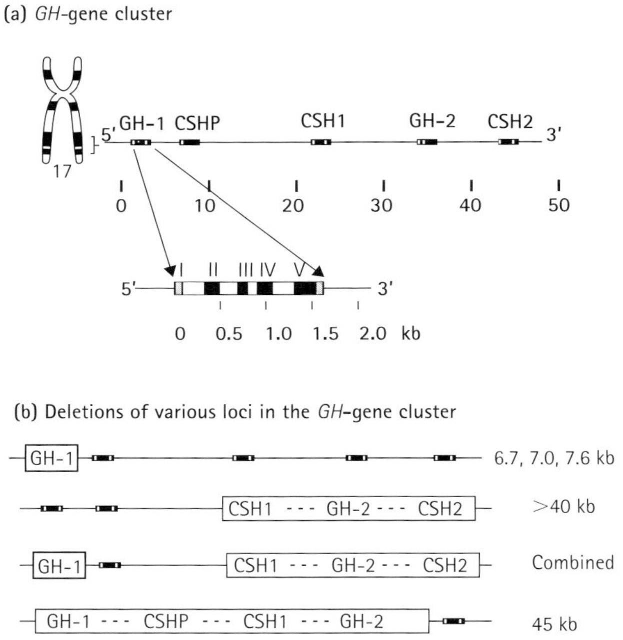

(a) *GH*-gene cluster

(b) Deletions of various loci in the *GH*-gene cluster

Figure 4.4 *GH* gene cluster and known deletions. (a) Schematic representation of the *GH* gene cluster and its localization on the long arm of chromosome 17. Exons, introns, and untranslated sequences are depicted by solid, open, and shaded rectangles, respectively. The sizes are indicated in kilobases (1 kb = 1000 base pairs). (b) The locations and sizes of the deletions are indicated at the lower panel.

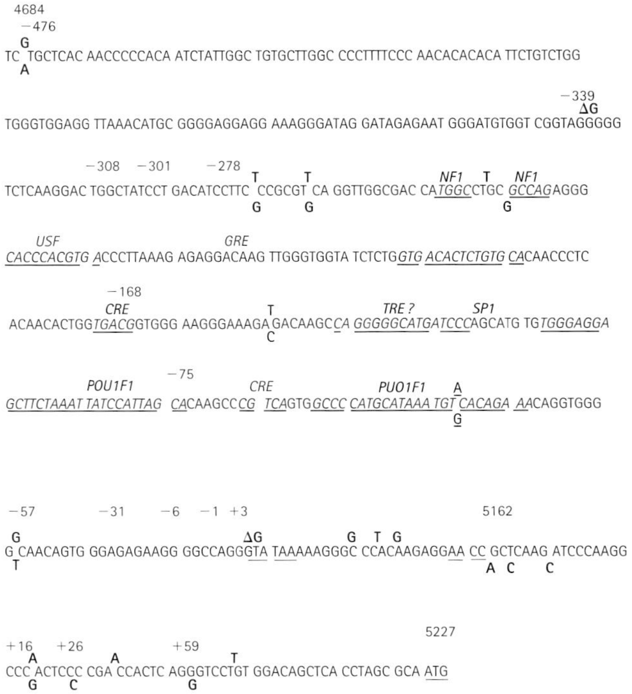

Figure 4.5 Structure of the 5′ untranslated and promoter region of the human *GH-1* gene. Transcription is regulated by proteins (trans-acting factors) that bind to regulatory (cis-acting) elements. The first nucleotide of the start site is designated +1, by convention, and the 5′ nucleotides are counted backwards from −1. The denoted known, putative or inferred binding sites for transcription factors are indicated. In addition, the TATA box, a Chi-like element and the ATG translational initiation sites are underlined. CRE: cAMP responsive elements; GRE: glucocorticoid responsive element; TRE: thyroid hormone responsive element; POU1F1: Pit1 (pituitary specific transcription factor); USF: upstream stimulatory factor; NF1: nuclear factor 1; SP1: specificity protein 1. Further, the polymorphic sites are indicated.

GH-N (product of *GH-1* gene) by 13 amino acids (aa). This hormone replaces pituitary GH in the maternal circulation during the second half of pregnancy.[74] The *CSH-1*, *CSH-2* genes encode proteins of identical sequences, whereas the CSHP encodes a protein that differs by 13 aa and contains a mutation (donor splice site of its second intron) that should alter its pattern of mRNA splicing and, therefore, the primary sequence of the resulting protein.[73] The extensive homology (92–98 percent) between the immediate flanking, intervening, and coding sequences of these five genes suggests that this multigene family arose through a series of duplicational events.[75] With the exception of *CSHP*, each gene encodes a 217 aa pre-hormone that is cleaved to yield a mature hormone with 191 aa and a molecular weight of 22 kDa. The expression of *GH-1* gene is controlled by cis- and trans-acting elements and factors, respectively. In Fig. 4.5, the 5′untranslated and the promoter region of the human *GH-1* gene is depicted. In addition, denoted known, putative or inferred binding sites of transcription factors are indicated.

Familial isolated growth hormone deficiency

Short stature associated with GH deficiency has been estimated to occur in about 1/4000 to 1/10 000 in various studies.[76–79] While most cases are sporadic and are believed to result from environmental cerebral insults or

developmental anomalies, 3–30 percent of cases have an affected first degree relative suggesting a genetic aetiology.[77,78] Since magnetic resonance examinations detect only in about 12–20 percent anomalies of either hypothalamus or pituitary gland in patients suffering from IGHD one might assume that many genetic defects may not be diagnosed and a significantly higher proportion of sporadic cases may have indeed a genetic cause.[80] Familial IGHD is associated with at least four Mendelian disorders (Table 4.4). These include two forms that have autosomal recessive inheritance (IGHD type IA, IB) as well as autosomal dominant (IGHD type 2) and X-linked (IGHD-3) forms.[81]

IGHD TYPE IA

IGHD type IA was first described by Illig[82] in three Swiss children with unusually severe growth impairment and apparent deficiency of GH. Affected individuals occasionally have short length at birth and hypoglycaemia in infancy but

Table 4.4   Isolated growth hormone deficiency

Category	Inheritance	GH–RIA	Candidate gene	Status
IGHD 1A	Recessive	Absent	hGH-1	Deletions/mutations frameshift
IGHD 1B	Recessive	Low	hGH-1	Splice site mutations
			GHRH	Unlikely
			GHRH-receptor	Mutations
			Trans-acting factors	Mutations/deletions
			Cis-acting elements	Mutations/deletions
IGHD 2	Dominant	Low	hGH-1	Splice site mutations
IGHD 3	X-linked	Low	Unknown	

uniformly develop severe growth retardation by the age of 6 months. Their initial good response to exogenous GH is hampered by the development of anti-GH antibodies leading to dramatic slowing of growth.[82,83]

GH-1 gene deletions

In 1981, Phillips *et al.* examined genomic DNA from these Swiss children reported and discovered using Southern blotting technique that the *GH-1* gene was missing.[84] Subsequently, additional cases of *GH-1* gene deletions have been described responding well to the GH treatment making the presence of anti-GH antibodies an inconsistent finding in IGHD IA patients with identical molecular findings (homozygosity for *GH-1* gene deletions).[85] The frequency of *GH-1* gene deletions as a cause of GH deficiency varies among different populations and the criteria and definition of short stature chosen. Analysing patients with severe IGHD (<-4 to -4.5 SDS) the prevalence reported was 9.4 percent (northern Europe; $n = 32$); 13.6 percent (Mediterranean; $n = 22$); 16.6 percent (Turkey; $n = 24$); 38 percent (Oriental Jews; $n = 13$); 12 percent (Chinese; $n = 26$); 0 percent (Japanese; $n = 10$) respectively.[86–89] The sizes of the deletions are heterogeneous with the most frequent (70–80 percent) being 6.7 kb.[86] The remaining deletions described include 7.6, 7.0, 45 kb, and a double deletion within the *GH* gene cluster (Fig. 4.4b). At the molecular level, these deletions involve unequal recombination and crossing over within the *GH* gene cluster at meiosis.[90,91] Interestingly, crossing over is reported to occur in 99 percent homologous regions (594 bp) flanking the *GH-1* gene, rather than in *Alu*-repeat sequences.[91] Although *Alu* repeats, which are frequent sites of recombination, are adjacent to the *GH-1* gene, they were not involved in any of the recombinational events studied. These highly homologous regions flanking the *GH-1* gene is currently used in a polymerase chain reaction (PCR) amplification method to screen for gene deletions[88] (Fig. 4.6). Inasmuch as the fusion fragments associated with the 6.7 kb deletions differ in the size of fragments produced by certain restriction enzymes (*Sma* I), homozygosity and heterozygosity for these deletions can easily be detected by enzyme digestion following PCR amplification.[92] The PCR approach is rapid, requires very small quantities of DNA, and can even be

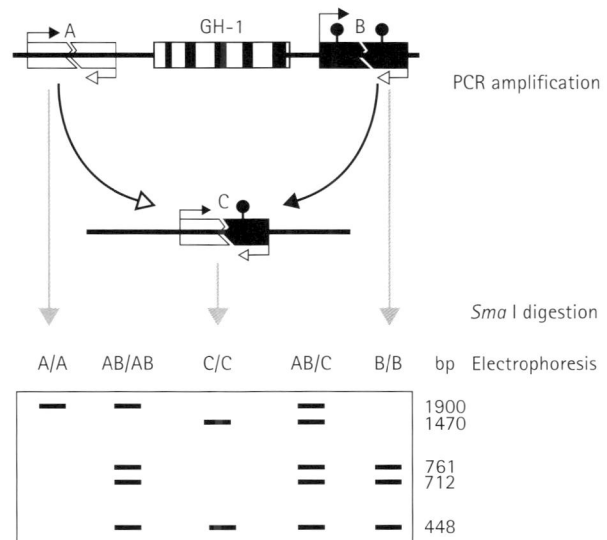

Figure 4.6   PCR amplification of homologous *GH-1* gene flanking sequences. PCR amplification of homologous sequences that flank *GH-1* gene using a single primer pair is shown. The two flanking sequences differ in terms of *Sma* I restriction sites (λ) that can be used for diagnostic purposes. DNA sequence analysis of the fusion fragments associated with *GH-1* gene deletions have shown that homologous recombination between sequences flanking GH-1 cause these deletions. Therefore, this PCR amplification based method is suitable for screening and prenatal diagnosis.

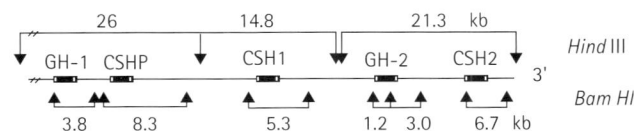

Figure 4.7   *GH*-gene cluster and restriction sites. Representation of the *GH*-gene cluster presenting the location of the restriction sites of *Hind* III and *Bam* HI.

done on filter paper spot of capillary blood samples. However, to detect heterozygosity for 7.0 or 7.6 kb deletions Southern blotting has to be performed using *Hind* III and *Bam* HI as restriction enzymes (Fig. 4.7).

Table 4.5   Mutational spectrum of growth hormone deficiency

Microdeletions				
Deficiency type	**Deletion**	**Codon**	**GH antibodies on treatment**	**References**
IA	TGcCTG	−10	Yes	93
IA	GGCcTGC	−12	Yes	Mullis unpublished
II	CGGggatggggagacctgtaGT	5′IVS-3 del+28 to +45	No	94
IA	GagTCTAT	55	No	95

Single base-pair substitutions in the *GH-1* gene coding region				
Deficiency type	**Mutation**	**Codon nucleotide**	**AB on treatment**	**References**
IA	TGG → TAG Trp → stop	−7	Yes	96
IA	GAG → TAG Glu → stop	−4	No	97
II	R183H	G6664A	No	98
II	V110F	G6191T	No	99
II	P89L	C6129T	No	100
II / bio-inactivity	CGC–TGC Arg → Cys	77	No	101 102

Single base-pair substitutions affecting mRNA splicing				
Deficiency type	**5′IVS-3**	**Δ exon 3**	**Origin**	**References**
II	GTGAGT → GTGAAT	Yes	Chile	103
II	GTGAGT → GTGACT	Yes	Turkey	Mullis unpublished
II	GTGAGT → GTGAGC	Yes	Turkey, Asia	104
II	GT → AT	Yes	Europe, America, Africa	105
II	GT → CT	Yes	Turkey	106
II	GT → TT	Yes	India	Mullis unpublished
II	GT → GC	Yes	Germany, Holland	99
	Exon splice enhancer	Yes		
II	ESE1m1: +1G→ T	Yes	Japan	107
II	ESE1m2: +5A→ G	Yes	Switzerland	108
	Intron splice enhancer	Yes		
II	ISEm1: IVS-3 +28 G → A	Yes		94
II	ISEm2: IVS-3 del28–45	Yes		94
	5′IVS-4			
IB	GT → CT	No	Saudi Arabia	96
IB	GT → TT	No	Saudi Arabia	109

GH-1 gene frameshift, and nonsense mutations

The frameshift and nonsense mutations diagnosed so far causing the different types of GH-deficiency are summarized in Table 4.5. It is worthwhile to stress that single-base pair deletions and nonsense mutations of the signal peptide result in no production of mature GH and are bound to produce anti-GH antibodies on exogenous replacement therapy.

IGHD TYPE IB

Patients with IGHD type IB are characterized by low but detectable levels of GH (<7 mU L^{-1}; <2.5 ng mL^{-1}), short

stature (<-2 SDS for age and sex), significantly delayed bone age, an autosomal recessive inheritance (two parents of normal height; two sibs affected), no demonstrable anatomic and/or endocrine cause for IGHD, and a positive response and immunological tolerance to treatment with exogenous GH. This subgroup of IGHD has been broadened and reclassified on the basis of the nature of their *GH* gene defects and now includes splicing site mutations of the *GH* gene; even an apparent lack of GH has been found by RIA. The phenotype of IGHD type IB, therefore, is more variable than IA. In one family, the children may resemble IGHD type IA, whereas in other families, growth during infancy is relatively normal and growth failure is not noted until mid-childhood. Similarly, GH may be lacking or simply low following a stimulation test. This heterogeneous phenotype suggests that there is more than one candidate gene causing the disorder. Possible candidate genes involved are noted in Table 4.4.

Splice site and nonsense mutations, frameshifts within the GH-1 gene

The *GH-1* gene has often been amplified and screened for small deletions and mutations which have been found and described (Table 4.5). However, generally speaking functional studies are necessary to prove the importance of all these alterations found in any gene. Therefore, for instance, all the mutations causing a suggested mRNA splicing error need transfection of the mutant gene into a cultured cell system allowing reverse transcription followed by cDNA sequencing. Thereafter, the impact of the changes of the amino acids encoded by the mutant genes can be studied. Studies with bovine GH mutants have shown that not only the stability and biological activity of the mutants may be altered but also the intracellular targeting of GH-protein products to the secretory granules important for secretion may be deranged.[110,111]

CANDIDATE GENES IN IGHD TYPE I B

Some of the components of the GH pathway are unique to GH, whereas others are shared by many others. In patients with IGHD, mutational changes in genes specific to GH are of importance and there is a need to focus on them.

GHRH gene

Workers at our laboratory and several others have tried to define any *GHRH* gene alterations and have failed so far.[112,113] Therefore, if *GHRH* mutations do cause IGHD in humans, they must be very rare.

GHRH-receptor gene

In 1992, Kelly Mayo cloned and sequenced the rat and human *GHRH-receptor* gene that provided the opportunity to examine the role of GHRH receptor in growth abnormalities that involve the GH axis.[114] Sequencing of the *GHRH-receptor* gene in the *little*-mouse (*lit/lit*) showed a single nucleotide substitution in codon 60 that changed aspartic acid to glycine (D60G) eliminating the binding of GHRH to its own receptor.[115] As the phenotype of IGHD type IB in humans has much in common with the phenotype of homozygous *lit/lit* mice including autosomal recessive inheritance, time of onset of growth retardation, diminished secretion of GH and IGF-I, proportional reduction in weight and skeletal size, and delay in sexual maturation, the *GHRH-receptor* gene was searched for alteration in these patients suffering from IGHD type IB.[116,117] In our laboratory, 65 children with IGHD type IB were studied of whom 12 did not respond to exogenous GHRH. None of the analyses revealed any structural abnormalities in these patients.[116]

However, it has to be mentioned that at that time this study was limited due to its ability to analyze only the sequence of the extracellular domain of the *GHRH-receptor* gene. The GHRH receptor is a member of a large family of hepta-helical transmembrane receptors that couple to G proteins upon receptor activation. Binding of GHRH to GHRH receptors expressed on the surface of somatotroph cells activates G_s and leads to a consequent increase in cAMP synthesis that induces cellular proliferation and GH secretion. Wajnrajch *et al.* reported a nonsense mutation similar to the *little* mouse in an Indian Moslem kindred.[117] Furthermore, in two villages in the Sindh area of Pakistan, Baumann reported another form of severe short stature caused by a point mutation in the *GHRH-receptor* gene resulting in a truncation of the extracellular domain of this receptor.[118] Individuals who are homozygous for this mutation are very short (-7.4 SDS) but normally proportioned. They appear of normal intelligence, and at least some are fertile. Biochemical testing revealed that they have normal levels of GHRH and GHBP, but undetectable levels of GH and extremely low levels of IGF-I. Later families from Sri Lanka, Brazil, United States, and Spain as well as Pakistan were reported.[119–122] Mutations in the *GHRH-receptor* gene have been described as the basis for a syndrome characterized by autosomal recessive IGHD and anterior pituitary hypoplasia, defined as pituitary height more than 2 SD below age-adjusted normal, which is likely due to depletion of the somatotroph cells (OMIM 139190). In a most recent report, however, a certain variability in anterior pituitary size even in siblings with the same mutation were described.[123]

Specific trans-acting factor to GH gene

Any alteration to the specific transcriptional regulation of the *GH-1* gene may produce IGHD type IB (Fig. 4.5). Mullis *et al.* have reported a heterozygous 211 bp deletion within the retinoic acid receptor α gene causing the phenotype of IGHD type IB.[124]

IGHD TYPE 2

Focusing on the autosomal dominant form of IGHD, type 2 (IGHD-2) is mainly caused by mutations within the first six base pairs of intervening sequences 3 (5′IVS-3),[125] which result in a missplicing at the mRNA level and the subsequent loss of exon 3, producing a 17.5 kDa hGH isoform.[106] This GH product lacks aa 32–71 (del32–71GH), which is the entire loop that connects helix 1 and helix 2 in the tertiary structure of hGH.[126,127] Skipping of exon 3 caused by *GH-1* gene alterations other than those at the donor splice site in 5′IVS-3 has also been reported in other patients with IGHD II. These include mutations in exon splice enhancer [ESE1 in exon 3 (E3)] (E3+ 1G → T: ESE1m1; E3+ 5A → G: ESE1m2) and within suggested intron splice enhancer (ISE) (IVS-3+ 28 G → A: ISEm1; IVS-3del+ 28–45: ISEm2) sequences.[94,105,107,108,125,128,129] Such mutations lie within purine rich sequences and cause increased levels of exon 3 skipped transcripts,[94,105,108,125,128,129] suggesting that the usage of the normal splicing elements (ESE1 at the 5′ end of exon 3 as well as ISE in intron 3) may be disrupted.[94,128,129] The first seven nucleotides in exon 3 (ESE1) are crucial for the splicing of GH mRNA[130] such that some nonsense mutations might cause skipping of one or even more exons during mRNA splicing in the nucleus. This phenomenon is called nonsense-mediated altered splicing (NAS); its underlying mechanisms are still unknown.[131] In addition to the above described splice site mutations that result in the production of del32–71 GH, three other mutations within the *GH-1* gene (missense mutations) are reported to be responsible for IGHD II, namely, the substitution of leucine for proline, histidine for arginine and phenylalanine for valine at aa positions 89 (P89V), 183 (R183H) and 110 (V110F), respectively.[98–100]

At the functional level, the 17.5 kDa isoform exhibits a dominant-negative effect on the secretion of the 22 kDa isoforms in both tissue cultures as well as in transgenic animals.[132–134] The 17.5 kDa isoform is initially retained in the endoplasmic reticulum, disrupts the Golgi apparatus, impairs both GH and other hormonal trafficking,[135] and partially reduces the stability of the 22 kDa isoform.[132] Furthermore, transgenic mice over-expressing the 17.5 kDa isoform exhibit a defect in the maturation of GH secretory vesicles and anterior pituitary gland hypoplasia due to a loss of the majority of somatotropes.[128,132,133] Trace amounts of the 17.5 kDa isoforms, however, are normally present in children and adults of normal growth and stature,[136] and heterozygosity for A731G mutation (K41R) within the newly defined ESE2 (which is important for exon 3 inclusion) led to approximately 20 percent exon 3 skipping resulting in both normal as well as short stature.[128,130] From the clinical point of view, severe short stature (< -4.5 SDS) is not present in all affected individuals, indicating that in some forms growth failure in IGHD II is less severe than one might expect.[99] It has been hypothesized that children with splice site mutations may be younger and shorter at diagnosis than their counterparts with missense mutations.[99] Furthermore, more recent *in vitro* and animal data suggest that both a quantitative and qualitative difference in phenotype may result from variable splice site mutations causing differing degrees of exon 3 skipping.[98,99,103,108,125,133,137–141] To summarize, these data suggest that the variable phenotype of autosomal dominant GHD may reflect a threshold and a dose dependency effect of the amount of 17.5 kDa relative to 22 kDa hGH.[133,134,137] Specifically, this has a variable impact on pituitary size, a variable impact on onset and severity of GHD, and, unexpectedly, that the most severe, rapid onset forms of GHD might be subsequently associated with the evolution of other pituitary hormone deficiencies.

IGHD TYPE *3*

This reported type is X-linked recessively inherited. In these families, the affected males were immunoglobulin- as well as GH-deficient.[142,143] Recent studies have shown that the long arm of chromosome X may be involved and that the disorder may be caused by mutations and/or deletions of a portion of the X-chromosome containing two loci, one necessary for normal immunoglobulin production, and the other for GH expression.[144] In addition, Durier *et al.*[145] reported an exon-skipping mutation in the *btk* gene of a patient with X-linked agammaglobulinemia and IGHD.

IGF–I DEFICIENCY AND GROWTH HORMONE INSENSITIVITY

Because IGF-I plays a pivotal role in growth, where it mediates most, if not all, of the effects of GH, in fact GHD could also be considered somehow as IGF-I deficiency (IGFD) (Table 4.6). Although IGFD can develop at any level of the GHRH–GH–IGF axis we would like to differentiate, however, between GHD (absent to low GH in circulation) and IGFD (normal to high GH in circulation).

A variety of studies have indicated that approximately 25 percent of children evaluated for idiopathic short stature (ISS) have primary IGFD presenting with abnormally low IGF-I in the face of normal to high GH in circulation.[146,147] In its purest and most dramatic forms, primary IGFD has been identified with three classes of molecular defects: (1) GH insensitivity (GHIS) resulting from mutations within the *GH-receptor* (*GHR*) gene primarily called Laron's syndrome;[148,149] (2) genetic defects affecting the GH-signaling pathway, mainly the Janus kinase 2 (JAK2) signal transducer and activator of transcription 5b (STAT5b);[150,151] and (3) deletions or mutations of the *IGF-I* gene itself.[152] Further, the concept of dysfunctional GH variants and/or bio-inactive GH molecules has been proposed for years[153] and opens an interesting platform to study the elements between GHD and IGFD, as some of these patients respond very well to

Table 4.6 Differential diagnosis of IGF-I deficiency and resistance

Growth hormone insensitivity
  (A) Primary GH insensitivity
    (i) dysfunctional GH/bio-inactive GH
    (ii) GH–receptor alteration
       Mutations/deletions of the extracellular domain of GHR
       Mutations/deletions of the transmembrane domain of GHR
       Mutations/deletions of the intracellular domain of GHR
    (iii) abnormal signal transduction
       JAK2/STAT5b/ERK
  (B) Secondary GH-insensitivity
    (i) malnutrition
    (ii) liver disease
    (iii) chronic illness
    (iv) anti-GH antibodies
Primary defects of IGF-I synthesis
Primary defects of IGF-I transport/metabolism/clearance
IGF-I resistance
  (A) Defects of IGF-I receptor type I
  (B) Post-receptor defects (signaling)

the exogenous GH treatment. In addition, there are reports on abnormal GHR-signaling in children with ISS in the absence of any *GHR-* or *GH-*gene alteration.[154,155]

Syndrome of bio-inactive growth hormone

The diagnosis 'syndrome of bio-inactive GH' has often been discussed and suggested in short children resembling the phenotype of IGHD but who had normal or even slightly elevated basal GH levels in combination with low IGF-I concentrations that increased after treatment with exogenous GH excluding the diagnosis of Laron syndrome. Takahashi *et al.* described two cases heterozygous for point mutations in the *GH-1* gene (R77C and D112G).[101,156,157] The R77C GH mutant bound with unusually high affinity to the GHBP and abnormally to the GHR. Further, it was able to inhibit tyrosine phosporylation in the GH signaling pathway, presumably acting in a dominant negative fashion as a GH antagonist, as IGF-I levels were not measurable following exogenous rhGH treatment. However, as the patient's father, who was also heterozygous for the same mutations, was phenotypically normal and of normal stature[101] many questions remain unanswered. The D112G mutant involved a single A to G substitution in exon 4[157] in a girl with short stature. The locus of the mutation was found within site 2 of the GH molecule in binding to the GHR/GHBP, which purportedly prevented dimerization of the GHR.[157] The patient presented with high levels of GH and low levels of IGF-I, but responded well to the rhGH, not only IGF-I increased but also the height velocity leading to an improved somatic growth (11 cm year^{-1} compared to 4.5 cm year^{-1} before therapy). Therefore, the authors claimed to report in this girl the first patient affected with a 'real' bio-inactive GH. In addition, in a recent report Millar *et al.* described several dysfunctional GH variants associated with a significantly reduced ability to activate GHR mediated JAK/STAT signal transduction.[137]

GH insensitivity and defects in the *GH–receptor* gene

Our understanding of the mechanism of action of GH has increased significantly since the characterization of the GH receptor (GHR) and demonstration of a partial gene deletion in two patients with Laron-type dwarfism by Godowski *et al.*[158] GHR is a transmembrane receptor, which is a member of the cytokine receptor superfamily. It has a soluble, circulating counterpart (GHBP) that consists of the extracellular domain and displays GH binding activity in humans.[159] *GHR* gene was characterized by Godowski *et al.* in 1989[158] who demonstrated that the coding and 3′ untranslated regions of the receptor are encoded by nine exons, numbered 2–10. Exon 2 corresponds to the secretion signal peptide; exons 3–7 encode the extracellular domain, 8 the transmembrane and 9–10 the cytoplasmic domain and the 3′ untranslated region.

Physiologically, the biological actions of GH are mediated through the activation of the GHR. As each of the GH has two highly specific binding sites, ensuring the binding of GH to the GHR a homodimer structure of the receptor is formed.[160] Dimerization of the GHR following GH binding is the first step and key event in the activation of target cells. Subsequently, tyrosine phosphorylation of JAK2 and STAT5 proteins plays a crucial role in the activation process, which ultimately results in gene transcription.

The GHR has been implicated in GH-insensitivity syndrome (GHIS), a rare autosomal-recessive GH-insensitive form of short stature first described in a group of Oriental Jewish children and reviewed by Laron, which is characterized by low serum concentrations of IGF-I and high levels of circulating GH.[148,161,162] In addition, GHIS is confirmed by the failure of exogenously administered GH to elevate levels of IGF-I or IGF-BP3 significantly. In contrast, GHBP was initially found to be absent, but more recent reports have suggested that some patients with GHIS may also have normal levels of GHBP.[158,159] Genetic and mutation analyses have verified the high molecular heterogeneity of this syndrome; to date, more than 50 different mutations in nearly 300 cases worldwide have been identified.[162–165] All classes of alterations have been reported: deletion, frameshift, nonsense, missense and splicing defects.[166] Of these, missense mutations are of particular interest as they have the potential to provide critical information on the structure–function relationship of the GHR and related molecules. Patients with atypical forms of GHIS have detectable plasma GH binding activity, associated with complete or partial GHIS.[146,167] However, molecular analyses of the phenotype with complete GHIS have revealed the existence of a missense mutation in the exoplasmic domain mainly located in exons 2–7 that impairs first receptor action by affecting GH binding and, therefore, second abolishes receptor homo-dimerization, thereby providing *in vivo* evidence for the critical role of the dimerization process in the growth-promoting action of GH.[168] Similarly, missense mutations in the cytoplasmic region, which would not be expected to affect GH-binding activity, should contribute to the identification of other important domains involved in signal transduction. The intracellular tyrosine kinase, Janus tyrosine kinase (JAK) 2, is associated with the cytoplasmic tail of GHR. After GH binding, two JAK2 molecules are brought into close proximity resulting in cross-phosporylation of both each other and tyrosine residues on the cytoplasmic tail on GHR. These phosphotyrosines act as docking points for cell signaling intermediates such as signal transducer and activator of transcription 5 (STAT5).[166] STAT5 binding to phosphorylated receptor tail then brings it into close proximity to JAK2, resulting in its own phosphorylation by JAK2. Phospo-STAT5 dimerizes and translocates to the nucleus in which it transactivates GH-responsive genes leading to the observed biological effects of GH [166] (Fig. 4.8).

Interestingly, one patient with GHIS was reported to have mutations located in the intracellular region.[169] Surprisingly, this patient, having very low serum GH binding activity,

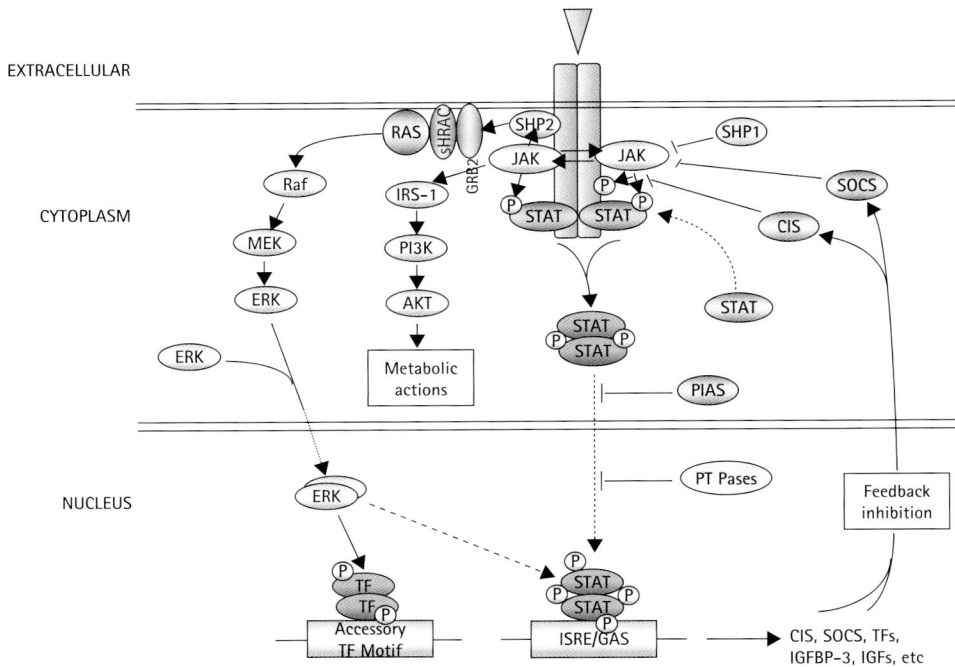

Figure 4.8   JAK/STAT signaling pathway following GH-receptor stimulation. (Adapted from Prof. Ron Rosenfeld, Stanford, CA.)

presented two mutations on a single GHR allele (C422F and P561T), whereas no other abnormality was detected on the remaining allele. The P561T mutation has already been excluded to be of any importance in causing the disorder by simply studying a sufficient large control group.[170] Therefore, most importantly, *in vitro* studies are required to test the functional consequences of all these identified missense mutations.

In theory, partial GHIS could encompass a wide range of distinct phenotypes with variable degrees of GH resistance.[146,171] Heterogeneity could result from a missense GHR mutation or from a quantitative GHR mRNA defect due to a mutation in the promoter, or to abnormal RNA maturation; this latter hypothesis was indeed recently confirmed.[164,172–174]

As previously mentioned, because GHBP is basically cleaved from the extracellular portion of the GHR, it is common knowledge that serum GHBP concentration is generally decreased in GHIS caused by any GHR gene defect in exons 2–7. There are, however, several cases of GHR defects reported associated with normal or raised GHBP levels in patients with mutations involving extracellular, transmembrane or intracellular domains. Duquesnoy *et al.* reported a D152H mutation in exon 6 causing positive GH-binding activity but abolished GHR homodimerization.[168] In contrast, in two subjects with severe GHIS caused by a 5′ splice donor site mutation within IVS-8, serum GHBP was massively increased, because the mutation resulted in a truncated GHR molecule.[175] In fact, complete exon 8 was skipped, producing a mutant GHR protein lacking transmembrane and intracellular domains. The authors predicted that this mutant protein would not be anchored in the cell membrane and would be measurable in the circulation as GHBP, hence explaining the phenotype of

severe GH resistance combined with elevated circulating GHBP.[175] Interestingly, a similar defect was reported by Silbergeld *et al.*[176] Analysis of the *GHR* gene performed in the proband revealed a G → T substitution at nucleotide 785-1 preceding exon 8 (3′ acceptor site). This mutation, which destroys the invariant dinucleotide of the splice acceptor site, is expected to alter GHR mRNA splicing and to be responsible for skipping exon 8.[176] Furthermore, two defects have been described which were associated with autosomal dominant GHIS.[177,178] First, a single G to C transversion in the 3′-splice acceptor site of intron 8 causing skipping of exon 9;[177] second, a G to A transversion at the +1 position of the 5′-donor splice site of intron 9 causing skipping of exon 9 and a premature stop codon in exon 10.[178] At the functional level it has been shown, that GH-induced tyrosine phosphorylation of STAT5 is inhibited and caused autosomal dominant GHIS.[179]

Evidence is accumulating that abnormalities in the intracellular signaling of GHR distal to the intracellular domain but proximal to IGF-I synthesis, can also cause GHIS.[180] In this report, Clayton *et al.* described two families with a defective signaling pathway. In the first (D152H mutation of *GHR* gene) neither STAT nor the mitogen-activated protein kinase (MAPK) pathways were activated, whereas in the second, GH activated STAT but failed to activate MAPK.[180]

Until recently, although several patients with a phenotype of GHIS and normal *GHR* gene have been described and no specific molecular down-stream defect of the GHR was identified[154] there is only one patient reported so far with the clinical and biochemical characteristics of GHIS presenting a homozygous missense mutation in the gene for STAT5b.[151] As it was shown in the patient suffering from a *IGF-I* gene defect the child experienced respiratory difficulties with increased oxygen requirements.[151,152]

Furthermore, mutations of the *GHR* gene were reported recently in a study on a highly selected group of patients with idiopathic short stature (ISS).[181] In this analysis, four of 14 children presented mutations in the region of the *GHR* gene that codes for the extracellular domain of the receptor. One of the four children with mutations was a compound heterozygote, with one mutation that reduced the affinity of the receptor for GH and a second mutation that may affect function other than ligand binding.[181] The remaining three patients had a heterozygous mutation in the *GHR* gene. However, it is of importance to stress that in one patient the mother presented the same heterozygous mutations but was of normal stature. Follow-up studies on the possible impact of heterozygous *GHR* gene mutations highlight the impact on short stature, especially in ISS.[182] Indeed, whereas many obligate carriers of GHIS have obtained normal height, others have not.[149,183] However, it may be a challenging concept that *GHR* gene mutations are responsible for about 5 percent of all ISS patients and it is important that these mutations should be considered when other causes of short stature have been eliminated. In addition, in order to broaden the possible scope abnormal GHR signaling may also underlie ISS even in the absence of *GHR* gene mutations.[154,184] Although until recently it had been assumed that GH signaling following GHR homodimerization was mediated primarily by the JAK/STAT pathway and that the ERK pathway does not induce hepatic IGF-I production,[185] a novel dysfunctional GH variant (Ile 179 Met) exhibiting a decreased ability to activate the extracellular signal regulated kinase (ERK) pathway resulting in short stature has been described.[186]

It could also be anticipated that, in some instances, the *GHR* gene is not involved in the GH-resistant phenotype, a hypothesis which can be tested by means of genetic linkage using the described intragenic GHR polymorphisms. This could help to identify other genes that control GHR expression or are required at different steps of the signal transduction pathway.[187] In this regard, the availability of a possible animal model (e.g., sex-linked dwarf chicken strains) for the Laron syndrome could open new ways in the identification of GH-inducible genes.[188]

Primary defects in IGF-I

IGF-I SYNTHESIS

Our laboratory and many others have searched intensively for gene alterations of the IGF-I gene causing GH resistance.[189,190] In 1996, Woods *et al.* reported a 15-year-old boy who had severe intrauterine and postnatal growth retardation, sensorineural deafness and mental retardation, and hyperactivity due to a homozygous deletion of exons 4 and 5 of the *IGF-I* gene.[152] Importantly, the parents were heterozygous for the same defect and possibly slightly affected as they were rather small and presented with lowish IGF-I levels. This report remains up to now the only confirmed case of an *IGF-I* gene defect.[191] This patient is of particular

interest in that he presents an unique opportunity to unravel the direct effects of GH from its indirect effects via IGF-I. Treatment for 1 year with IGF-I improved the patient's height velocity from 3.8 to 7.8 cm year^{-1}, normalized his GH levels and improved his insulin sensitivity.[192] In addition, focusing on the metabolic effects it has been shown that rhIGF-I improved body composition and normalized the insulin sensitivity.[193]

Furthermore, there is increasing evidence that IGF-I might be a major determinant of fetal growth. IGF-I knockout mice are born at 60 percent of their expected weight. This raises the possibility that defects of the *IGF-I* gene may contribute significantly to impaired fetal growth, which has been recently studied. However, Johnston *et al.*[184,194] concluded that *IGF-I* gene defects are likely only to be a very rare cause of impaired intrauterine growth.

IGF-I RESISTANCE

IGF-I receptor −/− mice were shown to be severely affected (birth weight 45 percent of normal weight) with the affected neonates dying from respiratory depression.[195,196] More than 50 mutations of the human insulin receptor gene have been reported to date.[197] In contrast, there is only one recent report on two patients with an IGF-I receptor (IGF-IR) gene alterations.[198] Patient 1 presented with a compound heterozygosity for missense mutations (R108Q and K115N) within the highly conserved, ligand binding domain of the *IGF-IR* gene resulting in high GH and IGF-I serum concentrations reflecting severe IGF-I resistance.[198] Patient 2 was heterozygous for the point mutation C to A leading to a stop codon (TAG; R59X) in exon 2.[198] This fact may point to interesting studies in the future. Patients who are haplo-insufficient for the *IGF-IR* gene because of an aneuploidy of chromosome 15 typically are dysmorphic and mentally as well growth retarded.[199] However, although the impact of the loss of contiguous genes on chromosome 15 is unclear, a clear gene-dosage on somatic growth was suggested in patient 2. In addition, the parents of patient 1 had marginal growth retardation at birth and an adult height substantially below the population mean. Further, many unexpected findings in these patients are awaiting an answer: (1) bone age less delayed than it is typical in GHD; (2) doubling of the height velocity on exogenous GH; (3) normal mental development; and (4) highly variable phenotype.[198]

IGF-I TRANSPORT AND CLEARANCE

Two possible clinical syndromes involving primary defects of IGF-I transport could theoretically present with growth failure.[12] The first would be an excess of IGFBPs, which might compete with the IGF-IR for binding and, therefore, inhibit IGF-I action. Further, in order to remain functionally in circulation, the normal formation of the ternary complex (acid-labile subunit, IGFBP and IGF) is necessary. Any defect at that level might have an impact on clearance as IGF peptides are not effectively bound and specific half-lives are changed. Along these lines, Barreca *et al.* reported a boy of short stature associated with high IGFBP-1 and high IGF-I levels responsive to exogenous rhGH treatment.[200] They speculated that the increased IGFBP-1 levels may inhibit: (1) the biological activity of IGF-I (IGF-I resistance); (2) the formation of the 150 kDa ternary complex (increased clearance); and (3) the feedback action on GH (increased GH levels) resulting in reduced stature.

AFRICAN PYGMIES

The cause of short stature in the African Pygmies is still unknown. Although resistance to GH action has been suggested by several investigators,[201] the suggestion that short stature in Pygmies is due to an abnormal GHR has not been substantiated, and the structure and DNA sequence of the *GHR* gene are indicated to be normal.[202] Hattori *et al.* studied IGF-I receptor expression and function in immortalized African Pygmy T cells, indicating that *IGF-I receptor* gene transcription and signaling may be the primary variation in the Pygmies.[203] These findings point not only to the IGF-I receptor as the locus governing short stature in the African Pygmies but also suggest that human stature may be generally controlled by expression of the IGF-I receptor.

CELL BIOLOGY AND POSTGENOMIC DEFECTS

As we have already entered the 'postgenomic' area it is most important to broaden our views and to focus, having defined the possible disorders at the DNA/RNA level, on function, and to go back and re-analyse the specific defects at the cellular level. As an example the autosomal dominant isolated growth hormone deficiency (IGHD type 2; IGHD 2) is stated.

Heterozygous *GH-1* gene mutations yielding an unfolded or misfolded GH protein do not have to cause ultimately GH deficiency. Some are dominant, others are recessive. This fact is of importance and suggests possible mechanisms in the secretory pathway. Furthermore, clinically IGHD 2 caused by variable gene defects may have the same phenotype. However, at the cellular level the disorder does have distinctive causes. Normally, secretory proteins are synthesized on polysomes attached to the ER and transported through its membrane into its lumen, where the proteins fold.[204] Vesicular or tubular structures transport folded proteins to the cis-region of the Golgi complex, and the proteins process through the stacks of the Golgi complex to the trans-side, after which the vesicles deliver secretory proteins to the cell surface.[205,206] The disorder might be caused at any (or all) of these different stages of the secretory process.[207–209] Proteins which are not properly folded are often retained in the ER and thereafter targeted for degradation by the ubiquitin–20S proteasome pathway.[210–212] Furthermore, the defect may be within the Golgi complex, as well as in the regulated secretory pathway, thus having an effect on the protein secretion.[213–216] All these

mechanisms are far from being confirmed and are still a major challenge to the whole scientific community focusing on the pathway of secretory proteins. Particularly interesting is the fact that identical phenotypes might be caused by different genotypes causing completely different defects at the cellular, and therefore functional level.

Acknowledgments

This work was supported by the Swiss National Science Foundation 3200-064623.01

KEY LEARNING POINTS

- The different components of the GH axis are discussed.
- The pituitary gland development and the clinically most important transcription factors and their impact on clinical phenotype are described.
- A special focus is on the various forms of isolated growth hormone deficiency as well as insulin-growth factor 1 deficiency.
- The impact of the cell biology is highlighted.

REFERENCES

● = Seminal primary article
◆ = Key review paper

1 Fluck C, Deladoey J, Rutishauser K, *et al.* Phenotypic variability in familial combined pituitary hormone deficiency caused by a PROP1 gene mutation resulting in the substitution of Arg–>Cys at codon 120 (R120C). *J Clin Endocrinol Metab* 1998; **83**: 3727–34.
2 Duquesnoy P, Roy A, Dastot F, *et al.* Human Prop-1: cloning, mapping, genomic structure. Mutations in familial combined pituitary hormone deficiency. *FEBS Lett* 1998; **437**: 216–20.
3 Deladoey J, Fluck C, Buyukgebiz A, *et al.* 'Hot spot' in the PROP1 gene responsible for combined pituitary hormone deficiency. *J Clin Endocrinol Metab* 1999; **84**: 1645–50.
4 Pfaffle RW, Blankenstein O, Wuller S, Kentrup H. Combined pituitary hormone deficiency: role of Pit-1 and Prop-1. *Acta Paediatr Suppl* 1999; **88**: 33–41.
5 Mullis PE. Transcription factors in pituitary development. *Mol Cell Endocrinol* 2001; **185**: 1–16.
6 Mullis PE. Transcription factors in pituitary gland development and their clinical impact on phenotype. *Horm Res* 2000; **54**: 107–19.
7 Dosen JS, Rosenfeld MG. Signaling mechanisms in pituitary morphogenesis and cell fate determination. *Curr Opin Cell Biol* 1999; **11**: 669–77.
◆ 8 Scully KM, Rosenfeld MG. Pituitary development: regulatory codes in mammalian organogenesis. *Science* 2002; **295**: 2231–5.

◆ 9 Pulichino AM, Vallette-Kasic S, Drouin J. Transcriptional regulation of pituitary gland development: binary choices for cell differentiation. *Curr Opin Endocrinol Diabetes* 2004; **11**: 13–17.

10 Dattani MT, Robinson IC. The molecular basis for developmental disorders of the pituitary gland in man. *Clin Genet* 2000; **57**: 337–46.

11 Parks JS, Brown MR. Transcription factors regulating pituitary development. *Growth Horm IGF Res* 1999; **9(Suppl B)**: 2–11.

◆ 12 Lopez-Bermejo A, Buckway CK, Rosenfeld RG. Genetic defects of the growth hormone-insulin-like growth factor axis. *Trends Endocrinol Metab* 2000; **11**: 39–49.

● 13 Szeto DP, Rodriguez-Esteban C, Ryan AK, *et al*. Role of the Bicoid-related homeodomain factor Pitx1 in specifying hindlimb morphogenesis and pituitary development. *Genes Dev* 1999; **13**: 484–94.

14 Vallette-Kasic S, Barlier A, Teinturier C, *et al*. PROP1 gene screening in patients with multiple pituitary hormone deficiency reveals two sites of hypermutability and a high incidence of corticotroph deficiency. *J Clin Endocrinol Metab* 2001; **86**: 4529–35.

15 Raetzman LT, Ward R, Camper SA. Lhx4 and Prop1 are required for cell survival and expansion of the pituitary primordia. *Development* 2002; **129**: 4229–39.

16 Andersen B, Pearse RV 2nd, Jenne K, *et al*. The Ames dwarf gene is required for Pit-1 gene activation. *Dev Biol* 1995; **172**: 495–503.

17 Ericson J, Norlin S, Jessell TM, Edlund T. Integrated FGF and BMP signaling controls the progression of progenitor cell differentiation and the emergence of pattern in the embryonic anterior pituitary. *Development* 1998; **125**: 1005–15.

18 Dasen JS, O'Connell SM, Flynn SE, *et al*. Reciprocal interactions of Pit1 and GATA2 mediate signaling gradient-induced determination of pituitary cell types. *Cell* 1999; **97**: 587–98.

◆ 19 Scully KM, Rosenfeld MG. Pituitary development: regulatory codes in mammalian organogenesis. *Science* 2002; **295**: 2231–5.

20 Keegan CE, Camper SA. Mouse knockout solves endocrine puzzle and promotes new pituitary lineage model. *Genes Dev* 2003; **17**: 677–82.

● 21 Pulichino AM, Vallette-Kasic S, Tsai JP, *et al*. Tpit determines alternate fates during pituitary cell differentiation. *Genes Dev* 2003; **17**: 738–47.

● 22 Dattani MT, Martinez-Barbera JP, Thomas PQ, *et al*. Mutations in the homeobox gene HESX1/Hesx1 associated with septo-optic dysplasia in human and mouse. *Nat Genet* 1998; **19**: 125–33.

23 Brickman JM, Clements M, Tyrell R, *et al*. Molecular effects of novel mutations in Hesx1/HESX1 associated with human pituitary disorders. *Development* 2001; **128**: 5189–99.

24 Carvalho LR, Woods KS, Mendonca BB, *et al*. A homozygous mutation in HESX1 is associated with evolving hypopituitarism due to impaired repressor-corepressor interaction. *J Clin Invest* 2003; **112**: 1192–201.

25 Hermesz E, Mackem S, Mahon KA. Rpx: a novel anterior-restricted homeobox gene progressively activated in the prechordal plate, anterior neural plate and Rathke's pouch of the mouse embryo. *Development* 1996; **122**: 41–52.

26 Tajima T, Hattorri T, Nakajima T, *et al*. Sporadic heterozygous frameshift mutation of HESX1 causing pituitary and optic nerve hypoplasia and combined pituitary hormone deficiency in a Japanese patient. *J Clin Endocrol Metab* 2003; **88**: 45–50.

27 Thomas P, Beddington RSP. Anterior primitive endoderm may be responsible for patterning the anterior neural plate in the mouse embryo. *Curr Biol* 1996; **6**: 1487–96.

28 Thomas PQ, Dattani MT, Brickman JM, *et al*. Heterozygous HESX1 mutations associated with isolated congenital pituitary hypoplasia and septo-optic dysplasia. *Hum Mol Genet* 2001; **10**: 39–45.

● 29 Wu W, Cogan JD, Pfaffle RW, *et al*. Mutations in PROP1 cause familial combined pituitary hormone deficiency. *Nat Genet* 1998; **18**: 147–9.

● 30 Sornson MW, Wu W, Dasen JS, *et al*. Pituitary lineage determination by the Prophet of Pit-1 homeodomain factor defective in Ames dwarfism. *Nature* 1996; **384**: 327–33.

31 Mendonca BB, Osorio MG, Latronico AC, *et al*. Longitudinal hormonal and pituitary imaging changes in two females with combined pituitary hormone deficiency due to deletion of A301,G302 in the PROP1 gene. *J Clin Endocrinol Metab* 1999; **84**: 942–5.

32 Rosenbloom AL, Almonte AS, Brown MR, *et al*. Clinical and biochemical phenotype of familial anterior hypo-pituitarism from mutation of the PROP1 gene. *J Clin Endocrinol Metab* 1999; **84**: 50–7.

33 Ingraham HA, Chen R, Mangalam HJ, *et al*. A tissue-specific transcription factor containing a homeodomain specifies a pituitary phenotype. *Cell* 1988; **55**: 519–29.

34 Li S, Crenshaw EB 3rd, Rawson EJ, *et al*. Dwarf locus mutants lacking three pituitary cell types result from mutations in the POU-domain gene pit-1. *Nature* 1990; **347**: 528–33.

35 Tatsumi K, Miyai K, Notomi T, *et al*. Cretinism with combined hormone deficiency caused by a mutation in the PIT-1 gene. *Nat Genet* 1992; **1**: 56–8.

36 Okamoto N, Wada Y, Ida S, *et al*. Monoallelic expression of normal mRNA in the PIT1 mutation heterozygotes with normal phenotype and biallelic expression in the abnormal phenotype. *Hum Mol Genet* 1994; **3**: 1565–8.

● 37 Pfaffle RW, DiMattia GE, Parks JS, *et al*. Mutation of the POU-specific domain of Pit-1 and hypopituitarism without pituitary hypoplasia. *Science* 1992; **257**: 1118–21.

38 Ohta K, Nobukuni Y, Mitsubuchi H, *et al*. Mutations in the Pit-1 gene in children with combined pituitary hormone deficiency. *Biochem Biophys Res Commun* 1992; **189**: 851–5.

39 Theill LE, Karin M. Transcriptional control of growth hormone expression and anterior pituitary development. *Endocr Rev* 1993: **14**: 670–89.

40 De Zegher F, Pernasetti F, Vanhole C, *et al*. A prismatic case: the prenatal role of thyroid hormone evidenced by fetomaternal Pit-1 deficiency. *J Clin Endocrinol Metab* 1995; **80**: 3127–30.

41 Brown MR, Parks JS, Adess ME, *et al*. Central hypothyroidism reveals compound heterozygous mutations in the Pit-1 gene. *Horm Res* 1998; **49**: 98–102.

42 Pfaffle R, Kim C, Otten B, *et al*. Pit-1: Clinical aspects. *Horm Res* 1996; **45(Suppl)**: 25–8.

43 Aarskog D, Eiken HG, Bjerknes R, Myking OL. Pituitary dwarfism in the R271W Pit-1 gene mutation. *Eur J Pediatr* 1997; **156**: 829–34.

44 Radovick S, Nations M, Du Y, *et al*. A mutation in the POU-homeodomain of Pit-1 responsible for combined pituitary hormone deficiency. *Science* 1992; **257**: 1115–8.

45 Rogol AD, Kahn CR. Congenital hypothyroidism in a young man with growth hormone, thyrotropin and prolactin deficiencies. *J Pediatr* 1976; **88**: 953–8.

46 Yoshimoto M, Aoki S, Baba T, *et al*. A severe case of pituitary dwarfism associated with prolactin and thyroid stimulating hormone deficiencies due to a transcription factor Pit1 abnormality. *J Jpn Pediatr Soc* 1988; **92**: 136–42.

47 Pernasetti F, Milner RD, al Ashwal AA, *et al*. Pro239ser: a novel recessive mutation of the Pit-1 gene in seven Middle Eastern children with growth hormone, prolactin, and thyrotropin deficiency. *J Clin Endocrinol Metab* 1998; **83**: 2079–83.

48 Fofanova OV, Takamura N, Kinoshita E, *et al*. Rarity of PIT-1 involvement in children from Russia with combined pituitary hormone deficiency. *Am J Med Genet* 1998; **77**: 360–5.

49 Blankenstein O, Mühleberg R, Kim C, *et al*. G. A new C-terminal located mutation (V272ter) in the Pit-1 gene manifestating with severe congenital hypothyroidism. *Horm Res* 2001; **56**: 81–6.

● 50 Salemi S, Besson A, Eble A, *et al*. New N-terminal located mutation (Q4ter) within the POU1F1-gene (PIT-1) causes recessive combined pituitary hormone deficiency and variable phenotype. *Growth Horm IGF Res* 2003; **13**: 264–8.

51 Sanchez-Garcia I, Rabbitts TH. The LIM domain: a new structural motif found in zinc-finger-like proteins. *Trends Genet* 1994; **10**: 315–20.

52 Bach I, Rhodes SJ, Pearse RV 2nd, *et al*. P-Lim, a LIM homeodomain factor, is expressed during pituitary organ and cell commitment and synergizes with Pit-1. *Proc Natl Acad Sci USA* 1995; **92**: 2720–4.

● 53 Netchine I, Sobrier ML, Krude H, *et al*. Mutations in LHX3 result in a new syndrome revealed by combined pituitary hormone deficiency. *Nat Genet* 2000; **25**: 182–6.

● 54 Machinis K, Pantel J, Netchine I, *et al*. Syndromic short stature in patients with a germline mutation in the LIM homeobox LHX4. *Am J Hum Genet* 2001; **69**: 961–8.

● 55 Rizzoti K, Brunelli S, Carmignac D, *et al*. SOX3 is required during the formation of the hypothalamo-pituitary axis. *Nat Genet* 2004; **36**: 247–55.

56 Laumonnier F, Ronce N, Hamel BC, *et al*. Transcription factor SOX3 is involved in X-linked mental retardation with growth hormone deficiency. *Am J Hum Genet* 2002; **71**: 1450–5.

57 Solomon NM, Nouri S, Warne GL, *et al*. Increased gene dosage at Xq26–q27 is associated with X-linked hypopituitarism. *Genomics* 2002; **79**: 553–9.

58 Collignon J, Sockanathan S, Hacker A, *et al*. A comparison of the properties of Sox-3 with Sry and two related genes, Sox-1 and Sox-2. *Development* 1996; **122**: 509–20.

59 Hamel BC, Smits AP, Otten BJ, *et al*. Familial X-linked mental retardation and isolated growth hormone deficiency: clinical and molecular findings. *Am J Med Genet* 1996; **64**: 35–41.

● 60 Winnier G, Blessing M, Labosky PA, Hogan BL. Bone morphogenetic protein-4 is required for mesoderm formation and patterning in the mouse. *Genes Dev* 1995; **9**: 2105–16.

● 61 Takuma N, Sheng HZ, Furuta Y, *et al*. Formation of Rathke's pouch requires dual induction from the diencephalon. *Development* 1998; **125**: 4835–40.

◆ 62 Treier M, Gleibermanm AS, O'Connell SM, *et al*. Multistep signaling requirements for pituitary organogenesis in vivo. *Genes Dev* 1998; **12**: 1691–704.

● 63 Meyers EN, Lewandoski M, Martin GR. An Fgf8 mutant allelic series generated by Cre-, Flp-mediated recombination. *Nat Genet* 1998; **18**: 2876–85.

● 64 Kimura S, Hara Y, Pineau T, *et al*. The T/ebp null mouse: thyroid-specific enhancer-binding protein is essential for the organogenesis of the thyroid, lung, ventral forebrain, and pituitary. *Genes Dev* 1996; **10**: 60–9.

● 65 Krude H, Schutz B, Biebermann H, *et al*. Choreoathetosis, hypothyroidism, and pulmonary alterations due to human NKX2-1 haploinsufficiency. *J Clin Invest* 2002; **109**: 475–80.

● 66 Pohlenz J, Dumitrescu A, Zundel D, *et al*. Partial deficiency of thyroid transcription factor 1 produces predominantly neurological defects in humans and mice. *J Clin Invest* 2002; **109**: 469–73.

● 67 Lanctôt C, Gauthier Y, Drouin J. Pituitary homeobox 1 (Ptx1) is differentially expressed during pituitary development. *Endocrinology* 1999; **140**: 1416–22.

● 68 Semina EV, Reiter R, Leysens NJ, *et al*. Cloning and characterization of a novel bicoid-related homeobox transcription factor gene, RIEG, involved in Rieger syndrome. *Nat Genet* 1996; **14**: 392–9.

● 69 Sheng HZ, Zhadanov AB, Mosinger B Jr, *et al*. Specification of pituitary cell lineages by LIM homeobox gen Lhx3. *Science* 1996; **272**: 1004–7.

● 70 Li H, Zeitler PS, Valerius MT, *et al*. Gsh-1, an orphan Hox gene, is required for normal pituitary development. *EMBO J* 1996; **15**: 714–24.

◆ 71 Sheng HZ, Moriyama K, Yamshita T, *et al*. Multistep control of pituitary organogenesis. *Science* 1997; **278**: 1809–12.

● 72 Bossé R, Fumagalli F, Jaber M, *et al*. Anterior pituitary hypoplasia and dwarfism in mice lacking the dopamine transporter. *Neuron* 1997; **19**: 127–38.

◆ 73 Hirt H, Kimelman J, Birnbaum MJ, *et al*. The human growth hormone gene locus: structure, evolution, and allelic variations. *DNA* 1987; **6**: 59–70.

74 Frankenne F, Closset J, Gomez F, *et al*. The physiology of growth hormones (GHs) in pregnant women and partial characterisation of the placental GH variant. *J Clin Endocrinol Metab* 1988; **66**: 1171–80.

◆ 75 Miller WL, Eberhardt NL. Structure and evolution of the growth hormone gene family. *Endocr Rev* 1983; **4**: 97–130.

76 Vimpani GV, Vimpani AF, Lidgard GP, *et al*. Prevalence of severe growth hormone deficiency. *BMJ* 1977; **ii**: 427–30.

77 Rona RJ, Tanner JM. Aetiology of idiopathic growth hormone deficiency in England and Wales. *Arch Dis Child* 1977; **52**: 197–208.

78 Lacey KA, Parkin JM. Causes of short stature: a community study of children in Newcastle upon Tyne. *Lancet* 1974; **I**: 42–5.

79 Lindsay R, Feldkamp M, Harris D, *et al*. Utah growth study: growth standards and the prevalence of growth hormone deficiency. *J Pediatr* 1994; **125**: 29–35.

80 Cacciari E, Zucchini S, Carla G, *et al*. Endocrine function and morphological findings in patients with disorders of the hypothalamo-pituitary area: a study with magnetic resonance. *Arch Dis Child* 1990; **65**: 1199–202.

◆ 81 Phillips III JA. Inherited defects in growth hormone synthesis and action. In: Scriver Ch, Beaudet AL, Sly WS, Valle D, eds. *The metabolic basis of inherited disease,* 7th ed. New York: McGraw-Hill, 1995: 3023–44.

82 Illig R. Growth hormone antibodies in patients treated with different preparations of human growth hormone (hGH). *J Clin Endocrinol Metab* 1970; **31**: 679–88.

83 Illig R, Prader A, Ferrandez A, Zachmann M. Hereditary prenatal growth hormone deficiency with increase tendency to growth hormone antibody formation ('A-type' of isolated growth hormone deficiency) [abstract]. *Acta Paediatr Scand* 1971; **60**: 60.

84 Phillips III JA, Hjelle B, Seeburg PH, Zachmann M. Molecular basis for familial isolated growth hormone deficiency. *Proc Natl Acad Sci USA* 1981; **78**: 6372–5.

85 Laron Z, Kelijman M, Pertzelan A, *et al*. Human growth hormone deletion without antibody formation or growth arrest during treatment: A new disease entity? *Isr J Med Sci* 1985; **250**: 999–1006.

86 Mullis PE, Akinci A, Kanaka C, *et al*. Prevalence of human growth hormone-1 gene deletions among patients with isolated growth hormone deficiency from different populations. *Pediatr Res* 1992; **31**: 532–4.

87 Parks JS, Meacham LR, McKean MC. Growth hormone (GH) gene deletion is the most common cause of severe GH deficiency among Oriental Jewish children [abstract]. *Pediatr Res* 1989; **25**: 90.

88 Vnencak-Jones CL, Phillips III JA, De Fen W. Use of polymerase chain reaction in detection of growth hormone gene deletions. *J Clin Endocrinol Metab* 1990; **70**: 1550–3.

89 Kamijo T, Phillips III JA, Ogawa M, *et al*. Screening for growth hormone gene deletions in patients with isolated growth hormone deficiency. *J Pediatr* 1991; **118**: 245–8.

90 Vnencak-Jones CL, Phillips III JA, Chen EY, Seeburg PH. Molecular basis of human growth hormone gene deletions. *Proc Natl Acad Sci USA* 1988; **85**: 5615–9.

● 91 Vnencak-Jones CL, Phillips III JA. Hot spots for growth hormone gene deletions in homologous regions outside Alu repeats. *Science* 1990; **250**: 1745–8.

92 Kamijo T, Phillips III JA. Detection of molecular heterogeneity in GH-1 gene deletions by analysis of polymerase chain reaction amplification products. *J Clin Endocrinol Metab* 1992; **74**: 786–9.

93 Duquesnoy P, Amselem S, Gourmelen M, *et al*. A frameshift mutation causing isolated growth hormone deficiency type IA. *Am J Hum Genet* 1990; **47**: A110.

94 Cogan JD, Prince MA, Lekhakula S, *et al*. A novel mechanism of aberrant pre-mRNA splicing in humans. *Hum Mol Genet* 1997; **6**: 909–12.

95 Igarashi Y, Ogawa M, Kamijo T, *et al*. A new mutation causing inherited growth hormone deficiency: a compound heterozygote of a 6.7 kb deletion and a two base deletion in the third exon of the GH-1 gene. *Hum Mol Genet* 1993; **2**: 1073–4.

96 Cogan JD, Phillips III JA, Sakati N, *et al*. Heterogeneous growth hormone (GH) gene mutations in familial GH deficiency. *J Clin Endocrinol Metab* 1993; **76**: 1224–8.

97 Wagner JK, Eble A, Cogan JD, *et al*. Allelic variations in the human growth hormone-1 gene promoter of growth hormone-deficient patients and normal controls. *Eur J Endocrinol* 1997; **137**: 474–81.

98 Deladoey J, Stocker P, Mullis PE. Autosomal dominant GH deficiency due to an Arg183His GH-1 gene mutation: clinical and molecular evidence of impaired regulated GH secretion. *J Clin Endocrinol Metab* 2001; **86**: 3941–7.

99 Binder G, Keller E, Mix M, *et al*. Isolated GH deficiency with dominant inheritance: new mutations, new insights. *J Clin Endocrinol Metab* 2001; **86**: 3877–81.

100 Duquesnoy P, Simon D, Netchine I, *et al*. *Familial isolated growth hormone deficiency with slight height reduction due to a heterozygote mutation in GH gene*. Program of the 80th Annual Meeting of The Endocrine Society. New Orleans, LA: The Endocrine Society; 1998: 2–202.

101 Takahashi Y, Kaji H, Okimura Y, *et al*. Brief report: short stature caused by a mutant growth hormone. *N Engl J Med* 1996; **334**: 432–6.

102 Chihara K. Identification of a growth hormone mutation responsible for short stature. *Acta Paediatr Suppl* 1996; **417**: 49–50.

103 Missarelli C, Herrera L, Mericq V, Carvallo P. Two different 5' splice site mutations in the growth hormone gene causing autosomal dominant growth hormone deficiency. *Hum Genet* 1997; **101**: 113–7.

104 Cogan JD, Phillips JA 3rd, Schenkman SS, *et al*. Familial growth hormone deficiency: a model of dominant and recessive mutations affecting a monomeric protein. *J Clin Endocrinol Metab* 1994; **79**: 1261–5.

105 Cogan JD, Ramel B, Lehto M, *et al*. A recurring dominant negative mutation causes autosomal dominant growth

hormone deficiency – a clinical research center study. *J Clin Endocrinol Metab* 1995; **80**: 3591–5.

106   Binder G, Ranke MB. Screening for growth hormone (GH) gene splice-site mutations in sporadic cases with severe isolated GH deficiency using ectopic transcript analysis. *J Clin Endocrinol Metab* 1995; **80**: 1247–52.

107   Takahashi I, Takahashi T, Komatsu M, *et al*. An exonic mutation of the GH-1 gene causing familial isolated growth hormone deficiency type II. *Clin Genet* 2002; **61**: 222–5.

108   Moseley CT, Mullis PE, Prince MA, Phillips JA 3rd. An exon splice enhancer mutation causes autosomal dominant GH deficiency. *J Clin Endocrinol Metab* 2002; **87**: 847–52.

109   Phillips JA 3rd, Cogan JD. Genetic basis of endocrine disease. 6. Molecular basis of familial human growth hormone deficiency. *J Clin Endocrinol Metab* 1994; **78**: 11–6.

110   Chen WY, Wight DC, Chen NY, *et al*. Mutations in the third alpha-helix of bovine growth hormome dramtically affect its intracellular distribution in vitro and growth enhancement in transgenic mice. *J Biol Chem* 1991; **266**: 2252–8.

111   McAndrew SJ, Chen NY, Wiehl P, *et al*. Expression of truncated forms of the bovine growth hormone gene in cultured mouse cells. *J Biol Chem* 1991; **266**: 20965–9.

112   Mullis PE, Patel M, Brickell PM, Brook CG. Isolated growth hormone deficiency: analysis of the growth hormone (GH) releasing hormone gene and the GH gene cluster. *J Clin Endocrinol Metab* 1990; **70**: 187–91.

113   Perez-Jurado LA, Phillips III JA, Francke U. Exclusion of growth hormone (GH)-releasing hormone gene mutations in family isolated GH deficiency by linkage and single strand conformation analysis. *J Clin Endocrinol Metab* 1994; **78**: 622–8.

● 114   Mayo K. Molecular cloning and expression of a pituitary-specific receptor for growth hormone-releasing hormone. *Mol Endocrinol* 1992; **6**: 1734–44.

● 115   Lin SC, Lin CR, Gukovsky I. Molecular basis of the little mouse phenotype and implications for cell type-specific growth. *Nature* 1993; **364**: 208–13.

116   Cao Y, Wagner JK, Hindmarsh PC, *et al*. Isolated growth hormone deficiency: Testing the little mouse hypothesis in man and exclusion of mutations within the extracellular domain of the growth hormone-releasing hormone receptor. *Pediatr Res* 1995; **38**: 962–6.

● 117   Wajnrajch MP, Gertner JM, Harbison MD, *et al*. Nonsense mutation in the human growth hormone receptor causes growth failure analogous to the little (lit) mouse. *Nat Genet* 1996; **12**: 88–90.

118   Baumann G, Maheshwari H. The Dwarfs of Sindh: severe growth hormone (GH) deficiency caused by a mutation in the GH-releasing hormone receptor gene. *Acta Paediatr Suppl* 1997; **423**: 33–8.

119   Maheshwari HG, Silverman BL, Dupuis J, Baumann G. Phenotype and genetic analysis of a syndrome caused by an inactivating mutation in the growth hormone-releasing hormone receptor: Dwarfism of Sindh. *J Clin Endocrinol Metab* 1998; **83**: 4065–74.

120   Netchine I, Talon P, Dastot F, *et al*. Extensive phenotypic analysis of a family with growth hormone (GH) deficiency caused by a mutation in the GH-releasing hormone receptor gene. *J Clin Endocrinol Metab* 1998; **83**: 432–6.

121   Salvatori R, Hayashida CY, Aguiar-Oliveira MH, *et al*. Familial dwarfism due to a novel mutation of the growth hormone-releasing hormone receptor gene. *J Clin Endocrinol Metab* 1999; **84**: 917–23.

122   Salvatori R, Fan X, Phillips JA 3rd, *et al*. Three new mutations in the gene for the growth hormone (GH)-releasing hormone receptor in familial isolated GH deficiency type IB. *J Clin Endocrinol Metab* 2001; **86**: 273–9.

123   Alba M, Hall CM, Whatmore AJ, *et al*. Variability in anterior pituitary size within members of a family with GH deficiency due to a new splice mutation in the GHRH receptor gene. *Clin Endocrinol (Oxf)* 2004; **60**: 470–5.

124   Mullis PE, Eblé A, Wagner JK. Isolated growth hormone deficiency is associated with a 211bp deletion within RAR ? gene [abstract]. *Horm Res* 1994; **41**: 61.

◆ 125   Mullis PE, Deladoey J, Dannies PS. Molecular and cellular basis of isolated dominant-negative growth hormone deficiency, IGHD type II: Insights on the secretory pathway of peptide hormones. *Horm Res* 2002; **58**: 53–66.

126   de Vos AM, Ultsch M, Kossiakoff AA. Human growth hormone and extracellular domain of its receptor: crystal structure of the complex. *Science* 1992; **255**: 306–12.

127   Cunningham BC, Ultsch M, De Vos AM, *et al*. Dimerization of the extracellular domain of the human growth hormone receptor by a single hormone molecule. *Science* 1991; **25**: 821–5.

128   Ryther RC, McGuinness LM, Phillips JA 3rd, *et al*. Disruption of exon definition produces a dominant-negative growth hormone isoform that causes somatotroph death and IGHD II. *Hum Genet* 2003; **113**: 140–8.

129   McCarthy EMS, Phillips III JA. Characterization of an intron splice enhancer that regulates alternative splicing of human GH pre-mRNA. *Hum Mol Gen* 1998; **7**: 1491–6.

130   Ryther RC, Flynt AS, Harris BD, *et al*. GH1 splicing is regulated by multiple enhancers whose mutation produces a dominant-negative GH isoform that can be degraded by allele-specific siRNA. *Endocrinology* 2004; **145**: 2988–96.

131   Dietz HC. Nonsense mutations and altered splice-site selections. *Am J Hum Genet* 1997; **60**: 729–30.

● 132   Lee MS, Wajnrajch MP, Kim SS, *et al*. Autosomal dominant growth hormone (GH) deficiency type II: the Del32-71-GH deletion mutant suppresses secretion of wild-type GH. *Endocrinology* 2000; **141**: 883– 90.

◆ 133   McGuinness L, Magoulas C, Sesay AK, *et al*. Autosomal dominant growth hormone deficiency disrupts secretory vesicles in vitro and in vivo in transgenic mice. *Endocrinology* 2003; **144**: 720–31.

● 134 Hayashi Y, Yamamoto M, Ohmori S, *et al*. Inhibition of growth hormone (GH) secretion by a mutant GH-I gene product in neuroendocrine cells containing secretory granules: an implication for isolated GH deficiency inherited in an autosomal dominant manner. *J Clin Endocrinol Metab* 1999; **84**: 2134–9.

● 135 Graves TK, Patel S, Dannies PS, Hinkle PM. Misfolded growth hormone causes fragmentation of the Golgi apparatus and disrupts endoplasmic reticulum-to-Golgi traffic. *J Cell Sci* 2001; **114**: 3685–94.

136 Lewis UJ, Sinha YN, Haro LS. Variant forms and fragments of human growth hormone in serum. *Acta Paediatrica Suppl* 1994; **399**: 29–31.

137 Millar DS, Lewis MD, Horan M, *et al*. Novel mutations of the growth hormone 1 (GH1) gene disclosed by modulation of the clinical selection criteria for individuals with short stature. *Hum Mutat* 2003; **21**: 424–40.

138 Fofanova OV, Evgrafov OV, Polyakov AV, *et al*. A novel IVS2 -2A>T splicing mutation in the GH-1 gene in familial isolated growth hormone deficiency type II in the spectrum of other splicing mutations in the Russian population. *J Clin Endocrinol Metab* 2003; **88**: 820–6.

139 Katsumata N, Matsuo S, Sato N, Tanaka T. A novel and de novo splice-donor site mutation in intron 3 of the GH-1 gene in a patient with isolated growth hormone deficiency. *Growth Horm IGF Res* 2001; **11**: 378–83.

140 Kamijo T, Hayashi Y, Seo H, Ogawa M. Hereditary isolated growth hormone deficiency caused by GH1 gene mutations in Japanese patients. *Growth Horm IGF Res Suppl* 1999; **B**: 31–6.

141 Kamijo T, Hayashi Y, Shimatsu A, *et al*. Mutations in intron 3 of GH-1 gene associated with isolated GH deficiency type II in three Japanese families. *Clin Endocrinol (Oxf)* 1999; **51**: 355–60.

142 Fleisher TA, White RM, Broder S, *et al*. X-linked hypogamma-globulinemia and isolated growth hormone deficiency. *N Engl J Med* 1980; **302**: 1429–39.

143 Sitz KV, Burks AW, Williams LW, *et al*. Confirmation of X-linked hypogamma-globulinemia with isolated growth hormone deficiency as a disease entity. *J Pediatr* 1990; **116**: 292–4.

144 Conley ME, Burks AW, Herrod HG, Puck JM. Molecular analysis of X-linked agammaglobulinemia and isolated growth hormone deficiency. *J Pediatr* 1991; **119**: 392–7.

145 Duriez B, Duquesnoy P, Dastot F, *et al*. An exon-skipping mutation in the btk gene of a patient with x-linked agammaglobulinemia and isolated growth hormone deficiency. *FEBS Lett* 1994; **346**: 165–70.

146 Attie KM, Carlsson LM, Rundle AC, Sherman BM. Evidence for partial growth hormone insensitivity among patients with idiopathic short stature. The National Cooperative Growth Study. *J Pediatr* 1995; **127**: 244–50.

147 Buckway CK, Guevara-Aguirre J, Pratt KL, *et al*. The IGF-I generation test revisited: a marker of GH sensitivity. *J Clin Endocrinol Metab* 2001; **86**: 5176–83.

● 148 Laron Z, Pertzelan A, Mannheimer S. Genetic pituitary dwarfism with high serum concentration of growth hormone: a new inborn error of metabolism? *Isr J Med Sci* 1966; **2**: 152–5.

● 149 Woods KA, Dastot F, Preece MA, *et al*. Phenotype: genotype relationships in growth hormone insensitivity syndrome. *J Clin Endocrinol Metab* 1997; **82**: 3529–35.

150 Hwa V, Little B, Kofoed EM, Rosenfeld RG. Transcriptional regulation of insulin-like growth factor-I by interferon-gamma requires STAT-5b. *J Biol Chem* 2004; **279**: 2728–36.

● 151 Kofoed EM, Hwa V, Little B, *et al*. Growth hormone insensitivity associated with a STAT5b mutation. *N Engl J Med* 2003; **349**: 1139–47.

● 152 Woods KA, Camacho-Hubner C, Savage MO, Clark AJ. Intrauterine growth retardation and postnatal growth failure associated with deletion of the insulin-like growth factor I gene. *N Engl J Med* 1996; **335**: 1363–7.

153 Kowarski AA, Schneider J, Ben-Galim E, *et al*. Growth failure with normal serum RIA-GH and low somatomedin activity: somatomedin restoration and growth acceleration after exogenous GH. *J Clin Endocrinol Metab* 1978; **47**: 461–4.

154 Salerno M, Balestrieri B, Matrecano E, *et al*. Abnormal GH receptor signaling in children with idiopathic short stature. *J Clin Endocrinol Metab* 2001; **86**: 3882–8.

155 Binder G, Benz MR, Elmlinger M, *et al*. Reduced human growth hormone (hGH) bioactivity without a defect of the GH-1 gene in three patients with rhGH responsive growth failure. *Clin Endocrinol (Oxf)* 1999; **51**: 89–95.

156 Takahashi Y, Chihara K. Clinical significance and molecular mechanisms of bioinactive growth hormone. *Int J Mol Med* 1998; **2**: 287–91.

157 Takahashi Y, Shirono H, Arisaka O, *et al*. Biologically inactive growth hormone caused by an amino acid substitution. *J Clin Invest* 1997; **100**: 1159–65.

● 158 Godowski PJ, Leung DW, Meacham LR, *et al*. Characterization of the human growth hormone receptor gene and demonstration of a partial gene deletion in two patients with Laron-type dwarfism. *Proc Natl Acad Sci USA* 1989; **86**: 8083–7.

● 159 Leung DW, Spencer SA, Cachianes G, *et al*. Growth hormone receptor and serum binding protein: purification, cloning and expression. *Nature* 1987; **330**: 537–43.

◆ 160 Wells JA. Binding in the growth hormone receptor complex. *Proc Natl Acad Sci USA* 1996; **93**: 1–6.

161 Laron Z, Parks JS. *Lessons from Laron Syndrome (LS) 1966–1992. A model of GH and IGF-I action and interaction*. Basel: Karger; 1993.

● 162 Laron Z. Growth hormone insensitivity (Laron syndrome). *Rev Endocr Metab Disord* 2002; **3**: 347–55.

163 Rosenfeld RG, Rosenbloom AL, Guevara-Aguirre J. Growth hormone (GH) insensitivity due to primary GH receptor deficiency. *Endocr Rev* 1992; **3**: 369–89.

164 Sobrier ML, Dastot F, Duquesnoy P, *et al*. Nine novel growth hormone receptor gene mutations in patients

with Laron syndrome. *J Clin Endocrinol Metab* 1997; **82**: 435–7.

165 Besson A, Salemi S, Eble A, *et al.* Primary GH insensitivity (Laron syndrome) caused by a novel 4 kb deletion encompassing exon 5 of the GH receptor gene: effect of intermittent long-term treatment with recombinant human IGF-I. *Eur J Endocrinol* 2004; **150**: 635–42.

◆ 166 Herrington J, Carter-Su C. Signaling pathways activated by the growth hormone receptor. *Trends Endocrinol Metab* 2001; **12**: 252–7.

167 Attie KM. Genetic studies in idiopathic short stature. *Curr Opin Pediatr* 2000; **12**: 400–4.

168 Duquesnoy P, Sobrier ML, Duriez B, *et al.* A single amino acid substitution in the exoplasmic domain of the human growth hormone receptor confers familial GH resistance (Laron syndrome) with positive GH-binding activity by abolishing receptor homodimerization. *EMBO J* 1994; **13**: 1386–95.

169 Kou K, Lajara R, Rotwein P. Amino acid substitutions in the intracellular part of the growth hormone receptor in a patient with the Laron syndrome. *J Clin Endocrinol Metab* 1993; **76**: 54–9.

170 Chujo S, Kaji H, Takahashi Y, *et al.* No correlation of growth hormone receptor gene mutation P561T with body height. *Eur J Endocrinol* 1996; **134**: 560–2.

◆ 171 Savage MO, Woods KA, Johnston LB, *et al.* Defects of the growth hormone receptor and their clinical implications. *Growth Horm IGF Res* 1999; **9(Suppl A)**: 57–61.

172 Johnston LB, Savage MO. Partial growth hormone insensitivity. *J Pediatr Endocrinol Metab* 1999; **12(Suppl 1)**: 251–7.

173 Amit T, Bergman T, Dastot F, *et al.* A membrane-fixed, truncated isoform of the human growth hormone receptor. *J Clin Endocrinol Metab* 1997; **82**: 3813–7.

174 Fisker S, Kristensen K, Rosenfalck AM, *et al.* Gene expression of a truncated and the full-length growth hormone (GH) receptor in subcutaneous fat and skeletal muscle in GH-deficient adults: impact of GH treatment. *J Clin Endocrinol Metab* 2001; **86**: 792–6.

175 Woods KA, Fraser NC, Postel-Vinay MC, *et al.* A homozygous splice site mutation affecting the intracellular domain of the growth hormone (GH) receptor resulting in Laron syndrome with elevated GH-binding protein. *J Clin Endocrinol Metab* 1996; **81**: 1686–90.

176 Silbergeld A, Dastot F, Klinger B, *et al.* Intronic mutation in the growth hormone (GH) receptor gene from a girl with Laron syndrome and extremely high serum GH binding protein: extended phenotypic study in a very large pedigree. *J Pediatr Endocrinol Metab* 1997; **10**: 265–74.

177 Ayling RM, Ross R, Towner P, *et al.* A dominant-negative mutation of the growth hormone receptor causes familial short stature. *Nat Genet* 1997; **16**: 13–4.

178 Iida K, Takahashi Y, Kaji H, *et al.* Growth hormone (GH) insensitivity syndrome with high serum GH-binding protein levels caused by a heterozygous splice site mutation of the GH receptor gene producing a lack of intracellular domain. *J Clin Endocrinol Metab* 1998; **83**: 531–7.

179 Iida K, Takahashi Y, Kaji H, *et al.* Functional characterization of truncated growth hormone (GH) receptor-(1–277) causing partial GH insensitivity syndrome with high GH-binding protein. *J Clin Endocrinol Metab* 1999; **84**: 1011–6.

180 Clayton PE, Freeth JS, Whatmore AJ, *et al.* Signal transduction defects in growth hormone insensitivity. *Acta Paediatr Suppl* 1999; **88**: 174–9.

● 181 Goddard AD, Covello R, Luoh SM, *et al.* Mutations of the growth hormone receptor in children with idiopathic short stature. *N Engl J Med* 1995; **333**: 1093–8.

182 Sanchez JE, Perera E, Baumbach L, Cleveland WW. Growth hormone receptor mutations in children with idiopathic short stature. *J Clin Endocrinol Metab* 1998; **83**: 4079–83.

183 Rosenbloom AL, Guevara-Aguirre J, Rosenfeld RG, Fielder PJ. Is there heterozygote expression of growth hormone receptor deficiency? *Acta Paediatr Suppl* 1994; **399**: 125–7.

184 Johnston LB, Pashankar F, Camacho-Hubner C, *et al.* Analysis of the intracellular signalling domain of the human growth hormone receptor in children with idiopathic short stature. *Clin Endocrinol (Oxf)* 2000; **52**: 463–9.

185 Shoba LN, Newman M, Liu W, Lowe WL Jr. LY. 294002, an inhibitor of phosphatidyl-inositol 3-kinase, inhibits GH-mediated expression of the IGF-I gene in rat hepatocytes. *Endocrinology* 2001; **142**: 3980–6.

186 Lewis MD, Horan M, Millar DS, *et al.* A novel dysfunctional growth hormone variant (Ile179Met) exhibits a decreased ability to activate the extracellular signal-regulated kinase pathway. *J Clin Endocrinol Metab* 2004; **89**: 1068–75.

187 Argetsinger LS, Campbell GS, Yang X, *et al.* Identification of JAK2 as a growth hormone receptor-associated tyrosine kinase. *Cell* 1993; **74**: 237–44.

188 Duriez B, Sobrier ML, Duquesnoy P, *et al.* A naturally occurring growth hormone receptor mutation: in vivo and in vitro evidence for the functional importance of the WS motif common to all members of the cytokine receptor family. *Mol Endocrinol* 1993; **7**: 806–14.

189 Lajara R, Galgani JP Jr, Dempsher DP, *et al.* Low prevalence of insulin-like growth factor I gene mutations in human growth disorders. *J Clin Endocrinol Metab* 1990; **70**: 687–92.

190 Mullis PE, Patel M, Brickell PM, Brook CGD. Constitutionally short stature: analysis of the Insulin-like growth factor-gene and the human growth hormone gene cluster. *Pediatr Res* 1991; **29**: 412–5.

◆ 191 Camacho-Hubner C, Woods KA, Clark AJ, Savage MO. Insulin-like growth factor (IGF)-I gene deletion. *Rev Endocr Metab Disord* 2002; **3**: 357–61.

192 Woods KA, Camacho-Hubner C, Gale EAM, *et al.* IGF-I gene deletion: effect of IGF-I therapy on insulin

sensitivity, body composition and linear growth. Horm Res 48, S2, 5th Joint Meeting of the ESPE and LWPES, Stockholm, 1997; abstract 239.

193 Woods KA, Camacho-Hubner C, Bergman RN, *et al.* Effects of insulin-like growth factor I (IGF-I) therapy on body composition and insulin resistance in IGF-I gene deletion. *J Clin Endocrinol Metab* 2000; **85**: 1407–11.

194 Johnston LB, Leger J, Savage MO, *et al.* The insulin-like growth factor-I (IGF-I) gene in individuals born small for gestational age (SGA). *Clin Endocrinol (Oxf)* 1999; **51**: 423–7.

195 Baker J, Liu JP, Robertson EJ, Efstratiadis A. Role of insulin-like growth factors in embryonic and postnatal growth. *Cell* 1993; **75**: 73–82.

196 Liu JP, Baker J, Perkins AS, *et al.* Mice carrying null mutations of the genes encoding insulin-like growth factor I (Igf-I) and type 1 IGF receptor (Igf1r). *Cell* 1993; **75**: 59–72.

197 Tritos NA, Mantzoros CS. Clinical review 97: Syndromes of severe insulin resistance. *J Clin Endocrinol Metab* 1998; **83**: 3025–30.

● 198 Abuzzahab MJ, Schneider A, Goddard A, *et al.* Intrauterine Growth Retardation (IUGR) Study Group. IGF-I receptor mutations resulting in intrauterine and postnatal growth retardation. *N Engl J Med* 2003; **349**: 2211–22.

199 Peoples R, Milatovich A, Francke U. Hemizygosity at the insulin-like growth factor I receptor (IGF1R) locus and growth failure in the ring chromosome 15 syndrome. *Cytogenet Cell Genet* 1995; **70**: 228–34.

● 200 Barreca A, Bozzola M, Cesarone A, *et al.* Short stature associated with high circulating insulin-like growth factor (IGF)-binding protein-1 and low circulating IGF-II: effect of growth hormone therapy. *J Clin Endocrinol Metab* 1998; **83**: 3534–41.

201 Baumann G, Shaw MA, Merimee TJ. Low levels of high-affinity growth hormone-binding protein in African Pygmies. *N Engl J Med* 1989; **320**: 1705–9.

202 Merimee TJ, Hewlett BS, Wood W, *et al.* The growth hormone receptor gene in African Pygmy. *Trans Assoc Am Physicians* 1989; **102**:163–169.

203 Hattori Y, Vera JC, Rivas CI, *et al.* Decreased Insulin-like growth factor I receptor expression and function in immortalized African Pygmy T cells. *J Clin Endocrinol Metab* 1996; **81**: 2257–63.

◆ 204 Dannies PS. Protein hormone storage in secretory granules: mechanisms for concentration and sorting. *Endocr Rev* 1999; 20: 3–21.

◆ 205 Dannies PS. Protein folding and deficiencies caused by dominant-negative mutants of hormones. *Vitam Horm* 2000; **58**: 1–26.

◆ 206 Dannies PS. Concentrating hormones into secretory granules: layers of control. *Mol Cell Endocrinol* 2001; **177**: 87–93.

207 Sferra TJ, Collins FS. The molecular biology of cystic fibrosis. *Annu Rev Med* 1993; **44**: 133–44.

208 Lomas DA, Evans DL, Finch JT, Carrell RW. The mechanism of Z α 1-antitrypsin accumulation in the liver. *Nature* 1992; **357**: 605–7.

209 Chessler SD, Byers PH. BiP binds type I procollagen pro ??chain with mutations in the carboxy-terminal propeptide synthesized by cells from patients with osteogenesis imperfecta. *J Biol Chem* 1993; **268**: 18226–33.

210 Ciechanover A. The Ubiquitin-Proteasome proteolytic pathway. *Cell* 1994; **79**: 13–21.

211 Schwartz AL, Ciechanover A. The Ubiquitin-Proteasome pathway and pathogenesis of human diseases. *Annu Rev Med* 1999; **50**: 57–74.

212 Arnold J, Dawson S, Fergusson J, *et al.* Ubiquitin and its role in neurodegeneration. *Prog Brain Res* 1998; **117**: 23–34.

213 Hurtley SM, Helenius A. Protein oligomerization in the endoplasmic reticulum. *Annu Rev Cell Biol* 1989; **5**: 277–307.

214 Ellgard L, Molinari M, Helenius A. Setting the standards: Quality control in the secretory pathway. *Science* 1999; **286**: 1882–8.

215 Wickner S, Maurizi MR, Gottesman S. Post-translational Quality Control: Folding, refolding and degrading proteins. *Science* 1999; **286**: 1888–93.

216 Thomas PJ, Qu BH, Pedersen PL. Defective protein folding as a basis of human disease. *Trends Biochem Sci* 1995; **20**: 456–9.

5

Nutrition and growth

J M KETELSLEGERS, V BEAULOYE, D MAITER, M MAES, L E UNDERWOOD, J P THISSEN

INTRODUCTION

Growth is a complex process, driven and controlled by many hormonal and metabolic interactions. The somatotroph axis plays a central role in this process (Fig. 5.1) and insulin growth factor-1 (IGF-I) and its binding proteins (Fig. 5.2) modulate the many peripheral hormone and metabolic signals to promote linear growth.[1]

Nutritional factors play a key role in the control of growth, as well as IGF-I and the IGF binding proteins (IGFBPs). Macronutrients provide the 'building blocks' and the energy required for growth and development, whereas micronutrients such as vitamins and minerals are essential for the regulatory pathways involved in growth. Nutrients also affect growth by interacting with functions of the somatotroph axis at many levels.

In this chapter, the influences of nutrients on growth and development are reviewed, with emphasis on the interactions between nutritional factors and the function of the somatotroph axis. Both human studies and data from animal experiments are discussed.

THE INFLUENCE OF NUTRIENTS ON GROWTH

The role of macronutrients

According to the World Health Organization, more than a third of the world's children are affected by protein-energy malnutrition and about 43 percent of children in developing

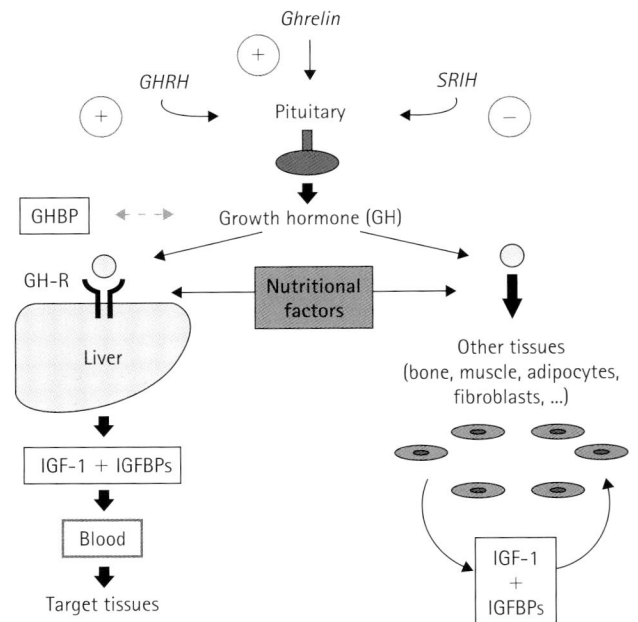

Figure 5.1 Overview of the GH/IGF-I axis. GHRH, growth hormone-releasing hormone; SRIH, somatotrophin release-inhibiting hormone; GH, growth hormone; GHBP, GH-binding protein; GH-R, GH receptor; IGF-I, insulin-like growth factor-1; IGFBPs, IGF-binding proteins.

countries (230 million) have growth retardation as a result of undernutrition.[2] Marasmus and kwashiorkor are associated with severe growth retardation. Marasmus, characterized by profound deficits in intake of both energy and

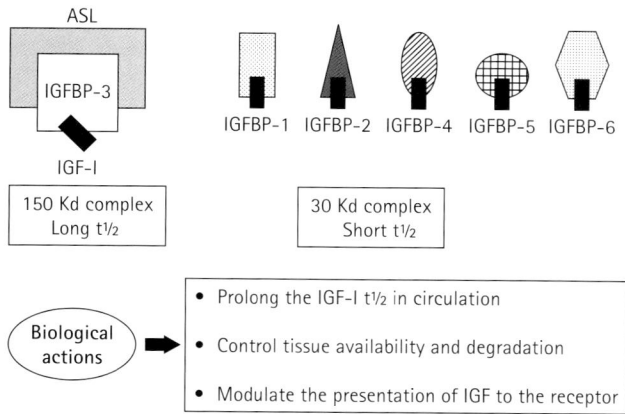

Figure 5.2 Overview of the structure and functions of the IGF-I binding proteins (IGFBPs).

protein, is often aggravated by chronic diarrhea resulting from malnutrition-induced alterations of the intestinal mucosa. In kwashiorkor, the energy deprivation is less severe, but the quantity and quality of dietary protein are inadequate, resulting in hypoalbuminemia and edema.

Besides the severe malnutrition of marasmus and kwashiorkor, milder states of undernutrition are encountered with high frequency in developing countries. Investigations of the Institute of Nutrition of Central America and Panama (INCAP) and the Nutrition Collaborative Research Support Program (CRSP), examining the effects of marginal nutrition,[3–5] concluded that undernutrition early in life causes growth stunting, and is accompanied by cognitive and behavioral deficits. These consequences of early malnutrition persist into later life. The effects of marginal nutrition on the somatotroph axis are not documented. The long-term effects of early severe malnutrition have recently been confirmed in a study of Senegalese preschool children, who had to undergo hospitalization for marasmus. At 5 years after nutritional rehabilitation, the post-marasmic children remained stunted with nutritional statuses significantly lower than control children.[6] Intervention studies suggest that protein-rich dietary supplements may have beneficial effects on growth, particularly when provided early in life. In a long-term intervention organized by the INCAP[5,7,8] raising energy and protein intakes by 10 percent and 40 percent, respectively, produced a significant improvement in growth in a group of children aged 15–36 months with inadequate dietary intake (severe stunting of growth was reduced from about 45 percent to 20 percent). In children between 3 and 7 years of age, nutritional supplementation had no beneficial effects on growth. Therefore, the effects of nutritional supplementation on growth coincide with an age at which growth velocities and growth deficits are greatest. Interestingly, the follow-up phase of the INCAP study conducted when the subjects were 11–27 years old shows that nutritional supplementation early in life had long-term benefits such as greater stature and fat-free mass, improved work capacity and enhanced intellectual performance. Beneficial effects of nutritional supplementation on

development of infants at risk for malnutrition have also been documented in other studies.[9,10] In a recent update, performed in Guatemala, a secular trend in growth in children from developing countries was confirmed. Most interestingly, the rate of child growth reflects, in part, the growth pattern of the mothers, including improvements to the pattern resulting from nutritional supplementation.[11] Also, in the same geographical area, it was shown that the improvement of the nutritional status of undernourished women and children may have positive long-term consequences, particularly on fasting plasma glucose.[12] In contrast, protein-energy supplementation in pregnancy or in early childhood does not seem to affect significantly blood pressure in young adults.[13] A recent update of the INCAP study has recently been presented.[14]

Most importantly, more studies are warranted to uncover more precisely the relations of changes in the various components of the somatotroph axis in the consequences of long-term nutritional interventions, particularly when initiated at a young age.

Another intervention study, carried out in Colombia,[15] shows that malnourished preschoolers (>3 years old) have improved growth when they are exposed to multifocal intervention for several years. It must be stressed, however, that this program included not only supplementary feeding, but also medical support and educational activities. It is difficult therefore to delineate the specific role of protein deficiency on linear growth, because the protein-rich diets that are used provide additional energy and micronutrients (minerals and vitamins).

In a cohort of 53 Dutch children, fed a macrobiotic diet based on whole-grain cereals, pulses and vegetables, significant growth retardation was recorded during the weaning period (6–18 months).[16,17] Growth in stature was related to the protein content of the diet, but not to energy intake. Deficiencies of vitamin B12, vitamin D, calcium, and riboflavin were also detected in the macrobiotic children. A follow-up study revealed that those children who had increased their consumption of fatty fish, dairy products or both grew in height more rapidly than those remaining on the macrobiotic diet.[16,17] Growth failure also occurs in children who restrict their energy intake because of fear of becoming obese.[18] In a recent cross-sectional study, focused on adults, Allen et al. found that in a cohort of 292 British women (99 meat eaters versus 92 vegan and 101 vegetarians; age: 20–70 years) a plant-based diet was associated with lower circulating total IGF-I and higher levels of IGFBP-1 and IGFBP-2.[19]

The impact of cow's milk upon linear growth in industrialized and developing countries has been reviewed extensively by Hoppe et al.[20] Several studies compared the growth and final outcome of breast-fed and formula-fed infants. In summary, infants fed formula based on cow's milk grow at a faster rate than breast-fed infants, even though the difference seems to be more significant for weight, some studies show a difference in linear growth.[21,22] This could be partially explained by differences in quality and amount of proteins in both types of infant feedings.[23] However, there seems to be no adverse effect of breast feeding on the long term, as some recent studies indicate that breast-fed infants are taller adults.[24,25] In a cohort of preschool children (12–36 months), in Central and South America, milk intake was associated with higher height-for-age Z-scores in all seven countries studied; in contrast, egg/fish/poultry intakes were only associated with height in one country.[26] A beneficial effect of milk and meat intake on linear growth was also observed in Mexican preschool children.[27] A putative effect of cow's milk on growth is likely to be related to baseline nutritional conditions, which are usually not precisely compared among studies. Therefore, it is of interest to mention that in a study performed in well-nourished Danish children (2.5 years old), height was positively associated with intakes of animal proteins and milk, but not intakes of vegetable proteins.[28] At a later age, the effects of nutrition on growth are more complex to define, given the confounding factor represented by the variability of the onset of puberty associated growth spurt. In this setting it is of interest to quote the classical Boyd Orr study, conducted in 1928 in Scotland, in which beneficial effects of whole or skimmed milk supplementation versus other sources of energy on height increase was clearly established in children between 5 and 14 years. These positive effects of milk were observed in the younger (5–6 years) as well as in the older group (13–14 years).[29] Again, possible poor basal nutrition may have to be taken into account to interpret these findings. Since the Boyd Orr study, many interventional or observational studies, in different areas of the world over the past decades until recent years have investigated the effects of milk on growth in school-age children. An extensive review of this literature, which is beyond the scope of this chapter, can be found in the report of Hoppe et al.[20] Several, but not all intervention studies concluded that there was a beneficial effect of cow's milk supplementation in school-age children, but that this association was not clear. Several observational studies in well-nourished populations show an association between the consumption of cow's milk and linear growth. One of these studies was performed on a cohort of 12 829 US children, aged 9–14 years, followed from 1996 to 1999.[30] It is also worth mentioning the NHANES 1999–2002 study, relating milk consumption and linear growth, particularly in pubertal children.[31] In another study, a significant positive effect of the consumption frequency of dairy products on catch-up growth, consistent with the concept that addition of moderate amounts of diary products to a vegan type of diet improved growth in children, especially girls.[32]

The role of micronutrients

Several minerals and vitamins also condition the organism for optimal growth and development.[33] Iron supplementation improves growth in stature and weight gain, particularly in anemic children. These responses might be mediated by increased appetite.[34]

Marginal chronic iron deficiency is difficult to uncover, since it precedes the overt reduction of hemoglobin. Ferritin is a good indicator of iron stores, but its interpretation is confounded by inflammatory states, which cause a significant increase of this parameter. More recently, increased levels of the soluble transferrin receptor (sTfR; a truncated form of the transferrin receptor) have been regarded as a more robust parameter for a marginal depletion of iron stores, as they are relatively independent of the inflammatory status and have shown their effectiveness for the diagnosis of iron deficiency in infants.[35,36]

We investigated the value of sTfR as a marker of marginal iron deficiency in early infancy. This study was performed in a poor rural area near Hanoi, Vietnam. This was a double-blind study which lasted for 6 months and included a total of 400 infants aged 6 to 8.5 months and who received a syrup supplemented with iron or a placebo. A total of 339 children completed the study. Mean hemoglobin levels at the beginning of the study were equivalent in both groups ($109 \, gL^{-1}$ and $108 \, gL^{-1}$; NS). After 6 months, hemoglobin rose in both groups, but the magnitude of this increase was significantly higher in the iron supplemented than in the placebo group ($133 \, g \, L^{-1}$ versus $118 \, g \, L^{-1}$ respectively; $p < 0.05$). At entry in the study, sTfR levels were equivalent in both groups. After 6 months sTfR significantly dropped by 28 percent ($p < 0.01$) but remained unchanged in the placebo group. Moreover, there was a highly significant inverse correlation between the changes in hemoglobin and sTfR ($r = 0.40$; $p < 0.01$) (Fig. 5.3). In conclusion, this interventional study demonstrates that young infants in some rural areas of Vietnam are marginally deficient in iron and that sTfR represents a valuable parameter to diagnose this condition and to monitor the effectiveness of iron supplementation. In this subpopulation with only marginal iron deficiency and no overt anemia,

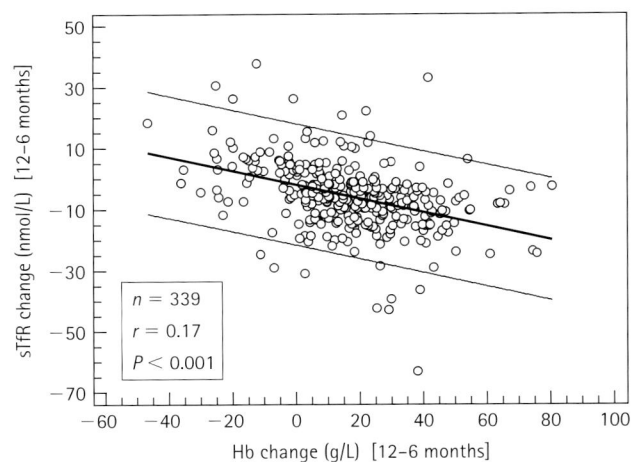

$n = 339$
$r = 0.17$
$P < 0.001$

Figure 5.3 Correlation between the changes in the soluble transferrin receptor and hemoglobin over a 6 month iron supplementation period in young infants (0.5–0.7 year) in a rural area near Hanoi, Vietnam, without overt anemia (mean hemoglobin: $108 \, g \, L^{-1}$).

there were no significant changes in the anthropometric parameters nor on IGF-I over that relatively short iron supplementation period. However, the impact of a prolonged fortification of nutrients in iron in such settings on growth and on the parameters of the somatotroph axis may be of importance, and remains to be evaluated.[37,38]

Copper deficiency also impairs weight gain of infants recovering from malnutrition.[39,40] The most common clinical manifestations of acquired copper deficiency are anemia, neutropenia, and bone abnormalities, but impaired growth may also occur.[41] The observed effects of vitamin A intervention on growth vary from one study to another.[42–44]

The role of zinc in growth and development was first recognized by Prazad[45,46] who described an association between dwarfism and hypogonadism in young Iranian adults with zinc deficiency caused by low-protein diets rich in phytate and fiber. Zinc supplementation is reported to improve height gain in some studies,[47–50] but not in others.[51–55] In industrialized countries, zinc supplementation in short, well-nourished children is reported to increase height velocity,[56–58] but such effects were not observed in all studies.[59,60] In several instances, the effects of zinc on growth were restricted to the male subjects, an observation that is poorly understood. In some studies, zinc supplementation caused weight gain, without stimulating growth.[61–63] Moreover, when zinc was provided to breast-fed infants (4–9 months old) from low income immigrant families in France, a significant increase in length was observed during a 3-month period of observation.[64] It is thus possible that individuals in wealthier countries may have mild zinc deficiency or that a segment of the population has relatively high zinc requirements.

THE INFLUENCE OF NUTRIENTS ON THE SOMATOTROPH AXIS: STUDIES IN HUMANS

The role of macronutrients

Growth-retarded children with marasmus or kwashiorkor have decreased bioactive somatomedin (IGF-I) in their serum[65–67] and decreased concentrations of IGF-I determined by radioreceptor assay or radioimmunoassay.[68] Low serum IGF-I levels in chronically malnourished individuals can be normalized by adequate nutritional rehabilitation, but the rapidity with which this occurs depends on chronological age, type of malnutrition, and quality of nutritional rehabilitation. The reduced serum IGF-I concentrations observed in children with marasmus or kwashiorkor are associated with normal or elevated GH levels, suggesting that there is resistance to the action of growth hormone.

Growth hormone insensitivity, suggested by the association of elevated growth hormone and reduced IGF-I, is also observed in some forms of malnutrition, such as adolescents with anorexia nervosa. In such patients, GHBP in serum is reduced.[69] As GHBP represents the extracellular moiety of the GH receptor that has been cleaved from the cell surface and released into the circulation, its reduction may be indicative of reduced somatogenic receptor numbers.

Studies of acute dietary restriction in healthy adults indicate that the somatotroph axis is under the control of nutrients. Fasting decreases serum immunoreactive IGF-I in adult humans within 24 h, resulting in levels reaching 10–15 percent of the prefast values by 10 days. IGF-I promptly returns to normal with reseeding.[70] The low serum IGF-I values in fasted humans are not the result of decreased growth hormone. Fasted humans have increased GH pulse frequency, increased 24 h integrated GH concentrations, and augmented pulse amplitude.[71] This disparity between growth hormone and IGF-I suggests that in fasting, as in anorexia nervosa, kwaskiorkor or marasmus, insufficient nutrient intake causes GH insensitivity. This is supported by the observation that growth hormone given exogenously to GH-deficient fasted subjects causes only a two-fold increment in serum IGF-I concentrations, whereas it produces a ten-fold increment in GH-deficient subjects who are fed normally.[72] Both energy and protein are important in regulation of IGF-I because each is essential for restoration of IGF-I after fasting.[73,74] The quality of dietary protein (content of essential amino acids) also regulates IGF-I.[75]

IGF-I is also a marker of choice for monitoring the response to nutritional rehabilitation. Thus in malnourished adults, the response of IGF-I to nutritional repletion was a much more sensitive index of acute directional changes in nutritional status than other plasma proteins, like prealbumin, transferrin, and retinal-binding protein.[76] Also, in Nigerian malnourished children (edematous and marasmic) (6–36 months), a treatment with mainly vegetable diet for an average of 19 days led to significant increases in somatomedin-C accompanied by a weight gain.[77]

Several lines of evidence suggest a link between animal protein intake, particularly cow's milk, and IGF-I, even though, in their extensive review Hoppe et al. point out that the overall literature contains some conflicting results, both in studies with children and adults.[20] However, the recent studies of this group point to a significant effect of milk proteins on IGF-I and growth. In a first cross-sectional study, Hoppe et al. observed that in 90 well-nourished Danish children (mean age: 2.5 years) circulating IGF-I was associated with intakes of animal protein and milk, but not with vegetable protein. Moreover, height of the infants was positively related to IGF-I and milk intake. Even though the ranges of dietary intakes and those of IGF-I levels were wide, the relations between those variables reached the level of significance.[28] In a 7 day interventional study the same group reported that in 8-year-old healthy boys, increased concentrations of IGF-I, as well as the IGF-I/IGFBP-3 ratios were higher (19 percent and 13 percent, respectively) after high skimmed milk intake than after increases in meat diets that provide similar amounts of proteins.[78] The mechanisms whereby milk proteins could stimulate IGF-I (and growth) remain to be determined. As pointed out by Hoppe et al. 'the active components in milk may be bioactive peptides, peptides formed in the gastrointestinal tract from degradation of milk proteins, a combination of certain amino acids, or a combination of proteins and minerals'.[20] Following these lines of reasoning it is of interest to underline that several bioactive peptides derived from milk proteins have been identified, with opiate, mineral binding, immunomodulatory or angiotensin-1 converting enzyme (ACE) inhibitory activities.[79] Of particular interest are the experimental and epidemiological observations that a number of studies have reported the antihypertensive action of milk peptides in spontaneous hypertensive rats and humans.[80-84] With Maes et al., we have reported that one of these peptides (seven amino acids), released by tryptic digestion from milk β-lactoglobulin, shows potential for intestinal absorption, has ACE-inhibitory activity and influences the release of the vasoconstrictor peptide, endothelin-1, from endothelial cells.[85] These observations support the concept that dietary peptides derived from milk proteins may interact with various endocrine systems.

The role of micronutrients

Micronutrients also play a role in the regulation of the somatotroph axis in humans. In a rural area of North Vietnam,[50] we have investigated the effect of zinc supplementation on growth-retarded children aged 4–36 months (Z score for height-for-age and weight-for-age < -2). In this double-blind study, zinc supplementation for 5 months improved cumulative weight and height gains compared with placebo-treated children, in whom growth declined (Fig. 5.4). The differences between the two groups were significant after 2–3 months. Plasma IGF-I concentrations increased significantly in zinc-treated subjects between 1 and 5 months, whereas they did not change in placebo-treated subjects (Fig. 5.4). The change in plasma IGF-I was correlated with the changes in height-for-age Z score ($p = 0.04$). The growth-promoting effect of zinc might therefore be mediated, at least in part, through changes in levels of circulating IGF-I and stimulation of the somatotroph axis (Fig. 5.5). Ninh et al. also evaluated the effects of zinc supplementation in a healthy unselected population of 5- to 7-month-old Vietnamese children, without overt growth stunting (double-blind study; zinc supplemented group: $n = 199$; placebo group: $n = 201$; time of intervention: 6 months).[37] There was a slight beneficial effect on weight gain (mixed time × treatment effect: $p < 0.01$) and a 10 percent increase in IGF-I, only in females (mixed time × sex effect: $p = 0.02$). These data contrasted with the overt beneficial effect of zinc supplementation in older infants with growth stunting.[50]

Nutrients also regulate the IGFBPs. Plasma concentrations of IGFBP-1 are rapidly suppressed after a meal, and exhibit marked increases after a brief fast.[86,87] These changes result mainly from the regulatory action of insulin on IGFBP-1 expression. In contrast, acute short-term dietary changes do not affect IGFBP-3. In states of prolonged severe malnutrition, such as anorexia nervosa, IGFBP-3 is decreased

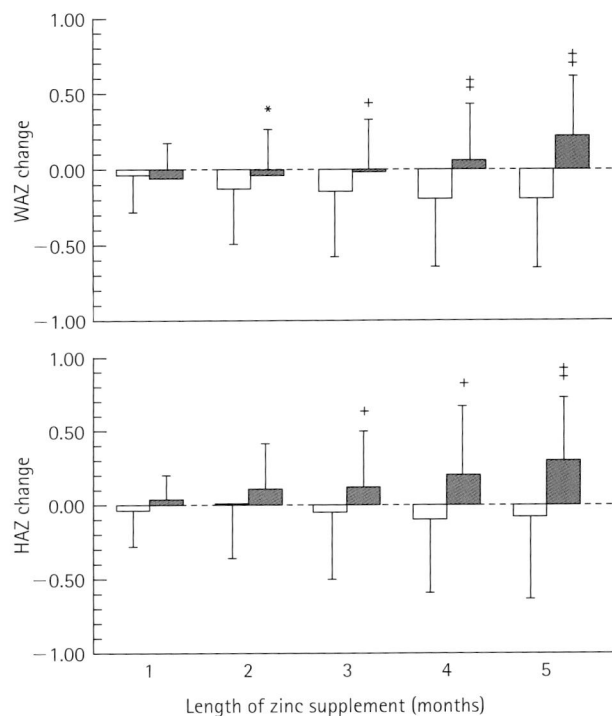

Figure 5.4 Effects on growth of 5 months of zinc supplementation in growth-retarded Vietnamese children. The data are shown as changes (mean ± SD) in the weight-for-age (WAZ) and height-for-age (HAZ) Z scores in placebo-treated (open bars; $n = 73$) and zinc-treated (solid bars; $n = 73$) groups. $^*p < 0.05$; $^†p < 0.01$; $^‡p < 0.001$ between the two groups (paired Student's t test). (Reproduced with permission from Ninh et al.[50] Copyright: The American Society for Clinical Nutrition.)

significantly, together with IGF-I, whereas IGFBP-1 and IGFBP-2 are markedly elevated.[69] A more recent study also emphasized the fact that in severe malnutrition (anorexia nervosa patients with BMI lower than $16.5 \, kg \, m^{-2}$) IGF-I and IGFBP-3 were reduced and IGFBP-2 increased as compared to control values. Interestingly, urinary excretion of C-terminal telopeptide of collagen type I, a marker for bone resorption was elevated and osteocalcin, a marker of bone formation was reduced. Intravenous hyperalimentation in some of the most severe patients rapidly increased the low IGF-I, followed by a progressive increase of osteocalcin (3–7 days), while increased bone resorption appeared to continue for at least 5 weeks.[88]

A reduction in energy (-50 percent) or protein (-30 percent) intake for 1 week, sufficient to reduce IGF-I and cause negative nitrogen balance in children and adults, also caused some changes in IGFBPs, which were dependent on age and type of nutritional restriction.[89] In particular, energy restriction decreased IGFBP-3 levels in children, but not in adults. Protein, but not energy, restriction increased IGFBP-2 levels in children and adults. Also, IGFBP-2 levels as high as twice the control values have been observed in undernourished Bangladeshi children.[90]

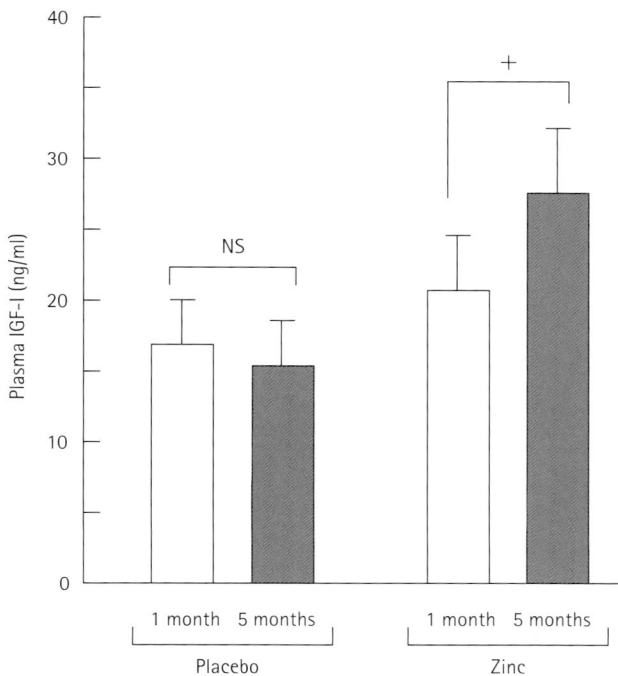

Figure 5.5 Effects on plasma IGF-I of 5 months of zinc supplementation in growth-retarded Vietnamese children. Plasma IGF-I concentrations after 1 and 5 months in placebo-treated ($n = 18$) and zinc-treated children ($n = 24$) are shown as means $\pm$ SEM. NS, $p > 0.05$; +, $p < 0.05$ (paired Student's t test). (Redrawn with permission from Ninh et al.[50] Copyright: The American Society for Clinical Nutrition.)

These fell to normal when the subjects were refed with a high-protein diet, but not a normal protein diet, indicating that IGFBP-2 is particularly dependent on protein intake and might be a good marker for monitoring the response of malnourished children to nutritional intervention.

MECHANISMS INVOLVED IN THE NUTRITIONAL CONTROL OF THE SOMATOTROPH AXIS: EXPERIMENTAL STUDIES

The role of energy and protein supply in young growing rats

ALTERATION OF GROWTH HORMONE SECRETION AND GROWTH HORMONE RESISTANCE

In humans and many animal species (guinea pig, sheep, cattle, and pig), reduced energy and protein intake are associated with elevated serum concentrations of growth hormone. The association of elevated levels of growth hormone with reduced IGF-I levels suggests that malnutrition produces a state of GH insensitivity. In rats, fasting causes a marked reduction of the pulsatile GH secretion, which

may participate in the fall of IGF-I levels.[91] However, administration of growth hormone to fasted or protein-deprived rats neither prevents growth stunting nor raises the IGF-I level in serum, giving further support to the argument favoring GH resistance.[92–94]

GROWTH HORMONE RECEPTOR AND POST-RECEPTOR DEFICITS

As the liver is the main source of IGF-I in serum, a loss of liver somatogenic receptors might explain the GH resistance in food deprived animals. In rats fasted for 3 days, liver GH-binding capacity is reduced to 25 percent of the control values. Refeeding restores GH binding to normal. These changes in liver GHRs are closely paralleled by changes in serum IGF-I.[95–98] The serum GHBP also closely follows the changes of liver GH binding capacity during fasting and refeeding.[99] Early studies have suggested that the reduction of GHR and GHBP during fasting is associated with impaired expression of the GHR/GHBP gene.[100,101] Several lines of evidence also indicate that the level of the GH receptor at the cell surface (receptor 'availability') is mainly regulated by the ubiquitin–proteasome pathway.[102,103] This proteolytic system has been shown to be up-regulated by fasting in skeletal muscle, and the expression of some of its components are partially down-regulated by IGF-I treatment of fasted rats.[104] It is therefore conceivable that GHR degradation is accelerated in fasting. Ligand-induced changes are also dependent on the pulsatility of GH exposure of the cell.[93]

If, in fasting, the reduced availability of GH receptors seems to play a role in GH resistance, the participation of a post-receptor deficit, distal to a loss of somatogenic receptors can not be excluded in other forms of undernutrition, and is in fact most likely to occur. Thus in protein-restricted rats, the role of liver GHRs in the decline in serum IGF-I is more questionable than in fasting. In 3- to 4-week-old pre-pubertal rats, feeding on a low-protein diet (5 percent casein) for 1 week caused an 80–90 percent reduction in serum IGF-I as compared with control rats fed an isocaloric 15 percent casein diet.[105] At the same time however, GH binding by liver was either decreased by only 30–40 percent (4-week-old rats) or unchanged (8-week-old rats). In adult rats (12 weeks), feeding a low protein diet for 1 week reduced serum IGF-I levels by 40 percent, without changing liver GHRs.[105]

The decrease in liver somatogenic receptors in pre-pubertal rats fed the low protein isocaloric diet could be prevented by continuous infusion of growth hormone. However, serum IGF-I levels remained low in the GH-treated protein restricted animals, despite normal liver GH binding capacity (Fig. 5.6).[106] These data, together with other experimental evidence,[94,107,108] strongly suggest that GH resistance in protein restriction results at least partially from defects distal to the binding of growth hormone with its receptor (post-receptor defect).

Total liver GH
binding sites

Serum IGF-I

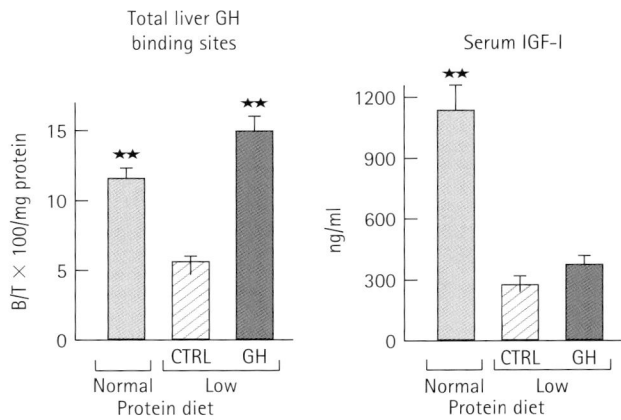

Figure 5.6 Effects of 1 week protein restriction in pre-pubertal rats, fed a low (P5) or normal (P15) protein diet and infused with GH (GH) or saline (CTRL) for 1 week. Total liver binding sites, as determined with labeled GH after removal of the endogenous/exogenous GH by $MgCl_2$ is shown on the left panel; serum IGF-I is represented in the right panel. (Redrawn with permission from Thissen et al.[106] Copyright: W.B. Saunders Co.)

NATURE OF THE GROWTH HORMONE RECEPTOR POST-DEFICITS IN NUTRIENTS DEPRIVATION

The mechanisms involved in the GH post-receptor defect caused by protein restriction have been investigated in several studies. Protein restriction causes impaired IGF-I gene expression at a pre-translational level. Northern blot analysis reveals that feeding pre-pubertal rats an isocaloric low-protein diet (5 percent casein) for 1 week causes a 40–60 percent decrease in IGF-I mRNA in liver, in comparison to the control animals receiving normal protein regimens (15 percent casein) (Fig. 5.7).[109] Reduced IGF-I mRNA levels in liver or other tissues (kidney, muscle, gut, and brain) have also been observed in fasting, protein restriction or neonatal food restriction.[100,101,110–114] Results of nuclear run-on studies, performed in fasted as well as protein-restricted animals, suggest that the diet-related decline in IGF-I mRNA levels is caused in part by a decreased transcription rate of the IGF-I gene.[100,101] In addition, protein restriction may cause decreased stability of the 7.5 kb IGF-I mRNA.[101,109]

Further studies have uncovered important mechanisms whereby nutrients control the IGF-I gene expression in response to GH. The major steps of the transduction cascade leading to the activation of GH, namely the induction of IGF-I gene expression, are now well documented (Figs 5.8 and 5.9).

Signal termination of the GH actions is mediated by a family of suppressors of cytokine signaling molecules (SOCS). They act as an intracellular negative feedback loop. Some members of the SOCS family (SOCS 1, 2, 3 and CIS) are induced by GH to varying degrees.[115–117] Recent investigations uncovered the central role of SOCS2 in growth and development. For instance, mice deficient in SOCS2 display excessive growth phenotype, dependent upon the presence of GH. This action was shown to

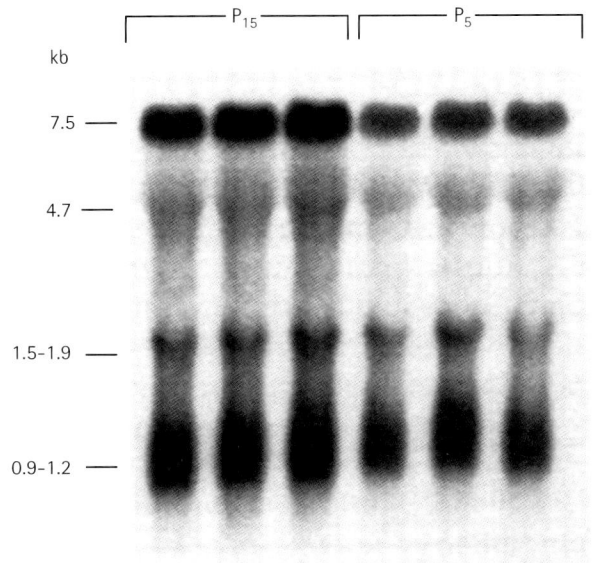

Figure 5.7 Northern blot analysis of liver IGF-I mRNA in three normally fed (P_{15}) and three protein-restricted (P_5) 4-week-old rats. Protein restricted diet was given for 1 week. Samples of liver RNA (20 pg) were loaded in each well. The blot was hybridized with a rat exon 3-specific IGF-I RNA probe. The signal obtained with hybridizing by a chicken Q-actin cDNA probe was equivalent in both groups. (Reproduced with permission from Thissen et al.[109] Copyright: W.B. Saunders Co.)

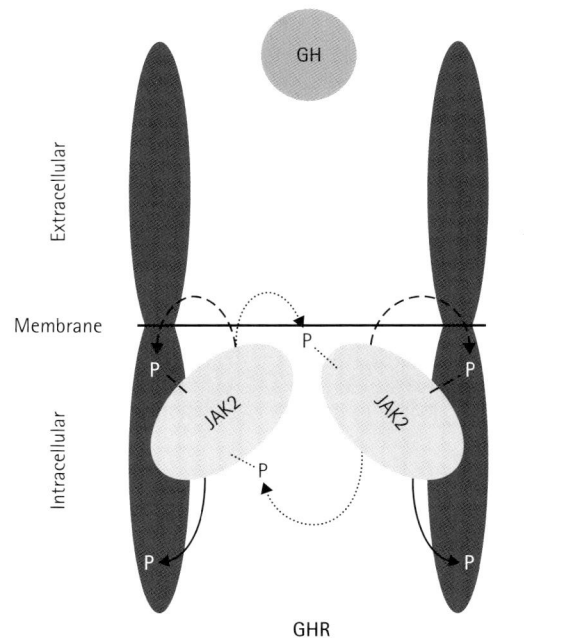

Figure 5.8 Model of GH activation of JAK2 tyrosine kinase. GH binding to two GHR molecules increases the affinity of each receptor for JAK2. The two receptor associated JAK2 molecules are in close proximity, so that each JAK2 can phosphorylate tyrosines of the other JAK2 molecule (····· arrows), thereby activating it. Activated JAK2 then phosphorylates itself (– – – arrows) and the cytoplasmic domain of the GHR (—— arrows) on tyrosines. These phosphotyrosines of the GHR and JAK2 form binding sites for signaling proteins.

be mediated by an interaction of SOCS2 with two phosphorylated tyrosines of the GH receptor.[118,119] Tyrosine phosphatases also play a role in termination of GH signaling.[120]

Given the extensive knowledge of the downstream signaling cascade induced by the interaction of GH with its receptor, we were led to investigate the impact of nutrients restriction on some of these transduction factor. We concentrated on the effects of fasting on the activation of the GH receptor, the JAK2/STAT5 factors and a member of the SOCS family. Beauloye et al.[121] observed that in well-fed

control rats, the liver GH receptor was rapidly phosphorylated by intraportal GH injection; in contrast, the receptor phosphorylation by GH was severely blunted and barely detectable in fasted rats, injected the same dose of GH. Also, fasting produced a significant decrease in the GH induced phosphorylation of liver JAK2 and STAT5 (Fig. 5.10). All these changes occurred without significant alterations of the GH receptor, JAK2 or STAT5 liver protein content. Moreover, the impairment of the JAK–STAT pathway in fasting was associated with an increased SOCS3 mRNA, suggesting the involvement in this signal termination factor in the negative effects of fasting. Glucocorticoids, highly stimulated in fasting do not appear to mediate these effects, as adrenalectomy failed to prevent the alterations of the JAK–STAT pathway caused by fasting. In these experiments, the lack of reduction of the GH immunoreactive GH receptor protein after fasting is not in accordance with the reduced binding sites availability in livers of fasted rats. This may suggest that the antibody used for the immunoblotting of the GH receptor do not distinguish between some partially altered forms of the receptor undergoing ubiquitin-mediated degradation (via coated pitts) and the intact receptor able to recognize the GH at the surface of the cell, clearly reduced after fasting.[108]

In addition to impaired transcription, evidence for translational stalling of the IGF-I mRNA has been observed in young protein-restricted rats. Indeed, pre-pubertal hypophysectomized rats, subjected for 1 week to a

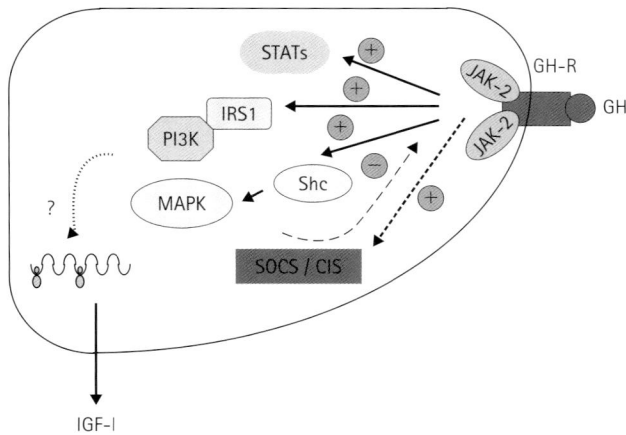

Figure 5.9 Schematic view of the signaling pathways involved in the stimulation of IGF-I production by GH in the hepatocyte.

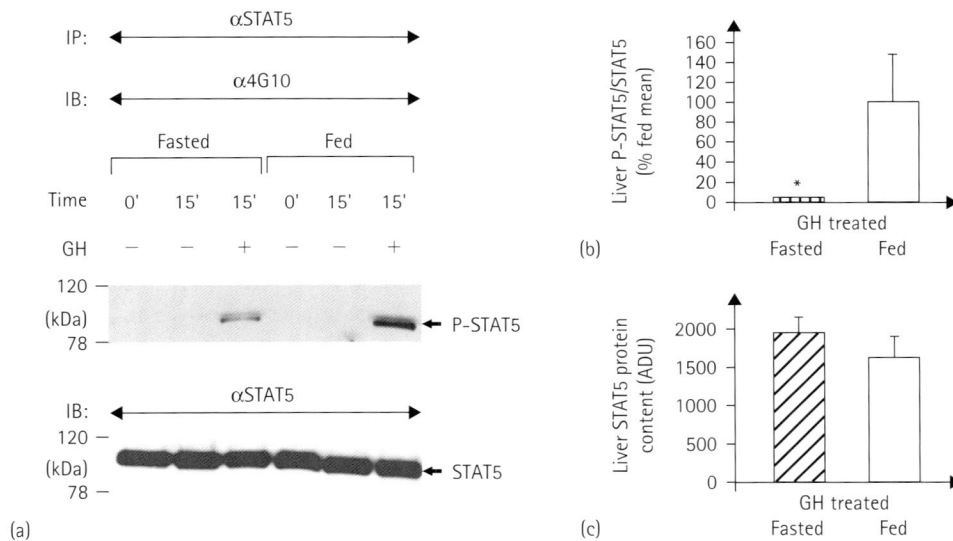

Figure 5.10 (a) Effects of fasting on GH-stimulated STAT5 tyrosine phosphorylation in rat liver. Liver extracts from rats sacrificed at time 0 or 15 min after injection of saline (−) or GH (+; 1.5 mg kg^{-1}) were prepared as described in Beauloye et al.[121] Tissue extracts were immunoprecipitated with αSTATSb antibody (1/250 dilution) and immunoblotted with an anti-phosphotyrosine antibody (a4G10; 1/10 000 dilution). The same blot was then stripped and incubated with αSTATSb antibody (1/1000) to check the amount of protein present. This αSTATSb antibody also partially recognized STATSa. (b) GH-stimulated STAT5 tyrosine phosphorylation after 15 min in fasted or fed rat livers from three independent experiments. Tissues extracts were immunoprecipitated with αSTATSb antibody and immunoblotted first with α4G10 then with αSTATSb as described above. (c) Densitometric analysis of P-STAT5 (top) and total STAT5 protein content (bottom) in the liver of GH-treated fasted (hatched bar) and fed rats (open bar). Phospho-protein signals were corrected for the specific protein levels present in the immunoprecipitate, and the ratios were normalized to the GH-stimulated fed mean, which was assigned a value of 100. Each data point represents the mean ± SEM for three rats expressed as a percentage stimulated fed mean (top) or as arbitrary densitometric units (ADU; bottom); *$p < 0.05$ versus fed rats. (Reproduced with permission from Beauloye et al.[121] Copyright: W.B. Saunders Co.)

low-protein diet, had a normal liver IGF-I mRNA response to a single injection of growth hormone. In contrast, the serum IGF-I response to growth hormone was severely blunted in the protein-restricted rats. Also, in intact young rats fed the low-protein diet, high doses of growth hormone (100 μg four times daily for 1 week) prevented the decrease in liver IGF-I mRNA, but not the fall of liver and serum IGF-I peptide. The discrepancy between normal abundance of liver IGF-I mRNA and reduced IGF-I peptide in liver or serum in the GH-treated, protein-restricted rats suggests that protein restriction causes impaired translation of the message.[109] Although the nature of this translational defect is not known, protein restriction does not affect binding of IGF-I mRNA to polysomes, suggesting that the initiation of translation is not affected.[122] Changes in the ribosome number could perhaps partly explain a translational stalling. In growing pigs, the increase in muscle protein synthesis induced by GH is due to an increase in ribosome number and not to a change in the processes that regulate translation initiation.[123] However, in a recent study, evaluating the effects of nutritional deprivation on signal transduction pathways influencing the translation apparatus in the rat diaphragm, it was observed that downstream effectors important in translation initiation were affected by nutritional deprivation.[124]

THE ROLES OF INSULIN AND AMINO ACID AVAILABILITY

In rats made diabetic with streptozotocin, serum IGF-I concentrations are low and return to normal with insulin treatment. Insulin deficiency causes GH refractoriness and a fall in IGF-I levels by reducing liver GHR and causing a GH post-receptor defect.[95,125,126] In primary cultures of hepatocytes, insulin stimulates the accumulation of IGF-I mRNA and increases somatogenic receptors.[127–129] Ingestion of a low protein diet reduces insulin and this could contribute to the reduction of IGF-I. It appears, however, that protein restriction can affect IGF-I independent of insulin, because in rats made diabetic with streptozotocin and treated with insulin, dietary protein restriction still reduced serum IGF-I levels, even though insulin levels are elevated.[130]

Support for a role of amino acids in regulating IGF-I has been obtained in primary cultures of rat hepatocytes.[131] When hepatocytes were incubated in a medium containing only 20 percent of the amino acid concentration of normal serum, IGF-I mRNA abundance decreased to 56 percent of control value after 24 h. Tryptophan appears to play a dominant role in the maintenance of IGF-I mRNA in cultured hepatocytes.[132,133]

CLEARANCE AND DEGRADATION OF IGF-I

Reduced serum IGF-I levels during dietary protein restriction may result from impaired production or accelerated clearance of IGF-I from the circulation. One week of protein restriction in 5-week-old rats accelerates serum clearance and degradation of IGF-I labeled with radioactive iodine.[134]

This effect could be explained by the observation that, in the protein-restricted rats, IGF-I binds preferentially to the rapidly cleared low molecular-weight IGFBPs (30 kDa), and less well to the long-lived, high-molecular-weight complex (150 kDa). These observations are consistent with the changes in IGFBPs that occur during protein restriction. Indeed, IGFBP-3, a component of the 150 kDa complex, is reduced two-fold in the protein-restricted rats.[135] In contrast, the liver abundance of the mRNA of IGFBP-1, a major component of the 30 kDa complex, is increased four- to six-fold in rats fed a low-protein diet.[136]

Increased IGF-I clearance is not the only cause of reduced IGF-I in serum, because endogenous production of IGF-I, calculated from steady-state serum levels and clearance data, was reduced by 29 percent during protein restriction.

EFFECTS OF NUTRIENTS ON THE GROWTH-PROMOTING AND ANABOLIC ACTIONS OF IGF-I

Several studies show that nutrient intake modulates the growth response to IGF-I. Young rats fed a low-protein diet and infused for 1 week with human recombinant IGF-I exhibited no stimulation of carcass growth (body weight, tail length, tibial epiphyseal width) despite normal serum IGF-I values. In contrast, growth of the spleen and kidney were enhanced (+45 percent and +28 percent, respectively), showing that the IGF-I resistance resulting from protein deprivation is organ specific.[137] Similarly, protein-energy deprivation in neonatal rats blocks the growth-stimulating effects of IGF-I.[138] This contrasts with the normal growth-promoting effects of exogenous IGF-I observed in intrauterine growth retarded pups that are nutritionally rehabilitated after birth.[139] The conclusions are therefore that normal IGF-I synthesis and adequate nutrition are necessary for optimal neonatal growth.

Fasting is associated with rapid decrease of circulating IGF-I, but also with a decrease of IGF-I content in several tissues, such as the skeletal muscle. The latter may contribute to reduced protein synthesis as well as increased protein degradation. We have observed that fasting was associated with a dramatic increase of the atrogin-1/MaAFbx muscle-specific ubiquitin–ligase, an enzyme implicated in muscle atrophy. Interestingly, injections of IGF-I into fasted rats, significantly attenuated this overexpression of the ubiquitin–ligase, suggesting that nutrient-induced changes in skeletal muscle tissue might regulate the antiproteolytic action of IGF-I.[104]

The effects of protein malnutrition during gestation

Restriction of energy and protein in pregnant rats reduces placental and fetal weight.[140,141] These manipulations mimic the human counterpart of symmetrical intrauterine growth retardation caused by chronic maternal malnutrition.[142] The effect of maternal malnutrition on fetal growth is probably related to changes in IGF-I expression.[143–145] When female rats are fed a low-protein diet throughout gestation

(5 percent casein versus 20 percent in controls), the birth-weight of the pups is significantly reduced (−15 percent) and levels of serum as well as liver IGF-I peptide, and liver IGF-I mRNA are decreased.[145] In contrast, protein deprivation during pregnancy did not influence neonatal IGF-II gene expression, or the relative abundance of the various IGFBP species, plasma insulin or GH levels. Fasting during late pregnancy results in decreased fetal weight and IGF-I levels.[146,147] Therefore, normal protein intake and some minimal energy intake are required for normal fetal growth and IGF-I expression late in pregnancy.

When female rats fed a low-protein diet from day 1 of gestation were sacrificed 2–3 days before term, growth of the fetuses was not affected, and fetal serum IGF-I peptide and liver IGF-I mRNA levels were normal. This suggests that the growth retardation and reduced IGF-I expression in pups born from protein-restricted mothers occurs in the last days of pregnancy, when fetal growth is rapid and utilization of maternal protein reserves is important.[148]

Protein restriction during gestation has long-lasting effects on post-natal growth of the offspring. Despite food rehabilitation during the suckling period, pups born from protein-malnourished mothers do not undergo immediate catch-up of growth.[148,149] Long-term rehabilitation is, however, associated with complete catch-up growth of tail length and organ weight, but not body weight.[150] These long-term effects of gestational protein malnutrition on the post-natal growth of the progeny are accompanied by parallel changes in serum and tissue IGF-I, supporting a role for IGF-I in the control of catch-up growth after intrauterine growth retardation.

The role of zinc in the regulation of growth and IGF-I

Young growing rats fed zinc-deficient diets have anorexia, a cyclical pattern of food intake and severe stunting of their growth.[151–153] The decreased growth rate results partly from the deficit in energy and protein intake. Comparison of zinc-deficient rats with pair-fed controls established that zinc deficiency is responsible for some of the growth retardation. Reduced circulating IGF-I concentrations in zinc-deprived rats, independent of the reduced food intake, has been observed in several studies.[153–157] This provides a possible mechanism for the growth retardation resulting from zinc deficiency. Such a mechanism is supported by the observation that the growth-stimulating effect of zinc supplementation in nutritionally deprived children might be mediated through increased IGF-I.

Several mechanisms may explain the reduction of IGF-I in zinc-deprived animals. Zinc deficiency reduces serum growth hormone.[158] In addition, GH resistance may be present, because exogenous growth hormone fails to raise IGF-I levels in zinc-deficient rats.[154,159] Zinc depletion also causes a decrease in liver GHR and serum GHBP,[153,160] and

this may participate in the GH insensitivity. The molecular mechanisms by which zinc controls the expression of the IGF-I and the GHR/GHBP genes remain unsettled. Even though zinc increases the affinity of human growth hormone for the prolactin receptor,[161] it has little effect on the binding of growth hormone to its own receptor. Zinc seems to play a role in the intracellular transduction pathways of several hormones and might activate protein kinase C which could play a role in the transduction of the GH signal.[162] Finally, zinc is an essential component of several of the 'zinc-finger' transcription factors.[163,164]

It is also possible that deficits in micronutrients cause impaired responsiveness to the growth-promoting effects of IGF-I. In addition to reducing IGF-I levels, zinc deficiency causes IGF-I resistance in rats.[50,165] Zinc is also implicated in some of the actions of IGF-I. Thus in an *in vitro* model of rat fibroblasts (Rat-1 cells), zinc chelation inhibits IGF-I mitogenic action. This inhibitory effect of zinc availability is associated with a marked decrease of the mitogen-activated protein kinase (MAPK) expression, a factor crucial for the IGF-I-induced mitogenic action in RAT-1 cells.[166]

NUTRITION AND INFLAMMATORY STATES

Clinical and epidemiological observations

Medical conditions accompanied by malnutrition, such as severe inflammatory bowel disease or celiac disease, can result in growth failure. Low levels of IGF-I have also been documented in such patients, and nutritional rehabilitation consistently increases serum IGF-I values.[158,167] In infants with renal disease, malnutrition together with electrolyte disturbances and metabolic acidosis contribute to reduced growth. This condition is associated with alterations in the somatotroph axis, such as diminished hepatic IGF-I production, low expression of liver GHRs suggested by low GHBP levels, and increased levels of low molecular weight IGFBPs.[168] Specific nutrients may influence growth and the GH–IGF-I axis in some situations. For example, in growth-retarded children receiving long-term total parenteral nutrition, supplementation with ornithine-2-oxoglutarate accelerates growth in stature and increases IGF-I levels.[169]

Epidemiologic studies also support the concept of the interaction between nutrition and infection.[170] Thus the INCAP studies recognized that any infection worsens nutritional status, with the most obvious effects of infection in poorly nourished children being on growth. In a rural area of Guatemala, it was also recognized that many neonatal deaths were attributable to the synergism between nutrition and infection. Conversely, the early INCAP studies uncovered the impact of infection on the nutritional status. Improving the nutritional status of underprivileged children lowers both morbidity and mortality and improved growth impaired by infection.

Interactions of inflammation with the somatotroph axis: experimental studies

As malnutrition favors inflammatory states, it of importance to consider their consequences on the somatotroph axis. Critical illness in humans is accompanied by elevated GH that fails to maintain normal IGF-I levels, suggesting GH resistance.[171] In rats, the endotoxin lipopolysaccharide (LPS) reduces GH secretion.[172] However, in LPS injected rats, the reduced IGF-I is not restored by GH administration, and this GH resistant state can be explained partially by a loss in liver GH receptors.[173] Several recent studies have shown that several inflammatory conditions such as LPS injection, sepsis, colitis and renal failure impairs GH-stimulated STAT5b phosphorylation and DNA binding activity in liver. The pathways leading to phosphorylation of the GH receptor associated JAK-2 tyrosine kinase phophorylating STAT5b are also impaired in inflammatory conditions, namely by pro-inflammatory cytokines.[174–178] Liver resistance to GH is also caused by two pro-inflammatory cytokines, released in inflammatory conditions, TNF-α and IL-1β. These cytokines blunt the expression of the IGF-I gene in primary cultures of hepatocytes.[175,179,180] Another potential mechanism implicated in the GH resistance consists of an upregulation of some members of the SOCS family, which inhibit the GH signaling, in particular STAT5 activation, through interactions with the cytoplasmic portions of the GH receptor and/or JAK-2. Several lines of evidence are in favor of the concept that IL-6 may contribute to the GH resistance of inflammation by induction of the members of the SOCS family.[181] It is also noteworthy that changes in the early stages of the signaling cascade of the GH message and activation of the signal termination mediators in inflammation are similar to those affected by nutrient deprivation, pointing towards interactions between these two conditions.

CONCLUSIONS

Adequate nutrient intake is essential for optimal growth and development. Marginal malnutrition is a common worldwide cause of growth retardation. Deficiencies of both macro- and micronutrients can lead to growth retardation. In developing countries, much of the growth retardation is likely to result from multiple deficiencies, with long-term deleterious consequences on developmental and work capacity performances. In Western countries, however, growth retardation may result from nutritional deficits related to specific dietary deficiencies, such as macrobiotic foods, or to pathological conditions. The relationships between chronic malnutrition and rehabilitation, with various parameters of the somatotroph axis should deserve further documentation.

In humans and animal models, nutrients play a predominant role in the control of the somatotroph axis. In particular, discordances between elevated GH and decreased IGF-I levels in chronic, severe malnutrition and

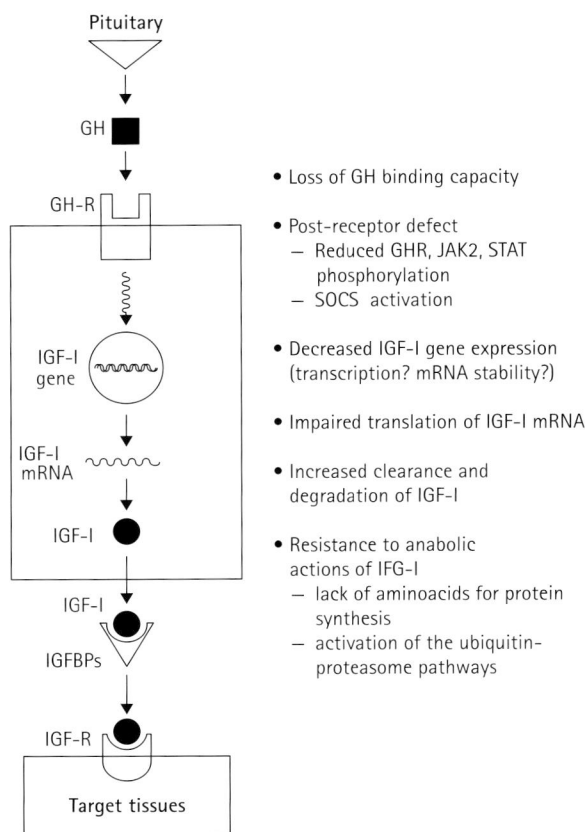

Figure 5.11 Overview of the mechanisms involved in the regulation of IGF-I in malnourished rats.

acute nutrient deprivation suggest that energy and protein restriction may cause GH insensitivity. The mechanisms by which nutrients control the various functions of the somatotroph axis have been studied in animals (Fig. 5.11).

In fasted rats, the hepatocyte GH-binding availability is reduced in parallel with the decrease in IGF-I, suggesting that GH resistance in this acute nutritional insult may result in part from decreased somatotroph receptors. It can be hypothesized that an activation of the GH-receptor targeted ubiquitin–proteasome pathway is involved in this loss of somatogenic receptors. A post-receptor defect in GH action is also present in acute nutrient deprivation. Thus in fasting, we observed that the GH resistance induces impaired activation of the JAK-2/STAT signaling cascade, associated with an activation of the signal termination factors (SOCS family).

A post-GH-receptor defect is also suggested to occur in chronic isocaloric protein restriction of growing rats, in which the liver GH binding capacity is normal (adult rats) or normalized by GH infusion (growing rats), but the IGF-I and the capacity to respond to GH are blunted. In protein-restricted pre-pubertal rats, liver IGF-I mRNA abundance is reduced, a consequence of impaired IGF-I gene expression (perhaps the expression of the post-receptor defect), most likely due to reduced transcription; indeed, message instability has not been ruled out. In addition, impaired translation of the IGF-I mRNA has been indirectly documented in the protein-restricted rats, because high doses of GH can muster the IGF-I mRNA levels without a concomitant increase in IGF-I.

Protein restriction also accelerates IGF-I clearance and attenuated expression of the biological actions of IGF-I on body weight and growth. Decreased IGF-I expression is also involved in the impaired fetal growth caused by maternal protein restriction during gestation.

Finally, macro- and micronutrient deficiencies can also induce a state of resistance to the anabolic and growth promotion effects of IGF-I. IGF-I resistance has been shown to occur in growing rats, submitted to an isocaloric, but protein-restricted diet, pointing to the essential role of protein supply early in growth. Micronutrients such as zinc also play a role in the regulation of the somatotroph axis. Zinc deficiency reduces GH secretion, GHR/GHBP and IGF-I gene expression, and attenuates the growth-promoting actions of IGF-I. Also, deficiencies of micronutrients, such as zinc, have been advocated to explain the impairment of mitogenic actions of IGF-I on connective tissue cells, by negative interaction with the MAP-kinase pathway.

The interaction between nutrient deficiencies, accelerated protein degradation and increased inflammatory states have often been underlined. Activation of specific ligases of the ubiquitin–proteasome complex (such as atrogin-1-MAFbx), observed in fasting, could be involved as factors favoring skeletal muscle proteolysis and therefore, impaired development. It is of importance to underline that alterations of GH dependent IGF-I gene activation pathways are under the negative control of pro-inflammatory cytokines, very often triggered in conditions of chronic malnutrition.

REFERENCES

1 Thissen JP, Ketelslegers JM, Underwood LE. Nutritional regulation of the insulin-like growth factors. *Endocr Rev* 1994; **15**: 80–101.
2 de Onis M, Monteiro C, Akre J, Glugston G. The worldwide magnitude of protein-energy malnutrition: an overview from the WHO Global Database on Child Growth. *Bull World Health Organ* 1993; **71**: 703–12.
3 Allen LH. The nutrition CRSP: what is marginal malnutrition, and does it affect human function? *Nutr Rev* 1993; **51**: 255–67.
4 Martorell R. Results and implications of the INCAP follow-up study. *J Nutr* 1995; **125(4 Suppl)**: 1127S–38S.
5 Martorell R, Habicht JP, Rivera JA. History and design of the INCAP longitudinal study (1969-77) and its follow-up (1988-89). *J Nutr* 1995; **125(4 Suppl)**: 1027S–41S.
6 Idohou-Dossou N, Wade S, Guiro AT, *et al.* Nutritional status of preschool Senegalese children: long-term effects of early severe malnutrition. *Br J Nutr* 2003; **90**: 1123–32.
7 Haas JD, Martinez EJ, Murdoch S, *et al.* Nutritional supplementation during the preschool years and physical work capacity in adolescent and young adult Guatemalans. *J Nutr* 1995; **125(4 Suppl)**: 1078S–89S.
8 Schroeder DG, Martorell R, Rivera JA, *et al.* Age differences in the impact of nutritional supplementation on growth. *J Nutr* 1995; **125(4 Suppl)**: 1051S–9S.
9 Super CM, Herrera MG, Mora JO. Long-term effects of food supplementation and psychosocial intervention on the physical growth of Colombian infants at risk of malnutrition. *Child Dev* 1990; **61**: 29–49.
10 Powell CA, Walker SP, Himes JH, *et al.* Relationships between physical growth, mental development and nutritional supplementation in stunted children: the Jamaican study. *Acta Paediatr* 1995; **84**: 22–9.
11 Stein AD, Barnhart HX, Wang M, *et al.* Comparison of linear growth patterns in the first three years of life across two generations in Guatemala. *Pediatrics* 2004; **113(3 Pt. 1)**: e270–5.
12 Conlisk AJ, Barnhart HX, Martorell R, *et al.* Maternal and child nutritional supplementation are inversely associated with fasting plasma glucose concentration in young Guatemalan adults. *J Nutr* 2004; **134**: 890–7.
13 Webb AL, Conlisk AJ, Barnhart HX, *et al.* Maternal and childhood nutrition and later blood pressure levels in young Guatemalan adults. *Int J Epidemiol* 2005; **34**: 898–904.
14 Grajeda R, Behrman JR, Flores R, *et al.* The human capital study 2002-04: tracking, data collection, coverage, and attrition. *Food Nutr Bull* 2005; **26(2 Suppl 1)**: S15–S24.
15 Perez-Escamilla R, Pollitt E. Growth improvements in children above 3 years of age: the Cali Study. *J Nutr* 1995; **125**: 885–93.
16 Dagnelie PC, Van Dusseldorp M, Van Staveren WA, Hautvast JG. Effects of macrobiotic diets on linear growth in infants and children until 10 years of age. *Eur J Clin Nutr* 1994; **48(Suppl 1)**: S103–11.
17 Dagnelie PC, Van Staveren WA. Macrobiotic nutrition and child health: results of a population-based, mixed-longitudinal cohort study in The Netherlands. *Am J Clin Nutr* 1994; **59(5 Suppl)**: 1187S–96.
18 Pugliese MT, Lifshitz F, Grad G, *et al.* Fear of obesity. A cause of short stature and delayed puberty. *N Engl J Med* 1983; **309**: 513–8.
19 Allen NE, Appleby PN, Davey GK, *et al.* The associations of diet with serum insulin-like growth factor I and its main binding proteins in 292 women meat-eaters, vegetarians, and vegans. *Cancer Epidemiol Biomarkers Prev* 2002; **11**: 1441–8.
20 Hoppe C, Molgaard C, Michaelsen KF. Cow's milk and linear growth in industrialized and developing countries. *Annu Rev Nutr* 2006; **26**: 131–73.
21 Dewey KG, Peerson JM, Brown KH, *et al.* Growth of breast-fed infants deviates from current reference data: a pooled analysis of US, Canadian, and European data sets. World Health Organization Working Group on Infant Growth. *Pediatrics* 1995; **96(3 Pt. 1)**: 495–503.
22 Michaelsen KF, Petersen S, Greisen G, Thomsen BL. Weight, length, head circumference, and growth velocity in a longitudinal study of Danish infants. *Dan Med Bull* 1994; **41**: 577–85.

23 Heinig MJ, Nommsen LA, Peerson JM, *et al.* Energy and protein intakes of breast-fed and formula-fed infants during the first year of life and their association with growth velocity: the DARLING Study. *Am J Clin Nutr* 1993; **58**: 152–61.

24 Martin RM, Smith GD, Mangtani P, *et al.* Association between breast feeding and growth: the Boyd-Orr cohort study. *Arch Dis Child Fetal Neonatal Ed* 2002; **87**: F193–201.

25 Victora CG, Barros F, Lima RC, *et al.* Anthropometry and body composition of 18 year old men according to duration of breast feeding: birth cohort study from Brazil. *BMJ* 2003; **327**: 901.

26 Ruel MT. Milk intake is associated with better growth in Latin America: evidence from the Demographic and Health surveys [Abstract]. *J FASEB* **17**: 2003.

27 Allen LH, Backstrand JR, Stanek EJ III, *et al.* The interactive effects of dietary quality on the growth and attained size of young Mexican children. *Am J Clin Nutr* 1992; **56**: 353–64.

28 Hoppe C, Udam TR, Lauritzen L, *et al.* Animal protein intake, serum insulin-like growth factor I, and growth in healthy 2.5-y-old Danish children. *Am J Clin Nutr* 2004; **80**: 447–52.

29 Orr JB. Milk consumption and the growth of school-children [Abstract]. *Lancet* 1928; **i**: 202–3.

30 Berkey CS, Rockett HR, Willett WC, Colditz GA. Milk, dairy fat, dietary calcium, and weight gain: a longitudinal study of adolescents. *Arch Pediatr Adolesc Med* 2005; **159**: 543–50.

31 Wiley AS. Does milk make children grow? Relationships between milk consumption and height in NHANES 1999–2002. *Am J Hum Biol* 2005; **17**: 425–41.

32 Van Dusseldorp M, Arts IC, Bergsma JS, *et al.* Catch-up growth in children fed a macrobiotic diet in early childhood. *J Nutr* 1996; **126**: 2977–83.

33 Allen LH. Nutritional influences on linear growth: a general review. *Eur J Clin Nutr* 1994; **48(Suppl 1)**: S75–89.

34 Lawless JW, Latham MC, Stephenson LS, *et al.* Iron supplementation improves appetite and growth in anemic Kenyan primary school children. *J Nutr* 1994; **124**: 645–54.

35 Mast AE, Blinder MA, Gronowski AM, *et al.* Clinical utility of the soluble transferrin receptor and comparison with serum ferritin in several populations. *Clin Chem* 1998; **44**: 45–51.

36 Vernet M, Doyen C. Assessment of iron status with a new fully automated assay for transferrin receptor in human serum. *Clin Chem Lab Med* 2000; **38**: 437–42.

37 Ninh NX, Nhien NV, Khan NC, *et al. Effects of zinc supplementation on growth and insulin-like growth factor-I (IGF-I) in healthy Vietnamese infants* [Abstract]. 83rd Annual Meeting of the Endocrine Society, Chicago, June 20-23, 2001.

38 Ninh NX, Goffinet C, Rybski J, Ketelslegers JM. The soluble transferrin receptor (sTfR) allows effective monitoring of iron supplementation therapy in young infants [Abstract]. *Clin Chem* 2001.

39 Castillo-Duran C, Uauy R. Copper deficiency impairs growth of infants recovering from malnutrition. *Am J Clin Nutr* 1988; **47**: 710–4.

40 Olivares M, Araya M, Uauy R. Copper homeostasis in infant nutrition: deficit and excess. *J Pediatr Gastroenterol Nutr* 2000; **31**: 102–11.

41 Olivares M, Uauy R. Copper as an essential nutrient. *Am J Clin Nutr* 1996; **63**: 791S–6S.

42 Ross AC, Gardner EM. The function of vitamin A in cellular growth and differentiation, and its roles during pregnancy and lactation. *Adv Exp Med Biol* 1994; **352**: 187–200.

43 Underwood BA. The role of vitamin A in child growth, development and survival. *Adv Exp Med Biol* 1994; **352**: 201–8.

44 Ramakrishnan U, Latham MC, Abel R. Vitamin A supplementation does not improve growth of preschool children: a randomized, double-blind field trial in south India. *J Nutr* 1995; **125**: 202–11.

45 Prazad AS, Halstedt JA, Nadimi M. Syndrome of iron deficiency anemia, hepatosplenomegaly, hypogonadism, dwarfism and geophagia. *Am J Med* 1961; **31**: 532–46.

46 Prazad AS, Miale A Jr, Farid Z, *et al.* Zinc metabolism in patients with the syndrome of iron deficiency anemia, hepatosplenomegaly, dwarfism, and hypogonadism. *J Lab Clin Med* 1963; **61**: 537–49.

47 Ronaghy HA, Reinhold JG, Mahloudji M, *et al.* Zinc supplementation of malnourished schoolboys in Iran: increased growth and other effects. *Am J Clin Nutr* 1974; **27**: 112–21.

48 Schlesinger L, Arevalo M, Arredondo S, *et al.* Effect of a zinc-fortified formula on immunocompetence and growth of malnourished infants. *Am J Clin Nutr* 1992; **56**: 491–8.

49 Castillo-Duran C, Garcia H, Venegas P, *et al.* Zinc supplementation increases growth velocity of male children and adolescents with short stature. *Acta Paediatr* 1994; **83**: 833–7.

50 Ninh NX, Thissen JP, Collette L, *et al.* Zinc supplementation increases growth and circulating insulin-like growth factor I (IGF-I) in growth-retarded Vietnamese children. *Am J Clin Nutr* 1996; **63**: 514–9.

51 Carter JP, Grivetti LE, Davis JT, *et al.* Growth and sexual development of adolescent Egyptian village boys. Effects of zinc, iron, and placebo supplementation. *Am J Clin Nutr* 1969; **22**: 59–78.

52 Golden BE, Golden MH. Effect of zinc on lean tissue synthesis during recovery from malnutrition. *Eur J Clin Nutr* 1992; **46**: 697–706.

53 Bates CJ, Evans PH, Dardenne M, *et al.* A trial of zinc supplementation in young rural Gambian children. *Br J Nutr* 1993; **69**: 243–55.

54 Cavan KR, Gibson RS, Grazioso CF, *et al.* Growth and body composition of periurban Guatemalan children in relation to zinc status: a longitudinal zinc intervention trial. *Am J Clin Nutr* 1993; **57**: 344–52.

55 Cavan KR, Gibson RS, Grazioso CF, *et al.* Growth and body composition of periurban Guatemalan children in relation to zinc status: a cross-sectional study. *Am J Clin Nutr* 1993; **57**: 334–43.

56 Walravens PA, Krebs NF, Hambidge KM. Linear growth of low income preschool children receiving a zinc supplement. *Am J Clin Nutr* 1983; **38**: 195–201.

57 Gibson RS, Vanderkooy PD, MacDonald AC, *et al.* A growth-limiting, mild zinc-deficiency syndrome in some southern

Ontario boys with low height percentiles. *Am J Clin Nutr* 1989; **49**: 1266–73.

58 Nakamura T, Nishiyama S, Futagoishi-Suginohara Y, *et al.* Mild to moderate zinc deficiency in short children: effect of zinc supplementation on linear growth velocity. *J Pediatr* 1993; **123**: 65–9.

59 Hambidge KM, Chavez MN, Brown RM, Walravens PA. Zinc nutritional status of young middle-income children and effects of consuming zinc-fortified breakfast cereals. *Am J Clin Nutr* 1979; **32**: 2532–9.

60 Krebs NF, Hambidge KM, Walravens PA. Increased food intake of young children receiving a zinc supplement. *Am J Dis Child* 1984; **138**: 270–3.

61 Gatheru Z, Kinoti S, Alwar J, Mwita M. Serum zinc levels in children with kwashiorkor aged one to three years at Kenyatta National Hospital and the effect of zinc supplementation during recovery. *East Afr Med J* 1988; **65**: 670–9.

62 Simmer K, Khanum S, Carlsson L, Thompson RP. Nutritional rehabilitation in Bangladesh – the importance of zinc. *Am J Clin Nutr* 1988; **47**: 1036–40.

63 Walravens PA, Hambidge KM, Koepfer DM. Zinc supplementation in infants with a nutritional pattern of failure to thrive: a double-blind, controlled study. *Pediatrics* 1989; **83**: 532–8.

64 Walravens PA, Chakar A, Mokni R, *et al.* Zinc supplements in breastfed infants. *Lancet* 1992; **340**: 683–5.

65 Grant DB, Hambley J, Becker D, Pimstone BL. Reduced sulphation factor in undernourished children. *Arch Dis Child* 1973; **48**: 596–600.

66 Hintz RL, Suskind R, Amatayakul K, *et al.* Plasma somatomedin and growth hormone values in children with protein-calorie malnutrition. *J Pediatr* 1978; **92**: 153–6.

67 Smith IF, Latham MC, Azubuike JA, *et al.* Blood plasma levels of cortisol, insulin, growth hormone and somatomedin in children with marasmus, kwashiorkor, and intermediate forms of protein-energy malnutrition. *Proc Soc Exp Biol Med* 1981; **167**: 607–11.

68 Soliman AT, Hassan AE, Aref MK, *et al.* Serum insulin-like growth factors I and II concentrations and growth hormone and insulin responses to arginine infusion in children with protein-energy malnutrition before and after nutritional rehabilitation. *Pediatr Res* 1986; **20**: 1122–30.

69 Counts DR, Gwirtsman H, Carlsson LM, *et al.* The effect of anorexia nervosa and refeeding on growth hormone-binding protein, the insulin-like growth factors (IGFs), and the IGF-binding proteins. *J Clin Endocrinol Metab* 1992; **75**: 762–7.

70 Clemmons DR, Klibanski A, Underwood LE, *et al.* Reduction of plasma immunoreactive somatomedin C during fasting in humans. *J Clin Endocrinol Metab* 1981; **53**: 1247–50.

71 Ho KY, Veldhuis JD, Johnson ML, *et al.* Fasting enhances growth hormone secretion and amplifies the complex rhythms of growth hormone secretion in man. *J Clin Invest* 1988; **81**: 968–75.

72 Merimee TJ, Zapf J, Froesch ER. Insulin-like growth factors in the fed and fasted states. *J Clin Endocrinol Metab* 1982; **55**: 999–1002.

73 Isley WL, Underwood LE, Clemmons DR. Changes in plasma somatomedin-C in response to ingestion of diets with variable protein and energy content. *JPEN J Parenter Enteral Nutr* 1984; **8**: 407–11.

74 Isley WL, Underwood LE, Clemmons DR. Dietary components that regulate serum somatomedin-C concentrations in humans. *J Clin Invest* 1983; **71**: 175–82.

75 Clemmons DR, Seek MM, Underwood LE. Supplemental essential amino acids augment the somatomedin-C/insulin-like growth factor I response to refeeding after fasting. *Metabolism* 1985; **34**: 391–5.

76 Clemmons DR, Underwood LE, Dickerson RN, *et al.* Use of plasma somatomedin-C/insulin-like growth factor I measurements to monitor the response to nutritional repletion in malnourished patients. *Am J Clin Nutr* 1985; **41**: 191–8.

77 Smith IF, Taiwo O, Payne-Robinson HM. Plasma somatomedin-C in Nigerian malnourished children fed a vegetable protein rehabilitation diet. *Eur J Clin Nutr* 1989; **43**: 705–13.

78 Hoppe C, Molgaard C, Juul A, Michaelsen KF. High intakes of skimmed milk, but not meat, increase serum IGF-I and IGFBP-3 in eight-year-old boys. *Eur J Clin Nutr* 2004; **58**: 1211–6.

79 Meisel H. Biochemical properties of peptides encrypted in bovine milk proteins. *Curr Med Chem* 2005; **12**: 1905–19.

80 Abubakar A, Saito T, Kitazawa H, *et al.* Structural analysis of new antihypertensive peptides derived from cheese whey protein by proteinase K digestion. *J Dairy Sci* 1998; **81**: 3131–8.

81 Maeno M, Yamamoto N, Takano T. Identification of an antihypertensive peptide from casein hydrolysate produced by a proteinase from Lactobacillus helvetius CP790. *J Dairy Sci* 1996; **79**: 1316–21.

82 Sipola M, Finckenberg P, Korpela R, *et al.* Effect of long-term intake of milk products on blood pressure in hypertensive rats. *J Dairy Res* 2002; **69**: 103–11.

83 Hata Y, Yamamoto M, Ohni M, *et al.* A placebo-controlled study of the effect of sour milk on blood pressure in hypertensive subjects. *Am J Clin Nutr* 1996; **64**: 767–71.

84 Seppo L, Jauhiainen T, Poussa T, Korpela R. A fermented milk high in bioactive peptides has a blood pressure-lowering effect in hypertensive subjects. *Am J Clin Nutr* 2003; **77**: 326–30.

85 Maes W, Van Camp J, Vermeirssen V, *et al.* Influence of the lactokinin Ala-Leu-Pro-Met-His-Ile-Arg (ALPMHIR) on the release of endothelin-1 by endothelial cells. *Regul Pept* 2004; **118**: 105–9.

86 Cotterill AM, Cowell CT, Baxter RC, *et al.* Regulation of the growth hormone-independent growth factor-binding protein in children. *J Clin Endocrinol Metab* 1988; **67**: 882–7.

87 Yeoh SI, Baxter RC. Metabolic regulation of the growth hormone independent insulin-like growth factor binding protein in human plasma. *Acta Endocrinol (Copenh)* 1988; **119**: 465–73.

88 Hotta M, Fukuda I, Sato K, *et al.* The relationship between bone turnover and body weight, serum insulin-like growth

factor (IGF) I, and serum IGF-binding protein levels in patients with anorexia nervosa. *J Clin Endocrinol Metab* 2000; **85**: 200–6.

89   Smith WJ, Underwood LE, Clemmons DR. Effects of caloric or protein restriction on insulin-like growth factor-I (IGF-I) and IGF-binding proteins in children and adults. *J Clin Endocrinol Metab* 1995; **80**: 443–9.

90   Pucilowska JB, Davenport ML, Kabir I, *et al*. The effect of dietary protein supplementation on insulin-like growth factors (IGFs) and IGF-binding proteins in children with shigellosis. *J Clin Endocrinol Metab* 1993; **77**: 1516–21.

91   Tannenbaum GS, Rorstad O, Brazeau P. Effects of prolonged food deprivation on the ultradian growth hormone rhythm and immunoreactive somatostatin tissue levels in the rat. *Endocrinology* 1979; **104**: 1733–8.

92   Phillips LS, Young HS. Nutrition and somatomedin. I. Effect of fasting and refeeding on serum somatomedin activity and cartilage growth activity in rats. *Endocrinology* 1976; **99**: 304–14.

93   Maiter D, Underwood LE, Maes M, *et al*. Different effects of intermittent and continuous growth hormone (GH) administration on serum somatomedin-C/insulin-like growth factor I and liver GH receptors in hypophysectomized rats. *Endocrinology* 1988; **123**: 1053–9.

94   Maiter D, Maes M, Underwood LE, *et al*. Early changes in serum concentrations of somatomedin-C induced by dietary protein deprivation in rats: contributions of growth hormone receptor and post-receptor defects. *J Endocrinol* 1988; **118**: 113–20.

95   Baxter RC, Bryson JM, Turtle JR. The effect of fasting on liver receptors for prolactin and growth hormone. *Metabolism* 1981; **30**: 1086–90.

96   Postel-Vinay MC, Cohen-Tanugi E, Charrier J. Growth hormone receptors in rat liver membranes: effects of fasting and refeeding, and correlation with plasma somatomedin activity. *Mol Cell Endocrinol* 1982; **28**: 657–69.

97   Maes M, Ketelslegers JM, Underwood LE. Low plasma somatomedin-C in streptozotocin-induced diabetes mellitus. Correlation with changes in somatogenic and lactogenic liver binding sites. *Diabetes* 1983; **32**: 1060–9.

98   Maes M, Underwood LE, Ketelslegers JM. Plasma somatomedin-C in fasted and refed rats: close relationship with changes in liver somatogenic but not lactogenic binding sites. *J Endocrinol* 1983; **97**: 243–52.

99   Mulumba N, Massa G, Ketelslegers JM, Maes M. Ontogeny and nutritional regulation of the serum growth hormone-binding protein in the rat. *Acta Endocrinol (Copenh)* 1991; **125**: 409–15.

100   Straus DS, Takemoto CD. Effect of fasting on insulin-like growth factor-I (IGF-I) and growth hormone receptor mRNA levels and IGF-I gene transcription in rat liver. *Mol Endocrinol* 1990; **4**: 91–100.

101   Straus DS, Takemoto CD. Effect of dietary protein deprivation on insulin-like growth factor (IGF)-I and -II, IGF

binding protein-2, and serum albumin gene expression in rat. *Endocrinology* 1990; **127**: 1849–60.

102   Strous GJ, dos Santos CA, Gent J, *et al*. Ubiquitin system-dependent regulation of growth hormone receptor signal transduction. *Curr Top Microbiol Immunol* 2004; **286**: 81–118.

103   Strous GJ, van Kerkhof P. The ubiquitin-proteasome pathway and the regulation of growth hormone receptor availability. *Mol Cell Endocrinol* 2002; **197**: 143–51.

104   Dehoux M, Van Beneden R, Pasko N, *et al*. Role of the insulin-like growth factor I decline in the induction of atrogin-1/MAFbx during fasting and diabetes. *Endocrinology* 2004; **145**: 4806–12.

105   Fliesen T, Maiter D, Gerard G, *et al*. Reduction of serum insulin-like growth factor-I by dietary protein restriction is age dependent. *Pediatr Res* 1989; **26**: 415–9.

106   Thissen JP, Triest S, Underwood LE, *et al*. Divergent responses of serum insulin-like growth factor-I and liver growth hormone (GH) receptors to exogenous GH in protein-restricted rats. *Endocrinology* 1990; **126**: 908–13.

107   Maes M, Amand Y, Underwood LE, *et al*. Decreased serum insulin-like growth factor I response to growth hormone in hypophysectomized rats fed a low protein diet: evidence for a postreceptor defect. *Acta Endocrinol (Copenh)* 1988; **117**: 320–6.

108   Thissen JP, Triest S, Maes M, *et al*. The decreased plasma concentration of insulin-like growth factor-I in protein-restricted rats is not due to decreased numbers of growth hormone receptors on isolated hepatocytes. *J Endocrinol* 1990; **124**: 159–65.

109   Thissen JP, Triest S, Moats-Staats BM, *et al*. Evidence that pretranslational and translational defects decrease serum insulin-like growth factor-I concentrations during dietary protein restriction. *Endocrinology* 1991; **129**: 429–35.

110   Emler CA, Schalch DS. Nutritionally-induced changes in hepatic insulin-like growth factor I (IGF-I) gene expression in rats. *Endocrinology* 1987; **120**: 832–4.

111   Bornfeldt KE, Arnqvist HJ, Enberg B, *et al*. Regulation of insulin-like growth factor-I and growth hormone receptor gene expression by diabetes and nutritional state in rat tissues. *J Endocrinol* 1989; **122**: 651–6.

112   Lowe WL Jr, Adamo M, Werner H, *et al*. Regulation by fasting of rat insulin-like growth factor I and its receptor. Effects on gene expression and binding. *J Clin Invest* 1989; **84**: 619–26.

113   Moats-Staats BM, Brady JL Jr, Underwood LE, D'Ercole AJ. Dietary protein restriction in artificially reared neonatal rats causes a reduction of insulin-like growth factor-I gene expression. *Endocrinology* 1989; **125**: 2368–74.

114   VandeHaar MJ, Moats-Staats BM, Davenport ML, *et al*. Reduced serum concentrations of insulin-like growth factor-I (IGF-I) in protein-restricted growing rats are accompanied by reduced IGF-I mRNA levels in liver and skeletal muscle. *J Endocrinol* 1991; **130**: 305–12.

115   Adams TE, Hansen JA, Starr R, *et al*. Growth hormone preferentially induces the rapid, transient expression of

SOCS-3, a novel inhibitor of cytokine receptor signaling. *J Biol Chem* 1998; **273**: 1285–7.

116 Tollet-Egnell P, Flores-Morales A, Stavreus-Evers A, *et al.* Growth hormone regulation of SOCS-2, SOCS-3, and CIS messenger ribonucleic acid expression in the rat. *Endocrinology* 1999; **140**: 3693–704.

117 Ram PA, Waxman DJ. SOCS/CIS protein inhibition of growth hormone-stimulated STAT5 signaling by multiple mechanisms. *J Biol Chem* 1999; **274**: 35553–61.

118 Greenhalgh CJ, Rico-Bautista E, Lorentzon M, *et al.* SOCS2 negatively regulates growth hormone action in vitro and in vivo. *J Clin Invest* 2005; **115**: 397–406.

119 Rico-Bautista E, Greenhalgh CJ, Tollet-Egnell P, *et al.* Suppressor of cytokine signaling-2 deficiency induces molecular and metabolic changes that partially overlap with growth hormone-dependent effects. *Mol Endocrinol* 2005; **19**: 781–93.

120 Feng GS, Hui CC, Pawson T. SH2-containing phosphotyrosine phosphatase as a target of protein-tyrosine kinases. *Science* 1993; **259**: 1607–11.

121 Beauloye V, Willems B, de C, V, Frank SJ, *et al.* Impairment of liver GH receptor signaling by fasting. *Endocrinology* 2002; **143**: 792–800.

122 Thissen JP, Underwood LE. Translational status of the insulin-like growth factor-I mRNAs in liver of protein-restricted rats. *J Endocrinol* 1992; **132**: 141–7.

123 Bush JA, Kimball SR, O'Connor PM, *et al.* Translational control of protein synthesis in muscle and liver of growth hormone-treated pigs. *Endocrinology* 2003; **144**: 1273–83.

124 Lewis MI, Bodine SC, Kamangar N, *et al.* Effect of severe short-term malnutrition on diaphragm muscle signal transduction pathways influencing protein turnover. *J Appl Physiol* 2006; **100**: 1799–806.

125 Maes M, Ketelslegers JM, Underwood LE. Low circulating somatomedin-C/insulin-like growth factor I in insulin-dependent diabetes and malnutrition: growth hormone receptor and post-receptor defects. *Acta Endocrinol Suppl (Copenh)* 1986; **279**: 86–92.

126 Maes M, Underwood LE, Ketelslegers JM. Low serum somatomedin-C in insulin-dependent diabetes: evidence for a postreceptor mechanism. *Endocrinology* 1986; **118**: 377–82.

127 Johnson TR, Blossey BK, Denko CW, Ilan J. Expression of insulin-like growth factor I in cultured rat hepatocytes: effects of insulin and growth hormone. *Mol Endocrinol* 1989; **3**: 580–7.

128 Tollet P, Enberg B, Mode A. Growth hormone (GH) regulation of cytochrome P-450IIC12, insulin-like growth factor-I (IGF-I), and GH receptor messenger RNA expression in primary rat hepatocytes: a hormonal interplay with insulin, IGF-I, and thyroid hormone. *Mol Endocrinol* 1990; **4**: 1934–42.

129 Boni-Schnetzler M, Schmid C, Meier PJ, Froesch ER. Insulin regulates insulin-like growth factor I mRNA in rat hepatocytes. *Am J Physiol* 1991; **260(6 Pt 1)**: E846–51.

130 Maiter D, Fliesen T, Underwood LE, *et al.* Dietary protein restriction decreases insulin-like growth factor I independent of insulin and liver growth hormone binding. *Endocrinology* 1989; **124**: 2604–11.

131 Thissen JP, Pucilowska JB, Underwood LE. Differential regulation of insulin-like growth factor I (IGF-I) and IGF binding protein-1 messenger ribonucleic acids by amino acid availability and growth hormone in rat hepatocyte primary culture. *Endocrinology* 1994; **134**: 1570–6.

132 Harp JB, Goldstein S, Phillips LS. Nutrition and somatomedin. XXIII. Molecular regulation of IGF-I by amino acid availability in cultured hepatocytes. *Diabetes* 1991; **40**: 95–101.

133 Phillips LS, Goldstein S, Pao CI. Nutrition and somatomedin. XXVI. Molecular regulation of IGF-I by insulin in cultured rat hepatocytes. *Diabetes* 1991; **40**: 1525–30.

134 Thissen JP, Davenport ML, Pucilowska JB, *et al.* Increased serum clearance and degradation of 125I-labeled IGF-I in protein-restricted rats. *Am J Physiol* 1992; **262(4 Pt 1)**: E406–11.

135 Clemmons DR, Thissen JP, Maes M, *et al.* Insulin-like growth factor-I (IGF-I) infusion into hypophysectomized or protein-deprived rats induces specific IGF-binding proteins in serum. *Endocrinology* 1989; **125**: 2967–72.

136 Lemozy S, Pucilowska JB, Underwood LE. Reduction of insulin-like growth factor-I (IGF-I) in protein-restricted rats is associated with differential regulation of IGF-binding protein messenger ribonucleic acids in liver and kidney, and peptides in liver and serum. *Endocrinology* 1994; **135**: 617–23.

137 Thissen JP, Underwood LE, Maiter D, *et al.* Failure of insulin-like growth factor-I (IGF-I) infusion to promote growth in protein-restricted rats despite normalization of serum IGF-I concentrations. *Endocrinology* 1991; **128**: 885–90.

138 Philipps AF, Persson B, Hall K, *et al.* The effects of biosynthetic insulin-like growth factor-1 supplementation on somatic growth, maturation, and erythropoiesis on the neonatal rat. *Pediatr Res* 1988; **23**: 298–305.

139 Muaku SM, Thissen JP, Gerard G, *et al.* Postnatal catch-up growth induced by growth hormone and insulin-like growth factor-I in rats with intrauterine growth retardation caused by maternal protein malnutrition. *Pediatr Res* 1997; **42**: 370–7.

140 McLeod KI, Goldrick RB, Whyte HM. The effect of maternal malnutrition on the progeny in the rat. Studies on growth, body composition and organ cellularity in first and second generation progeny. *Aust J Exp Biol Med Sci* 1972; **50**: 435–46.

141 Winick M. Nutrition, pregnancy, and early infancy. *The Placenta: Human and Animal.* New York: Praeger Publishers, 1982: 25–59.

142 Adair LS. Low birth weight and intrauterine growth retardation in Filipino infants. *Pediatrics* 1989; **84**: 613–22.

143 Pilistine SJ, Moses AC, Munro HN. Placental lactogen administration reverses the effect of low-protein diet on

maternal and fetal serum somatomedin levels in the pregnant rat. *Proc Natl Acad Sci USA* 1984; **81**: 5853–7.

144   Muaku SM, Underwood LE, Selvais PL, *et al.* Maternal protein restriction early or late in rat pregnancy has differential effects on fetal growth, plasma insulin-like growth factor-I (IGF-I) and liver IGF-I gene expression. *Growth Regul* 1995; **5**: 125–32.

145   Muaku SM, Beauloye V, Thissen JP, *et al.* Effects of maternal protein malnutrition on fetal growth, plasma insulin-like growth factors, insulin-like growth factor binding proteins, and liver insulin-like growth factor gene expression in the rat. *Pediatr Res* 1995; **37**: 334–42.

146   Davenport ML, D'Ercole AJ, Underwood LE. Effect of maternal fasting on fetal growth, serum insulin-like growth factors (IGFs), and tissue IGF messenger ribonucleic acids. *Endocrinology* 1990; **126**: 2062–7.

147   Straus DS, Ooi GT, Orlowski CC, Rechler MM. Expression of the genes for insulin-like growth factor-I (IGF-I), IGF-II, and IGF-binding proteins-1 and -2 in fetal rat under conditions of intrauterine growth retardation caused by maternal fasting. *Endocrinology* 1991; **128**: 518–25.

148   Naismith DJ, Morgan BL. The biphasic nature of protein metabolism during pregnancy in the rat. *Br J Nutr* 1976; **36**: 563–6.

149   Zeman FJ. Effect of protein deficiency during gestation on postnatal cellular development in the young rat. *J Nutr* 1970; **100**: 530–8.

150   Muaku SM, Beauloye V, Thissen JP, *et al.* Long-term effects of gestational protein malnutrition on postnatal growth, insulin-like growth factor (IGF)-I, and IGF-binding proteins in rat progeny. *Pediatr Res* 1996; **39(4 Pt 1)**: 649–55.

151   Williams RB, Mills CF. The experimental production of zinc deficiency in the rat. *Br J Nutr* 1970; **24**: 989–1003.

152   Giugliano R, Millward DJ. Growth and zinc homeostasis in the severely Zn-deficient rat. *Br J Nutr* 1984; **52**: 545–60.

153   Ninh NX, Thissen JP, Maiter D, *et al.* Reduced liver insulin-like growth factor-I gene expression in young zinc-deprived rats is associated with a decrease in liver growth hormone (GH) receptors and serum GH-binding protein. *J Endocrinol* 1995; **144**: 449–56.

154   Oner G, Bhaumick B, Bala RM. Effect of zinc deficiency on serum somatomedin levels and skeletal growth in young rats. *Endocrinology* 1984; **114**: 1860–3.

155   Bolze MS, Reeves RD, Lindbeck FE, Elders MJ. Influence of zinc on growth, somatomedin, and glycosaminoglycan metabolism in rats. *Am J Physiol* 1987; **252(1 Pt. 1)**: E21–6.

156   Cossack ZT. Effect of zinc level in the refeeding diet in previously starved rats on plasma somatomedin C levels. *J Pediatr Gastroenterol Nutr* 1988; **7**: 441–5.

157   Dorup I, Flyvbjerg A, Everts ME, Clausen T. Role of insulin-like growth factor-1 and growth hormone in growth inhibition induced by magnesium and zinc deficiencies. *Br J Nutr* 1991; **66**: 505–21.

158   Kirschner BS, Sutton MM. Somatomedin-C levels in growth-impaired children and adolescents with chronic inflammatory bowel disease. *Gastroenterology* 1986; **91**: 830–6.

159   Prazad AS, Oberleas D, Wolf P, Horwitz JP. Effect of growth hormone on nonhypophysectomized zinc-deficient rats and zinc on hypophysectomized rats. *J Lab Clin Med* 1969; **73**: 486–94.

160   McNall AD, Etherton TD, Fosmire GJ. The impaired growth induced by zinc deficiency in rats is associated with decreased expression of the hepatic insulin-like growth factor I and growth hormone receptor genes. *J Nutr* 1995; **125**: 874–9.

161   Cunningham BC, Bass S, Fuh G, Wells JA. Zinc mediation of the binding of human growth hormone to the human prolactin receptor. *Science* 1990; **250**: 1709–12.

162   Hubbard SR, Bishop WR, Kirschmeier P, *et al.* Identification and characterization of zinc binding sites in protein kinase C. *Science* 1991; **254**: 1776–9.

163   Klevit RE. Recognition of DNA by Cys2,His2 zinc fingers. *Science* 1991; **253**: 1367, 1393.

164   Chesters JK. Trace element-gene interactions. *Nutr Rev* 1992; **50**: 217–23.

165   Ninh NX, Maiter D, Verniers J, *et al.* Failure of exogenous IGF-I to restore normal growth in rats submitted to dietary zinc deprivation. *J Endocrinol* 1998; **159**: 211–7.

166   Lefebvre D, Boney CM, Ketelslegers JM, Thissen JP. Inhibition of insulin-like growth factor-I mitogenic action by zinc chelation is associated with a decreased mitogen-activated protein kinase activation in RAT-1 fibroblasts. *FEBS Lett* 1999; **449**: 284–8.

167   Lecornu M, David L, Francois R. Low serum somatomedin activity in celiac disease. A misleading aspect in growth failure from asymptomatic celiac disease. *Helv Paediatr Acta* 1978; **33**: 509–16.

168   Mehls O, Blum WF, Schaefer F, *et al.* Growth failure in renal disease. *Baillieres Clin Endocrinol Metab* 1992; **6**: 665–85.

169   Moukarzel AA, Goulet O, Salas JS, *et al.* Growth retardation in children receiving long-term total parenteral nutrition: effects of ornithine alpha-ketoglutarate. *Am J Clin Nutr* 1994; **60**: 408–13.

170   Scrimshaw NS. Historical concepts of interactions, synergism and antagonism between nutrition and infection. *J Nutr* 2003; **133**: 316S–21.

171   Van den Berghe G, de Zegher F, Veldhuis JD, *et al.* The somatotropic axis in critical illness: effect of continuous growth hormone (GH)-releasing hormone and GH-releasing peptide-2 infusion. *J Clin Endocrinol Metab* 1997; **82**: 590–9.

172   Soto L, Martin AI, Millan S, *et al.* Effects of endotoxin lipopolysaccharide administration on the somatotropic axis. *J Endocrinol* 1998; **159**: 239–46.

173   Defalque D, Brandt N, Ketelslegers JM, Thissen JP. GH insensitivity induced by endotoxin injection is associated with decreased liver GH receptors. *Am J Physiol* 1999; **276(3 Pt. 1)**: E565–72.

174 Mao Y, Ling PR, Fitzgibbons TP, *et al*. Endotoxin-induced inhibition of growth hormone receptor signaling in rat liver in vivo. *Endocrinology* 1999; **140**: 5505–15.

175 Bergad PL, Schwarzenberg SJ, Humbert JT, *et al*. Inhibition of growth hormone action in models of inflammation. *Am J Physiol Cell Physiol* 2000; **279**: C1906–17.

176 Schaefer F, Chen Y, Tsao T, *et al*. Impaired JAK-STAT signal transduction contributes to growth hormone resistance in chronic uremia. *J Clin Invest* 2001; **108**: 467–75.

177 Yumet G, Shumate ML, Bryant P, *et al*. Tumor necrosis factor mediates hepatic growth hormone resistance during sepsis. *Am J Physiol Endocrinol Metab* 2002; **283**: E472–81.

178 Yumet G, Shumate ML, Bryant DP, *et al*. Hepatic growth hormone resistance during sepsis is associated with increased suppressors of cytokine signaling expression and impaired growth hormone signaling. *Crit Care Med* 2006; **34**: 1420–7.

179 Wolf M, Bohm S, Brand M, Kreymann G. Proinflammatory cytokines interleukin 1 beta and tumor necrosis factor alpha inhibit growth hormone stimulation of insulin-like growth factor I synthesis and growth hormone receptor mRNA levels in cultured rat liver cells. *Eur J Endocrinol* 1996; **135**: 729–37.

180 Thissen JP, Verniers J. Inhibition by interleukin-1 beta and tumor necrosis factor-alpha of the insulin-like growth factor I messenger ribonucleic acid response to growth hormone in rat hepatocyte primary culture. *Endocrinology* 1997; **138**: 1078–84.

181 Denson LA, Held MA, Menon RK, *et al*. Interleukin-6 inhibits hepatic growth hormone signaling via upregulation of Cis and Socs-3. *Am J Physiol Gastrointest Liver Physiol* 2003; **284**: G646–54.

6

Endocrinology of growth: Central control

JULIE A CHOWEN, LAURA M FRAGO, JESÚS ARGENTE

INTRODUCTION

In 1940 Heatherington and Ranson reported that lesions of the entire ventral hypothalamus retarded longitudinal bone growth, demonstrating for the first time that the central nervous system (CNS) was involved in the control of growth hormone (GH) secretion from the anterior pituitary gland.[1] It was approximately 20 years later when Reichlin demonstrated that such lesions result in the depletion of pituitary GH content[2] and Frohman and Bernardis reported that more defined brain lesions, destroying only the ventral medial hypothalamic nucleus (VMH), also resulted in depletion of pituitary GH, circulating GH levels and growth retardation.[3] When electrical stimulation of the VMH was shown to increase plasma GH levels,[4] the hypothesis that this area of the brain was intimately involved in the control of GH secretion was consolidated. Although the race to isolate and identify the hypothalamic factors involved in controlling pituitary hormone synthesis and release began in the 1950s, the identity of many remained elusive for years.

We now know that hypothalamic neurons producing growth hormone-releasing hormone (GHRH) stimulate and those producing somatostatin (SS) inhibit GH synthesis and secretion by somatotrophs of the anterior pituitary. Indeed, the pulsatile secretion of GH,[5] fundamental for its physiological actions,[6] is generated by the episodic release of GHRH and SS into the portal vasculature.[7,8] The interaction of these two neuropeptides, as well as other factors discussed in more detail below, at the level of the somatotroph modulates the synthesis and release of GH into the circulation.

GROWTH HORMONE SECRETORY PATTERN

Growth hormone secretion is pulsatile in all species studied to date. Healthy men and women exhibit an ultradian GH secretory rhythm with an interpulse frequency of approximately 2 h.[9] In young women, overall or integrated GH levels are higher than in males of the same age and this is due to a higher pulse amplitude and baseline level.[9,10] The pattern of GH secretion is important for generating its physiological effects, with some GH dependent factors apparently more associated with baseline levels, while others are dependent on the pulse or peak of GH secretion.

In the adult rat, the GH secretory pattern is clearly sexually dimorphic. The adult male rat exhibits a GH secretory pattern with an interpulse interval of approximately 3 h superimposed on a low baseline level, while the female rat has more frequent, irregular bursts of GH release and an elevated baseline level.[11] This dimorphism has been associated with the difference in growth velocity and concentration of GH dependent factors seen between the sexes.[12] The episodic release of GH is regulated primarily at the hypothalamic level, as discussed below, and there are clear sexual dimorphisms in some of the systems that directly control GH secretion.[13–15]

The pulsatile pattern of GH secretion changes throughout development in both humans and the laboratory rat.[10,12,16] In humans, there is a peak in plasma GH levels at mid-gestation that then falls in the third trimester and into the neonatal period.[17] In pre-pubertal children, spontaneous GH secretion is very low during the waking hours, with GH secretory pulses increasing during sleep.[18] During pubertal development GH secretion increases, with this being primarily due to an increase in the pulse amplitude and not pulse frequency, which is then followed by a decrease in GH secretion to reach adult levels.[19,20] As individuals age, circulating GH levels continue to decrease, with this being primarily due to a decrease in pulse amplitude, but not pulse frequency.[10]

This GH secretory pattern can be modified by different pathological conditions that are discussed in various chapters of this text. However, one physiological situation where the pulsatile pattern of GH release is modified is the well established relationship between slow-wave sleep and GH secretion,[21–24] with GH release increasing significantly during sleep stages 3 and 4.[22] This increase is most likely related to both sleep itself and the ingrained circadian rhythm, as disruption of either decreases spontaneous GH secretion.[23–25] This correlation between GH secretion and sleep is most likely the result of altered cortical activity which subsequently modifies the hypothalamic GH control mechanisms.

THE HYPOTHALAMUS

The classical concept of neuroendocrine control of the pituitary postulates that the endocrine functions of the anterior pituitary are controlled by hypothalamic factors. These factors are present in hypothalamic neurons that project to the median eminence and end in contact with the hypothalamic hypophyseal portal vessels. This is indeed the circumstance for GH production, as many GHRH neurons in the arcuate nucleus and SS neurons in the periventricular nucleus (PeN) project to the hypophyseal portal vasculature[25,26] to directly modulate GH production by the somatotrophs of the anterior pituitary.

Although GHRH and SS neurons are directly involved in controlling GH secretion, many other hypothalamic neuropeptides and factors also play an important role in this process. Indeed, one of the functions of these two populations of neurons is to integrate incoming signals from other hypothalamic neurons and higher cortical areas, as well as circulating factors that feedback at the hypothalamic level, to control GH synthesis and secretion. Thus, it is the balance between numerous factors at the level of the hypothalamus and finally at the somatotroph, that will ultimately determine GH output from the anterior pituitary (Fig. 6.1).

Somatostatin

In 1973, the 14 amino acid GH-inhibiting peptide, somatostatin-14 (SS-14) was isolated and sequenced.[27] The 28 amino acid N-terminal-extended form of this tetradecapeptide (SS-28) was later isolated,[28–31] with a common 15 kDa polypeptide serving as the precursor for both isoforms.[31] The GH-inhibiting properties of SS were first demonstrated in pituitary cell cultures[27,32] and it is now believed that SS plays a determining role in the basal or interpulse level of GH secretion.[33,34] Although SS-14 is thought to be the predominant isoform involved in inhibiting GH secretion, SS-28 is also released from rat hypothalamic nerve endings in vitro[35] and is secreted into the hypophyseal portal system of rats in concentrations adequate for the inhibition of GH release.[36,37] Furthermore, on a molar basis the potency of SS-28 in inhibiting GH appears to be similar to, or even higher than that of SS-14,[38] which may be due to the fact that SS-28 binds to the pituitary with greater affinity than SS-14[39] and has a longer circulating half-life.[40]

Somatostatin is widely expressed throughout the brain and peripheral tissues.[41] In the CNS, SS-containing neurons are found in the neocortex, amygdala, hippocampus, olfactory bulb, throughout the hypothalamus, including the PeN, paraventricular nucleus (PVN), arcuate nucleus and ventromedial nucleus (VMN), as well as in many other brain areas.[42–44] The majority of SS projections to the median

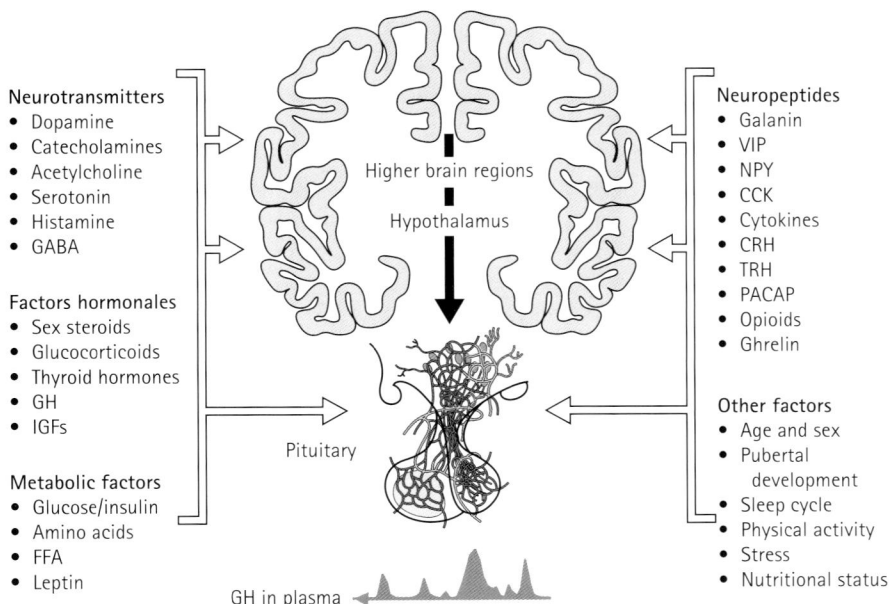

Figure 6.1 Schematic representation of the factors that can modulate the neuroendocrine control of growth hormone secretion.

eminence arise from the PeN[26,44] with these neurons playing a key role in the neuroendocrine control of pituitary function;[45] whereas in other areas of the CNS, SS is thought to act as a neuromodulator or neurotransmitter.[46,47] Hence, it is this population of SS neurons in the PeN that are most directly involved in the control of anterior pituitary hormones, including GH. These neurons interact with numerous other neuronal populations, including those expressing neuropeptide Y (NPY), γ-aminobutyric acid (GABA), corticotrophin-releasing hormone (CRH), GHRH, galanin and proopiomelanocortin (POMC),[48,49] all implicated in the control of GH secretion and possibly mediating their actions, at least in part, through modulation of SS release into the portal vasculature.

Five separate SS receptor (sstr1–5) genes have been identified, with sstr2 having two splice variants referred to as sstr2A and sstr2B. These receptors belong to the superfamily of G protein-coupled receptors and share the characteristic seven-transmembrane-segment topography. These five receptors share common signaling pathways such as inhibition of adenylyl cyclase, activation of phosphotyrosine phosphatase (PTP), and modulation of mitogen-activated protein kinase (MAPK). However, receptor specific mechanisms also exist as some subtypes are coupled to plasma membrane channels (e.g., inward rectifying K^+ channels or voltage-dependent Ca^{2+} channels), which modifies the cellular response. In both humans and laboratory animals, sstr2 and sstr5 are the subtypes most intimately involved in the regulation of GH secretion.[50–52]

Growth hormone–releasing hormone

The isolation of GHRH proved to be a formidable task, which in retrospect can be attributed to its miniscule concentration in the CNS and its susceptibility to biological inactivation during purification procedures. In 1982, human GHRH was ultimately purified and sequenced by two independent groups, each working with tissue from pancreatic islet adenomas from acromegalic subjects.[53,54] This peptide was shown to be present in three molecular forms, GHRH(1–44), GHRH(1–40), and GHRH(1–37).[53–55] In contrast, rat GHRH contains 43 amino acids and is structurally different from other GHRH peptides.[56] This hormone belongs to the family of brain–gut peptides that also includes glucagon, glucagon-like peptide (GLP)-1, GLP-2, vasoactive intestinal peptide (VIP), secretin, peptide histidine–methionine (PHM), glucose-dependent insulinotropic polypeptide (GIP) and pituitary adenylate cyclase-activating peptide (PACAP).[57,58] The rat GHRH gene spans nearly 10 kb of genomic DNA, contains five exons and encodes the 104 amino acid GHRH precursor.[59] The gene that codes for human GHRH, also of approximately 10 kb and containing five exons, is located on the long arm of chromosome 20 at band 20q11.2.[60]

Growth hormone-releasing hormone is produced by neurons located in the hypothalamic arcuate nucleus and ventromedial hypothalamic area, but those that project to the median eminence are primarily located in the arcuate nucleus.[61,62] In rats a small population of GHRH positive neurons have been described in the paraventricular nucleus and dorsomedial nucleus[25] and in humans in the periformical region and the periventricular zone.[61,63] A subset of GHRH neurons in the basal hypothalamus contain other neuropeptides or neuropeptide-producing enzymes such as the catecholamine synthesizing enzyme, tyrosine hydroxylase (TH), choline acetyltransferase (ChAT), GABA, or the neuropeptides neurotensin, galanin, or NPY.[64–68] It has been suggested that the co-release of these peptides with GHRH can modulate pituitary responsiveness and therefore GH secretion.[69]

The arcuate nucleus is located at the base of the hypothalamus, surrounding the ventral part of the third ventricle. In the rat brain, it is the third largest of the hypothalamic nuclei, extending rostral–caudally for approximately 2.8 mm.[70] The complex anatomical organization of this nucleus, with extensive afferents to and efferents from numerous other brain regions, indicates that it plays an important role in a variety of physiological functions. This is further evidenced by the number of neuropeptides and transmitters produced in this nucleus, including acetylcholine, dopamine, dynorphin, NPY, GHRH, SS, substance P, enkephalin, β-endorphin, ghrelin, galanin, amongst others.[42,61,62,65,67,71]

Growth hormone-releasing hormone appears to be involved in every facet of GH physiology as it stimulates the proliferation of somatotropes,[72] GH synthesis[73] and GH release.[53,54] After binding to specific GTP-linked receptors in the cell membrane of somatotrophs, various intracellular signaling mechanisms are activated including the adenylate cyclase–cAMP–protein kinase A, MAPK, Ca^{2+}, calmodulin, inositol phosphate–diacylglycerol–protein kinase C and the arachidonic acid–eicosanoic pathways.[74,75]

Generation of pulsatile growth hormone secretion

It is the coordinated interplay of GHRH and SS that orchestrates the pulsatile secretion of GH. As mentioned previously, GHRH is primarily responsible for the amplitude of the episodic event, whereas SS mainly determines the interpulse baseline GH level. Indeed, GHRH is indispensable for pulsatile GH secretion as this cannot be generated solely by removal of the inhibitory tone exerted by SS.[76] However, the inhibitory tone exerted by SS also contributes to GH pulse amplitude since release of SS's suppressive effects results in a rebound release of GH both in vivo and in vitro.[34,77] Therefore, to generate regular episodic release of GH, a reciprocal pattern of GHRH and SS release into the portal vasculature would be optimum. Such pattern is observed in the adult male rat where GHRH and SS are released in an episodic manner and 180° out of phase with each other.[7] Each GHRH pulse is preceded by a reduction in portal blood SS levels so that a burst of GH secretion occurs as a result of an increased stimulatory input and a concomitant reduction in the inhibitory tone exerted by SS.

To create this reciprocity between these two hypothalamic factors, it would be expected that SS and GHRH neurons communicate among themselves. Indeed, GHRH neurons form synapses on other GHRH neurons in the arcuate nucleus[78] and SS neurons form synapses on other SS neurons in the PeN,[79,80] with many SS neurons also expressing SS receptors.[81] In addition, numerous SS fibers lie in close approximation to GHRH perikarya and, although few in number, GHRH fibers can be found in close association with SS cell bodies,[82] raising the possibility for direct interaction between these two cell types. Furthermore, approximately 15% of GHRH mRNA containing neurons in the Arc expressing the sst1 receptor gene and 15% the sst2 receptor.[83] Experimental evidence suggests that GHRH stimulates SS secretion[84] and vice versa.[85,86]

At the level of the pituitary, GHRH and SS have noncompetitive antagonistic effects.[87] Through activation of the adenylate cyclase system, GHRH stimulates GH synthesis and secretion,[88] while SS suppresses cAMP levels. Of course numerous other factors are also involved in this process via modulation of GHRH or SS secretion or through a direct action at the level of the somatotroph.

OTHER HYPOTHALAMIC FACTORS

Neuropeptide Y

Neuropeptide Y, a member of the pancreatic polypeptide family, is the most abundant peptide in the CNS.[89] In addition to modulating food intake and energy balance, NPY inhibits GH secretion.[90–92] This inhibitory action of NPY may be mediated by stimulation of SS release,[92,93] which is supported by anatomical data demonstrating synaptic connections between NPY positive axons and SS neurons in the PeN.[94] Stimulation of SS release by NPY may be mediated in part by $\alpha 1$ and β-adrenergic receptor-mediated mechanisms.[92] Neuropeptide Y can also inhibit GHRH release.[93] Agouti related protein (AGRP), coexpressed in NPY neurons in the arcuate nucleus, does not appear to modulate GH secretion when injected i.c.v.[95]

As discussed below, circulating factors such as ghrelin, leptin, and GH itself may exert their hypothalamic effects, at least in part, through modulation of NPY secretion.[96,97] Indeed, NPY neurons in the arcuate nucleus express the GH receptor[98,99] and growth hormone secretagogue receptors (GHS) or ghrelin receptors.[100] Hence, these neurons play a fundamental role in integration of circulating metabolic signals to ultimately modify GH secretion through increasing SS and decreasing GHRH release.

Corticotropin-releasing hormone

Corticotropin-releasing hormone (CRH), involved in response of the CNS to stress, inhibits GH release and may be involved in decreased secretion of GH during some types of stress in the rat.[101–103] This effect is most likely mediated through modulation of both hypothalamic SS and GHRH neurons by CRH.[84,103] However, the effects of CRH on GH secretion in humans is less clear, as some authors report an inhibitory effect[104–106] and others no effect or a stimulatory effect.[107,108] The inhibitory effect of CRH(1–41) on GHRH-(1–29)-NH$_2$-induced GH release is not a result of ACTH or cortisol release, but most likely reflects a direct action of CRH on GH secretion, possibly via stimulation of somatostatin release.[106] Hence, the acute rise in GH following glucocorticoid administration could be explained in part by a rapid suppression of endogenous CRH.

Thyrotropin–releasing hormone

Under specific pathological situations TRH has been shown to stimulate GH release in humans.[109,110] In the laboratory rat, TRH has been shown to stimulate GH release in vitro and in vivo from pituitaries removed from hypothalamic control or during fetal and neonatal development.[49,111,112] These studies suggest a direct stimulatory effect of TRH at the level of the somatotroph, which expresses the TRH receptor.[113] At the level of the hypothalamus TRH may act to inhibit GH secretion most likely through modification of the somatostatinergc system.[101,109,114] Indeed, incongruencies in the literature regarding the effects of TRH on GH secretion in vivo may be related to the existing SS tone in the experimental paradigm.

Galanin

Galanin is a 29 amino acid peptide that is expressed throughout the CNS, but is highly concentrated in the hypothalamus, and stimulates GH secretion when administered either systemically or intraventricularly.[115–117] Not only does this peptide stimulate GH secretion, but it also stimulates release of GHRH[118] and potentiates the GHRH effects on GH secretion.[119,120] As mentioned above, galanin is co-expressed in GHRH neurons in the hypothalamus. This co-localization is sexually dimorphic with expression of galanin in GHRH neurons being higher in adult male rats compared to females.[68] Expression of galanin in these neurons is a target for GH feedback and is significantly reduced when GH is removed from the circulation.[98] In vitro galanin has been shown to stimulate both somatostatin and GHRH release in a dose-related manner and this was suggested to be mediated through a dopamine dependent mechanism.[121] Galanin may also directly affect somatostatin neurons in the PeN as they express galanin receptors.[98] In addition, the cholinergic,[122,123] catecholaminergic[124,125] and GABA[124] systems have all been proposed as mediators of galanin's effects on GH secretion.

Endogenous opioids

In the laboratory rat, both endogenous opioids and opiates, such as morphine, have been shown to stimulate GH secretion.[126,127] In humans this effect is less clear. Opioids may stimulate GH through GHRH release, as immunization with GHRH antiserum blocks the rise in GH induced by β-endorphin or morphine.[76] In addition, there are anatomical connections between β-endorphin containing terminals and somatostatin neurons in the rat hypothalamus.[128]

In laboratory rats, β-endorphin has been suggested to modulate GH through multiple opioid receptor subtypes, including δ, κ, and μ receptors.[129] In humans, the stimulatory effect of opioids on GH secretion appears to be mediated by μ receptors,[130] whereas the δ receptor subtype may mediate an inhibitory effect on GH secretion.[131] Some of the controversy regarding the effects of endogenous opioids on GH secretion could be due to differences in their acute or chronic effects.

Vasoactive intestinal peptide

Vasoactive intestinal peptide is found in both the pituitary and hypothalamus, with projections to the median eminence releasing this peptide into the portal vasculature.[132,133] When injected intracerebroventricularly, VIP stimulates GH secretion in rats, while systemic administration has no effect.[134,135] However, VIP has been shown to stimulate GH secretion from pituitaries *in vitro*,[135] but this may depend on the existing inhibitory tone exerted by SS.[136]

In humans, i.v. injection of VIP is reported to have no effect in normal human subjects, but stimulates GH secretion in patients with acromegaly.[137,138] In cultured pituitary adenomas from patients with acromegaly VIP stimulates GH release,[137] suggesting that this effect may be due to changes in the pituitary's response to this peptide.

Pituitary adenylate cyclase–activating peptide

Another member of the brain–gut family implicated in controlling GH secretion is PACAP. In addition to the gut, this 38 amino acid peptide is produced in a number of tissues including brain, pituitary, adrenal gland, reproductive tissue, and lung. Although produced in many brain areas, the highest concentration of PACAP is found in the hypothalamus. A dense network of PACAP positive fibers is found in the median eminence, suggesting that it is released into the portal vasculature.[139] Receptors for PACAP are found in somatotrophs of both rodents and humans and activation of these receptors increases cAMP production and Ca^{2+} release.[139] This in turn stimulates GH release and/or production depending upon the species or the experimental paradigm.[139–141] It is suggested that PACAP and GHRH work through the same intracellular signaling mechanism at the level of the somatotroph,[141] but PACAP may also have an indirect action on other pituitary cell types[142] or at the hypothalamic level through modulation of serotoninergic release of GH.[143]

Cytokines

Cytokines have emerged as a liaison between the neuroendocrine and immune systems. Intracerebroventricular injections of interleukin (IL)-1 and IL-2 have been shown to increase GH secretion[144–146] or to decrease GH secretion.[147,148] The inhibitory effect of IL-1 is suggested to be through the inhibition of GHRH, which is mediated by nitric oxide (NO) and stimulation of SS, also through NO.[149]

At the pituitary level, IL-1β, IL-2, and IL-6 were shown to stimulate GH secretion, but only IL-6 stimulated GH production.[150,151] Curiously, although IL-1β alone stimulated GH secretion, it inhibited galanin induced GH secretion, as did TGFα, while IL-6 potentiated the effect of other GH-releasing factors.[150] In addition, both IL-11 and ciliary neurotropic factor (CNTF) have been shown to stimulate GH release,[152] suggesting that many cytokines may have diverse effects on GH secretion. As cytokine receptors are expressed in the pituitary gland,[153] a direct effect of these factors is possible.

Insulin–like growth factor

The insulin-like growth factors (IGF-I and II) are mitogenic peptides that have a potent affect on cell growth and differentiation during both the prenatal and postnatal periods.[154–156] It was originally thought that GH promoted systemic growth by acting mainly on the liver to stimulate IGF-I production, which then reached target tissues via the circulation to activate mechanisms involved in tissue proliferation, growth and metabolism. Indeed, GH, after binding to its transmembrane receptor, initiates a signaling cascade leading to transcriptional regulation of the IGF-I and related genes.[157] However, it is now evident that not only does GH have independent actions that do not involve IGF-I production,[158] but IGF-I synthesis occurs in many tissues, including the hypothalamus, under the control of a variety of local and circulating factors, which may or may not include GH.[156,159–162] Furthermore, this local production of IGF-I may be directly responsible for some of the growth promoting effects of GH, indicating paracrine or autocrine effects, rather than or in addition to the classical endocrine mechanism via circulating growth factor.[162]

Data concerning the role of IGF-I in neuroendocrine control of GH secretion are controversial, although most suggest that it has an inhibitory effect. Some authors report that IGF-I does not modulate GH secretion via action at the hypothalamic level,[163,164] while others have demonstrated a direct inhibitory effect[165–168] through modulation of GHRH[165,166,168] and SS[166,168,169] neurons. Indeed, IGF-I administered i.c.v. mimics the negative feedback effects of GH, while immunoneutralization of hypothalamic IGF-I blocks GH feedback.[166] In addition, increasing circulating GH stimulates the production of IGF-I in the hypothalamus.[170] Hence, centrally produced IGF-I appears to be involved in the negative feedback control of GH secretion[166–169] and this may be mediated, at least in part, via GH induced production of hypothalamic IGF-I and subsequent modulation of SS and GHRH.[166] However, although the IGF-I receptor is expressed in the hypothalamus,[171] whether it is expressed in GHRH and SS neurons of postnatal animals remains to be demonstrated.

The role of circulating IGF-I on GH secretion and its effect on the anterior pituitary is discussed below.

Ghrelin

The isolation of a new hormone, ghrelin, was reported at the end of 1999.[172] This peptide is produced mainly by the stomach and will be discussed in detail below in the section regarding feedback effects of circulating hormones. However, Kojima et al.[172] reported that a ghrelin transcript could also be detected in brain by RT-PCR amplification. Subsequently, immunohistochemical analyses performed after colchicine treatments revealed that ghrelin-immunoreactive neurons are located in a theretofore uncharacterized group of neurons adjacent to the third ventricle between the hypothalamic dorsal, ventral, paraventricular and arcuate nuclei.[173] These neurons send efferents to key hypothalamic circuits, including those producing NPY, AGRP, POMC products, and CRH. Within the hypothalamus, ghrelin binds mostly to presynaptic terminals of NPY neurons, stimulates electrophysiological activity of arcuate NPY neurons and mimics the effect of NPY in the PVN.[173] Hence, it has been proposed that locally produced ghrelin may stimulate the release of orexigenic peptides and neurotransmitters, thus representing a novel regulatory circuit controlling energy homeostasis.[173] The role of these neurons in the control of GH secretion remains to be determined.

Classical neurotransmitters

The monoamine neurotransmitters include catecholamine (CA), dopamine (DE), norepinephrine (NE), epinephrine (E), histamine, and the indoleamines (5-HT) and can be found throughout the CNS.[174] Both the internal and external layers of the median eminence receive innervation from these systems. The hypothalamus receives NE projections from a ventral projection from the pons and medulla. One of the most important DA inputs to the median eminence arises from the tuberoinfundibulum. The major 5-HT projections to the hypothalamus and median eminence are received from the pontine raphe. The hypothalamus itself, including the arcuate nucleus and median eminence, is an important source of the acetylcholine synthesizing enzyme, CAT. Histamine is also produced in the hypothalamus, in particular in the arcuate, ventromedial and dorsomedial nuclei.

Specific amino acids also function as central neurotransmitters, including GABA, glycine, glutamate, and aspartate. GABAergic neurons are found in the hypothalamus and GAD has been located in different areas of this region. There is a GABAergic pathway that projects from the arcuate nucleus to the median eminence that is most likely involved in neuroendocrine control. Glutamate and aspartate are both found in high concentrations in many regions of the brain. In the hypothalamus, the arcuate, ventromedial and periventricular nuclei all have high concentrations of these amino acids, with projections to the median eminence.

CATECHOLAMINES

In both humans and rats GH secretion is stimulated through activation of the α-adrenergic receptor.[175,176] Pharmacological experiments show that when hypothalamic catecholamine stores are depleted, the decrease in GH secretion can be restored with the α_2-adrenergic receptor agonist clonidine, but not apomorphine, a DA agonist.[176] Likewise, inhibition of spontaneous GH secretion by specific inhibition of NE and E synthesis is also reestablished with clonidine administration.[177] Furthermore, selective inhibition of E synthesis, with no change in DA or NE stores in the hypothalamus, also reduced GH secretion and could be restored with clonidine, suggesting that E may be the most important catecholamine in the control of GH secretion.[178] Catecholamines appear to act through stimulation of GHRH release,[179–183] although chronic stimulation may inhibit GHRH production.[184] This chronic effect could be the result of a negative feedback effect of the increased GH secretion on GHRH production and not directly mediated by catecholamines. A decrease in hypothalamic SS content has also been reported after acute, but not chronic clonidine treatment.[183]

The responsiveness of GHRH and SS neurons to catecholamines may be developmentally regulated,[183] in addition to being dependent on the status of the hypothalamic secretory rhythm.[185] If clonidine is administered at the time of a spontaneous GH peak, it has no effect, while if given during a nadir GH release is stimulated. Furthermore, if clonidine is administered during the nadir before a GHRH challenge, the GH response is potentiated,[186] suggesting that SS neurons are involved in the response to clonidine. Furthermore, anatomical data support catecholamine innervation of SS neurons in the PeN.[187]

The role of α_1-adrenoceptors in stimulation of GH secretion is less clear and may be species related.[177,188–190] However, at least in the rat, these receptors mediate a negative effect on GH secretion.[177,190] This inhibitory response is most likely mediated through SS neurons as they receive NA afferents from the locus coeruleus[191] and activation of this region modulates GH secretion.[192] In humans, α_1-adrenoceptor agonists have been reported to stimulate GH secretion,[188] but there is little other evidence in the literature to support this finding.

The β-adrenergic receptor also mediates a negative effect on GH secretion. In humans, the GH response to

GHRH is inhibited by a β_2-adrenergic agonist.[193,194] Furthermore, activation of the β_2-adrenergic pathway not only inhibits the GH response to GHRH, but also to arginine and pyridostigmine, a cholinesterase inhibitor, and their interaction with GHRH.[194]

In humans, DA agonists increase GH release and the GH response to GHRH.[195] However, DA can blunt the GH response to other stimuli such as arginine or hypoglycemia.[196,197] These conflicting results may be explained by the fact that DA can release both GHRH and SS from rat hypothalamus.[118] The importance of DA to this system is exemplified by the fact that mice lacking the dopamine D2 receptor have decreased GH secretion, decreased number of somatotrophs and decreased response to GHRH. These mice are normal in size at birth, but are significantly smaller than littermates in postnatal life.[198] Furthermore, allelic variations in the D2 receptor gene have been suggested to play a role in some cases of idiopathic short stature in children.[199] Further evidence that DA has a direct effect on SS expression in the PeN comes from studies demonstrating that agonists of the D2/D3 receptors activate cFOS in these neurons, while D1 agonists do not.[200]

SEROTONIN

Serotonin has been shown to exert a stimulatory effect on GH release in rats, dogs and humans, although in sheep it may be inhibitory.[201–204] Many of the conflicting reports in the literature, especially regarding humans, may be due to the different 5-HT receptor agonists and antagonist employed, or the physiological situation of the patient or experimental animal. It is clear that in the beagle, the 5-HT(2C) and 5-HT(1D) receptors play a stimulatory role in GH secretion, the later possibly by acting through a decrease in hypothalamic SS release. However, 5-HT(2A) and 5-HT(3) receptors do not appear to be involved in the control of basal or GHRH-induced GH secretion.[204] In humans, 5-HT(1D) receptors have also been reported to have a stimulatory effect on GH secretion, possibly by inhibiting hypothalamic SS release,[201] while 5-HT(2) receptors may not be involved.[203,205] Indeed, serotoninergic inputs to SS neurons in the PeN have been described.[206]

Changes in the serotoninergic pathway are thought to mediate some of the aberrant GH responses in patients with depression, where depressed patients have a reduced GH response to clonidine.[202] Serotonin may also play a role in mediating the stimulatory effect of PACAP on GH secretion.[143] There is a close functional relationship between the adrenergic and serotoninergic pathways in the control of GH secretion, where an intact serotoninergic system may be fundamental for the response to adrenergic stimuli.[207]

ACETYLCHOLINE

The first clear demonstrations of the stimulatory effect of the central cholinergic system on GH release in humans[208] and in rats[209] were published in 1978. This effect is mediated through muscarinic receptors,[209–214] and probably also nicotinic mechanisms.[214] There is clear evidence that activation of muscarinic receptors is involved in endogenous opioid[213] and GHRH[212] stimulation of GH secretion, which may be mediated through the SS system.[215] The central cholinergic system may also be involved in the sleep-associated rise in GH release, as well as in the response to insulin-induced hypoglycemia.[214]

Muscarinic cholinergic receptors are found in the anterior pituitary[216] and acetylcholine modulates GH secretion directly at the level of the pituitary.[217–219] Although most studies indicate a stimulatory effect of acetylcholine at the pituitary level,[218–220] it is possible that acetylcholine can be inhibitory to GH secretion.[217,218] This differential response may depend on the concentration of dexamethasone present.[218] A synergistic stimulatory effect of acetylcholine and GHRH on GH release at the level of the pituitary has also been demonstrated in rats,[220] although this may not be true in humans.[212]

HISTAMINE

The role of histamine in the neural control of GH secretion in humans remains unclear. Although no effect or a stimulatory influence has been hypothesized in man,[221–223] the stimulatory effect may be associated with sleep.[222] However, in the rat histamine appears to have an inhibitory effect[224,225] that is mediated through both SS and GHRH, but with differential responses to acute or chronic treatment.[224] Histamine has also been shown to block the GH releasing effects of clonidine.[225]

AMINO ACIDS

Glutamate, which acts as an excitatory neurotransmitter in the CNS, stimulates GH secretion[226–229] through NMDA, kainate and AMPA receptors.[228,229] Glutamate can stimulate GH release directly at the level of the pituitary[227,228] with the majority of the input of glutamate to this gland coming from the hypothalamus. In pituitary cultures, SS inhibits the stimulatory effect of glutamate, suggesting an interaction of these two substances at the pituitary level to control GH secretion.[228]

The role of GABA in GH control remains controversial as both stimulatory and inhibitory effects have been reported. Indeed, GABA could play a dual role in GH control depending on the physiological state of the animal. γ-Aminobutyric acid injected either systemically or intraventricularly stimulates circulating GH concentrations in humans, rats and sheep.[124,230–234] However, no physiological effect was reported in pre-pubertal animals or in some studies on adult rats.[229,235] In adult rats, simultaneous injection of SS had no effect on GABA induced GH release,[234] although GABA antagonists inhibited GH stimulation induced by i.c.v. injection of SS.[236] GABA is suggested to inhibit SS release resulting in increased GH secretion[233] and has been shown to inhibit SS release in vitro.[237] Indeed, SS neurons in the PeN receive GABAergic inputs.[236] In addition, the stimulatory effect of GABA is inhibited by i.c.v. injection of GHRH antiserum.[238] Blockage of GABA blunts the opioid[238] and galanin[124] induced increases in GH and GABA releases galanin from the hypothalamus *in vitro*.[239] This amino acid may also be involved in the stimulation of GH release by GH secretagogues[240] and could activate the dopaminergic pathways in humans.[231]

The direct effect of GABA on GH release from the pituitary is less. In some studies in adult rats GABA had no effect,[232] while others report that GABA stimulated GH release from adult, as well as in neonatal rats.[241,242] However, somatotrophs express the GABA-C receptor subunit rho2 and demonstrate GABA-induced Cl-currents,[243] supporting an existing mechanism for response to this amino acid.

FEEDBACK CONTROL BY PERIPHERAL FACTORS

Growth hormone itself has a negative feedback action at the hypothalamus, stimulating SS and inhibiting GHRH synthesis.[244] Somatostatin neurons in the PeN express the GH receptor, suggesting a direct action on this neuropeptide system.[96,245] In contrast, GHRH neurons do not appear to express this receptor.[96,98] The negative feedback effect on this neuropeptide system is thought to occur, at least in part, via modulation of NPY neurons in the arcuate nucleus.[96,98,99] As NPY is intimately involved in metabolic control, this is one possible vinculum between the control of growth and metabolism. Other circulating factors involved in growth and metabolism, such as IGF-I, leptin, ghrelin, free fatty acids, and insulin, also modulate GH secretion at the level of the hypothalamus.

Growth hormone

Growth hormone feeds back at the level of the hypothalamus to inhibit its own synthesis and secretion. Hypophysectomy decreases hypothalamic SS content and mRNA levels and these are returned to normal with GH administration.[246,247] Furthermore, the effect of GH on central SS synthesis is specific to those neurons involved in regulating GH secretion.[247] Expression of the GH receptor in SS neurons of the PeN[245] indicates that this feedback can be directly exerted on this neuronal population.

The feedback mechanism of GH on GHRH is less clear. Hypophysectomy decreases GHRH immunoreactive levels, which are restored after GH treatment.[248] In contrast, GHRH mRNA levels are significantly increased in response to hypophysectomy, returning to control levels with GH replacement.[249] These data suggest that GH has a stimulatory effect on both GHRH synthesis and secretion. Hypophysectomy also reduces galanin mRNA expression in GHRH neurons, suggesting another mechanism of feedback at the hypothalamic level.[250] However, although the GH receptor is highly expressed in the arcuate nucleus, the vast majority of GHRH neurons do not express its mRNA.[251]

It was later demonstrated that NPY neurons in this area of the hypothalamus express the GH receptor[96,98,99] and have been implicated in the negative effect of GH on GHRH neurons.[96] Somatostatin receptor type-2 knock-out mice are refractory to the negative feedback effect of GH, even though GH can activate c-fos expression in PeN SS neurons in these animals.[252] Hence, the GH-mediated negative feedback involves signaling between periventricular and arcuate neurons with the signal being transduced specifically through SS subtype 2 receptors.[252]

Whether GH stimulates local production of IGF-I in the hypothalamus and if this is involved in some of its feedback effects at the level of the CNS remains controversial. The role of IGF-I in the control of GH secretion is addressed in the following section.

Insulin–like growth factor

Insulin-like growth factor 1 exerts a negative feedback effect on GH secretion via either direct actions at the pituitary level or indirect ones at the hypothalamic level, through stimulation of somatostatin (SS) and/or inhibition of GHRH release. Insulin-like growth factor was first identified and purified from blood and the best data at the time indicated that the liver was its major, if not sole, site of synthesis. However, in the early 1980s it was observed that explants from multiple fetal mouse tissues released immunoreactive IGF-I into the cultured media and that a large portion of this material was recognized by cell surface receptors specific for IGF-I.[159] It is now known that multiple human fetal and adult tissues synthesize IGF-I, including intestine, muscle, kidney, placenta, stomach, lung, heart, skin, pancreas, brain, testes, spleen, and adrenal and that its production may or may not be regulated by GH.[156,160,161,170,253] Hence, it was postulated that the actions of IGF-I are predominately local, being exerted either on the cells of origin (autocrine actions) or on nearby cells (paracrine actions) and that a significant part is dependent on GH regulation, at least postnatally.

As discussed above, IGF-I produced in the hypothalamus is most likely involved in the control of GH secretion. In addition, circulating IGF-I can also play an important role in this process as this growth factor is transported into cells of the hypothalamus[254] and this uptake is modulated by the hormonal status.[255] Recombinant human IGF-I (rhIGF-I) in humans inhibits spontaneous GH secretion, as well as the GH response to GHRH. The acute inhibitory effect of rhIGF-I on the GH response to GHRH may take place at the hypothalamic level, possibly via enhancement of SS release, and this effect can be inhibited by arginine.[256]

In primary pituitary cell cultures, IGF-I inhibits GH mRNA levels,[257,258] and secretion.[257] As all components of the IGF system are produced in the pituitary,[259] this factor could have both a paracrine and autocrine effect on anterior pituitary hormone production. In addition, a role for liver derived IGF-I in this process is exemplified by the fact that in liver IGF-I knock-out mice circulating GH levels are increased, with no change in hypothalamic GHRH, NPY or SS mRNA levels, although hypothalamic IGF-I expression is increased. These animals also have increased pituitary expression of GHRH and GHS receptors, as well as an increased GH response to these ligands.[260]

Ghrelin

Since the 1980s it has been known that small synthetic molecules called growth hormone secretagogues (GHSs) stimulate the release of GH from the pituitary. These exogenous substances act through the GHS receptor (GHS-R), a G protein-coupled receptor[261] and in 1999, Kojima et al.[172] reported the purification and identification from rat stomach of an endogenous ligand specific for this receptor. These authors[172] named this new GH-releasing peptide 'ghrelin' ('ghre' is the Proto-Indo-European root of the word 'grow'). Ghrelin consists of 28 amino acids in which the serine-3 residue is n-octanoylated. The acylated peptide specifically releases growth hormone (GH) both in vivo and in vitro, and O-n-octanoylation at serine-3 is essential for this activity. Human ghrelin is homologous to rat ghrelin apart from two amino acids.[262] Human pre-pro-ghrelin, isolated from a stomach cDNA library, consists of 117 amino acids, producing an mRNA of 0.62 kb, and the rat and human pre-pro-ghrelins are 82.9 percent identical.[262] In situ hybridization indicated that ghrelin mRNA is found in the stomach from the neck to the base of the oxyntic gland,[262] with ghrelin immuno-reactive cells having the same distribution.[262] In the secretory granules of X/A-like cells, a distinct endocrine cell type found in the submucosal layer of the stomach,[262,263] round, compact, electron-dense granules filled with ghrelin are found. In addition, ghrelin immunoreactive cells are also found in the small and large intestines.

Ghrelin, when injected intravenously, induces GH release, suggesting that circulating ghrelin may be involved in controlling the GH axis. Indeed, ghrelin strongly stimulates GH release in humans in a dose-dependent manner, being even more potent than GHRH[264] and this effect is mediated through the GHS receptor.[265] The lowest dose of ghrelin used in the experiments of Takaya et al.[264] ($0.2\,\mu g\,kg^{-1}$) led to massive GH release ($43.3 \pm 6.0\,ng\,mL^{-1}$), with minimum effects on ACTH or prolactin and no effect on serum LH, FSH or TSH levels. In addition to its role in regulating GH secretion, ghrelin is intimately involved in energy balance homeostasis and signals the hypothalamus when an increase in metabolic efficiency is necessary.[266] However, the role of this peptide in food intake and energy balance is beyond the scope of this chapter. (See van der Lely et al.[261] for a review of this subject.)

It is plausible that some of the effects of ghrelin on GH secretion, whether circulating or locally produced in the hypothalamus, are mediated via modulation of NPY neurons. After i.c.v. administration of ghrelin, Fos protein, a marker of neuronal activation, is found in NPY and AGRP neurons and augments NPY gene expression.[267] Indeed, as discussed above these neurons express the GHS-R and are thought to be involved in modulation of GHRH neurons in the arcuate nucleus. The mRNA for GHS-R is expressed in approximately 94 percent of the neurons expressing NPY, while only 20–25 percent of GHRH neurons are reported to express this receptor.[100] However, this indicates that ghrelin may have both direct and indirect effects on GHRH neurons, in addition to modulating SS neurons where approximately 30 percent also express this receptor.[100]

Howard et al.[268] cloned a G protein-coupled receptor of the pituitary and hypothalamus and showed it to be the target of GHSs, and hence ghrelin. Nucleotide sequence analysis revealed two cDNAs, apparently derived from the same gene, referred to as Ia and Ib. The full-length human Ia cDNA encodes a predicted polypeptide of 366 amino acids with seven transmembrane domains, a feature typical of G protein-coupled receptors, and a molecular mass of 41 kDa. This receptor is highly conserved across species, suggesting an essential biological function.[261] The type Ib receptor encodes a polypeptide of 289 amino acids with only five transmembrane domains and is derived by read-through of the intron. This produces an in-frame stop-codon so that the potential translation product has an identical N terminus with transmembrane domains 1–5, but lacking 6 and 7.

Binding of ligand to GHR 1a activates the phospholipase C signaling pathway, leading to increased inositol phosphate turnover and protein kinase C activation, followed by Ca^{2+} release from intracellular stores.[262,269] GHS-R activation also leads to an inhibition of K^+ channels, allowing the entry of Ca^{2+} through voltage-gated L-type, but not T-type channels.[270,271] Unlike GHSR 1a, GHSR 1b fails to bind and respond to some GHSs[268] and its functional role remains to be defined. The GHS-R 1a is expressed in the hypothalamus and anterior pituitary gland, where its expression is largely confined to somatotrophs and the arcuate nucleus,[100,268,272,273] consistent with its role in regulating GH release. In addition, detectable levels of GHS-R 1a mRNA are also found in various extrahypothalamic areas[273] indicating its involvement in as yet undefined non-endocrine actions.

Non-acylated ghrelin, which circulates in amounts far greater than the acylated form,[274] does not bind to hypothalamic or pituitary 1a receptors[275] and has no GH-releasing or other endocrine activities in rat,[172,276] although it may be involved in other aspects of ghrelin's actions.[274] In man, administration of non-acylated ghrelin does not induce changes in any hormonal parameters or in glucose levels, indicating that at least in humans, physiological concentrations of non-acylated ghrelin do not possess the endocrine activities of acylated ghrelin.[277]

Ghrelin might integrate the hormonal and metabolic response to fasting that, at least in humans, is connoted by a clear-cut increase in GH secretion coupled with inhibition of insulin secretion and activation of mechanisms devoted to maintaining glucose levels.[278,279] Ghrelin stimulates GH release, in part, directly at the level of the pituitary[280,281] via activation of cAMP production and accumulation, which is additive with the effects of GHRH. This increases intracellular

Ca^{2+} concentrations resulting in increased GH release, with this release being blocked by SS.[280,281] Hence, ghrelin may interact with intracellular mechanisms used by GHRH and SS to regulate GH release from somatotrophs. The pituitary itself produces ghrelin, and this production is augmented by GHRH and increases the somatotroph's GH response to GHRH.[282] Hence, the effect of ghrelin on GH secretion most likely involves both hypothalamic and pituitary mechanisms, with this peptide being produced either locally or arriving via the circulation. Indeed, in arcuate nucleus ablated rats, ghrelin's effect on food intake is totally abolished, while it continues to stimulate GH secretion, although to a significantly lower degree.[283]

Leptin

Leptin (from the Greek lepto meaning 'thin') was the name proposed by Halaas et al. for this fat-regulating hormone.[284] Leptin is a 16 kDa protein that plays a critical role in the regulation of body weight by inhibiting food intake and stimulating energy expenditure. This adipocyte-derived hormone suppresses feeding and stimulates thermogenesis and is proposed as a mediator of the negative feedback loop that controls body adiposity. This discovery led to a rapid revolution in the understanding of neurobiological mechanisms regulating obesity.[285] In addition to its effects on body weight, leptin has a variety of other functions, including the regulation of hematopoiesis, angiogenesis, wound healing, and immune and inflammatory responses.

Although evidence suggests that leptin may have a direct effect on GH release at the pituitary level,[286] most data indicate a hypothalamic mechanism. Intracerebroventricular administration of an antiserum to leptin decreased spontaneous GH secretion. However, while leptin itself had no effect in normally fed rats, it reversed the fasting induced decrease in GH secretion.[287,288] Leptin appears to inhibit the decrease in GH secretion induced by fasting through blockage of the inhibitory effect of NPY on this axis.[288] Leptin also accentuates the GH response to GHRH, which suggests a possible inhibition of hypothalamic SS release.[287] Indeed, leptin administered i.c.v. increases GHRH mRNA levels and decreases SS mRNA levels in the hypothalamus.[289] Leptin has high affinity transporters to cross the blood–brain barrier into the hypothalamus, as well as other brain areas.[290] The PI3K–PDE3B–cAMP pathway interacting with the JAK2–STAT3 pathways constitutes a critical component of leptin signaling in the hypothalamus.[291]

The leptin receptor (LEPR) is a single-transmembrane–domain receptor of the cytokine receptor family, with the highest homology to the IL-6, GCFS, and LIF receptors.[292] This receptor is expressed not only in the choroid plexus, but also in several other brain areas, including the hypothalamus.[292] The initial steps in leptin actions include activation of the JAK/STAT pathway. The STAT protein binds to phosphotyrosine residues in the cytoplasmic domain of the ligand-activated receptor, where they are subsequently phosphorylated. The activated STAT proteins dimerize and translocate to the nucleus where they bind DNA and activate transcription. In the hypothalamus, leptin injection activates STAT3 in a dose-dependent fashion.[293] In addition, Ghilardi et al.[294] cloned a long isoform of the wild type leptin receptor that is preferentially expressed in the hypothalamus and showed that it can activate STAT3, STAT5 and STAT6. Bates et al.[295] concluded that LEPR long form-STAT3 signaling mediates the effects of leptin on melanocortin production and body energy homeostasis, whereas distinct LEPR signals regulate NPY and the control of fertility, growth, and glucose homeostasis.

Glucocorticoids

It is well known that chronic treatment with glucocorticoids has an inhibitory effect on systemic growth. It is likely that glucocorticoids act at various levels, including pituitary, hypothalamus, and peripheral organs modulating GH synthesis, secretion, and action. In vitro, glucocorticoids increase the responsiveness of somatotrophs to GHRH[296] and decrease their responsiveness to SS most likely through modulation of receptor expression.[297] In the rat pituitary, glucocorticoids also modulate GH production at the transcriptional level with both negative and positive effects on GH expression, depending on the combination with other hormones and the time of exposure.[298] Señaris et al.[299] showed that in the rat, chronic treatment with dexamethasone decreases SS mRNA levels in the PeN and GHRH mRNA levels in the arcuate nucleus, with a decrease in GH receptor mRNA levels in both of these anatomical areas. However, in hypophysectomized rats, dexamethasone had no effect on SS mRNA levels, but decreases GHRH mRNA levels. These results suggest that the effect of dexamethasone on GHRH neurons is mediated directly at the level of the hypothalamus, while GH is responsible for mediating dexamethasone's effects on SS mRNA production.

Thyroid hormones

States of both hypo- and hyper-thyroidism result in reduced GH secretion.[300,301] As thyroid hormones stimulate GH production directly at the level of the pituitary,[119] this would explain the decrease in GH secretion in patients with hypothyroidism. In addition, responsiveness of the somatotroph to GHRH may also be modulated by thyroid hormones, possibly through decreasing GHRH receptor expression. The decrease in GH secretion due to hyperthyroid states could be mediated at the level of the hypothalamus either through IGF-I production or SS activity.[119,302]

Gonadal steroids

Changes in circulating levels of sex steroids modulate the synthesis, content and secretion of GH from the anterior pituitary,[12,303,304] which could be due to a direct action of gonadal steroids on the somatotroph and/or via modulation of the hypothalamic neuropeptides controlling GH secretion. While *in vitro* studies have shown that there may be no or only a slight effect of sex steroids on GH production at the pituitary level, the response of somatotrophs to hypothalamic factors may be modulated by the sex steroid environment.[258,305] Indeed, the ER is highly expressed in the anterior pituitary and estrogens have been demonstrated to have direct stimulatory effects through the proximal promoter region of GH gene.[298] In addition, the number of somatotrophs is permanently affected by the neonatal sex steroid environment.[306] However, the effect of sex steroids on this gland and other aspects of growth will be discussed in other chapters.

At the level of the hypothalamus, sex steroids also have both organizational and activational effects, at least in the

rat. Male rats have significantly more GHRH mRNA containing neurons than females, with no difference in the number of SS neurons in the PeN.[307] In addition, normal adult male rats have higher mean SS mRNA levels per neuron in the PeN and GHRH mRNA levels in the arcuate nucleus compared to females.[13,14,307] These differences in the number of GHRH neurons, SS and GHRH mRNA levels and GH secretion and growth pattern depend on exposure to sex steroids during both the neonatal and post-pubertal periods[12,303,307] (Fig. 6.2). Simonian *et al.*[308] demonstrated that the early organizational effects on SS neurons in the PeN are mediated through the ER, despite the fact that few or none of these neurons express this receptor, indicating mediation via another estrogen responsive cell type. *In vitro*, sex steroid effects on hypothalamic neuron survival are also mediated via the ER,[309] suggesting that the difference in GHRH

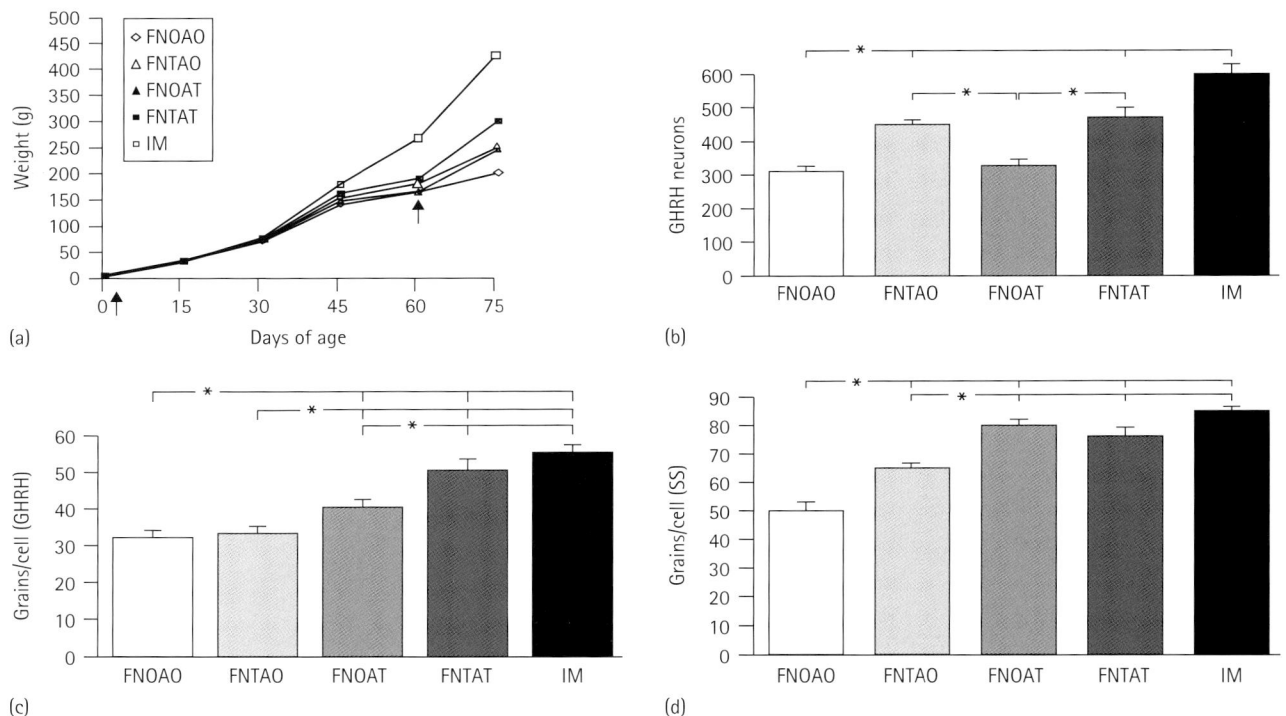

Figure 6.2 (a) Mean weight of rats throughout development. Normal males grow significantly faster than females beginning at puberty. Neonatal treatment of females with testosterone (T) results in an increased pubertal growth spurt, which then decreases after puberty if post-pubertal T is not received. (b) Mean number of growth hormone-releasing hormone (GHRH) neurons in the hypothalamus of adult rats. The number of GHRH neurons, as identified by *in situ* hybridization for GHRH mRNA, was counted in 10 anatomically matched sections throughout the arcuate nucleus and ventromedial hypothalamic area. There were significantly more GHRH neurons in adult male animals compared to adult females. If females received a single injection of T on the day of birth, the number of detectable GHRH neurons increased significantly. Treatment of female rats with T for 2 weeks with an implanted Silastic capsule from 60 to 75 days of age did not modify the number of GHRH neurons in the hypothalamus. The combination of neonatal and adult testosterone treatment did not have any significant impact on the number of GHRH neurons in comparison to neonatal treatment alone. (c) Relative mean levels of GHRH mRNA per neuron. Males have significantly more GHRH mRNA in the hypothalamus compared to females. Neonatal treatment with T had no significant effect, while adult T alone significantly increased GHRH mRNA levels in females, however, this increase was significantly greater if females received both neonatal and adult T. (d) Relative mean levels of somatostatin (SS) mRNA in the periventricular nucleus (PeN). Male rats have significantly more SS mRNA in the PeN compared to females. Both neonatal and adult T treatment significantly increased SS mRNA levels in female rats. FNOAO: normal female; FNTAO: female treated with testosterone neonatal; FNOAT: female treated with testosterone as an adult; FNTAT: female treated with testosterone both neonatally and as an adult; IM: intact male. (Modified from Chowen *et al.*[307].)

neuron number could involve estrogen promoted neuronal survival.

In the adult male animal, the stimulatory effect of testosterone on SS mRNA levels is mediated via the AR.[310] This effect is most likely direct as these neurons express the AR, with very few expressing the ER.[308,311] In contrast, the stimulatory effect of testosterone on GHRH mRNA levels is mediated through the ER[15] and these neurons express ERα[312] but not ARs.[313]

Glucose/insulin

Growth hormone secretion is modified in conditions of altered glucose metabolism or insulin secretion, such as obesity, diabetes or malnutrition. It is well established that GH release in humans is stimulated by hypoglycemia. Insulin injection stimulates GH release and decreases glucose levels, while intramuscular injection of glucagon increases GH, insulin and glucose levels.[314] This GH response most likely does not involve changes in circulating ghrelin, which is also modulated by insulin and glucose.[314,315] During hyperinsulinemic euglycemia, GH secretion did not change, but rose significantly after the onset of hypoglycemia and fell during the period of hyperglycemia.[315] However, hyperinsulinemia suppressed circulating ghrelin concentrations in the absence of hypoglycemia in these healthy subjects. No relationship between GH responses to hypoglycemia and ghrelin secretion supports studies showing that GHRH and SS are the critical intermediaries in this response. Jaffe et al.[316] demonstrated that the GH response to insulin-induced hypoglycemia is significantly suppressed by pretreatment with a GHRH antagonist. However, continuous infusion of GHRH does not sustain GH secretion, unlike prolonged hypoglycemia, suggesting that hypoglycemia (or insulin) may be suppressing SS.[317,318]

In rats, both hypo- and hyperglycemia suppress GH secretion[319,320] with this inhibitory effect most likely being mediated through stimulation of SS. Both acute hypo- and hyperglycemia stimulate SS mRNA levels, while only hyperglycemia stimulates GHRH mRNA levels.[320] Likewise, hypoglycemia stimulates the secretion of both GHRH and SS from hypothalamic fragments in vivo.[321] However, while GH secretion is reduced in diabetic rats, hypothalamic GHRH and SS mRNA levels are also reduced,[322,323] indicating a possible differential effect of acute and chronic hyperglycemia. In the diabetic rat the pituitary responsiveness to both SS and GHRH is also reduced,[323] as well as to the feedback effects of GH itself,[322] suggesting a possible pituitary involvement. Indeed, at the level of the pituitary, glucose does not alter basal GH release, but inhibits GHRH induced GH secretion,[324,325] while insulin inhibits basal GH secretion and mRNA levels.[326]

Amino acids

It has long been known that growth hormone secretion is stimulated by amino acids.[327–329] Although arginine is one of the most potent amino acids in the stimulation of GH secretion, lysine, ornithine, tyrosine, glycine, and tryptophan all release GH.[329] Stimulation of GH release in humans by L-arginine is suggested to occur through inhibition of SS secretion,[330,331] although the presence of GHRH is also important.[331] Blockage of α-adrenergic and cholinergic neurotransmission inhibits the arginine-induced GH secretion[213] and the response to arginine is modified by the sex steroid environment.[332] Nitric oxide (NO) is generated from both L- and D-arginine[333] and in rats, NO stimulates GHRH secretion and hence, GH. However, in humans there is no evidence to date that NO participates in GH stimulation by L-arginine.[334]

Fatty acids

Free fatty acids (FFAs) exert an inhibitory effect on the release of GH from the anterior pituitary,[335] with the increase in FFAs most likely being involved in the reduction in GH secretion in obese subjects.[336] Most evidence suggests that the effect of FFAs occurs at the level of the pituitary, possibly exerting a chronic inhibitory effect which blunts the response of this gland to other factors.[336,337] However, a possible hypothalamic site of action has been suggested by the fact that passive immunization with SS antiserum abolishes the in vivo inhibitory effect of FFAs.[338,339] Furthermore, in sheep SS levels in the portal blood increase in response to increased FFA levels.[340] In humans, inhibition of central cholinergic activation with pyridostigmine, which presumably reduces SS secretion, blocks the inhibitory effect of FFA on GH release,[339] again suggesting a possible effect of FFA at the hypothalamic level. However, in vitro, FFAs have been shown to increase GHRH release and inhibit SS release and production,[341] and whether this difference is due to the immature state of the hypothalamic neurons remains to be elucidated.

SUMMARY

It is clear that the neuroendocrine control of GH secretion is extremely complex. Although the basic regulatory mechanism comprised of somatostatin and GHRH neurons in the hypothalamus maintains its status as the primary orchestrator of GH secretion, these neurons receive a bombardment of information from neighboring cells, higher brain centers and circulating factors. They must constantly integrate these inputs to determine the final output to the anterior pituitary. Likewise, the somatotroph is inundated with information that must be deciphered and its response to specific inputs can be dramatically modified depending upon its immediate hormonal environment. Hence, it is difficult, if not impossible, to speak of the effect of one substance on GH secretion without taking into consideration many other factors at that precise moment.

KEY LEARNING POINTS

- Hypothalamic somatostatin and GHRH neurons constitute the main site of integration of signals arriving from within the hypothalamus, higher brain centers and the circulation to ultimately provide the main hypothalamic signal arriving to the somatotroph to control GH secretion.
- Brain derived peptides or neuropeptides affecting GH secretion include NPY, CRH, TRH, galanin, endogenous opioids, VIP, PACAP, interleukins, IGFs and ghrelin.
- Classical neuropeptides known to be involved in the control of GH secretion include catecholamines, serotonin, acetylcholine, histamine, glutamate, and GABA.
- Peripheral signals that feedback at the level of the hypothalamus to control GH secretion include GH itself, IGF-I, ghrelin, leptin, glucocorticoids, thyroid hormones, gonadal steroids, glucose, insulin, amino acids, and fatty acids.
- The effect of a specific factor on the release of GH may be modified by a number of physiological or pathophysiological situations including age, illness, stress, metabolic status, fasting, and sleep.

REFERENCES

- Seminal primary article
- Key review paper

- 1 Heatherington AW, Ranson, SW. Hypothalamic lesions and adiposity in the rat. *Anat Rec* 1940; **78**: 149–52.
  2 Reichlin S. Growth hormone content of pituitaries from rats with hypothalamic lesions. *Endocrinology* 1961; **69**: 225–30.
  3 Frohman LA, Bernardis LL. Growth hormone and insulin levels in weanling rats with ventromedial hypothalamic lesions. *Endocrinology* 1968; **82**: 1125–32.
  4 Frohman LA, Nernardis LL, Kant KJ. Hypothalamic stimulation of growth hormone secretion. *Science* 1968; **162**: 580–2.
  5 Quabbe HJ, Schilling E, Helge H. Pattern of growth hormone secretion during a 24-hour fast in normal adults. *J Clin Endocrinol Metab* 1966; **26**: 1173–7.
  6 Jansson JO, Carlsson L, Ekberg S, *et al.* Pulsatile growth hormone secretory pattern: autofeedback regulation and effects on growth factors. *Acta Paediatr Suppl Scand* 1990; **367**: 98–102.
- 7 Plotsky PM, Vale W. Patterns of growth hormone-releasing factor and somatostatin secretion into the hypophysial-portal circulation of the rat. *Science* 1985; **230**: 461–3.
- 8 Martin JB, Renaud LP, Brazeau P Jr. Pulsatile growth hormone secretion: suppression by hypothalamic ventromedial lesions and by long-acting somatostatin. *Science* 1974; **186**: 538–40.

  9 Winer LM, Shaw MA, Baumann G. Basal plasma growth hormone levels in man: new evidence for rhythmicity of growth hormone secretion. *J Clin Endocrinol Metab* 1990; **70**: 1678–86.
 10 Ho KY, Evans WS, Blizzard RM, *et al.* Effects of sex and age on the 24-hour profile of growth hormone secretion in man: importance of endogenous estradiol concentrations. *J Clin Endocrinol Metab* 1987; **64**: 51–8.
 11 Tannenbaum GS, Martin JB. Evidence for an endogenous ultradian rhythm governing growth hormone secretion in the rat. *Endocrinology* 1976; **98**: 562–70.
- 12 Jansson JO, Eden S, Isaksson O. Sexual dimorphism in the control of growth hormone secretion. *Endocr Rev* 1985; **6**: 128–50.
 13 Argente J, Chowen JA, Zeitler P, *et al.* Sexual dimorphism of growth hormone-releasing hormone and somatostatin gene expression in the hypothalamus of the rat during development. *Endocrinology* 1991; **128**: 2369–75.
 14 Chowen-Breed JA, Steiner RA, Clifton DK. Sexual dimorphism and testosterone-dependent regulation of somatostatin gene expression in the periventricular nucleus of the rat brain. *Endocrinology* 1989; **125**: 357–62.
 15 Zeitler P, Argente J, Chowen-Breed JA, *et al.* Growth hormone-releasing hormone messenger ribonucleic acid in the hypothalamus of the adult male rat is increased by testosterone. *Endocrinology* 1990; **127**: 1362–8.
 16 Gluckman PD, Grumbach MM, Kaplan SL. The neuroendocrine regulation and function of growth hormone and prolactin in the mammalian fetus. *Endocr Rev* 1981; **2**: 363–95.
 17 Kaplan SL, Grumbach MM, Shepard TH. The ontogenesis of human fetal hormones. I. Growth hormone and insulin. *J Clin Invest* 1972; **51**: 3080–93.
 18 Finkelstein JW, Roffwarg HP, Boyar RM, *et al.* Age-related change in the twenty-four-hour spontaneous secretion of growth hormone. *J Clin Endocrinol Metab* 1972; **35**: 665–70.
 19 Martha PM Jr, Gorman KM, Blizzard RM, *et al.* Endogenous growth hormone secretion and clearance rates in normal boys, as determined by deconvolution analysis: relationship to age, pubertal status, and body mass. *J Clin Endocrinol Metab* 1992; **74**: 336–44.
 20 Martha PM Jr, Rogol AD, Veldhuis JD, *et al.* Alterations in the pulsatile properties of circulating growth hormone concentrations during puberty in boys. *J Clin Endocrinol Metab* 1989; **69**: 563–70.
 21 Illig R, Stahl M, Henrichs I, Hecker A. Growth hormone release during slow-wave sleep. Comparison with insulin and arginine provocation in children with small stature. *Acta Paediatr Helv* 1971; **26**: 655–72.
 22 Holl RW, Hartman ML, Veldhuis JD, *et al.* Thirty-second sampling of plasma growth hormone in man: correlation with sleep stages. *J Clin Endocrinol Metab* 1991; **72**: 854–61.
 23 Van Cauter E, Kerkhofs M, Caufriez A, *et al.* A quantitative estimation of growth hormone secretion in normal man: reproducibility and relation to sleep and time of day. *J Clin Endocrinol Metab* 1992; **74**: 1441–50.

24 Radomski MW, Buguet A, Doua F, *et al.* Relationship of plasma growth hormone to slow-wave sleep in African sleeping sickness. *Neuroendocrinology* 1996; **63**: 393–6.

25 Merchenthaler I, Vigh S, Schally AV, Petrusz P. Immunocytochemical localization of growth hormone-releasing factor in the rat hypothalamus. *Endocrinology* 1984; **114**: 1082–5.

26 Merchenthaler I, Setalo G, Csontos C, *et al.* Combined retrograde tracing and immunocytochemical identification of luteinizing hormone-releasing hormone- and somatostatin-containing neurons projecting to the median eminence of the rat. *Endocrinology* 1989; **125**: 2812–21.

● 27 Brazeau P, Vale W, Burgus R, *et al.* Hypothalamic polypeptide that inhibits the secretion of immunoreactive pituitary growth hormone. *Science* 1973; **179**: 77–9.

28 Pradayrol L, Jornvall H, Mutt V, Ribet A. N-terminally extended somatostatin: the primary structure of somatostatin-28. *FEBS Lett* 1980; **109**: 55–8.

29 Esch F, Bohlen P, Ling N, *et al.* Primary structure of ovine hypothalamic somatostatin-28 and somatostatin-25. *Proc Natl Acad Sci USA* 1980; **77**: 6827–31.

● 30 Schally AV, Chang RC, Huang WY, *et al.* Isolation, structure, biological characterization, and synthesis of beta-[Tyr9]melanotropin-(9–18) decapeptide from pig hypothalami. *Proc Natl Acad Sci USA* 1980; **77**: 3947–51.

31 Zingg HH, Patel YC. Biosynthesis of immunoreactive somatostatin by hypothalamic neurons in culture. *J Clin Invest* 1982; **70**: 1101–9.

32 Krulich L, Dhariwal AP, McCann SM. Stimulatory and inhibitory effects of purified hypothalamic extracts on growth hormone release from rat pituitary in vitro. *Endocrinology* 1968; **83**: 783–90.

33 Steiner RA, Stewart JK, Barber J, *et al.* Somatostatin: a physiological role in the regulation of growth hormone secretion in the adolescent male baboon. *Endocrinology* 1978; **102**: 1587–94.

34 Tannenbaum GS, Epelbaum J, Colle E, *et al.* Antiserum to somatostatin reverses starvation-induced inhibition of growth hormone but not insulin secretion. *Endocrinology* 1978; **102**: 1909–14.

35 Kewley CF, Millar RP, Berman MC, Schally AV. Depolarization- and ionophore-induced release of octacosa somatostatin from stalk median eminence synaptosomes. *Science* 1981; **213**: 913–5.

36 Millar RP, Sheward WJ, Wegener I, Fink G. Somatostatin-28 is an hormonally active peptide secreted into hypophysial portal vessel blood. *Brain Res* 1983; **260**: 334–7.

37 Jacovidou N, Patel YC. Antiserum to somatostatin-28 augments growth hormone secretion in the rat. *Endocrinology* 1987; **121**: 782–5.

38 Meyers CA, Murphy WA, Redding TW, *et al.* Synthesis and biological actions of prosomatostatin. *Proc Natl Acad Sci USA* 1980; **77**: 6171–4.

39 Srikant CB, Patel YC. Receptor binding of somatostatin-28 is tissue specific. *Nature* 1981; **294**: 259–60.

40 Patel YC, Wheatley T. In vivo and in vitro plasma disappearance and metabolism of somatostatin-28 and somatostatin-14 in the rat. *Endocrinology* 1983; **112**: 220–5.

41 Patel YC, ed. *Somatostatin*. Philadelphia: Lippincott; 1990.

42 Bouras C, Magistretti PJ, Morrison JH, Constantinidis J. An immunohistochemical study of pro-somatostatin-derived peptides in the human brain. *Neuroscience* 1987; **22**: 781–800.

43 Vincent SR, McIntosh CH, Buchan AM, Brown JC. Central somatostatin systems revealed with monoclonal antibodies. *J Comp Neurol* 1985; **238**: 169–86.

44 Ishikawa K, Taniguchi Y, Kurosumi K, *et al.* Immunohistochemical identification of somatostatin-containing neurons projecting to the median eminence of the rat. *Endocrinology* 1987; **121**: 94–7.

45 Willoughby JO, Martin JB. Pulsatile growth hormone secretion: inhibitory role of medial preoptic area. *Brain Res* 1978; **148**: 240–4.

46 Reichlin S. Somatostatin (second of two parts). *N Engl J Med* 1983; **309**: 1556–63.

47 Reichlin S. Somatostatin. *N Engl J Med* 1983; **309**: 1495–501.

48 Bertherat J, Bluet-Pajot MT, Epelbaum J. Neuroendocrine regulation of growth hormone. *Eur J Endocrinol* 1995; **132**: 12–24.

49 Bluet-Pajot MT, Durand D, Drouva SV, *et al.* Further evidence that thyrotropin-releasing hormone participate in the regulation of growth hormone secretion in the rat. *Neuroendocrinology* 1986; **44**: 70–5.

50 Patel YC. Molecular pharmacology of somatostatin receptor subtypes. *J Endocrinol Invest* 1997; **20**: 348–67.

◆ 51 Hofland LJ, Lamberts SW. Somatostatin receptors in pituitary function, diagnosis and therapy. *Front Horm Res* 2004; **32**: 235–52.

52 Ren SG, Taylor J, Dong J, *et al.* Functional association of somatostatin receptor subtypes 2 and 5 in inhibiting human growth hormone secretion. *J Clin Endocrinol Metab* 2003; **88**: 4239–45.

● 53 Guillemin R, Brazeau P, Bohlen P, *et al.* Growth hormone-releasing factor from a human pancreatic tumor that caused acromegaly. *Science* 1982; **218**: 585–7.

● 54 Rivier J, Spiess J, Thorner M, Vale W. Characterization of a growth hormone-releasing factor from a human pancreatic islet tumour. *Nature* 1982; **300**: 276–8.

55 Spiess J, Rivier J, Vale W. Characterization of rat hypothalamic growth hormone-releasing factor. *Nature* 1983; **303**: 532–5.

56 Bohlen P, Wehrenberg WB, Esch F, *et al.* Rat hypothalamic growth hormone-releasing factor: isolation, sequence analysis and total synthesis. *Biochem Biophys Res Commun* 1984; **125**: 1005–12.

57 Campbell RM, Lee Y, Rivier J, *et al.* GRF analogs and fragments: correlation between receptor binding, activity and structure. *Peptides* 1991; **12**: 569–74.

58 Sherwood NM, Krueckl SL, McRory JE. The origin and function of the pituitary adenylate cyclase-activating polypeptide (PACAP)/glucagon superfamily. *Endocr Rev* 2000; **21**: 619–70.

59 Mayo KE, Cerelli GM, Rosenfeld MG, Evans RM. Characterization of cDNA and genomic clones encoding the precursor to rat hypothalamic growth hormone-releasing factor. *Nature* 1985; **314**: 464–7.

60 Pezzolo A, Gimelli G, Sposito M, *et al.* Definitive assignment of the growth hormone-releasing factor gene to 20q11.2. *Hum Genet* 1994; **93**: 213–4.

61 Bloch B, Gaillard RC, Brazeau P, *et al.* Topographical and ontogenetic study of the neurons producing growth hormone-releasing factor in human hypothalamus. *Regul Pept* 1984; **8**: 21–31.

62 Sawchenko PE, Swanson LW, Rivier J, Vale WW. The distribution of growth-hormone-releasing factor (GRF) immunoreactivity in the central nervous system of the rat: an immunohistochemical study using antisera directed against rat hypothalamic GRF. *J Comp Neurol* 1985; **237**: 100–15.

63 Bloch B, Brazeau P, Ling N, *et al.* Immunohistochemical detection of growth hormone-releasing factor in brain. *Nature* 1983; **301**: 607–8.

64 Ciofi P, Croix D, Tramu G. Colocalization of GHRF and NPY immunoreactivities in neurons of the infundibular area of the human brain. *Neuroendocrinology* 1988; **47**: 469–72.

65 Ciofi P, Croix D, Tramu G. Coexistence of hGHRF and NPY immunoreactivities in neurons of the arcuate nucleus of the rat. *Neuroendocrinology* 1987; **45**: 425–8.

66 Everitt BJ, Meister B, Hokfelt T, *et al.* The hypothalamic arcuate nucleus-median eminence complex: immunohistochemistry of transmitters, peptides and DARPP-32 with special reference to coexistence in dopamine neurons. *Brain Res* 1986; **396**: 97–155.

67 Meister B, Ceccatelli S, Hokfelt T, *et al.* Neurotransmitters, neuropeptides and binding sites in the rat mediobasal hypothalamus: effects of monosodium glutamate (MSG) lesions. *Exp Brain Res* 1989; **76**: 343–68.

68 Hohmann JG, Clifton DK, Steiner RA. Galanin: analysis of its coexpression in gonadotropin-releasing hormone and growth hormone-releasing hormone neurons. *Ann NY Acad Sci* 1998; **863**: 221–35.

69 Meister B, Hulting AL. Influence of coexisting hypothalamic messengers on growth hormone secretion from rat anterior pituitary cells in vitro. *Neuroendocrinology* 1987; **46**: 387–94.

70 Palkovits M, ed. *Sterotaxis map, cytoarchitectonic and neurochemical summary of the hypothalamic nuclei, rat.* Berlin: Springer Verlag; 1983.

71 Chronwall BM. Anatomy and physiology of the neuroendocrine arcuate nucleus. *Peptides* 1985; **6(Suppl 2)**: 1–11.

72 Billestrup N, Swanson LW, Vale W. Growth hormone-releasing factor stimulates proliferation of somatotrophs in vitro. *Proc Natl Acad Sci USA* 1986; **83**: 6854–7.

● 73 Barinaga M, Yamonoto G, Rivier C, *et al.* Transcriptional regulation of growth hormone gene expression by growth hormone-releasing factor. *Nature* 1983; **306**: 84–5.

74 Mayo KE, Miller T, DeAlmeida V, *et al.* Regulation of the pituitary somatotroph cell by GHRH and its receptor. *Recent Prog Horm Res* 2000; **55**: 237–67.

◆ 75 Mayo KE, Godfrey PA, Suhr ST, *et al.* Growth hormone-releasing hormone: synthesis and signaling. *Recent Prog Horm Res* 1995; **50**: 35–73.

● 76 Wehrenberg WB, Brazeau P, Luben R, *et al.* Inhibition of the pulsatile secretion of growth hormone by monoclonal antibodies to the hypothalamic growth hormone releasing factor (GRF). *Endocrinology* 1982; **111**: 2147–8.

77 Stachura ME. Influence of synthetic somatostatin upon growth hormone release from perifused rat pituitaries. *Endocrinology* 1976; **99**: 678–83.

78 Horvath S, Palkovits M. Synaptic interconnections among growth hormone-releasing hormone (GHRH)-containing neurons in the arcuate nucleus of the rat hypothalamus. *Neuroendocrinology* 1988; **48**: 471–6.

79 Alonso G, Tapia-Arancibia L, Assenmacher I. Electron microscopic immunocytochemical study of somatostatin neurons in the periventricular nucleus of the rat hypothalamus with special reference to their relationships with homologous neuronal processes. *Neuroscience* 1985; **16**: 297–306.

80 Epelbaum J, Tapia-Arancibia L, Alonso G, *et al.* The anterior periventricular hypothalamus is the site of somatostatin inhibition of its own release: an in vitro and immunocytochemical study. *Neuroendocrinology* 1986; **44**: 255–9.

81 Csaba Z, Simon A, Helboe L, *et al.* Targeting sst2A receptor-expressing cells in the rat hypothalamus through in vivo agonist stimulation: neuroanatomical evidence for a major role of this subtype in mediating somatostatin functions. *Endocrinology* 2003; **144**: 1564–73.

82 Willoughby JO, Brogan M, Kapoor R. Hypothalamic interconnections of somatostatin and growth hormone releasing factor neurons. *Neuroendocrinology* 1989; **50**: 584–91.

83 Tannenbaum GS, Zhang WH, Lapointe M, *et al.* Growth hormone-releasing hormone neurons in the arcuate nucleus express both Sst1 and Sst2 somatostatin receptor genes. *Endocrinology* 1998; **139**: 1450–3.

84 Mitsugi N, Arita J, Kimura F. Effects of intracerebroventricular administration of growth hormone-releasing factor and corticotropin-releasing factor on somatostatin secretion into rat hypophysial portal blood. *Neuroendocrinology* 1990; **51**: 93–6.

85 Murakami Y, Kato Y, Kabayama Y, *et al.* Involvement of hypothalamic growth hormone (GH)-releasing factor in GH secretion induced by intracerebroventricular injection of somatostatin in rats. *Endocrinology* 1987; **120**: 311–6.

● 86 Lumpkin MD, Gegro-Vilar A, McCann SM. Paradoxical elevation of growth hormone by intraventricular somatostatin: possible ultrashort-loop feedback. *Science* 1981; **211**: 1072–4.

87 Vale W, Vaughan J, Smith M, *et al.* Effects of synthetic ovine corticotropin-releasing factor, glucocorticoids, catecholamines, neurohypophysial peptides, and other

substances on cultured corticotropic cells. *Endocrinology* 1983; **113**: 1121–31.

88   Brazeau P, Ling N, Esch F, *et al.* Somatocrinin (growth hormone releasing factor) in vitro bioactivity; Ca^{++} involvement, cAMP mediated action and additivity of effect with PGE2. *Biochem Biophys Res Commun* 1982; **109**: 588–94.

89   Allen YS, Adrian TE, Allen JM, *et al.* Neuropeptide Y distribution in the rat brain. *Science* 1983; **221**: 877–9.

90   White JD. Neuropeptide Y: a central regulator of energy homeostasis. *Regul Pept* 1993; **49**: 93–107.

91   McDonald JK, Lumpkin MD, Samson WK, McCann SM. Neuropeptide Y affects secretion of luteinizing hormone and growth hormone in ovariectomized rats. *Proc Natl Acad Sci USA* 1985; **82**: 561–4.

92   Rettori V, Milenkovic L, Aguila MC, McCann SM. Physiologically significant effect of neuropeptide Y to suppress growth hormone release by stimulating somatostatin discharge. *Endocrinology* 1990; **126**: 2296–301.

93   Korbonits M, Little JA, Forsling ML, *et al.* The effect of growth hormone secretagogues and neuropeptide Y on hypothalamic hormone release from acute rat hypothalamic explants. *J Neuroendocrinol* 1999; **11**: 521–8.

94   Hisano S, Tsuruo Y, Kagotani Y, *et al.* Immunohistochemical evidence for synaptic connections between neuropeptide Y-containing axons and periventricular somatostatin neurons in the anterior hypothalamus in rats. *Brain Res* 1990; **520**: 170–7.

95   Tamura H, Kamegai J, Shimizu T, *et al.* The effect of agouti-related protein on growth hormone secretion in adult male rats. *Regul Pept* 2005; **125**: 145–9.

96   Minami S, Kamegai J, Sugihara H, *et al.* Growth hormone inhibits its own secretion by acting on the hypothalamus through its receptors on neuropeptide Y neurons in the arcuate nucleus and somatostatin neurons in the periventricular nucleus. *Endocr J* 1998; **45(Suppl)**: S19–26.

97   Carro E, Seoane LM, Senaris R, *et al.* Interaction between leptin and neuropeptide Y on in vivo growth hormone secretion. *Neuroendocrinology* 1998; **68**: 187–91.

98   Chan YY, Steiner RA, Clifton DK. Regulation of hypothalamic neuropeptide-Y neurons by growth hormone in the rat. *Endocrinology* 1996; **137**: 1319–25.

99   Kamegai J, Minami S, Sugihara H, *et al.* Growth hormone receptor gene is expressed in neuropeptide Y neurons in hypothalamic arcuate nucleus of rats. *Endocrinology* 1996; **137**: 2109–12.

100   Willesen MG, Kristensen P, Romer J. Co-localization of growth hormone secretagogue receptor and NPY mRNA in the arcuate nucleus of the rat. *Neuroendocrinology* 1999; **70**: 306–16.

101   Katakami H, Arimura A, Frohman LA. Involvement of hypothalamic somatostatin in the suppression of growth hormone secretion by central corticotropin-releasing factor in conscious male rats. *Neuroendocrinology* 1985; **41**: 390–3.

102   Ono N, Lumpkin MD, Samson WK, *et al.* Intrahypothalamic action of corticotrophin-releasing factor (CRF) to inhibit growth hormone and LH release in the rat. *Life Sci* 1984; **35**: 1117–23.

103   Mounier F, Pellegrini E, Kordon C, *et al.* Continuous intracerebroventricular administration of a corticotropin releasing hormone antagonist amplifies spontaneous growth hormone pulses in the rat. *J Endocrinol* 1997; **152**: 431–6.

104   Barbarino A, Corsello SM, Della Casa S, *et al.* Corticotropin-releasing hormone inhibition of growth hormone-releasing hormone-induced growth hormone release in man. *J Clin Endocrinol Metab* 1990; **71**: 1368–74.

105   Ghizzoni L, Vottero A, Street ME, Bernasconi S. Dose-dependent inhibition of growth hormone (GH)-releasing hormone-induced GH release by corticotropin-releasing hormone in prepubertal children. *J Clin Endocrinol Metab* 1996; **81**: 1397–400.

106   Raza J, Massoud AF, Hindmarsh PC, *et al.* Direct effects of corticotrophin-releasing hormone on stimulated growth hormone secretion. *Clin Endocrinol (Oxf)* 1998; **48**: 217–22.

107   Rolla M, Andreoni A, Bellitti D, *et al.* Corticotrophin-releasing hormone does not inhibit growth hormone-releasing hormone-induced release of growth hormone in control subjects but is effective in patients with eating disorders. *J Endocrinol* 1994; **140**: 327–32.

108   Delitala G, Tomasi P, Virdis R. Prolactin, growth hormone and thyrotropin-thyroid hormone secretion during stress states in man. *Baillieres Clin Endocrinol Metab* 1987; **1**: 391–414.

109   Harvey S. Thyrotrophin-releasing hormone: a growth hormone-releasing factor. *J Endocrinol* 1990; **125**: 345–58.

110   Kaltsas T, Pontikides N, Krassas GE, *et al.* Growth hormone response to thyrotrophin releasing hormone in women with polycystic ovarian syndrome. *Hum Reprod* 1999; **14**: 2704–8.

111   Andries M, Denef C. Gonadotropin-releasing hormone influences the release of prolactin and growth hormone from intact rat pituitary in vitro during a limited period in neonatal life. *Peptides* 1995; **16**: 527–32.

112   Welsh JB, Cuttler L, Szabo M. Ontogeny of the in vitro growth hormone stimulatory effect of thyrotropin-releasing hormone in the rat. *Endocrinology* 1986; **119**: 2368–75.

113   Konaka S, Yamada M, Satoh T, *et al.* Expression of thyrotropin-releasing hormone (TRH) receptor mRNA in somatotrophs in the rat anterior pituitary. *Endocrinology* 1997; **138**: 827–30.

114   Panerai AE, Gil-Ad I, Cocchi D, *et al.* Thyrotrophin releasing hormone-induced growth hormone and prolactin release: physiological studies in intact rats and in hypophysectomized rats bearing an ectopic pituitary gland. *J Endocrinol* 1977; **72**: 301–11.

• 115 Bauer FE, Ginsberg L, Venetikou M, *et al*. Growth hormone release in man induced by galanin, a new hypothalamic peptide. *Lancet* 1986; **2**: 192–5.

116 Bedecs K, Berthold M, Bartfai T. Galanin–10 years with a neuroendocrine peptide. *Int J Biochem Cell Biol* 1995; **27**: 337–49.

117 Ottlecz A, Samson WK, McCann SM. Galanin: evidence for a hypothalamic site of action to release growth hormone. *Peptides* 1986; **7**: 51–3.

118 Kitajima N, Chihara K, Abe H, *et al*. Effects of dopamine on immunoreactive growth hormone-releasing factor and somatostatin secretion from rat hypothalamic slices perifused in vitro. *Endocrinology* 1989; **124**: 69–76.

119 Giustina A, Wehrenberg WB. Influence of thyroid hormones on the regulation of growth hormone secretion. *Eur J Endocrinol* 1995; **133**: 646–53.

120 Sartorio A, Conti A, Monzani M, Faglia G. Galanin infusion restores the blunted GH responses to GHRH administration during GH treatment in children with constitutional growth delay. *J Endocrinol Invest* 1995; **18**: 109–12.

121 Aguila MC, Marubayashi U, McCann SM. The effect of galanin on growth hormone-releasing factor and somatostatin release from median eminence fragments in vitro. *Neuroendocrinology* 1992; **56**: 889–94.

122 Chatterjee VK, Ball JA, Davis TM, *et al*. The effect of cholinergic blockade on the growth hormone response to galanin in humans. *Metabolism* 1988; **37**: 1089–91.

123 Tanoh T, Shimatsu A, Murakami Y, *et al*. Cholinergic modulation of growth hormone secretion induced by galanin in rats. *Neuroendocrinology* 1991; **54**: 83–8.

124 Murakami Y, Kato Y, Shimatsu A, *et al*. Possible mechanisms involved in growth hormone secretion induced by galanin in the rat. *Endocrinology* 1989; **124**: 1224–9.

125 Cella SG, Locatelli V, De Gennaro V, *et al*. Epinephrine mediates the growth hormone-releasing effect of galanin in infant rats. *Endocrinology* 1988; **122**: 855–9.

126 Bruni JF, Van Vugt D, Marshall S, Meites J. Effects of naloxone, morphine and methionine enkephalin on serum prolactin, luteinizing hormone, follicle stimulating hormone, thyroid stimulating hormone and growth hormone. *Life Sci* 1977; **21**: 461–6.

127 Cocchi D, Santagostino A, Gil-Ad I, *et al*. Leu-enkephalin-stimulated growth hormone and prolactin release in the rat: comparison with the effect of morphine. *Life Sci* 1977; **20**: 2041–5.

128 Fodor M, Csaba Z, Epelbaum J, *et al*. Interrelations between hypothalamic somatostatin and proopiomelanocortin neurons. *J Neuroendocrinol* 1998; **10**: 75–8.

129 Janik J, Klosterman S, Parman R, Callahan P. Multiple opiate receptor subtypes are involved in the stimulation of growth hormone release by beta-endorphin in female rats. *Neuroendocrinology* 1994; **60**: 69–75.

130 Grossman A, Rees LH. The neuroendocrinology of opioid peptides. *Br Med Bull* 1983; **39**: 83–8.

131 degli Uberti EC, Salvadori S, Trasforini G, *et al*. Differential effects of deltorphin on arginine and galanin-induced growth hormone secretion in healthy man. *Regul Pept* 1995; **58**: 41–6.

132 Said SI, Porter JC. Vasoactive intestinal polypeptide: release into hypophyseal portal blood. *Life Sci* 1979; **24**: 227–30.

133 Arnaout MA, Garthwaite TL, Martinson DR, Hagen TC. Vasoactive intestinal polypeptide is synthesized in anterior pituitary tissue. *Endocrinology* 1986; **119**: 2052–7.

134 Muller EE. Neural control of somatotropic function. *Physiol Rev* 1987; **67**: 962–1053.

135 Bluet-Pajot MT, Mounier F, Leonard JF, *et al*. Vasoactive intestinal peptide induces a transient release of growth hormone in the rat. *Peptides* 1987; **8**: 35–8.

136 Enjalbert A, Epelbaum J, Arancibia S, *et al*. Reciprocal interactions of somatostatin with thyrotropin-releasing hormone and vasoactive intestinal peptide on prolactin and growth hormone secretion in vitro. *Endocrinology* 1982; **111**: 42–7.

137 Kato Y, Shimatsu A, Matsushita N, *et al*. Role of vasoactive intestinal polypeptide (VIP) in regulating the pituitary function in man. *Peptides* 1984; **5**: 389–94.

138 Chihara K, Kaji H, Minamitani N, *et al*. Stimulation of growth hormone by vasoactive intestinal polypeptide in acromegaly. *J Clin Endocrinol Metab* 1984; **58**: 81–6.

139 Rawlings SR, Hezareh M. Pituitary adenylate cyclase-activating polypeptide (PACAP) and PACAP/vasoactive intestinal polypeptide receptors: actions on the anterior pituitary gland. *Endocr Rev* 1996; **17**: 4–29.

140 Velkeniers B, Zheng L, Kazemzadeh M, *et al*. Effect of pituitary adenylate cyclase-activating polypeptide 38 on growth hormone and prolactin expression. *J Endocrinol* 1994; **143**: 1–11.

141 Goth MI, Lyons CE, Canny BJ, Thorner MO. Pituitary adenylate cyclase activating polypeptide, growth hormone (GH)-releasing peptide and GH-releasing hormone stimulate GH release through distinct pituitary receptors. *Endocrinology* 1992; **130**: 939–44.

142 Hart GR, Gowing H, Burrin JM. Effects of a novel hypothalamic peptide, pituitary adenylate cyclase-activating polypeptide, on pituitary hormone release in rats. *J Endocrinol* 1992; **134**: 33–41.

143 Yamauchi K, Murakami Y, Koshimura K, *et al*. Involvement of pituitary adenylate cyclase-activating polypeptide in growth hormone secretion induced by serotoninergic mechanisms in the rat. *Endocrinology* 1996; **137**: 1693–7.

144 Payne LC, Obal F Jr, Opp MR, Krueger JM. Stimulation and inhibition of growth hormone secretion by interleukin-1 beta: the involvement of growth hormone-releasing hormone. *Neuroendocrinology* 1992; **56**: 118–23.

145 Rettori V, Jurcovicova J, McCann SM. Central action of interleukin-1 in altering the release of TSH, growth hormone, and prolactin in the male rat. *J Neurosci Res* 1987; **18**: 179–83.

146 Atkins MB, Gould JA, Allegretta M, *et al*. Phase I evaluation of recombinant interleukin-2 in patients with advanced malignant disease. *J Clin Oncol* 1986; **4**: 1380–91.

147 Peisen JN, McDonnell KJ, Mulroney SE, Lumpkin MD. Endotoxin-induced suppression of the somatotropic axis is mediated by interleukin-1 beta and corticotropin-releasing factor in the juvenile rat. *Endocrinology* 1995; **136**: 3378–90.

148 Wada Y, Sato M, Niimi M, *et al.* Inhibitory effects of interleukin-1 on growth hormone secretion in conscious male rats. *Endocrinology* 1995; **136**: 3936–41.

149 McCann SM, Kimura M, Karanth S, *et al.* The mechanism of action of cytokines to control the release of hypothalamic and pituitary hormones in infection. *Ann NY Acad Sci* 2000; **917**: 4–18.

150 Mainardi GL, Saleri R, Tamanini C, Baratta M. Effects of interleukin-1-beta, interleukin-6 and tumor necrosis factor-alpha, alone or in association with hexarelin or galanin, on growth hormone gene expression and growth hormone release from pig pituitary cells. *Horm Res* 2002; **58**: 180–6.

151 Spangelo BL, Judd AM, Isakson PC, MacLeod RM. Interleukin-6 stimulates anterior pituitary hormone release in vitro. *Endocrinology* 1989; **125**: 575–7.

152 Perez Castro C, Carbia Nagashima A, Paez Pereda M, *et al.* Effects of the gp130 cytokines ciliary neurotropic factor (CNTF) and interleukin-11 on pituitary cells: CNTF receptors on human pituitary adenomas and stimulation of prolactin and GH secretion in normal rat anterior pituitary aggregate cultures. *J Endocrinol* 2001; **169**: 539–47.

153 Besedovsky HO, del Rey A. Immune-neuro-endocrine interactions: facts and hypotheses. *Endocr Rev* 1996; **17**: 64–102.

154 Jones JI, Clemmons DR. Insulin-like growth factors and their binding proteins: biological actions. *Endocr Rev* 1995; **16**: 3–34.

● 155 D'Ercole AJ, Underwood LE. Ontogeny of somatomedin during development in the mouse. Serum concentrations, molecular forms, binding proteins, and tissue receptors. *Dev Biol* 1980; **79**: 33–45.

● 156 Han VK, Lund PK, Lee DC, D'Ercole AJ. Expression of somatomedin/insulin-like growth factor messenger ribonucleic acids in the human fetus: identification, characterization, and tissue distribution. *J Clin Endocrinol Metab* 1988; **66**: 422–9.

◆ 157 LeRoith D, Werner H, Beitner-Johnson D, Roberts CT Jr. Molecular and cellular aspects of the insulin-like growth factor I receptor. *Endocr Rev* 1995; **16**: 143–63.

158 Wang J, Zhou J, Bondy CA. Igf1 promotes longitudinal bone growth by insulin-like actions augmenting chondrocyte hypertrophy. *FASEB J* 1999; **13**: 1985–90.

● 159 D'Ercole AJ, Applewhite GT, Underwood LE. Evidence that somatomedin is synthesized by multiple tissues in the fetus. *Dev Biol* 1980; **75**: 315–28.

160 Lowe WL Jr, Lasky SR, LeRoith D, Roberts CT Jr. Distribution and regulation of rat insulin-like growth factor I messenger ribonucleic acids encoding alternative carboxyterminal E-peptides: evidence for differential processing and regulation in liver. *Mol Endocrinol* 1988; **2**: 528–35.

161 Roberts CT Jr, Lasky SR, Lowe WL Jr, *et al.* Molecular cloning of rat insulin-like growth factor I complementary deoxyribonucleic acids: differential messenger ribonucleic acid processing and regulation by growth hormone in extrahepatic tissues. *Mol Endocrinol* 1987; **1**: 243–8.

◆ 162 Le Roith D, Bondy C, Yakar S, *et al.* The somatomedin hypothesis: 2001. *Endocr Rev* 2001; **22**: 53–74.

163 Minami S, Suzuki N, Sugihara H, *et al.* Microinjection of rat GH but not human IGF-I into a defined area of the hypothalamus inhibits endogenous GH secretion in rats. *J Endocrinol* 1997; **153**: 283–90.

164 Fletcher TP, Thomas GB, Dunshea FR, *et al.* IGF feedback effects on growth hormone secretion in ewes: evidence for action at the pituitary but not the hypothalamic level. *J Endocrinol* 1995; **144**: 323–31.

165 Uchiyama T, Kaji H, Abe H, Chihara K. Negative regulation of hypothalamic growth hormone-releasing factor messenger ribonucleic acid by growth hormone and insulin-like growth factor I. *Neuroendocrinology* 1994; **59**: 441–50.

166 Becker K, Stegenga S, Conway S. Role of insulin-like growth factor I in regulating growth hormone release and feedback in the male rat. *Neuroendocrinology* 1995; **61**: 573–83.

167 Aguila MC, Boggaram V, McCann SM. Insulin-like growth factor I modulates hypothalamic somatostatin through a growth hormone releasing factor increased somatostatin release and messenger ribonucleic acid levels. *Brain Res* 1993; **625**: 213–8.

● 168 Sato M, Frohman LA. Differential effects of central and peripheral administration of growth hormone (GH) and insulin-like growth factor on hypothalamic GH-releasing hormone and somatostatin gene expression in GH-deficient dwarf rats. *Endocrinology* 1993; **133**: 793–9.

169 Pazos F, Sanchez-Franco F, Balsa J, *et al.* Regulation of gonadal and somatotropic axis by chronic intraventricular infusion of insulin-like growth factor 1 antibody at the initiation of puberty in male rats. *Neuroendocrinology* 1999; **69**: 408–16.

170 Frago LM, Paneda C, Dickson SL, *et al.* Growth hormone (GH) and GH-releasing peptide-6 increase brain insulin-like growth factor-I expression and activate intracellular signaling pathways involved in neuroprotection. *Endocrinology* 2002; **143**: 4113–22.

171 Garcia-Segura LM, Rodriguez JR, Torres-Aleman I. Localization of the insulin-like growth factor I receptor in the cerebellum and hypothalamus of adult rats: an electron microscopic study. *J Neurocytol* 1997; **26**: 479–90.

● 172 Kojima M, Hosoda H, Date Y, *et al.* Ghrelin is a growth-hormone-releasing acylated peptide from stomach. *Nature* 1999; **402**: 656–60.

● 173 Cowley MA, Smith RG, Diano S, *et al.* The distribution and mechanism of action of ghrelin in the CNS demonstrates a novel hypothalamic circuit regulating energy homeostasis. *Neuron* 2003; **37**: 649–61.

174 Harmar AJ. Neuropeptides. In: Fluckiger E, Muller EE, Thorner MO, eds. *Transmitter molecules in the brain. Basic and clinical aspects of neuroscience*. Berlin: Springer-Verlag; 1987: 17–26.

175 Muller EE, Locatelli V, Ghigo E, *et al.* Involvement of brain catecholamines and acetylcholine in growth hormone deficiency states. Pathophysiological, diagnostic and therapeutic implications. *Drugs* 1991; **41**: 161–77.

176 Muller EE, Rolla M, Ghigo E, *et al.* Involvement of brain catecholamines and acetylcholine in growth hormone hypersecretory states. Pathophysiological, diagnostic and therapeutic implications. *Drugs* 1995; **50**: 805–37.

177 Krulich L, Mayfield MA, Steele MK, *et al.* Differential effects of pharmacological manipulations of central alpha 1- and alpha 2-adrenergic receptors on the secretion of thyrotropin and growth hormone in male rats. *Endocrinology* 1982; **110**: 796–804.

178 Terry LC, Crowley WR, Johnson MD. Regulation of episodic growth hormone secretion by the central epinephrine system. Studies in the chronically cannulated rat. *J Clin Invest* 1982; **69**: 104–12.

179 Muller EE, Pecile A, Felici M, Cocchi D. Norepinephrine and dopamine injection into lateral brain ventricle of the rat and growth hormone-releasing activity in the hypothalamus and plasma. *Endocrinology* 1970; **86**: 1376–82.

180 Cella SG, Locatelli V, De Gennaro V, *et al.* Pharmacological manipulations of alpha-adrenoceptors in the infant rat and effects on growth hormone secretion. Study of the underlying mechanisms of action. *Endocrinology* 1987; **120**: 1639–43.

181 Kabayama Y, Kato Y, Murakami Y, *et al.* Stimulation by alpha-adrenergic mechanisms of the secretion of growth hormone-releasing factor (GRF) from perifused rat hypothalamus. *Endocrinology* 1986; **119**: 432–4.

182 Miki N, Ono M, Shizume K. Evidence that opiatergic and alpha-adrenergic mechanisms stimulate rat growth hormone release via growth hormone-releasing factor (GRF). *Endocrinology* 1984; **114**: 1950–2.

183 Gil-Ad I, Laron Z, Koch Y. Effect of acute and chronic administration of clonidine on hypothalamic content of growth hormone-releasing hormone and somatostatin in the rat. *J Endocrinol* 1991; **131**: 381–5.

184 De Gennaro Colonna V, Zoli M, Settembrini BP, *et al.* Effects of single and short-term administration of clonidine on hypothalamic-pituitary somatotropic function of the adult male rat: an in situ hybridization study. *J Pharmacol Exp Ther* 1996; **276**: 795–800.

185 Devesa J, Lima L, Lois N, *et al.* Reasons for the variability in growth hormone (GH) responses to GHRH challenge: the endogenous hypothalamic-somatotroph rhythm (HSR). *Clin Endocrinol (Oxf)* 1989; **30**: 367–77.

186 Lanzi R, Lapointe M, Gurd W, Tannenbaum GS. Evidence for a primary involvement of somatostatin in clonidine-induced growth hormone release in conscious rats. *J Endocrinol* 1994; **141**: 259–66.

187 Liposits Z, Kallo I, Barkovics-Kallo M, *et al.* Innervation of somatostatin synthesizing neurons by adrenergic, phenylethanolamine-N-methyltransferase (PNMT)-immunoreactive axons in the anterior periventricular nucleus of the rat hypothalamus. *Histochemistry* 1990; **94**: 13–20.

188 Imura H, Kato Y, Ikeda M, *et al.* Effect of adrenergic-blocking or -stimulating agents on plasma growth hormone, immunoreactive insulin, and blood free fatty acid levels in man. *J Clin Invest* 1971; **50**: 1069–79.

189 Cella SG, Picotti GB, Muller EE. alpha2-Adrenergic stimulation enhances growth hormone secretion in the dog: a presynaptic mechanism? *Life Sci* 1983; **32**: 2785–92.

190 Cella SG, Picotti GB, Morgese M, *et al.* Presynaptic alpha 2-adrenergic stimulation leads to growth hormone release in the dog. *Life Sci* 1984; **34**: 447–54.

191 Mounier F, Bluet-Pajot MT, Durand D, *et al.* Alpha-1-noradrenergic inhibition of growth hormone secretion is mediated through the paraventricular hypothalamic nucleus in male rats. *Neuroendocrinology* 1994; **59**: 29–34.

192 Mounier F, Bluet-Pajot MT, Moinard F, *et al.* Activation of locus coeruleus somatostatin receptors induces an increase of growth hormone release in male rats. *J Neuroendocrinol* 1996; **8**: 761–4.

193 Ghigo E, Goffi S, Arvat E, *et al.* Pyridostigmine partially restores the GH responsiveness to GHRH in normal aging. *Acta Endocrinol (Copenh)* 1990; **123**: 169–73.

194 Ghigo E, Arvat E, Gianotti L, *et al.* Interaction of salbutamol with pyridostigmine and arginine on both basal and GHRH-stimulated GH secretion in humans. *Clin Endocrinol (Oxf)* 1994; **40**: 799–802.

195 Vance ML, Kaiser DL, Frohman LA, *et al.* Role of dopamine in the regulation of growth hormone secretion: dopamine and bromocriptine augment growth hormone (GH)-releasing hormone-stimulated GH secretion in normal man. *J Clin Endocrinol Metab* 1987; **64**: 1136–41.

● 196 Woolf PD, Lantigua R, Lee LA. Dopamine inhibition of stimulated growth hormone secretion: evidence for dopaminergic modulation of insulin- and L-dopa-induced growth hormone secretion in man. *J Clin Endocrinol Metab* 1979; **49**: 326–30.

197 Bansal S, Lee LA, Woolf PD. Dopaminergic modulation of arginine mediated growth hormone and prolactin release in man. *Metabolism* 1981; **30**: 649–53.

198 Diaz-Torga G, Feierstein C, Libertun C, *et al.* Disruption of the D2 dopamine receptor alters GH and IGF-I secretion and causes dwarfism in male mice. *Endocrinology* 2002; **143**: 1270–9.

199 Miyake H, Nagashima K, Onigata K, *et al.* Allelic variations of the D2 dopamine receptor gene in children with idiopathic short stature. *J Hum Genet* 1999; **44**: 26–9.

200 Cheung S, Johnson JD, Moore KE, Lookingland KJ. Dopamine receptor-mediated regulation of expression of Fos and its related antigens (FRA) in somatostatin neurons in the hypothalamic periventricular nucleus. *Brain Res* 1997; **770**: 176–83.

201 Mota A, Bento A, Penalva A, *et al.* Role of the serotonin receptor subtype 5-HT1D on basal and stimulated growth hormone secretion. *J Clin Endocrinol Metab* 1995; **80**: 1973–7.

202 Morris P, Hopwood M, Maguire K, *et al.* Blunted growth hormone response to clonidine in post-traumatic stress disorder. *Psychoneuroendocrinology* 2004; **29**: 269–78.

203 Tepavcevic D, Giljevic Z, Aganovic I, *et al.* Effects of ritanserin, a specific serotonin-S2 receptor antagonist, on the release of anterior pituitary hormones during insulin-induced hypoglycemia in normal humans. *J Endocrinol Invest* 1995; **18**: 427–30.

204 Valverde I, Penalva A, Dieguez C. Influence of different serotonin receptor subtypes on growth hormone secretion. *Neuroendocrinology* 2000; **71**: 145–53.

205 Tepavcevic D, Giljevic Z, Korsic M, *et al.* Effects of ritanserin, a novel serotonin-S2 receptor antagonist, on the secretion of pituitary hormones in normal humans. *J Endocrinol Invest* 1994; **17**: 1–5.

206 Kiss J, Csaky A, Halasz B. Demonstration of serotoninergic axon terminals on somatostatin-immunoreactive neurons of the anterior periventricular nucleus of the rat hypothalamus. *Brain Res* 1988; **442**: 23–32.

207 Conway S, Richardson L, Speciale S, *et al.* Interaction between norepinephrine and serotonin in the neuroendocrine control of growth hormone release in the rat. *Endocrinology* 1990; **126**: 1022–30.

208 Bruni JF, Meites J. Effects of cholinergic drugs on growth hormone release. *Life Sci* 1978; **23**: 1351–7.

209 Martin JB, Durand D, Gurd W, *et al.* Neuropharmacological regulation of episodic growth hormone and prolactin secretion in the rat. *Endocrinology* 1978; **102**: 106–13.

210 Casanueva FF, Betti R, Cella SG, *et al.* Effect of agonists and antagonists of cholinergic neurotransmission on growth hormone release in the dog. *Acta Endocrinol (Copenh)* 1983; **103**: 15–20.

211 Casanueva FF, Villanueva L, Diaz Y, *et al.* Atropine selectively blocks GHRH-induced GH secretion without altering LH, FSH, TSH, PRL and ACTH/cortisol secretion elicited by their specific hypothalamic releasing factors. *Clin Endocrinol (Oxf)* 1986; **25**: 319–23.

212 Casanueva FF, Villanueva L, Dieguez C, *et al.* Atropine blockade of growth hormone (GH)-releasing hormone-induced GH secretion in man is not exerted at pituitary level. *J Clin Endocrinol Metab* 1986; **62**: 186–91.

213 Casanueva FF, Villanueva L, Cabranes JA, *et al.* Cholinergic mediation of growth hormone secretion elicited by arginine, clonidine, and physical exercise in man. *J Clin Endocrinol Metab* 1984; **59**: 526–30.

214 Mendelson WB, Lantigua RA, Wyatt RJ, *et al.* Piperidine enhances sleep-related and insulin-induced growth hormone secretion: further evidence for a cholinergic secretory mechanism. *J Clin Endocrinol Metab* 1981; **52**: 409–15.

215 Locatelli V, Torsello A, Redaelli M, *et al.* Cholinergic agonist and antagonist drugs modulate the growth hormone response to growth hormone-releasing hormone in the rat: evidence for mediation by somatostatin. *J Endocrinol* 1986; **111**: 271–8.

216 Pinter I, Moszkovszkin G, Nemethy Z, Makara GB. Muscarinic M1 and M3 receptors are present and increase intracellular calcium in adult rat anterior pituitary gland. *Brain Res Bull* 1999; **48**: 449–56.

217 Carmeliet P, Denef C. Immunocytochemical and pharmacological evidence for an intrinsic cholinomimetic system modulating prolactin and growth hormone release in rat pituitary. *Endocrinology* 1988; **123**: 1128–39.

218 Carmeliet P, Baes M, Denef C. The glucocorticoid hormone dexamethasone reverses the growth hormone-releasing properties of the cholinomimetic carbachol. *Endocrinology* 1989; **124**: 2625–34.

219 Young PW, Bicknell RJ, Schofield JG. Acetylcholine stimulates growth hormone secretion, phosphatidyl inositol labelling, 45Ca2$^+$ efflux and cyclic GMP accumulation in bovine anterior pituitary glands. *J Endocrinol* 1979; **80**: 203–13.

220 Ingram CD, Bicknell RJ. Synergistic interaction in bovine pituitary cultures between growth hormone-releasing factor and other hypophysiotrophic factors. *J Endocrinol* 1986; **109**: 67–74.

221 Pontiroli AE, Viberti G, Vicari A, Pozza G. Effect of the antihistaminic agents meclastine and dexchlorpheniramine on the response of human growth hormone to arginine infusion and insulin hypoglycemia. *J Clin Endocrinol Metab* 1976; **43**: 582–6.

222 Valk TW, England BG, Marshall JC. Effects of cimetidine on pituitary function: Alterations in hormone secretion profiles. *Clin Endocrinol (Oxf)* 1981; **15**: 139–49.

223 Arvat E, Maccagno B, Ramunni J, *et al.* Effects of histaminergic antagonists on the GH-releasing activity of GHRH or hexarelin, a synthetic hexapeptide, in man. *J Endocrinol Invest* 1997; **20**: 122–7.

224 Grilli R, Sibilia V, Torsello A, *et al.* Role of the neuronal histaminergic system in the regulation of somatotropic function: comparison between the neonatal and the adult rat. *J Endocrinol* 1996; **151**: 195–201.

225 Netti C, Sibilia V, Guidobono F, Pecile A. Influence of brain histamine on growth hormone secretion induced by alpha-2-receptor activation. *Neuroendocrinology* 1993; **57**: 1066–70.

226 Veneroni O, Cocilovo L, Muller EE, Cocchi D. Delay of puberty and impairment of growth in female rats given a non competitive antagonist of NMDA receptors. *Life Sci* 1990; **47**: 1253–60.

227 Lindstrom P, Ohlsson L. Effect of N-methyl-D,L-aspartate on isolated rat somatotrophs. *Endocrinology* 1992; **131**: 1903–7.

228 Niimi M, Sato M, Murao K, *et al.* Effect of excitatory amino acid receptor agonists on secretion of growth hormone as assessed by the reverse hemolytic plaque assay. *Neuroendocrinology* 1994; **60**: 173–8.

229 Pinilla L, Gonzalez LC, Tena-Sempere M, Aguilar E. Interactions between GABAergic and aminoacidergic pathways in the control of gonadotropin and GH secretion

in pre-pubertal female rats. *J Endocrinol Invest* 2002; **25**: 96–100.

230   Vijayan E, McCann SM. Effects of intraventricular injection of gamma-aminobutyric acid (GABA) on plasma growth hormone and thyrotropin in conscious ovariectomized rats. *Endocrinology* 1978; **103**: 1888–93.

231   Cavagnini F, Benetti G, Invitti C, *et al*. Effect of gamma-aminobutyric acid on growth hormone and prolactin secretion in man: influence of pimozide and domperidone. *J Clin Endocrinol Metab* 1980; **51**: 789–92.

232   McCann SM, Vijayan E, Negro-Vilar A, *et al*. Gamma aminobutyric acid (GABA), a modulator of anterior pituitary hormone secretion by hypothalamic and pituitary action. *Psychoneuroendocrinology* 1984; **9**: 97–106.

233   Willoughby JO, Jervois PM, Menadue MF, Blessing WW. Activation of GABA receptors in the hypothalamus stimulates secretion of growth hormone and prolactin. *Brain Res* 1986; **374**: 119–25.

234   Spencer GS, Berry CJ, Bass JJ. Neuroendocrine regulation of growth hormone secretion in sheep. VII. Effects of GABA. *Regul Pept* 1994; **52**: 181–6.

235   Fiok J, Acs Z, Stark E. Possible inhibitory influence of gamma-aminobutyric acid on growth hormone secretion in the rat. *J Endocrinol* 1981; **91**: 391–7.

236   Murakami Y, Kato Y, Koshiyama H, *et al*. Involvement of alpha-adrenergic and GABAergic mechanisms in growth hormone secretion induced by central somatostatin in rats. *Brain Res* 1987; **407**: 405–8.

237   Stryker TD, Conlin T, Reichlin S. Influence of a benzodiazepine, midazolam, and gamma-aminobutyric acid (GABA) on basal somatostatin secretion from cerebral and diencephalic neurons in dispersed cell culture. *Brain Res* 1986; **362**: 339–43.

238   Murakami Y, Kato Y, Kabayama Y, *et al*. Involvement of growth hormone-releasing factor in growth hormone secretion induced by gamma-aminobutyric acid in conscious rats. *Endocrinology* 1985; **117**: 787–9.

239   Nishiki M, Murakami Y, Sohmiya M, *et al*. Effects of rat galanin and galanin message associated peptide (GMAP) on rat growth hormone secretion and stimulating effect of gamma-aminobutyric acid on galanin release from rat hypothalamus. *Neurosci Lett* 1997; **226**: 199–202.

240   Arvat E, Maccagno B, Ramunni J, *et al*. Effects of dexamethasone and alprazolam, a benzodiazepine, on the stimulatory effect of hexarelin, a synthetic GHRP, on ACTH, cortisol and GH secretion in humans. *Neuroendocrinology* 1998; **67**: 310–6.

241   Acs Z, Szabo B, Kapocs G, Makara GB. gamma-Aminobutyric acid stimulates pituitary growth hormone secretion in the neonatal rat. A superfusion study. *Endocrinology* 1987; **120**: 1790–8.

242   Anderson RA, Mitchell R. Effects of gamma-aminobutyric acid receptor agonists on the secretion of growth hormone, luteinizing hormone, adrenocorticotrophic hormone and thyroid-stimulating hormone from the rat pituitary gland in vitro. *J Endocrinol* 1986; **108**: 1–8.

243   Gamel-Didelon K, Kunz L, Fohr KJ, *et al*. Molecular and physiological evidence for functional gamma-aminobutyric acid (GABA)-C receptors in growth hormone-secreting cells. *J Biol Chem* 2003; **278**: 20192–5.

244   Zeitler P, Vician L, Chowen-Breed JA, *et al*. Regulation of somatostatin and growth hormone-releasing hormone gene expression in the rat brain. *Metabolism* 1990; **39(9 Suppl 2)**: 46–9.

245   Burton KA, Kabigting EB, Clifton DK, Steiner RA. Growth hormone receptor messenger ribonucleic acid distribution in the adult male rat brain and its colocalization in hypothalamic somatostatin neurons. *Endocrinology* 1992; **131**: 958–63.

246   Hoffman DL, Baker BL. Effect of treatment with growth hormone on somatostatin in the median eminence of hypophysectomized rats. *Proc Soc Exp Biol Med* 1977; **156**: 265–71.

247   Rogers KV, Vician L, Steiner RA, Clifton DK. The effect of hypophysectomy and growth hormone administration on pre-prosomatostatin messenger ribonucleic acid in the periventricular nucleus of the rat hypothalamus. *Endocrinology* 1988; **122**: 586–91.

248   Ganzetti I, De Gennaro V, Redaelli M, *et al*. Effect of hypophysectomy and growth hormone replacement on hypothalamic GHRH. *Peptides* 1986; **7**: 1011–4.

249   Chomczynski P, Downs TR, Frohman LA. Feedback regulation of growth hormone (GH)-releasing hormone gene expression by GH in rat hypothalamus. *Mol Endocrinol* 1988; **2**: 236–41.

250   Chan YY, Grafstein-Dunn E, Delemarre-van de Waal HA, *et al*. The role of galanin and its receptor in the feedback regulation of growth hormone secretion. *Endocrinology* 1996; **137**: 5303–10.

251   Burton KA, Kabigting EB, Steiner RA, Clifton DK. Identification of target cells for growth hormone's action in the arcuate nucleus. *Am J Physiol* 1995; **269(4 Pt 1)**: E716–22.

252   Zheng H, Bailey A, Jiang MH, *et al*. Somatostatin receptor subtype 2 knockout mice are refractory to growth hormone-negative feedback on arcuate neurons. *Mol Endocrinol* 1997; **11**: 1709–17.

253   D'Ercole AJ, Stiles AD, Underwood LE. Tissue concentrations of somatomedin C: further evidence for multiple sites of synthesis and paracrine or autocrine mechanisms of action. *Proc Natl Acad Sci USA* 1984; **81**: 935–9.

254   Reinhardt RR, Bondy CA. Insulin-like growth factors cross the blood-brain barrier. *Endocrinology* 1994; **135**: 1753–61.

255   Fernandez-Galaz MC, Torres-Aleman I, Garcia-Segura LM. Endocrine-dependent accumulation of IGF-I by hypothalamic glia. *Neuroreport* 1996; **8**: 373–7.

256   Gianotti L, Maccario M, Lanfranco F, *et al*. Arginine counteracts the inhibitory effect of recombinant human insulin-like growth factor I on the somatotroph responsiveness to growth hormone-releasing hormone in humans. *J Clin Endocrinol Metab* 2000; **85**: 3604–8.

257 Namba H, Morita S, Melmed S. Insulin-like growth factor-I action on growth hormone secretion and messenger ribonucleic acid levels: interaction with somatostatin. *Endocrinology* 1989; **124**: 1794–9.

258 Chowen JA, Gonzalez-Parra S, Garcia-Segura LM, Argente J. Sexually dimorphic interaction of insulin-like growth factor (IGF)-I and sex steroids in lactotrophs. *J Neuroendocrinol* 1998; **10**: 493–502.

259 Gonzalez-Parra S, Argente J, Chowen JA, *et al.* Gene expression of the insulin-like growth factor system during postnatal development of the rat pituitary gland. *J Neuroendocrinol* 2001; **13**: 86–93.

260 Wallenius K, Sjogren K, Peng XD, *et al.* Liver-derived IGF-I regulates GH secretion at the pituitary level in mice. *Endocrinology* 2001; **142**: 4762–70.

◆ 261 van der Lely AJ, Tschop M, Heiman ML, Ghigo E. Biological, physiological, pathophysiological, and pharmacological aspects of ghrelin. *Endocr Rev* 2004; **25**: 426–57.

◆ 262 Kojima M, Hosoda H, Matsuo H, Kangawa K. Ghrelin: discovery of the natural endogenous ligand for the growth hormone secretagogue receptor. *Trends Endocrinol Metab* 2001; **12**: 118–22.

263 Date Y, Kojima M, Hosoda H, *et al.* Ghrelin, a novel growth hormone-releasing acylated peptide, is synthesized in a distinct endocrine cell type in the gastrointestinal tracts of rats and humans. *Endocrinology* 2000; **141**: 4255–61.

264 Takaya K, Ariyasu H, Kanamoto N, *et al.* Ghrelin strongly stimulates growth hormone release in humans. *J Clin Endocrinol Metab* 2000; **85**: 4908–11.

265 Sun Y, Wang P, Zheng H, Smith RG. Ghrelin stimulation of growth hormone release and appetite is mediated through the growth hormone secretagogue receptor. *Proc Natl Acad Sci USA* 2004; **101**: 4679–84.

266 Tschop M, Smiley DL, Heiman ML. Ghrelin induces adiposity in rodents. *Nature* 2000; **407**: 908–13.

267 Nakazato M, Murakami N, Date Y, *et al.* A role for ghrelin in the central regulation of feeding. *Nature* 2001; **409**: 194–8.

● 268 Howard AD, Feighner SD, Cully DF, *et al.* A receptor in pituitary and hypothalamus that functions in growth hormone release. *Science* 1996; **273**: 974–7.

◆ 269 Smith RG, Van der Ploeg LH, Howard AD, *et al.* Peptidomimetic regulation of growth hormone secretion. *Endocr Rev* 1997; **18**: 621–45.

270 Chen C, Wu D, Clarke IJ. Signal transduction systems employed by synthetic GH-releasing peptides in somatotrophs. *J Endocrinol* 1996; **148**: 381–6.

◆ 271 Casanueva FF, Dieguez C. Neuroendocrine regulation and actions of leptin. *Front Neuroendocrinol* 1999; **20**: 317–63.

272 Shuto Y, Shibasaki T, Wada K, *et al.* Generation of polyclonal antiserum against the growth hormone secretagogue receptor (GHS-R): evidence that the GHS-R exists in the hypothalamus, pituitary and stomach of rats. *Life Sci* 2001; **68**: 991–6.

273 Guan XM, Yu H, Palyha OC, *et al.* Distribution of mRNA encoding the growth hormone secretagogue receptor in brain and peripheral tissues. *Brain Res Mol Brain Res* 1997; **48**: 23–9.

274 Hosoda H, Kojima M, Matsuo H, Kangawa K. Ghrelin and des-acyl ghrelin: two major forms of rat ghrelin peptide in gastrointestinal tissue. *Biochem Biophys Res Commun* 2000; **279**: 909–13.

275 Muccioli G, Papotti M, Locatelli V, *et al.* Binding of 125I-labeled ghrelin to membranes from human hypothalamus and pituitary gland. *J Endocrinol Invest* 2001; **24**: RC7–9.

276 Bowers CY. Unnatural growth hormone-releasing peptide begets natural ghrelin. *J Clin Endocrinol Metab* 2001; **86**: 1464–9.

277 Broglio F, Benso A, Gottero C, *et al.* Non-acylated ghrelin does not possess the pituitaric and pancreatic endocrine activity of acylated ghrelin in humans. *J Endocrinol Invest* 2003; **26**: 192–6.

278 Muller AF, Lamberts SW, Janssen JA, *et al.* Ghrelin drives GH secretion during fasting in man. *Eur J Endocrinol* 2002; **146**: 203–7.

279 Muller AF, Janssen JA, Hofland LJ, *et al.* Blockade of the growth hormone (GH) receptor unmasks rapid GH-releasing peptide-6-mediated tissue-specific insulin resistance. *J Clin Endocrinol Metab* 2001; **86**: 590–3.

280 Malagon MM, Luque RM, Ruiz-Guerrero E, *et al.* Intracellular signaling mechanisms mediating ghrelin-stimulated growth hormone release in somatotropes. *Endocrinology* 2003; **144**: 5372–80.

281 Yamazaki M, Nakamura K, Kobayashi H, *et al.* Regulational effect of ghrelin on growth hormone secretion from perifused rat anterior pituitary cells. *J Neuroendocrinol* 2002; **14**: 156–62.

282 Kamegai J, Tamura H, Shimizu T, *et al.* The role of pituitary ghrelin in growth hormone (GH) secretion: GH-releasing hormone-dependent regulation of pituitary ghrelin gene expression and peptide content. *Endocrinology* 2004; **145**: 3731–8.

283 Tamura H, Kamegai J, Shimizu T, *et al.* Ghrelin stimulates GH but not food intake in arcuate nucleus ablated rats. *Endocrinology* 2002; **143**: 3268–75.

● 284 Halaas JL, Gajiwala KS, Maffei M, *et al.* Weight-reducing effects of the plasma protein encoded by the obese gene. *Science* 1995; **269**: 543–6.

285 Harrold JA. Leptin leads hypothalamic feeding circuits in a new direction. *Bioessays* 2004; **26**: 1043–5.

286 Saleri R, Giustina A, Tamanini C, *et al.* Leptin stimulates growth hormone secretion via a direct pituitary effect combined with a decreased somatostatin tone in a median eminence-pituitary perifusion study. *Neuroendocrinology* 2004; **79**: 221–8.

287 Tannenbaum GS, Gurd W, Lapointe M. Leptin is a potent stimulator of spontaneous pulsatile growth hormone (GH) secretion and the GH response to GH-releasing hormone. *Endocrinology* 1998; **139**: 3871–5.

288 Vuagnat BA, Pierroz DD, Lalaoui M, *et al.* Evidence for a leptin-neuropeptide Y axis for the regulation of growth

hormone secretion in the rat. *Neuroendocrinology* 1998; **67**: 291–300.

289 Carro E, Senaris RM, Seoane LM, *et al.* Role of growth hormone (GH)-releasing hormone and somatostatin on leptin-induced GH secretion. *Neuroendocrinology* 1999; **69**: 3–10.

290 Zlokovic BV, Jovanovic S, Miao W, *et al.* Differential regulation of leptin transport by the choroid plexus and blood-brain barrier and high affinity transport systems for entry into hypothalamus and across the blood-cerebrospinal fluid barrier. *Endocrinology* 2000; **141**: 1434–41.

291 Zhao AZ, Huan JN, Gupta S, *et al.* A phosphatidylinositol 3-kinase phosphodiesterase 3B-cyclic AMP pathway in hypothalamic action of leptin on feeding. *Nat Neurosci* 2002; **5**: 727–8.

292 Tartaglia LA, Dembski M, Weng X, *et al.* Identification and expression cloning of a leptin receptor, OB-R. *Cell* 1995; **83**: 1263–71.

293 Vaisse C, Halaas JL, Horvath CM, *et al.* Leptin activation of Stat3 in the hypothalamus of wild-type and ob/ob mice but not db/db mice. *Nat Genet* 1996; **14**: 95–7.

294 Ghilardi N, Ziegler S, Wiestner A, *et al.* Defective STAT signaling by the leptin receptor in diabetic mice. *Proc Natl Acad Sci USA* 1996; **93**: 6231–5.

295 Bates SH, Stearns WH, Dundon TA, *et al.* STAT3 signalling is required for leptin regulation of energy balance but not reproduction. *Nature* 2003; **421**: 856–9.

296 Seifert H, Perrin M, Rivier J, Vale W. Binding sites for growth hormone releasing factor on rat anterior pituitary cells. *Nature* 1985; **313**: 487–9.

297 Schonbrunn A. Glucocorticoids down-regulate somatostatin receptors on pituitary cells in culture. *Endocrinology* 1982; **110**: 1147–54.

298 Iwasaki Y, Morishita M, Asai M, *et al.* Effects of hormones targeting nuclear receptors on transcriptional regulation of the growth hormone gene in the MtT/S rat somatotrope cell line. *Neuroendocrinology* 2004; **79**: 229–36.

299 Señaris RM, Lago F, Coya R, *et al.* Regulation of hypothalamic somatostatin, growth hormone-releasing hormone, and growth hormone receptor messenger ribonucleic acid by glucocorticoids. *Endocrinology* 1996; **137**: 5236–41.

300 Chernausek SD, Turner R. Attenuation of spontaneous, nocturnal growth hormone secretion in children with hypothyroidism and its correlation with plasma insulin-like growth factor I concentrations. *J Pediatr* 1989; **114**: 968–72.

301 Finkelstein JW, Boyar RM, Hellman L. Growth hormone secretion in hyperthyroidism. *J Clin Endocrinol Metab* 1974; **38**: 634–7.

302 Binoux M, Faivre-Bauman A, Lassarre C, *et al.* Triiodothyronine stimulates the production of insulin-like growth factor (IGF) by fetal hypothalamus cells cultured in serum-free medium. *Brain Res* 1985; **353**: 319–21.

303 Jansson JO, Ekberg S, Isaksson OG, Eden S. Influence of gonadal steroids on age- and sex-related secretory patterns of growth hormone in the rat. *Endocrinology* 1984; **114**: 1287–94.

◆ 304 Leung KC, Johannsson G, Leong GM, Ho KK. Estrogen regulation of growth hormone action. *Endocr Rev* 2004; **25**: 693–721.

305 Gonzalez-Parra S, Chowen JA, Garcia-Segura LM, Argente J. In vivo and in vitro regulation of pituitary transcription factor-1 (Pit-1) by changes in the hormone environment. *Neuroendocrinology* 1996; **63**: 3–15.

306 Gonzalez-Parra S, Argente J, Garcia-Segura LM, Chowen JA. Cellular composition of the adult rat anterior pituitary is influenced by the neonatal sex steroid environment. *Neuroendocrinology* 1998; **68**: 152–62.

307 Chowen JA, Argente J, Gonzalez-Parra S, Garcia-Segura LM. Differential effects of the neonatal and adult sex steroid environments on the organization and activation of hypothalamic growth hormone-releasing hormone and somatostatin neurons. *Endocrinology* 1993; **133**: 2792–802.

308 Simonian SX, Murray HE, Gillies GE, Herbison AE. Estrogen-dependent ontogeny of sex differences in somatostatin neurons of the hypothalamic periventricular nucleus. *Endocrinology* 1998; **139**: 1420–8.

309 Chowen JA, Torres-Aleman I, Garcia-Segura LM. Trophic effects of estradiol on fetal rat hypothalamic neurons. *Neuroendocrinology* 1992; **56**: 895–901.

310 Argente J, Chowen-Breed JA, Steiner RA, Clifton DK. Somatostatin messenger RNA in hypothalamic neurons is increased by testosterone through activation of androgen receptors and not by aromatization to estradiol. *Neuroendocrinology* 1990; **52**: 342–9.

311 Herbison AE. Sexually dimorphic expression of androgen receptor immunoreactivity by somatostatin neurones in rat hypothalamic periventricular nucleus and bed nucleus of the stria terminalis. *J Neuroendocrinol* 1995; **7**: 543–53.

312 Kamegai J, Tamura H, Shimizu T, *et al.* Estrogen receptor (ER)alpha, but not ERbeta, gene is expressed in growth hormone-releasing hormone neurons of the male rat hypothalamus. *Endocrinology* 2001; **142**: 538–43.

313 Fodor M, Oudejans CB, Delemarre-van de Waal HA. Absence of androgen receptor in the growth hormone releasing hormone-containing neurones in the rat mediobasal hypothalamus. *J Neuroendocrinol* 2001; **13**: 724–7.

314 Broglio F, Prodam F, Gottero C, *et al.* Ghrelin does not mediate the somatotroph and corticotrophin responses to the stimulatory effect of glucagon or insulin-induced hypoglycaemia in humans. *Clin Endocrinol (Oxf)* 2004; **60**: 699–704.

315 Flanagan DE, Evans ML, Monsod TP, *et al.* The influence of insulin on circulating ghrelin. *Am J Physiol Endocrinol Metab* 2003; **284**: E313–6.

316 Jaffe CA, DeMott-Friberg R, Barkan AL. Endogenous growth hormone (GH)-releasing hormone is required for GH responses to pharmacological stimuli. *J Clin Invest* 1996; **97**: 934–40.

317 Barbetti F, Crescenti C, Negri M, *et al.* Growth hormone does not inhibit its own secretion during prolonged hypoglycemia in man. *J Clin Endocrinol Metab* 1990; **70**: 1371–4.

318 Thorner MO, Chapman IM, Gaylinn BD, *et al.* Growth hormone-releasing hormone and growth hormone-releasing peptide as therapeutic agents to enhance growth hormone secretion in disease and aging. *Recent Prog Horm Res* 1997; **52**: 215–46.

319 Tannenbaum GS, Martin JB, Colle E. Ultradian growth hormone rhythm in the rat: effects of feeding, hyperglycemia, and insulin-induced hypoglycemia. *Endocrinology* 1976; **99**: 720–7.

320 Murao K, Sato M, Mizobuchi M, *et al.* Acute effects of hypoglycemia and hyperglycemia on hypothalamic growth hormone-releasing hormone and somatostatin gene expression in the rat. *Endocrinology* 1994; **134**: 418–23.

321 Baes M, Vale WW. Characterization of the glucose-dependent release of growth hormone-releasing factor and somatostatin from superfused rat hypothalami. *Neuroendocrinology* 1990; **51**: 202–7.

322 Busiguina S, Argente J, Garcia-Segura LM, Chowen JA. Anatomically specific changes in the expression of somatostatin, growth hormone-releasing hormone and growth hormone receptor mRNA in diabetic rats. *J Neuroendocrinol* 2000; **12**: 29–39.

323 Olchovsky D, Bruno JF, Wood TL, *et al.* Altered pituitary growth hormone (GH) regulation in streptozotocin-diabetic rats: a combined defect of hypothalamic somatostatin and GH-releasing factor. *Endocrinology* 1990; **126**: 53–61.

324 Renier G, Serri O. Effects of acute and prolonged glucose excess on growth hormone release by cultured rat anterior pituitary cells. *Neuroendocrinology* 1991; **54**: 521–5.

325 Barb CR, Kraeling RR, Rampacek GB. Glucose and free fatty acid modulation of growth hormone and luteinizing hormone secretion by cultured porcine pituitary cells. *J Anim Sci* 1995; **73**: 1416–23.

326 Yamashita S, Melmed S. Effects of insulin on rat anterior pituitary cells. Inhibition of growth hormone secretion and mRNA levels. *Diabetes* 1986; **35**: 440–7.

327 Besset A, Bonardet A, Rondouin G, *et al.* Increase in sleep related GH and Prl secretion after chronic arginine aspartate administration in man. *Acta Endocrinol (Copenh)* 1982; **99**: 18–23.

328 Isidori A, Lo Monaco A, Cappa M. A study of growth hormone release in man after oral administration of amino acids. *Curr Med Res Opin* 1981; **7**: 475–81.

329 Knopf RF, Conn JW, Floyd JC Jr, *et al.* The normal endocrine response to ingestion of protein and infusions of amino acids. Sequential secretion of insulin and growth hormone. *Trans Assoc Am Physicians* 1966; **79**: 312–21.

330 Alba-Roth J, Muller OA, Schopohl J, von Werder K. Arginine stimulates growth hormone secretion by suppressing endogenous somatostatin secretion. *J Clin Endocrinol Metab* 1988; **67**: 1186–9.

331 Hanew K, Utsumi A. The role of endogenous GHRH in arginine-, insulin-, clonidine- and l-dopa-induced GH release in normal subjects. *Eur J Endocrinol* 2002; **146**: 197–202.

332 Merimee TJ, Rabinowtitz D, Fineberg SE. Arginine-initiated release of human growth hormone. Factors modifying the response in normal man. *N Engl J Med* 1969; **280**: 1434–8.

333 Moncada S, Palmer RM, Higgs EA. Nitric oxide: physiology, pathophysiology, and pharmacology. *Pharmacol Rev* 1991; **43**: 109–42.

334 Fisker S, Nielsen S, Ebdrup L, *et al.* The role of nitric oxide in L-arginine-stimulated growth hormone release. *J Endocrinol Invest* 1999; **22(5 Suppl)**: 89–93.

335 Alvarez P, Isidro L, Peino R, *et al.* Effect of acute reduction of free fatty acids by acipimox on growth hormone-releasing hormone-induced GH secretion in type 1 diabetic patients. *Clin Endocrinol (Oxf)* 2003; **59**: 431–6.

336 Dieguez C, Carro E, Seoane LM, *et al.* Regulation of somatotroph cell function by the adipose tissue. *Int J Obes Relat Metab Disord* 2000; **24(Suppl 2)**: S100–3.

337 Alvarez CV, Mallo F, Burguera B, *et al.* Evidence for a direct pituitary inhibition by free fatty acids of in vivo growth hormone responses to growth hormone-releasing hormone in the rat. *Neuroendocrinology* 1991; **53**: 185–9.

338 Imaki T, Shibasaki T, Masuda A, *et al.* The effect of glucose and free fatty acids on growth hormone (GH)-releasing factor-mediated GH secretion in rats. *Endocrinology* 1986; **118**: 2390–4.

339 Penalva A, Gaztambide S, Vazquez JA, *et al.* Role of cholinergic muscarinic pathways on the free fatty acid inhibition of GH responses to GHRH in normal men. *Clin Endocrinol (Oxf)* 1990; **33**: 171–6.

340 Briard N, Rico-Gomez M, Guillaume V, *et al.* Hypothalamic mediated action of free fatty acid on growth hormone secretion in sheep. *Endocrinology* 1998; **139**: 4811–9.

341 Senaris RM, Lewis MD, Lago F, *et al.* Stimulatory effect of free fatty acids on growth hormone releasing hormone secretion by fetal rat neurons in monolayer culture. *Neurosci Lett* 1992; **135**: 80–2.

7

Peripheral hormone action

JEFF M P HOLLY

LOCAL TISSUE REGULATORS: GROWTH FACTORS

The regulation of tissue growth involves a complex interplay between many of the classic hormonal systems and a multitude of local signals. The local signals come under the general term 'cytokines', soluble products released from a cell that can then act on cells and modulate their function or activity. The term cytokine covers many different categories of signals used by cells for communication including those used by cells of the immune system originally known as the monokines or lymphokines, including the large family of interleukins. The other large category of cytokines are the peptide growth factors. These are subgrouped into a number of families: the insulin-like growth factors (IGFs), the epidermal growth factors (EGFs), the fibroblast growth factors (FGFs), the transforming growth factor-β (TGF-β) superfamily and the neurotrophic growth factors. The names of these families evolved in a historical manner that relates to cells or actions for which they were first recognised. These names can now seem inappropriate and even misleading for example, TGF-α is not related to TGF-β, but falls within the EGF family.

MODES OF OPERATION OF LOCAL REGULATORS

Conventionally hormones have been considered to be secreted from the ductless glands into the circulation to convey their signal to distant target tissues in an 'endocrine' manner. It was apparent that many of the cytokines conveyed their signals between cells in very different ways and other classifications of signaling were defined to describe the various modes of communication. Paracrine action, where factors secreted from one cell carry their signal to neighboring cells, is a term that encompasses most local tissue regulation. The term autocrine describes the secretion of cytokines that could stimulate functional responses in the same cells from which they were secreted.[1] Other terms describing variations of autocrine or paracrine signaling have also evolved. These include juxtacrine, in which the signal is not freely secreted, but is held on the surface and can stimulate receptors on the same or neighboring cells. This can involve the cytokine being produced as a propeptide with a transmembrane domain that becomes integrated into the plasma membrane where it can activate adjacent receptors within the membrane or on neighboring cells. The mature cytokine can also be shed from the surface by the action of specific proteinases and then act as a soluble signal as if secreted. Several members of the EGF family are produced in this way, as initially membrane proteins. Alternatively the cytokine could be retained on the surface either by a membrane anchor or by interacting with a cell surface docking protein. A number of growth factors including forms of platelet-derived growth factor (PDGF) and forms of vascular endothelial growth factor (VEGF) contain a conserved sequence of amino acids that form a cell surface retention sequence that ensures that they are retained at the cell surface by binding to specific binding proteins within the plasma membrane. There is also a variation of autocrine signaling called intracrine, in which the signal is never actually secreted or externalized, but conveys the signal within the cell.

In addition to these newly recognized modes of signaling for cytokines, it is now evident that many classical hormones are produced in many tissues other than the ductless glands with which they were historically associated. For example growth hormone (GH) is produced in the placenta and many other tissues in addition to the pituitary. These classical hormones can then have paracrine, autocrine and even intracrine actions in addition to their better known endocrine actions. In an analogous manner many local tissue growth factors are not restricted to only paracrine or autocrine modes of action, but in some instances they can operate in an endocrine mode. It should be noted that these classifications are somewhat arbitrary terms, which are used to help describe the various modes of action. They are not mutually exclusive and they mean nothing to the cell that actually receives the signal; the signal is generally interpreted by the cell in the same way regardless of how it arrives at the cell. There are some exceptions to this for growth factors that may act in an intracrine manner in addition to autocrine and paracrine modes following secretion. For example, forms of PDGF and VEGF can be localized with their receptors during routing of these proteins from the endoplasmic reticulum to the trans-Golgi network resulting in receptor activation and signaling. This can differ from the signaling that occurs from activation of receptors at the plasma membrane, due to differences in the presence of signaling components that can be coupled to the receptors at these different subcellular locations.

Most cytokines can not only operate via different modes of signaling, but they are also pluripotential; they can convey many different messages. Cells that possess the appropriate receptor can respond in many different ways. Most growth factors in addition to stimulating proliferation can also stimulate cell motility and migration, metabolism, specific differentiated functions and induce changes to the differentiated state of the cell. These actions are not necessarily mutually exclusive or independent and actions other than stimulation of mitogenesis can markedly influence tissue growth. For example, many cells proliferate more readily when not fully differentiated and stimulation of differentiation can result in a decrease in tissue growth. Most tissues are in a dynamic state with cells having a finite lifespan and continually dying through programmed cell death (apoptosis); tissue growth may therefore result not only from enhanced cell proliferation, but also a decrease in the rate of apoptosis (see Chapter 2). Tissue growth is also obviously an anabolic process that is dependent on increased fuel utilization and can be increased by stimulation of metabolism.

In addition to a number of the classical hormones there is evidence indicating that somatic growth regulation is also dependent upon important roles of growth factors including the IGFs and members of the FGF and TGF-β family.

INSULIN-LIKE GROWTH FACTORS

Consistent with their pluripotential nature, the IGFs were discovered from three independent lines of research. They were isolated from plasma as non-suppressible insulin-like activity,[2] as autocrine factors that could sustain the growth of cells in the absence of serum and termed 'multiplication-stimulating activity'[3] and as plasma intermediates of GH action.[4] This later observation arose from the demonstration that although epiphyseal cartilage was the prime target of the endocrine effects of growth hormone on skeletal growth, GH had no effect on cartilage growth measured *in vitro* as sulphate uptake. A GH-dependent factor with such activity was however identified in serum; this was originally called 'sulfation factor' and then later 'somatomedin'.[5] When subsequently purified and sequenced[6] it was clear that all of these actions were due to two related peptides which were members of the insulin gene family and in 1987 the nomenclature of IGF-I and IGF-II was adopted.[7]

IGFs: Peptides and receptors

Insulin-like growth factor-I (IGF-I) is a single chain polypeptide of 70 amino acids that is encoded from a complex gene on chromosome 12.[8] From this gene a number of transcripts are derived; these are differentially regulated in a tissue-specific manner, but all give rise to the same mature IGF-I peptide. The biological significance of the complexity at the gene level is still poorly understood. The other peptide, IGF-II, consists of 67 amino acids that are encoded on a single gene on chromosome 11, immediately downstream of the insulin gene. The IGFs share around 50 percent amino acid homology with each other and with proinsulin.

There are two specific cell surface receptors with which the IGFs interact. Most of the cellular actions of the IGFs have been attributed to binding to the IGF-I receptor (IGF-IR), which binds IGF-I with high affinity, IGF-II with a slightly lower affinity and has weak cross-reacting with insulin. This receptor shares 50–60 percent overall amino acid homology with the insulin receptor (IR), with the same heterotetrameric subunit structure and a cytoplasmic domain with tyrosine kinase activity that initiates the intracellular signal.[9] These receptors are so similar that in cells which express both, hybrid IGF-I/insulin receptors are formed by the dimerization of IGF-IR with IR. These hybrids are prevalent in many tissues and bind IGFs with high affinity although much is still to be learned regarding their physiological significance. The insulin receptor is also present in two differentially spliced forms, IR-A and IR-B, and the IR-A form binds IGF-II with high affinity and may account for many previously unexplained actions attributed to IGF-II specifically. It was originally considered that the IGF-IR mediated a growth response, whereas the insulin receptor mediated a metabolic response and that it was only at pharmacological levels that IGFs could cross-react with

IRs and elicit a metabolic response. It is now clear that these receptors are extremely similar and that differences in responses are more due to the context within which the receptor is activated rather than inherent differences in the receptors. In the important metabolic tissues the IR is activated on skeletal muscle myotubes and adipocytes; cells that respond metabolically, but which are terminally differentiated and therefore are not capable of further proliferation.

The other specific IGF receptor is the IGF-II/mannose-6-phosphate receptor (IGF-II/M6PR) a monomeric transmembrane protein that is structurally unrelated to IGF-IR or IR. This receptor binds IGF-II with high affinity, IGF-I with much lower affinity and does not bind insulin. This receptor has a well defined function, via its mannose-6-phosphate binding site, in trafficking newly formed enzymes from the endoplasmic reticulum to the lysosomes. It also has many other potential roles due to the large number of other molecules that it interacts with at the cell surface including retinoids and latent forms of TGF-β. This receptor appears to be a very pluripotential protein with many different actions, although it has no clear direct function in conveying IGF-mediated signals. In relation to the IGF-system, it is widely regarded as a scavenger receptor for the clearance of IGF-II and thus protecting the cell from excess exposure to IGF-I in the pericellular environment.

IGF-binding proteins

While the ligands and the receptors within the IGF and insulin systems are remarkably similar, there is an important distinction, which makes their physiology very different. Insulin is produced exclusively in the beta cells within pancreatic islets where it is stored and released in a controlled manner according to metabolic conditions. In contrast, the IGFs are produced within most, if not all, tissues within the body, but they are not stored within cells. Whereas insulin when secreted from the pancreas is then active to stimulate receptors within target tissues; the IGFs, however, when secreted are associated with high affinity soluble binding proteins. Virtually all of the IGF that is present within the body is tightly bound in high-molecular weight complexes that are formed with a family of six closely related proteins, named IGFBP-1 through to IGFBP-6[10] although the IGFs and their receptors are widely expressed, the pattern of IGFBPs produced and their processing vary from tissue to tissue and change developmentally within individual tissues. Each of the IGFBPs interacts with many other proteins in addition to IGFs, a number of the IGFBPs bind to components of the extracellular matrix (ECM) and retain an additional reservoir of IGF within the ECM. This complex array of IGFBPs and associated proteins therefore provide a means of conferring specificity on the actions of these ubiquitous pluripotential peptides (Table 7.1). The IGFBPs generally bind to the IGFs with affinities that are greater than that of the IGF-IR and the equilibrium therefore does not favor the IGFs interacting with and activating their signaling receptor. The affinity of binding can, however, be lowered by a variety of modifications to the IGFBPs; including changes in phosphorylation, specific interactions with proteoglycans and proteolytic cleavage. While the IGFs are relatively resistant to cleavage, the IGFBPs are very susceptible and cleavage by many general extracellular proteases has been described.[11] In addition, specific proteases that cleave individual IGFBPs have been reported. These enzymes generally do not destroy the IGFBP, but subtly modify it, decreasing its affinity for binding IGF. This provides a controlled mechanism for making IGFs available from IGFBPs for clearance, for interaction with other IGFBPs or for activation of cell receptors.

Considerable information has been obtained regarding the sites of production, the regulation and the properties of these IGFBPs; but there is still much to be learned before a coherent understanding of how they all interact to determine IGF activity throughout the body can be formulated. There

Table 7.1 Complexity of the principal growth factor families implicated in somatic growth regulation

Growth factor	Ligand	Binding protein/Accessory molecule	Receptor
IGF	IGF-I IGF-II (Insulin)	IGFBP-1 to IGFBP-6 ALS Matrix/cell surface proteoglycans	IGF-I receptor (signaling) IGF-II receptor (signaling)
FGF	FGF-1 to FGF-14 and FGF-16 to FGF-23	Matrix/cell surface proteoglycans	FGFR-1 to FGFR-4 (each receptor exists in multiple forms)
TGF-β	TGF-β1 to TGF-β3 BMP-2 to BMP-7 CDMPs Activins and inhibins Others	LAP TGF-β-binding protein Beta-glycan (type III receptor) IGF-II receptor Follistatin, noggin, chordin, others	Type I receptors (multiple forms) Type II receptors (multiple forms) (These interact to form multiple TGF-β/type I/type II receptor complexes

IGF, insulin-like growth factor; FGF, fibroblast growth factor; TGF, transforming growth factor; CDMP, cartilage-derived morphogenic protein; BMP, bone morphogenic protein; LAP, latency-associated peptide; ALS, acid labile substrate.

is, however, sufficient evidence to suggest clear roles for two of the IGFBPs. In addition, specific functions have been proposed for a number of the IGFBPs within individual tissues.

In contrast to most of the IGFBPs, the expression of IGFBP-1 is restricted to relatively few sites; primarily in the liver, but also in a few other tissues where rapid cell growth and tissue remodeling occurs, such as in the ovary, endometrium, and the decidua. Production of IGFBP-1 in the liver is tightly regulated by insulin, resulting in circulating concentrations that are dynamically regulated and synchronized to nutritional status. Increases in pancreatic insulin secretion rapidly suppress hepatic production of IGFBP-1 leading to decreasing levels in the circulation. This enables IGFBP-1 to function as an 'endocrine modulator' of systemic IGF actions, such that IGF activity complements that of insulin and tissue growth is only promoted when there is metabolic fuel available to sustain it and the signal to utilize the fuel. In the liver, IGFBP-1 is produced in the hepatocytes, the same cells that produce sex hormone-binding globulin (SHBG) and insulin regulates both in a synchronized manner. Circulating levels of both IGFBP-1 and SHBG decrease throughout puberty, coincident with an increase in insulin secretion enabling childhood growth and sexual maturation to be regulated in a co-ordinate manner according to metabolic status.[12]

The other IGFBP with a clear systemic role is IGFBP-3, which carries the vast majority of the IGF that is present in the circulation. When IGFBP-3 has an IGF molecule bound it can then associate with a further glycoprotein, known as the acid-labile subunit (ALS).[13] This ternary complex is around 150 kDa and is relatively retained within the vascular compartment, where it greatly extends the circulating half-life of the IGFs and therefore maintains a large circulating reservoir of IGF. In adult humans, total circulating IGF concentrations are around 100 nmol/l which is around 1000-fold higher than insulin concentrations and considerably higher than the concentrations of any other peptide growth factor, most of which are not normally found in the circulation in significant amounts other than in platelets. This large circulating reservoir enables the IGFs to act in an endocrine manner in addition to their autocrine and paracrine actions. The majority of the circulating IGF-I is produced from hepatocytes under GH regulation; the ALS is also produced from hepatocytes under GH regulation. In contrast IGFBP-3 production in the liver is from Kupfer cells which do not possess GH receptors, although circulating levels of IGFBP-3 are GH dependent. The circulating concentrations of each of the components of the IGF/IGFBP-3/ALS ternary complex are all interdependent due to their association being the predominant determinant of their clearance. The size of this circulating reservoir is primarily dependent upon GH status. The IGFs can be made available from this reservoir to the tissues by a number of potential mechanisms. Interactions with proteoglycans on the vascular endothelium can lead to disassociation of IGF/IGFBP-3 binary complexes from the

ALS in ternary complexes and these binary complexes can then pass out from the capillaries into the tissues. In the circulation specific proteolysis of IGFBP-3 can also occur which lowers the affinity with which the IGF is bound; the IGF can then re-equilibrate to other IGFBPs forming binary complexes which can then transport the IGF out into the tissues. An increase in proteolysis of circulating IGFBP-3 has been demonstrated in late pregnancy and in various catabolic states.

IGFs and growth

The original studies documenting the pattern of expression of IGFs and their receptors and the changes in circulating IGF concentrations during development, implied an important role in somatic growth regulation. The potential for IGF-I and, to a lesser extent, IGF-II to stimulate somatic growth was confirmed by studies in which the peptides were administered to laboratory animals and subsequently to humans.[14] Growth could be promoted by IGF-I even during fetal and early postnatal life when administration of GH had no such effect.[15] The administration of GH to young animals, however produced proportionate somatic growth, whereas the administration of IGF-I caused disproportionate growth of specific organs such as the spleen, kidney, and thymus.[16] These observations have to be interpreted with caution and a consideration of the experimental models. When GH is administered into the vasculature of experiment animals, this mimics its normal endocrine mode of action. Administration of IGF-I however cannot mimic the normal complex endocrine/paracrine/autocrine mode of action of this growth factor. In addition, systemic administration of IGF-I rapidly suppresses endogenous GH secretion and pancreatic insulin secretion; in these experiments IGF-I effects are therefore seen against a background of reduced GH and insulin levels, whereas in normal physiology it would generally act in concert with increased levels of both.

The important role that the IGFs play in somatic growth regulation have been confirmed by genetic manipulations in mice. Overexpression of human IGF-I in transgenic mice resulted in a 30 percent increase in body weight, which developed from 4 weeks of postnatal life;[17] whereas overexpression of IGF-II had no effect on skeletal growth.[18] Mice created with targeted disruption of the genes such that they do not express either the IGF-I gene or the IGF-II gene had reduced, but proportionate fetal growth, with birth weights that were 60 percent of normal, confirming a role for both as fetal growth regulators.[19–21] Survival and postnatal growth were normal in the mice lacking the IGF-II gene, but mice lacking the IGF-I gene had a marked increase in neonatal death rate and postnatal growth was reduced such that weight was down to 30 percent of normal at 8 weeks. This confirmed the role of IGF-I, but not IGF-II, as a postnatal growth regulator. The lack of IGF-I resulted in delays in long-bone ossification and sexual development.

Mice lacking both IGF-I and IGF-II had birthweights decreased further to 30 percent of normal and all died within minutes of birth. Mice lacking the IGF-IR were similar to the double IGF-I and IGF-II 'knock-out' except that fetal growth was slightly less compromised (45 percent normal birthweight), but again they died immediately after birth. Mice in which IGF-I and the IGF-IR were 'knocked out' were identical to those lacking the IGF-IR, implying that IGF-I has no additional effects that were not mediated by the IGF-IR. Mice lacking IGF-II and the IGF-IR were smaller, however, than those just lacking the IGF-IR (30 percent versus 45 percent normal birthweight) indicating that IGF-II has additional actions not mediated by the IGF-IR. Placental growth was only deficient in mice lacking IGF-II and this deficiency was apparently independent of IGF-I or IGF-IR. The recognition that IGF-II also acts via forms of the IR, helps to explain these observations. The phenotypes of these gene knockout studies reveal effects which are not compensated for by other regulators.

There have been a few reports of humans with genetic defects that complement these experimental mouse experiments. A patient homologous for a partial IGF-I gene deletion was reported with severe intrauterine growth retardation and postnatal growth failure.[22] The IGF-II gene is normally imprinted such that only the paternal allele is functional, whereas the maternal allele is inactive. Over-expression of IGF-II, as a result of either duplication of the paternal allele or relaxation of imprinting such that both parentally derived alleles are active, has been implicated in tissue overgrowth seen in some children with somatic overgrowth or with Beckwith–Wiedemann syndrome.[23] Local overexpression of IGF-II has also been reported in childhood solid tumors, particularly Wilms' tumor.[24] These observations are consistent with the data from mice indicating that IGF-II plays an important role in the regulation of growth in early life. In mice the IGF-II/ MGPR gene is also imprinted and exclusively expressed from the maternally derived allele. Most humans, however, express both alleles equally, although a few individuals may repress the paternal allele to a variable extent.[25] A few children with intrauterine growth retardation and postnatal growth failure have been identified to have mutations to the IGF-IR.[26] Although IGF-I is regarded as the classic cartilage growth regulator, much of the data that have been accumulated regarding this role had proceeded an appreciation of the complexities of the mode of operation of the IGF-system itself and its multiple interactions with other cytokines and hormones. Following the initial gene 'knock-out' studies that involved generalized knock-out of this gene, subsequent studies have used refined techniques to inactivate gene expression in a tissue specific manner. Targeted inactivation of the IGF-I gene just in the liver confirmed that this was the major source of IGF-I present in the circulation.[27,28] Despite the observed 75–80 percent reduction in circulating IGF-I concentration, the growth and development of these mice were essentially unaffected. These studies do not prove, however, that endocrine IGF-I does not have a role in somatic growth regulation and their interpretation is complex. These manipulations confirmed the importance of circulating IGF-I for feedback control at the pituitary gland, although the markedly elevated GH levels further complicate the interpretation of the deficiency in circulating IGF-I concentration. In the normal state the circulating reservoir of IGF is in such large excess that even an 80 percent reduction in concentration would still not reduce levels below that required for optimal activation of IGF-IR in target tissues. The complexity of these experimental models was further demonstrated when the inactivation of the ALS was reported.[29] Despite a smaller reduction in circulating IGF-I concentration (62 percent) these mice manifest mild postnatal growth retardation, being 13 percent smaller by 10 weeks. A lack of distinction between the role for liver-derived circulating IGF-I and locally produced IGF-I is not surprising as it seems clear that they would both combine to achieve the threshold for stimulating optimal growth in the tissues. A threshold of circulating IGF-I is suggested by mice with both ALS and hepatic IGF-I genes disrupted; these mice have even lower serum IGF-I concentrations than either single knock-out and reduced linear growth.[27] Local IGF-I synthesis within the epiphysical growth plate of the bones is also regulated by GH and by other hormones such as parathyroid hormone (PTH), steroids (including oestrogen and cortisol), thyroid hormones and vitamin D as well as by other local regulators including FGFs, TGF-β and PDGFs.[30] The relative importance of these compared with GH for determining the effects of IGF-I on growth is not clear. In addition, GH has been shown both to have direct effects and to modulate the production of other local growth factors such as basic FGFs[31] and again their relative importance compared with IGF-I, for mediating GH effects is unclear. In contrast to IGF-I, IGF-II appears to be less affected by systemic hormones and more dependent on local regulators,[32] but the relative contribution of IGF-II to overall growth is unclear. There are greater species differences in the physiology of IGF-II, than for IGF-I, between humans and rodents, which means the experimental models are less informative. Most of the IGFBPs are produced in skeletal tissue where they are regulated by hormones and local factors and most studies indicate that they generally restrict IGF effects in bone growth with the exception of IGFBP-5, which appears to potentiate IGF effects.[33] There is however evidence that IGFBP-2 can potentiate the effect of IGF-II on osteoblasts[34] and there is still much to be learned regarding how all of the components are integrated to regulate skeletal growth.

FIBROBLAST GROWTH FACTORS

Historically, the FGFs acquired their name from the description of a factor that stimulated mitogenesis of fibroblasts,[35] but the FGFs are now recognized to be pluripotential regulators of many cell types, affecting many aspects of cell function.

Complexities of ligands, receptors, and accessory molecules

Specificity is conferred on the pleiotropic FGFs by way of complex interactions between multiple components (see Table 7.1). In humans there are 22 known members of the FGF family (FGF1–14 and FGF16–23; human FGF-15 has not been identified) which range in size from 17 kDa to 34 kDa.[36] There is further heterogeneity because a number of FGFs exist in different forms, for several of the FGFs there are alternatively spliced forms derived from the same gene. Most of the FGFs have amino-terminal signal peptides and are secreted from cells via the conventional pathway, FGFs 9, 16, and 20 lack an obvious signal peptide, but are nevertheless secreted. FGF1 and FGF2 also lack signal peptides and are not secreted via the conventional pathway, although they are found outside of cells and are thought to be externalized via an alternative route. FGFs 11–14 lack signal peptide, and are thought to remain intracellular and act in an autocrine manner. At least a couple of the FGFs have nuclear-localization sequences and the proteins can be found in the nucleus where they could potentially affect transcription. The secreted or cytoplasmic ligands can interact with numerous high-affinity cell receptors, which are derived from four distinct genes, FGFR1–4. The receptors are transmembrane glycoproteins with extracellular immunoglobulin-like domains and cytoplasmic domains with intrinsic kinase activity. Multiple isoforms of these receptors are derived from alternative splicing which determines the number of extracellular immunoglobulin domains and the ligand specifying of the receptor. In addition to these high-affinity receptors, the FGFs also bind to heparan sulfate proteoglycans within the ECM and the cell surface. The cell surface glycosaminoglycans, such as the syndecans, act as 'accessory' co-factors that sequester FGFs and facilitate their interaction with the high affinity receptors and their subsequent dimerization that is required for activation. The variety of FGFs, FGFR isoforms, and proteoglycan co-factors which may all be expressed in a cell-specific and developmentally specific manner, provide for an extremely complex regulation system.

FGFs and somatic growth

The presence of FGFs within the growth plate implied that they could be important for skeletal (and hence somatic) growth and *in vitro* studies demonstrated that FGFs were potent stimulators of chondrocyte mitogenesis and matrix synthesis.[37] Their critical role was also indicated by experimental studies that demonstrated that the developmental defect in limb outgrowth caused by removal of the apical ectodermal ridge could be partially rescued by replacement with a bead soaked in FGF4.[38] The importance of FGFs for human skeletal growth was then verified by studies identifying the genetic defects leading to skeletal syndromes. Mutations in FGFR3 were identified as the cause of the vast

majority of cases of achondroplasia, the most common form of human dwarfism[39,40] and mutations in FGFRI and FGFR2 were described in a number of craniosynostosis syndromes.[41–43] A large number of mutations in these three FGF receptors have subsequently been described, although somewhat paradoxically only one mutation of a ligand, FGF23, has been associated with a human skeletal disorder, autosomal dominant hypophosphatemic rickets.[44] These observations were initially thought to indicate a loss of the growth promoting actions of FGFs that had been demonstrated with chondrocytes in culture. Subsequently, however, targeted disruption of the FGFR3 was shown to lead to skeletal overgrowth.[45,46] This seemed to be a contradiction and implied that the human syndromes may be caused by mutations that resulted in constitutively activated receptors and this was then confirmed for both FGFR2[47] and FGFR3.[48] Despite the FGFs stimulating the growth of chondrocytes, these *in vivo* findings suggested a role for FGFs as negative growth regulators. Skeletal growth, however, depends upon a balance of cell proliferation and differentiation. Cell proliferation ceases as a result of cell differentiation and ossification and the capacity of the bones to grow is lost when the epiphyses and sutures fuse. Although FGFs inhibit the terminal differentiation of chondrocytes grown in culture,[49] the administration of basic FGF *in vivo* directly into the growth plate accelerated vascular invasion and ossification of the growth plate cartilage[50] consistent with the phenotype observed with the receptor activity mutations in humans.

TRANSFORMING GROWTH FACTOR-β SUPERFAMILY

The human TGF-β superfamily includes over 30 genes. The three closely related proteins, TGF-β1, TGF-β2 and TGF-β3 share around 70–80 percent amino acid homology. The other members of the superfamily include the activins and inhibins, the growth and differentiation factors (GDF) which include the cartilage-derived morphogenic proteins (CDMP), the bone morphogenic proteins (BMP) and more distantly related proteins such as nodal and lefty.[51]

Complexities of ligands, receptors, and accessory molecules

Originally, TGF-β was identified as a factor secreted from sarcoma cells which induced anchorage-independent growth of normal cells and was named due to this transforming capability.[52] The BMPs were first identified as proteins purified from demineralized bone matrix that could induce the formation of ectopic cartilage and bone when implanted into rodents.[53] It is now recognized that these are all pleiotrophic peptides that regulate many different aspects of cell function in virtually every tissue. The original family member, TGF-β1, is produced as a 390 amino acid precursor which is cleaved into a C-terminal mature growth factor of

112 amino acids and an N-terminal peptide called the latency associated peptide (LAP). These remain associated in noncovalently linked complexes of disulfide-linked dimers of both the mature TGF-β and the LAP. The LAP can also be linked via disulfide bonds to a further peptide belonging to a family of latent TGF-β binding proteins (LT-BPs) which themselves exist as dimers. The LT-BPs are not structurally related to TGF-β or other growth factor binding proteins. The secreted product therefore comprises a large complex of around 220 kDa, which is not biologically active. This complex is found in many tissues and can be released from platelets and many cell types. In the circulation, TGF-β is also found completed with α_2-macroglobulin.

The generation of active growth factor from the large latent complexes is highly controlled. The TGF-β family members are highly conserved whereas the prodomains and LAP are poorly conserved and the BMPs appear to not be secreted in a latent complex. The LAP may be considered as a ligand trap, regulating access of the growth factor to the receptors. Although the BMPs are not secreted in a latent form, there are other ligand-binding antagonists that tightly regulate BMP activity including noggin, chordin, follistatin, cerberus, and sclerotin. Follistatin also regulates activin activity. A number of mechanisms for activating the latent TGF-β complexes have been described, including acidification and the action of various proteases. Within the LAP glycopeptide there are mannose-6-phosphate groups that enable the complex to bind to cell surface IGF-II/M6PR and it has been shown that addition of mannose-6-phosphate or antibodies against the IGF-II/M6PR can inhibit the activation of latent TGF-β,[54] suggesting that this may be a means for selective activation of the complex at the cell surface.

At the receptor level there are further complex interactions that provide additional controls on the signal. TGF-β peptides initiate cell signaling by assembling receptor complexes that then activate Smad transcription factors.[55] The TGF-β ligands bring together two receptors, a type I and a type II receptor, each of which has a small extracellular region, a single transmembrane domain and a cytoplasmic region with a serine/threonine kinase domain. The only known function of the type II receptors is to activate a type I receptor. The type I receptors phosphorylate and activate the Smads. Each of the TGF-β peptides may interact with several of the type I and type II receptors which are expressed in different combinations on different cells. Further control is provided by an additional group of membrane-anchored proteins, which act as accessory molecules or co-receptors and facilitate the delivery of the ligands to the signaling receptors. A proteoglycan called beta-glycan is also referred to as the TGF-β type III receptor. Beta-glycan binds to TGF-β and presents it to the type II receptor. The beta-glycan is then displaced from this complex by the type I receptor which is then activated and can transmit the intracellular signal. Beta-glycan also enables the activin antagonist, inhibin to bind to the activin receptor. Other related proteins such as endoglin may serve similar roles.

TGF-β and somatic growth

An important role for TGF-β in bone development and skeletal growth has been suspected since it was realized that, other than in platelets, the highest concentrations of TGF-β are found in bone[56] and the developing bone is one of the major sites of TGF-β expression in the fetus. Several members of the TGF-β superfamily, particularly the CDMPs and BMPs, appear to play a very important role in bone development. The CDMPs and BMPs are expressed in the embryo at sites and times that are consistent with an important role in the induction and development of cartilage and bone. Several mutations in the CDMP1 gene have been associated with human hereditary chondroplasias, confirming the importance of these peptides in skeletal development.[57] Mutations in noggin, which antagonizes BMP/GDF receptor binding, have been identified in hereditary synostosis with defects in joint morphogenesis.[58] The effects of TGF-β family members on skeletal growth and development are multiple and complex and still being elucidated.[59]

OTHER LOCAL REGULATORS

It has recently become clear that in addition to the conventional peptide growth factor family members there are other proteins that play a critical role in the local regulation of skeletal growth.

Indian hedgehog

Indian hedgehog (Ihh) belongs to a family of hedgehog proteins which play pivotal roles in embryonic development. Hedgehogs bind to a cell surface receptor called patched (Ptc), ligand binding to this receptor results in the release of a second membrane protein called smoothened (Smo), which has intrinsic intracellular activity that is inhibited when associated with Ptc. The binding of hedgehogs result in release of Smo which undergoes a conformational change to activate downstream signals. Ihh is expressed by chondrocytes in the growth plate, but exclusively the chondrocytes that are in transition from the proliferating zone into the hypertrophic zone. Mice in which Ihh was knocked out were dwarf and exhibited markedly reduced chondrocyte proliferation,[60] targeted inactivation of the gene for the signaling proteins Smo in cartilage confirmed its importance for chondrocyte proliferation.[61]

Parathyroid hormone–related peptide

Parathyroid hormone-related peptide (PTHrP) is expressed within the growth plate predominantly in the transitional zone between the proliferating and hypertrophic chondrocytes. PTHrP shares a common receptor with its related hormone PTH, the PTH/PTHrP receptor. Mice in which PTHrP was knocked out were dwarf and exhibited markedly accelerated chondrocyte differentiation that was virtually complete at birth[62] and PTH/PTHrP receptor knock-out mice demonstrated a similar, but more marked phenotype.[63] The relevance of this to human growth is demonstrated by the consequences of mutations to the PTH/PTHrP receptor; a constitutively activated receptor results in a metaphyseal chondrodysplasia and severe dwarfism[64] and homozygous inactivation of this receptor results in osteochondro-dysplasia also with associated dwarfism.[65]

Ihh/PTHrP feedback loop

These two local regulators form an integral feedback loop controlling the proliferation and differentiation of chond-rocytes within the growth plate and couples chondro-genesis to osteogenesis. Indeed in the Ihh knockout mice, PTHrP expression in the cartilage is virtually absent, indicating that Ihh is an important regulator of PTHrP.[60] There appears to be a feedback loop in which Ihh is expressed by chondrocytes in the transitional zone between the proliferating and the hypertrophic chondrocytes. Ihh activates adjacent chondrocytes and diffuses towards the periarticular perichondrium, where it stimulates expression of PTHrP expression. The PTHrP then diffuses toward the prehypertrophic zone and inhibits the differentiation of proliferating chondrocytes, thus reducing the number of cells capable of synthesizing Ihh.[63,66] Recently, it has become evident that Ihh extracellular diffusion and actions are dependent upon their ability to bind to heparan sulfate proteoglycans. Hedgehog proteins have lipid tails, which limits their ability to diffuse in the aqueous extracellular environment, and their movement appears to be facilitated by their ability to interact with proteoglycans. The ability of Ihh to stimulate chondrocyte proliferation has been shown to be completely lost in cells treated with heparinase (to remove cell surface proteoglycans) or with a neutralizing-antibody to the cell surface proteoglycan syndecan-3; in addition, cells overexpressing syndecan-3 become even more responsive to Ihh.[67] The ECM and cell surface proteglycans appear to be integral to the actions of Ihh in an analogous manner to their role in the actions of IGFs, FGF, and TGF-β family members.

GENERAL GROWTH FACTOR AVAILABILITY

As described above, it is now clear that a large number of different growth factors are involved in regulating the processes of cell differentiation, proliferation and matrix production that are involved in somatic growth. A common feature of the growth factors is that, unlike traditional hormones, they are not simply secreted in an active form, which can trigger receptors on target cells; in contrast they are either secreted in a latent form or they are immediately

sequestered into a complex that maintains them in an active state. For most of the growth factors there are large extra-cellular stores containing an excess of latent growth factor; a key determinant of activity is how the growth factor is then mobilized and activated. Interactions with extracellular proteases, specific components of the ECM or cell surface cofactors are generally involved in this activation process. Specific proteases can act on IGFBPs to release IGFs, on latent TGF-β complexes to release the active growth factor or act on the ECM to release growth factors such as FGF that are stored there or mobilize accessory molecules that can then facilitate growth factor actions. There has to be controlled proteolysis of the ECM for tissue growth, in order to overcome contact inhibition and to make room for cell proliferation. It is now apparent that such proteolysis and matrix remodeling is also important for mobilizing and activating local growth factors in an orchestrated regulation system. The production of matrix components and the production of extracellular proteases are themselves regulated by local growth factors.[37] The composition of the ECM, the specific proteases and inhibitors that are present, the combinations of growth factors and cell receptors all interact to determine the regulation of cell functions. Stimuli that affect any one of these components can trigger a cascade of growth factor actions. This complex network of local signals provides a framework whereby local factors and systemic signals can all be integrated to determine the rate of tissue growth.

INTERACTIONS BETWEEN SYSTEMIC HORMONES AND LOCAL CYTOKINES

While growth hormone clearly has an important role in somatic growth regulation, it is now evident that many, if not all, systemic hormones are involved and disturbances to most can lead to abnormal growth. The important metabolic hormones, including insulin, thyroid hormones and glucocorticoids, all have indirect effects by modulating the GH–IGF axis with effects on pituitary GH output and/or on hepatic IGF-I production. Insulin has a major role in regulating hepatic IGF-I production with a dual effect, modulating GH control by regulating levels of GH receptors on hepatocytes and also by direct effects on IGF-I gene expression.[68] Circulating insulin and IGF-I concentrations correlate closely throughout childhood, particularly through the pubertal growth spurt, when both rise coordinately.[69]

Growth hormone

The original somatomedin hypothesis suggested that hepatic IGF-I mediated the somatic growth-promoting effects of GH. This was revised when it was demonstrated that GH injected directly into the tibial growth plate of hypophysectomized rats resulted in unilateral bone growth.[70] Such growth could, however, be inhibited by antibodies to

IGF-I,[71] indicating that the local GH effect was at least partly mediated by IGF-I. The effects of GH and IGF-I within the growth plate depend on the stage of differentiation of the chondrocytes. Growth hormone acts on the pre-chondrocytes in the germinal cell layer,[72] whereas IGF-I production is localized more to the proliferative and hypertrophic chondrocytes.[73] This was consistent with the dual effector theory, originally suggested for GH effects on adipocytes, which proposed that GH acted to stimulate the differentiation of progenitor cells and IGF-I then stimulated their growth and clonal expansion.[74] As described in the sections above, it is now clear that both GH and IGF-I act in concert with many other regulators, which together determine somatic growth rates.

Thyroid hormones

Thyroid hormones have multiple direct and indirect effects on somatic growth. They act directly at the pituitary level to stimulate GH production and secretion, they can also affect IGFs both secondary to the increase in GH and also as a result of direct effects on IGF and IGFBP production locally.[75] Replacement of GH to hypothyroid rats normalized circulating IGF-I, but did not completely correct the growth deficiency indicating direct effects of the thyroid hormones.[76] Experiments with chondrocytes in culture also indicated separate effects with IGF-I stimulating proliferation and triiodothyronine (T3) inducing hypertrophic differentiation.[77] There is reciprocal regulation since the GH–IGF axis can also modulate thyroid hormone activity; IGF-I can potentiate the actions of thyroid stimulating hormone (TSH) on the thyroid gland and both GH and IGF-I can modulate the peripheral activity of thyroxine-5′-monodeiodinase which converts thyroxine (T4) to the more potent T3.[78] This enzyme has been reported to be active within the growth plate to regulate T3-inducible hypertrophic chondrocyte differentiation.[79]

Thyroid hormone status also has marked effects on the expression of both PTHrP and the PTH/PTHrP receptor within growth plates.[80] Hypothyroidism caused an increase in expression of PTHrP whereas in thyrotoxic rats the PTH/PTHrP receptor was undetectable. These observations suggest that disturbances to the Ihh/PTHrP feedback loop would underlie growth disorders in children with thyroid disorders.

Glucocorticoids

Glucocorticoids also have complex effects on growth with physiological levels and acute pharmacological adminis-tration enhancing pituitary GH output and growth, whereas chronic administration or pathological levels inhibit growth. This latter inhibitory effect is multifactorial with glucocorti-coids affecting GH secretion,[81] reducing IGF-I production in skeletal tissue,[82] affecting tissue sensitivity to GH and IGFs[83] and directly inhibiting cell proliferation.[84] Although the growth inhibiting effects of pharmacologically administered glucocorticoids are well recognized, the physiological role of glucocorticoids in regulating normal somatic growth is much less well understood. Again there is reciprocal regulation with the GH-IGF axis modulating glucocorticoid activity. Inactive cortisone is converted to active cortisol, mainly in liver and adipose tissue, by 11-β-hydroxysteroid dehydrogenase I and the activity of this enzyme has been reported to be inhibited by IGF-I.[85] Cortisol is inactivated by 11-β-hydroxysteroid dehydrogenase-2, which has been demonstrated to be active in osteoclasts and osteoblasts.[86]

Sex steroids

The effects of sex steroids on somatic growth are even more complex, but clearly important, particularly during the pubertal growth spurt. Their effects again are partly mediated by enhanced pituitary GH output and the resultant increase in IGF-I levels. Although it is also evident that sex steroids have a direct GH-independent effect on somatic growth because children with complete GH-insensitivity (Laron syndrome) have a pubertal growth spurt during sexual maturation.[87] During normal puberty, gonadal estradiol directly enhances pituitary GH secretion, although the effect of testosterone results at least partly from its aromatization to estradiol. Again there are reciprocal interactions because the IGFs increase steroidogenesis by potentiating the actions of gonadotrophins in the gonads and of ACTH in the adrenals. This provides a further means for integrating somatic growth and sexual maturation throughout puberty. In addition to these interactions, both estrogen and androgen receptors are present in cartilage and bone and the gonadal steroids have direct local effects on skeletal growth.[88,89] The estrogen receptor is expressed in the zones of the growth plate that also express Ihh and PTHrP and in the rat uterus estrogen has been reported to increase PTHrP expression[90] raising the possibility that estrogen may regulate the Ihh/PTHrP feedback loop. Supporting this it has been observed that both Ihh and PTHrP expression were increased in human growth plate during early puberty.[91] The epiphyseal cartilage also contains both 5-α-reductase and aromatase activity and so can convert testosterone to the more potent dihydrotestosterone and to estradiol. The administration of non-aromatizable androgens have been shown to stimulate the growth plate indicating that androgens have direct effects independent of estrogen. The effects of testosterone has been reported to increase cartilage expression of IGF-I and IGF-IR.[92,93] The proliferative effect of dihydrotestosterone on cultured chondrocytes has been associated with an increase in expression of IGF-I and to be blocked by IGF-I antibody.[94] The response of the cartilage to gonadal sex steroids varies with gender and with stage of development, the greatest response occurring during early puberty.[88]

Calciotrophic hormones

The regulation of skeletal growth is obviously linked to the homoeostasis of calcium and phosphorus levels which are coordinated by the calciotrophic hormones, PTH and vitamin D. In addition to systemic effects of PTH on calcium homeostasis and anabolic effects mediating GH,[95] PTH clearly has many direct local effects in the growth plate where it activates the same receptor as PTHrP.

In the intact growing male (but not female) rat, vitamin D has been generally found to be anabolic and to increase bone weight,[96] although these systemic effects may be as a result of altered calcium homeostasis or interactions with sex steroids. In contrast there have been reports indicating, in cultures of chondrocytes and osteoblasts, vitamin D reduces cell proliferation[97] and inhibits the release of IGF-I.[98] There have however also been reports that vitamin D enhances the production of IGFs and IGFBPs[99] and the proliferation of chondrocytes which could be prevented by an IGF-I antibody.[94] Vitamin D also has marked effects on chondrocyte differentiation, particularly acting on chondrocytes in the resting zone of the growth plate promoting their maturation into the growth zone.[100] Some of the previous conflicting reports of actions of vitamin D on chondrocyte growth factor production and proliferation may have been due to confounding effects of chondrocyte differentiation stage. Vitamin D has also been reported to inhibit PTH/PTHrP receptor expression by osteoblasts, but not by chondrocytes.[101] It has also been reported that retinoic acid upregulates Ihh expression by growth plate chondrocytes[102] and it is clear that there are many potential interacting effects of numerous nuclear receptor agonists on skeletal growth that have yet to be elucidated.

INTEGRATED REGULATION OF TISSUE GROWTH

It is evident from the previous sections that many hormonal systems are involved in regulating skeletal growth. All of these endocrine systems are integrated, they all inter-regulate each other and they all interact with the GH–IGF axis and with the network of local growth factors. These local growth factors are also regulated by each other and by other cytokines such as the inflammatory cytokines. Through experimental constraints of study design and interpretation most growth regulators have, to date, generally been examined individually or in pairs; the cells in the body are however always exposed to multiple signals. Not just the soluble secreted signals, but also via direct contacts with adjacent cells and also via the ECM. It is increasingly evident that most local growth factors operate intimately in conjunction with matrix proteins. These many signals can therefore be regarded as the letters of a very large alphabet that is used by the cells to communicate with each other. The meaning of each letter is determined by the context within which it appears, according to the other letters around

it. The cells' language comprises many different letters including hormones, cytokines, growth factors, and components of the ECM. The message conveyed by each signal is determined by the context within which it is received, as determined by the other concurrent signals. These signals are integrated to regulate cell proliferation, differentiation, matrix production and remodeling and cell death, processes that together determine tissue growth.

KEY LEARNING POINTS

- Pre- and postnatal growth are orchestrated by a large number of local growth factors and cytokines, many of which also integrate systemic hormonal signals.
- Regulation of cell growth, proliferation, differentiation, matrix production, and death all contribute to determine tissue and somatic growth.
- Over-activity of growth factors can cause growth failure if they promote premature cell differentiation.
- Most growth factor systems comprise large numbers of inter-related and interacting components that are independently regulated enabling integration of many inputs for determining growth.
- The responses to most growth factors and cytokines are dependent upon context. Context is determined by other soluble signals and the extracellular matrix.
- Tissue growth is controlled by counterbalancing regulators and feedback loops such as that of growth-plate chondrocytes involving Indian hedgehog and PTHrP.

REFERENCES

● = Seminal primary article

◆ = Key review paper

◆ 1 Sporn MB, Todaro GJ. Autocrine secretion and malignant transformation of cells. N Engl J Med 1980; 303: 878–80.

2 Froesch ER, et al. Non-suppressible insulin-like activity of human serum. II. Biological properties of plasma extracts with non-suppressible insulin-like activity. Biochim Biophys Acta 1966; 121: 360–74.

3 Dulak NC, Temin HM. Multiplication-stimulating activity for chicken embryo fibroblasts from rat liver cell conditioned medium: a family of small polypeptides. J Cell Physiol 1973; 81: 161–70.

● 4 Salmon WD Jr, Daughaday WH. A hormonally controlled serum factor which stimulates sulfate incorporation by cartilage in vitro. J Lab Clin Med 1957; 49: 825–36.

5 Daughaday WH, et al. Somatomedin: proposed designation for sulphation factor. Nature 1972; 235: 107.

6 Rinderknecht E, Humbel RE. The amino acid sequence of human insulin-like growth factor I and its structural homology with proinsulin. *J Biol Chem* 1978; **253**: 2769–76.

7 Daughaday WH, *et al.* On the nomenclature of the somatomedins and insulin-like growth factors. *J Clin Endocrinol Metab* 1987; **65**: 1075–6.

8 Sara VR, Hall K. Insulin-like growth factors and their binding proteins. *Physiol Rev* 1990; **70**: 591–614.

9 Czech MP. Signal transmission by the insulin-like growth factors. *Cell* 1989; **59**: 235–8.

10 Jones JI, Clemmons DR. Insulin-like growth factors and their binding proteins: biological actions. *Endocr Rev* 1995; **16**: 3–34.

11 Holly JM, *et al.* Proteases acting on IGFBPs: their occurrence and physiological significance. *Growth Regul* 1993; **3**: 88–91.

12 Holly JM, *et al.* Relationship between the pubertal fall in sex hormone binding globulin and insulin-like growth factor binding protein-I. A synchronized approach to pubertal development? *Clin Endocrinol (Oxf)* 1989; **31**: 277–84.

13 Baxter RC, Martin JL. Structure of the Mr 140,000 growth hormone-dependent insulin-like growth factor binding protein complex: determination by reconstitution and affinity-labeling. *Proc Natl Acad Sci USA* 1989; **86**: 6898–902.

14 Schoenle E, *et al.* Comparison of in vivo effects of insulin-like growth factors I and II and of growth hormone in hypophysectomized rats. *Acta Endocrinol (Copenh)* 1985; **108**: 167–74.

15 Philipps AF, *et al.* The effects of biosynthetic insulin-like growth factor-1 supplementation on somatic growth, maturation, and erythropoiesis on the neonatal rat. *Pediatr Res* 1988; **23**: 298–305.

16 Guler HP, *et al.* Recombinant human insulin-like growth factor I stimulates growth and has distinct effects on organ size in hypophysectomized rats. *Proc Natl Acad Sci USA* 1988; **85**: 4889–93.

17 Mathews LS, *et al.* Growth enhancement of transgenic mice expressing human insulin-like growth factor I. *Endocrinology* 1988; **123**: 2827–33.

18 Wolf E, *et al.* Skeletal growth of transgenic mice with elevated levels of circulating insulin-like growth factor-II. *Growth Regul* 1995; **5**: 177–83.

19 DeChiara TM, Efstratiadis A, Robertson EJ. A growth-deficiency phenotype in heterozygous mice carrying an insulin-like growth factor II gene disrupted by targeting. *Nature* 1990; **345**: 78–80.

20 Baker J, *et al.* Role of insulin-like growth factors in embryonic and postnatal growth. *Cell* 1993; **75**: 73–82.

21 Liu JP, *et al.* Mice carrying null mutations of the genes encoding insulin-like growth factor I (IGF-I) and type 1 IGF receptor (Igf1r). *Cell* 1993; **75**: 59–72.

22 Woods KA, *et al.* Intrauterine growth retardation and postnatal growth failure associated with deletion of the insulin-like growth factor I gene. *N Engl J Med* 1996; **335**: 1363–7.

23 Morison IM, *et al.* Somatic overgrowth associated with overexpression of insulin-like growth factor II. *Nat Med* 1996; **2**: 311–6.

24 Reeve AE, *et al.* Expression of insulin-like growth factor-II transcripts in Wilms' tumour. *Nature* 1985; **317**: 258–60.

25 Xu Y, *et al.* Functional polymorphism in the parental imprinting of the human IGF2R gene. *Biochem Biophys Res Commun* 1993; **197**: 747–54.

26 Abuzzahab MJ, *et al.* IGF-I receptor mutations resulting in intrauterine and postnatal growth retardation. *N Engl J Med* 2003; **349**: 2211–22.

27 Yakar S, *et al.* Circulating levels of IGF-I directly regulate bone growth and density. *J Clin Invest* 2002; **110**: 771–81.

28 Sjogren K, *et al.* Liver-derived insulin-like growth factor I (IGF-I) is the principal source of IGF-I in blood but is not required for postnatal body growth in mice. *Proc Natl Acad Sci USA* 1999; **96**: 7088–92.

29 Ueki I, *et al.* Inactivation of the acid labile subunit gene in mice results in mild retardation of postnatal growth despite profound disruptions in the circulating insulin-like growth factor system. *Proc Natl Acad Sci USA* 2000; **97**: 6868–73.

30 Canalis E, *et al.* Growth factors regulate the synthesis of insulin-like growth factor-I in bone cell cultures. *Endocrinology* 1993; **133**: 33–8.

31 Izumi T, *et al.* Administration of growth hormone modulates the gene expression of basic fibroblast growth factor in rat costal cartilage, both in vivo and in vitro. *Mol Cell Endocrinol* 1995; **112**: 95–9.

32 Gabbitas B, Pash J, Canalis E. Regulation of insulin-like growth factor-II synthesis in bone cell cultures by skeletal growth factors. *Endocrinology* 1994; **135**: 284–9.

33 Mohan S, *et al.* Studies on regulation of insulin-like growth factor binding protein (IGFBP)-3 and IGFBP-4 production in human bone cells. *Acta Endocrinol (Copenh)* 1992; **127**: 555–64.

34 Palermo C, *et al.* Potentiating role of IGFBP-2 on IGF-II-stimulated alkaline phosphatase activity in differentiating osteoblasts. *Am J Physiol Endocrinol Metab* 2004; **286**: E648–E57.

35 Gospodarowicz D. Localisation of a fibroblast growth factor and its effect alone and with hydrocortisone on 3T3 cell growth. *Nature* 1974; **249**: 123–7.

36 Ornitz DM, Itoh N. Fibroblast growth factors. *Genome Biol* 2001; **2**: REVIEWS3005.

37 Hill DJ, *et al.* Control of protein and matrix-molecule synthesis in isolated ovine fetal growth-plate chondrocytes by the interactions of basic fibroblast growth factor, insulin-like growth factors-I and -II, insulin and transforming growth factor-beta 1. *J Endocrinol* 1992; **133**: 363–73.

38 Niswander L, *et al.* FGF-4 replaces the apical ectodermal ridge and directs outgrowth and patterning of the limb. *Cell* 1993; **75**: 579–87.

39 Rousseau F, *et al.* Mutations in the gene encoding fibroblast growth factor receptor-3 in achondroplasia. *Nature* 1994; **371**: 252–4.

• 40 Shiang R, *et al*. Mutations in the transmembrane domain of FGFR3 cause the most common genetic form of dwarfism, achondroplasia. *Cell* 1994; **78**: 335–42.

41 Jabs EW, *et al*. Jackson–Weiss and Crouzon syndromes are allelic with mutations in fibroblast growth factor receptor 2. *Nat Genet* 1994; **8**: 275–9.

42 Muenke M, *et al*. A common mutation in the fibroblast growth factor receptor 1 gene in Pfeiffer syndrome. *Nat Genet* 1994; **8**: 269–74.

43 Reardon W, *et al*. Mutations in the fibroblast growth factor receptor 2 gene cause Crouzon syndrome. *Nat Genet* 1994; **8**: 98–103.

44 Wilkie AO, *et al*. FGFs, their receptors, and human limb malformations: clinical and molecular correlations. *Am J Med Genet* 2002; **112**: 266–78.

45 Deng C, *et al*. Fibroblast growth factor receptor 3 is a negative regulator of bone growth. *Cell* 1996; **84**: 911–21.

46 Colvin JS, *et al*. Skeletal overgrowth and deafness in mice lacking fibroblast growth factor receptor 3. *Nat Genet* 1996; **12**: 390–7.

47 Neilson KM, Friesel RE. Constitutive activation of fibroblast growth factor receptor-2 by a point mutation associated with Crouzon syndrome. *J Biol Chem* 1995; **270**: 26037–40.

48 Naski MC, *et al*. Graded activation of fibroblast growth factor receptor 3 by mutations causing achondroplasia and thanatophoric dysplasia. *Nat Genet* 1996; **13**: 233–7.

49 Kato Y, Iwamoto M. Fibroblast growth factor is an inhibitor of chondrocyte terminal differentiation. *J Biol Chem* 1990; **265**: 5903–9.

50 Baron J, *et al*. Induction of growth plate cartilage ossification by basic fibroblast growth factor. *Endocrinology* 1994; **135**: 2790–3.

◆ 51 Chang H, Brown CW, Matzuk MM. Genetic analysis of the mammalian transforming growth factor-beta superfamily. *Endocr Rev* 2002; **23**: 787–823.

• 52 Moses HL, *et al*. Transforming growth factor production by chemically transformed cells. *Cancer Res* 1981; **41**: 2842–8.

◆ 53 Wozney JM. The bone morphogenetic protein family and osteogenesis. *Mol Reprod Dev* 1992; **32**: 160–7.

54 Dennis PA, Rifkin DB. Cellular activation of latent transforming growth factor beta requires binding to the cation-independent mannose 6-phosphate/insulin-like growth factor type II receptor. *Proc Natl Acad Sci USA* 1991; **88**: 580–4.

◆ 55 Massague J, Blain SW, Lo RS. TGFbeta signaling in growth control, cancer, and heritable disorders. *Cell* 2000; **103**: 295–309.

56 Seyedin SM, *et al*. Purification and characterization of two cartilage-inducing factors from bovine demineralized bone. *Proc Natl Acad Sci USA* 1985; **82**: 2267–71.

57 Thomas JT, *et al*. A human chondrodysplasia due to a mutation in a TGF-beta superfamily member. *Nat Genet* 1996; **12**: 315–7.

58 Gong Y, *et al*. Heterozygous mutations in the gene encoding noggin affect human joint morphogenesis. *Nat Genet* 1999; **21**: 302–4.

59 Serra R, Chang C. TGF-beta signaling in human skeletal and patterning disorders. *Birth Def Res C Embryo Today* 2003; **69**: 333–51.

• 60 St-Jacques B, Hammerschmidt M, McMahon AP. Indian hedgehog signaling regulates proliferation and differentiation of chondrocytes and is essential for bone formation. *Genes Dev* 1999; **13**: 2072–86.

61 Long F, *et al*. Genetic manipulation of hedgehog signaling in the endochondral skeleton reveals a direct role in the regulation of chondrocyte proliferation. *Development* 2001; **128**: 5099–108.

62 Karaplis AC, *et al*. Lethal skeletal dysplasia from targeted disruption of the parathyroid hormone-related peptide gene. *Genes Dev* 1994; **8**: 277–89.

• 63 Lanske B, *et al*. PTH/PTHrP receptor in early development and Indian hedgehog-regulated bone growth. *Science* 1996; **273**: 663–6.

• 64 Schipani E, Kruse K, Juppner H. A constitutively active mutant PTH-PTHrP receptor in Jansen-type metaphyseal chondrodysplasia. *Science* 1995; **268**: 98–100.

65 Jobert AS, *et al*. Absence of functional receptors for parathyroid hormone and parathyroid hormone-related peptide in Blomstrand chondrodysplasia. *J Clin Invest* 1998; **102**: 34–40.

• 66 Vortkamp A, *et al*. Regulation of rate of cartilage differentiation by Indian hedgehog and PTH-related protein. *Science* 1996; **273**: 613–22.

67 Shimo T, *et al*. Indian hedgehog and syndecans-3 coregulate chondrocyte proliferation and function during chick limb skeletogenesis. *Dev Dyn* 2004; **229**: 607–17.

68 Holly JM, *et al*. The role of growth hormone in diabetes mellitus. *J Endocrinol* 1988; **118**: 353–64.

69 Smith CP, *et al*. Relationship between insulin, insulin-like growth factor I, and dehydroepiandrosterone sulfate concentrations during childhood, puberty, and adult life. *J Clin Endocrinol Metab* 1989; **68**: 932–7.

• 70 Isaksson OG, Jansson JO, Gause IA. Growth hormone stimulates longitudinal bone growth directly. *Science* 1982; **216**: 1237–9.

• 71 Schlechter NL, *et al*. Evidence suggesting that the direct growth-promoting effect of growth hormone on cartilage in vivo is mediated by local production of somatomedin. *Proc Natl Acad Sci USA* 1986; **83**: 7932–4.

72 Ohlsson C, *et al*. Growth hormone induces multiplication of the slowly cycling germinal cells of the rat tibial growth plate. *Proc Natl Acad Sci USA* 1992; **89**: 9826–30.

73 Nilsson A, *et al*. Regulation by GH of insulin-like growth factor-I mRNA expression in rat epiphyseal growth plate as studied with in-situ hybridization. *J Endocrinol* 1990; **125**: 67–74.

• 74 Green H, Morikawa M, Nixon T. A dual effector theory of growth-hormone action. *Differentiation* 1985; **29**: 195–8.

75 Schmid C, *et al*. Triiodothyronine (T3) stimulates insulin-like growth factor (IGF)-1 and IGF binding protein (IGFBP)-2 production by rat osteoblasts in vitro. *Acta Endocrinol (Copenh)* 1992; **126**: 467–73.

76   Nanto-Salonen K, *et al*. Mechanisms of thyroid hormone action on the insulin-like growth factor system: all thyroid hormone effects are not growth hormone mediated. *Endocrinology* 1993; **132**: 781–8.

77   Bohme K, *et al*. Induction of proliferation or hypertrophy of chondrocytes in serum-free culture: the role of insulin-like growth factor-I, insulin, or thyroxine. *J Cell Biol* 1992; **116**: 1035–42.

78   Jorgensen JO, *et al*. Growth hormone administration stimulates energy expenditure and extrathyroidal conversion of thyroxine to triiodothyronine in a dose-dependent manner and suppresses circadian thyrotrophin levels: studies in GH-deficient adults. *Clin Endocrinol (Oxf)* 1994; **41**: 609–14.

79   Miura M, *et al*. Thyroid hormones promote chondrocyte differentiation in mouse ATDC5 cells and stimulate endochondral ossification in fetal mouse tibias through iodothyronine deiodinases in the growth plate. *J Bone Miner Res* 2002; **17**: 443–54.

80   Stevens DA, *et al*. Thyroid hormones regulate hypertrophic chondrocyte differentiation and expression of parathyroid hormone-related peptide and its receptor during endochondral bone formation. *J Bone Miner Res* 2000; **15**: 2431–42.

81   Burguera B, *et al*. Dual and selective actions of glucocorticoids upon basal and stimulated growth hormone release in man. *Neuroendocrinology* 1990; **51**: 51–8.

82   McCarthy TL, Centrella M, Canalis E. Cortisol inhibits the synthesis of insulin-like growth factor-I in skeletal cells. *Endocrinology* 1990; **126**: 1569–75.

83   Luo JM, Murphy LJ. Dexamethasone inhibits growth hormone induction of insulin-like growth factor-I (IGF-I) messenger ribonucleic acid (mRNA) in hypophysectomized rats and reduces IGF-I mRNA abundance in the intact rat. *Endocrinology* 1989; **125**: 165–71.

84   Fagot D, Buquet-Fagot C, Mester J. Antimitogenic effects of dexamethasone in chemically transformed mouse fibroblasts. *Endocrinology* 1991; **129**: 1033–41.

85   Moore JS, *et al*. Modulation of 11beta-hydroxysteroid dehydrogenase isozymes by growth hormone and insulin-like growth factor: in vivo and in vitro studies. *J Clin Endocrinol Metab* 1999; **84**: 4172–7.

86   Cooper MS, *et al*. Expression and functional consequences of 11beta-hydroxysteroid dehydrogenase activity in human bone. *Bone* 2000; **27**: 375–81.

87   Laron Z, Sarel R, Pertzelan A. Puberty in Laron type dwarfism. *Eur J Pediatr* 1980; **134**: 79–83.

88   Corvol M, Blanchard O, Tsagris L. Bone and cartilage responsiveness to sex steroid hormones. *J Steroid Biochem Mol Biol* 1992; **43**: 415–8.

89   Vanderschueren D, Bouillon R. Androgens and bone. *Calcif Tissue Int* 1995; **56**: 341–6.

90   Paspaliaris V, Petersen DN, Thiede MA. Steroid regulation of parathyroid hormone-related protein expression and action in the rat uterus. *J Steroid Biochem Mol Biol* 1995; **53**: 259–65.

91   Kindblom JM, *et al*. Expression and localization of Indian hedgehog (Ihh) and parathyroid hormone related protein (PTHrP) in the human growth plate during pubertal development. *J Endocrinol* 2002; **174**: R1–6.

92   Maor G, Segev Y, Phillip M. Testosterone stimulates insulin-like growth factor-I and insulin-like growth factor-I-receptor gene expression in the mandibular condyle – a model of endochondral ossification. *Endocrinology* 1999; **140**: 1901–10.

93   Phillip M, *et al*. Testosterone stimulates growth of tibial epiphyseal growth plate and insulin-like growth factor-1 receptor abundance in hypophysectomized and castrated rats. *Endocrine* 2001; **16**: 1–6.

94   Krohn K, *et al*. 1,25(OH)2D3 and dihydrotestosterone interact to regulate proliferation and differentiation of epiphyseal chondrocytes. *Calcif Tissue Int* 2003; **73**: 400–10.

95   Hock JM, Fonseca J. Anabolic effect of human synthetic parathyroid hormone-(1-34) depends on growth hormone. *Endocrinology* 1990; **127**: 1804–10.

96   Ornoy A, *et al*. Gender-related effects of vitamin D metabolites on cartilage and bone. *Bone Miner* 1994; **27**: 235–47.

97   Saggese G, Federico G, Cinquanta L. In vitro effects of growth hormone and other hormones on chondrocytes and osteoblast-like cells. *Acta Paediatr Suppl* 1993; **82(Suppl 391)**: 54–60.

98   Linkhart TA, Keffer MJ. Differential regulation of insulin-like growth factor-I (IGF-I) and IGF-II release from cultured neonatal mouse calvaria by parathyroid hormone, transforming growth factor-beta, and 1,25-dihydroxyvitamin D3. *Endocrinology* 1991; **128**: 1511–8.

99   Chen TL, *et al*. Dexamethasone and 1,25-dihydroxyvitamin D3 modulation of insulin-like growth factor-binding proteins in rat osteoblast-like cell cultures. *Endocrinology* 1991; **128**: 73–80.

100 Boyan BD, *et al*. 24,25-(OH)(2)D(3) regulates cartilage and bone via autocrine and endocrine mechanisms. *Steroids* 2001; **66**: 363–74.

101 Amizuka N, *et al*. Vitamin D3 differentially regulates parathyroid hormone/parathyroid hormone-related peptide receptor expression in bone and cartilage. *J Clin Invest* 1999; **103**: 373–81.

102 Yoshida E, *et al*. Direct inhibition of Indian hedgehog expression by parathyroid hormone (PTH)/PTH-related peptide and up-regulation by retinoic acid in growth plate chondrocyte cultures. *Exp Cell Res* 2001; **265**: 64–72.

8

Normal fetal growth

LINDA B JOHNSTON

INTRODUCTION

Birth size in humans is influenced by environmental and genetic factors which can be fetal, placental, and parental in origin. Many environmental factors have been identified which influence birth size and some of these are listed in Table 8.1.

Table 8.1 Environmental factors often associated with poor fetal growth

Fetal
- Multiple gestation
- Congenital infection (herpes, rubella, toxoplasma, cytomegalovirus, syphilis)
- Rhesus disease
- Radiation injury

Placental
- Infection (bacterial, viral, parasitic)
- Infarction
- Reduced surface area
- Tumor (hydatidiform mole, chorioangioma)

Maternal
- Chronic disease (e.g., hypertension, renal failure, cardiac failure, SLE)
- Pregnancy-associated disease: pre-eclampsia, anemia, infection, antiphospholipid antibody syndrome
- Hypoxemia (altitude, cyanotic cardiac or pulmonary disease)
- Malnutrition
- Cigarette smoking
- Alcohol consumption
- Drug abuse (e.g., cocaine, heroin)
- Caffeine

GENETIC INFLUENCES

Epidemiological studies estimate that genetic factors contribute to over 50 percent birth size variance, with fetal genes having greater influence than maternal genes.[1,2] Familial trends in birth weight are well documented. The Scandinavian small for gestational age (SGA) study found that the odds ratio calculated for having an SGA mother and SGA father in families with two SGA births were 1.74 and 2.49.[3] A study of white and African–Americans found that the odds ratios for a low birth weight mother having a SGA child were 2.5 and 2.7 respectively, and this increased to 10.2 and 10.1 if there was also a low birth weight sibling.[4]

In terms of genetic influences on fetal growth, it is likely that there is interplay between parental, placental and fetal genetic and environmental factors, but the nature of these interactions has not yet been fully determined as there is limited knowledge of the specific genetic factors involved.

Mutations in the glucokinase gene which cause maturity onset diabetes of the young (MODY) type 2 have been shown also to influence birth size.[5] Hattersley and colleagues found that inheritance of a glucokinase gene mutation resulted in a mean reduction in birth weight of 533 g, equivalent to a fall from the 50th to the 25th birth weight centile.[6] If the mother was affected then the birth weight increased by a mean 601 g as a result of maternal hyperglycemia in pregnancy, equivalent to a rise from the 50th to the 85th centile in an unaffected child, or the 25th to the 50th centile in an affected child.[6] This study clearly demonstrates the interaction of the maternal and fetal genotypes.

The placenta is critically involved in transporting nutrition and acting as a barrier to infection and maternal corticosteroids. In the majority of cases the placenta is genetically identical to the fetus, but in 1–2 percent conceptuses and

20 percent of idiopathic, SGA, term deliveries confined placental mosaicism is observed.[7,8]

Human studies of fetal genes and animal models have shown significant influence of variation in insulin-like growth factor-I (IGF-I) and insulin pathway genes on fetal growth.[9–15] The human IGF-I gene defect cases had severe growth failure both pre- and postnatally as do patients with Silver–Russell syndrome.[13,16]

ENDOCRINE PHYSIOLOGY

The endocrine physiology of fetal growth is complex due to the interaction of maternal, placental, and fetal endocrine systems and nutritional factors which act on a background of varying degrees of maternal physical constraint. Fetal blood sampling and cord blood measurements have provided direct insight into human fetal endocrinology, although the former procedure is only undertaken in abnormal pregnancies because of the associated risk of fetal loss. Studies of normal and abnormal pregnancies in animal models have therefore provided most of the information on which our current understanding of the endocrinology of fetal growth is based.

Insulin

Insulin is generated by the fetal pancreas in response to the level of circulating fetal glucose and insulin receptors are detectable from late in the first trimester.[17,18] The majority of fetal glucose is derived from the maternal circulation by glucose transporter -1 (GLUT-1)-mediated transport across the placenta.[19] The levels of placental GLUT-1 and GLUT-3 expression are decreased after glucocorticoid administration and increased if the mother is diabetic, even if the diabetes is well controlled.[20,21] Thus maternal endocrine factors can have a significant influence on transplacental glucose flux.

The placenta utilizes a large proportion of the glucose and oxygen delivered by the uterine circulation and this varies according to gestation.[22,23] In situations where there is either maternal hypoglycemia or placental dysfunction, the fetus is capable of becoming catabolic in order to generate glucose and amino acids to fuel both fetal and placental demands.[22]

Serum insulin levels correlate with body weight in human newborns, fetal rats and fetal sheep and insulin infusions restore normal growth in pancreatectomized sheep fetuses.[24] Human fetuses with pancreatic agenesis are unable to produce insulin and have severe fetal growth retardation of late onset, from around 30 weeks.[25] Conversely, fetuses of diabetic mothers tend to hyperinsulinemia in response to maternal hyperglycemia with resultant increased lipogenesis. These fetuses have increased fat deposition and birth weights, but do not have increased linear growth.[26] These observations suggest that, in man, insulin is a major fetal growth factor, particularly in late gestation.

Table 8.2 Effects of gene knockouts on growth in mice

Gene knockout	Birth size (percent of wild-type)	Adult size (percent of wild-type)
IGF-I (−/−)	60	40
IGF-II (p−)	60	60
IGF1R (−/−)	45	Lethal
Insulin R (−/−)	90	Die in first few days
IRS1	Small	Smaller
Insulin (−/−)	Small	Lethal

Insulin-like growth factors: IGF–I and IGF–II

IGF-I and IGF-II are major fetal growth factors and complete deficiency of IGF-I as a result of partial gene deletion or bio-inactivity due to a point mutation causes severe intrauterine growth failure (see Table 8.2).[13,27–29]

IGF-II knockout mice have fetal growth retardation but have normal postnatal growth.[9] IGF-I knockouts, however, have both pre- and postnatal growth failure, being born at 60 percent expected size and reaching only 40 percent expected adult size.[27,28] These knockout animals have increased neonatal mortality which was felt to explain the lack of detection of IGF-I gene defects in human subjects. Only two patients are described with IGF-I gene defects, one with a partial gene deletion and the other with a point mutation.[13,29] They have strikingly similar phenotypes with severe pre- and postnatal growth failure, dysmorphic features, and developmental delay.

Type 1 IGF receptor gene knockout mice are born only 45 percent of expected size and all die shortly after birth with respiratory failure.[27,28] No homozygous IGF receptor gene defect has been described in man, however recently a compound heterozygous and two simple heterozygous defects have been reported in short SGA subjects.[14]

IGF-I and IGF-II act via the IGF type 1 receptor. Double knockouts of the IGF-I and IGF1R [Igf-1(−/−)/Igf1r (−/−)] have the same phenotype as the IGF1R knockout, but double knockouts of IGF-II and the IGF1R [Igf-2(p−)/Igf1r(−/−)] have a more severe phenotype.[27,28] This suggested that IGF-II could act through another receptor and it has more recently been demonstrated that this additional receptor is the insulin receptor.[9]

In humans, it has been observed that SGA fetuses and newborns have lower circulating levels of IGF-I.[30] Serum IGF-I levels correlate with fetal size and birth weight suggesting that IGF-I has a primary effect or mediates the influence of another factor on birth size. IGF-II levels do not correlate with birth size as well, but are reduced in SGA newborns.[30]

IGF-I and IGF-II act as fetal growth factors, probably working in paracrine, autocrine, and endocrine manners. IGF-II is the predominant growth factor in early (from week 6) and mid-gestation with a gradual switch to IGF-I, which is first found in the circulation around week 9, in late gestation.[28] This switch has been observed in many species and the reasons for it happening are not known.

IGF levels are influenced by nutritional, genetic and endocrine factors which is in contrast to postnatal life, when growth hormone (GH) is the main stimulus of IGF-I production. IGF-I is regulated by fetal glucose and to a lesser extent by insulin, independent of the glucose level.[26,31] Thus the reduction in IGF-I levels in SGA fetuses and newborns has hitherto been assumed to reflect adverse environmental factors, with reduced uteroplacental function being the predominant etiology. However, animal and human twin studies, in fetal and postnatal life, show that circulating IGF-I levels are strongly influenced by genetic background and correlate with birth size.[32–34]

IGF-II is widely expressed at levels five- to six-fold higher than in postnatal life and is less significantly influenced by nutrition than IGF-I.[31] Levels are decreased by glucocorticoids, which may in part explain the fall in IGF-II concentration in late gestation when cortisol rises.

IGFs are anabolic hormones. In sheep studies, fetal IGF-I infusions resulted in increased growth of the major organs and skeletal maturation and increased fetoplacental amino acid and glucose uptake.[35] Increasing maternal IGF-I levels resulted in increased fetoplacental uptake of substrates and increased lactate production.[35] In rats and mice, IGF-I therapy given to pregnant dams increases fetal growth, where GH and saline do not. In strains of mice bred to have low IGF-I levels, IGF-I therapy reverses the normal fetal growth constraint.[36] IGF-I may therefore regulate growth to some extent via its effects on nutrient supply.

The actions of the IGFs are modulated by the IGF binding proteins (IGFBPs), of which there are six with high affinity and four with low affinity.[37] The levels of IGF binding proteins are under a combination of nutritional and endocrine influences. IGFBP-3 protease activity increases in the last trimester and this may act to increase the biological actions of IGF-I during late gestation.[38] IGFBP-3 is reduced and IGFBP-1 and IGFBP-2 are increased in SGA fetuses and newborns.[30]

Growth hormone

Fetal GH appears to arise exclusively from the fetal pituitary and is detectable from week 10 of gestation.[18] Fetal GH levels are higher than adult levels in mid-gestation and fall towards term. Growth hormone is a major postnatal growth factor, but has only a minor effect on fetal growth. Infants with congenital GH or GH receptor deficiency are born around 1 SD shorter than population averages but there is hardly any effect on birth weight.[39,40]

Glucocorticoids

Activity of the fetal hypothalamic-pituitary-adrenal (HPA) axis can be detected by 8–12 weeks gestation.[41] The main role of the fetal HPA axis is to stimulate differentiation and tissue maturation of various vital organs in late gestation to ensure neonatal survival. In the lungs glucocorticoids increase compliance and surfactant production, in the liver there is enzyme induction and enhanced glycogen deposition to ensure a glucose supply after birth and there is villus proliferation and induction of digestive enzymes in the bowel.[42] Sheep fetuses which are adrenalectomized do not experience these effects and in addition have increased fetal growth in the last 2 weeks gestation but this is reversible with intrauterine corticosteroid replacement.[24] Glucocorticoids are therefore essential to tissue maturation but can also restrict growth.

The level of maternal glucocorticoid exposure in the fetal circulation is tightly controlled by 11-β-hydroxysteroid dehydrogenase type 2 (11-β-HSD2) which converts the active cortisol to the inactive cortisone. 11-β-HSD2 is expressed in fetal tissues (colon, gut, kidney, adrenal) and the placenta. Genetic defects of 11-β-HSD2 result in reduced birth weights and a syndrome of apparent mineralocorticoid excess with hypertension in postnatal life.[43] SGA fetuses have lower placental levels of 11-β-HSD2 resulting in increased exposure to maternal cortisol which may, in part, explain their growth retardation, particularly in late gestation.[44]

Thyroid hormones

Thyroid hormones regulate oxygen consumption by fetal tissues. In humans thyroxine can cross the placenta so congenital hypothyroidism does not result in severe growth restriction or developmental abnormalities, unless there is also untreated maternal hypothyroidism.[24,45]

Placental hormones: growth hormone and placental lactogen

The placenta expresses large amounts of the GH-V gene, one of the five genes in the GH cluster on chromosome 17. This GH variant differs from anterior pituitary GH by 13 amino acids and is constitutively expressed from mid-gestation.[46] It does not cross the placenta so is secreted into the maternal circulation where it suppresses pituitary GH and stimulates IGF-I production.[47] In pregnancies complicated by fetal growth retardation there is decreased GH production by the placenta and thus reduced maternal IGF-I levels.[23] However, deletion of the GH-V gene is compatible with normal fetal growth.[48]

The placental lactogen (PL) gene also forms part of the GH cluster on chromosome 17. PL is secreted into the maternal circulation from early in the first trimester and peaks in the last trimester.[47] Maternal levels have been correlated positively with fetal growth and birth weight but PL deficiency has also been reported not to result in a reduction in birth weight.[49] Thus its role is not clearly understood.

SUMMARY

The control of normal fetal growth is under both environmental and genetic influences. The exact genes involved and their interplay with other genes and environmental factors is the focus of intense study. Animal studies and human fetal blood sampling have demonstrated that insulin, IGF-I and IGF-II are the main fetal growth factors with GH contributing only a minor influence. These factors not only cause tissue growth directly but can also influence the partitioning of nutrients across the placental unit. Corticosteroids play an important role in tissue maturation but, where there is increased fetal exposure, may also restrict growth.

REFERENCES

1 Magnus P. Further evidence for a significant effect of fetal genes on variation in birth weight. *Clin Genet* 1984; **26**: 289–96.

2 Magnus P. Distinguishing fetal and maternal genetic effects on variation in birth weight. *Acta Genet Med Gemellol (Roma)* 1984; **33**: 481–6.

3 Magnus P, Bakketeig LS, Hoffman H. Birth weight of relatives by maternal tendency to repeat small-for-gestational-age (SGA) births in successive pregnancies. *Acta Obstet Gynecol Scand Suppl* 1997; **165**: 35–8.

4 Wang X, Zuckerman B, Coffman GA, Corwin MJ. Familial aggregation of low birth weight among whites and blacks in the United States. *N Engl J Med* 1995; **333**: 1744–9.

5 Velho G, Froguel P. Genetic, metabolic and clinical characteristics of maturity onset diabetes of the young. *Eur J Endocrinol* 1998; **138**: 233–9.

6 Hattersley AT, Beards F, Ballantyne E, *et al.* Mutations in the glucokinase gene of the fetus result in reduced birth weight. *Nat Genet* 1998; **19**: 268–70.

7 Lestou VS, Kalousek DK. Confined placental mosaicism and intrauterine fetal growth. *Arch Dis Child Fetal Neonatal Ed* 1998; **79**: F223–6.

8 Wilkins-Haug L, Roberts DJ, Morton CC. Confined placental mosaicism and intrauterine growth retardation: a case-control analysis of placentas at delivery. *Am J Obstet Gynecol* 1995; **172(1 Pt 1)**: 44–50.

9 Accili D, Nakae J, Kim JJ, *et al.* Targeted gene mutations define the roles of insulin and IGF-I receptors in mouse embryonic development. *J Pediatr Endocrinol Metab* 1999; **12**: 475–85.

10 Arends N, Johnston L, Hokken-Koelega A, *et al.* Polymorphism in the IGF-I gene: clinical relevance for short children born small for gestational age (SGA). *J Clin Endocrinol Metab* 2002; **87**: 2720.

11 Johnston LB, Dahlgren J, Leger J, *et al.* Association between insulin-like growth factor I (IGF-I) polymorphisms, circulating IGF-I, and pre- and postnatal growth in two European small for gestational age populations. *J Clin Endocrinol Metab* 2003; **88**: 4805–10.

12 Dunger DB, Ong KK, Huxtable SJ, *et al.* Association of the INS VNTR with size at birth. ALSPAC Study Team. Avon Longitudinal Study of Pregnancy and Childhood. *Nat Genet* 1998; **19**: 98–100.

13 Woods KA, Camacho-Hubner C, Savage MO, Clark AJ. Intrauterine growth retardation and postnatal growth failure associated with deletion of the insulin-like growth factor I gene. *N Engl J Med* 1996; **335**: 1363–7.

14 Abuzzahab MJ, Schneider A, Goddard A, *et al.* IGF-I receptor mutations resulting in intrauterine and postnatal growth retardation. *N Engl J Med* 2003; **349**: 2211–22.

15 Kawashima Y, Kanzaki S, Yang F, *et al.* Mutation at cleavage site of insulin-like growth factor receptor in a short-stature child born with intrauterine growth retardation. *J Clin Endocrinol Metab* 2005; **90**: 4679–87.

16 Gicquel C, Rossignol S, Cabrol S, *et al.* Epimutation of the telomeric imprinting center region on chromosome 11p15 in Silver–Russell syndrome. *Nat Genet* 2005; **37**: 1003–7.

17 Kaplan SA. The insulin receptor. *J Pediatr* 1984; **104**: 327–36.

18 Kaplan SL, Grumbach MM, Shepard TH. The ontogenesis of human fetal hormones. I. Growth hormone and insulin. *J Clin Invest* 1972; **51**: 3080–93.

19 Hahn T, Desoye G. Ontogeny of glucose transport systems in the placenta and its progenitor tissues. *Early Pregnancy* 1996; **2**: 168–82.

20 Hahn T, Barth S, Graf R, *et al.* Placental glucose transporter expression is regulated by glucocorticoids. *J Clin Endocrinol Metab* 1999; **84**: 1445–52.

21 Gaither K, Quraishi AN, Illsley NP. Diabetes alters the expression and activity of the human placental GLUT1 glucose transporter. *J Clin Endocrinol Metab* 1999; **84**: 695–701.

22 Evain-Brion D. Hormonal regulation of fetal growth. *Horm Res* 1994; **42**: 207–14.

23 Gluckman PD, Harding JE. The physiology and pathophysiology of intrauterine growth retardation. *Horm Res* 1997; **48(Suppl 1)**: 11–6.

24 Fowden AL. Endocrine regulation of fetal growth. *Reprod Fertil Dev* 1995; **7**: 351–63.

25 Lemons JA, Ridenour R, Orsini EN. Congenital absence of the pancreas and intrauterine growth retardation. *Pediatrics* 1979; **64**: 255–7.

26 Fowden AL. The role of insulin in prenatal growth. *J Dev Physiol* 1989; **12**: 173–82.

27 Liu JP, Baker J, Perkins AS, *et al.* Mice carrying null mutations of the genes encoding insulin-like growth factor I (Igf-I) and type 1 IGF receptor (Igf1r). *Cell* 1993; **75**: 59–72.

28 Baker J, Liu JP, Robertson EJ, Efstratiadis A. Role of insulin-like growth factors in embryonic and postnatal growth. *Cell* 1993; **75**: 73–82.

29 Walenkamp MJ, Karperien M, Pereira AM, *et al.* Homozygous and heterozygous expression of a novel insulin-like growth factor-I mutation. *J Clin Endocrinol Metab* 2005; **90**: 2855–64.

30 Giudice LC, de Zegher F, Gargosky SE, *et al.* Insulin-like growth factors and their binding proteins in the term and preterm human fetus and neonate with normal and extremes of intrauterine growth. *J Clin Endocrinol Metab* 1995; **80**: 1548–55.

31 Oliver MH, Harding JE, Breier BH, Gluckman PD. Fetal insulin-like growth factor (IGF)-I and IGF-II are regulated differently by glucose or insulin in the sheep fetus. *Reprod Fertil Dev* 1996; **8**: 167–72.

32 Hong Y, Pedersen NL, Brismar K, *et al.* Quantitative genetic analyses of insulin-like growth factor I (IGF-I), IGF-binding protein-1, and insulin levels in middle-aged and elderly twins. *J Clin Endocrinol Metab* 1996; **81**: 1791–7.

33 Morel PC, Blair HT, Ormsby JE, *et al.* Influence of fetal and maternal genotype for circulating insulin-like growth factor I on fetal growth in mice. *J Reprod Fertil* 1994; **101**: 9–14.

34 Verhaeghe J, Loos R, Vlietinck R, *et al.* C-peptide, insulin-like growth factors I and II, and insulin-like growth factor binding protein-1 in cord serum of twins: genetic versus environmental regulation. *Am J Obstet Gynecol* 1996; **175**: 1180–8.

35 Harding JE, Liu L, Evans PC, Gluckman PD. Insulin-like growth factor 1 alters feto-placental protein and carbohydrate metabolism in fetal sheep. *Endocrinology* 1994; **134**: 1509–14.

36 Gluckman PD, Morel PC, Ambler GR, *et al.* Elevating maternal insulin-like growth factor-I in mice and rats alters the pattern of fetal growth by removing maternal constraint. *J Endocrinol* 1992; **134**: R1–3.

37 Hwa V, Oh Y, Rosenfeld RG. The insulin-like growth factor-binding protein (IGFBP) superfamily. *Endocr Rev* 1999; **20**: 761–87.

38 Davenport ML, Pucilowska J, Clemmons DR, *et al.* Tissue-specific expression of insulin-like growth factor binding protein-3 protease activity during rat pregnancy. *Endocrinology* 1992; **130**: 2505–12.

39 Gluckman PD, Gunn AJ, Wray A, *et al.* Congenital idiopathic growth hormone deficiency associated with prenatal and early postnatal growth failure. The International Board of the Kabi Pharmacia International Growth Study. *J Pediatr* 1992; **121**: 920–3.

40 Woods KA, Dastot F, Preece MA, *et al.* Phenotype: genotype relationships in growth hormone insensitivity syndrome. *J Clin Endocrinol Metab* 1997; **82**: 3529–35.

41 Ng PC. The fetal and neonatal hypothalamic-pituitary–adrenal axis. *Arch Dis Child Fetal Neonatal Ed* 2000; **82**: F250–4.

42 Mesiano S, Jaffe RB. Developmental and functional biology of the primate fetal adrenal cortex. *Endocr Rev* 1997; **18**: 378–403.

43 White PC, Mune T, Agarwal AK. 11 beta-Hydroxysteroid dehydrogenase and the syndrome of apparent mineralocorticoid excess. *Endocr Rev* 1997; **18**: 135–56.

44 Stewart PM, Whorwood CB, Mason JI. Type 2 11 beta-hydroxysteroid dehydrogenase in foetal and adult life. *J Steroid Biochem Mol Biol* 1995; **55**: 465–71.

45 de Zegher F, Pernasetti F, Vanhole C, *et al.* The prenatal role of thyroid hormone evidenced by fetomaternal Pit-1 deficiency. *J Clin Endocrinol Metab* 1995; **80**: 3127–30.

46 Baumann G. Growth hormone heterogeneity: genes, isohormones, variants, and binding proteins. *Endocr Rev* 1991; **12**: 424–49.

47 Handwerger S, Freemark M. The roles of placental growth hormone and placental lactogen in the regulation of human fetal growth and development. *J Pediatr Endocrinol Metab* 2000; **13**: 343–56.

48 Simon P, Decoster C, Brocas H, *et al.* Absence of human chorionic somatomammotropin during pregnancy associated with two types of gene deletion. *Hum Genet* 1986; **74**: 235–8.

49 Nielsen PV, Pedersen H, Kampmann EM. Absence of human placental lactogen in an otherwise uneventful pregnancy. *Am J Obstet Gynecol* 1979; **135**: 322–6.

9

Growth in infancy and childhood

AMANDA J DRAKE, CHRISTOPHER J H KELNAR

INTRODUCTION

Somatic growth is a fundamental biologic process of childhood. A healthy, adequately nourished and emotionally secure child grows at a normal rate. On an individual basis, poor growth is a powerful indicator that all is not well with the child and is the 'final common pathway' for many organic and emotional problems of childhood. Growth monitoring is important in the early detection of suspected disease in children and of particular value in detecting a wide variety of endocrine abnormalities in which poor growth may be the earliest, or only, sign of a problem.[1,2]

A single measure of stature permits the assessment of current size and reflects previous growth; however, in a condition of recent onset, the duration of slow growth may not be long enough to cause short stature. Growth velocity, calculated from serial measures of height, represents the dynamics of growth much better than a single measure and a slowly growing child has a pathological disorder requiring diagnosis and, if possible, treatment.

In addition to identifying growth problems in the individual, in public health terms, anthropometric surveys are widely used to assess the prevalence of under- or overnutrition in a population and to identify groups with increased nutritional and health needs.[3–5] Additionally, they are a useful index of health and economic well-being in both developing and developed countries and are highlighting the marked effect of dietary changes on public health worldwide.[5–7] Since the nineteenth century there have been secular trends to increasing adult height,[8] with trends across Europe of between 1 and 3 cm per decade,[9]

necessitating periodic revision of growth standards. Additionally, meticulous data collection during the last century has been vital in establishing a link between growth in fetal life and early infancy and patterns of disease in adults.[10,11]

Although measurement of height is an important component of child health care and is an intrinsic part of pediatric care worldwide,[4] national practices vary markedly[3,12] and despite its widespread use in pediatric practice, little is known about the diagnostic performance of growth screening or monitoring in terms of its sensitivity and specificity for the detection of growth disorders and of its impact on child health.[12–14] In the UK, this has resulted in the most recent recommendations for height screening in childhood to be reduced to a single measurement at the age of 5 years.[15]

THE INFANCY–CHILDHOOD–PUBERTY MODEL OF GROWTH

The infancy–childhood–puberty (ICP) model of growth (Fig. 9.1) suggested by Karlberg et al.[16] is a mathematical model of the human growth curve that attempts to relate growth to the underlying dynamics of hormonal and other controls. The model suggests three additive components to growth, from the immediate post-natal period through to adult life.

The infancy component of this model is the initially rapid (but also rapidly decelerating) growth phase of the first 2–3 years of life and is a continuation of fetal growth.

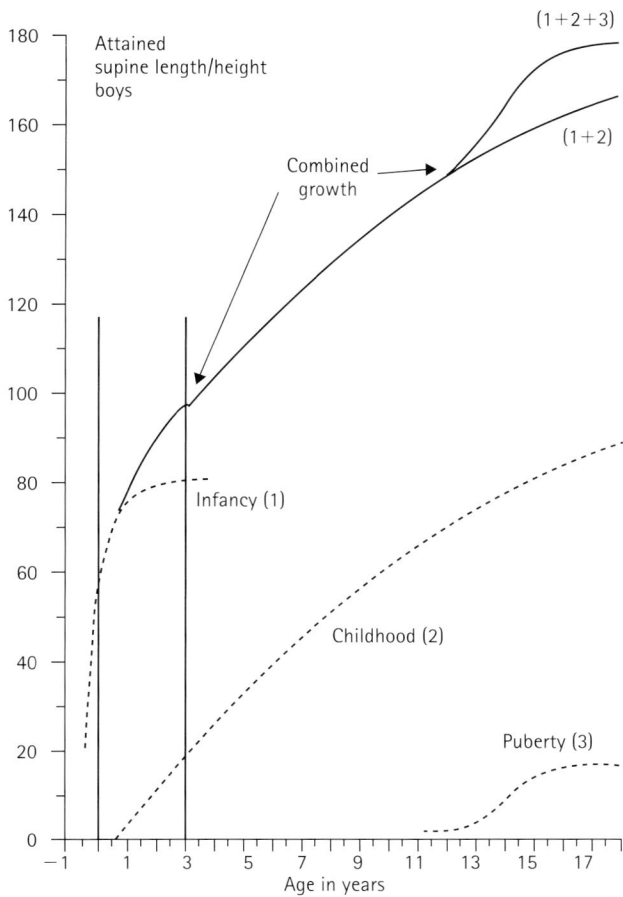

Figure 9.1   The infancy–childhood–puberty model of growth.

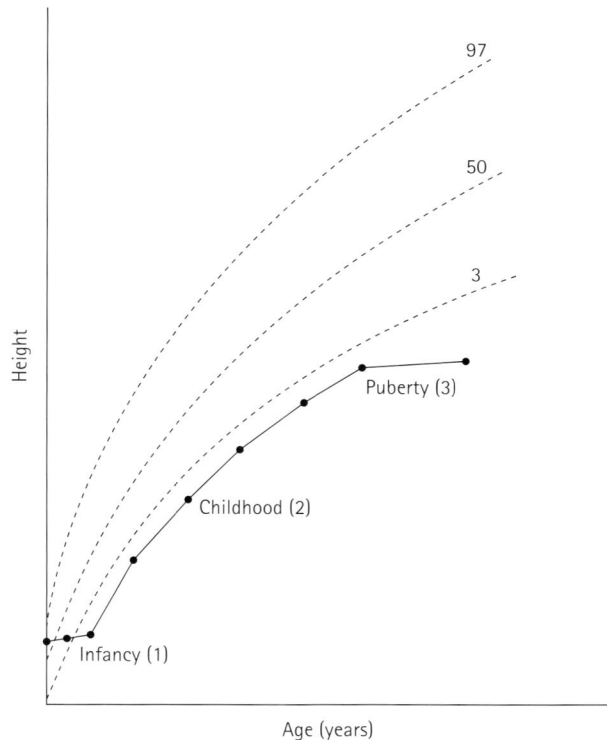

Figure 9.2   Growth in chronic renal failure originating in infancy.

It is largely nutritionally determined, although other factors are undoubtedly important.

Growth during this phase is extremely rapid; on average an infant will grow 25 cm in the first 12 months of life and will double the birth length by the age of 3–4 years. If growth is poor during the infancy phase, it is extremely difficult to make up later, even if growth is relatively normal in the childhood phase. This is well illustrated by infants who have early onset chronic illness, e.g., chronic renal failure (Fig. 9.2).

The childhood phase of growth assumes gradually more importance from about 6 months of age and becomes predominant from about 3 years of age. Many hormones influence skeletal and somatic growth in childhood including growth hormone (GH), thyroxine, glucocorticoids, androgens and estrogens, insulin and polypeptide growth factors, but the childhood component of the ICP growth model is primarily determined by GH secretion. The GH effect is sustained through puberty, but, in the absence of adequate sex steroid secretion, the pubertal component of the growth model will be blunted or absent.

It is the combined effect of these three components of the growth model that result in the pattern of growth culminating in the adult height.

ASSESSMENT OF GROWTH IN INFANCY AND CHILDHOOD

The ability to measure a child accurately and reproducibly is fundamental to growth assessment. Length and height measurements are often valueless and misleading because of inadequate apparatus and/or careless techniques. A single length or height measurement in any infant or child (growth screening) is an insensitive guide to the presence or absence of underlying pathology and of limited value – it tells you where that child is placed in terms of a normally distributed population – but only serial measurements (growth monitoring) and calculation of height velocity will tell you whether that child is currently growing normally.

Weight

Weight is easy to measure but it may fluctuate quite widely especially in early infancy, depending upon the contents of the stomach, bowel, and bladder and is additionally affected by minor illnesses. Because of these short-term variations, weight may be a poor indicator of growth when used in isolation. Additionally, mode of feeding affects weight gain in infancy; during the first 3–4 months of life, breast-fed infants gain weight more rapidly than those fed on formula milk. However, this trend is reversed thereafter, so that a longer duration of breast feeding is associated with a decline in weight for age and weight for length but not length for age.[17,18] In response to this, the World Health Organization is developing a growth chart based only on the growth of healthy children in optimal conditions.[19] Growth standards which describe how children *should* grow rather than how they *actually* grow would be a significant advance as they would reflect what is physiological rather than what is prevalent.[19]

Secular changes in weight have accompanied those in height over the last century[8,20] and whereas height appears to have stabilized, weight has continued to increase.[8] There has been a rapid increase in the prevalence of childhood obesity worldwide,[21–25] and thus routine growth assessment should include adiposity (see assessment using body mass index below).

Length

As length is not subject to the same short-term fluctuations as weight, it is a more reliable measure of infant and childhood growth. Length is measured supine in the first 12 to 18 months of life and can be measured even in a very small sick infant in an incubator using an appropriate measuring device (e.g., Pedobaby II). Height measurements using a stadiometer can be performed after a child is standing and certainly from the age of 2 years. Even in developing countries, 'length-for-age' at 3 months has been shown to be the best screening method to detect growth failure and better than weight in predicting subsequent stunting of growth.[26]

With accurate measurements, information on the normality of growth can be obtained over a 3 month period. Nevertheless, seasonal growth variation can occur – not every child grows at a consistent rate month by month – and measurement over 1 year is often necessary before growth velocity can be clearly seen to be abnormal. In addition, normal growth can be cyclical[27] with the rate varying over 2–3 years. Additionally, there may be marked diurnal variation in stature, which may significantly affect the accuracy of monitoring.[28]

The child who is growing with a height velocity consistently at or below 25th centile merits further investigation. In practice, during the middle years of childhood a child should grow at a rate of 4–7 cm year^{-1}; any child growing outside these limits requires further assessment.

Although from around 1 year until puberty, most children will track along the centile curves on a height chart,[29] infants commonly cross centiles before the age of 1 year. This phenomenon of catch-up or catch-down growth represents 'regression to the mean'[30] and the interpretation of weight velocity using conventional cross-sectional weight charts does not allow for this. Conditional reference charts use statistical methods to predict regression towards the mean and may be a more useful way of assessing weight gain in infants, comparing an infant's current weight with that predicted from their previous weight.[30]

Knemometry

Knemometry is the technique of choice for studying short-term longitudinal growth[31–34] as it allows precise, reproducible, non-invasive measurements of lower leg length in growing children, such that daily (or even within-day) and weekly fluctuations in leg length can be documented. Practically, it is possible to use knemometry in neonates and in cooperative children above about 4 years of age. Normal oscillatory cycles of growth over about 3 weeks have been demonstrated by knemometry, although more marked fluctuations have been shown during intercurrent illness, recovery from malnutrition,[35,36] or during the use of steroid therapy.[37,38] Knemometry ignores spinal growth and may be influenced by the hydration of soft tissues overlying bone.[39]

Body composition

Weight for height measurement does not distinguish between fat mass and lean body mass. Assessment of body composition, in particular total body fat and fat-free mass, can be very helpful in infancy and early childhood to assess the severity of growth and nutritional disorders (including obesity), and additionally, to evaluate treatment. Measurement of skinfold thickness is a useful clinical tool[40] and may be used to assess nutrition in young infants and older children; however, it can be difficult to do well and may not be as accurate in the young infant as water dilution techniques.[41] Additionally, care must be taken that prediction equations for skinfold thickness are valid for the population studied.[40,42] Waist circumference is easy to measure and may be better than body mass index (BMI) as a predictor of total body fat and cardiovascular risk factors.[43–45] Waist circumference is a highly sensitive and specific measure of upper body fat in young people,[46] and has increased over the past 10–20 years in British youth at a greater rate than BMI, particularly in females, suggesting that the accumulation of central body fat, associated with an increased risk of cardiovascular complications, has increased more steeply than whole-body fatness based on the measurement of height and weight.[46] The impact of this increase in waist measurement is unknown and the link between waist circumference, BMI and cardiovascular risk in young people requires further study. Centile charts are available for skinfold thickness and waist circumference. Arm circumference measurements have also been used in a number of studies and may be a useful measure of body composition in field studies.[47]

Non-invasive techniques such as total body electrical conductivity have allowed standards to be determined for total body fat and fat free mass in healthy infants.[48] Finally, dual-energy X-ray absorptiometry (DEXA) has become a preferred method for estimating whole-body composition in adults[49,50] and children.[51–53]

Body mass index

The use of body mass index (BMI), weight (in kg)/height^2, provides a practical clinical tool for identification of adults with different degrees of obesity which carry particular adverse risks, for example hypertension, hypercholesterolemia and type 2 diabetes. In adults, a simple definition of obesity is BMI $>30.0 \, kg \, m^{-2}$. However, in childhood, body mass index changes substantially, rising steeply in infancy, falling during preschool years and rising again after about 8 years into adulthood. Interpretation of BMI values in children therefore requires the use of age-related curves, and UK pediatric standards are available.[54] Although there are potential limitations of the use of BMI, including that it may underestimate the percentage of lean body mass by taking no account of variations in muscularity and may not be relevant for all ethnic groups,[55] studies have shown that the use of cut-off ranges for BMI is associated with high specificity and moderate sensitivity for identifying the fattest children, particularly when the cut-off is greater than the 90th centile.[56] These cut-offs are clinically meaningful: obesity defined in this way is associated with short- and long-term morbidity.[57–59]

The International Obesity Task Force has proposed that BMI offers a reasonable clinical measure of fatness in children and adolescents[55,60] and, using BMI data from a number of national surveys, has proposed an international definition of obesity.[61] The Scottish Intercollegiate Guidelines Network has recently published a guideline for the management of obesity in children and young people (www.sign.ac.uk/guidelines), recommending the use of the UK 1990 reference charts for BMI in the identification of childhood obesity. The guideline proposes that for clinical use overweight children are those with a BMI >91st centile and obese children are those with a BMI >98th centile for age and sex. However, for epidemiological (research) purposes, in order to remain consistent with definitions used in the current literature, the recommendation is that overweight is defined as BMI >85th centile and obesity >95th centile of the 1990 reference data for age and weight.

Interpretation

Care must be taken interpreting weight and length measurements particularly in infancy. For example, an infant who is below the 3rd centile for both weight and length may still be relatively 'fat'. Slow growth with >50th centile skin-fold measurements is characteristic of an endocrine disorder in childhood and increasing the calorie intake will not improve linear growth unless the underlying cause is identified. Infants with severe growth hormone insufficiency may present with poor weight gain, although longitudinal growth is more markedly affected. Thus, they are relatively fat and there is often a characteristic puckered or marbled appearance and texture to abdominal fat (Fig. 9.3).

Once accurate measurements have been made, use should be made of an appropriate growth chart. Useful reference manuals of normal physical measurements and characteristics are Buckler[62] and Hall et al.[63] The introduction in the UK of nine-centile growth charts, based on seven (largely cross-sectional) local growth surveys from diverse parts of the country between 1978 and 1990,[64] would be expected to help facilitate the appropriate referral of children with growth disorders following screening; however the usefulness of such charts may be limited by the introduction of a single height measurement at school entry. The lowest centile is the 0.4 line; only one normal child in 250 will fall below that line, which is a clear indicator for referral. The interval between each provided pair of centile lines is the same – two thirds of a standard deviation. Two percent of the normal population will have a height below the second centile. It is recommended that any child between the 2nd and 0.4 centiles is monitored to see whether their growth is normal. Versions are available for community and hospital use and should help to facilitate the appropriate referral of children with growth disorders. Similar updated growth charts based on cross-sectional data have been produced in other countries including the USA (www.cdc.gov/growthcharts) and the Netherlands.[65,66]

Revised charts based on the Tanner–Whitehouse growth standards (derived from a longitudinal study of south of England children in the 1960s) have been produced: the Buckler–Tanner longitudinal standards.[67] Height revision is adjusted to take account of the recent cross-sectional studies and of Buckler's 1990 longitudinal study of adolescent growth[68] (see also Chapter 10). For monitoring the growth pattern in an individual child such charts are preferable. Normal growth in a short or tall child suggests that familial factors are important in his or her stature – normal short parents or growth advance or delay. A persistently slowly growing child has a pathological disorder requiring diagnosis, and if possible, treatment. With conditions of recent onset, slow growth may not have occurred for sufficient time to cause short stature. Delay in diagnosis until a significant growth deficit has accrued often leads to significantly compromised adult height. Not all children complete their growth at the same age, and many normal children will take up to several years longer than their peers to reach their adult height. These children are likely to enter puberty later than their peer group, but in childhood they may appear relatively small for their parental heights and will have bone age delay. This normal variation is known as constitutional delay of growth and puberty. Disease specific reference charts have been developed to allow growth assessment in a number of common conditions which are associated with short stature (e.g., Down syndrome,[69] Turner syndrome,[70] achondroplasia[71]). Significant deviation from syndrome-specific centiles necessitates a search for additional pathology (e.g., hypothyroidism or Crohn's disease in girls with Turner syndrome).

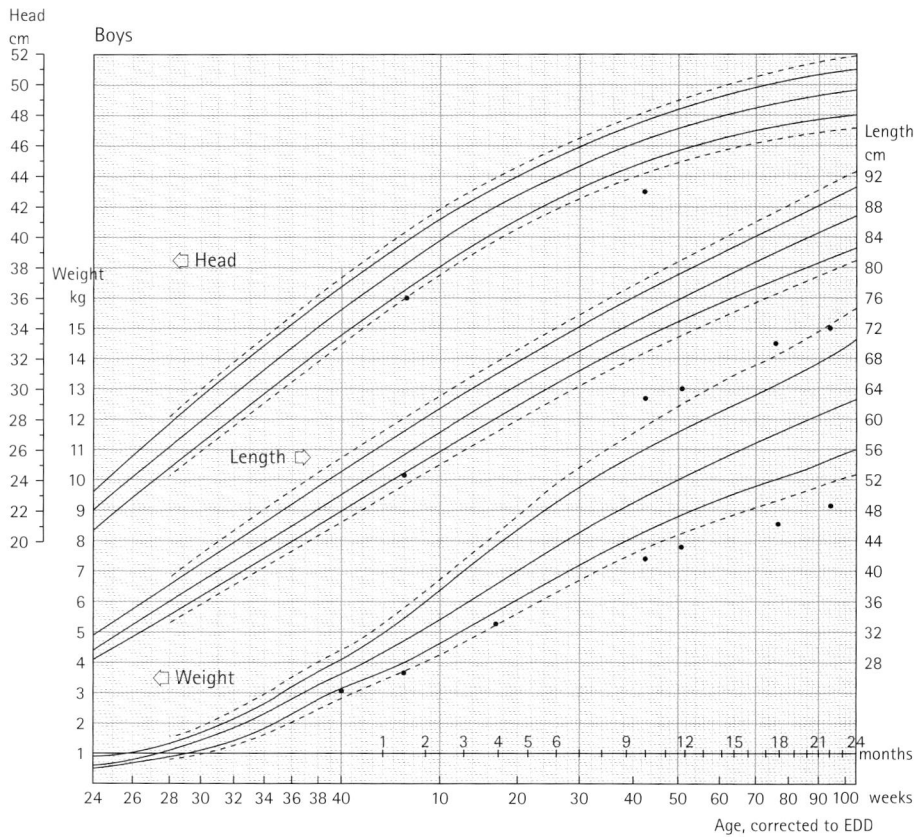

(a)

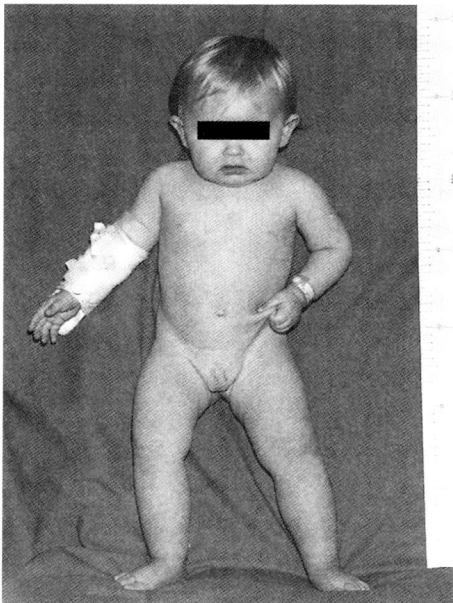

(b)

Figure 9.3 Growth chart and picture of child with growth hormone deficiency presenting in infancy.

The latest recommendations in the UK[15] suggest that routine growth monitoring to detect centile crossing has too low a sensitivity and specificity to be regarded as screening.[72] The book *Health for all Children*[15] recommends a minimum of weights at 2, 3, 4, 8 and 12–15 months, and at 3–4 years,

with height and weight at school entry. Routine growth monitoring is not recommended after the age of 5.[15] There is, however, considerable ongoing debate about how often measurements should be made in the school age child in order to identify those children in whom growth falters in

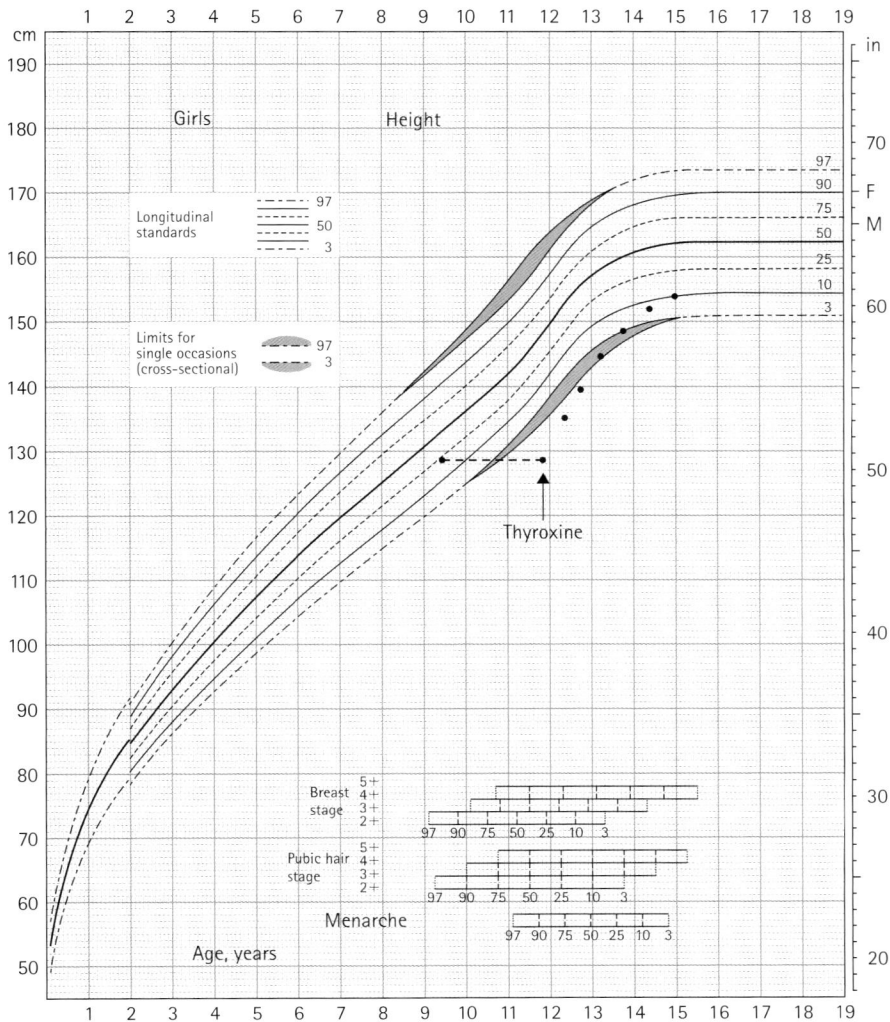

Figure 9.4 Growth chart of late presenting hypothyroidism.

mid-childhood (e.g., acquired hypothyroidism) and to detect the 25–50 percent of children whose growth disorder has not been identified by school entry (Fig. 9.4).

Influences on infant and childhood growth

Genetic influences affect growth *in utero*, during infancy and in childhood. Parental genetic contributions reduce the population standard deviation of height by about 30 percent; and 95 percent of the children of given parents will have a height prognosis within 8.5 cm of the mid-parental centile. However, environmental influences also have a major influence and may have an intergenerational effect on child health and growth. In 1986, Emanuel defined intergenerational influences as 'those factors, conditions, exposures and environments experienced by one generation that relate to the health, growth and development of the next generation'.[73] Epidemiological studies have suggested that there may be intergenerational effects on birth weight.[74–79] Additionally, in Britain,

despite the secular trend to increasing height across the population, the mean height of children from social class IV and V remained significantly less than that of those from social classes I and II in the 1980s, a situation which has remained unchanged for the past 100 years.[6] Thus, a child who is short, but an 'appropriate' height for his or her short parents, may in fact represent the consequence of poor nutrition or emotional deprivation continuing down the generations with no family member achieving their true genetic height potential. Finally, it is worth considering whether the short parent of a short child may have a heritable, but unrecognized and untreated growth disorder (e.g., a skeletal dysplasia, pseudohypoparathyroidism or growth hormone deficiency) before diagnosing familial short stature.

Prenatal influences

Many factors are important in determining size at birth. Epidemiological studies suggest that genetic factors account for 30–80 percent of birth weight variance[80] and genes may act to influence the growth of the fetus[81–83] and the placenta.[84,85] The genetic influence on birth weight is likely to be polygenic and candidate genes proposed to influence size at birth include the insulin-like growth factors.[81–86]

Although offspring birth weight is related to both maternal and paternal birth weight, many epidemiological studies have suggested that there is a greater influence of maternal than paternal birth size on offspring birth weight.[74,76–78,87,88] Indeed, a number have shown a matrilineal multigenerational effect on birth weight.[77,89] Although there is a significant relationship between paternal and offspring birth weight, this association is not as strong as that for maternal birth weight.[77,88,90,91] Maternal factors acting on the developing fetus may include maternal nutrition, maternal size,[92,93] hyperglycemia, hyperinsulinemia,[94] hypertension,[95,96] maternal health, and environmental factors including teratogens (especially smoking, alcohol, and drugs). Infants born to unusually large or small mothers will tend to regress towards their mid-parental centile after birth, but their growth pattern may cause concern if maternal details (and the relative size of the father) are not adequately assessed. Many placental factors are likely to have an influence on growth *in utero*, including placental size and function, vascular

abnormalities, hypoxia, and levels of placental growth hormone. Finally, in addition to genetic influences, fetal factors that can influence birth size include fetal hyperinsulinemia, intrauterine infection, chromosomal abnormalities and syndrome disorders. Infants born small for gestational age (SGA) must be assessed in detail, with particular reference to the pregnancy history. They may be symmetrically small (i.e., low birth weight, short length and small head circumference) or asymmetrically small (low birth weight but length and head circumference spared). Asymmetrically SGA infants have usually only had a relatively short period of inadequate growth *in utero*, often as a result of acute placental insufficiency, whereas those who are symmetrically small have had a much more prolonged insult or have an underlying 'fetal' reason for their poor growth, e.g., Silver–Russell syndrome. The pattern of intrauterine growth may be subsequently reflected in the growth pattern in infancy, and may influence whether the infant shows 'catch-up' growth during the early years of life. Although infants with late onset growth retardation have a better prognosis for catch-up growth,[97] there are as yet, no good prognostic tests in early infancy to differentiate those in whom catch up is not going to be adequate. In addition, the pre-term SGA infant may behave differently from his or her term counterparts in subsequent growth patterns (Fig. 9.5).

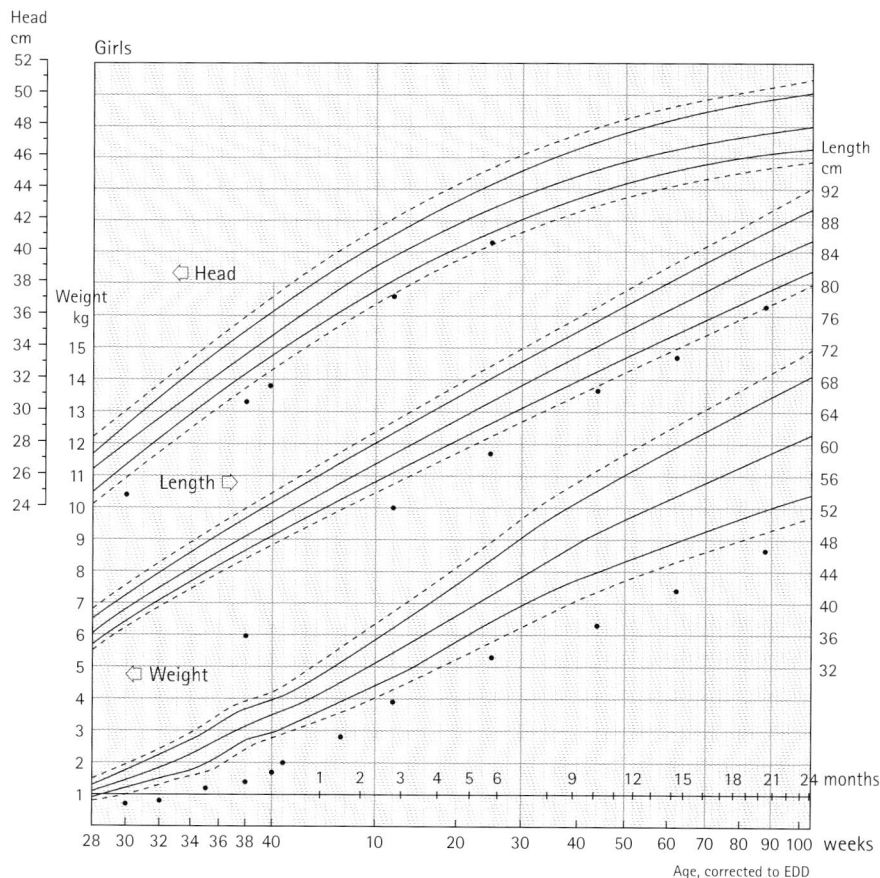

Figure 9.5 Growth chart of symmetrically small infant showing good catch up over first 2 years of life.

Growth factors are amongst the first products of the embryo and direct growth *in utero* and post-natally. Their actions coordinate with the developing endocrine system. Peptide growth factors, fibroblast growth factors, and epidermal growth factors are present in almost all tissues. Growth factors affect DNA synthesis and mitogenesis and act at different phases of the cell cycle. The insulin-like growth factors (IGFs) are bound to multiple IGF binding proteins (IGFBPs) of which at least six different species have been characterized. These binding proteins modulate IGF-I action, receptor binding and bioavailability[98] (see Chapters 7 and 29) and are expressed in a tissue-specific manner throughout human fetal life and early infancy.[99] Whereas IGF-II is the primary growth factor in embryonic growth, IGF-I becomes more important in late gestation,[100–102] although both growth factors are essential in fetal growth. Mice with targeted disruptions of IGF-I or IGF-II genes show severe growth restriction of prenatal onset.[103,104] IGF-II is imprinted and expressed from the paternal allele and in cases of isopaternal disomy in humans; IGF-II overexpression is associated with the Beckwith–Wiedemann overgrowth syndrome.[102] That IGF-I is essential for pre-natal growth in humans has been shown convincingly by the report of a patient with deletion of the IGF-I gene.[82] In contrast to post-natally, fetal insulin is the primary regulator of circulating IGF-I[105] and is sensitive to maternal nutrition. Most studies have shown that IGF-I levels are low in small for gestational age infants[106,107] and IGF-I gene polymorphisms may influence pre- and post-natal growth in some individuals.[108] In contrast, the macrosomic infants of diabetic and nondiabetic mothers have raised IGF-I levels.[109]

Nutritional influences on growth in infancy and childhood

Adequate nutrition is necessary to enable satisfactory growth to occur in infancy and early childhood. Indeed according to the ICP model of growth, nutrition is the prime influence affecting growth in the first years of life. Healthy eating guidelines are available for infants and young children (www.doh.gov.uk). Malnutrition may reflect either over- or undernutrition, and is a consequence of disturbance of energy and nutrient balance in terms of supply and demand. Undernutrition delays growth, but children subjected to an acute episode of starvation will recover as long as it is not too severe or long lasting. However, chronic malnutrition has much more severe effects and may compromise adult height. Undernutrition may be due to insufficient energy or nutrient intake, disordered digestion, absorption or metabolism, or excessive losses. The period of time when the child appears to be at most risk from malnutrition is from age 6 months to 3 years, coinciding with the infancy component of the ICP model of growth. Growth that is lost or poor during this period may not be regained in later childhood or during puberty.[110] In the developing world this is a particularly vulnerable time for young children; lactation may be declining, weaning occurs and is the time of most risk of infection. Growth faltering is widely prevalent in the developing world, with wide variations between countries and between regions.[110] The prevalence of low weight and height for age is highest in Asia, affecting one in every two children.[110] However, malnutrition is not only a problem of developing countries. Inadequate nutrition may be subtler in the developed world but a detailed dietary history is vital in any child who is not growing well (see Chapter 5) (Fig. 9.6).

Current UK (www.breastfeeding.nhs.uk) and WHO recommendations are that breast milk is sufficient as the sole energy source for the first 6 months of life and term infants should be exclusively breastfed from birth until about 6 months of age.[111] This is clearly important in the developing world in terms of prevention of infection etc. but may not be so crucial in developed countries. The infant and young child require diets with adequate protein,[112] carbohydrate and fat.[113] The WHO recommends that under 2 years of age, a child's diet contains 30–40

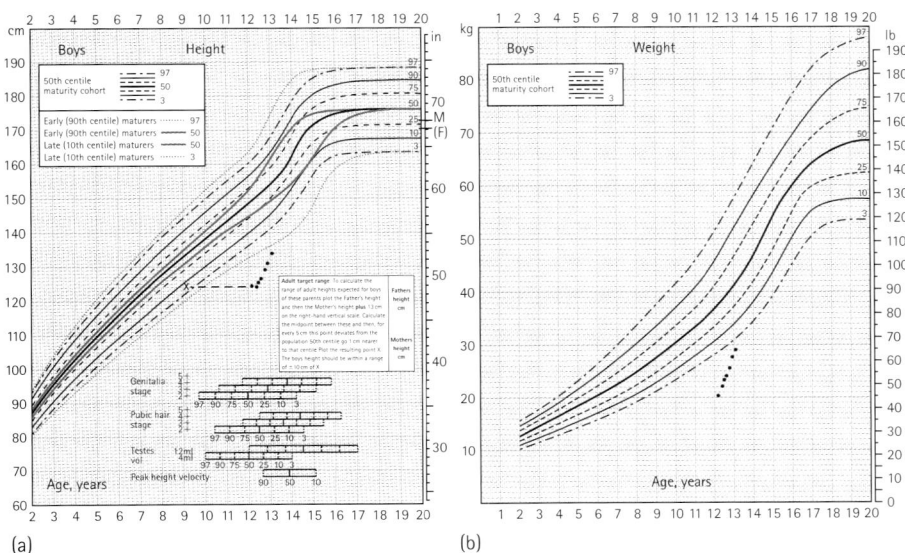

(a)   (b)

Figure 9.6 Growth chart of a malnourished child showing good catch-up growth following the resumption of normal nutrition.

percent of energy from fat and provides an amount of essential fatty acids similar to that found in human milk.[114] Beyond 2 years of age the WHO recommends more than 15 percent of energy from dietary fat. The American Academy of Pediatrics and the American Heart Association recommend no restrictions on dietary fat below the age of two years and that children over 2 years derive 30 percent energy from fat.[113] Recent reviews suggest that there is a wide variation in the dietary fat intake of children in Europe and in the USA.[113,115] Carbohydrate intake has increased as a result of the decrease in dietary fat, but instead of complex carbohydrates, carbohydrates with a higher glycemic index are being consumed which may be contributing to the epidemic of childhood obesity.[113,115]

Iron deficiency is the most widespread micronutrient deficiency among infants and young children, particularly associated with the early introduction of cow's milk into the diet[116] and improving iron status may have a major impact on motor and language development.[110,116] Studies have suggested that iron deficiency at 12 months of age, in a population of high birth weight, is associated with a faster growth rate and shorter breast feeding duration.[117] Iron deficiency per se may reduce growth rates; and supplementation may improve growth by mechanisms which remain

unclear, but which may include reduced morbidity, increased food intake and possibly a direct effect of iron.[116]

In an infant who is failing to thrive it is vital that a detailed feeding history is obtained as the growth of many such children can be improved by ensuring they have an appropriate diet.[118] It should also be remembered that conditions causing malabsorption e.g., celiac disease, may present with poor growth rather than gastrointestinal disturbance. Other chronic conditions can cause inappropriate loss of essential elements vital for growth. In particular, sodium is an important growth factor stimulating cell proliferation and protein synthesis and increasing cell mass, although the exact mechanism is not clearly understood. Salt 'wasting' conditions can lead to growth failure with subsequent improvement in growth with salt repletion.[119] This is characteristically seen in infants with salt-losing congenital adrenal hyperplasia in whom longitudinal growth may be poor if salt replacement is inadequate. Children with ongoing renal salt loss may also show poor longitudinal growth (Fig. 9.7).

Overfeeding in infancy and early childhood can also affect the growth patterns of later childhood and indeed adult body shape. Obesity in childhood often leads to relative tall childhood stature. Indeed it is the child who is

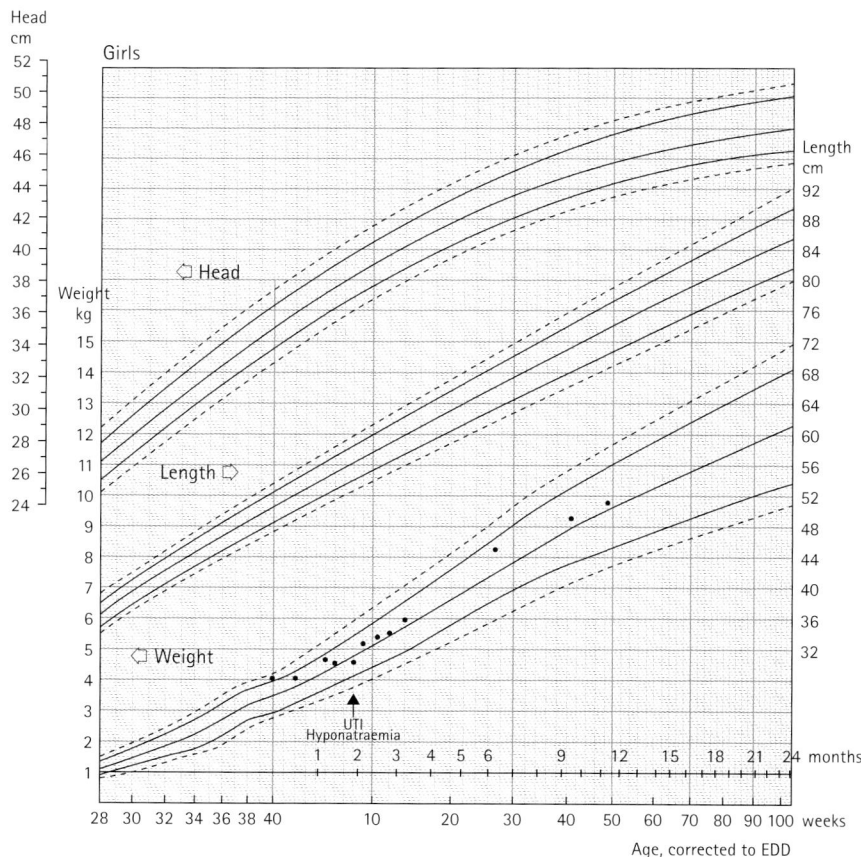

Figure 9.7　Growth chart of child with salt loss secondary to urinary tract infection.

'short and fat' who is more likely to have an underlying endocrinopathy. Not all obese children become obese adults and the timing of the development of their obesity, particularly in relation to BMI changes in the normal population, may be important.

Endocrine influences on infant and childhood growth

Endocrine influences on growth, particularly growth hormone, assume increasing importance in the childhood phase of growth. However, there is increasing evidence that growth hormone does influence growth in infancy. Growth hormone can be detected in the fetal circulation from around 10 weeks of gestation[120] and growth hormone receptors are present in chondrocytes, osteoblasts, fibroblasts and the epidermis from 15 weeks[121] and in hepatocytes from 30 weeks of gestation.[122] Although studies in animal models and in humans have suggested that growth hormone does not play a major role in fetal growth (reviewed in Ogilvy-Stuart[123]), studies over the last 10 years have shown that children with congenital growth hormone deficiency have birth lengths and weights below the mean and that some have severe prenatal growth failure.[123] Additionally, infants may have an excessive weight relative to length and progressive post-natal growth failure, sometimes noted relatively early in the post-natal period.[123–126] In the normal infant, growth hormone levels decline rapidly over the first 2 weeks of life and progressively during the first 2 years.[127] IGF-I levels are low throughout the first 15–18 months and gradually rise to adult levels thereafter.[128] During infancy, nutrition and endocrine factors are additive in promoting growth but there is a gradual change from the infancy component of the growth curve to the childhood component from the age of about 6

months and, from about 3 years of age, endocrine control of growth, particularly growth hormone secretion and action, becomes more important. Growth hormone secretion and action is described in detail elsewhere (see Chapter 7). There is an asymptotic relationship between growth rate and growth hormone secretion[129] and childhood growth appears to be growth hormone pulse–amplitude modulated. With-out adequate growth hormone secretion the childhood component of the growth model will be extremely blunted, and the child will become increasingly short compared to his or her peers. The differential diagnosis, investigation and management of the child with suspected GH insufficiency is discussed in Chapter 12 (Fig. 9.8).

Growth hormone secretion is pulsatile and controlled by the hypothalamus. Assessment of growth hormone secretion can be physiological (e.g., urinary GH, overnight GH profiling) or following pharmacological stimuli. Details of the evaluation of growth hormone secretion are discussed in Chapter 12. Secretory dynamics can be affected by other factors e.g., psychosocial deprivation (see later in this chapter and in Chapter 26) or cranial irradiation for brain tumours. The control of growth hormone secretion and its mode of action are complex. What matters in an individual child is not only growth hormone levels (however obtained and interpreted) (see Chapters 28 and 33), but also the biological action and translation of growth hormone secretion into signals at cellular level to promote growth which are less easy to quantify (see Chapters 7 and 29). Additionally, defects in the gene encoding the receptor have been identified in GH insensitivity syndrome (GHIS, Laron-type dwarfism) indicating that the receptor is required for normal growth (see Chapters 31 and 35). The most marked fluctuation of growth in childhood is the 'mid-childhood growth spurt'. During mid-childhood there is a steep rise in adrenal androgen secretion (known as 'adrenarche') coincident with the development of the

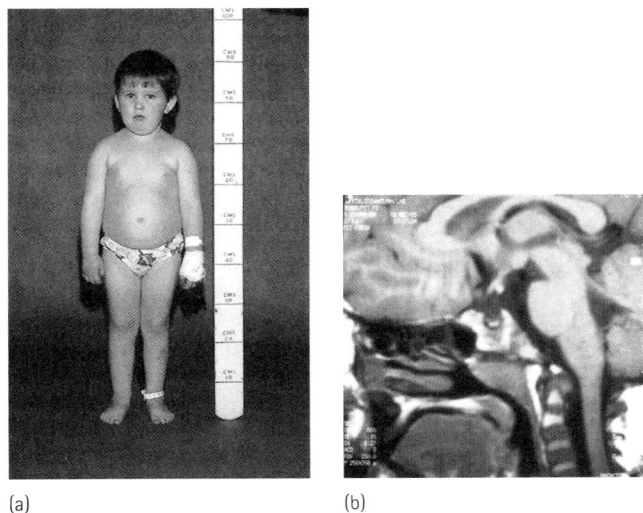

(a)

(b)

Figure 9.8 A child with a deficiency of growth hormone. Also shown is a magnetic resonance scan of his head.

adrenal zona reticularis. Adrenarche could be important for the triggering of normal puberty through a role for adrenal steroids in maturation of the central nervous system.[130,131] It occurs at the same time as the mid-childhood growth spurt and is also co-incident with the preadolescent fat spurt.[132] The mid-childhood growth spurt may reflect a direct bone and muscle response to the increased levels of adrenal androgens or may be due to an indirect effect of androgens on growth hormone secretion. Androgens are important in determining the pulsatile nature of growth hormone secretion in rats[133] and increased androgen levels may cause increased amplitude of growth hormone pulses.[134] At about the age of 7 years in children ('adrenarche') there is a change in the periodicity of growth hormone secretion[135] with the development of the characteristic dominant periodicity of about 200 min. There are also well documented positive correlations between blood pressure and age, with steep rises in systolic blood pressure coincident with rises in adrenal androgen levels at adrenarche in normal children followed longitudinally.[136] In some children, adrenarche is manifest as the growth of pubic and sometimes axillary hair before the age of 8, in the absence of other changes of puberty, a phenomenon termed 'exaggerated adrenarche'. Intriguingly, recent studies suggest that exaggerated adrenarche may not be a benign phenomenon and that children with exaggerated adrenarche are at risk of developing insulin resistance, dyslipidemia, and in girls, polycystic ovary syndrome (PCOS).[137–139] Observations suggest that exaggerated adrenarche may be part of the association between low birth weight and a number of cardiovascular risk factors (and see below).[140]

Adequate thyroxine levels are necessary for normal growth in infancy and childhood. Autoimmune hypothyroidism may first become manifest with slowing of height velocity. In infants with severe congenital hypothyroidism mean heights at 1 and 2 years are less than standards for healthy children but there is no difference by age 4 years.[141] Thyroid hormones are important both in mediating GH gene expression and in having direct effects on cartilage.[142]

Effects of chronic illness and psychosocial deprivation

Careful growth assessment often detects chronic disorders before there are specific symptoms and signs of the underlying condition. Conditions such as unrecognized or undertreated asthma, chronic renal failure or renal tubular acidosis, and conditions associated with malabsorption such as celiac disease or inflammatory bowel disease may first present at the growth clinic. Detailed history and careful clinical examination with appropriate investigations will lead to the appropriate diagnosis (see Chapter 12). A short thin child is more likely to have a chronic disorder than one who is slowly growing and fat who is more likely

to have an underlying endocrinopathy. Detailed discussions of the effects on growth of a variety of specific chronic conditions will be found in the appropriate chapters of this book. Psychosocial deprivation itself often causes poor growth.[143] It may mimic idiopathic hypopituitarism with abnormalities of growth hormone responses to conventional stimuli[144,145] and abnormal patterns of spontaneous growth hormone secretion.[146] These endocrine effects are readily reversible when the child is placed in a better environment.[146–148] If a child grows better whilst in hospital than at home, there should be strong suspicion of psychosocial problems occurring at home. Poor social and living conditions in early childhood may not only affect health and growth in infancy but also have far reaching consequences in adult life, e.g., the acquisition and persistence of *Helicobacter pylori* infection.[149] Psychosocial deprivation and emotional abuse can sometimes be extremely difficult to prove, e.g., in cases of fabricated illness (Munchausen syndrome by proxy, fictitious or falsified illness) (Fig. 9.9).[150]

Children with a history of non-organic failure to thrive have been found at the age of 5 years to be shorter and lighter than their matched controls.[151] The management of psychosocial growth failure is complex and requires a multidisciplinary approach. Early intensive home and community intervention can promote growth in children with non-organic failure to thrive, including fabricated illness.[152,153] The effects of psychosocial deprivation on growth are further discussed in Chapter 26.

LONG-TERM CONSEQUENCES OF GROWTH IN INFANCY AND CHILDHOOD

Many epidemiological studies in distinct populations in the UK and the rest of the world have demonstrated an association between low birth weight and the subsequent development of hypertension, insulin resistance, type 2 diabetes and cardiovascular disease.[154] Importantly, the association holds for the full range of birth weights, including those within the normal range. 'Early life programming' has been advanced as the mechanism underlying this association. This theory proposes that a stimulus or insult acting during critical periods of growth and development can permanently alter tissue structure and function, affecting fetal and childhood growth and increasing the risk of subsequent disease. Although the relative importance of genetic and environmental factors in the association between low birth weight and later disease remains unknown,[11,81,154,155] evidence from both human and animal studies suggests that many diseases of adult life can be induced by manipulating the environmental experience of the fetus.[156–159]

Additionally, infant nutrition may influence later disease risk.[160] Recent studies have demonstrated that preterm infants randomly assigned human milk versus formula milk showed benefits in terms of lipid profile, blood pressure,

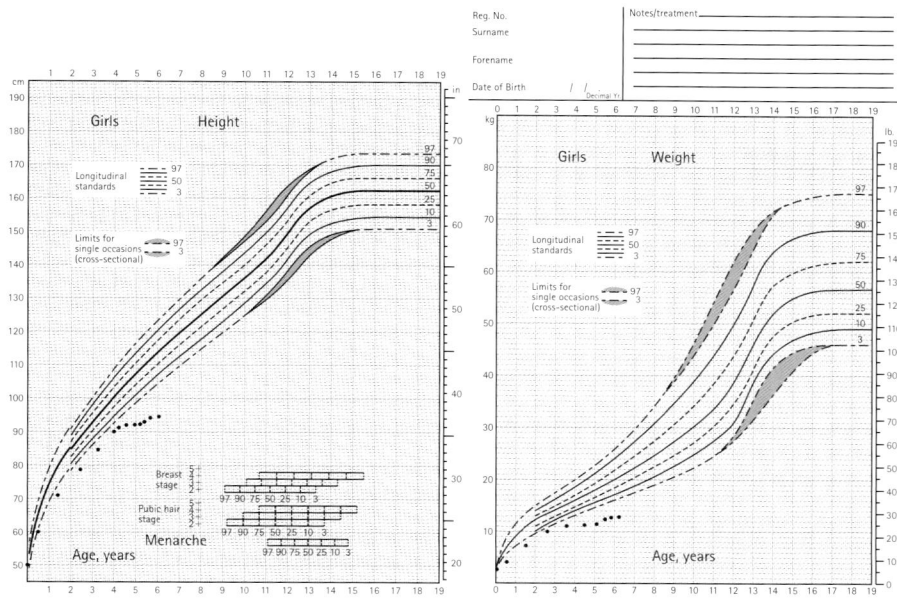

(a)

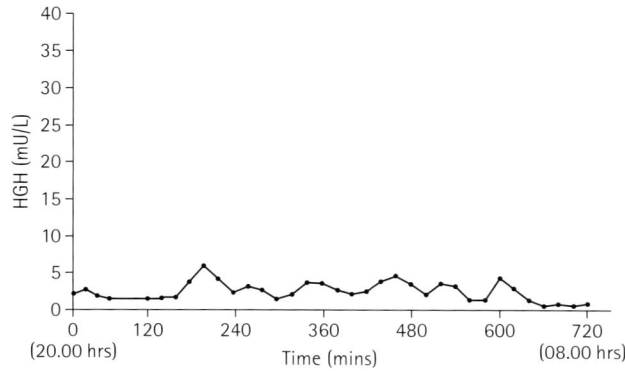

(b)

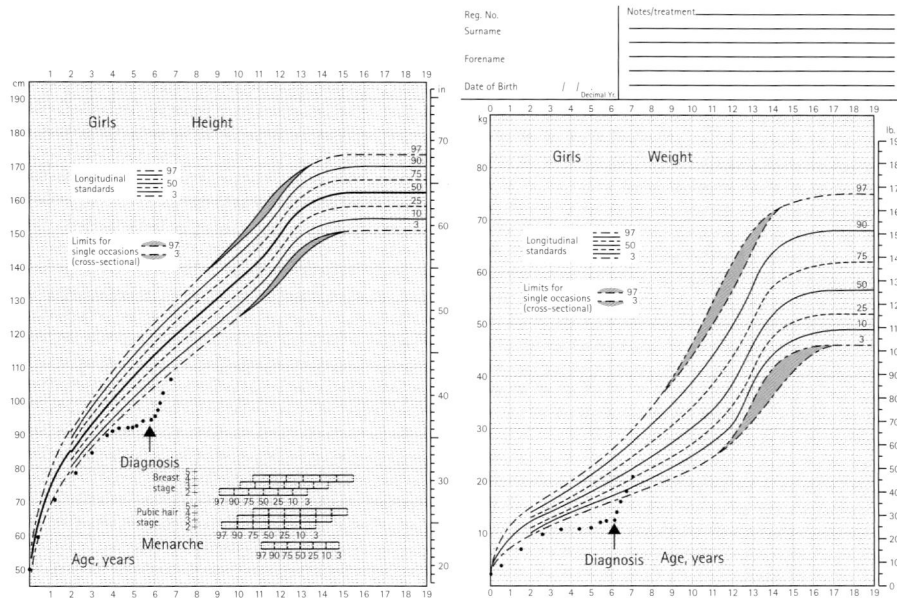

(c)

Figure 9.9   Growth chart of girl who was a victim of fabricated illness.

leptin resistance and insulin resistance,[160–162] whilst term, small-for-gestational age babies fed a growth-promoting formula showed higher diastolic blood pressure 6–8 years later.[160] Further, nutritional supplementation in infancy has been associated with higher blood pressure in adults.[163]

Moreover, the post-natal environment may interact with that experienced *in utero*, to further influence the phenotype, such that catch-up growth in childhood and the subsequent development of obesity appear to be important factors modifying the risk of later disease associated with low birth weight.[164–170] Fetal growth and the management of the pregnancy with a growth retarded fetus are discussed respectively in Chapter 8.

CONCLUSIONS

The technique and interpretation of measurement of growth in infancy and childhood requires care and skill. Poor growth is the final common pathway for many organic and emotional problems of childhood. The ICP model of the growth curve can be used as a basis to reveal the major influences on growth in infancy and childhood, particularly nutritional in infancy, endocrine in childhood and the additional influence of sex steroids during puberty. Growth *in utero*, infancy, and childhood has long-reaching effects not only on adult height but also on morbidity and mortality in adulthood. This chapter constitutes a background for the many aspects of the control and pathophysiology of growth which are discussed in detail in many of the other chapters of this volume.

KEY LEARNING POINTS

- Growth monitoring is important in the early detection of suspected disease in children and of particular value in detecting a wide variety of endocrine abnormalities.
- Growth monitoring practises vary widely and little is known about the diagnostic performance of growth screening or monitoring in terms of its sensitivity and specificity for the detection of growth disorders and of its impact on child health.
- The ability to measure a child accurately and reproducibly is fundamental to growth assessment.
- Many factors influence infant and childhood growth including genetic, pre- and post-natal environmental influences, nutrition, endocrine factors, the presence of other chronic diseases and psychosocial deprivation.
- Growth *in utero*, infancy, and childhood has long-reaching effects not only on adult height but also on morbidity and mortality in adulthood.

REFERENCES

● = Seminal primary article
◆ = Key review paper
✳ = First formal publication of a management guideline

1 Kelnar CJH. Growth. *Med Int* 1993; **21**: 217–23.
2 Kelnar CJH. Normal childhood and pubertal growth. In: Kelnar CJH, ed. *Childhood and Adolescent Diabetes*. London: Chapman and Hall, 1995: 47–74.
◆ 3 de Onis M, Wijnhoven TMA, Onyango AW. Worldwide practices in child growth monitoring. *J Pediatr* 2004; **144**: 461–5.
4 de Onis M, Blossner M. The World Health Organization Global Database on Child Growth and Malnutrition: methodology and applications. *Int J Epidemiol* 2003; **32**: 518–26.
5 Pinchinat S, Enel C, Pison G, *et al*. No improvement in weight-for-age of young children in southern Senegal, 1969–1992, despite a drastic reduction in mortality. Evidence from a growth monitoring programme. *Int J Epidemiol* 2004 Dec; 33(6): 1202–8.
● 6 Floud R, Gregory A, Wachter K. *Height, Health and History: Nutritional Status in the United Kingdom 1750–1980*. Cambridge: Cambridge University Press, 1990.
7 Popkin BM. The nutrition transition and obesity in the developing world. *J Nutr* 2001; **131**: 871S–3.
8 Cole TJ. Secular trends in growth. *Proc Nutr Soc* 2000; **59**: 317–24.
9 Cole TJ. Assessment of growth. *Best Prac Res Clin Endocrinol Metab* 2002; **16**: 383–98.
● 10 Barker DJ, Gluckman PD, Godfrey KM, *et al*. Fetal nutrition and cardiovascular disease in adult life. *Lancet* 1993; **341**: 938–41.
● 11 Barker DJ, Osmond C. Infant mortality, childhood nutrition, and ischaemic heart disease in England and Wales. *Lancet* 1986; **1**: 1077–81.
12 van Buuren S, van Dommelen P, Zandwijken GRJ, *et al*. Towards evidence based referral criteria for growth monitoring. *Arch Dis Child* 2004; **89**: 336–41.
13 Hindmarsh PC, Cole TJ. Height monitoring as a diagnostic test. *Arch Dis Child* 2004; **89**: 296–7.
◆ 14 Garner P, Panpanich R, Logan S. Is routine growth monitoring effective? A systematic review of trials. *Arch Dis Child* 2000; **82**: 197–201.
15 Hall DMB. *Health for all Children*, 4th ed. Oxford: Oxford University Press, 2003.
16 Karlberg J, Engstron I, Karlberg P, Fryer JG. Analyses of linear growth using a mathematical model. *Acta Paediatr Scand Suppl* 1987; **76**: 478–88.
◆ 17 Dewey KG, Peerson JM, Brown KH, *et al*. Growth of breast-fed infants deviates from current reference data: a pooled analysis of US, Canadian, and European data sets. World Health Organization Working Group on Infant Growth. *Pediatrics* 1995; **96**: 495–503.
18 Hediger ML, Overpeck MD, Ruan WJ, Troendle JF. Early infant feeding and growth status of US-born infants and children aged 4–71 mo: analyses from the third National

Health and Nutrition Examination Survey, 1988–1994. *Am J Clin Nutr* 2000; **72**: 159–67.

19 Wright CM. Growth charts for babies. *BMJ* 2005; **330**: 1399–400.

20 Liestol K, Rosenberg M. Height, weight and menarcheal age of schoolgirls in Oslo – an update. *Ann Hum Biol* 1995; **22**: 199–205.

21 Lobstein T, Baur L, Uauy R. Obesity in children and young people: a crisis in public health. *Obes Rev* 2004; **5(Suppl 1)**: 4–85.

22 Reilly JJ. Assessment of childhood obesity: national reference data or international approach? *Obes Res* 2002; **10**: 838–40.

● 23 Reilly JJ, Dorosty AR. Epidemic of obesity in UK children. *Lancet* 1999; **354**: 1874–5.

24 Chinn S, Rona RJ. Prevalence and trends in overweight and obesity in three cross sectional studies of British children, 1974–94. *BMJ* 2001; **322**: 24–6.

25 Flegal KM. Epidemiologic aspects of overweight and obesity in the United States. *Physiol Behav* 2005; **86**: 599–602.

26 Ruel MT, Rivera J, Habicht JP. Length screens better than weight in stunted populations. *J Nutr* 1995; **125**: 1222–8.

27 Butler GE, McKie M, Ratcliffe SG. The cyclical nature of prepubertal growth. *Ann Hum Biol* 1990; **17**: 177–98.

28 Voss LD, Bailey BJR. Diurnal variation in stature: is stretching the answer? *Arch Dis Child* 1997; **77**: 319–22.

29 Rudolf MCJ, Cole TJ, Krom AJ, *et al.* Growth of primary school children: a validation of the 1990 references and their use in growth monitoring. *Arch Dis Child* 2000; **83**: 298–301.

30 Cole TJ. Conditional reference charts to assess weight gain in British infants. *Arch Dis Child* 1995; **73**: 8–16.

31 Valk IM, Langhout-Chabloz AME, Smals AGH, *et al.* Accurate measurement of the lower leg length and ulnar length and its application in short term growth measurement. *Growth* 1983; **47**: 53–66.

32 Hermanussen M, Geiger-Benoit K, Burmeister J, Sippell WG. Knemometry in childhood: accuracy and standardisation of a new technique of lower leg measurement. *Ann Hum Biol* 1988; **15**: 1–16.

33 Wales JK, Milner RD. Knemometry in assessment of linear growth. *Arch Dis Child* 1987; **62**: 166–71.

34 Ahmed SF, Wallace WH, Kelnar CJH. Knemometry in childhood: a study to compare the precision of two different techniques. *Ann Hum Biol* 1995; **22**: 247–52.

35 Doherty CP, Crofton PM, Sarkar MAK, *et al.* Malnutrition, zinc supplementation and catch-up growth: changes in insulin-like growth factor I, its binding proteins, bone formation and collagen turnover. *Clin Endocrinol* 2002; **57**: 391–9.

36 Doherty CP, Sarkar MA, Shakur MS, *et al.* Linear and knemometric growth in the early phase of rehabilitation from severe malnutrition. *Br J Nutr* 2001; **85**: 755–9.

37 Wolthers OD, Pedersen S. Short term linear growth in asthmatic children during treatment with prednisolone. *BMJ* 1990; **301**: 145–8.

38 Wolthers OD, Hansen M, Juul A, *et al.* Knemometry, urine cortisol excretion, and measures of the insulin-like growth factor axis and collagen turnover in children treated with inhaled glucocorticosteroids. *Pediatr Res* 1997; **41**: 44–50.

39 Ahmed SF, Wardhaugh BW, Duff J, *et al.* The relationship between short-term changes in weight and lower leg length in children and young adults. *Ann Hum Biol* 1996; **23**: 159–62.

40 Reilly JJ. Assessment of body composition in infants and children. *Nutrition* 1998; **14**: 821–5.

41 Kabi N, Forsum E. Estimation of total body fat and subcutaneous adipose tissue in full-term infants less than three months old. *Pediatr Res* 1993; **34**: 448–54.

42 Ellis KJ. Selected body composition methods can be used in field studies. *J Nutr* 2001; **131**: 1589S–95.

43 Freedman DS, Serdula MK, Srinivasan SR, Berenson GS. Relation of circumferences and skinfold thicknesses to lipid and insulin concentrations in children and adolescents: the Bogalusa Heart Study. *Am J Clin Nutr* 1999; **69**: 308–17.

44 Maffeis C, Pietrobelli A, Grezzani A, *et al.* Waist circumference and cardiovascular risk factors in prepubertal children. *Obes Res* 2001; **9**: 179–87.

45 Taylor RW, Jones IE, Williams SM, Goulding A. Evaluation of waist circumference, waist-to-hip ratio, and the conicity index as screening tools for high trunk fat mass, as measured by dual-energy X-ray absorptiometry, in children aged 3–19 y. *Am J Clin Nutr* 2000; **72**: 490–5.

46 McCarthy HD, Ellis SM, Cole TJ. Central overweight and obesity in British youth aged 11–16 years: cross sectional surveys of waist circumference. *BMJ* 2003; **326**: 624–6.

47 Shaikh S, Mahalanabis D. Empirically derived new equations for calculating body fat percentage based on skinfold thickness and midarm circumference in preschool Indian children. *Am J Hum Biol* 2004; **16**: 278–88.

48 de Bruin NC, van Velthoven KA, De Ridder M, *et al.* Standards for total body fat and fat-free mass in infants. *Arch Dis Child* 1996; **74**: 386–99.

49 Prior BM, Cureton KJ, Modlesky CM, *et al.* In vivo validation of whole body composition estimates from dual-energy X-ray absorptiometry. *J Appl Physiol* 1997; **83**: 623–30.

50 Kohrt WM. Preliminary evidence that DEXA provides an accurate assessment of body composition. *J Appl Physiol* 1998; **84**: 372–7.

51 Goulding A, Gold E, Cannan R, *et al.* DEXA supports the use of BMI as a measure of fatness in young girls. *Int J Obes Relat Metab Disord* 1996; **20**: 1014–21.

52 Taylor RW, Gold E, Manning P, Goulding A. Gender differences in body fat content are present well before puberty. *Int J Obes Relat Metab Disord* 1997; **21**: 1082–4.

53 Goran MI, Gower BA, Treuth M, Nagy TR. Prediction of intra-abdominal and subcutaneous abdominal adipose tissue in healthy pre-pubertal children. *Int J Obes Relat Metab Disord* 1998; **22**: 549–58.

❊ 54 Cole TJ, Freeman JV, Preece MA. Body mass index reference curves for the UK, 1990. *Arch Dis Child* 1995; **1995**: 25–9.

55 Bellizzi MC, Dietz WH. Workshop on childhood obesity: summary of the discussion. *Am J Clin Nutr* 1999; **70**: 173S–5.

56 Reilly JJ, Dorosty AR, Emmett PM. Identification of the obese child: adequacy of the body mass index for clinical practice and epidemiology. *Int J Obes Relat Metab Disord* 2000; **24**: 1623–7.

57 Whitaker RC, Wright JA, Pepe MS, *et al.* Predicting obesity in young adulthood from childhood and parental obesity. *N Engl J Med* 1997; **337**: 869–73.

58 Freedman DS, Dietz WH, Srinivasan SR, Berenson GS. The relation of overweight to cardiovascular risk factors among children and adolescents: The Bogalusa Heart Study. *Pediatrics* 1999; **103**: 1175–82.

59 Morrison JA, Barton BA, Biro FM, *et al.* Overweight, fat patterning, and cardiovascular disease risk factors in black and white boys. *J Pediatr* 1999; **135**: 409–10.

60 Dietz WH, Bellizzi MC. Introduction: the use of body mass index to assess obesity in children. *Am J Clin Nutr* 1999; **70**: 123S–5.

61 Cole TJ, Bellizzi MC, Flegal KM, Dietz WH. Establishing a standard definition for child overweight and obesity worldwide: international survey. *BMJ* 2000; **320**: 1240–3.

62 Buckler JMH. *A Reference Manual of Growth and Development,* 2nd edn. Oxford: Blackwell Science, 1997.

63 Hall DB, Foster-Iskenius UG, Allanson JE. *Handbook of Normal Physical Measurements.* Oxford: Oxford Medical Publications, 1989.

❊ 64 Freeman JV, Cole TJ, Chinn S, *et al.* Cross sectional stature and weight reference curves for the UK, 1990. *Arch Dis Child* 1995; **73**: 17–24.

65 Gerver WJM, de Bruin R. *Paediatric Morphometrics: A Reference Manual.* Maastricht: University Press Maastricht, 2001.

66 Fredriks AM, Van Buuren S, Burgmeijer RJF, *et al.* Continuing positive secular growth change in the Netherlands 1955-1997. *Pediatr Res* 2000; **47**: 316–23.

❊ 67 Buckler JMH, Tanner JM. *Tanner–Whitehouse Revised Growth and Development Record. British Longitudinal Standards.* Welwyn Garden City: Castlemead Publications, 1996.

68 Buckler JMH. *A Longitudinal Study of Adolescent Growth.* London: Springer Verlag, 1990.

69 Cronk CE, Crocker AC, Pueschel SM, *et al.* Growth charts for children with Down syndrome: 1 month to 18 years of age. *Pediatrics* 1988; **81**: 102–10.

70 Lyon AJ, Preece MA, Grant DB. Growth curve for girls with Turner syndrome. *Arch Dis Child* 1985; **60**: 932–5.

71 Horton WA, Rotter JI, Rimoin DL, *et al.* Standard growth curves for achondroplasia. *J Pediatr* 1978; **93**: 435–8.

72 Hall DMB. Growth monitoring. *Arch Dis Child* 2000; **82**: 10–5.

73 Emanuel I. Maternal health during childhood and later reproductive performance. *Ann N Y Acad Sci* 1986; **477**: 27–39.

● 74 Ounsted M, Ounsted C. Rate of intra-uterine growth. *Nature* 1968; **220**: 599–600.

75 Johnstone F, Inglis L. Familial trends in low birth weight. *BMJ* 1974; **3**: 659–61.

76 Klebanoff MA, Graubard BI, Kessel SS, Berendes HW. Low birth weight across generations. *JAMA* 1984; **252**: 2423–7.

77 Emanuel I, Filakti H, Alberman E, Evans SJ. Intergenerational studies of human birthweight from the 1958 birth cohort. 1. Evidence for a multigenerational effect. *Br J Obstet Gynaecol* 1992; **99**: 67–74.

78 Hennessy E, Alberman E. Intergenerational influences affecting birth outcome. I. Birthweight for gestational age in the children of the 1958 British birth cohort. *Paediatr Perinat Epidemiol* 1998; **12(Suppl 1)**: 45–60.

79 Collins JW, Wu SY, David RJ. Differing intergenerational birth weights among the descendants of US-born and foreign-born whites and African Americans in Illinois. *Am J Epidemiol* 2002; **155**: 210–6.

80 Johnston LB, Clark AJL, Savage MO. Genetic factors contributing to birth weight. *Arch Dis Child Fetal Neonatal Ed* 2002; **86**: F-a2–3.

● 81 Dunger DB, Ong KK, Huxtable SJ, *et al.* Association of the INS VNTR with size at birth. ALSPAC Study Team. Avon Longitudinal Study of Pregnancy and Childhood. *Nat Genet* 1998; **19**: 98–100.

● 82 Woods KA, Camacho-Hubner C, Savage MO, Clark AJ. Intrauterine growth retardation and postnatal growth failure associated with deletion of the insulin-like growth factor I gene [Comment]. *New Engl J Med* 1996; **335**: 1363–7.

● 83 Hattersley AT, Beards F, Ballantyne E, *et al.* Mutations in the glucokinase gene of the fetus result in reduced birth weight. *Nat Genet* 1998; **19**: 268–70.

● 84 Constancia M, Hemberger M, Hughes J, *et al.* Placental-specific IGF-II is a major modulator of placental and fetal growth. *Nature* 2002; **417**: 945–8.

85 Reik W, Constancia M, Fowden A, *et al.* Regulation of supply and demand for maternal nutrients in mammals by imprinted genes. *J Physiol* 2003; **547**: 35–44.

86 Lindsay RS, Dabelea D, Roumain J, *et al.* Type 2 diabetes and low birth weight: the role of paternal inheritance in the association of low birth weight and diabetes. *Diabetes* 2000; **49**: 445–9.

87 Emanuel I, Leisenring W, Williams MA, *et al.* The Washington State Intergenerational Study of Birth Outcomes: methodology and some comparisons of maternal birthweight and infant birthweight and gestation in four ethnic groups. *Paediatr Perinat Epidemiol* 1999; **13**: 352–69.

88 Alberman E, Emanuel I, Filakti H, Evans SJ. The contrasting effects of parental birthweight and gestational age on the birthweight of offspring. *Paediatr Perinat Epidemiol* 1992; **6**: 134–44.

89 Klebanoff MA, Schulsinger C, Mednick BR, Secher NJ. Preterm and small-for-gestational-age birth across generations. *Am J Obstet Gynecol* 1997; **176**: 521–6.

90 Klebanoff MA, Mednick BR, Schulsinger C, *et al.* Father's effect on infant birth weight. *Am J Obstet Gynecol* 1998; **178**: 1022–6.

91 Magnus P, Gjessing HK, Skrondal A, Skjaerven R. Paternal contribution to birth weight. *J Epidemiol Community Health* 2001; **55**: 873–7.

92 Cawley RH, McKeown T, Record RG. Parental stature and birth weight. *Ann Hum Genet* 1954; **6**: 448–56.

93 Emanuel I. Invited commentary: an assessment of maternal intergenerational factors in pregnancy outcome. *Am J Epidemiol* 1997; **146**: 820–5.

94 Breschi MC, Seghieri G, Bartolomei G, *et al.* Relation of birthweight to maternal plasma glucose and insulin concentrations during normal pregnancy. *Diabetologia* 1993; **36**: 1315–21.

• 95 Churchill D, Perry I, Beevers D. Ambulatory blood pressure in pregnancy and fetal growth. *Lancet* 1997; **349**: 7–10.

96 Ferrer RL, Sibai BM, Mulrow CD, *et al.* Management of mild chronic hypertension during pregnancy: a review. *Obstet Gynecol* 2000; **96(5 Pt 2)**: 849–60.

97 Harding JE, McCowan LME. Perinatal predictors of growth patterns to 18 months in children born small for gestational age. *Early Hum Dev* 2003; **74**: 13–26.

98 Duan C. Specifying the cellular responses to insulin-like growth factor (IGF) signals: roles of IGF binding proteins. *J Endocrinol* 2002; **175**: 41–54.

99 Funk B, Kessler U, Eisenmenger W, *et al.* The expression of insulin-like growth factor binding proteins is tissue specific during human fetal life and early infancy. *Acta Endocrinol* 1992; **127**: 107–14.

100 Le Roith D, Bondy C, Yakar S, *et al.* The somatomedin hypothesis: 2001. *Endocr Rev* 2001; **22**: 53–74.

101 Haig D, Graham C. Genomic imprinting and the strange case of the insulin-like growth factor II receptor. *Cell* 1991; **64**: 1045–6.

102 Gluckman PD, Pinal CS. Regulation of fetal growth by the somatotrophic axis. *J Nutr* 2003; **133**: 1741S–6.

103 Baker J, Liu JP, Robertson EJ, Efstratiadis A. Role of insulin-like growth factors in embryonic and postnatal growth. *Cell* 1993; **75**: 73–82.

104 Liu JP, Baker J, Perkins AS, *et al.* Mice carrying null mutations of the genes encoding insulin-like growth factor I (Igf-I) and type 1 IGF receptor (Igf1r). *Cell* 1993; **75**: 59–72.

105 Oliver MH, Harding JE, Breier B, Gluckman PD. Fetal insulin-like growth factor (IGF)-I and IGF-II are regulated differently by glucose or insulin in the sheep fetus. *Reprod Fertil Dev* 1996; **8**: 167–72.

106 Beck Jensen RB, Chellakooty M, Vielwerth S, *et al.* Intrauterine growth retardation and consequences for endocrine and cardiovascular diseases in adult life: does insulin-like growth factor-I play a role? *Horm Res* 2003; **60(Suppl 3)**: 136–48.

107 Boyne MS, Thame M, Bennett FI, *et al.* The relationship among circulating insulin-like growth factor (IGF)-I, igf-binding proteins-1 and -2, and birth anthropometry: A prospective study. *J Clin Endocrinol Metab* 2003; **88**: 1687–91.

108 Johnston LB, Dahlgren J, Leger J, *et al.* Association between insulin-like growth factor I (IGF-I) polymorphisms, circulating igf-I, and pre- and postnatal growth in two european small for gestational age populations. *J Clin Endocrinol Metab* 2003; **88**: 4805–10.

109 Wiznitzer A, Reece EA, Homko C, *et al.* Insulin-like growth factors, their binding proteins, and fetal macrosomia in offspring of nondiabetic pregnant women. *Am J Perinatol* 1998; **15**: 23–8.

110 Lutter CK, Rivera JA. Nutritional status of infants and young children and characteristics of their diets. *J Nutr* 2003; **133**: 2941S–9.

111 Michaelson KF, Weaver LT, Branca F, *et al.*, eds. *Feeding and Nutrition of Infants and Young Children.* Copenhagen: WHO Regional Publications, 2000.

112 Raiha NC, Axelsson IE. Protein nutrition during infancy. An update. *Pediatr Clin North Am* 1995; **42**: 745–64.

113 Butte NF. Fat intake of children in relation to energy requirements. *Am J Clin Nutr* 2000; **72**: 1246S–52.

114 FAO/WHO. *Fats and Oils in Human Nutrition.* Rome: FAO, 1994.

115 Slyper AH. The pediatric obesity epidemic: causes and controversies. *J Clin Endocrinol Metab* 2004; **89**: 2540–7.

116 Booth IW, Aukett MA, Logan S. Iron deficiency anaemia in infancy and early childhood – Commentary. *Arch Dis Child* 1997; **76**: 549–54.

117 Thorsdottir I, Gunnarsson BS, Atladottir H, *et al.* Iron status at 12 months of age – effects of body size, growth and diet in a population with high birth weight. *Eur J Clin Nutr* 2003; **57**: 505–13.

118 Maggioni A, Lifschitz F. Nutritional management of failure to thrive. *Pediatr Clin North Am* 1995; **42**: 791–810.

119 Haycock GB. The influence of growth in infancy. *Pediatr Nephrol* 1993; **7**: 871–5.

120 Kaplan SL, Grumbach MM, Shepard TH. The ontogenesis of human fetal hormones. 1. Growth hormone and insulin. *J Clin Invest* 1972; **51**: 3080–93.

121 Werther GA, Haynes K, Waters MJ. Growth hormone (GH) receptors are expressed on human fetal mesenchymal tissues – identification of messenger ribonucleic acid and GH-binding protein. *J Clin Endocrinol Metab* 1993; **76**: 1638–46.

122 Hill DJ, Riley SC, Bassett NS, Waters MJ. Localization of the growth hormone receptor, identified by immunocyto-chemistry, in second trimester human fetal tissues and in placenta throughout gestation. *J Clin Endocrinol Metab* 1992; **75**: 646–50.

123 Ogilvy-Stuart AL. Growth hormone deficiency (GHD) from birth to 2 years of age: diagnostic specifics of ghd during the early phase of life. *Horm Res* 2003; **60(Suppl 1)**: 2–9.

124 Gluckman PD, Gunn AJ, Wray A, et al. Congenital idiopathic growth hormone deficiency associated with prenatal and early postnatal growth failure. The International Board of the Kabi Pharmacia International Growth Study. J Pediatr 1992; **121**: 920–3.

125 Carel J-C, Huet F, Chaussain J-L. Treatment of growth hormone deficiency in very young children. Horm Res 2003; **60(Suppl 1)**: 10–7.

126 Wit JM, van Unen H. Growth of infants with neonatal growth hormone deficiency. Arch Dis Child 1992; **67**: 920–4.

127 Leger J, Noel M, Limal JM, Czernichow P. Growth factors and intrauterine growth retardation. II. Serum growth hormone, insulin-like growth factor (IGF) I, and IGF-binding protein 3 levels in children with intrauterine growth retardation compared with normal control subjects: prospective study from birth to two years of age. Study Group of IUGR. Pediatr Res 1996; **40**: 101–7.

128 Giudice LC, de Zegher F, Gargosky SE, et al. Insulin-like growth factors and their binding proteins in the term and preterm human fetus and neonate with normal and extremes of intrauterine growth. J Clin Endocrinol Metab 1995; **80**: 1548–55.

129 Hindmarsh PC, Smith PJ, Brook CG, Matthews DR. The relationship between height velocity and growth hormone secretion in short prepubertal children. Clin Endocrinol 1987; **27**: 581–91.

130 Ducharme JR, Forest MG, De Peretti E, et al. Plasma adrenal and gonadal sex steroids in human pubertal development. J Clin Endocrinol Metab 1976; **42**: 468–76.

131 Stirling HF, Kelnar CJ. Adrenarche. Growth Matters 1990; **1**: 6–8.

✳ 132 Tanner JM, Whitehouse RH. Clinical longitudinal standards for height, weight, height velocity, weight velocity, and stages of puberty. Arch Dis Child 1976; **51**: 170–9.

133 Millard WJ, Politch JA, Martin JB, Fox TO. Growth hormone-secretory patterns in androgen-resistant (testicular feminized) rats. Endocrinology 1986; **119**: 2655–60.

134 Eakman GD, Dallas JS, Ponder SW, Keenan BS. The effects of testosterone and dihydrotestosterone on hypothalamic regulation of growth hormone secretion. J Clin Endocrinol Metab 1996; **81**: 1217–23.

135 Hindmarsh PC, Brook CGD. Normal growth and its endocrine control. In: Brook CGD, ed. Clinical Paediatric Endocrinol. Oxford: Blackwell Scientific Publications, 1989: 57–73.

136 Kelnar CJ. Adrenal steroids in childhood [MD Thesis]. Cambridge: University of Cambridge, 1985.

137 Ibanez L, Valls C, Ferrer A, et al. Sensitization to insulin induces ovulation in nonobese adolescents with anovulatory hyperandrogenism. J Clin Endocrinol Metab 2001; **86**: 3595–8.

138 Ibanez L, Dimartino-Nardi J, Potau N, Saenger P. Premature adrenarche – normal variant or forerunner of adult disease? Endocr Rev 2000; **21**: 671–96.

139 Ibanez L, Potau N, Chacon P, et al. Hyperinsulinaemia, dyslipaemia and cardiovascular risk in girls with a history of premature pubarche. Diabetologia 1998; **41**: 1057–63.

● 140 Ibanez L, Potau N, de Zegher F. Recognition of a new association: reduced fetal growth, precocious pubarche, hyperinsulinism and ovarian dysfunction. Ann Endocrinol 2000; **61**: 141–2.

● 141 Grant DB. Growth in early treated congenital hypothyroidism. Arch Dis Child 1994; **70**: 464–8.

142 Burch WM, Van Wyk JJ. Triiodothyronine stimulates cartilage growth and maturation by different mechanisms. Am J Physiol 1987; **252**: E176–82.

143 Annecillo C, Money J. Abuse or psychosocial dwarfism: an update. Growth Genet Horm 1985; **1**: 1–4.

● 144 Powell GF, Brasel A. Emotional deprivation and growth retardation simulating idiopathic hypopituitarism. I. Clinical evaluation of this syndrome. New Engl J Med 1967; **276**: 1271–8.

● 145 Powell GF, Brasel A, Raiti S, Blizzard RM. Emotional deprivation and growth retardation simulating idiopathic hypopituitarism. II. Endocrinologic evaluation of this syndrome. New Engl J Med 1967; **276**: 1279–83.

146 Albanese A, Hamill G, Jones J, et al. Reversibility of physiological growth hormone secretion in children with psychosocial dwarfism. Clin Endocrinol 1994; **40**: 687–92.

147 Stanhope R, Adlard P, Hamill G, et al. Physiological growth hormone (GH) secretion during the recovery from psychosocial dwarfism: a case report. Clin Endocrinol 1988; **28**: 335–9.

148 Thomas BC, Stanhope R. Long-term growth data and growth hormone secretion in 65 patients with psycho-social dwarfism. Pediatr Res 1993; **33(suppl)**: 312.

149 Fall CHD, Goggin PM, Hawtin P, et al. Growth in infancy, infant feeding, childhood living conditions, and Helicobacter pylori infection at age 70. Arch Dis Child 1997; **77**: 310–4.

150 Lyall EG, Stirling HF, Crofton PM, Kelnar CJ. Albuminuric growth failure. A case of Munchausen syndrome by proxy. Acta Paediatr 1992; **81**: 373–6.

151 Reif S, Beler B, Villa Y, Spirer Z. Long-term follow-up and outcome of infants with non-organic failure to thrive. Isr J Med Sci 1995; **31**: 483–9.

152 Berg B, Jones DPH. Outcome of psychiatric intervention in factitious illness by proxy (Munchausen's syndrome by proxy). Arch Dis Child 1999; **81**: 465–72.

153 Black MM, Dubowitz H, Hutcheson J, et al. A randomized clinical trial of home intervention for children with failure to thrive. Pediatrics 1995; **95**: 807–14.

154 Barker D. In utero programming of chronic disease. Clin Sci 1998; **95**: 115–28.

155 Hattersley AT, Tooke JE. The fetal insulin hypothesis: An alternative explanation of the association of low birthweight with diabetes and vascular disease. Lancet 1999; **353**: 1789–92.

156 Langley-Evans SC, Phillips GJ, Benediktsson R, et al. Protein intake in pregnancy, placental glucocorticoid

metabolism and the programming of hypertension in the rat. *Placenta* 1996; **17**: 169–72.

● 157   Nyirenda MJ, Lindsay RS, Kenyon CJ, *et al.* Glucocorticoid exposure in late gestation permanently programs rat hepatic phosphoenolpyruvate carboxykinase and glucocorticoid receptor expression and causes glucose intolerance in adult offspring. *J Clin Invest* 1998; **101**: 2174–81.

158   Doyle LW, Ford GW, Davis NM, Callanan C. Antenatal corticosteroid therapy and blood pressure at 14 years of age in preterm children. *Clin Sci* 2000; **98**: 137–42.

● 159   Edwards CR, Benediktsson R, Lindsay RS, Seckl JR. Dysfunction of placental glucocorticoid barrier: a link between the fetal environment and adult hypertension? *Lancet* 1993; **341**: 355–7.

160   Singhal A, Lucas A. Early origins of cardiovascular disease: is there a unifying hypothesis? *Lancet* 2004; **363**: 1642–5.

161   Singhal A, Cole TJ, Lucas A. Early nutrition in preterm infants and later blood pressure: two cohorts after randomised trials. *Lancet* 2001; **357**: 413–9.

162   Singhal A, Fewtrell M, Cole TJ, Lucas A. Low nutrient intake and early growth for later insulin resistance in adolescents born preterm. *Lancet* 2003; **361**: 1089–97.

163   Martin RM, McCarthy A, Davey Smith G, *et al.* Infant nutrition and blood pressure in early adulthood: the Barry Caerphilly Growth Study. *Am J Clin Nutr* 2003; **77**: 1489–97.

164   Ong KK, Ahmed ML, Emmett PM, *et al.* Association between postnatal catch-up growth and obesity in childhood: prospective cohort study. *BMJ* 2000; **320**: 967–71.

165   Lithell HO, McKeigue PM, Berglund L, *et al.* Relation of size at birth to non-insulin dependent diabetes and insulin concentrations in men aged 50–60 years. *BMJ* 1996; **312**: 406–10.

166   Leon DA, Koupilova I, Lithell HO, *et al.* Failure to realise growth potential in utero and adult obesity in relation to blood pressure in 50 year old Swedish men. *BMJ* 1996; **312**: 401–6.

167   Forsen T, Eriksson J, Tuomilehto J, *et al.* The fetal and childhood growth of persons who develop type 2 diabetes. *Ann Intern Med* 2000; **133**: 176–82.

168   Eriksson JG, Forsen T, Tuomilehto J, *et al.* Catch-up growth in childhood and death from coronary heart disease: longitudinal study. *BMJ* 1999; **318**: 427–31.

169   Eriksson JG, Forsen T, Tuomilehto J, *et al.* Early adiposity rebound in childhood and risk of type 2 diabetes in adult life. *Diabetologia* 2003; **46**: 190–4.

170   Law CM, Shiell AW, Newsome CA, *et al.* Fetal, infant, and childhood growth and adult blood pressure: a longitudinal study from birth to 22 years of age. *Circulation* 2002; **105**: 1088–92.

10

Growth at adolescence

JOHN M H BUCKLER

INTRODUCTION

Adolescence is a phase of life during which many dramatic changes occur, physical, sexual, behavioral, and psychological, which transform a dependent, immature child into a mature self-sufficient adult. One of the most striking of these changes is physical growth, later and more marked in boys than in girls, comprising a dramatic acceleration but followed by a slowing down and ultimate cessation. This phase contributes, in a relatively short time, a substantial amount of ultimate stature. Although this basic pattern of growth is invariable in healthy children, there is great variability in certain aspects between individuals, notably in timing, so that no particular pattern of growth can be described as 'normal'. To ascribe a precise chronological age range to adolescence would be misleading and the characteristics of the growth of each adolescent are specific to that individual. Interpretation of growth in adolescence is much more complex than for pre-pubertal children.

Knowledge of adolescent growth patterns demands longitudinal observations but, owing to their duration and practical difficulties, reliable studies of this kind are few and far between. Many of the data described in this chapter are the outcome of a longitudinal study[1,2] and observations of Tanner et al.[3] but references to comparable reports from other countries are included in these and other publications.[4,5]

THE AVERAGE PATTERN OF PUBERTAL GROWTH

Comparison of boys and girls

The median patterns of growth in height and height velocity, weight and weight velocity, comparing boys and girls,

are shown in Fig. 10.1.[1] Growth in these parameters is similar before the onset of puberty, but girls are earlier by about 2 years in all aspects of puberty: onset, age of peak height velocity, and completion of growth. As a result of the earlier growth spurt, girls are slightly taller than boys for a period of two years or so at an average age of 11.5–13.5 years, with a maximum difference of 2.5 cm at 12.5 years; they are also heavier between average ages of 11 and 14 years, with a maximum difference of 3.5 kg at age 13 years. As growth continues for longer in boys and is of greater magnitude (peak height velocities averaging 9.8 cm year^{-1} at an average age of 14.1 years in boys, compared with 8.1 cm at 12.1 years in girls, and peak weight velocities of 8.6 kg for boys and 8.0 kg for girls at similar ages), ultimate height and weight for men are considerably greater than for women; in this study the sex difference of median values at age 18 was 13.5 cm and 11.0 kg, respectively.

Relationship of height velocity changes to other physical changes of puberty

The changes of growth velocity at puberty are dependent fundamentally on changes in circulating hormone levels and are therefore associated with the other secondary sexual characteristics. Although the precise ages vary greatly between individuals, there is an overall correlation in the timing of the components of height velocity and other physical changes of puberty. Some of these are shown in a very simplified way for an average boy and girl in Fig. 10.2.[6] The average duration of the majority of pubertal growth is 6 years in both boys and girls, although a trivial increase in stature can continue for longer, particularly in boys,[7] with the peak height velocity about 2 years after the start of acceleration.

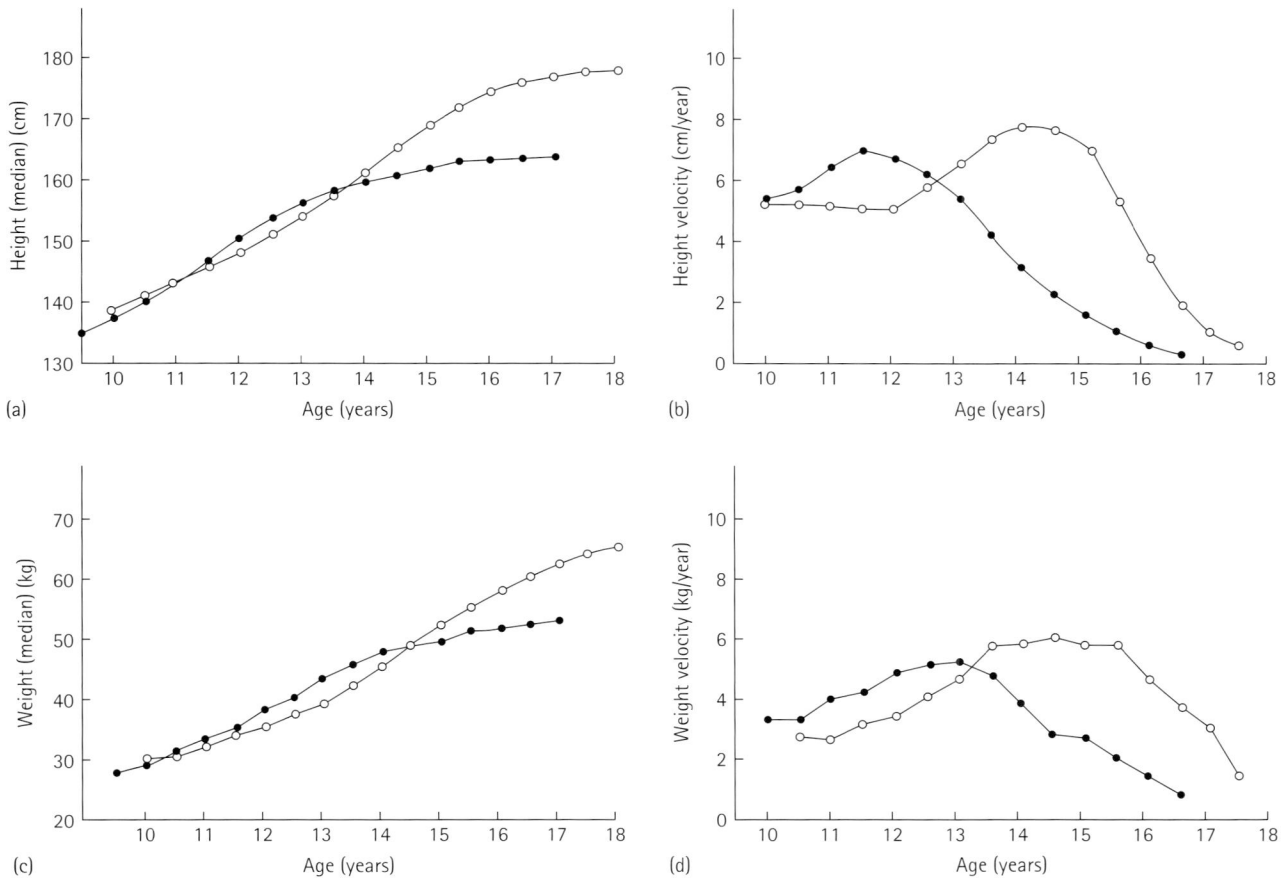

Figure 10.1 Median values for boys (○—○) and girls (●—●) for (a) height, (b) height velocity, (c) weight, (d) weight velocity.[1]

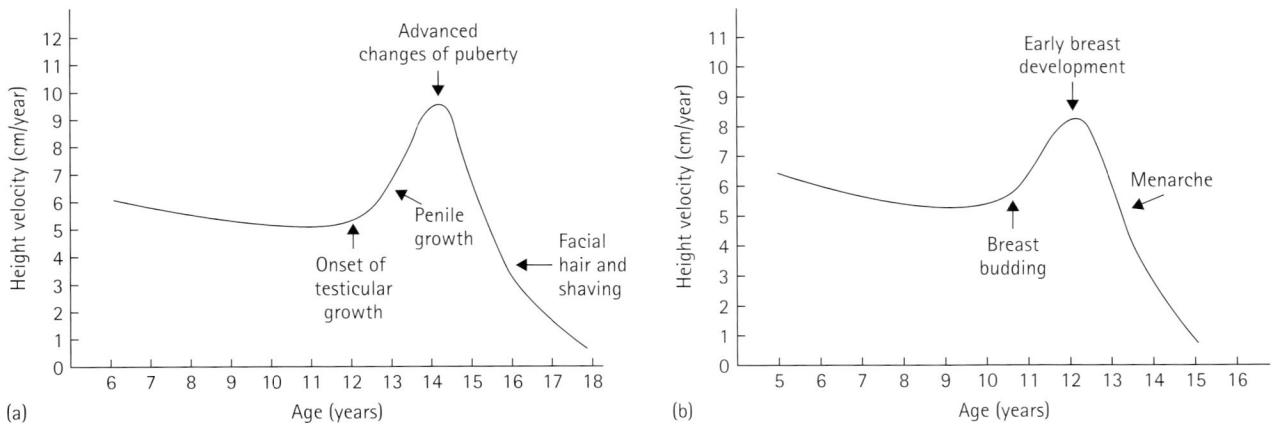

Figure 10.2 Schematic representation of the relationship of some secondary sexual features to height velocity: (a) boys, (b) girls.

In most boys the first, and frequently unrecognized, sign of puberty is enlargement of the testicles; this is a reliable indicator that puberty is imminent, even though it may precede the development of other more generally accepted signs such as genital growth and pubic hair by as much as a year, and peak height velocity by an average of 1.7 years. This sign of early testicular growth usually coincides with the onset of acceleration of stature. Other signs of puberty are usually quite advanced before height velocity begins to slow down, so these pubertal features do not as such preclude the possibility of significant further growth, although the development of marked facial hair is a late feature indicating that growth in stature is virtually complete.

Peak height velocity in girls is at an earlier phase of overall pubertal development, only about a year after the first feature, which, in over 90 percent of girls, is the onset of breast development. The menarche occurs on average a

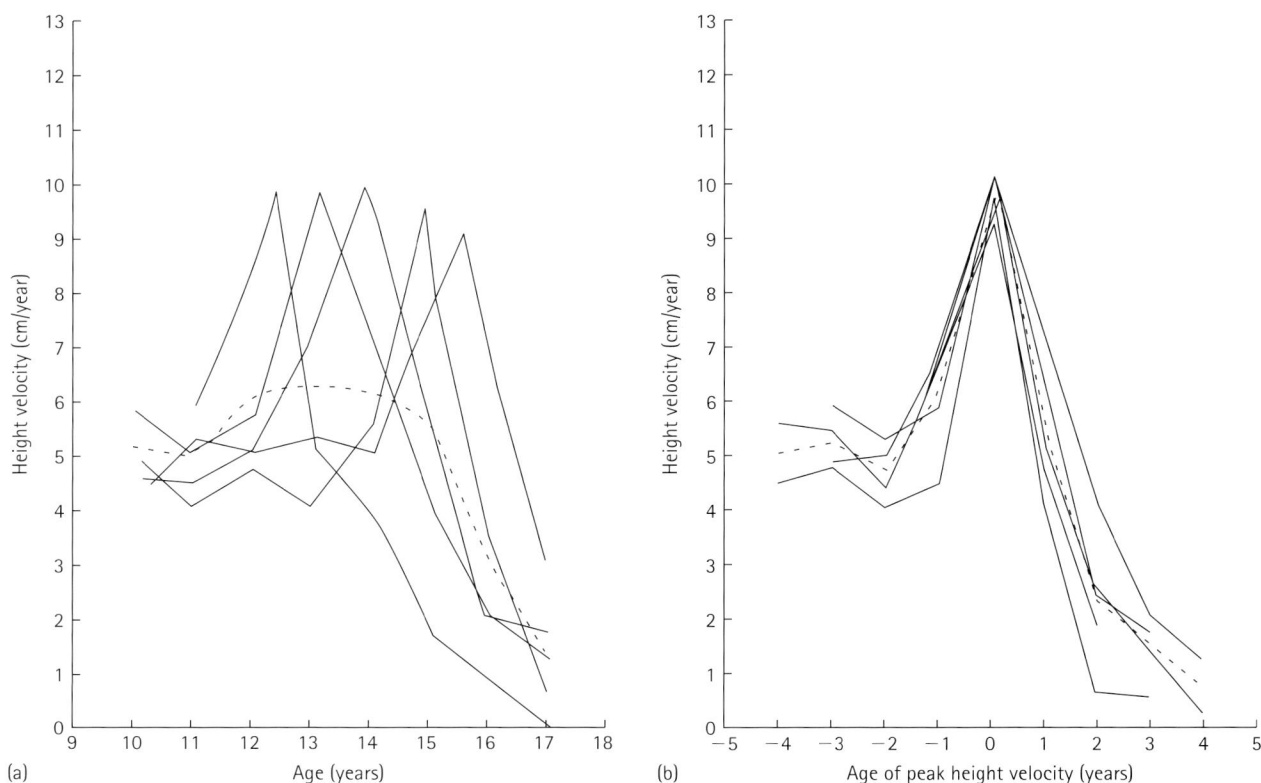

Figure 10.3 Height velocity curves for five normal boys plotted on the basis of (a) chronological age, (b) age of peak height velocity (PHV). Individual curves (−); mean curve (−−) − based on data of Buckler.[1]

year after the age of most rapid growth, at a stage when the pubertal process is advanced and there is only, on average, 5 cm of residual growth. These observations are based on Buckler[1] in which more detailed information can be found.

Interpretation of centile charts: cross−sectional and longitudinal data

What has been written so far depicts the growth of a child going through puberty at an average age. In practice, however, the age range is vast. Combining the values of height of boys or of girls with different tempos of growth produces a growth curve that does not represent the growth of the individual. This important aspect of growth was highlighted by Boas[8] as long ago as 1932 and by Shuttleworth[9] and has been stressed on many occasions by Tanner.[10] Figure 10.3 illustrates, in a similar way to the work of these authors, that the 'shapes' of height velocity curves of individuals are very similar with a wide variation in the age of pubertal growth, yet any attempt to combine the data of such children to produce an average velocity curve based on chronological age is misleading, not being typical of the growth of any of them. For this reason cross-sectional studies, such as the British growth charts reported by Freeman et al.[11] although acceptable for screening purposes, are inappropriate and misleading when interpreting the growth

of individuals through the years when puberty is to be considered, and standards typifying the longitudinal growth of individuals must then be used.[5,12] Centile charts should show this typical growth pattern but also give an indication of the spread of ages at which pubertal growth occurs in the overall population. Thus the growth of any individual should parallel that shown by the growth curve of a child of average age, although it will almost certainly deviate from the pre-pubertal centile line of this average child, upwards or downwards, depending on whether puberty is earlier or later than average. This is illustrated in Fig. 10.4 which shows the growth of two brothers, one earlier than average and the other later than average in the timing of puberty. These are presented on the background of the longitudinal style height centile chart.[12] Despite being of similar height before puberty, the early developing boy was about 16 cm taller than the late developer at the age of 14, yet the late developer ended up 3 cm taller than his brother when fully grown. (It is not apparent, however, why both these brothers achieved much higher ultimate height centiles than they started on.)

Body components

Growth of components of the body does not occur in parallel. This is most strikingly demonstrated when the growth

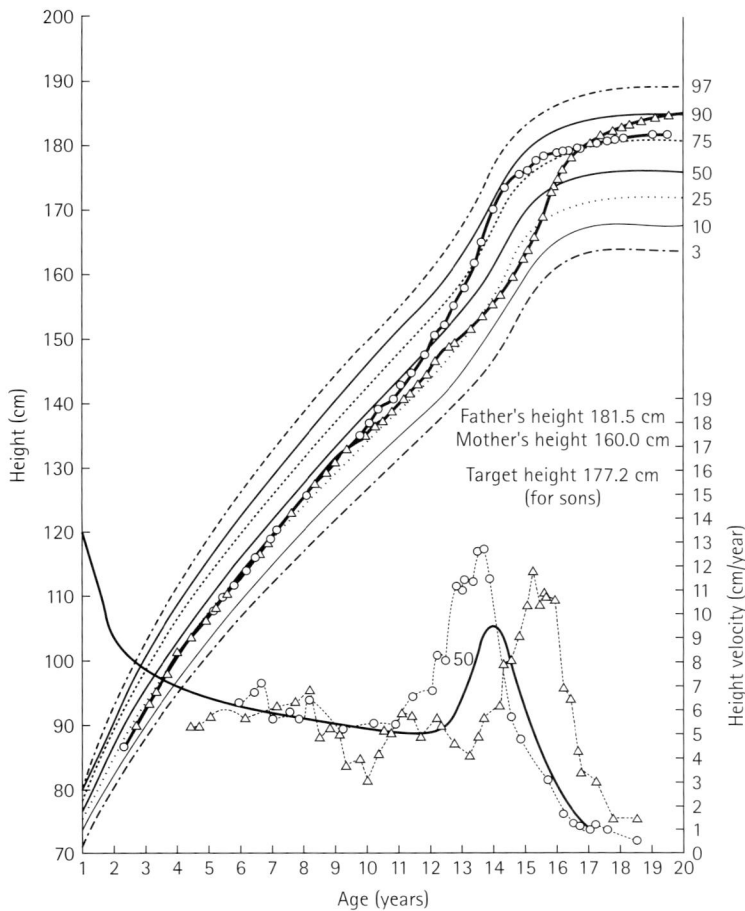

Figure 10.4 Height and height velocities of two brothers. (Modified from Buckler.[1])

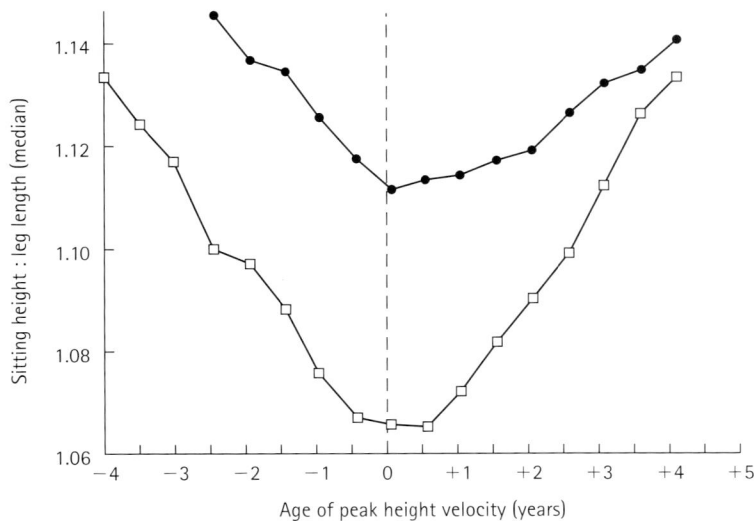

Figure 10.5 Median values for sitting height to leg length ratios for boys (□—□) and girls (●—●).[1]

of the trunk is compared with that of the limbs. The most rapid growth of the limbs precedes that of the trunk, being predominantly in the first 'half' of puberty before the age of overall peak height velocity, whereas growth in the trunk is more after the age of peak height velocity. Thus the ratio of sitting height (an effective indicator of trunk and head height) to (sub-ischial) leg length alters greatly throughout

the course of puberty, being at its lowest value at the actual age of overall peak height velocity. These changes are more marked in boys than girls, as shown in Fig. 10.5 in which age is presented in terms of peak height velocity rather than actual chronological age. This was achieved by combining the data of all the subjects, using the age of peak height velocity as the common factor, thus matching them up on

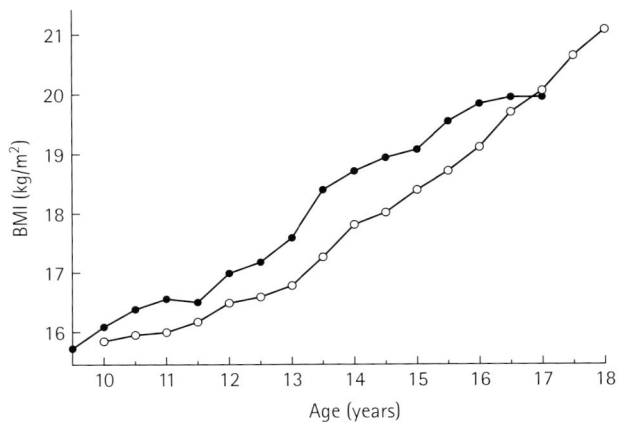

Figure 10.6 Median values for body mass index for boys (○—○) and girls (●—●) plotted against chronological age.[1]

the basis of similar pubertal status rather than using chronological age which would bear no consistent relationship to pubertal development.

Growth in the width of the trunk, as indicated by biacromial and bi-iliac diameters, parallels that of overall stature in timing. As with most features of pubertal growth, that across the shoulders is much greater in boys than in girls, although later. However, the bi-iliac diameter is among the few bony measurements that is as great in the adult woman as in the man.

Throughout puberty weight changes are dramatic, proportionately more so than height changes. For this reason indices relating weight to height, such as body mass index (BMI = weight in kilograms divided by the square of height in meters), increase rapidly through the course of puberty (Fig. 10.6). Interpretation of this index must be cautious at these ages and, strictly speaking, should be related to the stage of pubertal development, as that is what is responsible for the changing values. Bini et al.[13] reported that BMI values were significantly higher in postmenarcheal girls than girls of a similar age premenarcheal. It must not be concluded that the rise in BMI during the years of adolescence is a reflection of the increase of fatness, which would usually be the case in adults. Though there is an increase in the percentage body weight that is fat over these years, from 16 percent to 19 percent in boys and from 17 percent to 25 percent in girls,[1] Figure 10.7 shows that in terms of actual weight this is predominantly the result of increases in lean body mass (muscle and bone) rather than of fat. Skin-fold measurements throughout puberty are greater in girls than in boys, and their increase is more marked in girls and the distribution different, but in both sexes there is a change in distribution of fat which becomes more evident on the trunk.[1] The major factor accounting for much greater overall weight gain through puberty, and ultimate greater BMI, shown by boys when compared with girls is the predominance of muscle and bone.

A failure to recognize that an increase in BMI is a normal and expected finding at puberty has resulted in unjustified

conclusions linking obesity with puberty in those children who undergo puberty at an early age. The implications of obesity in adolescence are well known. Adolescence is one of the critical periods when there is increased risk of developing persistent obesity and its complications, risks that are greater for females than for males. About 30 percent of obese adult women were obese in adolescence whereas only 10 percent of obese adult men had the onset in teenage.[14] Although obesity as reported is commonly associated with advancement in puberty, such progression in puberty in itself will increase BMI, an increase which is not necessarily due to increasing fatness.[15] Adair and Gordon-Larsen[16] reported that early maturation in girls (based on the age of menarche) increased the risk twofold of being overweight as judged by a BMI at or above the 85th centile for age and sex. This chance might not, however, have been as high if it had been compared with older girls, who were postmenarcheal.

Hormonal changes related to growth at puberty

At puberty and prior to it, circulating levels of many hormones increase. These involve gonadotrophins, androgens, estrogens, growth hormone (GH), insulin-type growth factor-I (IGF-I), and leptin. The hormonal changes are inter-related and complex and for normal growth all constituents have to contribute appropriately.[17]

Growth hormone secretion increases dramatically through the course of puberty; boys in late puberty have two to three times the output of pre-pubertal boys.[18] This rise is GH is paralleled by a rise in testosterone from the growing testes, which may be the trigger for it, following the stimulus of increased output of gonadotrophins from the hypothalamus. One of the earliest tests for imminent puberty in boys is the rise in early morning serum or salivary testosterone levels.[19] GH, IGF-I, and testosterone promote growth independently but also potentiate each other, and for full growth the appropriate increase of all components is necessary.[20–22] Late in puberty and in adulthood, levels of GH and IGF-I fall, despite maintained high levels of testosterone, but by then growth potential is reduced, ultimately to zero, due to epiphyseal fusion, probably the consequence of very high androgen and estrogen levels. Evidence has been produced that estrogen in girls and boys – in the latter following aromatization of testosterone – is the likely sex steroid stimulus which increases the secretory activity of the GH axis at puberty.[22,23]

In recent years it has become evident that leptin plays an important role in providing a link between nutrition, energy balance, maturation, and aspects of pubertal growth. Longitudinal studies have suggested that leptin is important in the normal regulation of childhood weight gain, initiation of puberty, the development of secondary sexual characteristics and body composition. It is strongly associated with BMI.[24,25] Leptin levels rise gradually through childhood

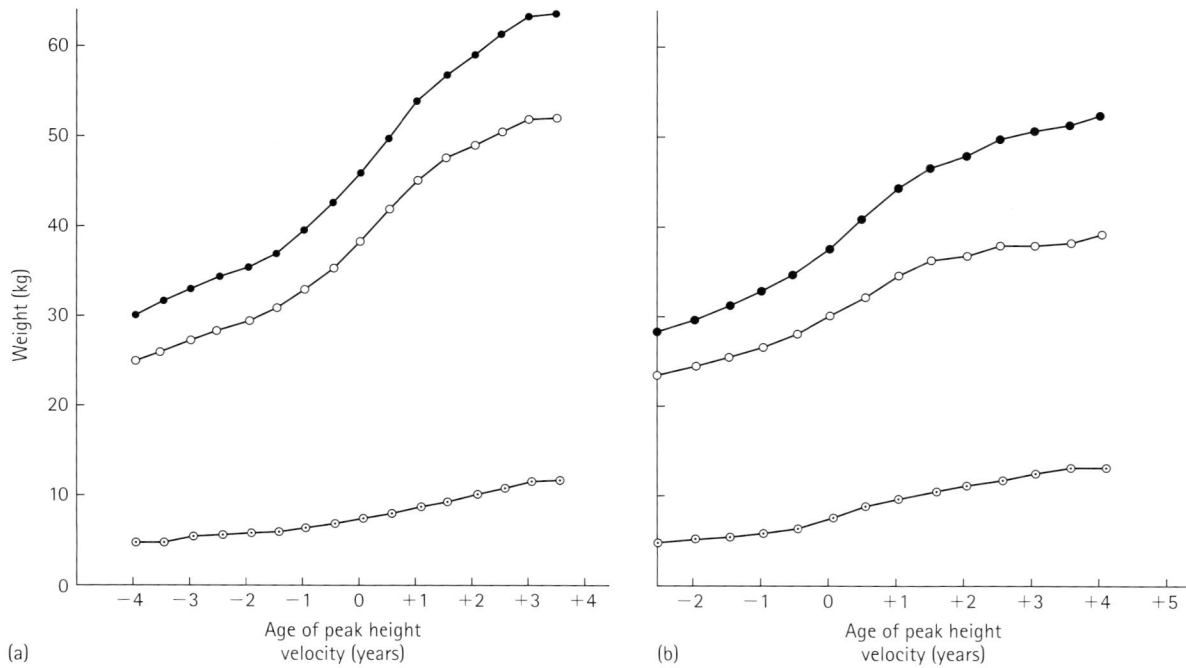

Figure 10.7   Median values for total body weight (●─●), lean body mass (○─○) and body fat (dot within open circle) for (a) boys and (b) girls, plotted against age based on that of peak height velocity (PHV).[1]

and notably just before puberty. This suggests a threshold effect reflecting the quantity of fat stores (as indicated by BMI) which triggers the pubertal activation of the hypothalamus.[26–28] Leptin is necessary for normal pubertal maturation to proceed but is not sufficient on its own. The absence of elevated leptin levels may be associated with delayed puberty. As puberty progresses, leptin levels continue to rise in girls, but fall in boys, which suggests a link with sex related differences in body composition at puberty. In both sexes leptin levels are positively related to fat mass and inversely related to fat free mass.[27] The sustained increase in leptin levels in females reflects the greater pubertal gain of fat compared with boys (perhaps linked with preparation for childbearing and lactation).

NORMAL VARIATIONS IN GROWTH IN PUBERTY

Timing

In assessing characteristics of growth around adolescence, the criterion of overall timing of puberty has frequently been the age of peak height velocity (PHV).[1,3] This has the advantage that it can be identified with greater precision than other features of puberty, but it can only be used retrospectively. Analysis of data has, however, shown poor correlation between the age of PHV and the age of onset of puberty – as defined in girls by the first signs of breast development (B2) and in boys by the onset of testicular growth to a size greater than 4 mL (G2) – Tanner stage

2.[10,29] Though the age of the appearance of the first feature of puberty may be difficult to define precisely, the benefits of its use in relation to the timing of puberty in preference to PHV are obvious. Decisions about the course of puberty, possible management of early and late developers and predictions for ultimate outcome are of greater value the earlier they are made.

In the relatively small numbers in the longitudinal study of adolescent growth of normal children,[1] the age range found for pubertal development is probably typical of that of the overall population. The mean age of the appearance of first signs of puberty (G2) in 128 boys was 12.2 years; 10 percent of the boys reached G2 before 11.2 years and 10 percent after 13.2 years. The comparable figures for the group of 83 (B2) girls were respectively 11.1 years, 10.0 years and 12.3 years. The mean age of menarche was 13.5 years; 10 percent were before 12.0 years and 10 percent after 14.9 years.

In boys there was very little difference in stature at a comparable pre-pubertal chronological age, whatever the actual timing of puberty may have been, or in the ultimate stature or weight between the groups, although with a difference in stature of 15 cm or more at an age of about 14 years between the early and late developers, based on age at PHV (Fig. 10.8a,c). Early developing girls tended, however, to be taller and heavier pre-pubertally than late developers, and remained heavier into adult life although with little difference in adult stature (Fig. 10.8b,d). The total increment in stature from pre-puberty to adulthood was similar in boys whatever the timing of their puberty, but, in contrast, early developing girls, who were more commonly

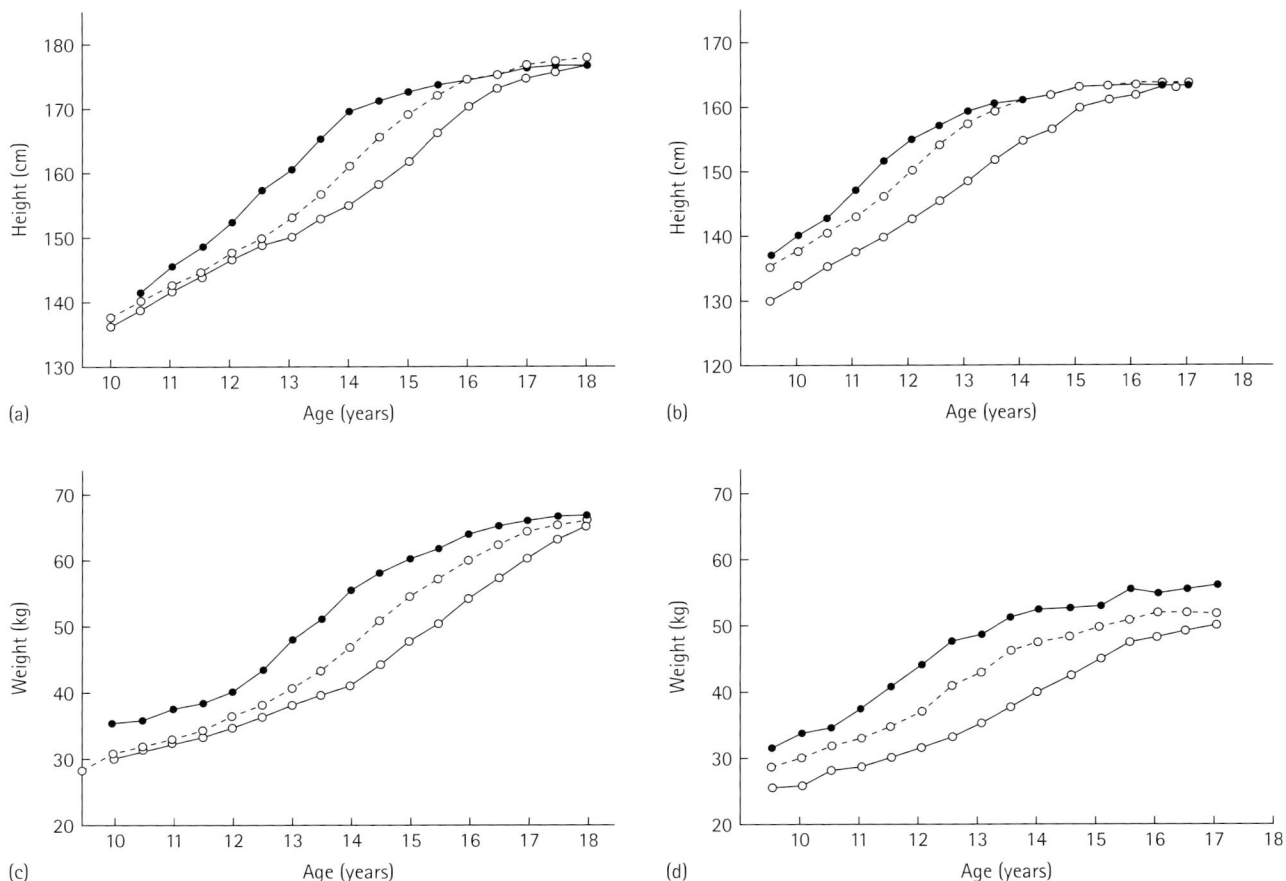

Figure 10.8 Comparison of the growth of early (●—●), average age (○---○) and late (○—○) developers: (a) boys' height; (b) girls' height; (c) boys' weight; and (d) girls' weight. Median values for the sub-groups based on the age of peak height velocity (PHV).[1]

of greater weight and taller at the onset, increased their stature less over the course of puberty.[1]

In this study there was little difference in BMI of boys at comparable stages of puberty, whatever the timing of their puberty as assessed by the age of onset. In contrast, the later girls passed through puberty the less was their weight at comparable stages, and the lower their BMI (which was probably a reflection of less fatness). As a corollary, boys did not show any marked relationship in the timing of puberty to the degree of fatness, whereas in girls the level of fatness (as indicated by skin folds) was closely related to the timing of all stages of puberty, these being progressively advanced in relation to the degree of fatness.

The increase in stature in both boys and girls through the course of puberty is greater the younger the age at which puberty starts but this is fully compensated by the greater pre-pubertal growth in the later developers. There is little difference in the ultimate stature of early, average-aged and late developers. This is shown in Fig. 10.9 based on the data from the longitudinal growth study,[1] but categorizing the timing of pubertal development on the basis of an equal division of the age range of appearance of the first signs of puberty in the subjects of the study (separately

for boys and girls).[29] The proportion of growth that occurs at early and late stages of puberty in boys and girls differs according to the timing of puberty. Early developing boys and girls have a greater proportion of their growth in puberty before the age of PHV compared with late developers (Fig. 10.10).

Figure 10.9 shows also the increments of weight according to the timing of puberty. The weight gain through the course of puberty is greater the younger the age of its onset in girls but not boys. The ultimate weight at the completion of puberty is slightly less the later the timing of development. This is in contrast to the finding with stature. This difference in weight gain is predominantly linked to weight gain in the early phases of puberty (Fig. 10.10).

As growth in the legs is the component of stature that predominates in the earlier stages of puberty, and in later stages the trunk, later developers have lesser sitting height:leg length ratios than early developers because they have a longer time during which the legs can grow (Fig. 10.11). Gasser et al.[30] confirmed in a longitudinal study from infancy to adulthood that only leg length (out of height, leg length, sitting height, arm length, bi-iliac and bihumeral width) showed a smaller adult size for early maturers.

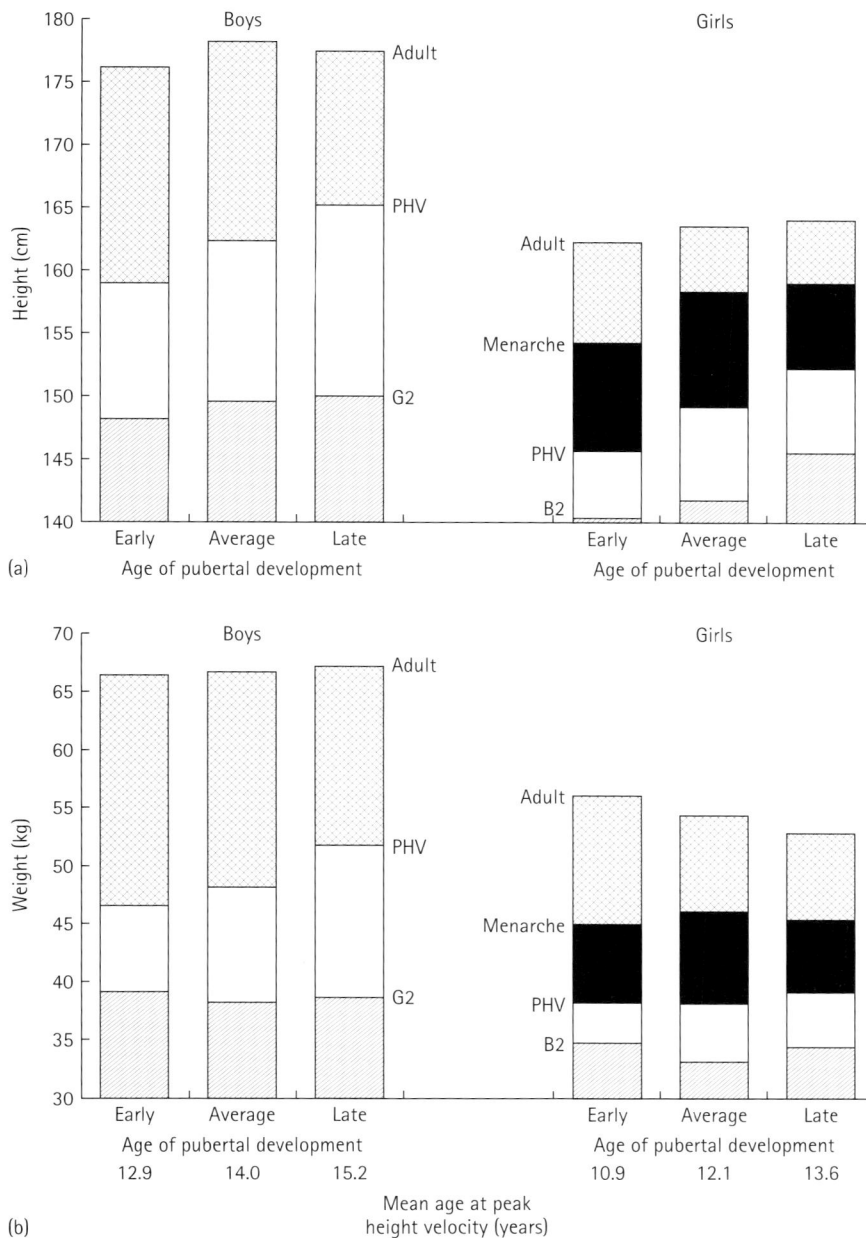

Figure 10.9 Histograms showing (a) height, and (b) weight in boys and girls as median values for early, average age and late developers (as assessed by the age of G_2/B_2) from the data of Buckler.[1] Each histogram shows the height achieved at the first sign of puberty (genital stage G_2 in boys and breast stage B_2 in girls[10]), at the time of peak height velocity (PHV), at the age of menarche in girls, and when fully grown (adult).

Factors influencing the timing and course of puberty

The variation in the timing of puberty in a healthy population is multifactorial, and whatever the cause this will have implications with regard to growth.[6]

NUTRITION

Among these factors nutrition is most noteworthy; thin and undernourished children, and notably girls, being delayed in puberty compared with those who are fatter. Underweight in the adolescent age group may be due to anorexia, chronic diseases, poverty or self induced restriction (in the extreme form, anorexia nervosa). This impaired nutritional status has a powerful adverse effect on overall growth at any age as well as delaying the onset of adolescence and the associated growth spurt and at a later stage, in girls, the menarche. Conversely, obesity (unless due to a pathological cause) is associated with tall stature in prepubertal and early pubertal years, although not with increased adult stature. There is no direct correlation shown between childhood BMI gain and final height. The temporary increase in height gain in childhood will be compensated by an earlier puberty and lessened overall height gain in adolescence.[31]

Laron[32] showed in a study of Israeli boys and girls that at all ages up to 14 years, obese subjects were taller and had

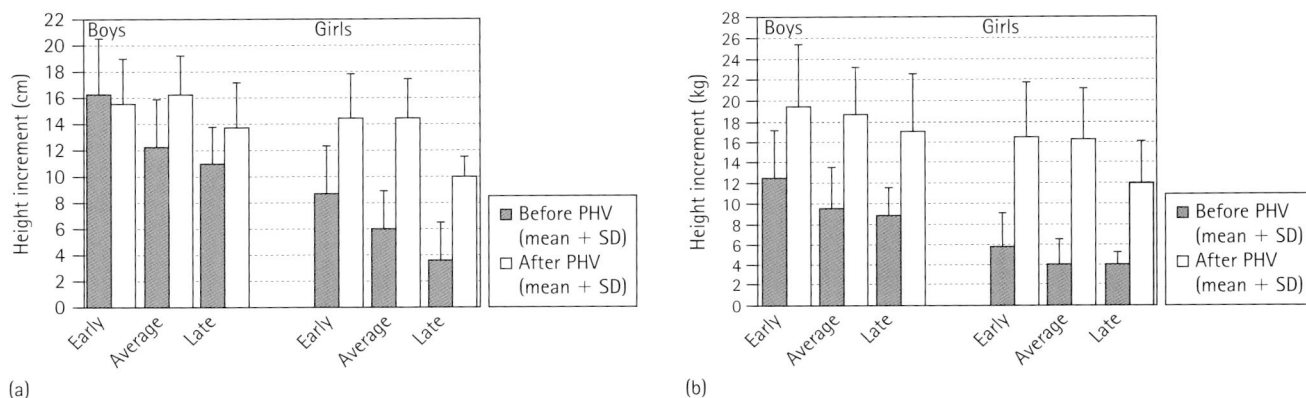

Figure 10.10 The increase in (a) height and (b) weight observed in boys and girls from the onset of puberty to adult height before and after the age of peak height velocity (PHV). The subjects are grouped according to the timing of onset of puberty as early, average aged or late.

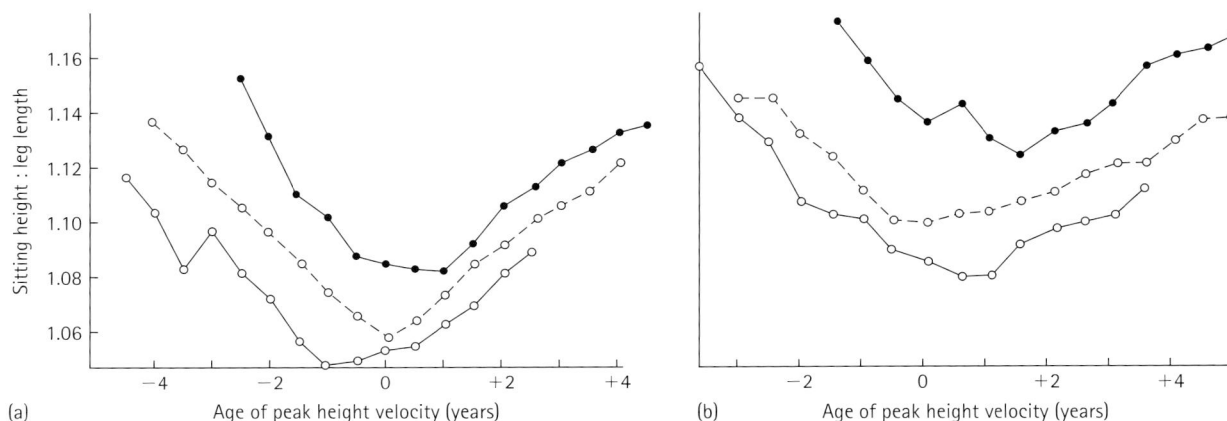

Figure 10.11 Comparison of the sitting height to leg length ratios for early (●—●), average age (○——○) and late (○—○) developers, (a) boys, (b) girls. Median values for sub-groups (based on the timing of PHV).[1]

advanced bone age compared with age matched controls. The obese boys did not, however, show any advancement in the appearance or progress of the features of puberty. Though Laron did not find advancement of puberty in obese girls either, many authors have reported that early maturing girls are consistently heavier than their later maturing counterparts.[15,16,33–35] Wang[34] reported an opposite effect between girls and boys. There was a higher prevalence of overweight in early maturing girls, but early maturing boys tended to be thinner. This sex difference may be related to the different patterns of leptin production through puberty in girls and boys.

SIZE AT BIRTH

Recent reports have indicated that size at birth is significant in relation to subsequent timing of puberty. Karlberg[33] concluded that children, both boys and girls, who were shorter and/or thinner at birth had earlier timing of puberty. Delemarre-van de Waal et al.[36] also showed that

fetal and early postnatal growth failure might have persistent consequences for growth and pubertal development in later life but found that in boys the association of low birthweight was with late development, though confirming the earlier onset of puberty and menarche in girls who had low birthweight. Adair,[37] evaluating the timing of puberty in girls by the age of menarche, reported that birthweight per se was not correlated with timing of menarche, but girls who were long and thin at birth reached menarche on average 6 months earlier than those who were short and thin. This effect of thinness was greatest in those who gained weight most rapidly in the first 6 months of life. Rapid post-natal growth seems to potentiate the effects of size at birth and is related independently to earlier pubertal maturation.

FAMILIAL INFLUENCES

There are familial and racial influences on the timing of puberty and the genetic effect is indicated by twin studies.[38–41]

SECULAR TRENDS

The secular trends in height and adolescent development indicate the influence of environmental factors on this genetic potential. The secular trend towards earlier puberty is less marked than the secular trend in adolescent growth and the two are not as closely connected as might be expected.[33] The increase in height of children over the last century (about 1–2 cm per decade) is largely the result of the earlier onset of the GH dependent phase of growth in earlier life. The age when this increase in growth rate occurs correlates with final height, but is not related to age of PHV during puberty. The gain in adult stature is less than that earlier in childhood partly due to an earlier achievement of the ultimate adult height through earlier bone maturation. The secular trend in the timing of puberty, which had been advancing worldwide over the last century at a rate of about a year per generation[10] is slowing down in recent years in many Western countries, though continues in many underdeveloped countries.[42]

GENERAL HEALTH

The state of general physical and mental health and well-being is of great importance in relation to the achieving of normal growth and progress through puberty. Almost any chronic disorder with or without associated undernutrition will delay puberty and slow down growth. Psychosocial neglect and abuse can have similar adverse effects, which may not readily be recognized, particularly as general physical health and nutrition may appear to be satisfactory.

PHYSICAL ACTIVITY

Physical activity has been shown to have an important role in normal growth, well-being and development and particularly bone development. Moderate activity is beneficial in every way. Extreme competitive sporting activities, however, markedly delay puberty and slow down growth, particularly in girls. This is usually reported in terms of delay in menarche, because intense physical activity of almost any kind – distance running, swimming, ballet dancing, skating, gymnastics, rowing, and weight lifting – have all been associated with primary amenorrhea, the delay being about 5 months per year of training, as well as commonly causing secondary amenorrhea in those who had already reached the menarche.[43–45] Theinz et al.[46] reported that gymnasts undergoing heavy training (unlike swimmers) advanced through puberty without a normal pubertal growth spurt, so that full adult height was not achieved, though catch-up could occur if exercise stopped at a sufficiently early stage. Georgopoulos et al.[47] however, reported that the elite rhythmic athletes in their study compensated for a loss of pubertal growth spurt by a late acceleration of linear growth and, despite a delay in skeletal maturation, achieved their genetic potential.

These adverse effects of excessive physical exercise are probably the result of strict weight control and high energy expenditure,[48,49] perhaps exacerbated by psychological stress. They are much more commonly seen in girls than boys, though they have been reported in male wrestlers.[50]

Prediction of ultimate stature

Residual growth depends primarily on the state of the epiphyses, because when epiphyses fuse to the shaft of long bones, with the obliteration of the growth plate, no further growth is possible. Methods of predicting adult stature depend, therefore, on estimation of bone age, because it is this rather than chronological age that is the indicator of residual growth. There are numerous methods recommended[51–53] with differing methods of bone age assessment. The one most widely advocated in the UK is that of Tanner et al.[53]

One of the problems of bone age assessment is that, inevitably, standards were based on cross-sectional observations. In practice, bone age estimations on the same individual undertaken repeatedly over the years of puberty do not show increments of 1 year bone age per year of chronological age, because bone age accelerates and deviates from a cross-sectional-based centile in a way similar to that for height.[1] This is normal, but may be interpreted as indicative of some pathology. This fact does, however, result in bone ages becoming increasingly retarded in children with delayed puberty (the standards being based on those with puberty at an average age) with a rapid catch-up when puberty occurs and, conversely, a rapid acceleration and progressive advancement of bone age in those children going into puberty at an age ahead of average. There is a great approximation and range of possible outcomes with standard methods of height prediction based on bone ages. Some concept of likely residual growth can also be gained from noting the pubertal status of an individual in terms of secondary sexual characteristics once puberty is under way.[54] This is clearly not possible before that time because, on physical grounds (without radiology), there is little indication when puberty is likely to start.

IMPLICATIONS WITH REGARD TO GROWTH DEPENDENT ON THE TIMING OF PUBERTY

The process of adolescence involves many aspects, all inter-related and occurring in parallel. Of these, growth is merely one but a very important one and, although an atypical growth pattern may be the only cause of concern, the associated stress and psychological upset are often the cumulative outcome of the atypical timing of other parallel aspects as well, i.e. delayed or precocious appearance of secondary sexual characteristics, menstruation, physical strength, sexual drive, etc. The many behavioral, emotional and psychological features that are to be expected in 'normal' adolescence may be exaggerated when the timing of puberty is atypical. It is natural, as at any age, to treat a child in accordance with the age that height and appearance suggest rather than what the age actually is. These stresses may be enormous, but particularly when associated with teasing and taunting which result in a lack of self-esteem and a poor concept of the individual's real worth. The magnitude of emotional stress will depend on the attitude of the family (including an awareness of family history) and friends and those at school, the degree of previous self-confidence and ability in intellectual and physical roles, and the nature of the underlying 'cause' if one is identifiable. Crowne et al.[55,56] reviewed the outcomes of untreated constitutional delay in growth and puberty in 43 boys and 23 girls attending their clinics. These patients retrospectively completed psychological questionnaires which showed no significant difference in self-esteem, marital or employment status between the patient and control groups, although most had felt that growth delay had affected their success at school, work or socially, and about half would have preferred treatment to advance their growth spurt.

There is a very important place in treatment for counselling, including explanation and discussion of the background and etiology, and consideration of such factors as undernutrition (anorexia) and excessive competitive exercise, as well as frank pathologies. Reassurance, if appropriate, with regard to the ultimate outcome in terms of stature, weight, physique, physical and sexual function and performance is fundamental.

LONG–TERM IMPLICATIONS OF PUBERTY OCCURRING AT AN EARLY OR LATER THAN AVERAGE AGE

With adequate support and appropriate treatment the psychological effects of the severe emotional stress are transient, but if not properly handled they can be long lasting. Excluding extremes of precocious and delayed development, the variations in timing of puberty do not have any marked adverse effect on ultimate physical size and general health. Sperlich et al.[57] considered final height in boys with untreated constitutional growth delay, including a review of 10 previous reports, and showed that there was only a small deficit in final height in such patients when compared with predicted values based on bone age assessment. However, although their heights were within the normal range, they did end up short of stature. All but one study showed that final height was lower than target height (based on parental heights) by between 1.7 and 7.7 cm. A more recent report[58] increased the listed reports to 17 on boys and 10 on girls with untreated constitutional delay in growth and puberty. A deficit in final height compared with target height occurred in all but two of the male subject groups and ranged from 1.7 to 10.9 cm and in girls

groups there was a deficit also in 8 out of the 10 ranging from 0.7 to 9.0 cm. The vast majority of the boys in these studies were over 2 standard deviations (SD) below average height at the time of presentation and in many studies this was a prerequisite for the classification of 'constitutional delay of growth and puberty'. In many cases there was a background of familial short stature as well as familial developmental delay, but these reports imply that this was not enough to account fully for the degree of ultimate shortness. Uriarte et al.[59] showed that prolonged delay in puberty (6 years or more) in men with isolated hypogonadotrophic hypogonadism is associated with a modest increase of about 5 cm of adult height, the increase correlating with the duration of pubertal delay. On this basis, boys with constitutional delay in puberty should grow taller rather than shorter. Early treatment to induce puberty might therefore be expected to be detrimental to ultimate height, but although few studies have satisfactory long-term follow-up to adult height, which is clearly of utmost importance,[60] such adverse effects do not seem to occur as a result of treatment, except when dosage is too high.[61]

Hormone treatment is often the appropriate course (with gonadotrophins or sex steroids) to initiate puberty when this is delayed, with dramatically rapid effects on stature, progress in puberty, well-being and morale. That this does not appear to have any adverse effect on the ultimate outcome is illustrated in Fig. 10.12 which shows the outcome for children who have attended the author's growth clinic, comparing the boys in whom puberty was triggered off with a short course of gonadotrophin with those who were untreated.[58] Figure 10.12 includes for comparison the normal unselected children in the longitudinal study[1] and, as previously indicated, there was little difference in ultimate heights in relation to the timing of puberty. Unfortunately, no information about parental height was available for these children, but there was no reason to suspect that target heights would not have matched the adult heights of these healthy, unselected schoolchildren. The children referred to clinic because of delayed puberty proved to be much shorter in stature than those in the study group and although a familial component contributed, because parental heights were shorter than average, this was not the only factor as these children ended up with statures considerably below their target heights. The degree to which puberty was delayed was greater than in the late developing subgroup of the longitudinal study, but not dramatically so, and the explanation is more likely to have been due to the fact that they were of short stature throughout, increasing the concern that led to referral.

BONE MINERALIZATION

Factors that adversely influence or delay bone growth during the growing years, such as delay in puberty, may

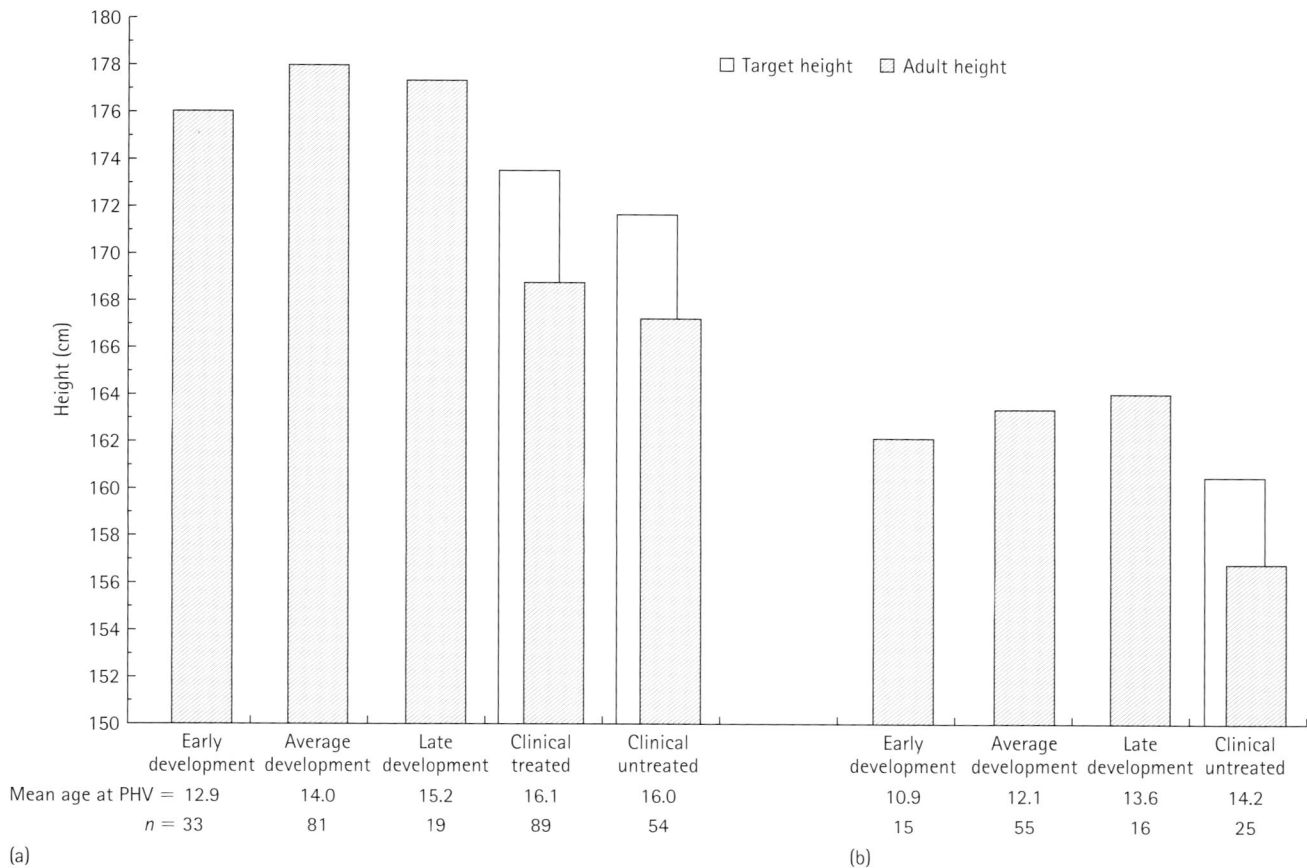

	Early development	Average development	Late development	Clinical treated	Clinical untreated		Early development	Average development	Late development	Clinical untreated
Mean age at PHV =	12.9	14.0	15.2	16.1	16.0		10.9	12.1	13.6	14.2
n =	33	81	19	89	54		15	55	16	25

(a)   (b)

Figure 10.12   Adult heights for (a) boys and (b) girls subdivided into early, average age and late developers according to the timing of onset of puberty (data from Buckler[1]), contrasted with children with delayed puberty referred to a growth clinic.

increase the likelihood of adverse effects of bone loss in later life. Bone mass is accumulated steadily during childhood and rapidly in adolescence, with an increase in bone mineral content and density at the same time as an increase in bone growth and body mass, reaching a peak after the end of puberty. About 90 percent of the peak bone mineral density is achieved by the end of the second decade, and about a quarter of adult bone is laid down during the 2 years spanning peak bone growth velocity.[49] Mineral status is consistently correlated with pubertal staging and with androgen and estrogen levels.[62–69] Measures that promote bone deposition in youth may lessen the effects of bone loss in later life. Situations in which puberty is delayed show a lower degree of bone development and mineralization than average, whether the delay is constitutional, resulting from undernutrition (notably in anorexia nervosa) or an endocrine deficiency, but in all is probably dependent on low levels of estrogen and androgen.[70] In constitutional delay of growth and puberty, bone mineral content is only about 66 percent of that of age matched controls.[62] Weight bearing physical activity is associated with more rapid mineralization in pre-pubertal chidren,[71] which will help to prevent bone disorders in later life.[72] The exercise induced

bone mineralization is maturity dependent with a critical time period during early and mid puberty. This has been termed a 'window of opportunity' to achieve peak bone mass that should occur during puberty.[49]

Extreme athletic activity causes loss of bone as a result of secondary hypogonadism, manifested in girls by delayed menarche or secondary amenorrhea, which overrides the benefit of exercise,[49,73–75] and may be exaggerated by being underweight.

Hormone treatment to bring on puberty is associated with a parallel increase in bone mineralization in both sexes.[74,76,77] There is evidence to suggest, however, that in boys with delayed puberty, even if hormone insufficiency is ultimately corrected and puberty does progress satisfactorily, there may be suboptimal mineralization in adult life with an increased risk of later osteoporosis and fractures.[49,78] As yet, however, it is not known whether early androgen supplementation in boys with delayed puberty would protect them from later osteoporosis.

In females similar effects also occur. Scoliosis, stress fractures and osteopenia are common in ballet dancers, related to amenorrhea but particularly if menarche has been delayed.[79] The loss may be irreversible.[75] Many dancers begin their training early in life before puberty, which will consequently be delayed, and pubertal deposition of bone may be decreased so that at maturation bone density is lower than normal. Hypoestrogenic amenorrhea from any cause is associated with decreased bone density and stress fractures in young women, but as yet it is uncertain just how early hormone deficit needs correcting to avoid long-term osteopenia in adult life. These observations provide added impetus for assessing the need for earlier treatment to initiate puberty in those in whom it is delayed.

KEY LEARNING POINTS

- The range of timing of puberty within the normal healthy population is considerable.
- The mean ages of appearance of comparable changes of adolescence are earlier in girls than boys by 1–2 years.
- Changes in height velocity relate to other changes of adolescence in a basically consistent way.
- Stature and height velocity should be interpreted on the basis not of chronological age but of 'physiological' or 'pubertal' age.
- BMI increases dramatically as puberty progresses, due primarily to increase in lean body mass rather than fatness, and the use of BMI in assessing fatness can be misleading in the teenage years.
- Marked delay in adolescence is frequently associated with emotional and psychological upsets as with delay in bone mineralization and long-term undermineralization and often justifies hormone treatment to speed up the onset of puberty.

REFERENCES

◆ = Key review paper

1 Buckler J. *A Longitudinal Study of Adolescent Growth*. London: Springer Verlag, 1990.
2 Buckler JMH, Wild J. Longitudinal study of height and weight at adolescence. *Arch Dis Child* 1987; **62**: 1224–32.
3 Tanner JM, Whitehouse RH, Marubini E, Resele LF. The adolescent growth spurt of boys and girls of the Harpenden Growth Study. *Ann Hum Biol* 1976; **3**: 109–26.
4 Eveleth PB, Tanner JM. *Worldwide Variation in Human Growth*, 2nd edn. Cambridge: Cambridge University Press, 1990.
5 Buckler JMH. *A Reference Manual of Growth and Development*, 2nd edn. Oxford: Blackwell Scientific Publications, 1997.
6 Buckler JMH. *Growth Disorders in Children*. London: BMJ Publishing Group, 1994.
7 Roche AF, Davila GH. Late adolescent growth in stature. *Pediatrics* 1972; **50**: 874–80.
8 Boas F. Studies in growth. *Hum Biol* 1932; **4**: 307–50.
9 Shuttleworth FK. The physical and mental growth of girls and boys aged 6–19 in relation to age at maximum growth. *Monogr Soc Res Child Dev* 1939; **4**: No. 3; 1–291.
10 Tanner JM. *Growth at Adolescence*, 2nd edn. Oxford: Blackwell Scientific Publications, 1962.
11 Freeman JV, Cole TJ, Chinn S, *et al*. Cross sectional stature and weight reference curves for the UK. *Arch Dis Child* 1990; **73**: 17–24.
12 Buckler JMH, Tanner JM. *Growth and Development Record, British Longitudinal Standards*. Welwyn Garden City: Castlemead Publications, 1996.
13 Bini V, Celi F, Berioli MG, *et al*. Body mass index in children and adolescents according to age and pubertal stage. *Eur J Clin Nutr* 2000; **54**: 214–8.
14 Dietz WH. Critical periods in childhood for the development of obesity. *Am J Clin Nutr* 1994; **59**: 955–9.
15 Lin-Su K, Vogiatzi MG, New MI. Body mass index and age at menarche in an adolescent clinic population. *Clin Pediatr* 2002; **41**: 501–7.
16 Adair LS, Gordon-Larsen P. Maturational timing and overweight prevalence in US adolescent girls. *Am J Public Health* 2001; **91**: 642–4.
17 Houchin LD, Rogol AD. Androgen replacement in children with constitutional delay of puberty: the case for aggressive therapy. *Bailliere's Clin Endocrinol Metab* 1998; **12**: 427–40.
18 Martha PM, Gorman KM, Blizzard RM, *et al*. Endogenous growth hormone secretion and clearance rates in normal boys, as determined by deconvolution analysis: relationship to age, pubertal status and body mass. *J Clin Endocrinol Metab* 1992; **74**: 336–44.
19 Butler GE, Walker RF, Walker RV, *et al*. Salivary testosterone levels and progress of puberty in the normal boy. *Clin Endocrinol* 1989; **30**: 587–96.
20 Cara JF, Rosenfield RL, Furlanetto RW. A longitudinal study of the relationship of plasma somatomedin-C concentration to the pubertal growth spurt. *Am J Dis Child* 1987; **141**: 562–4.
21 Martha PM, Rogol AD, Veldhuis JD, *et al*. Alternatives in the pulsatile properties of circulating growth hormone concentrations during puberty in boys. *J Clin Endocrinol Metab* 1989; **69**: 563–70.
22 Keenan BS, Richards GE, Ponder SW, *et al*. Androgen stimulated pubertal growth: the effects of testosterone and dihydrotestosterone on growth hormone and insulin-like growth factor-1 in the treatment of short stature and delayed puberty. *J Clin Endocrinol Metab* 1993; **76**: 996–1001.
23 Veldhuis JD, Metzger, DL, Martha PM, *et al*. Estrogen and testosterone, but not a nonaromatizable androgen, direct network integration of the hypothalamo-somatrope (growth hormone)–insulin-like growth factor 1 axis in the human: evidence from pubertal pathophysiology and sex steroid hormone replacement. *J Clin Endocrinol Metab* 1997; **82**: 3414–20.
24 Mantzoros CS, Moschos S, Avramopoulos I, *et al*. Leptin concentrations in relation to body mass index and the tumor necrosis factor-μ system in humans. *J Clin Endocrinol Metab* 1997; **82**: 3408–13.

◆ 25 Ong KK, Ahmed ML, Dunger DB. The role of leptin in human growth and puberty. *Acta Paediatr Suppl* 1999; **88**: 95-8.

26 Mantzoros CS, Flier JS, Rogol AD. A longitudinal assessment of hormonal and physical alterations during normal puberty in boys: V: Rising leptin levels may signal the onset of puberty. *J Clin Endocrinol Metab* 1997; **82**: 1066-70.

27 Ahmed ML, Ong KK, Morrell DJ, *et al.* Longitudinal study of leptin concentrations during puberty: Sex differences and relationship to changes in body composition. *J Clin Endocrinol Metab* 1999; **84**: 899-905.

28 Gill MS, Hall CM, Tillman V, Clayton PE. Constitutional delay in growth and puberty (CDGP) is associated with hypoleptinaemia. *Clin Endocrinol* 1999; **50**: 721-6.

29 Buckler JMH, Green M. Growth variability in normal adolescence. *Acta Meda Auxolog* 1999; **31**: 109-23.

30 Gasser T, Sheehy A, Molinari L, Largo RH. Growth of early and late maturers. *Ann Hum Biol* 2001; **28**: 328-36.

31 He Q, Karlberg J. BMI in childhood and its association with height gain, timing of puberty and final heights. *Pediatr Res* 2001; **49**: 244-51.

32 Laron Z. Is obesity associated with early sexual maturation? *Pediatrics* 2004; **113**: 171-2.

33 Karlberg J. Secular trends in human development. *Horm Res* 2002; **57(Suppl 2)**: 19-30.

34 Wang Y. Is obesity associated with early sexual maturation? A comparison of the association in American boys versus girls. *Pediatrics* 2002; **110**: 903-10.

35 Wang Y. Is obesity associated with early sexual maturation? *Pediatrics* 2004; **113**: 172.

36 Delemarre-Van de Waal HA, Van Coeverden SCCM, Engelbregt MJL. Factors affecting onset of puberty. *Horm Res* 2002; **57(Suppl 2)**: 15-18.

37 Adair LS. Size at birth predicts age at menarche. *Pediatrics* 2001; **107**: 765 (E59).

38 Sklad M. The rate of growth and maturing of twins. *Acta Genet Med Gemellolog* 1977; **26**: 221-37.

◆ 39 Carter CO, Marshall WA. The genetics of adult stature. In: Falkner F, Tanner JM, eds. *Human Growth: A Comprehensive Treatise*, Vol. 1. New York, London: Plenum Press, 1978: 299-305.

40 Sharma JC. The genetic contribution to pubertal growth and development studied by longitudinal growth data on twins. *Ann Hum Biol* 1983; **10**: 163-71.

41 Kapprio J, Rimpela A, Winter T, *et al.* Common genetic influences on BMI and age at menarche. *Hum Biol* 1995; **67**: 739-53.

42 Liu YX, Wikland KA, Karlberg J. New reference for the age at childhood onset of growth and secular trend in the timing of puberty in Swedish. *Acta Paediatr* 2000; **89**: 637-43

43 Heath H. Athletic women, amenorrhea and skeletal integrity. *Ann Intern Med* 1985; **102**: 258-60.

44 Baxter-Jones ADG, Helms P, Baines-Preece J, Preece M. Menarche in intensively trained gymnasts, swimmers and tennis players. *Ann Hum Biol* 1994; **21**: 407-15.

45 Malina RM. Physical growth and biological maturation of young athletes. *Exerc Sport Sci Revi* 1994; **22**: 389-433.

46 Theinz GE, Howald H, Weiss U, Sizonenko PC. Evidence for a reduction of growth potential in adolescent female gymnasts. *J Pediatr* 1993; **122**: 306-13.

47 Georgopoulos NA, Markou KB, Theodoropoulou A, *et al.* Height velocity and skeletal maturation in elite female rhythmic gymnasts. *J Clin Endocrinol Metab* 2001; **86**: 5159-64.

◆ 48 Rogol AD, Clark PA, Roemmich JN. Growth and pubertal development in children and adolescents: effects of diet and physical activity. *Am J Clin Nutr* 2000; **72**: 5215-85.

◆ 49 Eliakim A, Beyth Y. Exercise training, menstrual irregularities and bone development in children and adolescents. *J Pediatr Adolesc Gynecol* 2003; **16**: 201-6.

50 Roemmich JN, Sinning WE. Sport – seasonal changes in body composition, growth, power and strength of adolescent wrestlers. *Int J Sport Med* 1996; **17**: 92-9.

51 Bayley N, Pinneau SR. Tables for predicting adult height from skeletal age: revised for use with the Greulich–Pyle hand standards. *J Pediatr* 1952; **40**: 423-41.

52 Roche AF, Wainer H, Thissen D. Predicting adult stature for individuals. *Monogr Paediatr* 1975; **3**: 1-114.

53 Tanner JM, Whitehouse RH, Cameron N, *et al. Assessment of Skeletal Maturity and Prediction of Adult Height*, 2nd ed. London: Academic Press, 1983.

54 Green M, Buckler JMH. Prediction of adult stature of children delayed in puberty. *Acta Med Auxolog* 2001; **33**: 13-8.

55 Crowne EC, Shalet SM, Wallace WHB, *et al.* Final height in boys with untreated constitutional delay in growth and puberty. *Arch Dis Child* 1990; **65**: 1109-12.

56 Crowne EC, Shalet SM, Wallace WHB, *et al.* Final height of girls with untreated constitutional delay in growth and puberty. *Eur J Paediatr* 1991; **150**: 708-12.

57 Sperlich M, Butenandt O, Schwarz HP. Final height and predicted height in boys with untreated constitutional growth delay. *Eur J Pediatr* 1995; **154**: 627-32.

58 Buckler JMH, Green M. Observations on growth and adult height in boys and girls delayed in puberty. *Acta Med Auxolog* 2001; **33**: 1-12.

59 Uriarte MM, Baron J, Garcia HB, *et al.* The effect of pubertal delay on adult height in men with isolated hypogonadotrophic hypogonadism. *J Clin Endocrinol Metab* 1992; **74**: 436-40.

60 Kelnar CJH. Treatment of the short sexually immature adolescent boy. *Arch Dis Child* 1994; **71**: 285-7.

61 Martin MM, Martin ALA, Mossman RL. Testosterone treatment of constitutional delay in growth and development: effect of dose on predicted versus definitive height. *Acta Endocrinol* 1986; **279(Suppl)**: 147-52.

62 Krabbe S, Christiansen C, Rodbro P, Transbol I. Effect of puberty on rates of bone growth and mineralisation. *Arch Dis Child* 1979; **54**: 950-3.

63 Krabbe S, Transbol I, Christiansen C. Bone mineral homeostasis, bone growth and mineralisation during years

of pubertal growth; a unifying concept. *Arch Dis Child* 1982; **57**: 359–63.

64   Bonjour J, Theinz G, Buchs B, *et al.* Critical years and stages of puberty for spinal and femoral bone mass accumulation during adolescence. *J Clin Endocrinol Metab* 1991; **73**: 555–63.

65   Katzman DK, Bachrach LK, Carter DR, Marcus R. Clinical and anthropometric correlates of bone mineral acquisition in healthy adolescent girls. *J Clin Endocrinol Metab* 1991; **73**: 1332–4.

66   Lloyd T, Rollings N, Andon MB, *et al.* Determinants of bone density in young women. I: Relationships among pubertal development, total body bone mass and total body bone density in premenarcheal females. *J Clin Endocrinol Metab* 1992; **75**: 383–7.

67   Theinz GE, Buchs B, Rizzoli R, *et al.* Longitudinal monitoring of bone mass accumulation in healthy adolescents: Evidence for a marked reduction after 16 years of age at the levels of lumbar spine and femoral neck in female subjects. *J Clin Endocrinol Metab* 1992; **75**: 1060–5.

◆ 68   Houchin LD, Rogol AD. Androgen replacement in children with constitutional delay of puberty: the case for aggressive therapy. *Bailliere's Clin Endocrinol Metab* 1998; **12**: 427–40.

◆ 69   Rogol AD, Roemmich JN, Clark PA. Growth at puberty. *J Adolesc Health* 2002; **31**: 192–200.

70   Dhuper S, Warren MP, Brooks-Gunn J, Fox R. Effects of hormonal status on bone density in adolescent girls. *J Clin Endocrinol Metab* 1990; **71**: 1083–8.

71   Slemenda CW, Reister TK, Hui SL, *et al.* Influences on skeletal mineralization in children and adolescents: Evidence for varying effects of sexual maturation and physical activity. *J Pediatr* 1994; **125**: 201–7.

◆ 72   Lucas JA, Lucas PR, Vogel S, Gamble GD, *et al.* Effect of sub-elite competitive running on bone density, body composition and sexual maturity of adolescent females. *Osteoporosis Int* 2003; **14**: 848–56.

73   Drinkwater BL, Nilson K, Chestnut CH III, *et al.* Bone mineral content of amenorrheic and eumenorrheic athletes. *New Engl J Med* 1984; **311**: 277–81.

74   Herengroeder AC. Bone mineralization, hypothalamic amenorrhea and sex steroid therapy in female adolescents and young adults. *J Pediatr* 1995; **126**: 683–9.

◆ 75   Warren MP, Stiehl AL. Exercise and female adolescents: Effects on the reproductive and skeletal systems. *J Am Med Wom Assoc* 1999; **54**: 115–20.

76   Finkelstein JS, Klibanski A, Neer RM, *et al.* Increases in bone density during treatment of men with idiopathic hypogonadotrophic hypogonadism. *J Clin Endocrinol Metab* 1989; **69**: 776–83.

77   Bertelloni S, Baroncelli GI, Battini R, *et al.* Short term effect of testosterone treatment on reduced bone density in boys with constitutional delay of puberty. *J Bone Miner Res* 1995; **10**: 1488–95.

78   Finkelstein JS, Neer RM, Biller BMK, *et al.* Osteopenia in men with a history of delayed puberty. *New Engl J Med* 1992; **326**: 600–4.

79   Warren MP, Brooks-Gunn J, Hamilton LH, *et al.* Scoliosis and fractures in young ballet dancers. Relation to delayed menarche and secondary amenorrhea. *New Engl J Med* 1986; **314**: 1348–53.

11

Growth references

STEF VAN BUUREN

MOTIVATION FOR GROWTH REFERENCES

What is a growth reference?

A growth reference describes the variation of an anthropometric measurement within a group of individuals. A reference is a tool for grouping and analyzing data and provides a common basis for comparing populations.[1]

A well known type of reference is the age-conditional growth diagram. The traditional height-for-age (HfA) diagram shows how height varies both within and across age. Figure 11.1 is the official Dutch diagram of height and weight for Dutch boys aged 1–21 years.[2,3] In the HfA diagram, the vertical distance of shaded area in the graph delineates the variation in heights between −2 and +2 standard deviations (SD). The interval between the −2 and +2 SD curves contains about 95.4 percent of all individuals of the same age in the reference sample. The graph at the top displays the variation of weight as a function of height. For reasons that will be discussed in the section 'Detection of growth disorders' on p. 174, the shaded area is chosen here between the −1 and +1 SD curves.

Anthropometry is an extraordinarily good tool for gauging health and well-being in both individuals and in populations.[4] Height and weight are cheap and easy to measure, and provide an almost universal appraisal for assessing children's well-being. Height is one of the very few positive health indicators. A secular shift in height is a sensitive indicator of socio-economic and socio-medical changes, and thus allows comparisons of the health status of different populations. In fact, secular shifts in height may provide a better and more relevant measure for the detection and evaluation of possible changes in living conditions than such vague concepts as 'income per capita' and 'national product'.[5] Weight is clearly relevant for evaluating both undernutrition and obesity. Both are important problems on a global level. Besides height and weight, many other useful anthropometric measures exist, but the present chapter will concentrate on height, weight and derivates thereof.

Uses of growth references

Growth references are useful at both the population and the individual level. At the population level, growth references can assist in estimating prevalence, in determining causes of disease, in identifying groups at risk, in monitoring trends, and in evaluating the effects of interventions. On the individual level, growth references are indispensable tools for screening, diagnosis, monitoring and prognosis of growth-related diseases.[6] Table 11.1 provides an overview of typical questions that one might ask from growth references. In addition to these health-related applications, growth references are also needed in ergonomic design, for

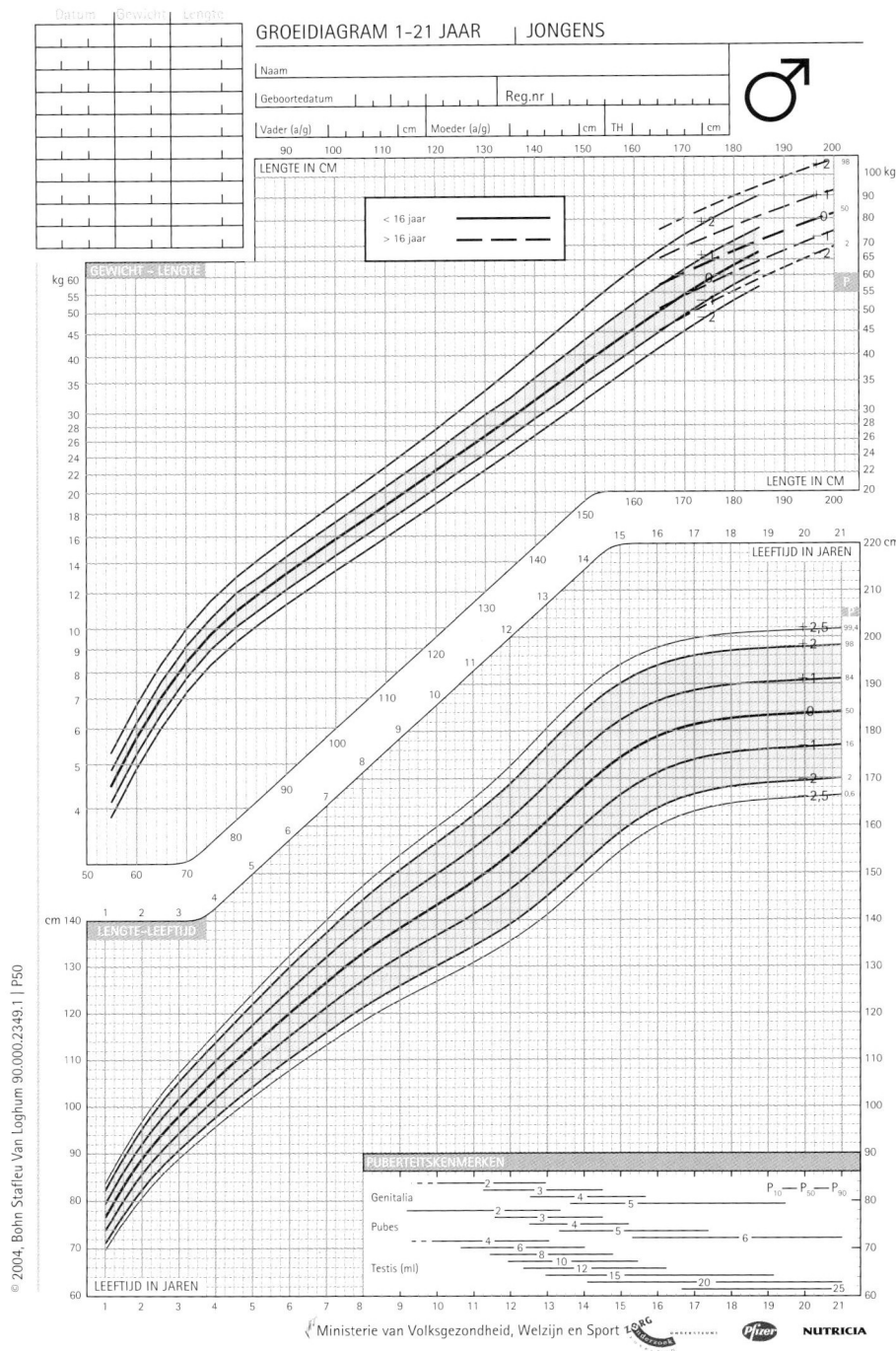

Figure 11.1 Growth diagram of height-for-age, weight-for-height and pubertal development of Dutch boys 1–21 years.

deriving safety guidelines, for establishing appropriate matches between garment size and the client population, for determining construction requirements, and so on.

Standards and references

A subtle but important distinction exists between the concept of a 'reference' and a 'standard'. A growth reference simply describes the variation of some measure within a reference population, often conditional on age and sex.

A growth standard, on the other hand, delineates the variation that is considered to be normal, optimal, or healthy. Standards embrace the notion of a norm or desirable target, and thus involve a value judgment.[1] The distinction between (normative) standards and (descriptive) references is often blurred because standards are frequently derived from references, but the conceptual distinction is important.

Clinical practice requires standards. A basic clinical question is: Is this child normal? Answering this question involves comparing the individual child to a standard. It is not always obvious which reference should be selected as a

Table 11.1 Typical questions whose answers require growth references

Individual	
Screening	Is this child's diet inadequate?
	Does this child need supplementary food, or treatment for disease?
	Is this child overweight?
	Does this child need to be referred because of a growth problem?
Diagnosis	Does this child have organic diseases?
	Is there 'failure to thrive' because of an underlying disease?
	What causes this child's overweight?
	Does an infection cause stunted growth?
Monitoring	What are the effects of increased physical exercise for this obese child?
	What are the effects of improvements in nutrition?
	What are the effects of improved health care on individual growth?
Prediction	How will this child grow in future?
	What is the risk that this child will develop a growth-related disease?
	What final height will this child attain?
Population	
Prevalence	How many people are overweight?
	What is the proportion of people in each height category?
	What is the optimal height of chairs in public transport?
Causes	What is the impact of infectious epidemic on growth?
	Can differences in growth be attributed to socio-economic differences?
Targeting	What parts of the population have the greatest need for interventions?
	How should resources be allocated?
Monitoring	At what year did the global obesity epidemic start?
	How did the height distribution evolve over the last century?
Evaluation	How many children were saved because of the nutritional aid program?
Prediction	How tall will people be in the year 2020?
	What is the impact of overweight on the prevalence of future chronic diseases?

standard. The WHO recommends choosing 'references that resemble, as far as possible, true standards, so that the same deviation from the reference data has the same biological meaning'.[1] Breast-feeding is an example where this occurs. Breast-feeding is associated with positive health outcomes, and considerable evidence exists that growth of infants with exclusive breast-feeding is different from that of formula-fed infants.[7–9] This evidence motivated the development of separate references for exclusively breast-fed infants.

In many situations however, there is no cut-and-dried answer. Evidence is often scant or inconsistent, so it might be unclear what reference to use as a standard. Body mass index (BMI) provides an example where a (descriptive) reference might not be a good standard. Like in the rest of the industrialized world, the prevalence of overweight and obesity in the Netherlands substantially increased between 1980 and 1997.[10,11] The Dutch references for BMI in 1997 accurately describe the growth expected in the 1997 population, but since a rise in BMI brings additional health risks, the 1997 references should not be used as some optimal standard. A better alternative is to base BMI standards on references from populations that existed before the recent obesity epidemic. Examples of such references include the IOTF international criteria for overweight and obesity[12] and the references for (serious) underweight in Dutch children.[13]

ISSUES IN STUDY DESIGN

References are constructed from data obtained from a sample of the reference population. Various choices in the study design affect the ability to construct appropriate references. In general, major choices in study design depend on the following questions:

- Will longitudinal references be needed?
- What is the statistical precision required at each age?
- What are the costs of recruitment and management of the reference sample?
- What resources are available for data collection and statistical analysis?
- In which settings will the references be used?
- When should the new references become available?

Cross-sectional and longitudinal studies

A cross-sectional growth study is a study in which children of different ages are measured once at the same point of time. Cross-sectional studies are relatively easy to carry out. References obtained from cross-sectional studies are perfectly suited for evaluating the status of a child encountered in a situation where only one measurement is made, such as a screening study. Repeated cross-sectional studies provide very sensitive information about changes in the health status of the population. Secular changes of growth are among the most striking biological consequences of social and economic development.[5]

Cross-sectional studies, however, do not provide adequate information for following growth of an individual child over time, in particular at ages where the growth rate is high, as in infancy and during puberty.[4,14] The reason is that references derived from cross-sectional studies do not allow for the child's tempo of growth. Though it is possible to infer the average rate of growth from the difference of average size at increasing age, a cross-sectional study cannot be used to estimate the variability between children in the amount of growth over time. To do so requires a longitudinal study, i.e., a study where children are measured at two or more occasions. In longitudinal data, the growth rate between the occasions is directly observed for each child. This information can be used to construct longitudinal references that portray the variability in growth between children over time.

Longitudinal studies are generally more difficult to manage, but may be efficient if the amount of effort to identify and locate the individuals in the reference sample is large.[15] A longitudinal study takes more time, so if important secular trends occur, references obtained from longitudinal studies may be outdated by the time they are published. On the other hand, it may be more efficient to use a longitudinal design if the costs of managing the cohort are small. Having multiple measurements per individual not only increases the precision of the growth references, but also allows for the construction of longitudinal references.

A mixed longitudinal design represents a compromise between a cross-sectional and a longitudinal design. A mixed design requires more sophisticated statistical methods: individuals are measured more than once, but not throughout the entire age range. Mixed longitudinal designs are quite popular. Examples of recent, large scale mixed longitudinal studies include the Euro-Growth study[16,17] and the WHO Multicentre Growth Reference Study.[18,19] The mixed longitudinal study combines the advantages of the cross-sectional and longitudinal designs, but may have less precision than an exclusively cross-sectional or longitudinal study. In addition, a mixed design is often more difficult to analyze.

Sample size

Sample size is the most important factor affecting the precision of the reference values. Other relevant determinants include the study design, the timing of measurement and the method of curve fitting.[15] The simplest advice is to have at least 200 individuals per age and sex group.[20] Assuming a normal distribution with a standard deviation of 7 cm, the standard error of the mean is equal to $7/\sqrt{200} = 0.5$ cm. Thus, a sample size of 200 is adequate to detect a secular shift in

Table 11.2 Ninety-five percent confidence intervals for the correlation coefficient for sample sizes of $N = 100$ and $N = 200$

Correlation	$N = 100$	$N = 200$
0.99	0.985–0.993	0.987–0.992
0.95	0.926–0.967	0.934–0.962
0.90	0.854–0.932	0.870–0.924
0.80	0.716–0.861	0.744–0.845
0.70	0.584–0.788	0.621–0.764

mean height of about 1.9 cm with a type I error rate of 5 percent and a power of 80 percent. The standard errors of a given percentile can be obtained by multiplying the standard error of the mean by a fixed constant that depends on the centile value only.[21] Under normality, these multiplication factors are 1.25 for P50, 1.74 for P90, 1.81 for P95, and 2.51 for P97. So for a sample size of 200, the standard error of 97th centile is equal to $2.5 \times 0.5 = 1.2$ cm.

Goldstein[22] argued that the assumption of normality ceases to provide good estimates for the extreme percentiles, even for variables like height. Using a simple ranking method free of the normality assumption leads to sample sizes that are about twice as high to achieve the same precision. Other specialized ways of calculating sample size have been proposed, dealing with the slope of the median curve, the correlation between measurements, and the precision of the median curve overall.[15]

In longitudinal designs, the primary parameter of interest is the correlation between measurement occasions. The precision of the correlation coefficient depends on both sample size and the expected correlation coefficient. Table 11.2 contains the 95 percent confidence interval for the correlation for various samples sizes and correlations.

The use of neighboring information across age by smoothing methods can drastically increase precision of the overall percentile curves. One could potentially base sample size calculations on the precision of the smoothed curves, but this does not seem to have been practiced yet.

A related question is how the sample should spread across the age range. Traditionally, oversampling at the ages of high growth rates has been used in order to capture accurately the pattern of growth. Approximate sampling fractions per sex are known.[22] As an example, the Fourth Dutch Growth Study[2] constructed age groups such that the population for ages 0–2 years and around puberty were oversampled. In order to improve precision at the edges when using smoothing methods, enough children should be sampled at the extreme ages of the intended references. The WHO Multicentre Growth Study applied a four-fold increase of the sample size at birth, and extended the sample to month 71, whereas the final chart should stop at an earlier age.[19]

Inclusion criteria

Inclusion criteria articulate the reference population. For normative references, the population should live in a healthy environment and contain no overtly sick or very few clinically sick individuals. Eligibility criteria in the WHO Multicentre Growth Study include, amongst others, socio-economic status that does not constrain growth, low mobility of the population, mothers willing to follow feeding recommendations, term birth, single birth, no maternal smoking, and birth weight $>1500\,g$.[19]

Inclusion criteria like these take care that children in the reference sample are raised in an healthy environment. Note however their use makes the reference unsuitable as a descriptive reference. Children not living in a healthy environment are systematically missing from the sample, leading to a picture that may be too positive. If descriptive references are wanted also (for example in order to monitor progress on the population level) one could measure all children meeting in the population, and temporarily set aside the data from ineligible children when calculating normative references.

DISTANCE REFERENCES

Uses of distance references

The diagrams in Figure 11.1 summarize the distribution of attained size in a known reference population at different ages. A chart of attained size is known as a distance chart. Distance charts are often constructed from cross-sectional data. A distance chart can be legitimately used:

- To compare attained growth between two different populations.
- To compare attained growth of the same population at different occasions.
- To detect aberrant individual growth using a single observation located in an extreme centile.

It is tempting to classify a sequence of measurements of one particular person that 'cross centiles' rapidly over time as unusual. However, the distance chart is inappropriate for assessing longitudinal patterns. The implicit assumption is that children should grow parallel along the centile curves, and that deviations from this pattern indicate unusual growth. Yet, this is not true.[23] The curve of the cross-sectional 50th centile is not the curve actually followed by any individual, even the individual who is at the 50th percentile before puberty, at the 50th percentile after puberty, and who has a spurt at the average time at the average intensity.[4] The distance chart contains no information about changes in centiles from one age to another. Several authors have emphasized this point,[4,24,25] but the use of the distance diagram as a tool for monitoring longitudinal measurements is nevertheless widespread.

A number of methods for constructing reference charts (cf. next section) allow the calculation of a standard deviation score (SDS), or z-score, for each individual measurement. This score is normally distributed with mean 0 and variance 1, and indicates the relative position of attained size at a given age. For a normally distributed measurement SDS can be calculated as $Z = (X - M)/S$, where X is attained size, M is the mean according to the reference at age T, and where S is the corresponding standard deviation. The SDS can also be calculated for other (e.g., skewed) distributions, but the precise method depends on the fitting model that is used to construct the references.

Methods for creating distance references

Producing centile charts has been labeled as 'something of a black art'.[26] This section briefly reviews about 30 methods for fitting centile curves that have been proposed over the last 30 years. The material presented here draws upon more extensive reviews by Wright and Royston[27] and Borghi et al.[28]

The major task in centile construction is to smooth the reference distribution in two directions simultaneously, between age and within age. Borghi et al.[28] used and extended a classification of methods for references originally put forward by Cole. In this classification, methods are distinguished on the following characteristics:

- Estimating centiles separately versus estimating them together. Methods that estimate centiles together can be further classified according to the distributional assumptions made.
- Recoding data into age groups versus treating age as continuous.
- The type of age-smoothing method.

BASIC METHOD

The basic method for deriving distance references consists of three main steps:

- Classify the observations into age groups.
- Calculate the empirical distribution function from the ordered values of size at each age, and estimate the desired set of centile values, e.g., the 3, 10, 25, 50, 75, 90, 97 centiles, per age group.
- For each desired centile, smooth the centile values across age to form an age-dependent curve. Smoothing can be done by splines functions,[29] kernel regression[30,31] or by eye.[32,33]

This method is simple to understand and provides an accurate estimate of the shape of the size distribution across age if the sample size is large. On the other hand, it is not without problems. First of all, creating age groups will bias the variance upwards if the measurements are taken from children whose exact ages differ from the midpoint age.

Healy[34] proposed to reduce the variance by a factor $b^2/12$, where b is the average amount of growth occurring during the interval. Even if all children would be measured at the same exact calendar age, estimating centiles from the empirical distribution function sounds easier than it actually is. Care is needed in computing extreme centiles, as some interpolation is needed. The algorithms implemented in SPSS and SAS can give odd results, producing estimates that are too extreme, irrespective of the interpolation algorithm used. The S-Plus function quantile does not have this problem.[35] Finally, because the method does not use neighboring information, the influence of sample fluctuations can produce centile curves that could potentially cross each other.[36]

DISTRIBUTIONAL ASSUMPTIONS

The basic method can be improved by incorporating the assumption that size measurements within an age group follow some distribution. This assumption facilitates assessment of asymptotic behaviors and provides simple formulas for calculating SD scores. Of course, these advantages will only be realized if the assumed distribution fits the data. Methods have been developed using the normal distribution,[37] possibly obtained after applying a Box–Cox transformation,[26,38] a square-root transformation,[39] or a variance stabilizing transformation.[40]

AGE AS A CONTINUOUS VARIABLE

Another type of improvement involves using age as a continuous variable. Koenker and Bassett[41] proposed to estimate a given regression quantile directly from the data, conditional on one or more co-variates. The method is elegant because it combines both within and across age variation into one optimization function. The method estimates quantile curves separately, which could unfortunately result in curves that touch or cross each other. The method has been adapted in several ways to prevent quantile crossing.[42–44] Related nonparametric methods have been developed by Wellek and Merz,[45] Rossiter,[46] Gasser et al.[47] and Gannoun et al.[48] The HRY method[49] estimates each centile through a moving window using a high-order polynomial function. Constraints are applied to the coefficients of the polynomial so that these vary smoothly with the percentiles, thereby ensuring commonality on the centiles so that the curves do not cross. A problem with this procedure is that a fixed polynomial may not be sufficiently flexible if smoothing is applied to a wide age range. Pan and Goldstein developed extensions that improved upon the original formulation of the HRY model.[50,51]

DISTRIBUTIONAL ASSUMPTIONS AND AGE AS A CONTINUOUS VARIABLE

Many methods have been developed that incorporate both improvements. Methods differ in the type of the assumed age-conditional distribution, and can be broadly classified into three groups:

- Methods assuming a normal distribution
- Methods assuming a normal distribution after transformation
- Methods assuming a non-normal distribution.

In the first group, Aitkin[52] proposed to use maximum likelihood estimation of a linear model for the mean and a log–linear model for the variance. Altman[53] modeled the absolute residuals about the fitted mean as a function of age.

The group of methods assuming normality after a transformation is quite large. By far, the most popular method is the extended LMS method by Cole and Green.[54] The LMS method assumes that the age-conditional distribution is normal after a Box–Cox[55] type of transformation. An age-dependent L-curve models skewness, the M-curve portrays how the median attained size varies with age, and the S-curve describes in what way the coefficient of variation depends on age. The L-, M- and S-curves are fitted by maximum penalized likelihood. Centiles are calculated in the transformed scale, and then back-transformed into the original scale. Similar methods have been proposed by Wade and Ades[56] who used a parametric smoothing method, Thompson and Theron[57] who assumed the four-parameter family of Johnson's distribution[58] to model kurtosis, and Royston[59] who applied a shifted-logarithmic transformation. The method of Tango[60] finds transformations for both size and age such that after transformation size is a linear function of age with constant variance. If successful, the normal model can be applied on the transformed data to obtain centile curves. Royston and Wright[61,62] proposed a parametric variant of the LMS method, called the 'fractional polynomials and exponential transformation' (FPET) method. The distribution of size can be an exponential distribution with three parameters, or a modulus–exponential distribution with four parameters (which models kurtosis). The parameters of the chosen three- or four-parameter distribution are estimated by maximum likelihood. Yee[63] replaced the Box–Cox transformation by the more general Yeo–Johnson transformation[64] towards normality, which amongst others, allows for negative values of size and potentially results in better normal approximations.

Several methods based on non-normal distributions have been developed. Sorribas et al.[65] proposed a parametric method based on the flexible S-distribution. This method smooths the parameters of the distribution across age. Yee[63] pioneered the use of the Box–Cox transformation towards a gamma distribution, which leads to computational benefits. Rigby and Stasinopoulos[66] generalize the LMS method so that the distribution after the Box–Cox transformation is a t-distribution instead of the normal. This allows to model leptokurtosis, i.e., a higher mean and thicker tails than the normal distribution. In another generalization of the LMS method, the same authors apply the

Box–Cox power exponential distribution, which models skewness and both leptokurtosis and platykurtosis.[67]

CHOOSING A METHOD

By now, the reader may be left somewhat bewildered by the wide array of possibilities. What method should be used in practice? The short answer is: the LMS method. The LMS method is easy to understand, fits reasonably well for many anthropometric measures, provides closed formula for calculating SD scores, comes with good model fitting tools, and has been applied by so many authors that it has become the *de facto* standard. On the other hand, the LMS method is not without weaknesses. It assumes that there is no kurtosis, which may not be true. Evidence is accumulating that kurtosis can have a significant effect on the location of the extreme centiles.[68] Nonparametric methods do not make any distributional assumption, but this comes at the expense of a loss of precision and the capability to calculate SD scores. Methods using other transformations (FPET, Yeo–Johnson, Tango, Johnson family) or distributions (S-, t- or BCPE distributions) may give more accurate descriptions of the data while accounting for kurtosis. The LMS method is limited to single covariates, and is cumbersome to apply if the analysis sample must split into groups, e.g, in modeling the weight-for-height (WfH) relationship for different age groups. The methods of Royston and Wright, Yee, and Rigby and Stasinopoulos can be used with multiple covariates.

Some comparisons of methods have been published,[27,69–71] but the performance of the more recent methods has not yet been evaluated. The WHO is currently working on a comparison involving the methods of the Box–Cox, the Box–Cox t, the Box–Cox power exponential, the FPET method, and the Johnson family of distributions. More comparative work is needed to infer whether the newer methods would actually make a difference in practice.

VELOCITY REFERENCES

Standards based on longitudinal data are required when the same child is to be seen on more than one occasion. Conventionally, velocity is calculated as $V = (X_2 - X_1)/(T_2 - T_1)$, where X_1 and X_2 are the attained size at ages T_1 and T_2. Velocity can be expressed as gain in cm years^{-1}, or kg month^{-1}. Low velocity appears on the distance chart as downwards centile crossing.

An alternative is to define velocity in the rate of change in SDS per time, i.e., $W = (Z_2 - Z_1)/(T_2 - T_1)$, where Z_1 and Z_2 are the SDS corresponding to X_1 and X_2. This measure standardizes the velocity scale to SDS per year, but does not standardize the distribution of W itself. The distribution of W depends on T_1 and T_2. This implies that a deflecting curve with a slope of -1 SDS year^{-1} can indicate dramatic growth stunting during childhood, while the same deflection could fall within the normal range during

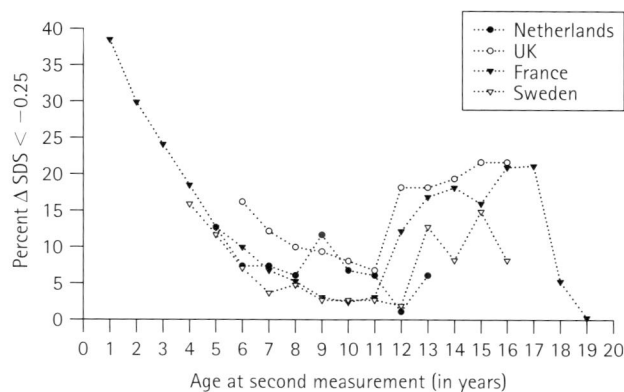

Figure 11.2 Expected percentage in the reference population having an SDS velocity below -0.25 SDS year^{-1}. The measurement interval is one year.

infancy. Interpretations of W that fail to take the age dependency into account might lead to misleading inferences.[72,73] Figure 11.2 provides an indication of the percentages of the children whose velocity is lower than -0.25 SDS year^{-1}, as calculated from several longitudinal studies.[24,74–76] Note the strong dependency on age.

Cole discussed a velocity measure whose distribution is independent of age: $Z_g = (Z_2 - Z_1)/\text{SD}(Z_2 - Z_1)$, where $\text{SD}(Z_1 - Z_2) = \sqrt{(2 - 2r)}$, and where r is the correlation between Z_1 and Z_2 in the reference population.[77] Z_g has a standard normal distribution for all pairs of (T_1, T_2), and for that reason Z_g is preferable over W. Depending on the value of r, the conclusions emanating from both indices can be quite different.

CONDITIONAL REFERENCES

The interpretation of change over time is affected by regression to the mean.[78] An individual with an extreme size on T_1 can expect a less extreme size on T_2. The strength of the effect is determined by the correlation coefficient. Regression to the mean is crucial in the interpretation of repeated observations. A child in a low centile at T_1 will have a greater expected velocity than one of the same age starting from a higher centile. Velocity references do not take this effect into account, and are thus intrinsically flawed.[23]

Healy[79] suggested that conditioning on previous observations may overcome the problem. Cameron[75] and Berkey et al.[80] have put this idea to practice. A conditional reference adjusts the population reference for another variable. In longitudinal data, past observations evidently make up relevant information to condition on.[81] Cole[24,77] proposed the conditional gain score $cZ_g = (Z_2 - rZ_1)/\sqrt{(1 - r^2)}$, which improves upon Z_g since it properly accounts for regression to the mean.

Conditioning may also involve multiple factors. For example, Thompson and Fatti[82] proposed a weight chart for women that adjusted the overall location of the references to individual characteristics like height, age, and parity. Clearly, the idea of conditioning can be exploited to develop screening and monitoring tools that might have elevated sensitivity and specificity for detecting growth-related diseases.[15]

Table 11.3 summarizes indices for age-related references, illustrating the pros and cons of each index. It will be clear that the methodology also applies to references that are conditional on other factors, such as weight or parental height.

Velocity and conditional indices rely on two measurements instead of one. A disadvantage is that both are sensitive to measurement error, especially if the period $T_2 - T_1$ is short. Of these two, the conditional SDS gain is less sensitive to measurement error, and should therefore be preferred. The variance of the conditional SDS gain is always lower than that of the SDS gain, especially for small r.

Methods for estimating conditional references have been described by Cameron et al.,[75] Berkey et al.,[80] Wright et al.,[83] Cole,[24] Royston,[81] Gasser et al.,[47] Pan and Goldstein,[84,85] Thompson and Fatti,[82] Fatti et al.,[86] Wade and Ades,[87] and Reinhard and Wellek.[88] It may not be so easy to get the correlation between Z_1 and Z_2 from a tabulated reference. In daily practice, the observation ages T_1 and T_2 may not be sufficiently close to the tabulated reference age intervals. It is not yet clear what the best way is to approximate r in such cases.

This section concentrated on conditional velocity reference, where conditioning is applied to one or more previous observations. Conditional distance references are also possible, and that type of references is in fact older. Examples include references that condition on parental height[89] and sibling births weight.[90]

MODEL EVALUATION

It is crucial that models used to estimate reference intervals fit the data extremely well.[91] Yet, relatively little research has been done on methods for evaluating and improving the fit of the model. References can be fitted in a variety of ways, but all approaches need to specify in some way the amount of smoothness that provides a reasonable trade-off between parsimony of the curves and the fidelity to the data. This section discusses various ways to gauge this trade-off. Let us distinguish among the following approaches.[35]

Visual inspection of the shape of the reference curves

Experienced researchers may recognize the appropriateness of a given set of reference curves based on subtle features in the shape, like a 'pubertal belly' in cross-sectional data. In general, substantial exposure to reference curves is needed to develop the necessary skills.

Centiles plotted onto the individual data points

This type of plot is useful for inspecting outliers and for detecting gaps in the data and gross errors in the model, but its resolution is too limited to be helpful in choosing among different models. Attained size can be visualized in

Table 11.3 Indices for individual attained size and growth, to be used in conjunction with age-related distance, velocity and conditional references

Definition	Name	Advantages	Disadvantages
Distance			
X_1	Attained size at age T_1	Simple	Interpretation depends on age and sex
Z_1	Standard deviation score (SDS) at T_1	Comparable across age and sex, has standard normal distribution	Provides no information about growth over time
Velocity			
$V = (X_2 - X_1)/(T_2 - T_1)$	Velocity	Easy to calculate	Interpretation depends on age and sex
$W = (Z_2 - Z_1)/(T_2 - T_1)$	Velocity in SD scale	Adjusts velocity for age and sex	Distribution still depends on age
$Z_g = (Z_2 - Z_1) / \sqrt{(2 - 2r)}$	Standardized gain score (SDS gain)	Comparable across age and sex, has standard normal distribution for all T_1 and T_2	Does not account for regression to the mean, requires correlation between Z_1 and Z_2
Conditional			
$cZ_g = (Z_2 - rZ_1) / \sqrt{(1 - r^2)}$	Conditional SDS gain	As Z_g, but accounts for regression to the mean	Requires correlation between Z_1 and Z_2

both the original and in the SD scale, but the latter possibility offers a higher resolution.

Empirical and fitted centiles plotted on top of each other

This is an old and quite accurate technique in which the observations are divided into age groups. Empirical centiles are computed for each group, and these are plotted together with the fitted curves. If everything is right, the fitted curves should be close to the point estimates (i.e., within sampling error). Various choices are possible for the vertical scale (raw, standardized for mean and/or standard deviation). A disadvantage of the raw data plot is that if the standard deviation changes with age, the same distance means different things at different ages. Van Wieringen[5] pioneered a standardized graph under the heading of 'graphical graduation', which plots empirical and fitted centiles in deviations from the median on the original scale.

Observed and expected counts

Healy et al.[49] suggested comparing observed and expected frequencies of observations within defined centile and age groups, a method now known as the grid test.[91] Suppose that observations are grouped into centile groups divided by the 5th, 50th, and 95th centile curves and grouped according to age. If the model fits well, we would expect to observe about 5, 45, 45 and 5 percent of the cases in each group. The difference can be summarized by a chi-squared statistic, which can be tested for statistical significance. Although intuitively appealing, the grid test lacks statistical power because of the severe data reduction steps.[91] Metcalfe[92] defended the grid test by arguing that the grid test may detect aberrant patterns near the extremes that more powerful statistical tests may fail to pick up.

Statistical tests applied to the distribution of the SD score

In all models that assume a normal distribution, the SD score should be normally distributed at all ages. A mix of clearly non-normal age-conditional SD scores can make up a marginal distribution that is close to normality. Therefore, global tests that do not account for the age-conditional nature of the SD score are uninformative and should not be used.[35] Royston and Wright[91] developed a series of age-conditional Q-tests, which summarize how much the SD score deviates from the normal in the mean, spread, skewness and kurtosis. Likelihood ratio tests are also used to fit models, though it is not entirely clear what should be taken as the appropriate reference distribution.[67] Statistical tests are very useful in signaling that there is a problem, but may be less able to tell at what age the problem occurs.

Quantile–quantile plot (Q–Q plot) of the SD scores

Q–Q plots[93] can be applied if the measurements are supposed to follow a known distribution. The display plots the quantiles of the theoretical distribution (on the horizontal axis) against those of the empirical distribution (on the vertical axis). The Q–Q plot for normal data, also known as the normal probability plot, is best known, but it can be adapted to other distributions. The plot yields insight into structural characteristics (e.g., skewness, kurtosis) of empirical deviations from the assumed distribution. A detrended Q–Q plot is obtained if each empirical quantile is subtracted from its corresponding unit normal quantile. The detrended plot is sensitive to subtle deviations.[94] Global Q–Q plots across the entire age range are not informative, and should thus be split according to age.

Worm plot

The worm plot[35] consists of a collection of detrended Q–Q plots, each of which applies to a successive age group. The vertical axis of the worm plot portrays, for each observation, the difference between its location in the theoretical and empirical distributions. The data points in each plot form a worm-like string. The shape of the worm indicates how the data differ from the assumed underlying distribution, and when taken together, suggests useful modifications to the model. A flat worm indicates that the data follow the assumed distribution in that age group. So the aim of the model fitting process is to 'tame the worms'. Figure 11.3 is the end result of fitting height distribution of boys. All worms are reasonably flat and are within chance variation, so the model fits quite well.

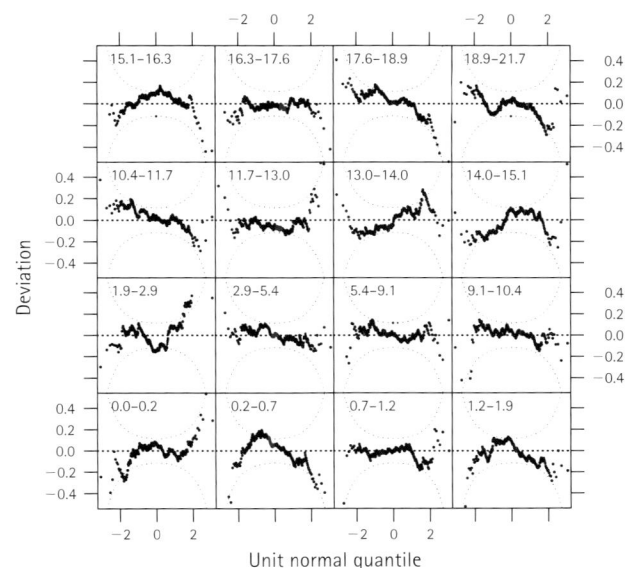

Figure 11.3 Worm plot of the final LMS model (0/10/6r) fitted to height of Dutch boys 1–21 years.

Pan and Cole compared the behavior of the worm plot, the Q test and the Likelihood ratio test by fitting LMS models to data from the Third Dutch Growth Study.[33] They concluded that all are useful tools for testing goodness of fit, and suggested in what ways they complement each other.

Outliers also influence the fit. Tango[95] proposed a method for identifying outliers. Kapitula and Bedrick[96] proposed a diagnostic for measuring the influence of individual cases on the estimated centile curves within the context of FPET model.[61]

DETECTION OF GROWTH DISORDERS

The growth diagram is widely used in pediatric practice, but not much is known about its performance in detecting growth disorders.[97] A growth diagram defines the specificity of a single height measurement, but its sensitivity is unknown for even the most frequent diseases. This is unfortunate because it precludes an informed discussion about referral criteria. Referral criteria have been developed and evaluated,[98–101] but this has not prevented the appearance of widely different guidelines. For example, the recent UK guideline[102] is based on just one universal height measurement at age five, whereas the Dutch consensus guidelines[103] consist of multiple referral criteria covering infancy, childhood and adolescence. All in all, current practice differs among practitioners, and practices are not founded on evidence.

This issue was recently addressed by a new methodology for estimating sensitivity, specificity and median referral age for referral rules.[104] Turner syndrome was taken as a target disease. Three basic rules were investigated: (1) height SDS below a given cut point; (2) height SDS below a cut point but corrected for parental height; and (3) height SDS velocity below a given cut point. Using two longitudinal data sets, one for Turner syndrome and one reference, it was found that the parentally adjusted rule is superior to both of the others, with sensitivity near 70 percent and a specificity of 99.4 percent. Turner syndrome is, in some sense, an 'ideal condition' to show the methodology,[105] but the principle can be adapted to other disorders covered by the chapters of this book.

Implementing new screening protocols using growth references requires careful consideration of the current setting. An example is the new Dutch protocol for detecting overweight and obesity.[106] Both overweight and obesity are defined in terms of BMI, yet existing practice in the Netherlands is based on the WfH chart. It was considered undesirable to replace the WfH chart by the BMI diagram, as that would create a new obligation to calculate BMI for every child. The solution to this dilemma was to continue using WfH, and calculate BMI only for children that have a WfH SDS over +1 SD. For this reason, the 'normal range' on the Dutch WfH chart was chosen to be between −1 and +1 SD (cf. Figure 11.1). Figure 11.4 is a flow chart of the new protocol.

INDIVIDUALIZING REFERENCES

Growth references typically take the form of age-conditional reference ranges by sex. These references portray the growth expected over all members of the reference population. Increased heterogeneity among these members will lead to more variability in the references, and thus to a lower level of precision for the growth expected for an individual member.

It is often useful to eliminate unwanted variation from the population standards. Factors that can account for considerable variability between members are: individual growth history, parental height, premature birth, region, ethnicity, age of pubertal onset, being part of a twin, breast feeding, presence of a disease, and the level of education. One can condition on one or more factors. In practice, this can involve selecting subgroups from the reference population, and adapting the reference data to reflect the characteristics of this subgroup. The results may be a narrower, more precise, reference that is tailored to the characteristics of the individual.

Conditioning is not always good, and should only be done if the subgroup reference fits the purpose of the applied context. An example where this may not be true is parental weight. Creating a reference from the subgroup of children with overweight parents is likely to shift the weight distribution upwards. Using this individualized reference in a normative way may miss children that actually are at risk, leading to a loss of potential health gains.

MISCELLANEOUS TOPICS

Synthetic growth charts

Growth references require large and costly studies. When resources are limited, synthetic growth reference charts[107] can help in providing quick-and-dirty growth charts. For boys, a synthetic height reference can be constructed using samples from the population at the ages of 0, 2, 6, 14, and 18 years. The remaining ages of the reference can be interpolated according to the known shape of the distance diagram. Synthetic growth charts for body weight have also been developed.[108] Little is known about the accuracy of these synthetic charts, but the idea is interesting and may stimulate the realization of gross savings in periodical updates of reference values.

Chart design issues

Traditionally, the reference diagram plots a set of percentiles against age, usually the P3, P10, P25, P50, P75, P90 and P97.

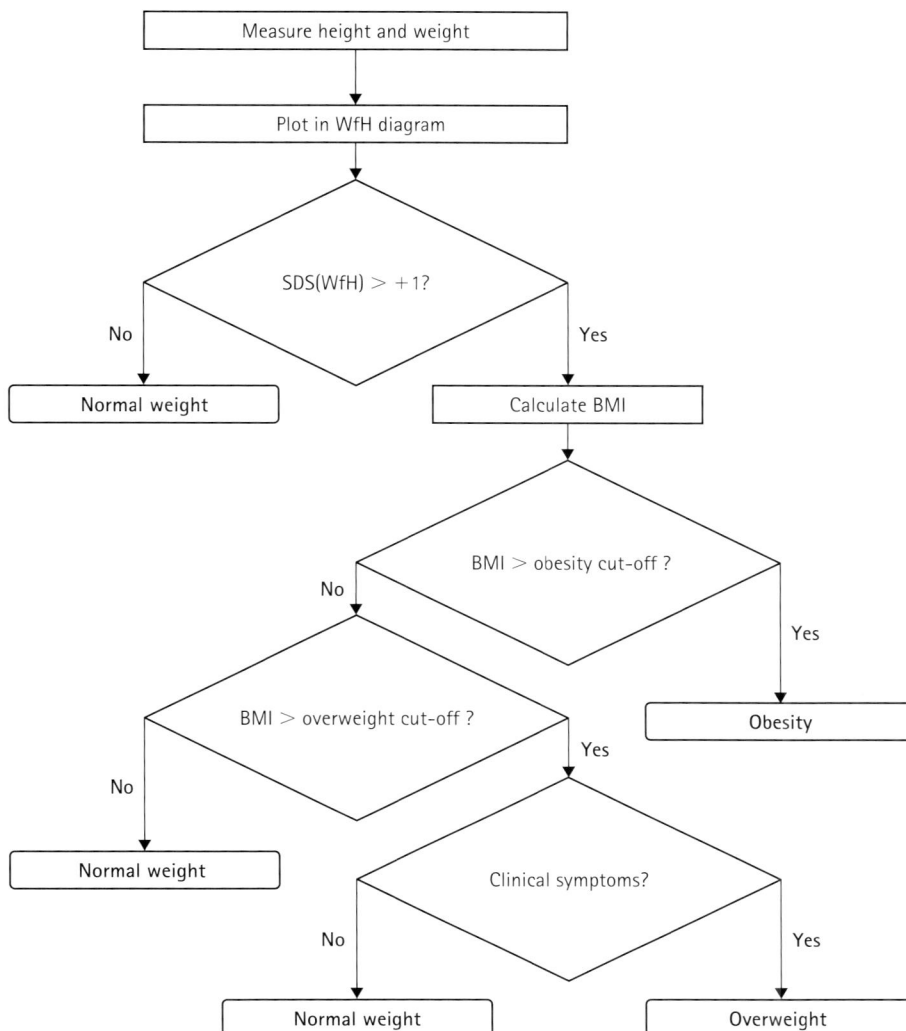

Figure 11.4 Flow chart of the new Dutch protocol for identifying overweight and obesity.

The extreme centile lines are sometimes combined with P5 and P95 curves.[109] Though percentiles are easy to understand, a difference on the percentile scale is meaningless. The clinical implication of 'losing 10 percentile points' can be very different, depending on the location on the scale. If a child migrates from P50 to P40, there is probably little reason for concern. On the other hand, migrating from P11 to P1 can have profound clinical significance. The SD score does not have this problem, can be calculated outside the extreme centile curves, and be visually interpolated from the diagram. The British[110] reference uses a spacing of 2/3 SD, whereas the Dutch diagrams apply an intercurve spacing of 1 and 1/2 SD. A drawback is that SD-based charts are less intuitive to the uninitiated.

The traditional growth chart design fails to use 90 percent of the rectangular graphic area. There are few toddlers with a height of 180 cm or adults with a height of 60 cm. It is therefore more efficient and more informative to plot the SDS against age. Sorva et al.[111] developed a format in which normal growth is shown as a horizontal line and any deviation from this indicates abnormal change in growth. Thus far, such charts seem to have been used only in Finland. Figure 11.5 plots a chart for Dutch boys 0–24 months. The curved lines can be interpreted as height contours, so the name 'meridian chart' seems appropriate for this type of display.

The effective display of conditional references is a major challenge. Cole[112,113] developed ways to enrich the distance diagram with velocity information by means of overlays. Given the importance of monitoring growth, more work along these lines is needed. Chart design issues are heavily tied to growth diagrams on paper. The use of computerized

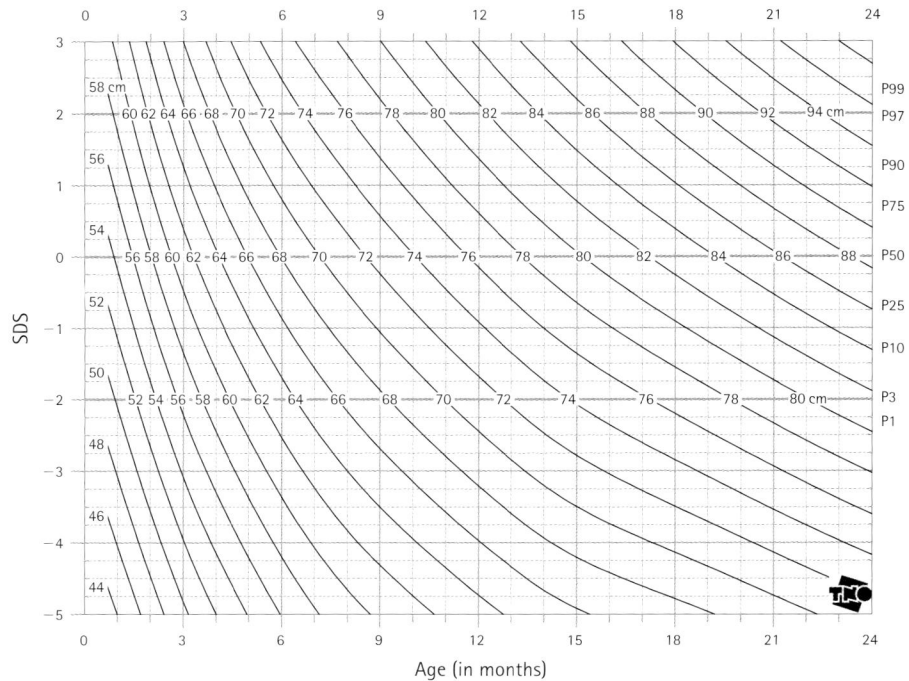

Figure 11.5 Meridian chart of height of Dutch boys aged 0–24 months based on data from the Third Dutch Growth Study. Instruction: At the appropriate age, find the meridian (cm) line that equals the measurement, and mark the location. If necessary, interpolate between the two nearest meridian lines.

systems for presenting and using growth diagrams will have a major impact of the type of design decisions that need to be made.

Non-continuous outcomes

Relatively little work has been done on the construction of age-related references for non-continuous measures. Non-continuous measures that are of interest include: pubertal stages, indicators of motor and mental development, visual acuity, developmental milestones, clinical grades, and so on.

Figure 11.6 shows how the probability of attaining pubertal stages G2–G5 of Dutch boys stages varies with ages.[114] These probabilities were modeled separately for each stage as a continuous, nonlinear function of age by a generalized additive logistic model.[115] The probability of passing P10, P50 and P90 can be read off from the curve (except for P10 of G2), and used in the reference diagram as in Fig. 11.1.

Figure 11.7 is a collection of reference diagrams of menarche probability of Dutch girls, where probability is modeled by an additive logistic model with two main factors. The first is age, the second is either weight, height or BMI, in both raw and standardized forms. A vertical course of the lines means that menarche probability is indifferent to the factor. So, the top-left plot indicates that higher weight is associated with an increase of menarche probability, but

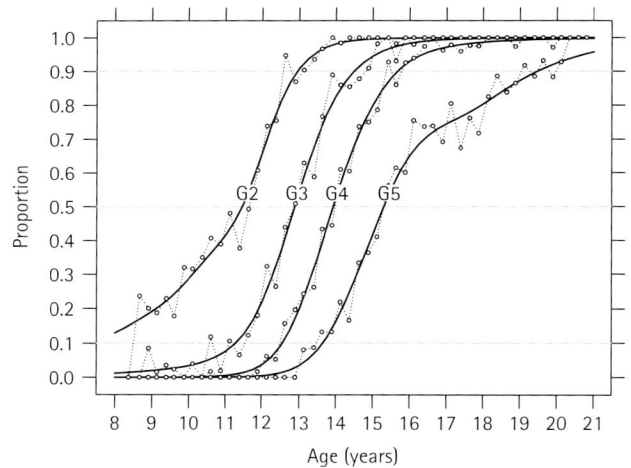

Figure 11.6 Empirical probabilities and fitted reference curve of genital stages G2–G5 for Dutch boys 8–21 years (Data: Fourth Dutch Growth Study).

that weights beyond 60 kg do not further increase the menarche probability, irrespective of age.

Wade et al.[116,117] estimated references for ordinal outcomes using a fully parametric proportional odds model with asymmetric logistic models per cumulative category. More work on non-continuous outcomes would be useful.

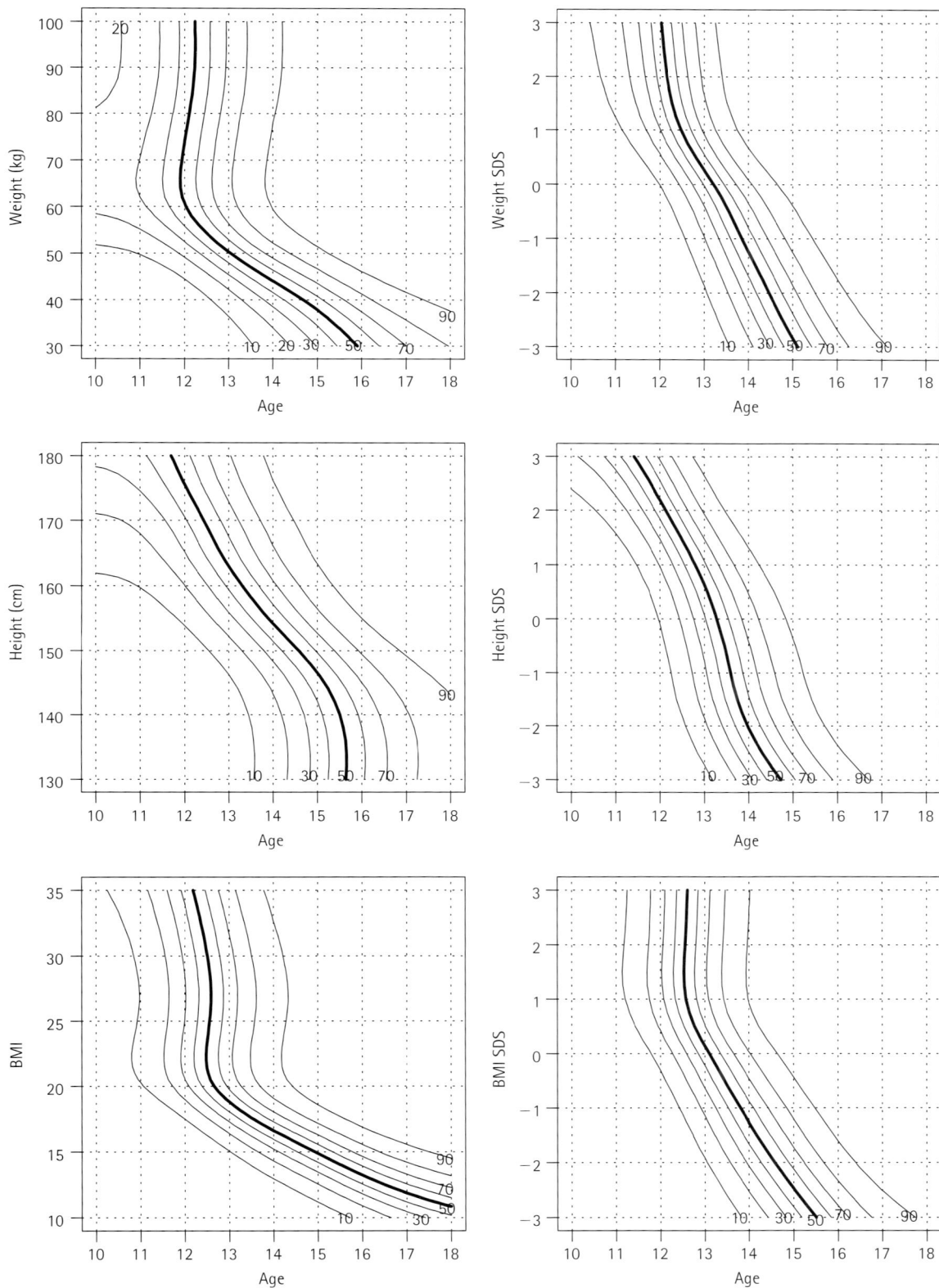

Figure 11.7   Reference chart of menarche probability as a function of age and weight (kg and SDS), height (cm and SDS) or BMI (kg m^{-2} and SDS) (Data: Fourth Dutch Growth Study).

KEY LEARNING POINTS

- Growth references describe anthropometric variation within a group of individuals. Standards delineate variation that is considered normal, optimal or healthy.
- Growth references are valuable for answering a wide variety of questions on both the individual and population level.
- References can be classified as distance, velocity and conditional. Distance references are informative about attained size only, whereas velocity and conditional references describe the process of growth over time.
- The best current methods for fitting age-conditional references treat age as continuous and assume a distribution per age.
- Good tools like Q-tests and worm plots exist to evaluate the quality of a fitted growth model.
- Detecting growth disorders by a growth diagram requires information about its sensitivity, specificity and referral time distribution.
- More work is needed on diagnostic performance, on methods for individualizing references, on synthetic growth charts, on computerized systems, and on non-continuous outcomes.

REFERENCES

- Seminal paper
- Review paper

1 World Health Organization. *Report of WHO Expert Committee: Physical Status – The Use and Interpretation of Anthropometry.* WHO Technical report no. 854. Geneva, Switzerland: World Health Organization, 1995.
2 Fredriks AM, van Buuren S, Burgmeijer RJF, *et al.* Continuing positive secular growth change in The Netherlands 1955–1997. *Pediatr Res* 2000; **47**: 316–23.
3 Fredriks AM, van Buuren S, Burgmeijer RJF, *et al. Groeidiagrammen* (derde druk) (*Growth Diagrams*, 3rd edn.) Houten: Bohn, Stafleu, Van Loghum, 2004.
- 4 Tanner JM. Use and abuse of growth standards. In: Falkner F, Tanner JM, eds. *Human Growth: A Comprehensive Treatise*, 2nd edn, vol. 3. New York: Plenum Press, 1986: 95–109.
- 5 Van Wieringen JC. *Seculaire groeiverschuiving* (Secular Growth Shift). Leiden, Netherlands: Institute for Preventive Medicine, TNO, 1972.
6 World Health Organization. An evaluation of infant growth: the use and interpretation of anthropometry in infants. *Bull WHO* 1995; **73**: 165–74.
7 World Health Organization Working Group on Infant Growth. *An evaluation of infant growth.* Report WHO/NUT/94.8. Geneva, Switzerland: World Health Organization, 1994.

8 Cole TJ, Paul AA, Whitehead RG. Weight reference charts for British long-term breastfed infants. *Acta Paediatr* 2002; **91**: 1296–300.
9 De Onis M, Onyango AW. The Centers for Disease Control and Prevention 2000 growth charts and the growth of breastfed infants. *Acta Paediatr* 2003; **92**: 413–9.
10 Cole TJ, Roede MJ. Centiles of body mass index for Dutch children aged 0–20 years in 1980 – A baseline to assess recent trends in obesity. *Ann Hum Biol* 1999; **26**: 303–8.
11 Fredriks AM, van Buuren S, Wit JM, Verloove-Vanhorick SP. Body index measurements in 1996–7 compared with 1980. *Arch Dis Child* 2000; **82**: 107–12.
12 Cole TJ, Bellizzi MC, Flegal KM, Dietz WH. Establishing a standard definition for child overweight and obesity worldwide: international survey. *BMJ* 2000; **320**: 1240–3.
13 van Buuren S. Afkapwaarden van de 'body mass index' (BMI) voor ondergewicht van Nederlandse kinderen. (Body-mass index cut-off values for underweight in Dutch children). *Nederlands Tijdschrift voor de Geneeskunde* 2004; **148**: 1967–72.
14 Healy MJR. Statistics of growth standards. In: Falkner F, Tanner JM, eds. *Human Growth: A Comprehensive Treatise*, 2nd edn, vol. 3. New York: Plenum Press, 1986: 47–58.
- 15 Frongillo EA. Univariate and bivariate growth references. In: Hauspie RC, Cameron N, Molinari L, eds. *Methods in Human Growth Research.* Cambridge: Cambridge University Press, 2004: 261–86.
16 Haschke F, van't Hof MA, and the Euro-Growth Study Group. Euro-Growth references for length, weight, and body circumferences. *J Pediatr Gastroenterol Nutr* 2000; **31**: S14–38.
17 Van't Hof MA, Haschke F, Darvay S and the Euro-Growth Study Group. Euro-Growth References on increments in length, weight, head- and arm circumference during the first three years of life. *J Pediatr Gastroenterol Nutr* 2000; **31**: S39–47.
18 De Onis M, Victora CG, Garza C, *et al.* A new international growth reference for young children. In: Dasgupta P, Hauspie RC, eds. *Perspectives in Human Growth, Development and Maturation.* Dordrecht, The Netherlands: Kluwer Academic Publishers, 2001: 45–53.
19 De Onis M, Garza C, Victora CG, *et al.* The WHO multicentre growth reference study: Planning, study design, and methodology. *Food Nutr Bull* 2004; **25**: S15–26.
- 20 Waterlow JC, Buzina R, Keller W, *et al.* The presentation and use of height and weight data for comparing nutritional status of groups of children under the age of 10 years. *Bull WHO* 1977; **55**: 489–98.
21 Kendall M, Stuart A, Ord JK. *Kendall's Advanced Theory of Statistics. Vol. I: Distribution Theory.* London: Charles Griffin, 1980.
22 Goldstein H. Sampling for growth studies. In: Falkner F, Tanner JM, eds. *Human Growth: A Comprehensive Treatise*, 2nd edn, vol. 3. New York: Plenum Press, 1986: 59–78.
23 Cole TJ. Growth and development. In: Armitage P, Colton T, eds. *Encyclopedia of Biostatistics.* New York: Wiley, 1998: 1790–7.

● 24 Cole TJ. Growth charts for both cross-sectional and longitudinal data. *Stat Med* 1994; **13**: 2477–92.

25 Preece MA. Standardization of growth. *Acta Paediatr Scand* 1989; **349**: 57–64.

26 Cole TJ. Fitting smoothed centile curves to reference data, *J R Stat Soc A* 1988; **151**: 385–418.

◆ 27 Wright EM, Royston P. A comparison of statistical methods for age-related reference intervals. *J R Stat Soc A* 1997; **160**, 47–69.

◆ 28 Borghi E, de Onis M, Garza C, *et al.* Methods for constructing the WHO child growth references: Recommendations of a statistical advisory group. *Stat Med* 2006; **25**: 247–65.

29 Hamill PVV, Drizd TA, Johnson CL, *et al. NCHS Growth Curves for Children Birth to 18 Years.* Vital and Health Statistics Series 11, No 165. Washington DC: National Center for Health Statistics, 1977.

30 Gasser T, Köhler W, Müller H-G, *et al.* Velocity and acceleration of height growth using kernel estimation. *Ann Hum Biol* 1984; **11**: 397–411.

31 Guo S, Roche AF, Baumgartner RN, *et al.* Kernel regression for smoothing percentile curves: reference data for calf and subscapular skinfold thicknesses in Mexican Americans. *Am J Clin Nutr* 1990; **51**: 908S–16.

32 Van Wieringen JC, Wafelbakker F, Verbrugge HP, de Haas JH. *Growth Diagrams 1965 Netherlands. Second National Survey on 0–24-year-olds.* Groningen: Wolters-Noordhoff, 1971.

33 Roede MJ, van Wieringen JC. Growth diagrams 1980: Netherlands third nation-wide survey, *Tijdschrift voor Sociale Gezondheidszorg* 1985; **63(Suppl)**.

34 Healy MJR. The effect of age-grouping on the distribution of a measurement affected by growth. *Am J Phys Anthropol* 1962; **20**: 49–50.

35 van Buuren S, Fredriks AM. Worm plot: A simple diagnostic device for modeling growth reference curves. *Stat Med* 2001; **20**: 1259–77.

36 Jones MC. Discussion of 'Fitting smoothed centile curves to reference data' by TJ Cole. *J R Stat Soc* 1988; **151**: 412–3.

37 Tanner JM, Whitehouse RH, Takaishi M. Standards from birth to maturity for height, weight, height velocity, and weight velocity: British children, 1965; Part I. *Arch Dis Child* 1966; **41**: 454–71.

38 Van 't Hof MA, Wit JM, Roede MJ. A method to construct age references for skewed skinfold data, using Box–Cox transformations to normality. *Hum Biol* 1985; **57**: 131–9.

39 Niklasson A, Ericson A, Fryer JG, *et al.* An update of the Swedish reference standards for weight, length and head circumference at birth for given gestational age (1977–1981). *Acta Paediatr Scand* 1991; **80**: 756–62.

40 Chinn S. A new method for calculation of height centiles for preadolescent children. *Ann Hum Biol* 1992; **19**: 221–32.

● 41 Koenker RW, Bassett G Jr. Regression quantiles. *Econometr* 1978; **46**: 33–50.

42 He X. Quantile curves without crossing. *Am Stat* 1997; **51**: 186–92.

43 Heagerty PJ, Pepe MS. Semiparametric estimation of regression quantiles with application to standardizing weight for height and age in US children. *Appl Stat* 1999; **48**: 533–51.

44 Ducharme GR, Gannoun A, Guertin MC, Jéquier JC. Reference values obtained by kernel-based estimation of quantile regressions. *Biometrics* 1995: **51**: 1105–16.

45 Wellek S, Merz E. Age-related reference ranges for growth parameters. *Methods Inf Med* 1995; **34**: 523–8.

46 Rossiter JE. Calculating centile curves using kernel density estimation methods with application to infant kidney lengths. *Stat Med* 1991; **10**: 1693–701.

47 Gasser T, Molinari L, Roos M. Methodology for the establishment of growth standards. *Horm Res* 1996; **45(Suppl 2)**: 2–7.

48 Gannoun A, Girard S, Guinot C, Saracco J. Reference curves based on non-parametric quantile regression. *Stat Med* 2002; **21**: 3119–35.

49 Healy MJR, Rasbash J, Yang M. Distribution-free estimation of age-related centiles. *Ann Hum Biol* 1988; **15**: 17–22.

50 Pan H, Goldstein H, Yang Q. Non-parametric estimation of age-related centiles over wide age ranges. *Ann Hum Biol* 1990; **17**: 475–81.

51 Goldstein H, Pan H. Percentile smoothing using piecewise polynomials, with covariates. *Biometrics* 1992; **48**: 1057–68.

52 Aitkin M. Modelling variance heterogeneity in normal regression using GLIM. *Appl Stat* 1987; **36**: 332–9.

53 Altman DG. Construction of age-related reference centiles using absolute residuals. *Stat Med* 1993; **12**: 917–24.

● 54 Cole TJ, Green PJ. Smoothing reference centile curves: the LMS method and penalised likelihood. *Stat Med* 1992; **11**: 1305–19.

● 55 Box GEP, Cox DR. An analysis of transformations. *J R Stat Soc B* 1964; **26**: 211–52.

56 Wade AM, Ades AE. Age-related reference ranges – significance tests for models and confidence intervals for centiles. *Stat Med* 1994; **13**: 2359–67.

57 Thompson ML, Theron GB. Maximum likelihood estimation of reference centiles. *Stat Med* 1990; **9**: 539–48.

58 Johnson NL. Systems of frequency curves generated by methods of translation. *Biometrika* 1949; **36**: 149–76.

59 Royston P. Constructing time-specific reference ranges. *Stat Med* 1991; **10**: 675–90.

60 Tango T. Estimation of age-specific reference ranges via smoother AVAS. *Stat Med* 1998; **17**: 1231–43.

61 Wright EM, Royston P. Simplified estimation of age-specific reference intervals for skewed data. *Stat Med* 1997; **16**: 2785–803.

62 Royston P, Wright EM. A method for estimating age-specific reference intervals ('normal ranges') based on fractional polynomials and exponential transformation. *J R Stat Soc A* 1998; **161**: 79–101.

63 Yee TW. Quantile regression via vector generalized additive models. *Stat Med* 2004; **34**: 2295–315.

64 Yeo I-K, Johnson RA. A new family of power transformations to improve normality and symmetry. *Biometrika* 2000; **87**: 954–9.

65 Sorribas A, March J, Voit EO. Estimating age-related trends in cross-sectional studies using S-distributions. *Stat Med* 2000; **19**: 697–713.

66 Rigby RA, Stasinopoulos DM. Generalized additive models for location, scale and shape (with discussion). *Appl Statist* 2005; **54**: 507–34.

67 Rigby RA, Stasinopoulos DM. Smooth centiles curves for skew and kurtotic data modelled using the Box–Cox power exponential distribution. *Stat Med* 2004; **23**: 3053–76.

◆ 68 Pan H, Cole TJ. A comparison of goodness of fit tests for age-related reference ranges. *Stat Med* 2004; **23**: 1749–65.

69 Moussa MAA. Estimation of age-specific reference intervals from skewed data. *Methods Info Med* 2002; **42**: 147–53.

70 Bonellie SR, Raab GM. A comparison of different approaches for fitting centile curves to birthweight data. *Stat Med* 1996; **15**: 2657–67.

71 Pere A. Comparison of two methods for transforming height and weight to normality. *Ann Hum Biol* 2000; **27**: 35–45.

72 Van Buuren S, Fredriks AM. Methoden voor het objectiveren van groeiafbuiging (in Dutch) (Objective methods for growth deflection). In: Wit JM, ed., *De Vierde Landelijke Groeistudie; Presentatie nieuwe groeidiagrammen.* Leiden: Boerhaave Commissie, 1998: 91–101.

73 Van Buuren S, Fredriks AM, Verkerk PH. Consensus 'Diagnostiek kleine lichaamslengte bij kinderen'. *Nederlands Tijdschrift voor de Geneeskunde* 1999; **143**: 1585–6.

74 Prahl-Andersen B, Kowalksi CJ, Heijendael P. *A Mixed-Longitudinal Interdisciplinary Study of Growth and Development: Nijmegen Growth Study.* San Francisco: Academic Press, 1979.

75 Cameron N. Conditional standards for growth in height of British children from 5.0 to 15.99 years of age. *Ann Hum Biol* 1980; **7**: 331–7.

76 Karlberg J. *Modelling of Human Growth.* [Dissertation] Gotenburg, 1987.

77 Cole TJ. Conditional reference charts to assess weight gain in British infants. *Arch Dis Child* 1995; **73**: 8–16.

● 78 Galton F. Regression towards mediocrity in hereditary stature. *J Anthropol Inst* 1886; **15**: 246–63.

● 79 Healy MJR. Notes of the statistics of growth standards. *Ann Hum Biol* 1974; **1**: 41–46.

80 Berkey CS, Reed RB, Valadian I. Longitudinal growth standards for pre-school children. *Ann Hum Biol* 1983; **10**: 57–67.

81 Royston P. Calculation of unconditional and conditional reference intervals for foetal size and growth from longitudinal measurements. *Stat Med* 1995; **14**: 1417–36.

82 Thompson ML, Fatti LP. Construction of multivariate centile charts for longitudinal measurements. *Stat Med* 1997; **16**: 333–45.

83 Wright CM, Matthews JNS, Waterston A, Aynslay-Green A. What is the normal rate of weight gain in infancy? *Acta Paediatr* 1994; **83**: 351–6.

84 Pan H, Goldstein H. Multi-level models for longitudinal growth norms. *Stat Med* 1997; **16**: 2665–78.

85 Pan H, Goldstein H. Multi-level repeated measures growth modelling using extended spline functions. *Stat Med* 1998; **17**: 2755–70.

86 Fatti LP, Senaoana EM, Thompson ML. Bayesian updating in reference centiles charts. *J R Stat Soc A* 1998; **161**: 103–15.

87 Wade AM, Ades AE. Incorporating correlations between measurements into the estimation of age-related reference ranges. *Stat Med* 1998; **17**: 1989–2002.

88 Reinhard I, Wellek S. Age-related reference regions for longitudinal measurements of growth characteristics. *Methods Info Med* 2001; **40**: 132–6.

89 Tanner JM, Goldstein H, Whitehouse RH. Standards for children's height at ages 2 to 9 years, allowing for heights of parents. *Arch Dis Child* 1970; **45**: 755–62.

90 Tanner JM, Lejarrage H, Healy MJR. Within-family standards for birthweight, a revision. *Lancet* 1972; **ii**: 1314–5.

91 Royston P, Wright EM. Goodness-of-fit statistics for age-specific reference intervals. *Stat Med* 2000; **19**: 2943–62.

92 Metcalfe C. Letter to the editor. *Stat Med* 2002; **21**: 3749–50.

93 Hoaglin DC. Using quantiles to study shape. In: Hoaglin DC, Mosteller F, Tukey JW, eds. *Exploring Data Tables, Trends, and Shapes.* New York: Wiley, 1985: 417–59.

94 Friendly M. *SAS System for Statistical Graphics,* 1st edn. Cary, NC: SAS Institute, 1991.

95 Tango T. Estimation of normal ranges in clinical laboratory data. *Stat Med* 1986; **5**: 335–46.

96 Kapitula LR, Bedrick EJ. Diagnostics for the exponential normal growth curve model. *Stat Med* 2005; **24**: 95–108.

97 Garner P, Panpanich R, Logan S. Is routine growth monitoring effective? A systematic review of trials. *Arch Dis Child* 2000; **82**: 197–201.

98 Hindmarsh PC. Monitoring children's growth: Abnormal growth should also be defined by the crossing of height centiles [Letter]. *BMJ* 1996; **312**: 122.

99 Mulligan J, Voss LD, McCaughey ES, *et al.* Growth monitoring: testing the new guidelines. *Arch Dis Child* 1998; **79**: 318–22.

100 Voss LD. Changing practice in growth monitoring. *BMJ* 1999; **318**: 344–5.

101 Hall DMB. Growth monitoring. *Arch Dis Child* 2000; **82**: 10–5.

102 Hall DMD, Elliman D. *Health for all Children,* 4th edn. Oxford: Oxford University Press, 2003.

103 De Muinck Keizer-Schrama SMPF. Consensus 'Diagnostiek kleine lichaamslengte bij kinderen' (Dutch consensus guidelines for short stature). *Nederlands Tijdschrift voor de Geneeskunde* 1998; **142**: 2519–25.

104 van Buuren S, van Dommelen P, Zandwijken GRJ, *et al.* Towards evidence based referral criteria for growth monitoring. *Arch Dis Child* 2004: **89**: 336–41.

105 Hindmarsh PC, Cole TJ. Commentary: Height monitoring as a diagnostic test. *Arch Dis Child* **89**: 296–7.

106 Bulk-Bunschoten AMW, Renders CM, van Leerdam FJM, HiraSing RA. *Signalering Overgewicht in de Jeugdgezondheidszorg*. Amsterdam: VuMC, 2004.

107 Hermanussen M, Burmeister J. Synthetic growth reference charts. *Acta Paediatr* 1999; **88**: 809–14.

108 Hermanussen M, Meigen C. Synthetic standards for body weight. *Homo* 2003; **54**: 142–56.

109 Kuczmarski RJ, Ogden CK, Gummer-Strawn LM, *et al*. CDC Growth Charts: United States. Hyattsville, MD: National Center for Health Statistics. Available from hhtp://www.cdc.gov/growthcharts/.

110 Cole TJ, Freeman JV, Preece MA. British 1990 growth reference centiles for weight, height, body mass index and head circumference fitted by maximum penalized likelihood. *Stat Med* 1998; **17**: 407–29.

111 Sorva R, Perheentupa J, Tolppanen EM. A novel format for a growth chart. *Acta Paediatr Scand* 1984; **73**: 527–9.

112 Cole TJ. 3-in-1 weight monitoring chart. *Lancet* 1997; **349**: 1020–30.

113 Cole TJ. Presenting information on growth distance and conditional velocity in one chart: practical issues of chart design. *Stat Med* 1998; **17**: 2697–707.

114 Mul D, Fredriks AM, van Buuren S, *et al*. Pubertal development in The Netherlands 1965–1997. *Pediatr Res* 2000; **50**: 479–86.

115 Hastie TJ, Tibshirani RJ. *Generalized Additive Models*. London: Chapman and Hall, 1990.

116 Wade AM, Ades AE, Salt AT, *et al*. Age-related standards for ordinal data: modelling the changes in visual acuity from 2 to 9 years of age. *Stat Med* 1995; **14**: 257–66.

117 Wade AM, Salt AT, Proffitt RV, *et al*. Likelihood-based modelling of age-related normal ranges for ordinal measurements: changes in visual acuity through early childhood. *Stat Med* 2004; **23**: 3623–40.

PART 2

GROWTH ASSESSMENT

12

Abnormal growth: Definition, pathogenesis, and practical assessment

MALCOLM D C DONALDSON, WENDY PATERSON

INTRODUCTION

Growth can be defined simply as increase in size, and is closely linked with development, that is, increase in specialization and skills. Growth and development can be subdivided into somatic growth, secondary sexual development, neurodevelopment, and psychological, social and educational development. In this chapter we examine indices of somatic growth and development, define abnormal growth, and consider the mechanisms for normal variant and abnormal growth patterns. Finally we outline a practical strategy for the assessment of abnormal growth.

MEASURES OF SOMATIC GROWTH

The principal parameters of somatic growth are supine length or height (which measure the skeleton), weight (measuring all tissues) and head circumference (reflecting brain growth).[1]

Assessment of supine length or height can be refined by measuring the upper and lower segments. This is done by measuring sitting height which, when subtracted from the standing height, gives the subischial leg length.[1–3] Other measures of skeletal growth are less commonly used and include arm span, length and size of hands, feet and limbs, and measurement of biacromial and bi-iliac diameter.[4]

Weight can be measured easily, and the degree of fatness crudely expressed as body mass index (BMI) (see below). Measurement of skin-fold thickness using the subscapular and triceps areas gives an index of fatness.[5] More specialized techniques are needed to accurately measure the body composition. Methods such as isotope dilution and bioelectrical impedance are not routinely available, but can be performed in specialist centers.[6] More recently, dual energy X-ray absorptiometry (DEXA) scanning has become available in many centers.[7] This technique is of value in assessing bone mineral content and density, fat free mass (e.g., muscle and bone), and fat mass.[7–9]

Measurement of head circumference gives a useful guide to normal growth and development until the age of about 2 years by which time the head has nearly achieved its adult size. Measures of facial structure such as the distance between the inner canthi are commonly used by dysmorphologists, and may be of value in the growth clinic in selected cases.

ESSENTIAL SKILLS FOR GROWTH ASSESSMENT

Table 12.1 lists the requirements for the assessment of growth. It is important that the measurement of children is

Table 12.1 Techniques required for growth and pubertal assessment

1   Accurate measurement of supine length (children aged >
    2 years), standing height, sitting height and weight
2   Measurement of parent and sibling heights
3   Calculation of decimal age
4   Calculation of body surface area
5   Calculation of height velocity
6   Calculation of midparental height and target range
7   Pubertal staging
8   Assessment of skeletal maturity (bone age)
9   Pelvic ultrasonography
    - uterine length, fundocervical ratio
    - presence/absence of endometrial echo
    - ovarian volume; number and size of follicles

widely taught and practiced, and for medical undergraduates and trainee nurses to be proficient not only in measurement techniques, but also in plotting data on the growth chart, and interpreting the information. Most of these skills will be within the scope of all healthcare professionals who deal with children, including family practitioners, school nurses and health visitors. However, some skills, assessment of skeletal maturity and pelvic ultrasonography for example, are best carried out by a few professionals who have a particular interest in the field.

MEASUREMENT OF LENGTH, HEIGHT, SITTING HEIGHT, AND WEIGHT

This is described in detail elsewhere (see Chapter 13) and will be dealt with only briefly here. Measurement of supine length requires time, patience, and at least two people, if the result is to be meaningful, and is the preferred measurement for children who are less than 2 years of age, or who are unable to stand unsupported.[2] In the best hands, measurement of supine length in small children has significant inter- and intraobserver variation, but if done carefully the result is of value whereas poor technique will yield information that is useless or (worse) misleading. Standing height measurement is much easier, although with younger children assistance may be required to keep the child straight and the heels on the ground. Sitting height measurement is usually confined to orthopedic and growth clinics. It is valuable in the recognition of children with disproportionate short stature and essential in the growth monitoring of childhood cancer survivors who may have received treatment (e.g., craniospinal radiotherapy) affecting segmental growth.[10] Weight should be measured with nothing on but the vest in children of less than 2 years of age because clothing (especially diapers/nappies) will materially affect the result. In older children, clothing is generally less important and only shoes and heavy outer garments need be removed.

Measurement of parental and sibling heights

Self-reported heights are unreliable and inadequate for clinical practice.[11] It is therefore highly desirable to measure both parents at the first clinic visit unless, of course, the child is adopted. Usually there is no problem, but sometimes the situation is delicate and requires tact and diplomacy. Occasionally, parents do not take kindly to being measured, and not infrequently the father is not the natural father but may not necessarily divulge this fact in front of the child. Often one parent is absent at the first clinic visit, in which case he or she should be measured at a later date.

Although measurement of siblings is not standard practice, there is a case for building this into routine growth assessment because family patterns are of value in making the distinction between normal and abnormal growth.[12]

Calculation of decimal age

In the table of decimals of year, printed on the back of the Buckler–Tanner 1995, Age 2–20 years (Castlemead Publications) and Child Growth Foundation Four-in-One Birth-20 years Decimal (Harlow Printing) height charts, each day is expressed as a fraction of the year in decimal format.[13] Thus if a child was born on 13 November 1981, his date of birth in decimals is expressed as 81.866. To calculate his decimal age at any particular date his birth date is subtracted from the actual date. For example, if the date is 10 January 1992 (92.025) the child's decimal age will be $92.025 - 81.866 = 10.159$ years.

Calculation of surface area

This can be calculated using the weight-based formula

$$\text{surface area} = \frac{(\text{weight} \times 4) + 7}{\text{weight} + 90}$$

where the surface area is in m^2 and the weight is in kg. This is the DuBois formula based on height and weight.[14] Alternatively, there is a height/weight nomogram from which surface area can be calculated.

Calculation of height velocity

This is calculated by dividing the difference in height (cm) by the difference in interval (years). For example, a child born on 28 March 1972, measuring 132.6 cm on 3 February 1981 and 138.2 cm on 4 January 1982 will have decimal ages at these times of 9.772 and 8.854 so that the height velocity (in cm year^{-1}) is

$$\frac{138.2 - 132.6}{9.772 - 8.854} = \frac{5.6}{0.918} = 6.1.$$

The workings do not need to be shown but the interval must be indicated when recording the height velocity. Although it is common practice in growth clinics to calculate height velocity over periods of 6 months to 1 year, the inherent error in height measurement (even when carried out by a single, trained observer using accurate equipment) is compounded by calculation of height velocity, particularly over short time intervals.[15] Caution must therefore be exercised in interpretation of height velocity, and the interval used should not be less that 6 months.

Calculation of midparental height and target range (Fig. 12.1)

For a worked example of this, please refer to the Appendix on page 674.

For boys, the father's height should be indicated at the right-hand side of the growth chart. As the mother's height must be plotted on a male chart, it is necessary to correct this (by adding the mean difference between adult male and female heights) to give the equivalent centile position. The midparental height (MPH), i.e., the mean of father's height and mother's corrected height, should then be plotted. Finally, target range is calculated as the MPH $+/-2$ SD (two standard deviation (SD) confidence limits).

For girls the same procedure applies, except that the mother's height is plotted directly and the father's height is corrected by subtracting the mean difference between adult male and female heights.[12] If at a later date reported heights are replaced with measured heights, the MPH and target range should be recalculated.

The formulae quoted for calculating MPH and target range vary from country to country, according to the type of growth chart used. In the UK, in the case of the Child Growth Foundation charts, a correction factor of 14 cm is applied, with the 2 SD confidence limits expressed as 10 cm for males and 8.5 cm for females. For the Buckler–Tanner charts, the correction factor is 13 cm and the 2 SD confidence limits are 10 cm for males and 9 cm for females.

With normal parents and physiological children their final heights will be normally distributed around the MPH, with only a 5 percent probability of falling outside the target range. In other words calculation of MPH and target range creates a growth curve specific to the child and family, with MPH representing the 50th centile, while the upper and lower ends of the target range correspond to the 2nd and 98th centiles.

From the age of 2 years, a normal child will have tracked onto his or her predestined centile and will remain on this centile until the time of puberty.[16] Thus the pre-pubertal height centile of most normal children will fall within the target range centiles. By contrast a child whose height centile is outside the target range centiles may have a growth disorder (see also Chapter 13).

Pubertal staging in boys and girls

This is a delicate area, but with tactful handling and proper explanation neither patient nor family should be upset.

The ideal situation is for girls to be examined by a female doctor or nurse and for boys to be examined by a male, but this is not always practicable. It is prudent to have a chaperone present (e.g., a parent or other member of staff) when examining the child.

Tanner's system of staging is well described and will not be discussed in detail.[17] The authors would stress the importance of careful testicular palpation in order to determine the volume, because simple inspection may be misleading especially in the early stages of puberty. Testicular volume can be assessed using the Prader orchidometer. Measurement of testicular length and breadth with a tape measure (multiplying these parameters to determine the volume) is more practical for physicians who do not routinely have orchidometers at their disposal. Penile development can be recorded by measuring the length and circumference of the penis and this is particularly helpful in monitoring progress through puberty.

In girls of normal or low weight the assessment of breast development is straightforward. However, in obese girls the distinction between stage 1 and 3 breast development can be difficult and in some cases pubertal status can only be determined by further investigation, such as pelvic ultrasonography and gonadotrophin-stimulation testing.

Bone age estimation and height prediction

The Tanner and Whitehouse system[18,19] is most commonly used in the UK, whereas Greulich and Pyle,[20] with Bayley–Pinneau[21] tables are more commonly used in the rest of Europe and North America. Whatever system of bone age assessment is adopted, it is important that it is done by someone experienced in the technique, the ideal situation being for a single observer to be used. Bone age is plotted on the growth chart by taking the height of the child on the date of the radiograph, and entering this as height for bone age. The height for chronological age and height for bone age are then linked by a dotted line (Fig. 12.1). In healthy children, the height for bone age is more representative of true height status than height for chronological age and should fall within the target range centiles. A rough final height estimate can be made by extrapolating the height centile for bone age to adult height, but this model is unreliable if bone age delay is in excess of two years. It is important to stress that final height cannot be predicted from height centile for bone age in children with endocrine disorders such as precocious puberty and growth hormone (GH) deficiency. Although height prediction is possible from early childhood, the authors have found it of most practical value from around the age of 10 years in girls and 11 in boys, and have demonstrated its accuracy and clinical utility in boys with physiological delay in puberty.[22] Other uses for bone age are in aiding diagnosis because marked delay or advance may indicate pathology. Sequential bone age estimation is important in monitoring treatment with growth hormone, oxandrolone, sex steroids, and hydrocortisone.

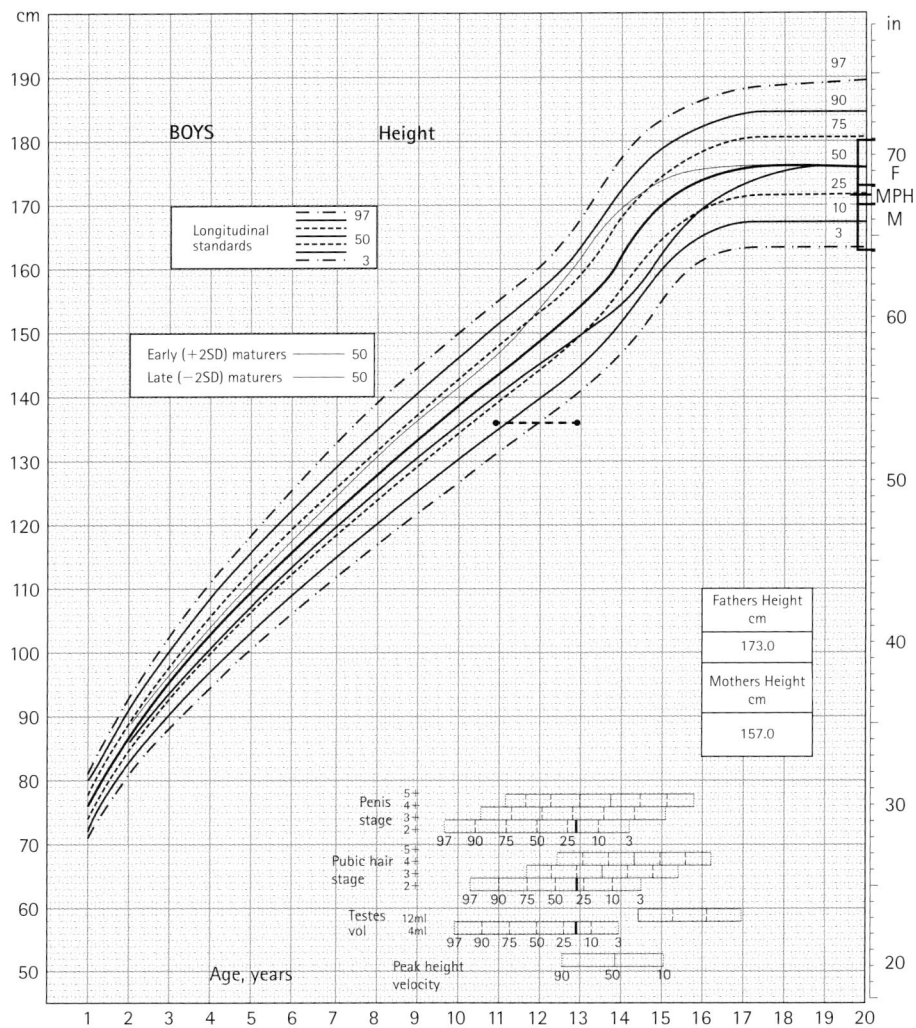

Figure 12.1   Growth chart (boy) showing height, height for bone age, midparental height and target range, and pubertal stages. (Reproduced with permission of Castlemead Publications.)

Pelvic ultrasonography

As for bone age estimation, pelvic ultrasonography should be done by an experienced observer. The parameters we use are uterine length, cervicofundal ratio, endometrial echo, ovarian volume, and the number and size of ovarian follicles.[23] The uterine changes reflect estrogen secretion and are reasonably reproducible. The authors have found ovarian size and morphology to be less helpful; indeed in a control study one or both ovaries were not identified in 15 percent of pre-pubertal control children.[23]

EXPRESSION OF GROWTH STATUS AND CHANGES IN GROWTH RATE

Plotting growth data accurately

Measurement of height and weight can be expressed in absolute values of centimeters and kilograms but it is more

helpful to put them into context as height or weight centile for chronological age (Fig. 12.1). A ball-point pen should be used to achieve a distinct small dot – not dots with circles, crosses and, above all, not crosses with circles! As mentioned previously, two types of growth chart are currently available in the UK. The Child Growth Foundation (1995) charts incorporate the nine centiles (0.4th to 99.6th) devised by T.J. Cole and cover the period from birth (including pre-term data) until 20 years of age.[24] They were constructed from cross-sectional data only. The Buckler–Tanner (1995) charts, a revised version of the former Tanner–Whitehouse (1975) charts, retain the familiar seven-centile format (3rd to 97th) and range from 2 to 20 years. They incorporate both cross-sectional and longitudinal data.[24–28]

Skeletal maturity

Skeletal maturity (bone age) can be expressed on the growth chart as height centile for bone age (see Fig. 12.1).

Bone age can also be expressed as a ratio of chronological age and bone age (CA:BA). Change in bone age can be expressed as bone age advance per chronological age (e.g., 2.3/2 years).

Puberty

Pubertal stages can be documented and expressed on the growth chart (see Fig. 12.1).

Height status

Height status for chronological age and bone age can be expressed as standard deviation scores according to the formulae:[13]

$$\frac{\text{child's height} - \text{mean height for age}}{1 \text{ SD for age}}$$

and

$$\frac{\text{height of child} - \text{mean height for bone age}}{1 \text{ SD for bone age}}.$$

The advantage of height standard deviation scores (height SDS) is that height data on groups of children of different age and sex can be pooled in a way that would not be possible using raw data.

Plotting height velocity

Height velocity is expressed as centimeters per year, as shown previously. Height velocity SDS can be derived from standard tables using the formula:[13]

$$\frac{\text{height velocity of child} - \text{mean height velocity for age}}{1 \text{ SD for age}}.$$

Adjustments must be made for the pubertal stage of the child and the age at which peak height velocity occurred. Height velocity SDS is of some value in the statistical analysis of groups of children, but its usefulness is limited by the disproportionate effect of small measurement errors on the SDS value. For individual children, especially those with particular growth problems (e.g., GH deficiency, precocious puberty, adrenal hyperplasia), it is best to use height velocity charts.[13] The height velocity value for each clinic visit is expressed as a horizontal bar spanning the time interval. By joining the midpoints the dynamics of the child's growth are represented (Fig. 12.2).

Weight status

Weight status should be expressed in relation to height, either by comparing height and weight centiles or by calculating body mass (Quetelet's) index according to the formula

$$\frac{\text{weight}}{\text{height}^2}$$

where weight is in kilograms and height is in meters. Overweight and obesity can be defined using the nine-centile UK chart devised by Cole et al.[29] as BMI above the 91st and 98th centiles, respectively, while BMI below the 2nd centile denotes a child who is significantly underweight (Fig. 12.3). Weight velocity charts exist, but are rarely used.

Recognition of normal growth and its variants

The following are factors that influence growth:

- Age
- Sex
- Race
- Nutrition
- Birth weight
- Parental heights
- Puberty
- Skeletal maturity
- Chronic disease
- Specific growth disorders
- Socioeconomic status
- Emotional factors

These all need to be considered when assessing the individual child. Normal growth has been covered in Chapters 8 and 9, and only the key points will be reiterated here, which can be summarized as follows:

1. Growth can be divided into three phases: the infantile phase which represents a continuation of intrauterine growth and is dependent more on nutrition, insulin, insulin-like growth factors (IGFs), and thyroxine than on growth hormone; the childhood phase of growth which is predominantly GH dependent and decelerating, particularly in the latter stages; and the pubertal phase which is sex steroid and GH dependent and ends with the attainment of adult final height.[30]
2. Birth size is influenced by the intrauterine environment while height during childhood is partially influenced by the parental heights together with the child's general health and nutrition. The authors describe the phenomenon of 'catch-up' or 'lag-down' growth,[16] whereby a newborn infant grows towards his or her genetically determined height centile, as tracking, and this is achieved by 2 years. Thereafter the child should stay on the same height centile until puberty.

cm/yr

GIRLS — Height velocity

Longitudinal whole-year centiles
when peak velocity occurs at average age — 97 / 50 / 3
when peak velocity occurs at early and late limits of age (entire curves fall within shaded limits) — 97 / 50 / 3

Published by
Castlemead Publications
Swains Mill, 4A Crane Mead
Ware, Herts SG129PY
A division of Ward's Publishing Services
Chart prepared by J.M. Tanner and
R. H. Whitehouse
University of London Institute of Child Health
for the
Hospital for Sick Children Great Ormond street
London WCI
© Castlemead Publication 1984
All rights are reserved No part of this chart may be reproduced, stored in a retrieval system or transmitted in any form or by any means, electronic, electrostatic, magnetic tape, mechanical photocopying, recording or otherwise without permission in writing from the copyright owner. All enquiries should be addressed to the publisher
Printed in England by Print Direction.

Age, years

97 90 75 50 3 10 25

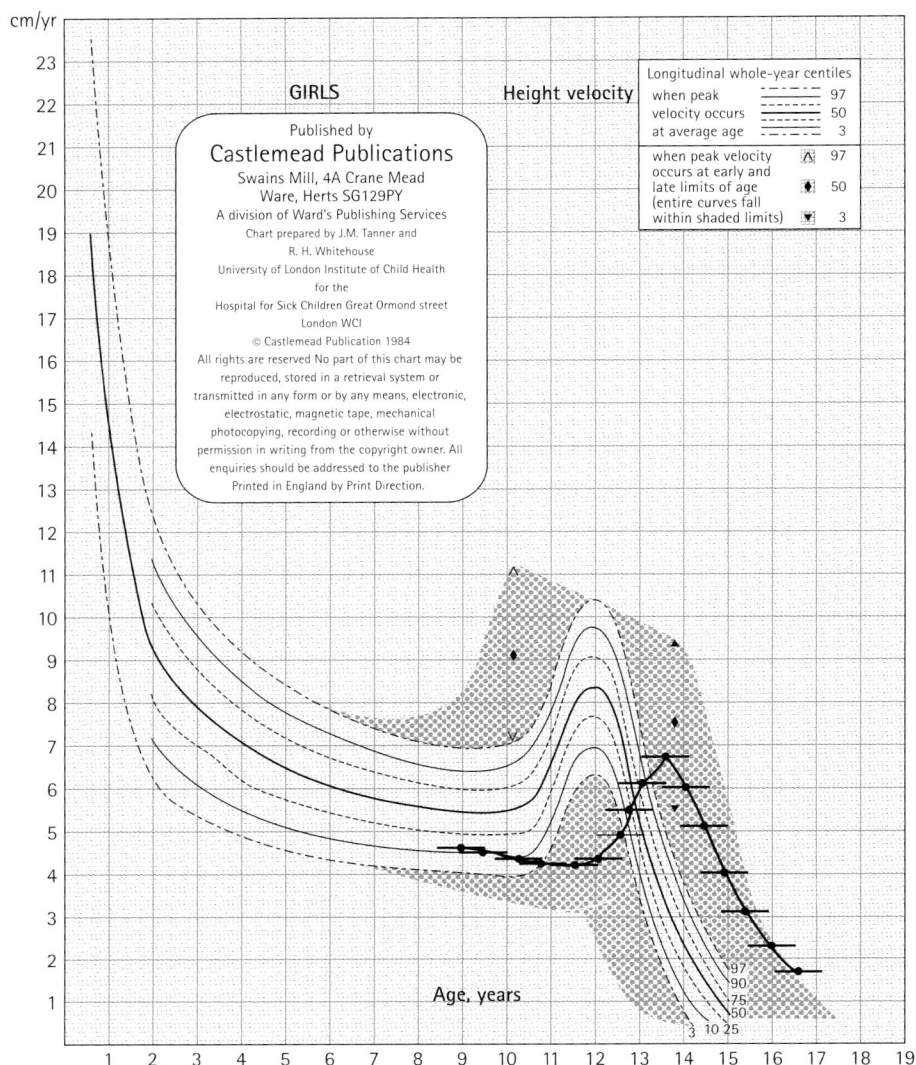

Figure 12.2   Height velocity chart of a girl with constitutional delay in growth and adolescence, showing 'rolling' height velocities. (Reproduced with permission of Castlemead Publications.)

3. The discrepancy between height centile during childhood and height centile in adulthood is accounted for by the variation in onset, intensity and duration of puberty. It is therefore not abnormal for a pubertal child to cross centiles.[28]

4. There is an inherent tendency for short children to have bone age delay and to show delay in adolescence with subsequent catch-up growth (Fig. 12.4). In these children the childhood phase of growth will be pronounced and consequently the degree of pre-pubertal deceleration will be more marked.

5. Tall children have an inherent tendency towards bone age advance with earlier adolescence and catch-down growth so that final height centile is less than childhood centile, i.e., a mirror image of the short child (Fig. 12.4).

6. A normal child will, from the age of 2 years onwards, usually grow within the parental target range centile. However, children with physiological delay or advance in growth may lie outside the parental target range, but in these cases the height centile for bone age will be within the target range (Fig. 12.5).

7. In normal children and adolescents, it is possible to carry out prediction of final adult height based on skeletal maturity, chronological age and actual height. However, the correlation between actual final adult height and predicted adult height for the individual can never be certain because so many variables are involved in determining the outcome of growth, the most important of which is puberty.

DEFINITION OF ABNORMAL GROWTH

Abnormal growth can be broadly defined as a disturbance in the normal process of linear growth, commensurate weight gain, and secondary sexual development such that

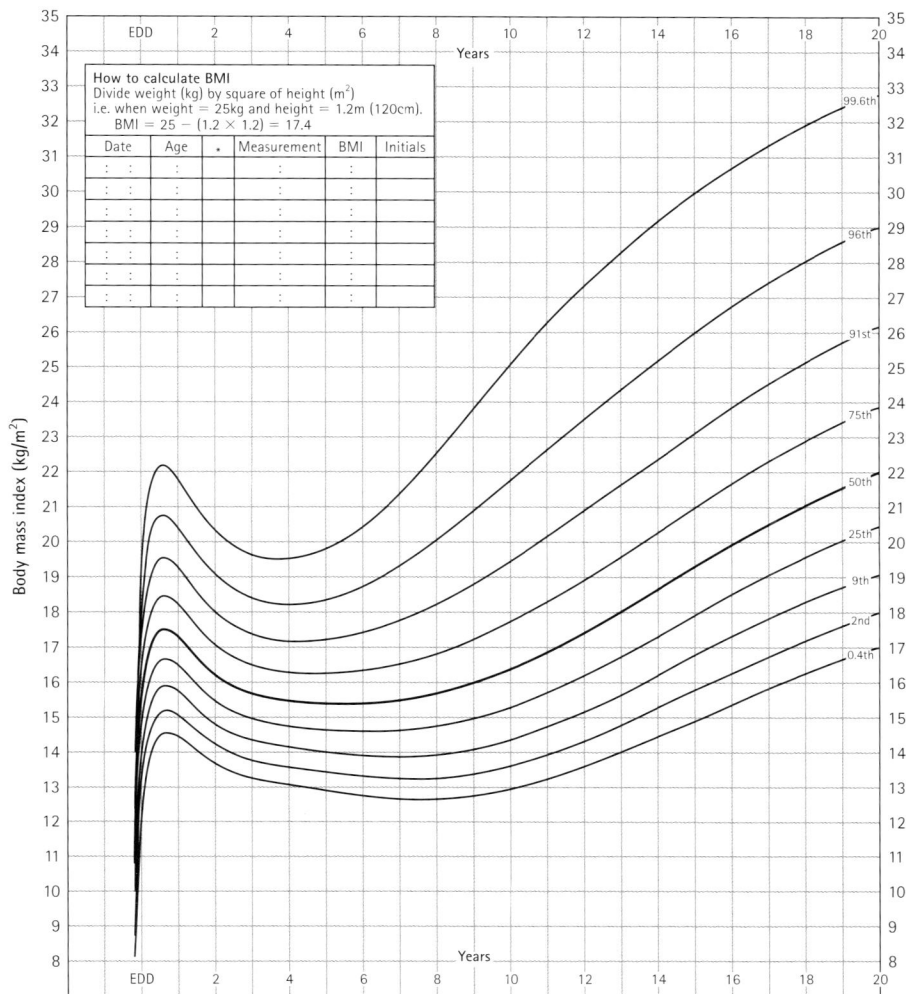

Figure 12.3 Body mass index chart (boy). EDD, estimated date of delivery. (Reproduced with permission of the Child Growth Foundation.)

the individual faces problems whether in childhood, adolescence or adulthood of a physical, psychological or social nature. Perhaps the most obvious example of abnormal growth is that of growth failure (from causes such as skeletal dysplasia and GH deficiency), resulting in a reduction in adult height with psychosocial consequences. Abnormalities of growth during childhood may lead to important problems in adult life, for example, the possible association between insulin resistance during childhood (secondary to simple obesity) and the development of polycystic ovarian disease in adolescence and adulthood.[31,32]

DEFINITION AND TYPES OF COMMON GROWTH PROBLEMS

If a boy of 14 is below the 3rd centile for height, in only the earliest stages of puberty, and enduring considerable teasing at school, there is clearly a problem. However, in the great majority of cases such delay in growth and adolescence

will be a normal variant, and not a growth abnormality. It is helpful therefore to think in terms of growth problems rather than concentrating purely on abnormal growth. A growth problem can be defined as an alteration in growth from the normal pattern sufficient to cause concern to the child, parent or doctor.

The following are the types of growth problem commonly encountered in children:

- Short stature
- Failure to thrive
- Growth failure
- Tall stature
- Obesity
- Delayed puberty
- Sexual precocity

The term 'short stature' simply means that the child's height is below the 2nd or 3rd centile for age (roughly equivalent to 2 SD below the mean). It says nothing about

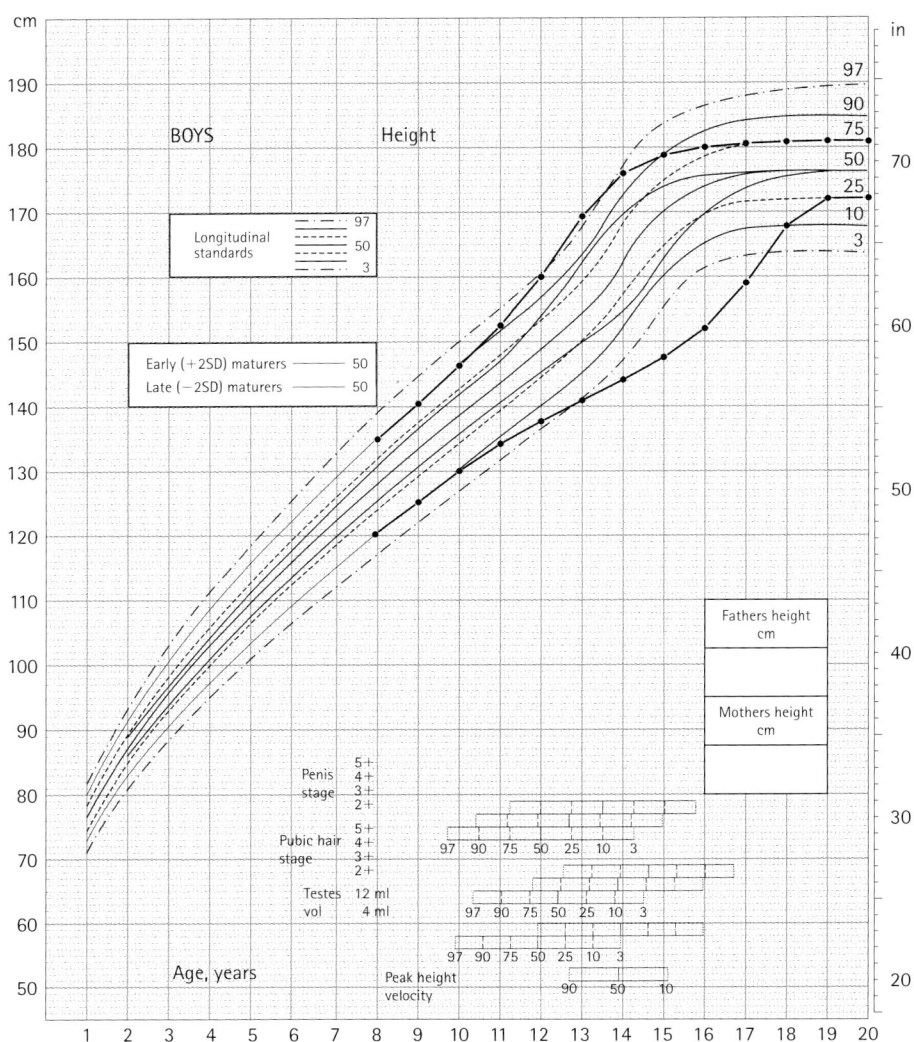

Figure 12.4 Growth chart (boy) showing the classic pattern of short stature and delayed adolescence in one individual, tall stature and advanced puberty in another. Note that adult heights for both subjects are closer to the mean than their childhood heights. (Reproduced with permission of Castlemead Publications.)

the underlying cause and is not itself a growth abnormality; indeed most children with short stature are normal. Growth failure is defined as the failure of a child to achieve and maintain a height velocity that is normal for age and maturity. Growth failure by definition is abnormal, but it can be difficult clinically to distinguish between slow growth caused by abnormality and slow growth caused by a more pronounced deceleration in the childhood component of the growth curve than usual, a situation commonly encountered in constitutional delay (see Fig. 12.5).[33] Failure to thrive or weight faltering are terms usually applied to infants and pre-school children and denote a failure to gain weight at an appropriate rate so that the child is thin. The term 'failure to thrive' must be used carefully. Some children are referred to the growth clinic with 'failure to thrive' because their weight is below the 3rd centile, when in fact they are short and normally nourished. Failure to thrive can be subdivided into organic and

non-organic, the latter being likely unless there are pointers in the clinical history and examination to suggest disease. Obesity has already been mentioned, and can be defined as weight more than three major centiles above height on the new nine-centile growth chart,[34] or body mass index above the 98th centile.[29] Tall stature is defined as height above the 97th or 98th centile (roughly equivalent to 2 SD above the mean).

The terms used to describe advanced secondary sexual development can cause confusion. In this chapter the term 'sexual precocity' is used to describe early sexual development of any etiology in children. The term 'precocious puberty' is defined as normal puberty, mediated by the hypothalamus, occurring abnormally early: before the age of 8 years in girls and 9 years in boys. The term 'early (or advanced) puberty' refers to normal puberty occurring between the ages of 8 and 10 years in girls and 9 and 11 years in boys.

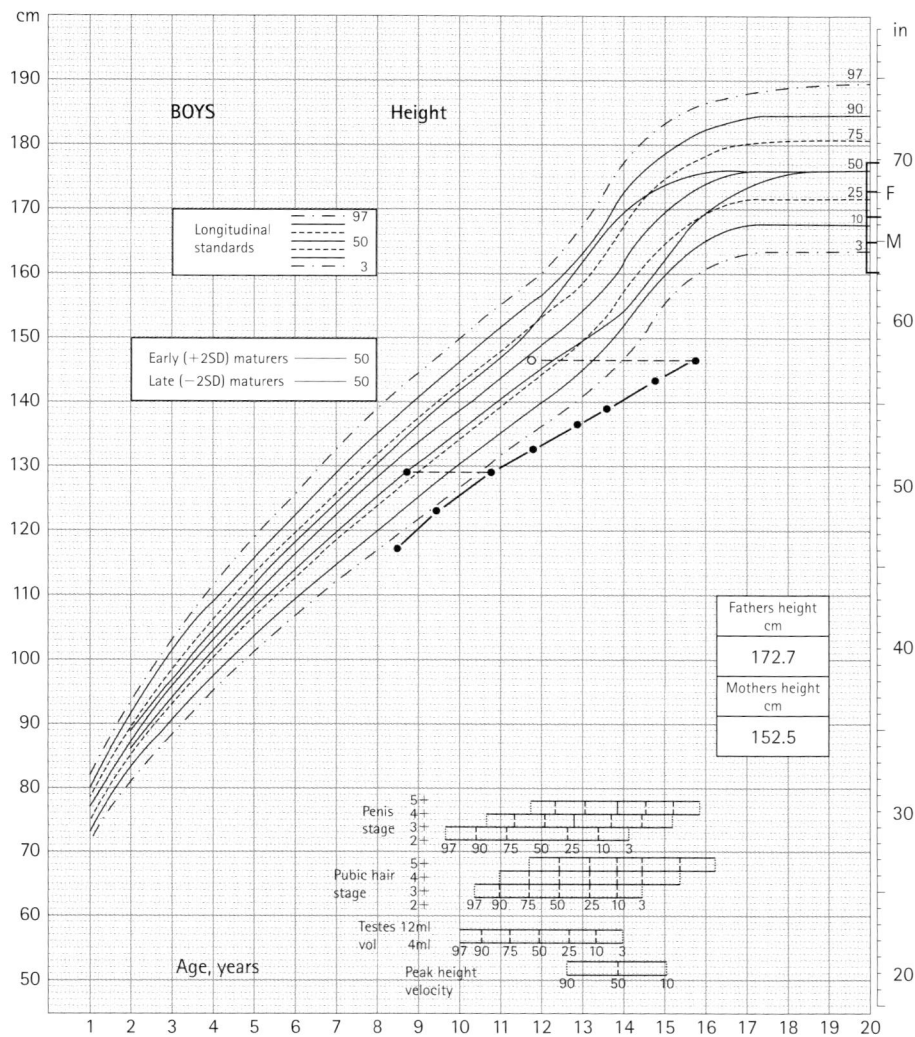

Figure 12.5 Height for chronological age is outside the parental target range centiles but height for bone age is within the target range in this child with constitutional delay. (Reproduced with permission of Castlemead Publications.)

There is no satisfactory definition of delayed puberty. A working definition is delay in the appearance and/or progression of secondary sexual characteristics sufficient to cause concern to the boy or girl, family or physician. The absence of any secondary sexual development in a girl aged 14 years and a boy aged 15 years obviously carries a higher risk of pathology, but this is not a particularly helpful dictum in clinical practice.

CLINICAL ASSESSMENT OF CHILDREN WITH GROWTH PROBLEMS

History taking and examination

By taking a thorough history and conducting a good general examination most growth problems can be managed without recourse to investigations other than assessment of skeletal maturity and, sometimes, pelvic ultrasonography. As short stature is by far the most common problem referred to the growth clinic, it is used here as a model for describing the history taking and examination.

Presenting complaint

It is important at the outset of the consultation to establish exactly who it is that feels there to be a problem and what the nature of the problem is. Usually, it is the family who seek medical referral, but in some instances children are referred by the school doctor or family practitioner for an endocrine opinion following the detection of short stature. Height may be the principal concern but sometimes it is more the child's build and weight. In adolescents with pubertal delay the lack of secondary sexual development may be of equal or greater concern than the height.

History of presenting complaint

This can be divided into three components. First, the pattern of growth should be determined. Second, an enquiry as to any symptoms of ill health, which might have led to the short stature, should be made. Third, a sensitive history is required to determine what, if any, consequences the short stature is having in terms of emotional distress and disadvantage.

Ideally, the pattern of growth will have been established by previous measurements, but this is not always the case. The obvious starting question in short stature is whether or not the child has always been small, to which the answer is usually 'yes'. Parents should be asked to pinpoint the age at which they noticed their child to be small: this may be by the end of the first year or at primary school entry, or (in the case of delayed adolescence) from the age of 10 years onwards. An idea of growth rate can be obtained by asking if the child is growing steadily and keeping up with his peer group, or becoming relatively shorter with age. This question is not as useful as one would hope because parental perception of their child's height velocity is often inaccurate. Not infrequently parents will assert that their child has completely stopped growing although measurements refute this.

On the other hand, if the child is growing out of his clothes this is crude confirmation that growth is proceeding at a reasonable rate. In delayed adolescence both parents and child will notice a widening gap between patient and peer group.

With regard to accompanying symptoms that may suggest ill health, it is usually best to start by asking if the child is well despite being short. If the answer is a vigorous 'yes' then a complete review of systems is probably unnecessary. However, vague symptoms such as tiredness and lack of energy require careful evaluation. Table 12.2 lists the standard review of systems that is used at the authors' hospital in Glasgow. Endocrine-related questions include headache, polydipsia, nocturia, cold intolerance and energy level.

The psychological effects of short stature have been the subject of considerable debate for many years.[35–37] It could be argued that questions about psychological distress should be left until the end of the consultation, but in practice it is helpful to get an early idea of the extent of the problem. The clinician must steer a course between being dismissive about small size and treating the problem as if it were a major disaster. It may be helpful to phrase the question thus:

> We see a lot of short boys and girls in this clinic. We know that some get very upset about their size and find it difficult to manage at school, join in activities and so on, but we also know that others don't seem to mind at all. However, we usually find that most people's feelings are somewhere in the middle. Where do you think you would put yourself?

This is an important moment in the consultation. Some children will burst into tears and say how dreadful they are

Table 12.2 Review of systems in children with suspected chronic disease

Gastrointestinal
  Appetite
  Eating habits
  Weight status
  Vomiting
  Abdominal pain
  Diarrhea/constipation

ENT
  Persistent and troublesome upper respiratory, ear, and throat infections
  Otitis media with effusion and intermittent deafness
  Snoring

Respiratory tract
  History of asthma
  Troublesome cough, wheeze or breathlessness
  Night sweats

Cardiovascular system
  History of cardiac problem or heart murmur
  Genitourinary system
  Polyuria and polydipsia; nocturia and enuresis; history of urinary tract infection; itching; pallor; lack of energy; history of cryptorchidism/orchidopexy

Central nervous system
  Headache
  Problems with balance
  Deterioration in vision; development of squint
  Hearing loss

feeling. More often than not the child will tend to understate his or her distress. Sometimes the parents will intervene and say that the child is doing less well academically than previously, avoiding outside activities and having a restricted social life.

Medical history

With a very complicated patient it is helpful to peruse the notes before consultation and list the problems, operations and hospital admissions in chronological order. The birth place, birth weight, gestation, and mode of delivery should be noted, and also whether there were any neonatal problems including jaundice and hypoglycemia. If the child was small for gestational age (birth weight below the 2nd or 3rd centile) details of health during the pregnancy should be sought including cigarette and alcohol consumption and problems with high blood pressure.

It is important to ask the parents if the child has asthma, which is very common in the general population and an important factor in delayed puberty.[38] A history of previous or continuing problems with recurrent middle ear infection and effusion in a girl with short stature should always raise suspicion of Turner syndrome.

Family history

A good family history is of great value and can avoid absurd situations where one child is singled out for rigorous endocrine investigation and perhaps treatment whereas siblings of comparable short stature are never even seen in the clinic. A family tree should be constructed, obtaining the first name, age, and height of each family member. As stated above, parents should be measured in the clinic and asked if each sibling is tall, average or short in comparison with his or her peer group, also how tall he or she is in relation to the patient. This is important because younger siblings can be as tall or taller than the patient, a concern that might not have been expressed at the start of the consultation.

Having established the family structure and heights, the clinician should then enquire about puberty. In women the simplest question to ask is about menarche and the answer is usually reliable. No such milestone exists for men, and considerable patience is required to elicit useful information. A good question to ask about delayed puberty is 'were you late in growing compared with your friends, or did you keep growing after you left school?' There may be a history of delayed puberty in second-degree relatives.

Social and developmental history

The educational and social history is valuable both in terms of diagnosis and management. For example mild to moderate educational difficulties may be part of an underlying dysmorphic syndrome while specific difficulty with mathematics in a girl may indicate Turner syndrome. A particularly troubled social situation in a child with short stature and growth failure may point to a psychosocial element.

The name of the school that the child attends, the class he or she is in, and whether this is age appropriate should be established. The child can be asked if he or she finds the work easy, difficult or average compared with the class, and the parents can be asked about school reports and how they would rate their child in ability. If it seems that the child is below average then enquiry should be made as to whether there is extra help with certain subjects. School attendance is an important index of child and adolescent health, and parents can be asked to estimate the number of days or weeks missed during a school term or academic years.

Details of housing, employment, and social difficulties may be appropriate. If the home situation is obviously problematic it is easier to carry out this part of the interview in the child's absence.

EXAMINATION

The process of examination begins before the child has entered the room by plotting the height, weight, and parental heights. It is important to ensure that the child's appearance

tallies with the growth chart! If not then the measurements may be wrong or the data incorrectly transcribed. During the consultation the clinician will have gained an impression of the child's build, demeanor, color, general health and, where appropriate, signs of dysmorphism.

The distinction between true dysmorphism and exaggerations of normal features (e.g., big nose, large ears etc.!) is not difficult in practice. Dysmorphic children usually have a constellation of recognizable anomalies, e.g., small chin, malar hypoplasia, simple/low set/posteriorly rotated ears, long philtrum, etc., which, in combination with problems such as short/tall stature and learning difficulties, suggest one of a multitude of syndromes.[39] The appreciation that a child is dysmorphic should be followed by a careful assessment of cardiovascular system (given the increased incidence of cardiac malformation in conditions such as Down, Noonan, Turner and Williams syndromes).

The clinician should conduct a full general examination, looking for signs of chronic disease including anemia, jaundice, and finger clubbing. With reference to children with short stature the following are important:

- *Hands.* Features of dysmorphism such as incurving of the little finger (clinodactyly) and (in girls) the slightly puffy fingers, tapering distal phalanges, hyperconvex nails and increased nail folds typical of Turner syndrome.
- *Face.* Dysmorphic features.
- *Neck.* Presence of goiter.
- *Skin.* Café-au-lait patches with or without axillary freckling are features of neurofibromatosis, which is often associated with short stature.
- *Cardiovascular system.* The blood pressure should always be checked. In girls, especially, the femoral pulses must be palpated.
- *Respiratory system.* The chest shape should be carefully examined for chronic deformity as a result of conditions such as asthma and cystic fibrosis.
- *Abdomen.* Inspection for abdominal distension (e.g., from malabsorption) and palpation for organomegaly and masses (e.g., resulting from Crohn's disease).
- *Central nervous system.* Examination of the fundi in every case. Where a pituitary lesion is suspected visual fields and pupillary reactions must be examined.
- *Pubertal status.* See above

CLINICAL DIAGNOSIS IN CHILDREN WITH GROWTH PROBLEMS

Once the history taking and examination have been completed the clinician should resist the temptation to carry out any investigations before writing down the most likely clinical diagnosis. With a combination of careful history and examination, and application of the essential skills in growth assessment mentioned earlier in this chapter, the correct clinical diagnosis can be made at the first consultation for most new referrals.

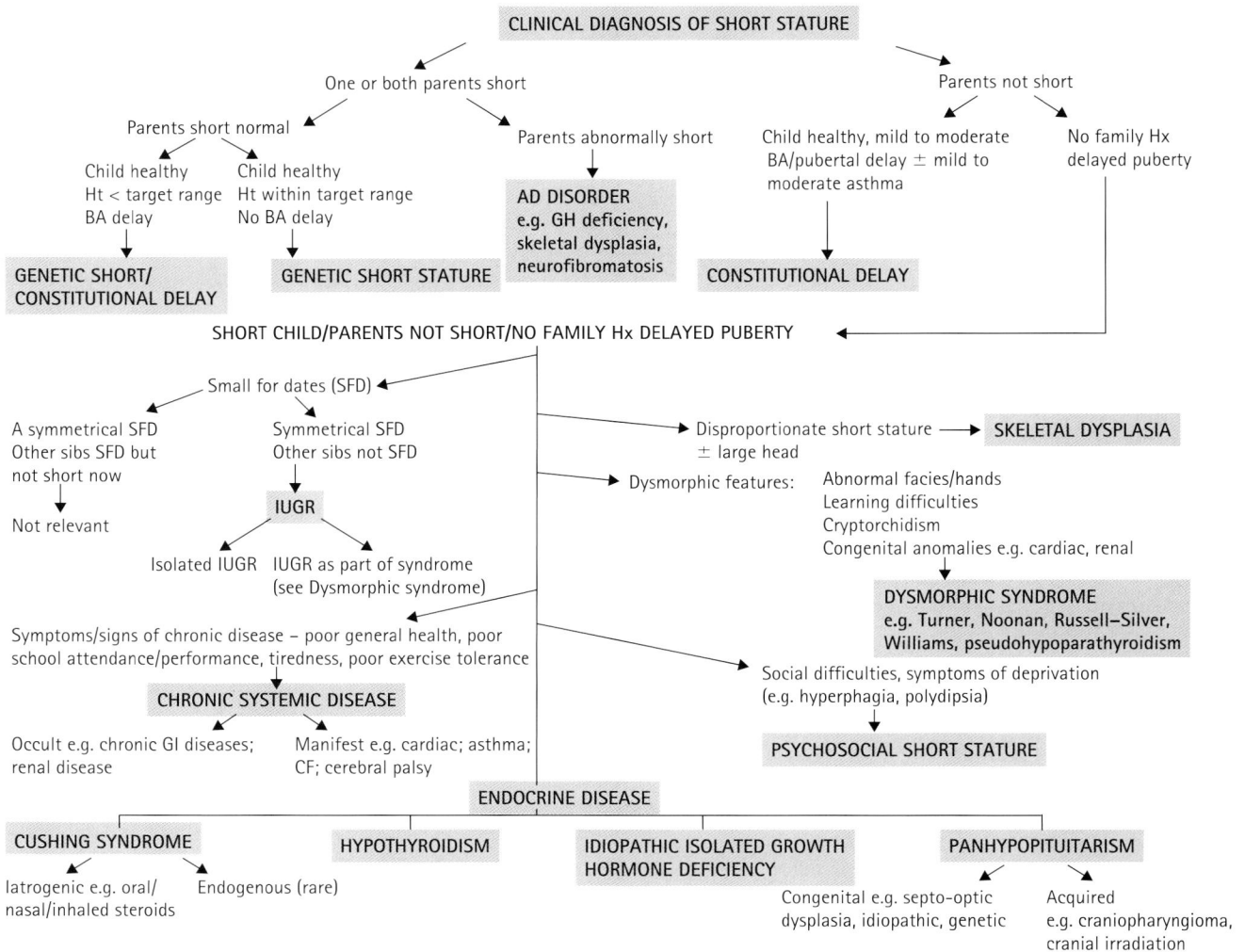

Figure 12.6 Flow chart to enable clinical diagnosis of children with short stature. AD, autosomal dominant; BA, bone age; CF, cystic fibrosis; GI, gastrointestinal; IUGR, intrauterine growth retardation.

Figures 12.6 to 12.10 show flow charts for establishing the clinical diagnosis in children presenting with five of the common growth problems: short stature, growth failure, tall stature, delayed puberty, and sexual precocity (obesity and failure to thrive are primarily nutritional problems and beyond the scope of this chapter). The following points should be made about these flow charts:

1. Their purpose is to establish a working diagnosis at the end of the first consultation. By definition, therefore, they do not mention growth surveillance yet this is obviously a crucial adjunct to investigation.
2. For tall and short stature and growth failure, in the UK the only initial investigation incorporated is bone age, which can be considered as an extension of the clinical measurements. In certain cases of delayed puberty determination of karyotype and gonadotrophins may be required to achieve a working diagnosis, and for sexual precocity the measurement of gonadotrophins before and after stimulation with luteinizing hormone-releasing hormone (LHRH) may be essential. With

these exceptions, the flow charts rely on clinical assessment only.
3. An inherent shortcoming in these flow charts is their failure to take into account the multifactorial nature of growth problems. For instance, a child may be short as a result of a combination of short parents, social and emotional difficulties, poor nutrition and a chronic disorder such as asthma.

Bearing these caveats in mind, each growth problem will be briefly considered.

SHORT STATURE (SEE FIG. 12.6)

Most short children have either normal genetic short stature, constitutional delay or a combination of the two. Caution must be exercised in making the diagnosis of normal genetic short stature when one of the parents is particularly short, and in this instance the possibility of a dominant growth disorder should be considered such as one of the

DIAGNOSIS AND PRACTICAL INVESTIGATION OF GROWTH FAILURE

Height trajectory crossing centile lines or deviating from lowest centile

Recheck measurement

Previous/current measurement incorrect → **MEASUREMENT ERROR**

Measurement correct → Check plotting of measurement

Incorrect → **TRANSCRIPTION ERROR**

Correct

Child <9yr OR deceleration too pronounced to attribute to physiological delay

Child 9–14 yr → **?PERIPUBERTAL/EARLY PUBERTAL CHILD WITH PHYSIOLOGICAL DECELERATION DUE TO CONSTITUTIONAL DELAY**

GROWTH FAILURE

History of asthma

No history of asthma

Asthma now mild Not on inhaled steroids

Irrelevant/coincidental

Asthma moderate/severe ± on inhaled steroids

ASTHMA-RELATED CONSTITUTIONAL DELAY

CHRONIC ASTHMA CAUSING GROWTH FAILURE

GROWTH FAILURE SECONDARY TO INHALED STEROIDS

Symptoms/signs suggestive of chronic disease

Ix FOR CHRONIC DISEASE e.g. celiac, inflammatory bowel, chronic renal failure

Dysmorphism/learning difficulties/short stature

DYSMORPHIC SYNDROME e.g. Turner, skeletal dysplasia

Growth failure despite weight gain/obesity

HYPOTHYROIDISM CUSHING'S SYNDROME

Social difficulties ± hyperphagia, polydipsia, enuresis

PSYCHOSOCIAL GROWTH FAILURE

GROWTH HORMONE DEFICIENCY

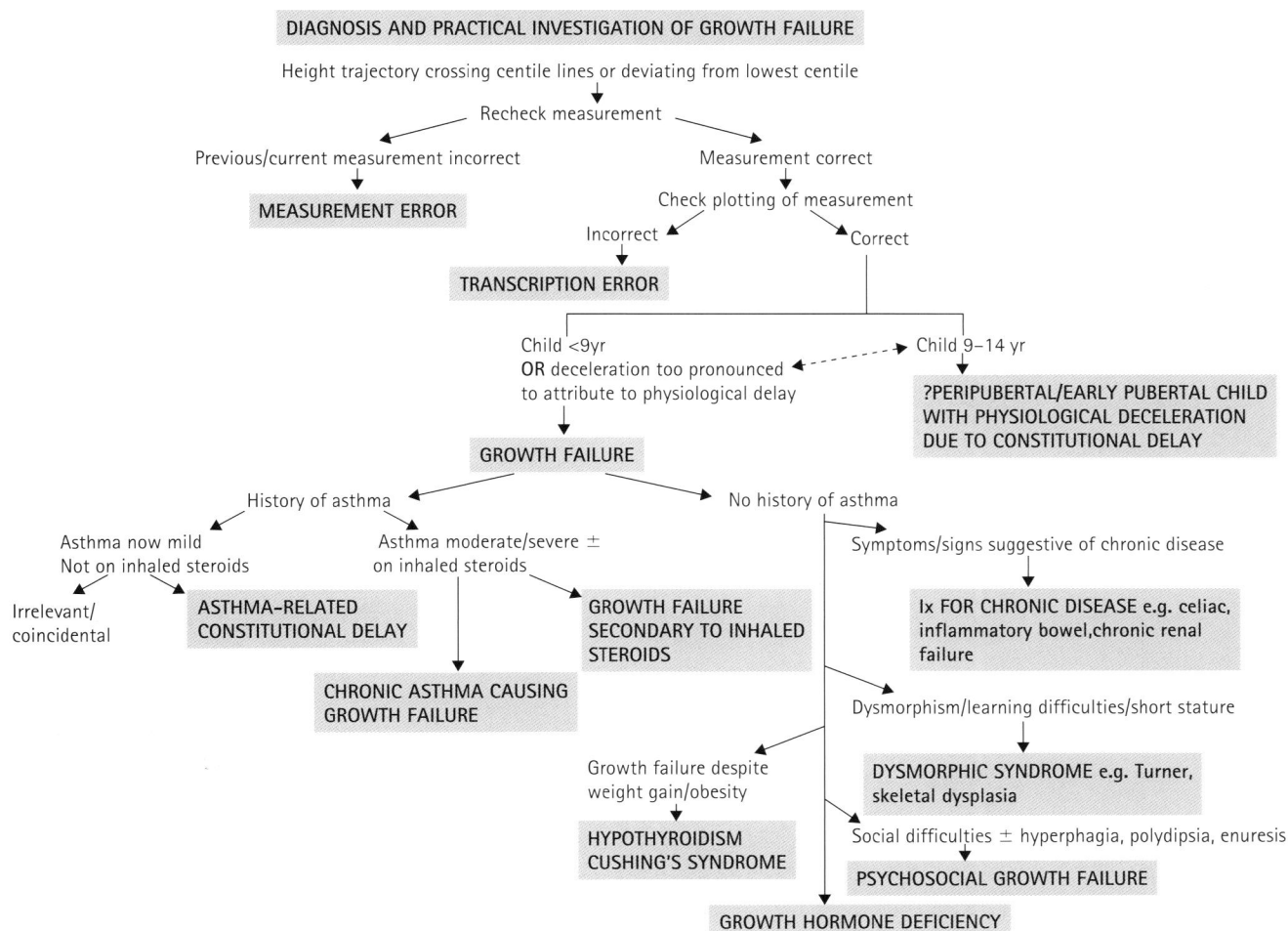

Figure 12.7   Flow chart to enable clinical diagnosis of children with growth failure.

skeletal dysplasias, autosomal dominant growth hormone deficiency and neurofibromatosis.[40] Less commonly, a child will be short despite normal-sized parents and no family history of delayed puberty, requiring careful evaluation. Smallness for gestational age (SGA) is a potential cause of short stature during childhood. However it should be remembered that most children with SGA show catch-up growth, so SGA cannot be automatically assumed to be the main contributory factor. The prevalence of dysmorphic syndromes in children with short stature has already been mentioned, and a wide range of syndromes including Turner, Williams, Noonan, Russell–Silver and Prader–Willi syndromes have been diagnosed on clinical assessment in the authors' growth clinic. Skeletal dysplasia, often indeterminate in nature, is an important cause of inappropriate short stature and important clinical clues include large head, increased lumbar lordosis, limb and spine disproportion, and advance in skeletal maturity. Although chronic disease is a potent cause of short stature, affected children rarely present with this. However, certain conditions, including inflammatory bowel disease, celiac disease and chronic renal failure, are notoriously silent and may present to the growth clinic with short stature, slow growth and delayed puberty.

The importance of socioeconomic and emotional deprivation in causing short stature has been underestimated in the past, and there is now clear evidence that severe deprivation may result in functional hypopituitarism: the polydipsic, hyperphagic, growth failure syndrome.[41] Unfortunately, this is often diagnosed retrospectively when the child has shown a poor response to GH therapy.

Endocrine causes of short stature form a small but important minority of referrals. Iatrogenic short stature caused by steroid therapy is not usually a diagnostic problem, whereas endogenous steroid excess is extremely rare. However, the authors have recently seen a number of children with short stature and growth failure resulting from the systemic effect of steroid nose-drops, and this may be a more important factor in short stature than has been previously recognized.[42] Rarely, inhaled steroids taken for asthma can cause short stature[43] (see Figs 12.13 and 12.14). Hypothyroidism is an uncommon cause of short stature because congenital hypothyroidism is treated from birth as a result of neonatal screening, while children with acquired hypothyroidism will have growth failure rather than short stature (unless they had borderline short stature predating the onset of hypothyroidism).

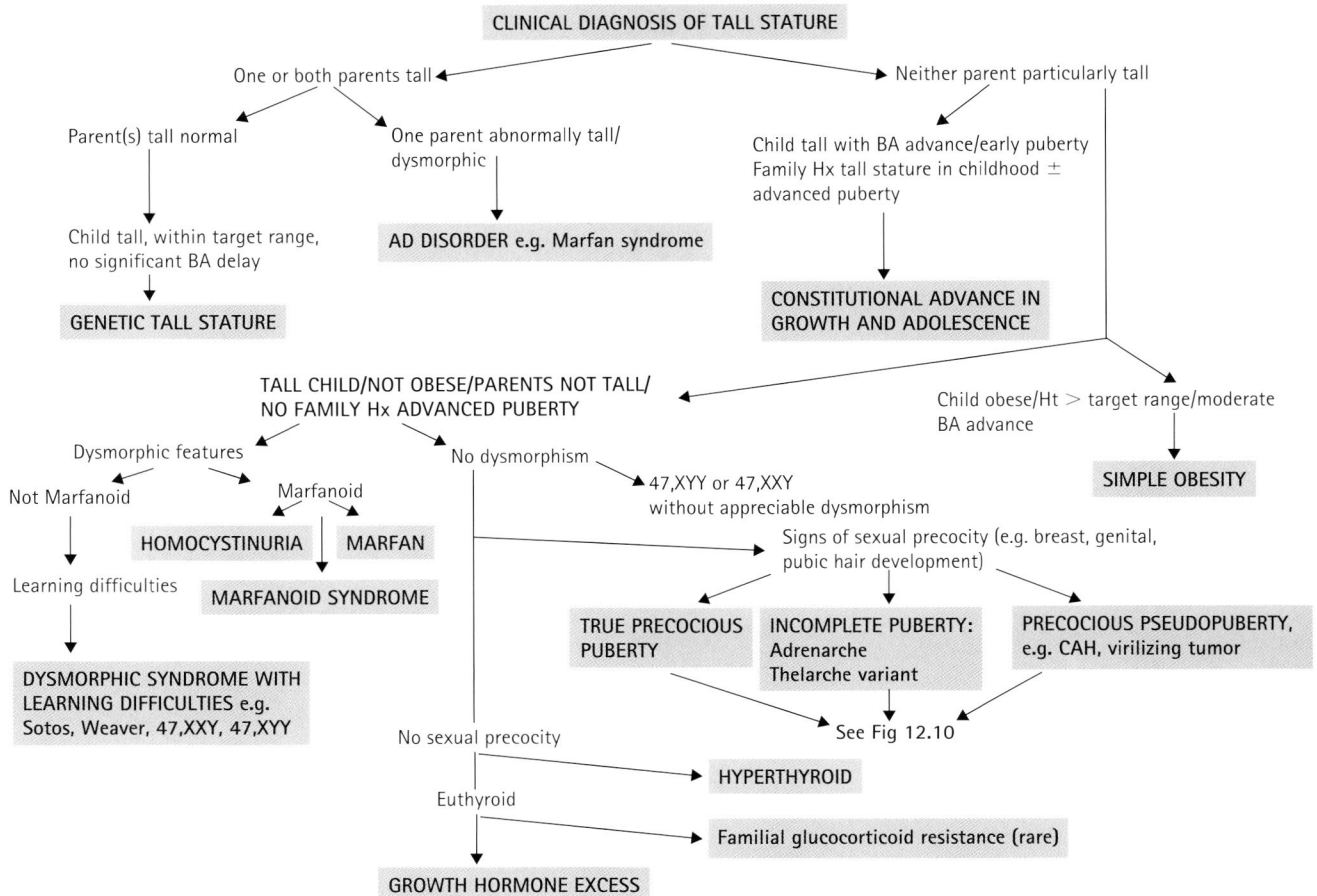

Figure 12.8 Flow chart to enable clinical diagnosis of children with tall stature. AD, autosomal dominant; BA, bone age; CAH, congenital adrenal hyperplasia.

The diagnosis of GH deficiency is secure if there are associated multiple anterior pituitary deficiencies and/or relevant clinical associations, e.g., neonatal jaundice and hypoglycemia, optic nerve hypoplasia, previous cranial irradiation, and craniopharyngioma.[44]

By contrast, the diagnosis of idiopathic isolated GH deficiency is much less clear and, even after careful evaluation of height status, height velocity, parental heights, bone age and stimulated GH levels, the distinction between isolated GH deficiency and constitutional delay/genetic short stature may still be difficult.[45]

More recently, research has focused on the molecular basis of idiopathic short stature (ISS).[46,47] For example, SHOX (short stature homeobox-containing gene) deletions have been identified in around 2 percent of children investigated for ISS.[48,49] Another significant area of study is the identification of molecular defects of the GH–IGF axis. Children investigated for ISS often have low or low/normal IGF-I levels in the context of normal GH secretion, suggesting GH insensitivity.[50,51] The most common etiology of GH insensitivity is a mutation or deletion of the gene for the growth hormone receptor (GHR). The severity of the defect varies widely, with poor correlation between genotype and clinical and biochemical phenotype in GH insensitivity

syndrome.[52] In addition, there have been reports of dysfunctional mutations in the GH gene (GH1), IGF-I mutations and genetic defects affecting components of the GH signaling pathway.[53–56] Other candidate genes include IGF receptors, IGF binding proteins and the IGF signaling cascade, while epiphyseal unresponsiveness to IGFs and other growth factors comprise another area of potential research.[47]

Investigation of short stature

If initial assessment suggests that the child may have an underlying disorder, day-case admission for screening investigations of short stature is indicated. Table 12.3 shows the short stature screening protocol used in the authors' hospital in Glasgow. Note that it is important to exclude systemic disorders such as celiac disease before subjecting children to endocrine stimulation testing.

Detailed endocrine assessment is required in a minority of the children referred with short stature. Protocols for combined pituitary assessment comprise insulin or clonidine, LHRH and thyrotrophin-releasing hormone (TRH) stimulation. In children under 5 years of age, arginine may be used in preference to clonidine or insulin, in which case

CLINICAL DIAGNOSIS OF DELAYED PUBERTY

Boy or girl with delayed/absent secondary sexual development

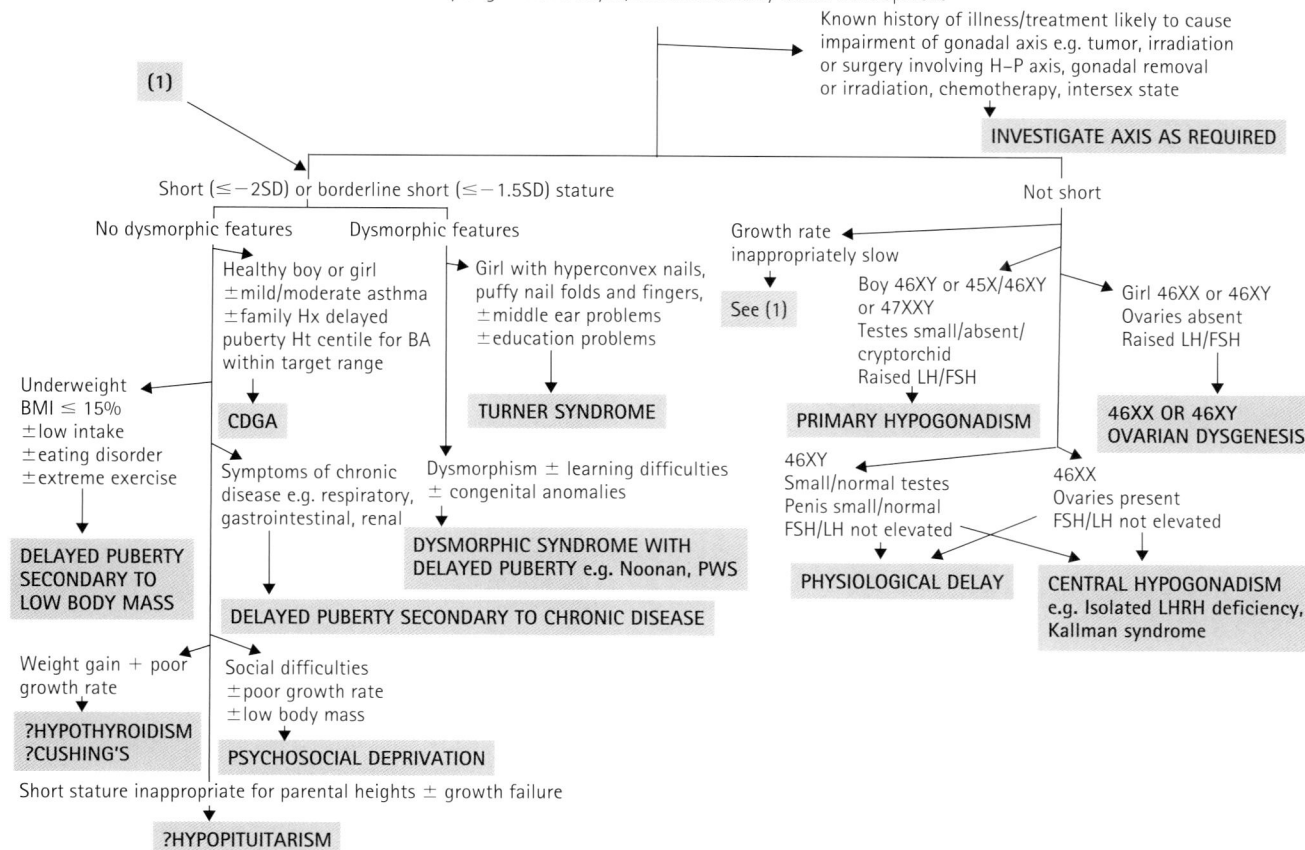

Known history of illness/treatment likely to cause impairment of gonadal axis e.g. tumor, irradiation or surgery involving H–P axis, gonadal removal or irradiation, chemotherapy, intersex state

INVESTIGATE AXIS AS REQUIRED

(1)

Short (≤ −2SD) or borderline short (≤ −1.5SD) stature

Not short

No dysmorphic features   Dysmorphic features

Growth rate inappropriately slow

Healthy boy or girl ±mild/moderate asthma ±family Hx delayed puberty Ht centile for BA within target range

Girl with hyperconvex nails, puffy nail folds and fingers, ±middle ear problems ±education problems

See (1)

Boy 46XY or 45X/46XY or 47XXY Testes small/absent/ cryptorchid Raised LH/FSH

Girl 46XX or 46XY Ovaries absent Raised LH/FSH

Underweight BMI ≤ 15% ±low intake ±eating disorder ±extreme exercise

CDGA

TURNER SYNDROME

PRIMARY HYPOGONADISM

46XX OR 46XY OVARIAN DYSGENESIS

46XY Small/normal testes Penis small/normal FSH/LH not elevated

46XX Ovaries present FSH/LH not elevated

Symptoms of chronic disease e.g. respiratory, gastrointestinal, renal

Dysmorphism ± learning difficulties ± congenital anomalies

DYSMORPHIC SYNDROME WITH DELAYED PUBERTY e.g. Noonan, PWS

PHYSIOLOGICAL DELAY

CENTRAL HYPOGONADISM e.g. Isolated LHRH deficiency, Kallman syndrome

DELAYED PUBERTY SECONDARY TO LOW BODY MASS

DELAYED PUBERTY SECONDARY TO CHRONIC DISEASE

Weight gain + poor growth rate

Social difficulties ±poor growth rate ±low body mass

?HYPOTHYROIDISM ?CUSHING'S

PSYCHOSOCIAL DEPRIVATION

Short stature inappropriate for parental heights ± growth failure

?HYPOPITUITARISM

Figure 12.9 Flow chart to enable clinical diagnosis of children with delayed puberty. BA, bone age; BMI, body mass index; CDGA, constitutional delay in growth and adolescence; FSH, follide-stimulating hormone; LH, luteinizing hormone; LHRH, luteinizing hormone releasing hormone; PWS, Prader–Willi syndrome.

tetracosactrin (Synacthen) should be given concurrently. The diagnosis of GH deficiency should not be made purely on the basis of low peak GH values after stimulation, but also in the clinical context. High resolution pictures of the hypothalamo-pituitary area can now be achieved with modern magnetic resonance imaging (MRI) scanners, and we have found this investigation most valuable in cases where pituitary insufficiency is suspected.

GROWTH FAILURE (SEE FIG. 12.7)

Growth failure is by definition abnormal and requires investigation. However, it is important to distinguish growth failure from artefact caused by measurement and transcription errors. Although growth failure in prepubertal children does not cause diagnostic confusion, in children with constitutional delay it can be difficult to distinguish between physiological deceleration and growth failure (see Fig. 12.5). Care must be exercised to examine height velocity in context. Figure 12.11 shows the growth chart of a boy who appeared to have typical constitutional delay, but then failed to show a

growth response to puberty and was subsequently found to have panhypopituitarism caused by a small craniopharyngioma. The importance of chronic disease and social deprivation in causing short stature has been discussed above, and such conditions can only be discovered by a meticulous initial history and examination combined with astute follow-up.

Dysmorphic syndromes, especially Turner syndrome, may present with growth failure from 5 years onwards (Fig. 12.12). Although obvious skeletal dysplasias do not pose diagnostic difficulty, more subtle degrees of hypochrondroplasia may be more difficult to detect.

Hypothyroidism can be diagnosed from growth failure, but more commonly the symptoms are pallor, weight gain and tiredness accompanied by features of myxoedema. Cushing syndrome is extremely rare, and most children referred with this as a possible diagnosis have simple obesity. However, the combination of obesity, short stature relative to the parental heights, and growth failure should always raise the possibility of Cushing syndrome including iatrogenic causes such as nasal drops and inhaled steroids.

Special mention should be made of growth deceleration in children with asthma.[43] It is well recognized that asthma

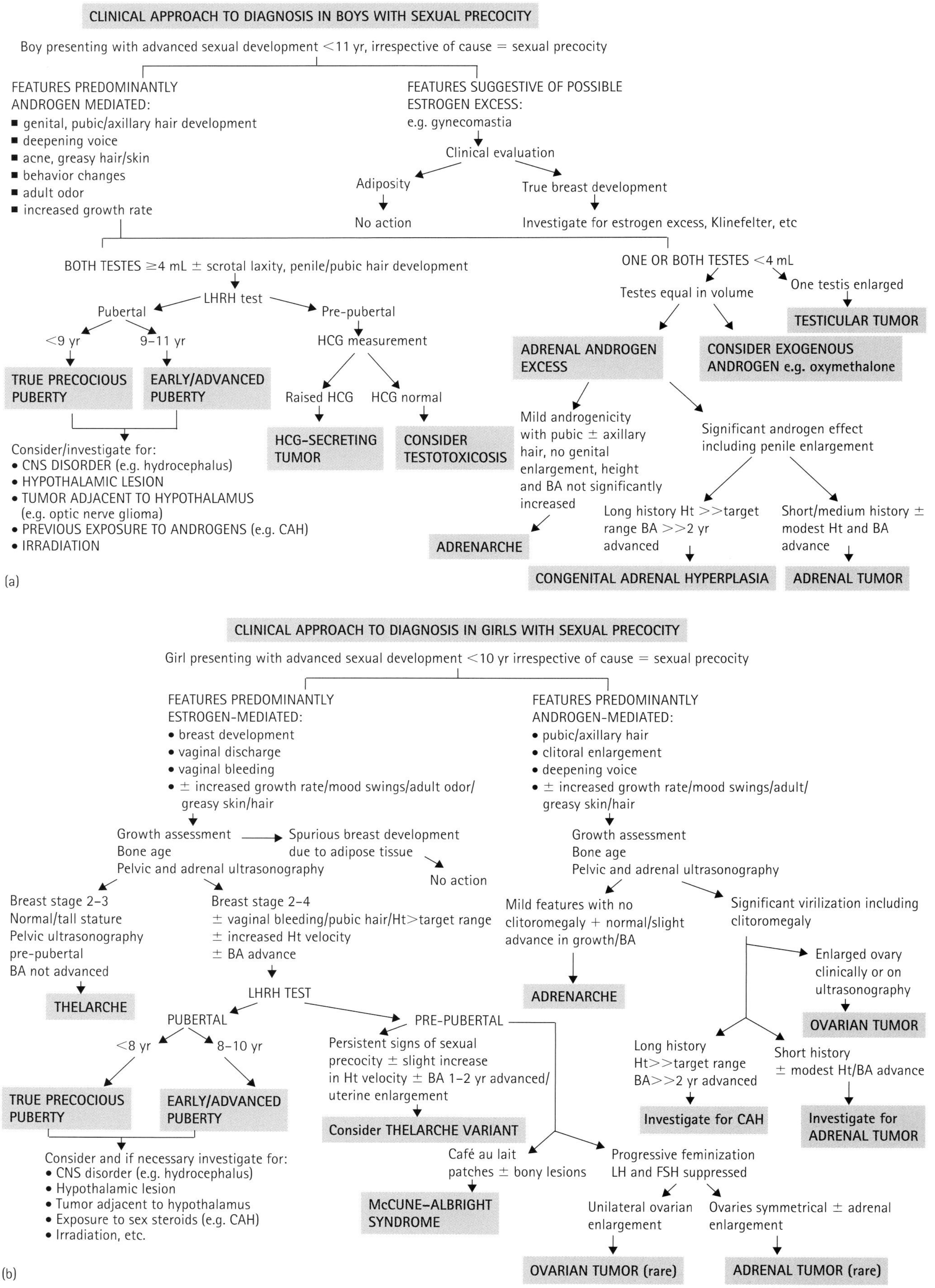

CLINICAL APPROACH TO DIAGNOSIS IN BOYS WITH SEXUAL PRECOCITY

Boy presenting with advanced sexual development <11 yr, irrespective of cause = sexual precocity

FEATURES PREDOMINANTLY ANDROGEN MEDIATED:
- genital, pubic/axillary hair development
- deepening voice
- acne, greasy hair/skin
- behavior changes
- adult odor
- increased growth rate

FEATURES SUGGESTIVE OF POSSIBLE ESTROGEN EXCESS:
e.g. gynecomastia

Clinical evaluation

Adiposity → No action

True breast development → Investigate for estrogen excess, Klinefelter, etc

BOTH TESTES ≥4 mL ± scrotal laxity, penile/pubic hair development

LHRH test

Pubertal
- <9 yr → **TRUE PRECOCIOUS PUBERTY**
- 9–11 yr → **EARLY/ADVANCED PUBERTY**

Consider/investigate for:
- CNS DISORDER (e.g. hydrocephalus)
- HYPOTHALAMIC LESION
- TUMOR ADJACENT TO HYPOTHALAMUS (e.g. optic nerve glioma)
- PREVIOUS EXPOSURE TO ANDROGENS (e.g. CAH)
- IRRADIATION

Pre-pubertal

HCG measurement
- Raised HCG → **HCG-SECRETING TUMOR**
- HCG normal → **CONSIDER TESTOTOXICOSIS**

ONE OR BOTH TESTES <4 mL

Testes equal in volume

One testis enlarged → **TESTICULAR TUMOR**

ADRENAL ANDROGEN EXCESS

CONSIDER EXOGENOUS ANDROGEN e.g. oxymethalone

Mild androgenicity with pubic ± axillary hair, no genital enlargement, height and BA not significantly increased → **ADRENARCHE**

Significant androgen effect including penile enlargement
- Long history Ht >>target range BA >>2 yr advanced → **CONGENITAL ADRENAL HYPERPLASIA**
- Short/medium history ± modest Ht and BA advance → **ADRENAL TUMOR**

(a)

CLINICAL APPROACH TO DIAGNOSIS IN GIRLS WITH SEXUAL PRECOCITY

Girl presenting with advanced sexual development <10 yr irrespective of cause = sexual precocity

FEATURES PREDOMINANTLY ESTROGEN-MEDIATED:
- breast development
- vaginal discharge
- vaginal bleeding
- ± increased growth rate/mood swings/adult odor/greasy skin/hair

FEATURES PREDOMINANTLY ANDROGEN-MEDIATED:
- pubic/axillary hair
- clitoral enlargement
- deepening voice
- ± increased growth rate/mood swings/adult/greasy skin/hair

Growth assessment / Bone age / Pelvic and adrenal ultrasonography → Spurious breast development due to adipose tissue → No action

Breast stage 2–3 / Normal/tall stature / Pelvic ultrasonography pre-pubertal / BA not advanced → **THELARCHE**

Breast stage 2–4 / ± vaginal bleeding/pubic hair/Ht>target range / ± increased Ht velocity / ± BA advance

LHRH TEST

PUBERTAL
- <8 yr → **TRUE PRECOCIOUS PUBERTY**
- 8–10 yr → **EARLY/ADVANCED PUBERTY**

Consider and if necessary investigate for:
- CNS disorder (e.g. hydrocephalus)
- Hypothalamic lesion
- Tumor adjacent to hypothalamus
- Exposure to sex steroids (e.g. CAH)
- Irradiation, etc.

PRE-PUBERTAL

Persistent signs of sexual precocity ± slight increase in Ht velocity ± BA 1–2 yr advanced/uterine enlargement → **Consider THELARCHE VARIANT**

Café au lait patches ± bony lesions → **McCUNE–ALBRIGHT SYNDROME**

Progressive feminization LH and FSH suppressed
- Unilateral ovarian enlargement → **OVARIAN TUMOR (rare)**
- Ovaries symmetrical ± adrenal enlargement → **ADRENAL TUMOR (rare)**

Growth assessment / Bone age / Pelvic and adrenal ultrasonography

Mild features with no clitoromegaly + normal/slight advance in growth/BA → **ADRENARCHE**

Significant virilization including clitoromegaly

Enlarged ovary clinically or on ultrasonography → **OVARIAN TUMOR**

- Long history Ht>>target range BA>>2 yr advanced → **Investigate for CAH**
- Short history ± modest Ht/BA advance → **Investigate for ADRENAL TUMOR**

(b)

Figure 12.10 Flow chart to enable clinical diagnosis of children with sexual precocity. BA, bone age; CAH, congenital adrenal hyperplasia; CNS, central nervous system; FSH, follicle-stimulating hormone; HCG, human chorionic gonadotrophin; LH, luteinizing hormone; LHRH, luteinizing hormone releasing hormone.

Table 12.3 Screening investigations in cases of short stature

Child arrives at 9 a.m., fasted
  Application of anesthetic cream, if indicated
Blood
  Chromosomes
  Full blood count and film, ferritin, red cell folate (screening for
    chronic gastrointestinal disease, e.g. malabsorption)
  Tissue transglutaminase (TTG) antibodies (screening for celiac
    disease)
  Creatinine, urea and electrolytes, calcium and phosphate
    (screening for renal disease, parathyroid hormone resistance)
  IGF-I (screening for growth hormone deficiency)
  Thyroid function tests
  Cortisol (screening for adrenal insufficiency) NB a basal cortisol
    $>100\,nmol\,L^{-1}$ is a prerequisite before an insulin tolerance
    test can be carried out
  Prolactin
  Basal gonadotrophins (if Turner syndrome suspected)
Urine
  Ward analysis for pH, protein, blood, and ketones
  Clean catch urine for culture
  Early morning urine osmolality
  Child allowed food and drink
Diagnostic imaging
  Bone age (this is best performed at the clinic)
  Pelvic and renal ultrasonography

Note: additional investigations such as skeletal survey (looking for dysplasias), clinical photographs, and genetic testing for specific disorders (e.g., chromosome 22 deletion, PTPN11 mutation in Noonan syndrome etc) can be carried out after discussion with radiology and genetic colleagues.

is associated with constitutional delay and delayed puberty, even when the condition is mild. Chronic asthma is also a potent cause of slow growth. Frank growth failure in response to inhaled steroids is usually seen with high dose treatment (Fig. 12.13). We have occasionally seen growth failure in association with modest doses of inhaled steroids when no other factor could be invoked (Fig. 12.14).

Investigation of growth failure

Growth failure secondary to a known cause (e.g., chronic renal failure, steroid therapy) does not require specific investigation and efforts should be directed towards treating the underlying problem. In cases where an underlying chronic disease has been ruled out a full endocrine assessment is merited including pituitary function stimulation testing and neuroimaging with MRI.

TALL STATURE (SEE FIG. 12.8)

It is unusual to reach the end of a new patient consultation without having achieved a correct working diagnosis. As with short stature, it is necessary to establish whether or not one or both parents are tall and if so whether there is a dominant growth abnormality such as Marfan syndrome. Some children clearly have normal genetic tall stature, others have constitutional advance in growth in adolescence and others a combination of the two.

Children with simple obesity usually have heights in the upper half of the target range centiles, so that if the parents are moderately tall, the child him- or herself may well be above the 97th centile for height.

Children whose tallness is out of context with the family patterns, and in whom obesity cannot be invoked as the main cause, must be assessed in terms of dysmorphic features and learning difficulties, and sexual precocity. Although dysmorphism may occur in Klinefelter syndrome (47,XXY) and the 47,XYY syndrome, the clinical features are often subtle or absent.

Tall stature is unlikely to be the presenting symptom in sexual precocity (see below), but all children with tall stature must have careful assessment of secondary sexual characteristics.

Although thyrotoxicosis is a potent cause of tall stature, it is again rare for children to present with tallness as the principal complaint.[57] The same is true of familial glucocorticoid resistance caused by adreno-corticotrophic hormone (ACTH) receptor defect.[58]

By contrast, GH excess, although very rare, can present with unexplained tall stature and enhanced height velocity. It is important to examine the fundi and test the visual fields of inexplicably tall children, to exclude the presence of a pituitary adenoma.

Investigation of tall stature

The following investigations may be appropriate if clinical examination, bone age and pelvic ultrasonography indicate that the tall stature is not genetic/constitutional in nature:

- Chromosomes
- DNA for genetic studies and urine for homocystinuria if Marfan syndrome or homocystinuria is suspected.
- Thyroxine (T_4), triiodothyronine (T_3), thyroid-stimulating hormone (TSH) if hyperthyroidism is suspected.
- IGF-I measurement, and GH response to an oral glucose load, if GH excess is suspected. If IGF-I is $>400\,\mu g\,L^{-1}$ or if GH fails to suppress below $5\,mU\,L^{-1}$, an overnight GH profile with 20 min sampling is indicated.

DELAYED PUBERTY (SEE FIG. 12.9)

The cause of delayed puberty will be obvious in certain adolescents, for example, those with a history of testicular or ovarian irradiation, craniopharyngioma, etc. In these subjects investigation may be required to determine the extent of gonadal impairment, rather than to determine the cause.

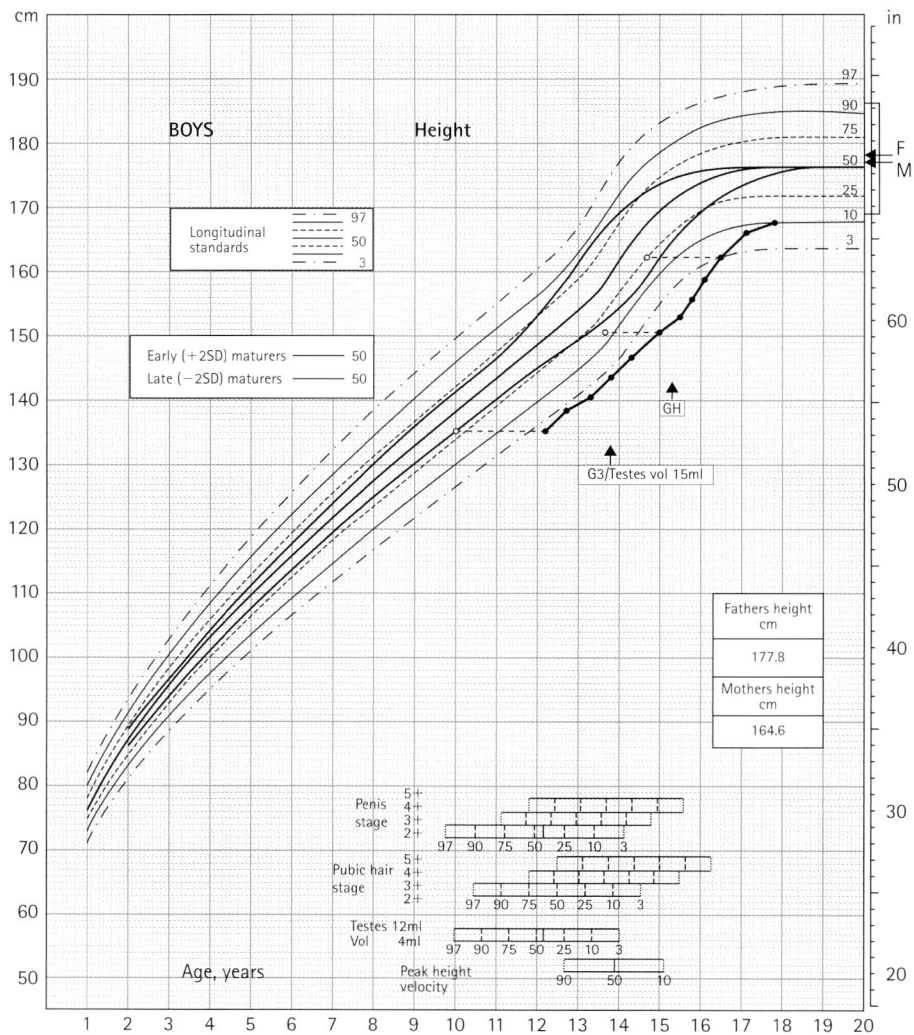

Figure 12.11 This boy shows a growth pattern typical of constitutional delay but was found to have hypopituitarism as a result of a small craniopharyngioma. (Reproduced with permission of Castlemead Publications.)

In adolescents without an obvious reason for delayed puberty, a distinction must be made between the short adolescent with delayed puberty, in whom constitutional delay is by far the most likely diagnosis, and in the subject with normal or tall stature in whom there is a higher chance of finding pathology.

Delayed puberty in short boys and girls

This is most likely to be caused by constitutional delay if there are no symptoms or signs of dysmorphism or disease, and especially if there is a family history of delayed puberty. Commonly there is a history of mild-to-moderate asthma.[38]

Eating disorders can cause delayed puberty, and may range from obvious anorexia nervosa[59] to milder forms of food refusal and obsession.

Social difficulties may cause both short stature and growth failure (see above), with attendant delay in bone age and secondary sexual development. It is important to remember that these problems may coexist, for example, so that a child may have short stature and delayed puberty resulting from a combination of positive family history, poor diet with low body mass and chronic asthma treated with inhaled steroids.

Chronic disease, especially inflammatory bowel disease, chronic renal failure, chronic conditions requiring steroid therapy, cystic fibrosis, etc. commonly cause delayed puberty. Although delayed puberty is seldom the presenting feature in most chronic diseases, conditions such as inflammatory bowel disease, celiac disease and chronic renal failure are occasionally discovered in the growth clinic.

Dysmorphic syndromes may be associated with delayed puberty, the classic example being Turner syndrome with ovarian dysgenesis. In the authors' experience Turner syndrome girls rarely have the florid dysmorphic features such as neck webbing and the classic facial appearance. The diagnosis is more likely to be reached by recognizing the

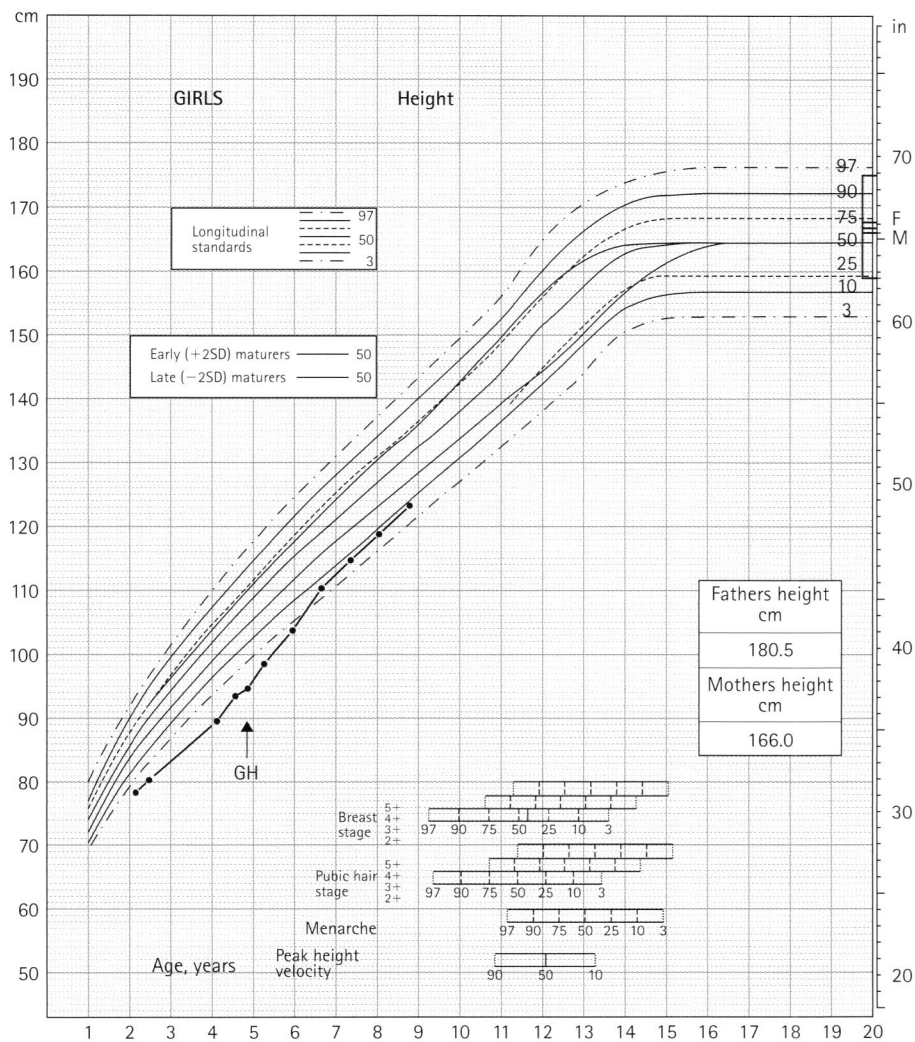

Figure 12.12 Note the growth deceleration in early childhood in this girl with Turner syndrome and the mismatch between her height and the parental target range. (Reproduced with permission of Castlemead Publications.)

combination of mismatch between the girl's height centile and the target height (see Fig. 12.12), pubertal failure, the presence of subtle features including puffy nail folds and fingers with hyperconvex nails, wide carrying angle, high palate, and increase in nevi.[60] Other dysmorphic syndromes such as Noonan syndrome are also commonly associated with delayed puberty.

More rarely delayed puberty is caused by endocrine disease, such as hypopituitarism with gonadotrophin deficiency, hypothyroidism, and Cushing syndrome.

Delayed puberty in boys and girls who are not short

Constitutional delay is still the most likely cause in these individuals. However, if the growth rate is inappropriate, acquired growth failure caused by chronic disease, social difficulties or endocrine disorders (including tumors adjacent to the pituitary gland) should be considered.

Hypogonadism, either central or peripheral, should be considered in boys with hypoplastic genitalia or cryptorchidism and in both sexes if puberty is particularly delayed, or incomplete. Investigations include chromosome analysis, measurement of gonadotrophins before and after gonadotrophin-releasing hormone (GnRH) stimulation, testosterone response to human chorionic gonadotrophin (hCG) stimulation in boys and pelvic ultrasonography in girls, formal testing of the sense of smell, and in selected cases DNA for molecular genetic analysis, e.g., KAL-1 mutation for Kallmann's syndrome.

The distinction between central hypogonadism and physiological delay in puberty is not always possible during the adolescent years. In doubtful cases, the best option is to give sex steroid replacement therapy until puberty is complete, fully reinvestigating the gonadal axis once off therapy. In the authors' experience, unless the external genitalia are abnormal, imaging of the pituitary area with MRI has shown a lesion, or there is impaired sense of smell with olfactory hypoplasia/absence caused by Kallmann

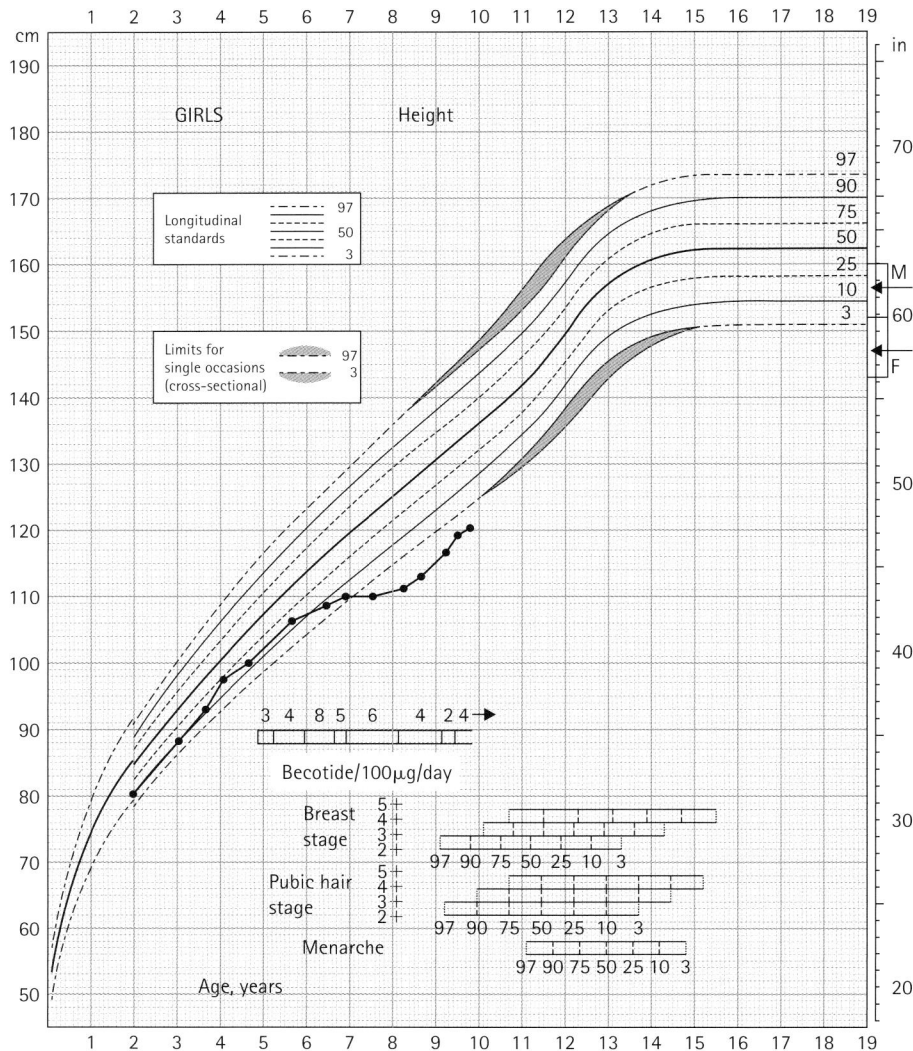

Figure 12.13 Growth failure is attributable to relatively high doses of inhaled steroids in this girl with asthma. (Reproduced with permission of Castlemead Publications.)

syndrome,[61] most doubtful cases turn out to have physiological delay.

SEXUAL PRECOCITY (SEE FIG. 12.10)

The history and examination must establish whether the child's symptoms and signs reflect predominant androgen or estrogen effect. The distinction is not always clear cut, because true precocious puberty in girls will often be accompanied by the development of pubic and axillary hair. Symptoms of androgen excess include the development of pubic and axillary hair, acne, greasy hair and skin, adult body odor, enlargement of the male genitalia, and in girls enlargement of the clitoris. Symptoms and signs of estrogen excess include breast development, vaginal discharge, menstrual bleeding, and mood swings. Common to both androgen and estrogen excess are increase in growth rate, and sexually oriented 'teenagerish' behavior.

Boys with sexual precocity (see Fig. 12.10a) very rarely have estrogen excess, and the majority with apparent breast development have simple obesity, gynecomastia of unknown cause or puberty-related gynecomastia.

The finding of significant androgen excess in any boy below 11 years of age demands further investigation, but the cause can usually be deduced by careful clinical examination of the genitalia. Obvious enlargement of both testes is virtually diagnostic of true central precocious puberty, whereas symmetrical but lesser enlargement raises the possibility of an hCG-producing tumor or activating LH-receptor defect (testotoxicosis).[62] Unilateral testicular enlargement is suggestive of a Leydig's cell tumor. If both testes are pre-pubertal in volume the cause must be either adrenal or drug induced. In this situation mild androgenicity with pubic and axillary hair but no development of the genitalia is almost always the result of adrenarche,[63] whereas more significant androgen effect will reflect either adrenal hyperplasia or tumor. These latter conditions can

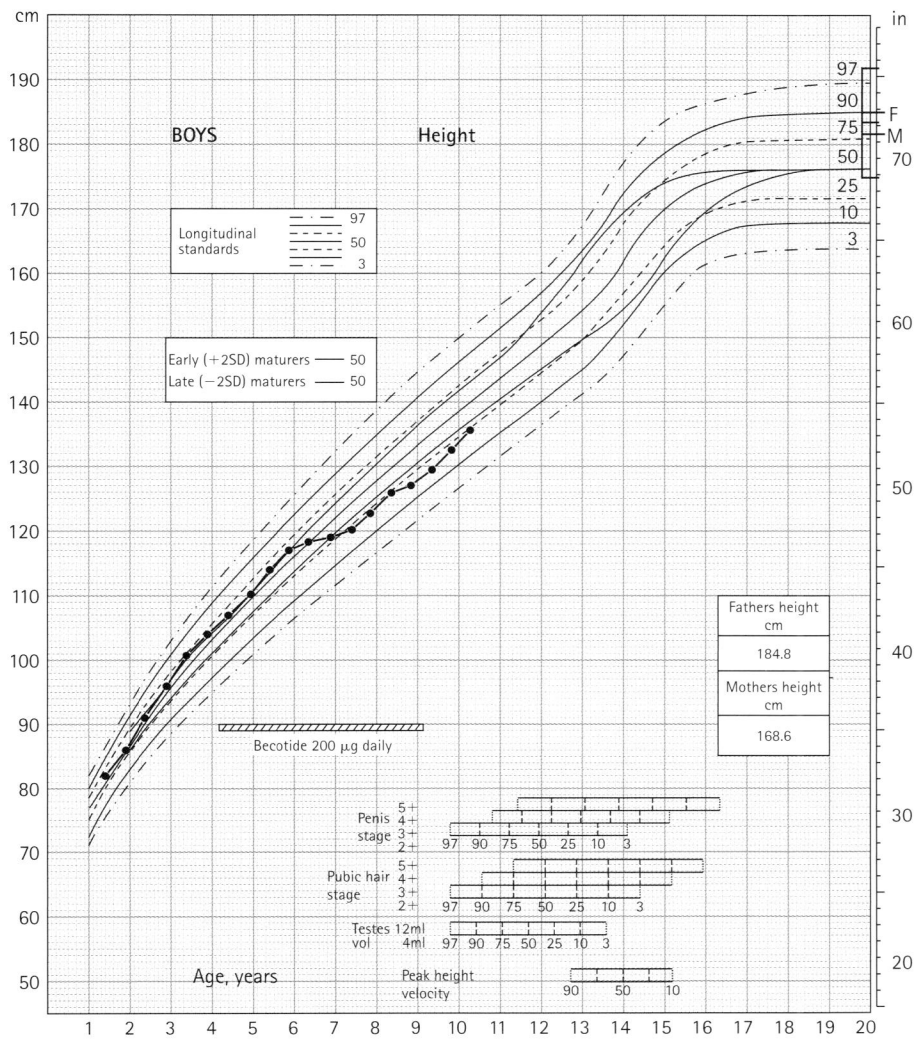

Figure 12.14 This boy with asthma exhibits an idiosyncratic growth response to a relatively low dose of inhaled steroids. (Reproduced with permission of Castlemead Publications.)

be distinguished by the length of the history and the degree of tall stature.

Girls with sexual precocity (see Fig. 12.10b) are easy to categorize if the problem is mainly androgen-mediated. Again, isolated pubic and axillary hair development with little or no bone age advancement is almost always the result of adrenal puberty (adrenarche), whereas virilization with enlargement of the clitoris will be caused by either adrenal hyperplasia or an androgen-producing tumor (adrenal or ovarian).

The cause of sexual precocity in girls with predominantly estrogen-mediated symptoms and signs is more difficult to establish, and often it is not possible to make a diagnosis on purely clinical grounds. Even after investigation, months or even years of surveillance may be required before a final diagnosis can be reached. In mild cases of sexual precocity, e.g., premature thelarche, investigations may be waived. Usually, however, the clinician should request bone age and pelvic ultrasound assessment. Premature thelarche is probable in girls of 2 years or less with isolated breast development and normal height status. Girls aged 9 years or more with breast development are very likely to be in the earliest stages of true puberty and again investigation is rarely required unless the clinician is considering giving suppressive treatment. In other girls day-case assessment is usually necessary, comprising a GnRH stimulation test, measurement of plasma steroids under basal conditions and 24 h urine for steroid analysis. On the basis of this assessment the three principal diagnoses of thelarche, thelarche variant[64] and precocious/early puberty are usually made. Very rarely estrogen-mediated sexual precocity is caused by a feminizing adrenal or ovarian tumor. We have seen this in one girl who had an adrenal adenoma mimicking true central precocious puberty so that secondary sexual development was typical and even the ovaries were enlarged on ultrasonography, regressing when the tumor was removed. The McCune–Albright syndrome may be indistinguishable from thelarche or thelarche variant in terms of the sexual precocity and laboratory investigations.[65] In these cases the diagnosis is usually made on discovery of bony lesions and café-au-lait patches.

KEY LEARNING POINTS

- A thorough understanding of normal growth and puberty is a prerequisite for the assessment of growth disorders.
- With a careful history, good auxology, and appropriate examination, the correct clinical diagnosis of growth problems can usually be made without resorting to extensive investigations.
- Height prediction in children with normal variant short and tall stature is helpful provided that the assessment of skeletal age (bone age) is carried out by an experienced observer.
- Day-case admission for endocrine assessment is necessary in a minority of short, tall and pubertally delayed children but is more likely to be required when there is growth failure or sexual precocity.
- It is likely that advances in molecular genetics will result in specific diagnoses in an increasing proportion of children currently labeled as having idiopathic short stature.

REFERENCES

● = Seminal primary article
◆ = Key review paper

1 Tanner JM, Kelnar CJH. Physical growth, development and puberty. In: Campbell AGM, McIntosh N, eds. *Forfar and Arneil's Textbook of Paediatrics*, 4th edn. Edinburgh: Churchill Livingstone, 1992: 389–445.

● 2 Tanner JM, Whitehouse RH, Takaishi M. Standards from birth to maturity for height, weight, height velocity and weight velocity: British children 1965, Part I. *Arch Dis Child* 1966; **41**: 454–71.

3 Tanner JM, Whitehouse RH. Clinical longitudinal standards for height, weight, height velocity, weight velocity, and stages of puberty. *Arch Dis Child* 1976; **51**: 170–9.

4 Hall JG, Froster-Iskenius UG, Allanson JE. *Handbook of Normal Physical Measurements*. Oxford: Oxford University Press, 1989.

5 Tanner JM, Whitehouse RH. Revised standards for triceps and subscapular skinfolds in British children. *Arch Dis Child* 1975; **50**: 142–5.

6 Laman TG. Advances in body composition assessment. In: *Current Issues in Exercise Science Series*, Monograph 3. Champaign, Illinois: Human Kinetics Publishers, 1992.

7 Goran MI, Driscoll P, Johnson R, *et al*. Cross-calibration of body-composition techniques against dual-energy X-ray absorptiometry in young children. *Am J Clin Nutr* 1996; **63**: 299–305.

8 Bachrach LK. Dual energy X-ray absorptiometry (DEXA) measurements of bone density and body composition: promise and pitfalls. *J Pediatr Endocrinol Metab* 2000; **13(Suppl 2)**: 983–8.

◆ 9 Sanchez MM, Gilsanz V. Pediatric DXA bone measurements. *Pediatr Endocrinol Rev* 2005; **2(Suppl 3)**: 337–41.

● 10 Shalet SM, Gibson BE, Swindell R, Pearson D. Effect of spinal irradiation on growth. *Arch Dis Child* 1987; **62**: 461–4.

11 Cizmecioglu F, Doherty A, Paterson WF, *et al*. Measured versus reported parental height. *Arch Dis Child* 2005; **90**: 941–2.

12 Tanner JM, Goldstein H, Whitehouse RH. Standards for children's height at ages 2–9 years allowing for height of parents. *Arch Dis Child* 1970; **45**: 755–62.

● 13 Tanner JM, Whitehouse RH, Takaishi M. Standards for birth to maturity for height, weight, height velocity and weight velocity: British children, 1965, Part II. *Arch Dis Child* 1966; **45**: 613–35.

14 DuBois D, DuBois EF. A formula to estimate the approximate surface area if height and weight are known. *Arch Intern Med* 1916; **17**: 863–71.

15 Voss L, Walker J, Lunt H, *et al*. The Wessex Growth Study: First Report. *Acta Paediatr Scand Suppl* 1989; **349**: 65–72.

16 Smith DW, Truog W, Rogers JE, *et al*. Shifting linear growth during infancy: illustration of genetic factors in growth from fetal life through infancy. *J Pediatr* 1976; **89**: 225–30.

17 Tanner JM. *Growth at Adolescence*, 2nd edn. Oxford: Blackwell Scientific, 1962.

18 Tanner JM, Whitehouse RH, Cameron N, *et al*. *Assessment of Skeletal Maturity and Prediction of Adult Height (TW2 Method)*, 2nd edn. London: Academic Press, 1983.

19 Tanner JM, Healy MJR, Goldstein H, Cameron N. *Assessment of Skeletal Maturity and Prediction of Adult Height (TW3 Method)*, 3rd edn. London: WB Saunders, 2001.

20 Greulich WW, Pyle SI. *Radiographic Atlas of Skeletal Development of the Hand and Wrist*, 2nd edn. Stanford, California: Stanford University Press, 1959.

21 Bayley N, Pinneau SR. Tables for predicting adult height from skeletal age: revised for use with the Greulich–Pyle hand standards *J Pediatr* 1952; **40**: 423–41. (Published errata appear in *J Pediatr* 1952; **41**: 371.)

22 Kelly BP, Paterson WF, Donaldson MDC. Final height outcome and value of height prediction in boys with constitutional delay in growth and adolescence treated with intramuscular testosterone 125 mg per month for 3 months. *Clin Endocrinol* 2003; **58**: 267–72.

● 23 Griffin IJ, Cole TJ, Duncan KA, *et al*. Pelvic ultrasound measurements in normal girls. *Acta Paediatr Scand* 1995; **84**: 536–43.

● 24 Freeman JV, Cole TJ, Chinn S, *et al*. Cross sectional stature and weight reference curves for the UK, 1990. *Arch Dis Child* 1995; **73**: 17–24.

25 Roche AF, Davila GH. Late adolescent growth in stature. *Pediatrics* 1972; **50**: 872–80.

26 Lindgren G. Growth of schoolchildren with early, average and late ages of peak height velocity. *Ann Hum Biol* 1978; **5**: 253–67.

27 Tanner JM, Davies PSW. Clinical longitudinal standards for height and height velocity for North American children. *J Pediatr* 1985; **107**: 317–29.

28 Buckler JMH. *A Longitudinal Study of Adolescent Growth*. London: Springer-Verlag, 1990.

29 Cole TJ, Freeman JV, Preece MA. Body mass index reference curves for the UK, 1990. *Arch Dis Child* 1995; **73**: 25–9.

30 Tse WY, Hindmarsh PC, Brook CGD. The infancy–childhood–puberty model of growth: clinical aspects. *Acta Paediatr Scand Suppl* 1989; **356**: 38–43.

31 Nobels F, Dewailly D. Puberty and polycystic ovarian syndrome. The insulin/insulin-like growth factor hypothesis. *Fertil Steril* 1992; **58**: 655–63.

32 Legro RS. Detection of insulin resistance and its treatment in adolescents with polycystic ovary syndrome. *J Pediatr Endocrinol Metab* 2002; **15(Suppl 5)**: 1367–78.

33 Stanhope R, Brook CGD. Disorders of puberty. In: Brook CGD, ed. *Clinical Paediatric Endocrinology*, 2nd edn. Oxford: Blackwell Scientific, 1989.

34 Hulse JA. Referral criteria for growth screening. *J Med Screen* 1995 **2**: 168–70.

35 Law CM. The disability of short stature. *Arch Dis Child* 1987; **62**: 855–9.

36 Sandberg DE, Voss LD. The psychosocial consequences of short stature: a review of the evidence. *Best Pract Res Clin Endocrinol Metab* 2002; **16**: 449–63.

37 Erling A. Why do some children of short stature develop psychologically well while others have problems? *Eur J Endocrinol* 2004; **151(Suppl 1)**: 535–9.

38 Balfour-Lynn L. Growth and childhood asthma. *Arch Dis Child* 1986; **61**: 1049–55.

39 Jones KL. *Smith's Recognizable Patterns of Human Malformation*, 6th edn. Philadelphia: WB Saunders Company, 2005.

40 North KN. Neurofibromatosis type 1: review of the first 200 patients in an Australian clinic. *J Child Neurol* 1993; **8**: 395–402.

41 Skuse D, Albanese A, Stanhope R, *et al.* A new stress-related syndrome of growth failure and hyperphagia in children, associated with reversibility of growth hormone insufficiency. *Lancet* 1996; **348**: 353–8.

42 Findlay CA, MacDonald JF, Wallace AM, *et al.* Childhood Cushing's syndrome, betamethasone nose drops and repeat prescriptions. *BMJ* 1998; **317**: 739–40.

43 Shaw NJ, Fraser NC, Weller PH. Asthma treatment and growth. *Arch Dis Child* 1997; **4**: 284–6.

44 DeVile, CJ, Grant DB, Hayward RD, Stanhope R. Growth and endocrine sequelae of craniopharyngioma. *Arch Dis Child* 1996; **75**: 108–14.

45 Price DA, Johnston DI, Betts PR, *et al.* Biosynthetic human growth hormone in the UK: an audit of current practice. *Arch Dis Child* 1994; **71**: 266–71.

46 Kant SG, Wit JM, Breuning MH. Genetic analysis of short stature. *Horm Res* 2003; **60**: 157–65.

47 Rosenfeld RG, Hwa V. Toward a molecular basis for idiopathic short stature [Editorial]. *J Clin Endocrinol Metab* 2004; **89**: 1066–7.

48 Rappold GA, Fukami M, Niesler B, *et al.* Deletions of the homeobox gene *SHOX* (Short Stature Homeobox) are an important cause of growth failure in children with short stature. *J Clin Endocrinol Metab* 2002; **87**: 1402–6.

49 Binder G, Ranke MB, Martin DD. Auxology is a valuable instrument for the clinical diagnosis of SHOX haploinsufficiency in school-age children with unexplained short stature. *J Clin Endocrinol Metab* 2003; **88**: 4891–6.

50 Attie KM, Carlsson LMS, Rundle AC, Sherman BM. Evidence for partial growth hormone insensitivity among patients with idiopathic short stature. *J Pediatr* 1995; **127**: 244–50.

51 Buckway CK, Guevara-Aguirre J, Pratt KL, *et al.* The IGF-I generation test revisited: a marker of GH sensitivity. *J Clin Endocrinol Metab* 2001; **86**: 5176–83.

52 Woods KA, Dastot F, Preece MA, *et al.* Phenotype: genotype relationships in growth hormone insensitivity syndrome. *J Clin Endocrinol Metab* 1997; **82**: 3529–35.

53 Lewis MD, Horan M, Millar DS, *et al.* A novel dysfunctional growth hormone variant (Ile179Met) exhibits a decreased ability to activate the extracellular signal-regulated kinase pathway. *J Clin Endocrinol Metab* 2004; **89**: 1068–75.

54 Takahashi Y, Kaji H, Okimura Y, *et al.* Short stature caused by a mutant growth hormone. *New Engl J Med* 1996; **334**: 432–6.

55 Woods KA, Camacho-Hubner C, Savage MO, Clark AJL. Intrauterine growth retardation and postnatal growth failure associated with deletion of the insulin-like growth factor I gene. *New Engl J Med* 1996; **335**: 1342–9.

56 Kofoed EM, Hwa V, Little B, *et al.* Growth hormone insensitivity associated with a STATb mutation. *New Engl J Med* 2003; **349**: 1139–47.

57 Buckler JMH, Willgerodt H, Keller E. Growth in thyrotoxicosis. *Arch Dis Child* 1986; **61**: 464–71.

58 Clark AJL, Cammas FM, Watt A, *et al.* Familial glucocorticoid deficiency: One syndrome, but more than one gene. *J Mol Med* 1997; **75**: 394–9.

59 El Kholy M, Job JC, Chaussain JL. Growth of adolescents with anorexia nervosa. *Arch Françaises Pediatr* 1986; **43**: 35–40.

60 Ranke MB, Saenger P. Turner's syndrome. *Lancet* 2001; **358**: 309–14.

61 Fuerxer F, Carlier R, Iffenecker C, *et al.* Magnetic resonance imaging of the olfactory sulci in Kallmann syndrome. *J Neuroradiol* 1996; **23**: 223–30.

62 Rosenthal IM, Refetoff S, Rich B, *et al.* Response to challenge with gonadotrophin-releasing hormone agonist in a mother and her two sons with a constitutively activating mutation of the luteinizing hormone receptor – a clinical research center study. *J Clin Endocrinol Metab* 1996; **81**: 3802–6.

63 Forest MG. Adrenal puberty or adrenarche. *Andrologie* 1997; **7**: 165–86.

64 Stanhope R, Brook CGD. Thelarche variant: a new syndrome of precocious sexual maturation? *Acta Endocrinol* 1990; **123**: 481–6.

65 Foster CM. Endocrine manifestations of McCune–Albright syndrome. *Endocrinologist* 1993; **3**: 359–64.

13

Practical auxology and skeletal maturation

JERRY K H WALES

INTRODUCTION

Auxology is the study of growth – from the Greek, 'auxien', meaning to increase, a term coined by Paul Godin in 1919. The methodology and landmarks used were first laid out in the 'International Agreement for the Unification of Anthropometric Measurements to be made on the Living Subject' by the Congress of Prehistoric Anthropology and Archaeology in 1912. Tanner in the UK and Prader in Switzerland further refined the techniques from the second half of the twentieth century.

Growth proceeds until epiphyseal fusion occurs (firstly in the long bones and later in the spine) under the influence of sex hormones, particularly estrogen. An estimation of remaining growth potential in a normal child can be made from assessment of skeletal maturity coupled with clinical information about health, current height, parental height, past growth and stage of puberty.

The correct measuring techniques will be described in this chapter along with an estimate of their reliability in hospital-based studies, and finally, a description of the methods of estimating skeletal maturity will be given.

Table 13.1 demonstrates the complementary information that may be obtained from each measurement described below.

RELIABILITY OF MEASUREMENTS

Detailed measurements of a child can give an immense amount of information when properly performed and charted. An inaccurate measurement may be due to errors of installation and mechanical problems with the measuring device (machine error); to problems with technique (operator error) or with the child (patient error). Finally, any data collected may be mis-transcribed or mis-plotted. These

Table 13.1 Auxological methods for measuring body compartments

	Water	Fat	Muscle	Bone	Brain
Weight	+	+	+	+	
Height/Sitting height				+ Bone length	
Skin fold	+	+			
Impedance	+				
DEXA scan	+ (independently)	+ (independently)	+ (independently)	+ Bone mass (independently)	
OFC					+
Span/segment				+ Bone length	

errors are remarkably common[1,2] and although they can never be eliminated they can be minimized by using trained auxologists with access to good-quality, well-maintained equipment and appropriate charts or computerized growth records.

The technical error, or precision of an instrument, can be tested by repeated measurement of a single subject by a single observer 'blinded' to previous measurements. This error should ideally be quoted for each instrument used in any single-observer growth studies.

In clinical practice and with some study designs it is more common to have multiple measurers and subjects. By allowing each observer to measure a number of subjects on the same occasion, and comparing their results, an assessment of accuracy that includes both machine and operator error can be derived. Cameron[3] recommends the estimation of the 'percentage reliability' (PR) as being one of the most meaningful values to allow the comparison of techniques and of growth studies. This is calculated as follows:

$$PR = \frac{d^2/2N}{x} \times 100$$

where x is the overall mean value of the measurements, d the difference between the measurements of an individual by two observers and N the number of duplicate measurements. The values for PR given below are derived from analysis of data collected by Wales and Milner,[4] and are comparable to the values given by Johnston et al.[5] and Malina et al.[6]

MEASUREMENTS

Weight

This is an apparently simple measurement that is often performed very badly. All scales should be regularly calibrated and serviced. One still sees records of babies weighed in wet nappies, or children weighed fully clothed. A wet disposable nappy can weigh as much as 450 g, the same as an infant of 6 months may be expected to gain in about 6 weeks. 'Baby-gros', socks, and boots all add to this inaccuracy.

An infant should be weighed naked. A struggling subject's weight can be approximated by setting electronic scales to zero whilst mother stands on them (usually achieved by turning the device on), and then handing her the infant.

In older children 'the minimal clothing compatible with modesty', usually vest and pants should be worn during weighing as indoor clothing (sports shoes and jeans) weighs around 1.5 kg, compared with a mean weight gain in mid-childhood of 2–3 kg/year.

For body weight the PR is 1.8 percent. This renders futile any attempt to measure true nutritional weight gain at intervals of less than a week and certainly invalidates the practice of 'test weighing' before and after breast feeds.[7] More frequent weighing may of course be vital to monitor the progress of pathological conditions related to fluid retention or loss.

Length and height

Under the age of 2 years, and in children with motor disability, it is usual to record supine length (Fig. 13.1). This requires two people, often the mother plus auxologist. The head is held against the headboard with the face in a horizontal plane. The hips and knees are gently extended and the feet rolled down onto the movable footboard brought up to touch the soles of the feet held at 90°.

Standing height should be measured using a ruler such as a purpose-made stadiometer. There are many proprietary devices but they must all be checked for correct installation and calibrated against a solid object of known length. The child should be positioned in bare feet (socks do not add to the height significantly but can obscure curled toes), with the heels and buttocks in the same vertical plane as the measuring instrument. A command such as 'stand like a soldier' usually results in a stiff child with their face pointing upwards, and should be avoided. The arms should fall relaxed at the sides, and the face should be horizontal (the 'Frankfurt plane' with the outer canthus and upper ear level). The subject should be asked to take a breath in, and then out whilst the auxologist exerts *gentle* upward traction on the mastoid processes (Fig. 13.2). It has been shown that the 'stretch' technique where the traction is sufficient to slightly lengthen the spine is unnecessary and may result in increased inter-observer error.[8] Height is then read to the nearest completed millimeter at the end of the breath.

If repeated measurements of height are taken to establish a growth velocity then ideally they should be performed at the same time of day (to avoid errors due to spinal compression; on average the height measured in the morning is

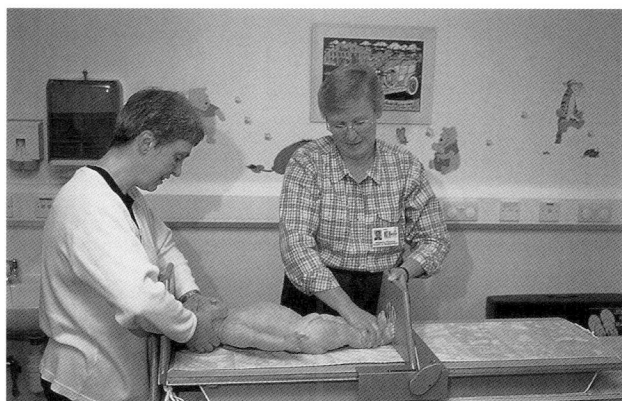

Figure 13.1 Measurement of supine length in an infant. Two operators; head with face in horizontal plane, touching headboard, legs gently extended and feet rolled down footplate to obtain reading.

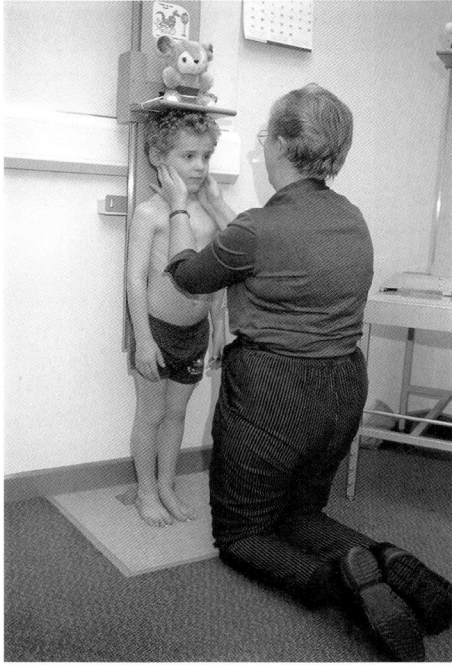

Figure 13.2   Measurement of height. Feet, buttocks, and occiput in same vertical plane. Head in Frankfurt plane, gentle stretch.

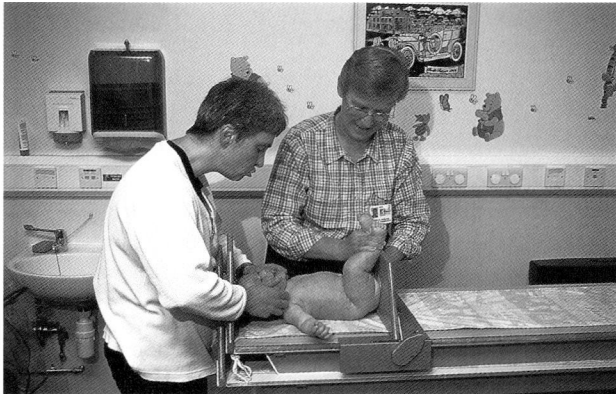

Figure 13.3   Measurement of crown–rump length. Two operators; head with face in horizontal plane, touching headboard, back flattened as legs flexed and buttocks touching footplate.

8 mm more than the afternoon value)[9] and by the same person, using the same equipment, to minimize measurement error.

The standard error of measurement of height on a single occasion in the hands of a trained auxologist is in the order of 0.2 cm and the PR for multiple measurers is 0.37 percent.

Crown–rump length or sitting height

The estimation of the length of the back and head can be of great benefit in establishing the relative proportions of the body. In an infant the legs are flexed at 90° and the footboard brought into contact with the buttocks (Fig. 13.3).

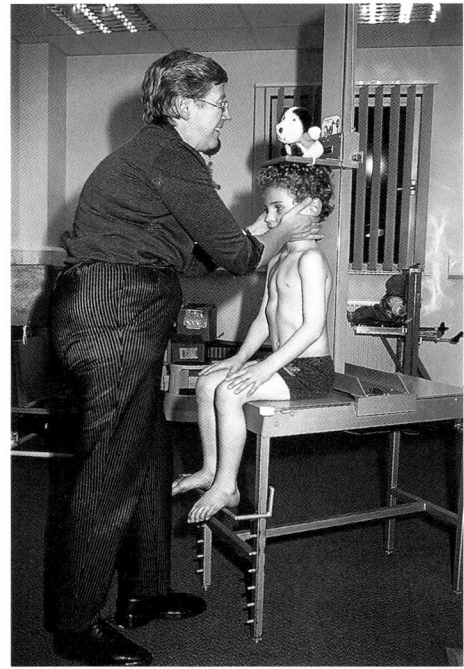

Figure 13.4   Measurement of sitting height. Buttocks and occiput in same vertical plane, sitting with hands in lap. Head in Frankfurt plane, gentle stretch.

In an older child, using a specially designed instrument with the feet resting on a bar, the arms folded loosely in the lap and a similar gentle stretch technique to the one described above, it is possible to obtain precise estimates of sitting height (Fig. 13.4). A simpler method uses a hard seat of known height and horizontal top placed under the height stadiometer or measures the child sitting on the floor, legs extended.

The reading is again taken to the nearest 0.1 cm. The PR of this method is 0.86 percent and it is thus less accurate than measurement of standing height. The Tanner and Whitehouse standards for sitting height and hence derived leg length were obtained using a Harpenden anthropometer, which is a caliper-like device that is now seldom used. This was a difficult technique which has resulted in differences between the standards published by Tanner and Whitehouse[10] and current UK standards obtained conventionally.[11]

Crown-rump length or sitting height may then be subtracted from standing height to derive sub-ischial leg length. By plotting both values on a chart subtle abnormalities such as mild skeletal dysplasias (short legs) or collagen abnormalities (short backs) may be suspected. The 'longer-legs-than-back' shape is also typical of children with delayed puberty and may help in confirming the diagnosis.

Measurement of linear growth over periods of less than 3 months

Pediatricians normally monitor the growth of their patients at relatively infrequent intervals, and for relatively brief periods of the child's growth-span. At this level the healthy child will tend to follow a centile channel determined (after the first 2 years of life) by his or her genetic background. Because of the error inherent in any measurement of height it is impracticable to measure growth at intervals of much less than 12 weeks with conventional stadiometry. However, true understanding of the dynamics that underlie the attainment of final height must rely on detailed longitudinal measurements of individuals when deviations from the smooth lines of a mathematically constructed centile chart become apparent.[12] Montbeillard's son is the classic example, the Count demonstrating that there was apparently periodic acceleration and deceleration in the growth rate of his child as early as 1777. Some of these changes in rate were associated with the season of the year, others were unexplained.[13,14] The more closely we look at growth in an individual the more nonlinearity is seen. The multiple small events throughout the body that control growth, from cell division upwards through the 58 epiphyses between the heel and head all summate to gain in height, but growth cannot be a truly 'linear' process.

A number of radiographic studies on short-term bone growth have been made in humans. Green and Anderson[15] showed that the distal ends of the fibula and tibia grew at different rates, i.e., different parts of the skeleton grow and mature at different rates despite a similar hormonal milieu. The same authors[16] also demonstrated that the proximal end of the femur elongated at half the rate of the distal portion around puberty, so the same conclusions apply even within a single bone. Using radio-stereogrammetry Aronson and Selvick showed a fluctuating pattern of growth in four different children before and after various therapies.[17]

Nonradiological measurement of short-term growth in stable aggregates of bones began with ulnar condylography[18] but evolved into the measurement of the lower leg as knemometry ('kneme' is Greek meaning the lower leg). Knemometry in children is precise (mean SD of measurement 0.09 mm, PR 0.1 percent) and observer independent.[4] The lower legs of healthy children appear to grow at a steady rate then show unexplained leaps in growth (or 'saltations'). These events have also been observed at a whole-body level.[19] There are also clear slowings or small shrinkages followed by catch-up growth that can be associated with even minor catabolic stress or steroid administration.[4,20] Shrinkage here is presumably due to compression of nongrowing bone and cartilage and a possible shift in the balance between bone deposition and resorption with illness that can account for the growth arrest or Harris' lines seen on plain radiographs. The neonatal knemometer is also precise (mean SD of measurement 0.3 mm), allowing for observations of leg growth occurring over 2–3 days even in the premature infant, but unlike the bigger knemometer is highly dependent on the use of an experienced observer.[21] As in older children 'negative' growth, or shrinkage, may occur, especially at times of catabolic stress and with steroid treatment.[22] This nonlinearity defeats any attempts to predict long-term growth from short-term observations either of one bone or the whole body.[23]

Adiposity

Body weight comprises elements of bony skeleton, muscle and organ tissue. Determination of adiposity either directly or indirectly requires measurement of whole body or subcutaneous fat stores. Direct measurement of whole-body fat depends on complex densitometry or isotope dilution techniques that are not suitable for routine use.

ARM, HIP, AND WAIST CIRCUMFERENCE

Indirect assessment of subcutaneous fat stores may be estimated simply but crudely by measurement of the upper arm circumference and this measurement is much used in the rapid determination of nutritional status in areas of undernutrition[24] and waist and hip circumferences (also expressed as a waist/hip ratio) as a measure of overnutrition.[25]

Mid upper arm circumference (MUAC) is measured at a point half way between elbow and shoulder. Waist circumference is measured between the lower ribs and the ischial ridge, at the level of the umbilicus at the end of a normal expiration. Hip circumference is measured at the level of both greater trochanters. Standards exist for waist and hip circumference and the waist–hip ratio.[25,26]

SKIN–FOLD THICKNESS

Subcutaneous fat is not distributed evenly over the body surface or between the sexes and changes its distribution with age. Other commonly used estimations of adiposity are the measurement skin-fold thickness. The skin-fold calipers used to perform these measurements must be standardized as to the constant pressure exerted by, and the area of, the caliper tips. The UK charts, for instance,[27] are designed for use with the Holtain™ calipers (Holtain Ltd, Crosswell, Crymych, UK) with values of $10\,g\,mm^{-2}$ and $55\,mm^2$, respectively. It is not possible to compare studies or values using other caliper designs directly. Four sites are often chosen, of which the first two are in most common use. The triceps skin-fold (Fig. 13.5) is determined with the left arm loose at the side and a fold raised between the measurer's thumb and forefinger at the midpoint of the dorsum of the upper arm. The calipers are applied and after the reading has stabilized (4 or 5 s), the reading is made. The sub-scapular skin-fold is raised at the tip of the shoulder blade, on the left, with the arms again relaxed at the sides. The biceps skin-fold is determined as for the triceps skin-fold but on the ventral aspect of the upper arm. The supra-iliac fold is found at the maximum height of the iliac crest. The skin-fold thicknesses give an estimation of the amount of subcutaneous fat, and its distribution by plotting these values on a standard chart

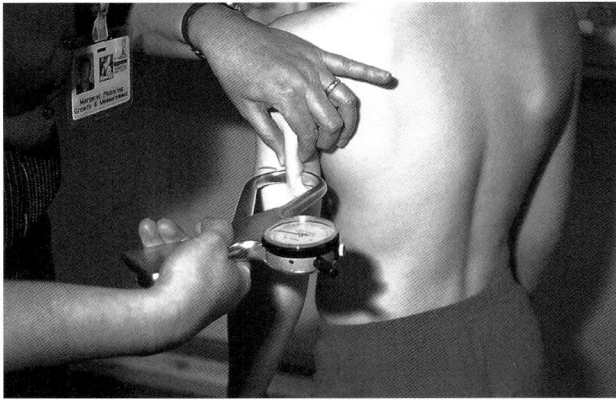

Figure 13.5 Measurement of triceps skin-fold. Left arm gently at side, fold raised at mid-point of dorsum of upper arm. Standard Holtain™ calipers in use, Holtain Limited, Crymych, UK.

(noting that the value of skin-fold thicknesses within a population is not normally distributed and requires logarithmic transformation) and may be used in various equations to estimate total body adiposity. Whole-body subcutaneous fat may be estimated in a baby by the method of Dauncey et al.[28] using two skin-fold values as the fat thickness covering a cylindrical representation of the body calculated from a simple geometrical formula that incorporates measurement of head circumference, length, crown rump length, chest circumference and limb length. In the older child and young adult the formulae of Durnin and Rahaman[29] or Forbes and Amirhakimi[30] or Parizkova,[31] may be used though their validity for the young child is not proven. These formulae depend on regression calculations of skin-fold thickness against directly measured adiposity.

All the above estimations suffer from the inherent difficulty of accurate skin-fold measurement (PR triceps, 3.5 percent; sub-scapular, 7.8 percent), the limited number of sites sampled over the body surface and the difficulty in knowing the amount of uncompressed fat (as opposed to two folds of skin and some subcutaneous tissue and muscle fascia) that is contained in the skin-folds. It is also very difficult to raise an adequate skin-fold in the severely obese individual.

OTHER TECHNIQUES FOR MEASURING FAT MASS

Bioelectrical impedance

Bioelectrical impedance devices for estimation of total fat mass are frequently marketed to professionals and the public, and values are thus often quoted by parents. The devices are fairly inexpensive and portable. They measure conductance of a small electrical charge through body water and, by a derived formula estimate lean body mass (and hence, by subtraction, fat mass). They are extremely sensitive to error from malpositioned electrodes, sweat and diet, and the formulae built in to the software of many devices are not suitable for use in childhood. They should

not be used outside carefully controlled clinical studies[32] where appropriate formulae have been calculated for the reference population.

Dual X-ray absorption (DEXA) scanning

Although not a non-invasive direct technique DEXA scanning has become a standard pediatric method that allows for calculation of lean body mass and fat mass by measuring the attenuation of photon energy passing through nonbony tissue. It allows for a precise measurement of body composition, though the values produced by different manufacturers' devices can be large,[32] so single devices must be used for longitudinal studies. Whole-body and regional magnetic resonance imaging (MRI) and computed tomography (CT) scanning have also been used to measure fat mass but the availability of the former and the radiation dose of the latter limit their applicability in pediatrics.

Body mass index

BMI is a value calculated from height and weight that can be used as an estimate of relative obesity or, more rarely, thinness. The formula is weight (in kilograms)/height (in meters)^2. For adults cut-off values can be used to define, e.g., obesity = BMI > 30; but the relationship of height to weight in a growing child means that appropriate age and sex specific centile charts must be used. The International Obesity Task Force (IOTF) has produced extrapolated cut-offs from an adult BMI of 30 and 25 available on the UK childhood BMI chart.[33] As stated above, weight is a combination of many tissues, and so the formula does not relate directly to adiposity in the very muscular or edematous child, though this rarely is a problem clinically. The height denominator is squared, thus magnifying measurement error and increasing the reliability on an accurate measurement.

Head circumference

The 'lasso' (Lasso-o™ available from the UK Child Growth Foundation) as illustrated (Fig. 13.6) is an ideal device for measuring head circumference. It allows for a relatively constant force to be applied when measuring the deformable skull of an infant. In any case a nonstretchable paper or metal tape should be used and NOT a sewing aid-type cloth measure that can stretch by more than 1 cm at 0.5 m with repeated use.

Three estimations should be made of the maximum occipito-frontal circumference (OFC) and the average recorded. In children with a very abnormal head shape such as ex-premature babies with plagiocephaly it may not be possible to obtain meaningful readings.

Span and segment measurements

It is sometimes helpful to directly assess other body sizes and their relationships, descriptions of technique, and

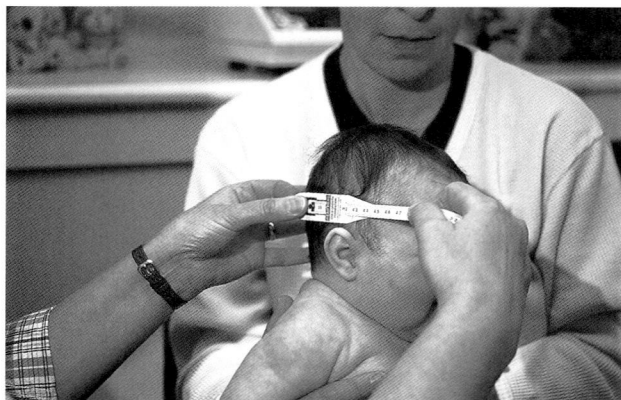

Figure 13.6 Measurement of head circumference (occipito-frontal circumference; OFC). Using a non-stretchable lasso (Lasso-o™ Child Growth Foundation, UK).

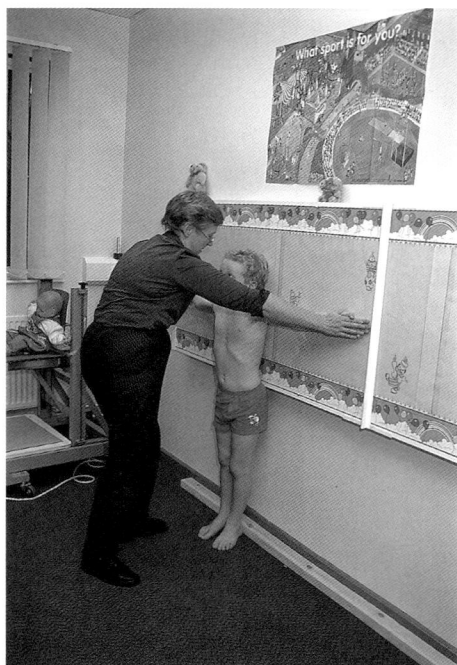

Figure 13.7 Measurement of span. Arms horizontal, fingers touching fixed and moveable vertical rule.

standard centile charts exist for almost every imaginable parameter for use in particular in the diagnosis of dysmorphic syndromes; for instance, inter-canthal distance, penile length etc.[34]

Measurement of span is the most likely to be of use in the endocrine clinic, for instance in Marfan syndrome or as an approximate surrogate for height in the wheelchair bound. It may be estimated by measuring the fingertip to fingertip distance with the arms held horizontally (Fig. 13.7). The normal relationship of span to height is span = height ± 3.5 cm. In common with many forensic techniques used to estimate height from body fragments the technique is good for group data but less precise at estimating the height on an individual.

In short-limbed conditions and if hemihypertrophy is suspected then direct measurement of limb segments using a specially designed anthropometer or a metal builder's tape measure may be of help.

GROWTH CHARTS

Up-to-date standards for height, sitting height, weight, BMI and head and waist circumference are available for many populations. Standards should be up-dated regularly to take secular changes in growth into account, and ideally ethnic sub-groups should be compared to appropriate charts, though this is not always possible. Most commonly used charts are sex-specific and show the measured parameter on the vertical axis and age on the horizontal. It is common to use decimal age scales when longitudinal data are required as it allows for easier calculation of height velocity (see below). Charts incorporating a decimal age scale have a decimal calendar that allows subtraction of a birthdate (e.g., 28 July 1997 = 1997.570) from the clinic date (e.g., 15 October 2004 = 2004.786) to calculate age = 7.22 years and time from last clinic visit when, for example, 6.34 years = 0.88.

Almost all vertical scales are linear except for skin-fold thickness where a vertical logarithmic axis is used and in some charts extending into premature infancy where a non-linear age axis allows expansion of data in the early months.

Many charts use 'centile' lines spaced at varying intervals depending on the design of the chart. A common lay-out is to use the 0.4th, 2nd, 9th, 25th and 50th centile with corresponding values above the mean to give nine centile lines, smoothed by a statistical method known as LMS.[35] Thus only 1/250 children would fall below the 0.4th or above the 99.6th centile in a normal population, which may form the basis for a referral protocol.

Charts of height and weight in many named syndromic conditions have been published, and should be used where necessary. There are also charts of limb length, height and OFC in many of the skeletal dysplasias.

The measured value should be plotted as a simple dot and other values, such as bone age (see below) plotted in a different color or a square symbol.

PARENTAL SIZE

Ideally both parents should have measurements of height, weight and, if relevant, head circumference recorded directly, as reported size can vary greatly from reality.[36] Overweight individuals are poor reporters of weight[37] and so any derived value, such as body mass index, calculated solely on reported values is doubly suspect. A large number of children are referred unnecessarily with 'big heads' when they are merely taking after one or both parents.

Whenever a standard centile chart is used, of whatever construction, it is possible to rapidly estimate the expected genetic potential of the subject, for height or OFC, by plotting the centile value of each parent on the right-hand *y*-axis. The mid-parental centile can then be drawn. Alternatively, for height only, the following simple calculations may be performed:

Target height (in centimeters) boy:
[(father's height + mother's height)/2} + 7
Target height (in centimeters) girl:
[(mother's height + father's height)/2] − 7

If a secular trend is expected, for example if the economic situation of the child is much better than that of the parents in their youth, one can add 4.5 cm to the target height.[38] In 95 percent of the cases the final height of the child is expected to be within the target height ± 10 cm for boys and 8.5 cm for girls, the so-called 'target range'. The centile position of the target height can then be compared to the centile position of the present height of the child.

As growth is a longitudinal process, change of height with time is even more important than absolute height at a point. The final evaluation of growth in any parameter is made by connecting consecutive measurements on the growth chart and visually assessing any deviation upwards or downwards through the centile lines.

Growth rate can also be evaluated by calculating a velocity that can be compared with published height and weight velocity curves. Velocity is calculated by the formula

$$\frac{\text{height 1} - \text{height 2}}{\text{interval, in years}}$$

Hence in the example given above, with two measurements separated by 0.88 year a difference in height of 6.7 cm would equal a velocity of 6.7/0.88 = 7.6 cm/year.

Because measurement error is magnified when two separately obtained values are used to calculate a velocity, (95 percent confidence interval (CI) for velocity estimated from two measurements 1 year apart = $\pm q \times \sqrt{2}$ (where *q* is 2SD of measurement, i.e., around 0.2 cm). For a 3 month interval the CI is four times this value. The use of this calculation is dependent on accurate measurements and improved by long intervals between estimates. The design of the reference charts[39] means that optimal information will come from yearly estimations of height velocity (and in clinical practice a minimum period of 6 months).

SDS or *Z* score

To allow more precise quantification of any normally distributed parameter for which standards exist it is common to use the standard deviation score (SDS or *Z* score), especially for values that lie outside the normal centile range. This technique allows comparison of the parameters for children of different age and sex.

$$\text{SDS} = \frac{x - \bar{x}}{\text{SD}}$$

where *x* is the measured value; $\bar{x}$ the mean, and SD the standard deviation for a given population. In a normally distributed population the SDS will have a mean of 0 and a SD of 1. A SDS of −1 to +1 includes 68.26 percent and −2 to +2 includes 95.44 percent of the population, respectively. Only 0.13 percent of a population will have a SDS of more or less than 3.

SKELETAL MATURITY

Growth occurs at a different 'tempo' in individuals, there being both fast and slow developers. The concept of assessing developmental maturity by the differential ossification of the bones of the wrist was introduced first by Pryor.[40] Several means of assessing this maturity exist, but the three most commonly used are the Gruelich and Pyle (G&P),[41] the Tanner and Whitehouse methods versions 2 and 3 (TW2 & TW3)[42,43] and the Fels[44] methods, all working from an X-ray of the left hand and wrist. There are also methods for assessing maturity of other aggregates of bones in the knee, ankle, foot, and dental age. There may be very little relation between, for instance, dental age and bone age as assessed by a wrist radiograph[45] and there may be differential maturation of different areas of the skeleton,[46] so a single method must be used in any centre and in longitudinal studies. The maturation of the skeleton as assessed by these methods has a relatively poor correlation between stages of pubertal development[47] and the rate of change of maturation varies between different stages of puberty.[48]

The large number of bones in the hand and wrist, the relative lack of overlapping structures and the relatively low dose of radiation required have made the hand and wrist the most usual target for methods of assessment of skeletal maturity (Fig. 13.8).

The standard populations used to create the reference radiographs were of normal children of relatively selected populations. The Gruelich and Pyle series was relatively 'advanced' for its time, probably because the population was from a relatively well-off socio-economic group. The longitudinal series used for the Tanner and Whitehouse methods (2 and 3) were collected over 20 years before the early 1980s. Population comparisons from modern China show a relative 'delay' of 6–18 months; modern Japanese children a 'delay' of only 3–6 months in comparison to the TW3 reference. In contrast some ages of Argentinean and Italian children have a slight 'advance' in comparison to the TW3 reference.[43]

The assignment of a bone age may be used to give an estimate of final height ('prediction'), first proposed by Bayley then refined for use with the G&P method by Bayley and Pinneau[49] and further by Roche et al.[50] (RWT method) for use with the G&P system using equations incorporating bone age, height, weight and parental height. The TW3 method uses present height + (RUS score)x + y where x and y are constants varying according to the age of the child to predict adult height. (The RUS score is referred to below.)

It must be remembered that all the reference data were collected on healthy children. The systems were not intended to be used in children with short stature caused by ill-health or drug administration or in children with syndromic short or tall stature. A 'delay' in bone age in a child may not relate

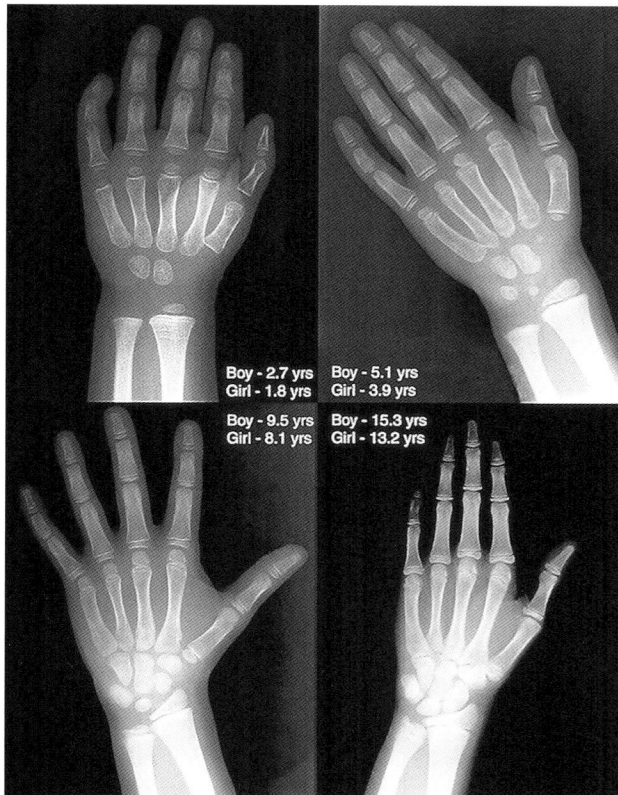

Figure 13.8   Bone maturation at four ages.

to improved height potential if caused by steroids or renal failure. Any attempt at predicting height in children with an advanced bone age due to sexual precocity will produce huge errors as given in Table 13.2.[51] For children with simple delayed puberty and modest bone age delay (up to 3 years) the TW3 method underestimates final height by 2.5 cm in a boy and 2 cm in a girl, though the range was −2 to +8 cm.[43] In simple familial tall stature the TW2 method underestimated final height in boys by 2–5 cm in teenage years.[52]

The radiograph used for assessment must be taken in a standard manner with the hand placed lightly flat on the film cassette to avoid any rotation, with the thumb at about 30° to the fingers and must include all the bones of the hand and wrist. All too often radiographs taken in 'inexperienced' units omit the epiphyses at the wrist, or even several fingers. The exposure of the film must be sufficient to reveal the anterior and posterior detail of the bone modeling.

The G&P technique allots a 'bone age' by comparison of the ossification centers to a standard atlas. The film is compared to a series of plates and the allocated age is that of the closest match. The standard stages of maturation are thus discontinuous but are being applied to a continuous process. It is also evident that even within a single individual there may be considerable discrepancies between the apparent maturity of bones of the same wrist (up to 20 months). An 'overall' age is often estimated for speed and simplicity rather than taking the time-consuming average of bone maturity (which is necessary for the RWT height prediction method). These cautions mean that in clinical practice outside research-based studies the method is rather subjective and poorly reproducible.[53]

The TW3 method gives a maturity score by examining characteristics of each ossification center of 20 bones in the hand and wrist excluding the 2nd and 4th rays. Each bone is assessed and allocated a letter indicating its individual maturity. A sum of scores produces a total skeletal maturity score. A smaller sample of 13 bones excluding the carpal bones produces an RUS score (radius, ulna, and short bones) that may be used in equations to predict final height, as indicated above.

Table 13.2   Comparison of adult height prediction (AHP) and final height (FHt) in six groups of patients

Group (n)	AHP/FHt r^2	FHt −AHP range (cm)	FHt −AHP mean (cm)	Percent final values in TW2 range
1 (66)	0.95	−7.7 to +7.2	−0.58	86
2 (26)	0.62	−9.1 to +15	+1.21	70
3 (35)	0.69	−10.8 to +7.7	−3.40	51
4 (41)	0.21	−41.0 to +7.0	−6.60	59
5 (26)	0.71	−16 to +7.0	−0.50	77
6 (55)	0.77	−14.5 to +10.5	−1.18	76

All estimations were performed by a single professional auxologist.
Group 1: Short patients with no eventual pathological diagnosis; 2: GHD patients before therapy commenced; 3: Turner syndrome; 4: congenital adrenal hyperplasia; 5: cystic fibrosis; 6: diabetes mellitus.

The Fels method is also bone-specific but uses some different maturity indicators to the TW3 method. A computerized scoring program allows for the fact that some stages of maturation of a bone last longer than others and provide less information about maturity and hence weights the overall score appropriately. The system gives poor agreement with the TW2 method during adolescence.[54]

Because of the limitations of the three main scoring systems outlined above there have been attempts to devise computerized assessment systems (CASAS, computer-assisted skeletal age scores) using either digitized images of individual bones matched to a template and analyzed by a complex mathematical transformation or automatic analysis of scanned images to assess bone staging.[55] These two methods allow for a continuous scoring more akin to real life as all the characteristics of the bones are assessed simultaneously. The first method has been used to score with reasonable accuracy children with Turner syndrome, where manual scoring is poorly predictive.[56] A recent development is to use a new series of digital standards and computer assessment over the internet to allow for web-based bone age assessment.[57] These advanced techniques are still in use in only a small number of centers and further information as to their financial and time-cost and reliability will emerge in the future.

SUMMARY

Good-quality measurements, correctly plotted on appropriate charts, coupled with parental heights, an estimate of bone maturation and past readings are the 'temperature chart' of chronic disease, giving more information, non-invasively, than any other technique in pediatrics. It is therefore essential that trained personnel are used to record data using well maintained and calibrated equipment. New technology should be evaluated and incorporated locally where appropriate. Any studies of growth should assess and quote the exact techniques and equipment used and inter- and intra-observer measurement error.

KEY LEARNING POINTS

- Measurements of height, weight and other anthropometric parameters form the cornerstone of pediatric diagnosis.
- Parental size must be measured to assess the child's genetic growth potential.
- Appropriate charts must be used and the data plotted correctly.
- Longitudinal changes provide a non-invasive means of following a child's health or disease process.
- Short-term growth measurements provide information about the basic biology of growth.

- Skeletal maturity may, if accurately scored, and in conjunction with an assessment of stage of sexual maturation provide information about growth potential in the normal child.
- New technologies for assessment of skeletal maturity are emerging.

REFERENCES

● = Seminal primary article
◆ = Key review paper

● 1 Voss LD, Wilkin TJ, Bailey BJ, Betts PR. The reliability of height and height velocity in the assessment of growth (the Wessex Growth Study). *Arch Dis Child* 1991; **66**: 833–7.
● 2 Voss LD, Bailey BJ, Cumming K, et al. The reliability of height measurement (the Wessex Growth Study). *Arch Dis Child* 1990; **65**: 1340–4.
3 Cameron N. The methods of auxological anthropometry. In: Falkner F, Tanner JM, eds. *Human Growth. A Comprehensive Treatise*, 2nd edn. New York, London: Plenum Press, 1986.
● 4 Wales JKH, Milner RDG. Knemometry in assessment of linear growth. *Arch Dis Child* 1987; **62**: 166–71.
5 Johnston FE, Hamill PVV, Lemeshow S. Skinfold thickness of children 6–1 years. *United States Vital Health Statistics* 1972; **11(120)**: 1–60.
6 Malina RM, Hamill PVV, Lemeshow S. Selected body measurements of children 6–11 years. *United States Vital Health Statistics* 1973; **11(123)**: 1–48.
7 Whitfield MF, Kay R, Stevens S. Validity of routine clinical test weighing as a measure of intake in breast fed infants. *Arch Dis Child* 1981; **56**: 919–21.
8 Voss LD. Bailey BJ. Diurnal variation in stature: is stretching the answer. *Arch Dis Child* 1997; **77**: 319–22.
9 Whitehouse RH, Tanner JM, Healy MJR. Diurnal variation in stature and sitting height in 12–14-year-old boys. *Ann Hum Biol* 1974; **1**: 103–6.
10 Tanner JM, Whitehouse Rh. *Standards for Sitting Height and Sub-ischial Leg Length From Birth to Maturity: British Children 1978*. Ware: Castlemead Publications, 1979.
11 Dangour AD, Schilg S, Hulse JA, Cole TJ. Sitting height and subischial leg length centile curves for boys and girls from Southeast England. *Ann Hum Biol* 2002; **29**: 290–305.
◆ 12 Wales JKH. A brief history of the study of human growth dynamics. *Ann Hum Biol* 1998; **25**: 175–84.
13 Scammon RE. The first seriatim study of human growth. *Am J Phys Anthropol* 1927; **10**: 329–36.
14 Togo M. Time-series analysis in human growth studies. In: Hauspie R, Lindgren G, Falkner F, eds. *Essays on Auxology*. Welwyn Garden City: Castlemead Publications, 1995.
15 Green WT, Anderson M. Experiences with epiphyseal arrest in correcting discrepancy in length of the lower

extremities in infantile paralysis. *J Bone Joint Surg* 1947; **29A**: 659–75.

16 Green WT, Anderson M. Epiphyseal arrest for the correction of discrepancies in length of the lower extremities. *J Bone Joint Surg* 1957; **39**: 853–72.

17 Aronson AS, Selvik G. X-ray stereophotogrammetry, a method for high accuracy analysis of growth rate. *Acta Paediatr Scand Suppl* 1988; **343**: 186–7.

18 Valk IM. Ulnar length and growth in twins with a simplified technique for ulnar measurement using a condylograph. *Growth* 1972; **36**: 291–309.

● 19 Lampl M, Veldhuis JD, Johnson ML. Saltation and stasis: A model of human growth. *Science* 1992; **258**: 801–3.

20 Wales JKH, Milner RDG. Variation in lower leg growth with alternate day steroid treatment. *Arch Dis Child* 1988; **63**: 981–3.

21 Gibson AT, Pearse RG, Wales JKH. Knemometry and the assessment of growth in premature babies. *Arch Dis Child* 1993; **69**: 498–504.

22 Gibson AT, Pearse RG, Wales JKH. Growth retardation after dexamethasone administration: assessment by knemometry. *Arch Dis Child* 1993; **69**: 505–9.

◆ 23 Wales JKH, Gibson AT. Short-term growth – rhythms, chaos or noise? *Arch Dis Child* 1994; **71**: 84–89.

24 Jeliffe DB. *The Assessment of the Nutritional Status of the Community.* WHO Monograph 53. Geneva: World Health Organization, 1966.

25 Fredriks AM, van Buuren S, Wit JM, Verloove-Vanhorick SP. Body mass index measurements in 1996–7 compared with 1980. *Arch Dis Child* 2000; **82**: 107–12.

26 McCarthy HD, Jarrett KV, Crawley HF. The development of waist circumference percentiles in British children aged 5.0–16.9 y. *Eur J Clin Nutr* 2001; **55**: 902–7.

27 Tanner JM, Whitehouse RH. Revised standards for triceps and subscapular skinfolds in British children. *Arch Dis Child* 1975; **50**: 142–5.

28 Dauncey MJ, Gandy G, Gairdner D. Assessment of total body fat in infancy from skinfold thickness measurements. *Arch Dis Child* 1977; **52**: 223–7.

29 Durnin JVGA, Rahaman MM. The assessment of the amount of fat in the human body from measurements of skinfold thickness. *Br J Nutr* 1967; **21**: 681–9.

30 Forbes GB, Amirhakimi GH. Skinfold thickness and body fat in children. *Hum Biol* 1970; **42**: 401–18.

31 Parizkova J. Total body fat and skinfold thickness in children. *Metabolism* 1961; **10**: 794–807.

◆ 32 Ellis KJ. Human body composition: in vivo methods. *Physiol Rev* 2000; **80**: 649–80.

33 Child Growth Foundation. *Boys & Girls BMI Chart.* South Shields: Harlow Printing, 2003.

34 Hall JG, Froster-Iskenius UG, Allanson JE. *Handbook of Normal Physical Measurements.* Oxford: Oxford University Press, 1989.

● 35 Cole TJ. The LMS method for constructing normalized growth standards. *Eur J Clin Nutr* 1990; **44**: 45–60.

36 LeJarraga H, Laspuir M, Adamo P. Validity of reported parental height in outpatient growth clinics in Buenos Aires city. *Ann Hum Biol* 1995; **22**: 163–6.

37 Wang Z, Patterson CM, Hills AP. A comparison of self-reported and measured height, weight and BMI in Australian adolescents. *Aust NZ J Public Health* 2002; **26**: 473–8.

38 Fredriks AM, van Buuren S, Burgmeijer RJ, *et al.* Continuing positive secular growth change in The Netherlands 1955–1997. *Pediatr Res* 2000; **47**: 316–23.

● 39 Tanner JM, Whitehouse RH. Clinical longitudinal standards for height, weight, height velocity, weight velocity and stages of puberty. *Arch Dis Child* 1976; **51**: 170–9.

40 Pryor JW. Time of ossification of the bones of the hand of the male and female and union of epiphyses with the diaphyses. *Am J Phys Anthropol* 1925; **8(Old Series)**: 401–10.

41 Greulich WW, Pyle SI. *Radiographic Atlas of Skeletal Development of the Hand and Wrist,* 2nd edn. Stanford: Stanford University Press, 1959.

● 42 Tanner JM, Whitehouse RH, Marshall WA, *et al.* *Assessment of Skeletal Maturity and Prediction of Adult Height (TW2 Method).* London: Academic Press, 1975.

● 43 Tanner JM, Healy MJR, Goldstein H, Cameron N. *Assessment of Skeletal Maturity and Prediction of Adult Height (TW3 Method).* London: WB Saunders, 2001.

● 44 Roche AF, Chumlea W, Thissen D. *Assessing the Skeletal Maturity of the Hand-Wrist: FELS method.* Springfield, Illinois: Charles C Thomas, 1988.

45 Vallejo-Bolanos E, Espana-Lopez AJ, Munoz-Hoyos A, Fernandez-Garcia JM. The relationship between bone age, chronological age and dental age in children with isolated growth hormone deficiency. *Int J Paediatr Dent* 1999; **9**: 201–6.

46 Roche AF. Differential timing of maximum length increments among bones within individuals. *Hum Biol* 1974; **46**: 145–57.

47 Benso L, Vannelli S, Pastorin L, *et al.* Main problems associated with bone age maturity evaluation. Horm Res 1996; **45(Suppl 2)**: 42–8.

48 Buckler JMH. Skeletal age changes in puberty. *Arch Dis Child* 1984; **59**: 115–9.

● 49 Bayley N, Pinneau SR. Tables for predicting adult height from skeletal age; revised for use with Greulich and Pyle hand standards. *J Pediatr* 1952; **40**: 423–41.

50 Roche AF, Wainer H, Thissen D. *Predicting Adult Stature for Individuals.* Monographs in Paediatrics, vol. 3. Basel: Karger, 1975.

51 Pickering M, Wales JKH. TW2 height prediction in the endocrine clinic. *Humanobiol Budapest* 1994; **24**: 22.

52 de Waal WJ, Greyn-Fokker MH, Stijnen T, *et al.* Accuracy of final height prediction and effect of growth-reductive therapy in 362 constitutionally tall children. *J Clin Endocrinol Metab* 1996; **81**: 1206–16.

53 Gilli G. The assessment of skeletal maturation. *Horm Res* 1996; **45(Suppl 2)**: 49–52

54 van Lenthe FJ, Kemper HC, van Mechelen W. Skeletal maturation in adolescence: a comparison between the Tanner–Whitehouse 2 and the Fels method. *Eur J Pediatr* 1998; **157**: 798–801.

55 Cox LA. Tanner–Whitehouse method of assessing skeletal maturity: problems and common errors. *Horm Res* 1996; **45(Suppl 2)**: 52–5

56 Schwarze CP, Arens D, Haber HP, *et al*. Bone age in 116 untreated patients with Turner's syndrome rated by a computer-assisted method (CASAS). *Acta Paediatr* 1998; **87**: 1146–50.

57 Van Teunenbroek A, De Waal W, Roks A, *et al*. Computer-aided skeletal age scores in healthy children, girls with Turner syndrome, and in children with constitutionally tall stature. *Pediatr Res* 1996; **39**: 360–7.

14

Endocrine assessment and principles of endocrine testing

P C HINDMARSH

INTRODUCTION

There are a wide number of tests available for assessing growth hormone (GH) secretion. A considerable amount of attention has been paid to the underlying mechanisms assessed by the tests, how the samples should be collected and what type of measurement should be performed. Less attention has been paid to the mathematical assumptions underlying the performance of diagnostic tests. The statistical theory behind many tests is complex as they do not follow an all-or-nothing law. Rather than being left with a clear-cut answer to the initial diagnostic question, the clinician is left with a series of probabilities as to whether or not the patient is likely to have the condition in question.

Clinical diagnosis identifies patient symptoms and signs that result from the underlying disorder in a number of ways. First, pattern recognition would say that the person looks so obviously panhypopituitary that there is no other likely explanation. Second, clinical algorithms can be applied to the problem. Figure 14.1 shows a possible approach to short stature. Finally, the gather-all approach could be used and all possible data collected. This is expensive and seldom productive, not least because no thought has gone into formulating a hypothesis about what actually was wrong. In practice most clinicians, however, settle for a list of potential diagnoses and use investigation to limit the length of the list.

It is possible to create an artificial gulf between what has gone on before the elucidation of symptoms and signs and what is about to happen, the performance of a test. This is unhelpful because the possibility of the presence of the disorder before testing has an important influence on the probability of the individual having the disorder after the completion of the test. This chapter reviews the principles underlying the diagnostic process using the paradigm of growth hormone (GH) testing in short children to elucidate the diagnosis of GH deficiency (GHD).[1]

CLINICAL OBSERVATIONS

Failure of physical growth is an important sign of systemic disease but also the hallmark of endocrine disease, because pituitary, thyroid, adrenal, and gonadal hormones are all involved in the process. Initially, the categorization of an individual child depends on clinical evaluation and growth assessment and not on laboratory investigations, which should not be employed until and unless auxological data indicate them to be necessary. The diagnosis of GHD is made by exclusion of other possible explanations for poor growth before accepting that the likely diagnosis is GHD.[1] This is important because, although growth in childhood is predominantly GH dependent,[2,3] GH probably represents the final common pathway for the mediation of the growth process and is modulated by a number of other factors (Fig. 14.2).

It is likely that a child with a potential growth or endocrine disorder undergoes clinical examination and anthropometric assessment. The principles of the latter have been well described elsewhere.[4–6] The accuracy of the examination and precision of the anthropometry are crucial determinants for

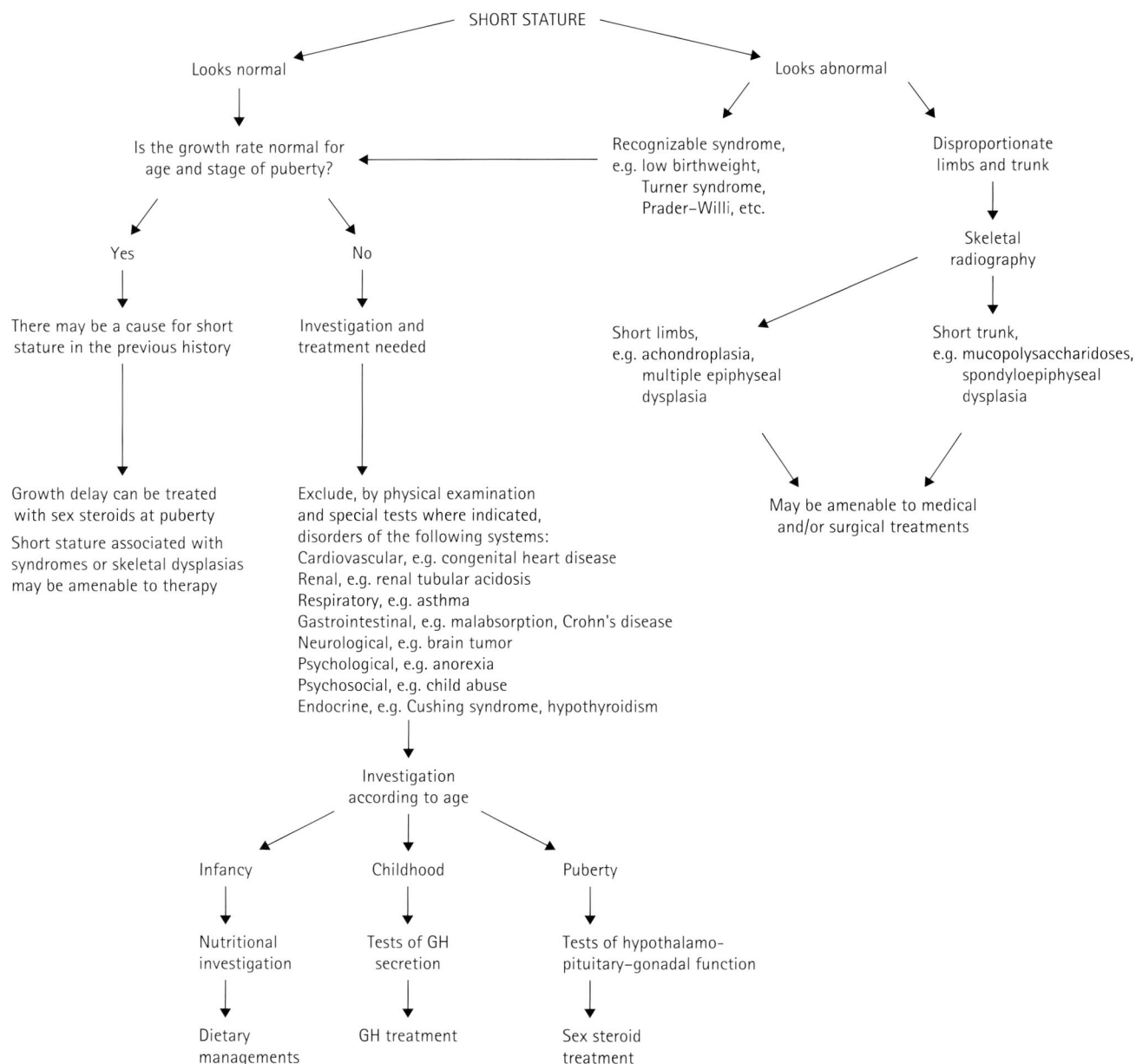

Figure 14.1   Algorithm for the assessment of short stature.

diagnosis.[6] Conventional approaches to growth disorders list features seen in association with certain conditions but the power of clinical observation in determining the diagnosis is rarely discussed. Nor is the magnitude and cause of diagnostic error considered. Could a simple assessment of key clinical points improve diagnostic certainty to the point where testing is unhelpful? No test will help if the degree of uncertainty is high and, equally, if the degree of certainty is high, why test?

EVALUATION OF CLINICAL POINTS IN THE PRESENTATION OF GROWTH HORMONE DEFICIENCY

Several texts describe the characteristic clinical picture of GHD – a short plump child with a round immature face.

Birth weight is usually normal and poor growth is apparent from about six months of age.[7–9] GHD may be isolated or associated with other pituitary hormone deficiencies. Small genitalia may suggest gonadotrophin deficiency. Hypoglycemia in the newborn period is often a feature of ACTH deficiency. Prolonged neonatal jaundice raises the question of thyroxine (unconjugated) or cortisol (conjugated hyperbilirubinemia) deficiency. Given these features, it might be possible on the basis of pattern recognition to ascribe the diagnosis of GHD to a patient with a high degree of certainty.

If, however, we simply restricted the assessment to obesity as a feature problems would arise. Testing the GH axis would yield a large number of individuals with a poor GH response, because obesity per se is associated with blunted GH responses to various stimuli.[10,11] What is demonstrated is the poor performance of obesity alone as a diagnostic criterion

Neurotransmitters, glucose, amino acids,
lipids, sleep, temperature

Hypothalamus   Growth hormone-releasing ········· Somatostatin
hormone

+ve   −ve   +ve   −ve

Pituitary   Growth hormone

Bone   Cell differentiation

IGF-I
synthesis

Clonal expansion

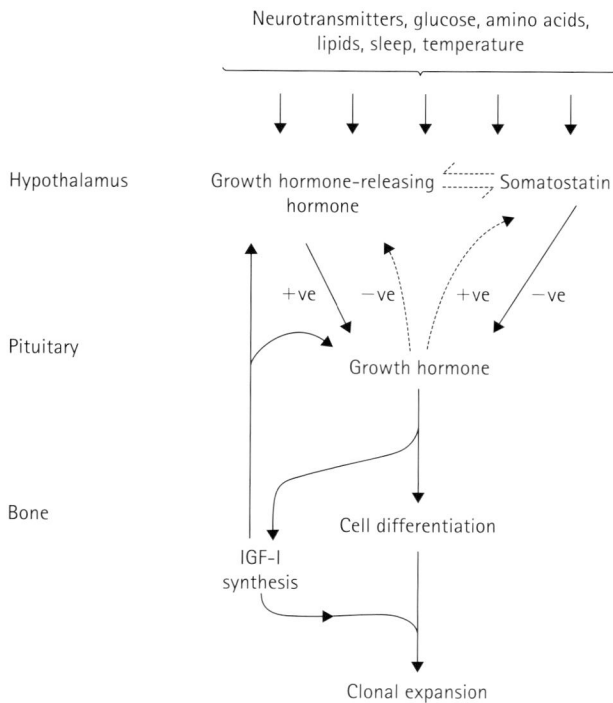

Figure 14.2   The growth hormone cascade.

for GHD. Individuals who are GHD are often obese but the converse is clearly not the case.

What is required from the clinical standpoint is some assessment of the strength of various symptoms and signs in making the diagnosis of GHD. This might be achieved by introducing additional clinical information into the diagnostic model. At this juncture, a note of caution needs to be sounded: little is known of the sensitivity and specificity of many of the clinical observations, either alone or in combination. The prevalence of many of the clinical features within the general population is unknown, which heightens the problem. Even the presence of specific features or combination of features will increase only slightly the likelihood of disease if they are relatively insensitive. However, as will be seen below, it is still possible for the clinicians to come out with 'best estimate' for the probability that the individual has a particular condition or not. An understanding of the growth process is essential as it will impact directly on the probability of disease presence.

Growth during the first year of life is largely dependent on nutrition, and poor growth during this time is most likely to be the result of nutritional or gastrointestinal problems.[12] The manifestation of GHD as a result of GH gene deletion is early and poor growth can be detected as early as the sixth month of postnatal life.[7-9] With advancing age, more GH has to be secreted to maintain concentrations of GH sufficient for growth, so idiopathic isolated pituitary GHD may present at any time. It is the degree of deficiency that dictates when the individual comes to medical attention and the majority of cases of GHD in childhood, other than those secondary to cranial irradiation for leukemia or brain tumors, could well be detected before the age of 5 years.[13,14]

Assessing a child's growth by single or multiple measurements does not lead immediately to confirmation of the diagnosis because GH plays such a central role in the control of childhood growth.[2,3] There are many chronic illnesses in childhood that influence GH secretion, such as celiac disease,[15] asthma, and the treatment of a number of chronic inflammatory diseases with exogenous glucocorticoids, all of which influence growth, if not GH secretion.[16]

Because of the multiple non-endocrine causes for poor growth, the clinician will tend to rule out the more common causes and then embark on a series of investigations to confirm or refute the hypothesis that the individual has GHD. The concept of testing an hypothesis reflects the need to account for degrees of certainty or uncertainty with respect to the underlying diagnosis. This is particularly important because techniques will now be described to evaluate and quantify the degree of certainty or uncertainty.

CREATING THE ENVIRONMENT FOR THE TEST

Analysis of hormones in the circulation may use single or multiple samples. Variations in hormone secretion take place on a day to day basis and need not be confined to short time intervals, e.g., changes in gonadotrophins during the menstrual cycle. The majority of tests conducted in pediatric practice take place at a fixed time of the day. In the execution and interpretation of these tests, consideration needs to be given to the physiology of the hormone studied and the sampling interval chosen for the collection of blood samples. Finally, the test will only be as good as the framework within which the question is set.

Hormone physiology

Many of the analytes measured in clinical endocrine practice do not have a circadian rhythm or are complexed in the serum to binding proteins. In such situations, it is generally assumed that there are no long-term variations, although this may not always be the case (see reproducibility section below). Cortisol, the gonadotrophins, GH, and insulin are the best known of the hormones that pulse.[17-20] The implication of pulsatile secretion assumes great importance when assessing the performance of diagnostic tests.[21] Efficiency, sensitivity and specificity will all be dependent to some extent on the repeatability and reproducibility of the tests under study and the pulsatile system will influence both of these in a number of ways.

Most endocrine tests are conducted over short periods of time and their results are often extrapolated to longer time frames. GH provocation tests used to assess the GH secretory state in children are performed over a 2 h period and the results are then compared to height velocity measurements obtained over a longer period of time, often 1 year. That there is a relationship is perhaps surprising; that there are high false positive and negative rates, perhaps not.

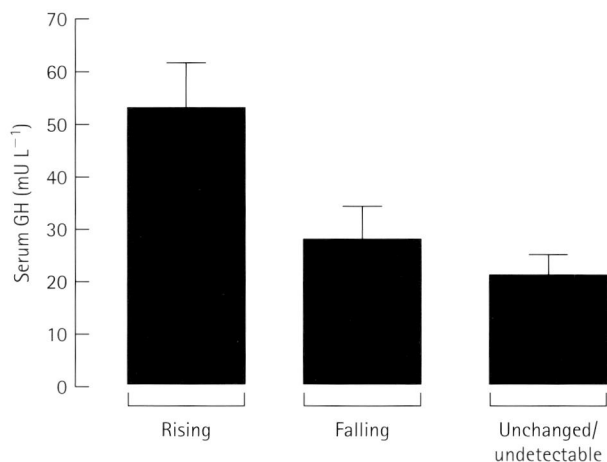

Figure 14.3 Growth hormone response to exogenous growth hormone-releasing hormone depending upon whether pre-administration growth hormone levels are rising, falling or unchanged. Modified from Suri et al.[30]

Hormone pulsatility may also influence diagnostic tests if the test itself (e.g., the stimulus applied) is influenced by oscillations within the system under study. It has been recognized for a long time that the GH response to insulin-induced hypoglycemia is heavily influenced by the serum GH concentration measured at the commencement of the study. If it is measurable, a rise in GH in response to the hypoglycemic stimulus is less likely.[22]

Understanding hormone physiology is therefore essential both in defining the circadian rhythm and the variability of the hormone concentration under study and also in beginning to understand from the pattern of secretion what the underlying regulatory processes are. In the example quoted above of the GH response to insulin-induced hypoglycemia, it is clear that the GH response at any point in time is going to be heavily dependent on the interplay between the hypothalamic regulatory proteins involved in GH release, namely GH-releasing hormone and somatostatin.[23] Figure 14.3 shows the effect of differing states of GH secretion before the application of a stimulus (GHRH) and how the response to the same exogenous stimulus varies. Subsequent studies have demonstrated that somatostatin, in particular, is a key determinant of the amount of GH released as a result of GHRH stimulation. Attempts have been made to take control of this variable[24] by pre-treatment with somatostatin. GHRH combined with arginine is an alternative approach.[25] The GH secretagogues were thought initially to overcome many of these limitations because of their potent GH-releasing qualities but suffer the same problems of reproducibility.[26] The importance of the trough concentration, a reflection of somatostatin exposure, in determining GH responsivity and growth has been demonstrated (Table 14.1).[27]

Other hormones and environmental factors influence the amount of GH that may be released. Both thyroxine and cortisol alter GH gene transcription and these need to be

Table 14.1 Mean peak growth hormone response (mU L^{-1}) to insulin-induced hypoglycemia with respect to peak and trough growth hormone concentrations in 24 h physiological profiles of GH secretion

	Low peaks	High peaks	Total
Low troughs	13.0	28.2	22.0
High troughs	7.6	21.4	13.9
Total	9.8	25.1	

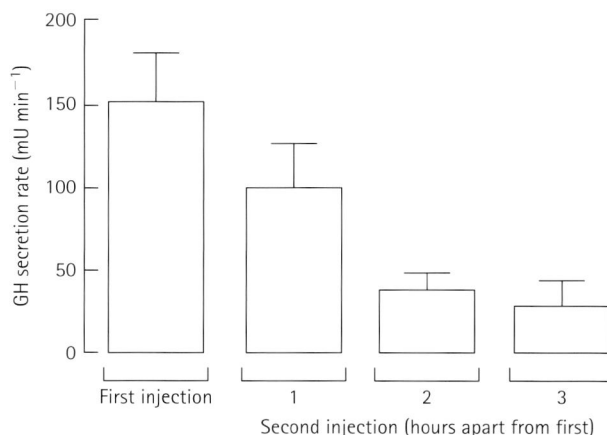

Figure 14.4 Effect of differing time intervals on the growth hormone response to repeated growth hormone releasing hormone administration. Modified from Suri et al.[30]

normal before undertaking a diagnostic study.[28] Similarly, the presence of high plasma concentrations of glucose or free fatty acids may influence responsivity.[29] Alterations in sex steroid concentrations during puberty (or the menstrual cycle) modify the GH response to GHRH.

Endocrine systems are subject to feedback from target tissues and this influences not only in the interpretation of single provocation tests but also where second tests are performed in rapid succession to the first. A diminished response to GHRH can be observed if the second stimulus is applied one, two or three hours after the first (Fig. 14.4).[30] The implication of doing two tests on the same day, often following each other, are immense, because the cut-off that might be implied to determine normality or not may not be the same for the second test as for the first, especially if the second stimulus is different from the first.

In assessing the results of endocrine evaluations, it is generally assumed that the single or multiple samples measured are relatively stable, at least over short periods. A thyroxine measurement on one day should be similar to one measured the next day or week. Whilst this may be true generally, it cannot be assumed. When important changes are postulated to be taking place, for example in a disease process, some knowledge of the inherent variability within the measurement system is required. In endocrine practice,

Table 14.2 Within-individual coefficients of variation for pituitary hormones

	Coefficient of variation (%) Mean (range)
Mean 24-h serum GH concentration	35 (9–58)
Mean 24-h serum LH concentration	19 (5–29)
Serum IGF-I concentration	21 (14–34)
Serum testosterone concentration	13 (8–19)

we are well aware of the errors incurred in the measurement of hormones and the between- and within-assay coefficients of variation greatly aid the interpretation of hormone measurements. In the short term, a number of studies have demonstrated variability within and between individuals in terms of endocrine tests.[31–34] Group data are usually reproducible but problems can arise if it is assumed that individual oscillatory profiles are consistent from day to day. Table 14.2 summarizes data relating to intra-individual coefficients of variation in 24 h hormone profiles measured over 1 year.[32] These observations add an additional dimension to the comparison of studies obtained under one series of circumstances with a set obtained under another series of circumstances, particularly if they are separated by long periods of time.

Finally, it is clear from studies of acromegaly and Cushing disease, as well as physiological observations, that alterations in the exposure of target organs to the stimulating hormone greatly influences the end organ response. Diagnosis of Cushing disease or acromegaly centers on establishing persistent elevation in cortisol or GH concentrations but it is not necessary for this elevation to be great. More important is that there is no respite from persistent exposure to elevated levels. From basic principles, analysis of hormone pulsatility tells the clinician that the chances of documenting the problem will be increased by increasing sample numbers. Taking a midnight and early morning cortisol sample limits the probability of confirming the presence of disease, particularly when the variability in these parameters in the normal population is taken into account. A series of samples may be required.

Sampling interval

The concept of generating false information by inappropriate sampling intervals is known as aliaising.[35] Determining the correct sampling interval is part of the process involved in minimizing this problem. Knowledge of the half-life of the hormone is essential to determine the correct sampling interval. Using sampling intervals that are greater than the half-life of the hormone will lead to the potential for missing a response when it takes place. Taking a large number of frequent samples will alleviate the problem but must be offset by the discomfort to the patient, the practicality and expense. Sampling intervals need to be close to the half-life of the hormone under study but should not exceed it.

Independent marker of stimulus application

In considering provocation tests, the situation may arise where no response is observed: a possible explanation is that the strength of the stimulus was insufficient to provoke hormone release. In such a situation, it is valuable to have an independent marker of stimulus application. In the insulin-induced hypoglycemia test, this marker is glucose and the attainment of adequate hypoglycemia. In the glucagon test, it may be the release of glucose. In other tests, there may be no independent markers so that doubt may be cast on the reliability of the nonresponse (e.g., clonidine).

How much stimulus to apply

Conventional endocrine tests use standard dosing schedules of the stimulus. These are usually adjusted for body size but all tend to generate a maximal response. This is reasonable if the investigator wishes to determine what is available under maximal stimulation (e.g., stress and cortisol release) but may not equate to the amount of hormone released to produce a target organ effect. Physiological studies of hormone release might be more meaningful than provocative studies. Rather than enter a debate in depth, it is probably more productive to consider what is actually required of the test in the first instance.

GHRH tests are often used to show whether or not the gland is capable of releasing GH. However, more subtle questions might need to be asked, such as whether the gland has changed in its sensitivity to GHRH. A similar situation might be encountered in determining whether an individual has a degree of hormone insensitivity. Using the classic IGF-I generation test is unlikely to unravel the complexity of target tissue responsivity. These dose–response range take three forms: insensitive (reduced gradient of the dose-response curve), resetting (no change in gradient) but can still respond to a maximal stimulation, and those who cannot, no matter how high the stimulus, achieve a maximal response (resistance).[36]

Is the test response reasonable?

Consideration needs to be given to the magnitude of the response to the stimulus. It is preferable that the response allows discrimination to be made between the normal and pathological situation. The response should be greater than the background hormone level in the unstimulated state. A rise greater than three times the coefficient of variation of the assay at that concentration might be closer but whatever value is chosen the hormone concentration should be easily measurable and responsive. Low but consistent responses seen in the heat (pyrogen) test are not helpful.[37]

PRINCIPLES OF DIAGNOSTIC TESTING

The aim of any diagnostic test is to progress the clinical history and examination to the point where the care of the patient is altered. There is a vast and bewildering literature on GH testing but the clinician can be guided by asking the questions detailed in Table 14.3.

Several of the points are considered further in this chapter but the first two deserve special mention. First, it is unusual in endocrinology for there to be a diagnostic 'gold standard'. The anterior pituitary is not accessible and molecular biology is not sufficiently advanced to give definitive answers. Care needs to be taken in ascribing the role of a gold standard. It may change with time but, more importantly, if it is infallible, no test, no matter how good, will ever surpass it. So, comparing the insulin tolerance test (ITT – the gold standard) with 24 h profiles will always lead to the conclusion that the ITT is better; there could be no other conclusion.[38]

Second, the test must be well validated by application to large numbers of individuals with and without the condition. The temptation is to use the extremes but this may lead to a considerable overestimate of sensitivity and specificity[39] which may not be borne out in field studies.[40,41]

Normal ranges and cut-off values

Normal values in pediatric practice are hard to obtain and performing many of the tests on normal children is unethical. Furthermore, standards would be needed for tall, normal and short children because their GH secretion differs.[3] In addition, both age and pubertal stage influence GH secretion[3] as does body composition.[10,11] Values for these would also have to be included.

The classic approach of defining normal data in terms of a Gaussian distribution does not come without hazard. Endocrine testing rarely fits this distribution and, even if it did, it would imply that the lowest and highest 2.5 percent of values are abnormal and that all diseases have the same frequency – clearly unlikely. Creating upper and lower limits does not help either. It is more appropriate to identify a range of diagnostic test results beyond which the disorder of GHD is likely.

Table 14.3　Underlying principles of assessing tests

1.　Has there been an independent blind comparison with the diagnostic 'gold standard'?
2.　Was the test conducted in a wide range of patients with and without the condition?
3.　Is the test reproducible?
4.　What was the definition of normal in the test situation?
5.　How might the test interact with others in a diagnostic sequence?
6.　Does the test entail risk or reduce risk for the patient?

Most decisions on placing the value have been empirical rather than statistical. In practice, cut-off values could be chosen at an absolute extreme. If 100 short children were studied and GH sufficiency or deficiency was defined by a peak response of less than $5\,\mathrm{mU\,L^{-1}}$, only 3–5 percent might have a response at this level. When testing the next 100 children, one or two normal individuals might have such a response. They will be outliers but they are important because the more patients studied, the greater the chance of finding outliers.

Moving the cut-off to more extreme values to exclude these patients restricts the population of treatable individuals. Relaxing the criteria interposes normal individuals into the diagnosis zone. Placing the cut-off is based partly on clinical judgement and can be greatly assisted by generating a series of receiver operator curves (ROCs) for different tests. As there is no disadvantage, apart from financial cost, in falsely labeling someone with GHD and treating them, a relaxed cut-off would be acceptable.

Specificity and sensitivity

Two principles operate when using diagnostic tests:[21] the first is that probability is a useful marker of diagnostic uncertainty. This is when the sensitivity (ability to detect a target disorder when present or true positive rate) and specificity (ability to identify correctly the absence of the disorder or true negative rate) become important. If both were 85 percent, 15 percent of patients with disease would have a negative result (false negative) and 15 percent without disease would have a positive result (false positive). Abnormal results would occur in patients with and without disease. Whatever the result, new information has been generated that may or may not influence decision making. The second principle is that diagnostic tests should be obtained only when they can alter the management of the case, that is if the test result alters the probability of the disease. Sensitivity and specificity are important components of test performance and Table 14.4 shows how they are calculated.

Table 14.4　Test results in 100 individuals with respect to a diagnosis of GH insufficiency

Test result	Growth hormone insufficiency		Total
	Present	Absent	
Positive	20	10	30
Negative	5	65	70
Total	25	75	100

$$\mathrm{Sensitivity} = \frac{20}{25} = 80\%$$

$$\mathrm{Specificity} = \frac{65}{75} = 87\%$$

Sensitivity and specificity indicate how the test compares with the gold standard. But this is not quite what is required: in the clinical situation, it is more useful to know what a positive or negative test result means. Table 14.4 can yield more as it shows that 20 of 30 individuals (66 percent) with a positive test have GHD (positive predictive value) and 65 of 70 (93 percent) with negative test do not (negative predictive value). The test can be used to generate these predictive values, which may or may not help strengthen the diagnosis.

Predictive values are easy to calculate but they are not constant and they change with the number of patients who have the target disorder. Applying the test to a different population than the one used to find the value in Table 14.4 might yield different results. For example, these results might have come from an endocrine service where the prevalence of the condition would be expected to be higher than a community growth screening programme. If, in the latter, prevalence was 5 percent (probably less, given the data in the Ohio Growth Study[42]) and the sensitivity and specificity were unchanged, then the positive predictive value would be 29 percent and the negative predictive value 99 percent – excellent for exclusion, but not for diagnosis.

Pre- and post-test probability

The relationship between the probability of disease after the results of diagnostic tests are known (the post-test probability) and pre-test probability test of disease depends on the sensitivity and specificity of the test as shown in Fig. 14.5. There are two important points to note: the first is that the more certain the clinician is of the diagnosis before the test is performed, the less effect the confirmatory test has on the probability of disease. The obverse is also true. The second point is that tests will have major effects on probability of disease in the intermediate zone. Testing is not likely to be beneficial if the pre-test probability is very high or low. This is one reason why screening for GH secretory problems in short children purely on the basis of biochemical tests is unhelpful.

One problem that clinicians face is how to define the pre-test probability of the condition. Given the paucity of information on the prevalence of symptoms and signs associated with GHD in the general population, it is difficult at first sight to see how this can be achieved. There are a number of possible ways. The easiest is where a consensus is obtained from practising clinicians. This approach has been used in a slightly different manner in the area of clinical trials where the issue is when to stop the clinical trial. Clinicians in this situation were asked prior to the study at what point they would accept that one treatment had a greater effect than another (e.g., 5 percent, 10 percent or 50 percent improvement). By obtaining this information it was possible to determine a pre-trial estimate of the level of improvement that would be required to convince sceptic clinicians compared to the enthusiasts for the study.

Such a balance is useful and could be achieved in GHD by presenting a series of clinical scenarios to experienced clinicians and asking them to rate the probability that the individual has GHD.

A second approach is to use pre-existing disease data sets. Recent studies have improved on the estimates of pre-test probability by using combinations of anthropometric data such as height, height velocity and parental height to identify cases for further evaluation.[43] Although applied to Turner syndrome the strengths of the approach are that they provide better estimates of pre-test likelihood of disease presence than hithertofore and also allow comparison of the performance of different screening rules.

Clinicians are often faced with the situation where they feel really sure the patient has the condition but the test does not confirm this. Table 14.5 analyses this concept. Here, specificity and sensitivity have been fixed and the effects on post-test probability are considered. In the situation of 90 percent pre-test probability that the patient is GH deficient, then, even if the test is negative in the individual, there is still a 67 percent probability (down 23 percent) that they have the condition, so treatment would still be justified. When the pre-test probability was 5 percent (very certain

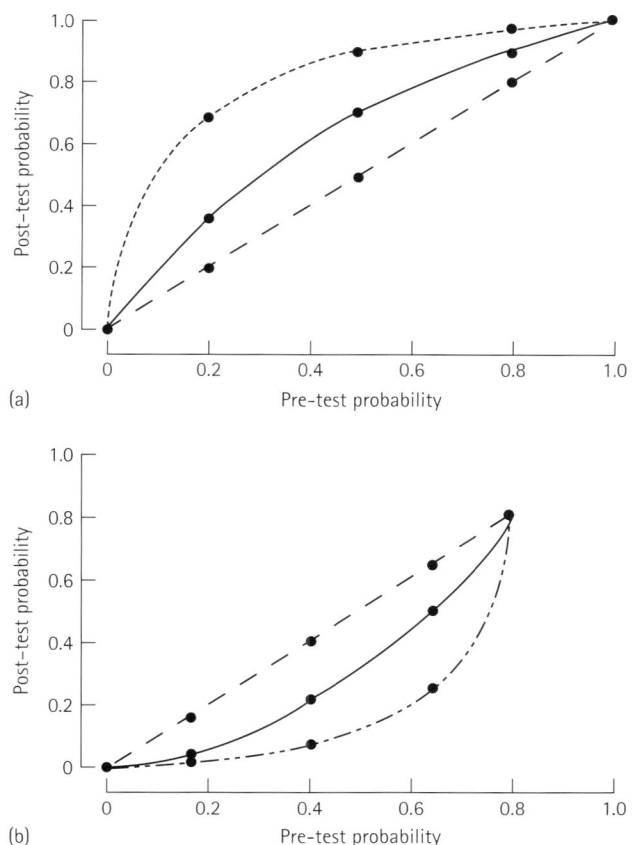

(a)

(b)

Figure 14.5 Plot of the relationship between pre- and post-test probability of disease presence and the effect of different sensitivity and specificity of the tests. (a) Test positive; (b) test negative. ——, line of identity; —, 60 percent sensitivity or specificity; ————, 80 percent sensitivity or specificity.

Table 14.5 Growth hormone test results in situations of differing pre-test certainty

Pre-test probability (%)	Post-test probability	
	Test positive	Test negative
90	98 (+8)	67 (−23)
50	87 (+37)	19 (−32)
5	25 (+20)	1 (−4)

Change from pre-test probability in parenthesis.

that the patient does not have GHD) and the test is positive, all the result says is that the patient has a 1 in 4 chance of having the condition, so we would probably not treat. In the middle ground, certainty in either direction is dramatically improved.

Multiple tests

Table 14.5 could have been made much larger by introducing different pre-test probabilities. There comes a point, however, when post-test probability changes to a level where a decision has to be made to stop and either accept or reject the proposal that the condition is present. The decision to stop investigation and to treat or not depends on how convinced the clinician is of the diagnosis, the benefits and risks of the therapy and the potential yield and risks of further tests. There are two ways to assist this situation: conduct another test or use a more sophisticated analysis rather than a simple positive or negative.

The former is problematic in the GH field because the methodology assumes that the results of the two tests are independent. The data about this are mixed. In normal individuals, undergoing repeat GHRH tests, dependence cannot be assumed.[30] Where repeat tests have been done in children, concordance was seen 50 percent of the time, a value close to that calculated for independent events using a test with a 70–85 percent efficiency. Another important issue is whether the test might change in individuals as they age. There is evidence that the clonidine test is less effective in releasing GH in young adults compared to that seen in children.[44] Whether the magnitude of the response to other stimuli can be assumed to remain unchanged is unknown.

Assuming that the two tests are done (on different days) and that they are dependent, the results could resemble Table 14.6. Here again, it has been assumed the condition can be identified correctly by some other method. Results from these two tests can be combined and we can constrain the results so that both tests are positive and called positive; if both are negative or one or other is negative, then this is called negative (Table 14.7). The bottom of Table 14.7 shows the situation where both tests are negative.

The assumption that both tests need to be positive maximizes specificity and avoids falsely labeling normal

Table 14.6 Results of applying two tests assessing growth hormone (GH) secretion, insulin-induced hypoglycemia, and clonidine to patients with and without GH insufficiency

Clonidine	Insulin-induced hypoglycemia	
	Positive	Negative
Patients with GH insufficiency		
Positive	55	10
Negative	15	20
Patients without GH insufficiency		
Positive	10	5
Negative	25	60

Replot on whether GH insufficiency present or absent and constraining both tests either to be positive or negative.

Test result	GH insufficiency	
	Present	Absent
*Both tests positive for diagnosis		
Both positive	55	10
One or both negative	45	90
Both tests negative to exclude		
†Both positive	80	40
One or both negative	20	60

*Sensitivity 55%; specificity 90%.
†Sensitivity 80%; specificity 60%.

Table 14.7 Information from Table 14.6 using different test combinations to define diagnosis

	Growth hormone insufficiency		Cut-off
	Present	Absent	
Both positive	55	10	Sensitivity 55% Specificity 90%
One positive	25	30	
Both negative	20	60	Sensitivity 80% Specificity 60%

children but it misses a lot of treatable individuals. Insisting that both tests are negative maximizes sensitivity, minimizes misdiagnoses but falsely labels a lot more normal children.

The construction of complex tables is an extension of these concepts but uses different levels of test result rather than having to rely on absolute cut-off values. Table 14.7 shows how data from Table 14.6 can be used to produce three levels; we could demand that both tests are positive to give a sensitivity of 55 percent and a specificity of 90 percent, whilst both or only one is positive should give a sensitivity of

Table 14.8 Effect of applying different peak growth hormone (GH) cut-off values in response to insulin-induced hypoglycemia for diagnosis of GH insufficiency.

GH concentration (mU L^{-1})	Efficiency (%)	Sensitivity (%)	Specificity (%)
10	63	51	79
13.5	20	64	70
20	68	82	49

80 percent and a specificity of 60 percent. Table 14.8 gives an example of different cut-off values to define GH insufficiency/deficiency.[45] This would then serve as a base to allow post-test probability to be calculated giving an idea of how the diagnosis is changing.

More complex calculations can be used to produce probability ratios. These express the odds that a given level of diagnostic test result would be expected in a patient with GHD as opposed to one without the diagnosis. For a positive test, the likelihood ratio is sensitivity divided by (1 − specificity). So, for Table 14.6, people with a positive GH test are 6.2 times as likely to come from patients with GHD as from normal. The likelihood ratio for a negative test is false negative rate divided by specificity. This technique is independent of disease prevalence and can be applied at multiple cut-off levels. The most important value is that it allows for a sequence of tests to be created and a decision tree constructed.[46]

One final area needs to be considered and this brings together the issue of two tests with pre-test probability. Several recent publications have suggested that individuals who were originally diagnosed as GHD do not appear to have the biochemical abnormality when the test is repeated later.[47,48] This has led to statements being made that these individuals are no longer GHD. Two issues are worth considering: first, the population studied during the second test is not the same as that during the first as on the first round those thought unlikely to have the condition have been excluded. If the absolutist approach were to be used, some of those not re-tested may have abnormal test results. A change of stance has taken place.

Second, it is worth rehearsing the scenario that has led to the second test. The child was initially evaluated because of concerns over short stature and poor growth. At that point a test was conducted because the clinician required an answer with which to rule in or rule out the diagnosis. Taking the situation depicted in Table 14.5, let us assume that the initial pre-test probability was 50 percent so that, having obtained a positive test, the post-test probability of the child having the condition rose to 87 percent. This value now forms the pre-test probability for the second test, not the 50–50 situation which the clinician faced prior to investigation. Information has been collected which influences the probability of the disease process being present. When the clinician comes to apply the second test,

Table 14.5 shows that the post-test probability of the condition being present after the second test resides in the top line (98 percent of the test if the test is positive and 67 percent if the test is negative). It does not lie on the second line, which is the position that many clinicians have adopted by simply considering the second test not to be influenced by the acquisition of prior information.

The concept of acquisition of information during the course of evaluation is important. Clinical history and examination, along with the initial endocrinological investigation, changes the likelihood of disease presence. The situation does not stop at this point since additional information may be acquired such as that obtained from neuro-imaging. For example, the presence of pituitary hypoplasia in a patient with GHD would significantly increase the likelihood of disease, whereas the clinician might be sceptical of the GH test results in a situation where pituitary size was normal. This is because somatotroph mass makes up at least 50 percent of the size of the anterior pituitary. Neuro-imaging may then be an important contributor to altering likelihood of disease.

The growth response to intervention with GH therapy is also a component of assessment and this is where the predictive models that have been derived[49,50] can be extremely important. If the response to intervention behaves along classical lines expected for severe GHD, this strengthens the likelihood that the individual has the condition. What is created is a huge decision tree whose branched structure represents all these pieces of information. The challenge to endocrinologists is to determine the strengths of the various components.

CONCLUSIONS

Careful clinical assessment coupled with detailed anthropometric measurement are the keystone for the evaluation of any endocrinological disorder. The clinical features of endocrine disorders are not always pathognomonic. The presence of findings or a combination of findings that are specific but insensitive increase the likelihood of disease only slightly. In many situations in endocrine practice, there is no gold standard for diagnosis. In such a situation the application of probability to testing a hypothesis is essential. In the field of GH, the specificity and sensitivity of any of the tests of GH secretion are only 80 percent, so the clinician should expect false positive and false negative results. Careful consideration of test results in the light of probability theory needs to be made in order to maximize diagnostic certainty. The evaluation of an individual should not stop at the point that treatment is initiated, since ongoing information should be acquired from the response to GH therapy. Second tests of endocrine function need to be carefully constructed and interpreted in the light of probability theory. It is important at all stages to recognize that there are no absolutes and the clinician may operate effectively only when the likelihood of disease being present or absent is expressed in terms of probability.

KEY LEARNING POINTS

- It is unusual to have 'gold standards' for the assessment of endocrine tests.
- Knowledge of test sensitivity and specificity are essential to aid test interpretation.
- Bayesian concepts of probability are useful for clinical decision making.
- When pre-test probability is low or high, no test, no matter how sensitive and specific, will alter post-test probability.
- Multiple testing needs to be considered as a complex statistical process.

REFERENCES

● = Seminal primary article

1 Milner RDG, Russell-Fraser T, Brook CGD, *et al.* Experience with human growth hormone in Great Britain: the report of the MRC working Party. *Clin Endocrinol* 1979; **11**: 15–38.

2 Hindmarsh PC, Smith PJ. Brook CGD, Matthews DR. The relationship between height velocity and GH secretion in short prepubertal children. *Clin Endocrinol* 1987; **27**: 581–91.

3 Albertsson-Wikland K, Rosberg S. Analysis of 24-hour growth hormone profiles in children: relation to growth. *J Clin Endocrinol Metab* 1988; **67**: 493–500.

4 Tanner JM, Hiernaux J, Jarman S. Growth and physique studies. In: Weiner JS, Iounie JA, eds. *Human Biology: A Guide to Field Methods.* Oxford: Blackwell Scientific Publications, 1969.

5 Cameron N. *The Measurement of Human Growth.* London: Croom Helm, 1984.

6 Cox LA, Savage MD. Practical auxology: techniques of measurement and assessment of skeletal maturity. In: Kelnar CJH, Savage MD, Stirling HF, Saenger P, eds. *Growth Disorders: Pathophysiology and Treatment.* London: Chapman and Hall, 1998.

7 Goossens M, Brauner R, Czernichow P, *et al.* Isolated growth hormone deficiency Type 1A associated with a double deletion in the human growth hormone gene cluster. *J Clin Endocrinol Metab* 1986; **62**: 712–16.

8 Wit JM, Van Unen H. Growth of infants with neonatal growth hormone deficiency. *Arch Dis Child* 1982; **67**: 920–4.

9 Huet F, Carel J-C, Nivelon J-L, Chaussain J-L. Long term results of GH therapy in GH-deficient children treated before 1 year of age. *Eur J Endocrinol* 1999; **140**: 29–34.

10 Rahim A, O'Niell P, Shalet SM. The effect of body composition on hecretin-induced growth hormone release in normal elderly subjects. *Clin Endocrinol* 1988; **49**: 659–64.

11 Iranmanesh A, Lizaralde G, Veldhuis JD. Age and relative adiposity are specific negative determinants of the pregnancy and amplitude of growth hormone (GH) secretory

bursts and the half-life of endogenous GH in healthy men. *J Clin Endocrinol Metab* 1991; **73**: 1081–8.

12 Marcovitch H. Failure to thrive. *BMJ* 1994; **308**: 35–8.

13 Herber SM, Milner RDG. Growth hormone deficiency presenting under age 2 years. *Arch Dis Child* 1984; **59**: 557–60.

14 Gluckman PD, Gunn A-J, Wray A. Congenital idiopathic growth hormone deficiency associated with early postnatal growth failure. *J Pediatr* 1992; **121**: 920–3.

15 Vanderschuren-Lodeweyckx M, Wolter R, Mulla A, *et al.* Plasma growth hormone in coeliac disease. *Acta Pediatr (Helv)* 1973; **28**: 349–57.

16 Crowley S, Hindmarsh PC, Matthews DR, Brook CGD. Growth and the growth hormone axis in prepubertal children with asthma. *J Pediatr* 1995; **126**: 297–303.

17 Krieger DT. Rhythms in CRF, ACTH and corticosteroids. In: Krieger DT, ed. *Endocrine Rhythms.* New York: Raven Press, 1979.

18 Clayton RN, Royston JP, Chapman J, *et al.* Is changing hypothalamic activity important for control of ovulation? *BMJ* 1987; **295**: 7–12.

19 Hunter WM, Friend JAR, Strong JA. The diurnal pattern of plasma growth hormone concentration in adults. *J Endocr* 1966; **34**: 139–46.

20 Goodner CJ, Walike BC, Koerker DJ, *et al.* Insulin, glucogen and glucose exhibit synchronous sustained oscillations in fasting monkeys. *Science* 1977; **195**: 177–9.

21 Sox HC Jr. Probability theory in the use of diagnostic tests. *Ann Int Med* 1986; **104**: 60–6.

22 Youlton R, Kaplan SL, Grumbach MM. Growth and growth hormone. IV. limitations of the growth hormone response to insulin and arginine in the assessment of growth hormone deficiency in children. *Pediatrics* 1969; **43**: 989–1004.

● 23 Devesa J, Lima L, Lois N, *et al.* Reasons for the variability in growth hormone (GH) responses to GHRH challenge: the endogenous hypothalamic–somatotroph rhythm (HSR). *Clin Endocrinol* 1989; **30**: 367–77.

24 Tzanela M, Guyada H, Van Vliet G, Tannenbaum GS. Somatostatin pretreatment enhances growth hormone responsiveness to GH-releasing hormone: a potential new diagnostic approach to GH deficiency. *J Clin Endocrinol Metab* 1996; **81**: 2487–94.

25 Bernasconi S, Volta C, Cozzini A, *et al.* GH response to GHRH, insulin, clonidine and arginine after GHRH pretreatment in children. *Acta Endocrinol* 1992; **126**: 105–8.

26 Massoud AF, Hindmarsh PC, Matthews DR, Brook CGD. The effect of repeated administration of hexarelin, a growth hormone releasing peptide, and growth hormone releasing hormone (GHRH) on growth hormone (GH) responsivity. *Clin Endocrinol* 1996; **44**: 555–62.

27 Achermann JC, Brook CGD, Robinson ICAF, *et al.* Peak and trough growth hormone (GH) concentrations influence growth and serum like growth factor-1 (IGF-I) concentrations in short children. *Clin Endocrinol* 1999; **50**: 8046–50.

28 Pringle PJ, Stanhope R, Hindmarsh P, Brook CGD. Abnormal pubertal development in primary hypothyroidism. *J Clin Endocrinol* 1988; **28**: 479–86.

29 Cordido F, Fernandez T, Martinez T, *et al.* Effect of acute pharmacological reduction of plasma free fatty acids on growth hormone (GH) releasing hormone-induced GH secretion in obese adults with and without hypopituitarism. *J Clin Endocrinol Metab* 1998; **83**: 4350–4.

30 Suri D, Hindmarsh PC, Matthews DR, *et al.* The pituitary gland is capable of responding to two successive doses of growth hormone releasing hormone (GHRH). *Clin Endocrinol* 1991; **34**: 13–7.

31 Donaldson DL, Holowell JG, Pan F, *et al.* Growth hormone secretion profiles: variation on consecutive nights *J Pediatr* 1989; **115**: 51–6.

32 Saini S, Hindmarsh PC, Matthews DR, *et al.* Reproducibility of 24hour serum growth hormone profiles in man. *Clin Endocrinol* 1991; **34**: 455–62.

33 Bridges NA, Hindmarsh PC, Pringle PJ, *et al.* Cortisol, androstenedione, dehydroepidrosterone sulphate and 17 hydroxyprogesterone responses to low dose of (1-24)ACTH. *J Clin Endocrinol Metab* 1998; **83**: 3750–3.

34 Rasmuson S, Olsson T, Hagg E. A low dose ACTH test to assess the function of the hypothalamic–pituitary–adrenal axis. *Clin Endocrinol* 1996; **44**: 151–6.

35 Matthews DR, Hindmarsh PC. Hormone pulsatility. In: Brook CGD, Hindmarsh PC, eds. *Clinical Paediatric Endocrinology.* Oxford: Blackwell Science, 2001.

36 Hindmarsh PC. Standard and low-dose IGF-I generation tests and spontaneous growth hormone secretion in children with idiopathic short stature. *Clin Endocrinol* 2004; **60**: 161–2.

37 Fisher S, Jorgensen JD, Orskov H, Christiansen JS. GH stimulation tests: evaluation of GH responses to heat test versus insulin-tolerance test. *Eur J Endocrinol* 1998; **139**: 605–10.

38 Rose SR, Ross JL, Uriarte M, *et al.* The advantages of measuring stimulated as compared with spontaneous growth hormone levels in the diagnosis of growth hormone deficiency. *N Engl J Med* 1988; **319**: 201–7.

39 Blum WF, Ranke MB, Kietzmann K, *et al.* A specific radioimmunoassay for the growth hormone (GH)-dependent somatomedin-binding protein: its use for diagnosis of GH deficiency. *J Clin Endocrinol Metab* 1990; **70**: 1292–8.

40 Tillman V, Buckler JM, Kibirge MS, *et al.* Biochemical tests in the diagnosis of childhood growth hormone deficiency. *J Clin Endocrinol Metab* 1997; **82**: 531–5.

41 Mitchell H, Dattani MT, Nanduri V, *et al.* Failure of IGF-I and IGFBP-3 to diagnose growth hormone insufficiency. *Arch Dis Child* 1999; **80**: 443–7.

● 42 Lindsay R, Feldkamp M, Harris D, *et al.* Utah Growth Study: growth standards and the prevalence of growth hormone deficiency. *J Pediatr* 1994; **125**: 29–35.

43 Van Buuren S, van Dommelen P, Zandwijken GRJ, *et al.* Towards evidence based referral criteria for growth monitoring. *Arch Dis Child* 2004; **89**: 336–41.

44 Rahim A, Toogood A, Shalet SM. The assessment of growth hormone status in normal young adult males using a variety of provocative tests. *Clin Endocrinol* 1996; **45**: 557–62.

45 Dattani MT, Pringle PJ, Hindmarsh PC, Brook CGD. What is a normal stimulated growth hormone concentration? *J Endocr* 1992; **133**: 447–50.

46 Sackett DL, Haynes RB, Guyatt GH, Tugwell P. *Clinical Epidemiology: A Basic Science for Clinical Medicine,* 2nd edn. Boston: Little-Brown, 1991: 144.

47 Wacharasindhu S, Cotterill AM, Comacho-Hubner C, *et al.* Normal growth hormone secretion in growth hormone insufficient children re-tested after completion of linear growth. *Clin Endocrinol* 1986; **45**: 553–6.

48 Tauber M, Houlin P, Pienkowski C, *et al.* Growth hormone (GH) retesting and auxological data in 131 GH-deficient patients after completion of treatment. *J Clin Endocrinol Metab* 1997; **82**: 352–6.

49 Tanner JM, Whitehouse RH, Hughes PC, Vince FP. Effects of human growth hormone treatment for 1–7 years on growth of 100 children with growth hormone deficiency, low birth weight, inherited smallness, Turner's syndrome and other complaints. *Arch Dis Child* 1971; **46**: 745–82.

50 Ranke MB, Lindberg A. Approach to predicting the growth response during growth hormone treatment. *Acta Paediatr* 1996; **85(Suppl 147)**: 64–5.

15

Radiologic and imaging assessment of the skeletal dysplasias

RALPH S LACHMAN

INTRODUCTION

The skeletal dysplasias (bone dysplasias) are a group of approximately 160 well-defined disorders of which about 50 are often lethal in the perinatal period. When dealing with postnatal growth problems, which is the major thrust of this text, one must therefore take into account about 110 non-lethal skeletal dysplasias, and their radiologic assessment.

PROPORTIONATE SHORT STATURE

One cannot consider the radiologic evaluation of the bone dysplasias without also considering the general radiologic assessment of short stature. When faced with the problem of short stature in the pediatric age group, the clinical determination of whether proportionate or disproportionate short stature is being dealt with is crucial. When confronted with proportionate short stature the differential diagnosis, as a general rule, consists of constitutional delay, familial short stature and perhaps a small group of endocrinopathies. Their clinical (radiologic) assessment usually warrants a left hand and wrist for bone age determination. A complete 'genetic' skeletal survey is not necessary in those cases and even contraindicated, as the role of the pediatric radiologist and pediatric specialist is to try to keep ionizing radiation doses to patients as low as possible.

However, should the patient in question have normal proportions and be dysmorphic or manifest multiple congenital anomalies on clinical evaluation, then one of the dysmorphology syndromes is present and a genetic skeletal survey is appropriate (Table 15.1). This genetic skeletal survey should be modified, if possible, by assessing the clinical features present and if necessary consulting a text such as the *Radiology of Syndromes, Metabolic Disorders, and Skeletal Dysplasias*[1] to tailor the radiographic investigation to a specific diagnosis. It may even be necessary to use other imaging modalities in the work-up of this group of patients. These include ultrasonography of varying organs, especially the kidneys for those that might manifest a renal abnormality, a nuclear medicine (isotopic) study of bones, kidneys, liver and/or spleen for example, and even computed tomography (CT) or magnetic resonance imaging (MRI) studies of the brain and other body parts,

Table 15.1 Genetic skeletal survey (unmodified): For short stature (multiple anomaly and/or dysmorphology) syndromes

- Skull: posteroanterior (PA) or Caldwell view and lateral
- Spine: anteroposterior (AP) and lateral
- Chest: (thorax): AP (rib technique)
- Pelvis and hips: AP
- Long bones: (all four) AP
- Hands and feet: (all four) AP

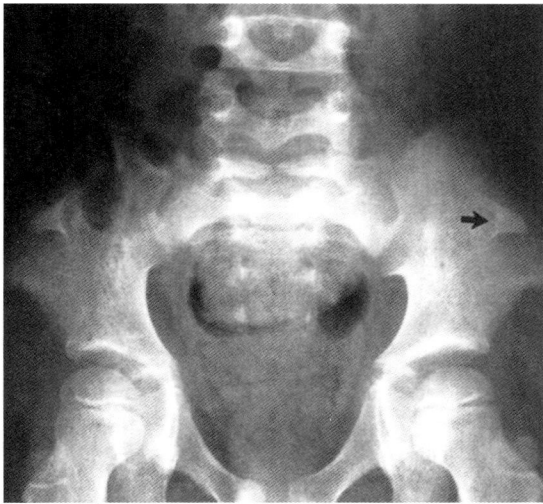

Figure 15.1 Nail–patella syndrome (osteoonychodysplasia): iliac horns (arrow).

Table 15.2 Skeletal dysplasia skeletal survey

- Skull: Caldwell, Towne and lateral
- Spine: Thoracic and lumbar – AP and lateral; cervical (separate) lateral
- Chest (thorax): AP (rib technique)
- Pelvis and hips: AP
- Long bones: (all four) AP
- Hands and feet: (all four) AP

depending upon the signs and symptomatology derived and the diagnoses that these are directed towards, for example, a patient has short stature and clinical absence of or small palpated patellas as well as dystrophic and hypoplastic nails. This individual's primary radiologic work-up can be modified to an anteroposterior (AP) view of the pelvis (looking for iliac horns) and an AP and lateral view of both knees and feet to determine whether this patient manifests either the nail–patella syndrome or the rare patella–aplasia–coxa vara–tarsal synostosis syndrome (Fig. 15.1).

DISPROPORTIONATE SHORT STATURE: CLINICAL ASSESSMENT

The radiologic analysis of the skeletal dysplasias is generally the assessment of disproportionate short stature. If the patient is disproportionate, he/she might still have an endocrinopathy such as severe hypothyroidism (cretinism) which can produce the secondary changes of a skeletal dysplasia. However, almost all patients with disproportionate short stature have a primary skeletal dysplasia. Therefore, it is extremely important that, before ordering any radiographic studies for diagnosis, the clinical assessment not only of established short stature but of a disproportion in that stature be determined. This evaluation includes sitting height (trunk), span, extremity and hand measurements, among others. The disproportion may consist of trunkal shortening, extremity shortening and even segments of extremity shortening such as rhizomelia (short upper arms [humeri] and thighs [femurs]), mesomelia (short middle segments – radii/ulnae [forearms], and tibiae/fibulae [shanks]) and acromelia (short hands and feet). Many forms of skeletal dysplasia will have combinations of the above. Once this disproportion is established it is necessary

to assess the condition radiologically to establish the true diagnosis for correct genetic counseling and management.

IMAGING STUDIES FOR THE SKELETAL DYSPLASIAS

The diagnosis of almost all of the skeletal dysplasias still relies to a major degree on the radiologic findings. The skeletal dysplasia skeletal survey is listed in Table 15.2. It basically consists of the evaluation of all the bones including skull, spine, 'flat' bones, and extremities. It is important that certain areas (such as the spine) be evaluated in two views (AP and lateral) for diagnostic completeness. Once the diagnosis is established of certain of these conditions, it may become necessary for management to obtain other special imaging studies. This is especially true of the skeletal dysplasias that have neurologic complications.[2] An example of this is the group of type II collagenopathies which manifest upper cervical spine problems such as C1–2 subluxation/ dislocation and will need lateral flexion/extension views of the cervical spine; if clinically warranted they may need MRI evaluation of the cord and subarachnoid space for subsequent cervical spine fusion, if necessary (Fig. 15.2). There are a number of other forms of skeletal dysplasia that will also require this more extensive evaluation.

Another bone dysplasia, achondroplasia, which is the most common non-lethal skeletal dysplasia, may also require special imaging studies. As achondroplasia represents a defect in enchondral bone formation, there is a special effect upon the base of the skull – especially the foramen magnum – resulting in obstruction in this region to the flow of cerebrospinal fluid (CSF), as well as upon venous drainage which results in hydrocephalus uncommonly but, more importantly, in sleep apnea and sudden infant death syndrome in early infancy secondary to brainstem compression. The achondroplastic infant may require CT or MRI evaluation for foramen magnum size measurements as well as MRI studies of the brain (posterior fossa) and upper cervical cord region, including special CSF flow studies across the foramen magnum (Fig. 15.3). The indications for those studies depend upon clinical symptomatology and evaluation.

Again, as in the evaluation of the dysmorphologic, proportionate, short stature patient, certain patients with skeletal dysplasias may warrant other imaging studies of non-osseous structures for diagnosis and management.

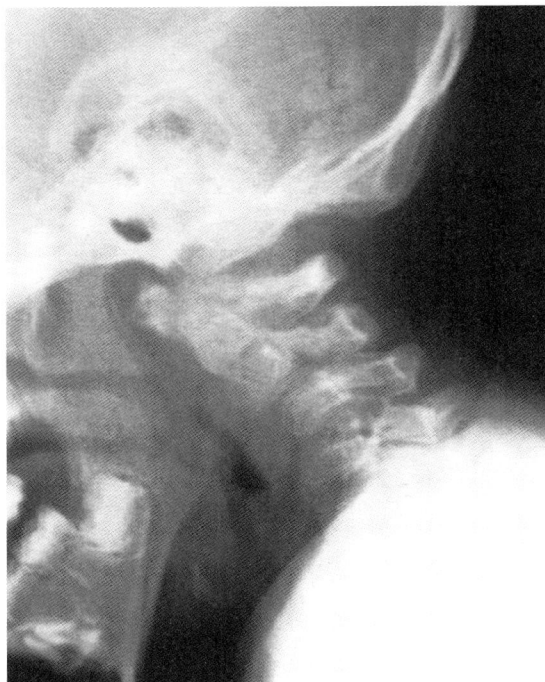

(a)

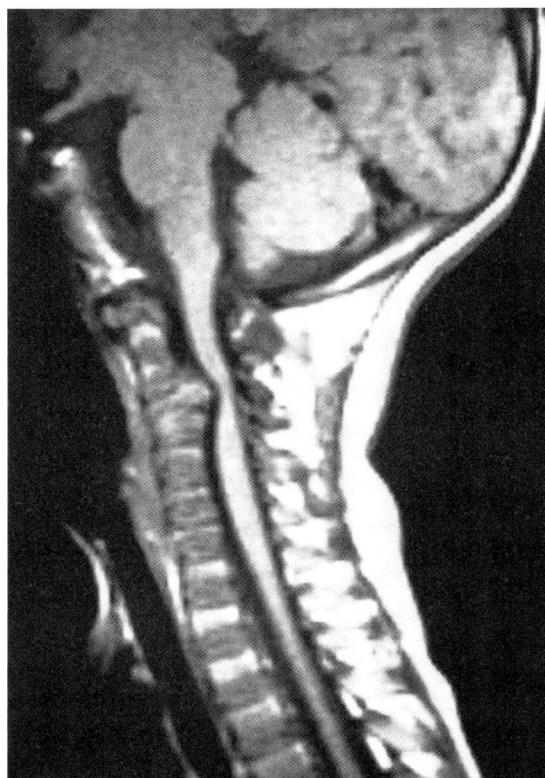

(b)

Figure 15.2   Spondyloepiphyseal dysplasia congenita:
(a) flexion film revealing C2–3 subluxation. (b) Magnetic
resonance imaging (MRI) shows cervical cord impingement and
secondary thinning.

Examples of these include echocardiography in chondroectodermal dysplasia (Ellis–van Creveld dysplasia) with a consideration of associated congenital heart disease; intravenous urography (IVU) or renal ultrasonography in acrodysplasia with retinitis pigmentosa and nephropathy (Saldino–Mainzer dysplasia) for kidney evaluation; cervical cord region MRI is used in acromesomelic dysplasia for cervical cord syrinx – a newly identified association.

STEPWISE RADIOLOGIC ANALYSIS OF THE SKELETAL DYSPLASIAS

The history of the delineation and classification of specific skeletal dysplasias reveals that the radiologic assessment has played a major role up to and including the present time. This is apparent because most of the skeletal dysplasias may have distinctive radiologic features (such as stippled ossification centers), are dense or osteopenic bone disorders, or have pathophysiologic abnormalities at or near the developing growth plates. An organized evaluation of the radiographs in the skeletal dysplasia survey includes the following steps.

Step 1

An assessment is made again about whether or not there is disproportion, this time from a radiologic point of view. A quick look at the films will decide whether or not there is significant generalized platyspondyly (flattening and/or end-plate irregularity) present which contributes to short trunkedness. Then a look at the extremities to try to ascertain whether rhizomelia, mesomelia, and/or acromelia is present will be helpful. It should be noted that clinical rhizomelia etc. are not always confirmed by the radiologic findings because the visual evaluation is guided by the skin creases and folds rather than the underlying bone length, and a significantly curved long bone may appear much shorter externally than radiologically.

If the femora and humeri are very shortened compared with the other segments, this constitutes rhizomelia and this is very important for confirming the specific diagnosis of, for example, the rhizomelic form of chondrodysplasia punctata (a peroxisomal enzyme abnormality) (Fig. 15.4). On the other hand, very significant mesomelia alone (shortened and/or deformed radius/ulna, tibia/fibula – extremity middle bones) suggests a group of specific disorders loosely classified as the mesomelic dysplasias.

Acromelia is found in many disorders but is important to recognize because if, for example, it is associated with a particular form of vertebral abnormality, then the specific diagnosis of spondyloperipheral dysplasia can be made.[3] Of course, acromelia may be present by itself and one might be dealing with a variety of disorders, including skeletal dysplasias such as acrodysostosis, and acromicric dysplasia, or non-skeletal dysplasia brachydactyly of any sort, especially

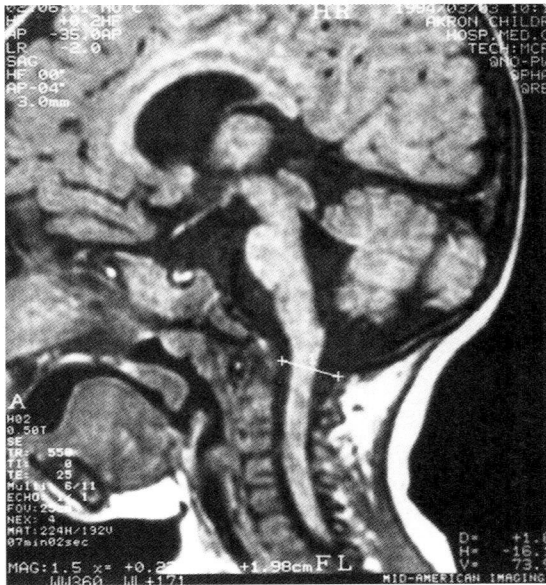

(a)

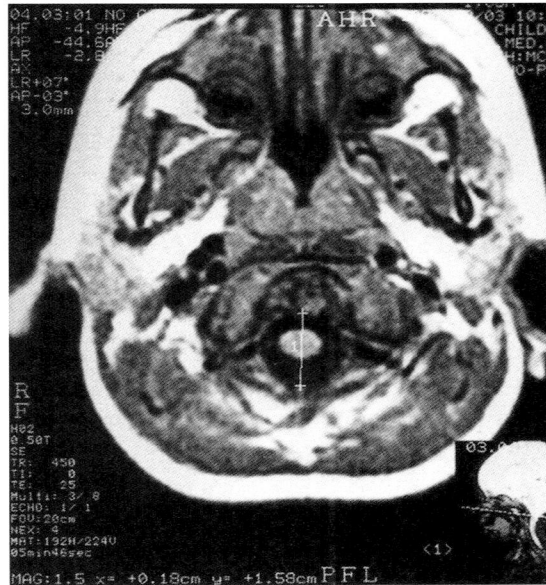

(b)

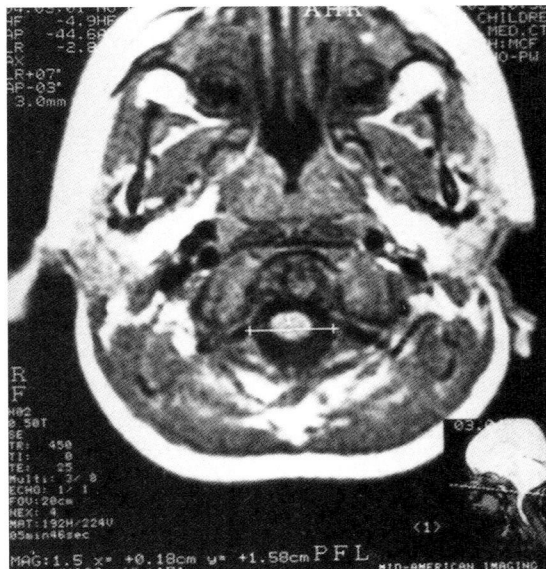

(c)

Figure 15.3   Achondroplasia: MRI of foramen magnum region with measurements (three dimensions).

brachydactyly type E, pseudohypoparathyroidism with cyclic AMP and GMP abnormalities or even a chromosomal disorder (Turner's syndrome). However, acromelia is found as part of other types of shortening in many specific skeletal dysplasias (i.e., achondroplasia and hypochondroplasia), whereas the lack of significant hand and foot shortening is important in many specific and non-specific forms of spondyloepiphyseal dysplasia (Fig. 15.5).

Step 2

Next, an overall assessment of epiphyseal ossification is made. If the ossified epiphyses are very small and/or irregular for

age, then an epiphyseal dysplasia of some sort is present. Should the metaphyses be widened, flared and/or irregular, the diagnosis of a metaphyseal chondrodysplasia is entertained. Finally, if diaphyseal abnormalities are present, such as widening and/or cortical thickening or marrow space expansion, the implication is that this represents a diaphyseal dysplasia of some sort. Combinations of the aforementioned abnormalities with or without platyspondyly were ascribed not only to specific disorders early on but also nonspecific types of disorders (i.e., spondyloepiphyseal dysplasia congenita [SEDC], a specific type II collagenopathy and the group of spondyloepimetaphyseal or spondylometa-epiphyseal dysplasias [SEMD]). This rough estimation of type of disorder helps in narrowing down to

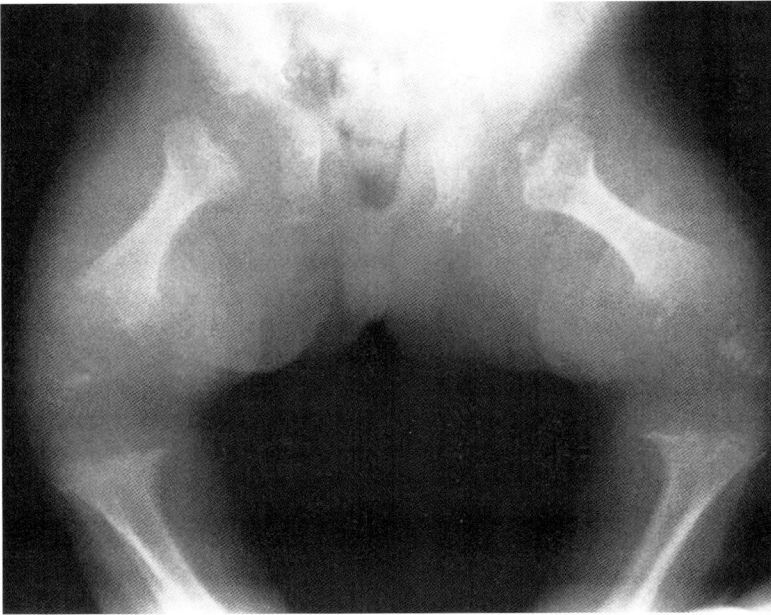

Figure 15.4 Rhizomelic chondrodysplasia punctata: hips and lower extremity radiographs revealing punctate epiphyseal calcifications and severe femoral shortening (rhizomelia).

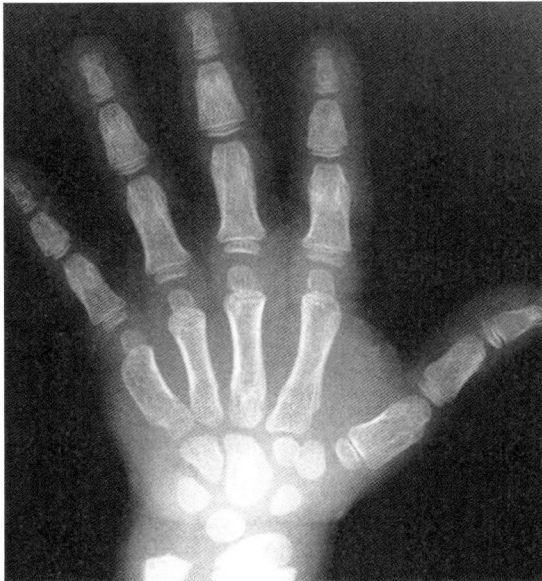

Figure 15.5 Hypochondroplasia: hand and wrist radiograph shows generalized brachydactyly (shortened metacarpals and proximal, middle and distal phalanges).

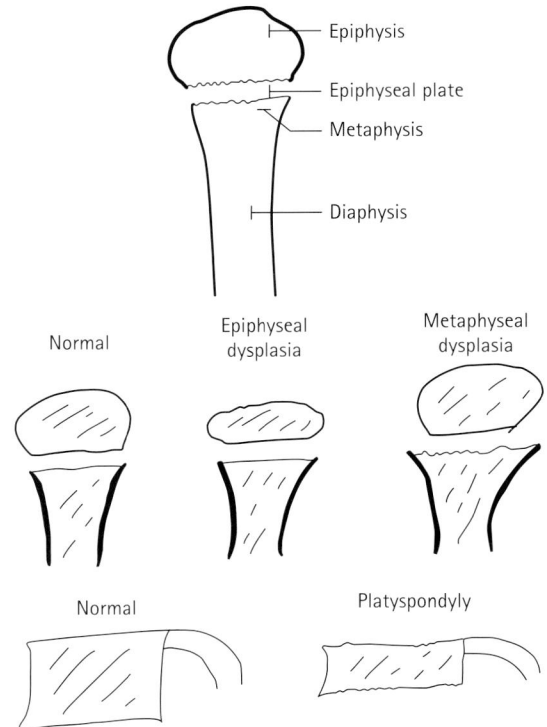

Figure 15.6 Artistic rendition of the growth plate (epiphyseal plate) region of a still growing (pediatric) tubular bone: epiphyseal, metaphyseal and spondylic (vertebral body) abnormalities.

a specific (well-described) entity. Figure 15.6 shows a crude depiction of these radiologic manifestations. If only the spine (vertebral bodies) is affected with no significant changes in any of the growth plate regions, then the patient is manifesting brachyolmia. Which one of the three well-described types of brachyolmia is present will be ascertained by the type of vertebral involvement and other clinical findings.[4] At this point, it is important to re-emphasize that, although the radiology may play a major role in the diagnosis, other clinical manifestations are often very important to make a correct and complete diagnosis.

The more precise evaluation of all the skeletal structures available in the skeletal dysplasia survey should then be performed. This then results perhaps in the recognition of a specific well-described skeletal dysplasia from the previous broad categorization into a non-specific group, which is so important for genetic counseling, i.e., the Jansen-type of metaphyseal chondrodysplasia (the most severe metaphyseal chondrodysplasia) within the large group of about 20 metaphyseal dysplasias that are well described (Fig. 15.7). Another possibility is that a single pathognomonic finding will give a precise diagnosis, i.e., the snail-shaped iliac bones of Schneckenbecken's (snail-pelvis) dysplasia (Fig. 15.8).

Step 3

This next step is more difficult and requires someone with either a fair amount of expertise with the skeletal dysplasia or at least significant radiologic experience, preferably in the pediatric portion of radiologic imaging. It is necessary to be able to recognize normal variations from pathologic abnormalities in the growing skeleton. An assessment needs to be made of all the skeletal structures. The author believes that this is best performed in an organized fashion, dealing with each bone separately. Although every portion of every structure is looked at for any possible abnormal feature, concentration is especially on certain abnormalities that specifically relate to the skeletal dysplasias. It is necessary also to recognize pathognomonic and singular findings that suggest a specific diagnosis or a narrow group of differential diagnosis disorders which may then lead to a specific diagnosis by other features.

SKELETAL SECTIONAL RADIOLOGIC ANALYSES TO DIAGNOSE SPECIFIC SKELETAL DYSPLASIAS

After all the pathologic findings in every area have been established, then a gamut search of some or all of these, in conjunction with the clinical findings, may lead to the specific diagnosis; or, if the 'group' of dysplasias has been established, then often the specific disorder diagnosis can be made by referring to a differential diagnosis table.[1]

Skull

An evaluation of the craniofacial relationship will reveal micro- or macrocephaly, or any more localized abnormality such as dolichocephaly. Midface hypoplasia can be determined as well. Mandibular abnormalities such as micrognathia, antegonial notching or loss of the mandibular angle can be ascertained separately. Tooth abnormalities such as dentinogenesis imperfecta and hypoplasia may be seen; either hypo- or hypertelorism may occur. Bone density increased at the skull base or generalized increased skull density can be determined (this, for example, is very important in the craniotubular skeletal dysplasias). Certain characteristic skull changes may be discovered such as an

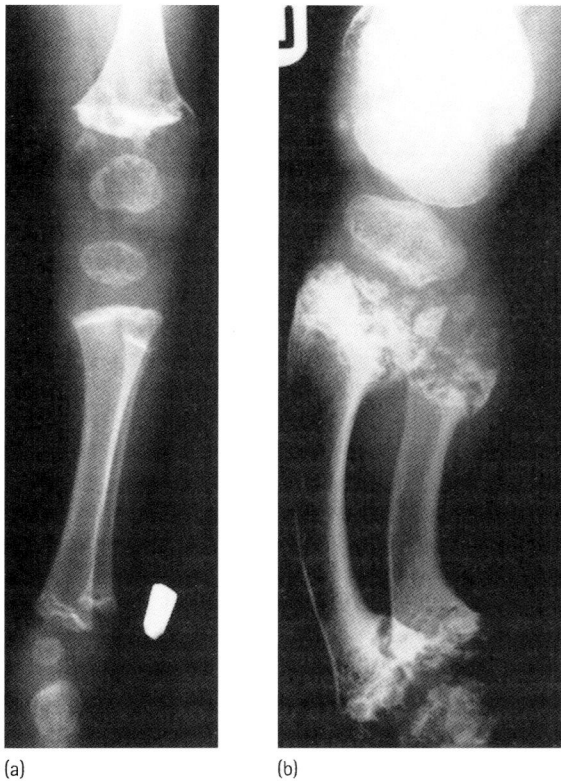

(a)   (b)

Figure 15.7 Metaphyseal chondrodysplasia, Jansen type: (a) at age 9 months, lower extremity film (knees and ankles) shows severe metaphyseal flaring, irregularity, sclerosis and growth plate widening with 'fairly' normal epiphyses. (b) At age 8 years, marked progression of the metaphyseal abnormalities.

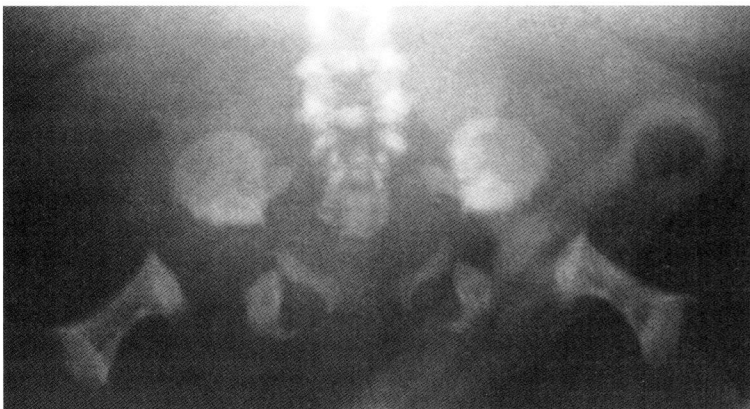

Figure 15.8 Schneckenbecken dysplasia: pelvic radiograph shows the characteristic snail shape of the iliac wings, with the head extruded toward the sacrum; 'dumb-bell' femurs are also seen.

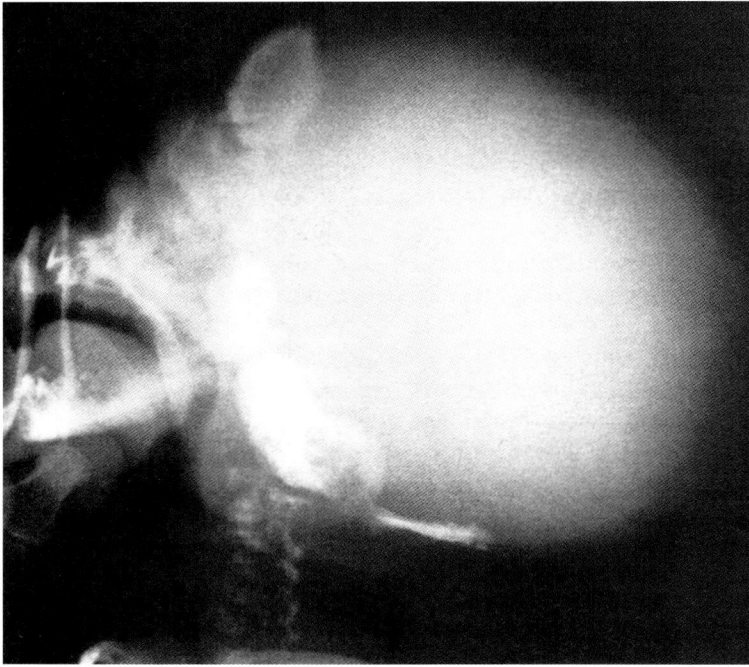

Figure 15.9 Hypophosphatasia, perinatal lethal type: lateral skull film exhibits characteristic dense ossification of frontal bone center, occipital bone center, and base of skull in a background of osteoporotic (poorly ossified) convexity of the remainder of the skull.

excess number of wormian bones, *kleeblattschadel* (cloverleaf skull) or even the beaten copper appearance of increased intracranial pressure (after suture closure). Premature craniosynostosis may be noted.

An analysis of the cranial base includes abnormality in size of foramen magnum, ossification defects anterior to the mendosal suture and platybasia. Sella turcica changes, especially an abnormal J-shaped sella, may be important. Intracranial calcifications of varying structures may be ascertained. Other specific skull abnormalities such as an encephalocele, generalized poor ossification or even island-like ossifications (as in hypophosphatasia) may occur (Fig. 15.9).[5] The frontal sinus may be protuberant (as in frontometaphyseal dysplasia). The sutures may be abnormally widened and the anterior fontanelle may be persistently open or enlarged far beyond its proper time of closure (as in pycnodysostosis or cleidocranial dysplasia among others). It should be noted that some of these described skull changes can also be otherwise clinically determined.

Spine

The spine is a very important structure for skeletal dysplasia analysis. Quite a bit more than just vertebral body flattening (platyspondyly) may be ascertained. Spine shape (scoliosis, kyphosis, lordosis, and gibbus) can be important. Vertebral body abnormalities including segmentation defects, absence or hypoplasia may be encountered. Coronal and sagittal clefts play an important role in several disorders (Fig. 15.10). Wedging and shape abnormalities of vertebrae must

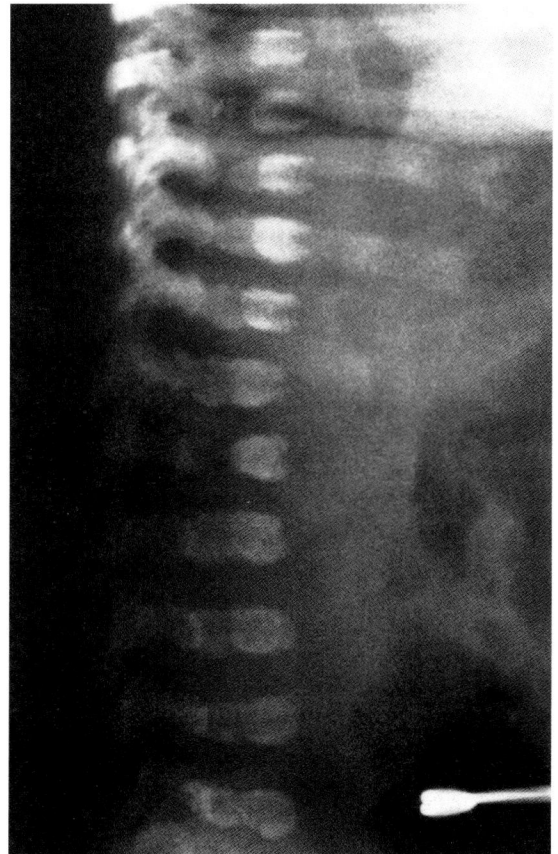

Figure 15.10 Kniest's dysplasia, newborn: lateral spine radiograph showing coronal (mid and posterior) clefts of the thoracic and lumbar vertebrae.

be recognized. Also, some miscellaneous peculiarities are important such as punctate calcifications (stippling), end-plate sclerosis and/or irregularity as well as humped vertebral bodies. Analysis of the anterior portion of vertebrae may reveal superior/anterior notching (inferior beaking) or a central tongue, as seen in the mucopolysaccharidoses (MPS).

The posterior elements of the spine also cannot be forgotten. Absence of these elements and interpediculate narrowing can be important findings. Special attention is paid to the cervical spine, appreciating not only ossification defects in this region but also C1–2 subluxation (dislocation) and cervical kyphosis.

Pelvis

The pelvis has been useful from the early years' descriptions of the skeletal dysplasias. Although the pelvic shape of many disorders is not as pathognomonic as previously thought, it is an extremely helpful area to analyze. Iliac wing shape changes as well as characteristic iliac abnormalities (African elephant ear – achondroplasia; apophyseal crest irregularity/sclerosis–Dyggve–Melchior–Clausen dysplasia; arched or snail-shaped) are looked for. The greater sacrosciatic notches may be narrowed, widened or even absent. Acetabular roof changes also contribute to the overall shape of the 'pelvis' (irregular, trident [three-pronged], hypoplastic, notched or flattened). The ischia and pubic bone development may also play a contributory role. Are they hypoplastic or enlarged? Are they vertical in inclination or are they even absent?

Thorax/upper limb girdle

The upper limb girdle and thorax can be quite significant. The shape of the chest may be of some help, but the ribs, on the other hand, demand strict analysis. Is there anterior and/or posterior rib flaring or cupping present? Are the ribs shortened (Fig. 15.11)? Rib width, including thickened, thinned, paddle (oar)-shaped, rib gaps, rib fusions, waviness (irregularity), may be a significant feature. Rib fractures and especially beading play a role in several skeletal dysplasias (osteogenesis imperfecta [OI] type II, achondrogenesis type IA, and pychnoachondrogenesis). The clavicles may be elongated, handlebar shaped or contain a 'lateral hook'. They may be hypoplastic, absent, resorbed, short, thickened or even comma-shaped. Scapula abnormalities in the skeletal dysplasias have recently been investigated (Fig. 15.11).[6] A diagnostic finding in campomelic dysplasia is the absence of the body of the scapula (Fig. 15.12).

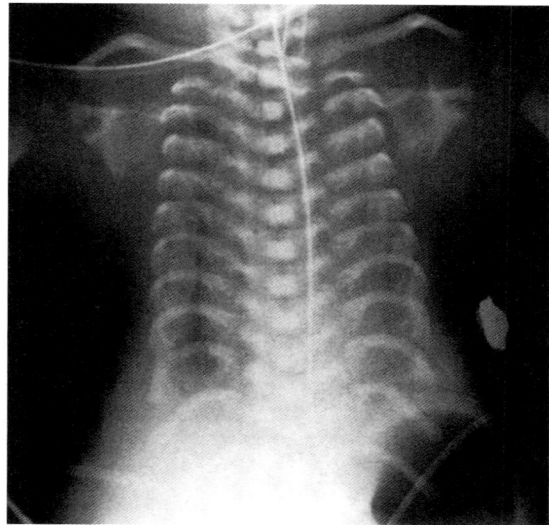

Figure 15.11   Short rib polydactyly dysplasia, type III, newborn: thoracic (chest) radiograph reveals very short ribs, an asphyxiated appearing thorax with marked lung hypoplasia, elongated (handlebar) clavicles and abnormal scapulae.

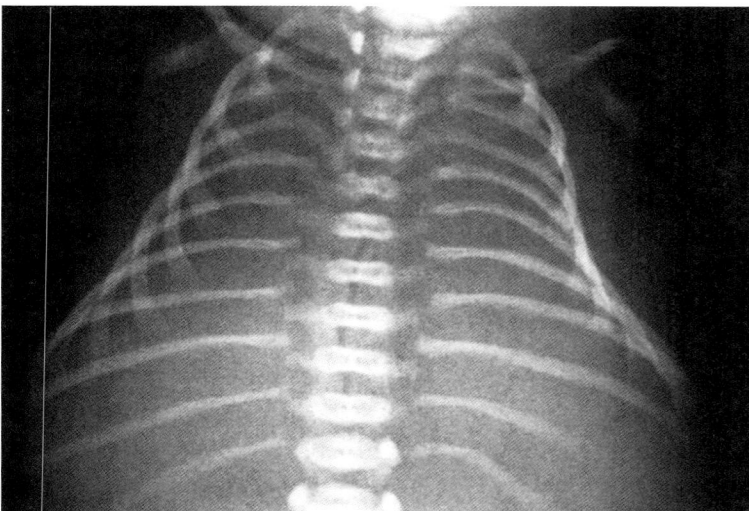

Figure 15.12   Campomelic dysplasia: thoracic (chest) radiograph revealing absence of the body of both scapulae, 11 ribs and absent thoracic vertebral pedicles.

Hands and feet

A meticulous search of abnormalities in the hands is crucial. For example, brachydactyly (shortened tubular bones of the hand) as well as the sites of involvement are often key:

- Is it confined to the metacarpals?
- Are all the metacarpals affected or just several?
- Which of the phalanges are shortened?

Also, metacarpal and phalangeal width may be significant. The shape of the proximal portion of the metacarpals may have considerable diagnostic significance (rounded, cupped, pseudoepiphyses, flattened, sucked candy appearance [resorbed] or even pointed – as in the MPS dysplasias) (Fig. 15.13). Metacarpal and phalangeal metaphyseal abnormalities as well as first ray abnormalities (first metacarpal, multangulum majus [greater multangular] navicular and radius) can be diagnostically helpful, i.e., the ovoid first metacarpal of diastrophic dysplasia (Fig. 15.14). Carpal number and abnormalities must be sought (Fig. 15.4). The same is true of the epiphyses of the tubular bones of the hand (cone-shaped, irregular, small, irregularly ossified, precociously ossified (large) or prematurely fused, Thieman's epiphyses, ivory, stippled or flattened). Interphalangeal fusions may be important as well as osteolysis in any region, especially acro (and/or carpal). Specific phalangeal anomalies may be encountered, some of which are almost diagnostic of certain disorders (clinodactyly, Kirner's deformity, delta phalanx, parchesipiece shaped, dislocated, round, half/quarter moon shaped, coffin [tombstone] shaped, dumbbell, bifid terminal phalanges). Even more important is the presence or absence of polydactyly and which type is present (preaxial, postaxial, unilateral, bilateral or intra-axial). Although osseous syndactyly is apparent, soft tissue syndactyly is a clinical finding.

The foot evaluation, although often not as rewarding as that of the hand with many more normal variations, must be performed. Minimal analysis should include shape of the foot, ossification abnormalities of tarsal bones and again the presence of polydactyly and type.

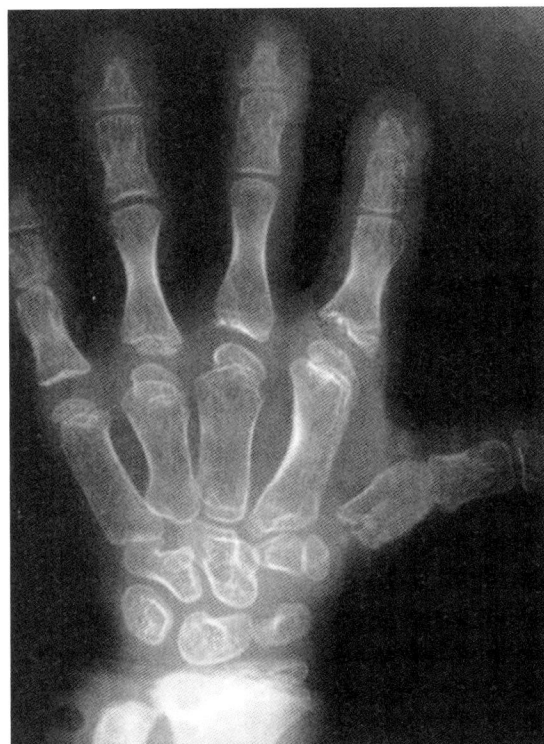

Figure 15.14 Diastrophic dysplasia: radiograph of hand demonstrating the 'hitchhiker thumb' with an 'ovoid' first metacarpal, generalized epiphyseal hypoplasia and extra-carpal ossification centers.

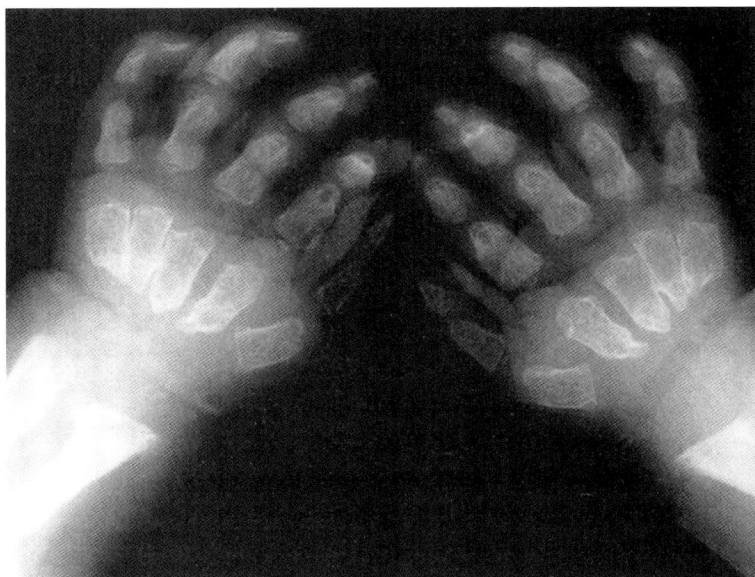

Figure 15.13 Mucopolysaccharidosis type I–H (Hurler): radiograph of hands exhibiting proximal metacarpal pointing, generalized brachydactyly and short tubular bone expansion.

Soft tissues and other organs

Calcification in soft tissues and other body organs are important radiologic clues. Also, other organ abnormalities available on imaging studies should not be ignored.

Upper and lower extremity long bones

An analysis of the long bone regions is best broken down into two parts. First, a consideration of generalized long-bone abnormalities which included the previous superficial appraisal of epiphyseal, metaphyseal and diaphyseal changes in all regions, and specific characteristic abnormalities including campomelia (bent bone[s]), periosteal cloaking, moth-eaten bones, ice cream cone epimetaphyses and dysostosis multiplex (MPS changes). Second, an accurate detailed appraisal of all the long bones individually. A selective perusal of all areas of the humerus, elbow region, radius and ulna, as well as the femur, tibia, and fibula.

For each long bone the size, in general, is appreciated (absent, hypoplastic, long). The epiphyses are analyzed. Are they absent or hypoplastic appearing, stippled, irregularly calcified, increased in osseous density (avascular necrosis), decreased in density, cloud effect, cone epiphyses, preconsciously ossified or enlarged? Do the epiphyses have irregular contours and where? Are there abnormalities of the epiphyseal plates themselves (widened, chevron deformity, narrow, abnormally or precociously fused)?

The metaphyses are then evaluated (flaring, cupping, irregularity with ossification defects, sclerotic infractions [fragmented/spurs], cloud effect, rounded, central spur [ball in], V groove, slanted, Erlenmeyer flask-like changes).

Diaphyseal abnormalities looked for include: under-modeling at bone ends (clubbed); overmodeled (constricted); increased thickness – generalized; thick or thin cortex; shortened or elongated; angulated (bent); marrow changes; fractures; tapering (proximal/distal); and chromosome appearance – as in the perinatal (lethal) form of hypophosphatasia.

Periosteal changes may also be helpful and at times diagnostic (periosteal new bone formation, subperiosteal bone resorption and periosteal cloaking – as in mucolipidosis type II) (Fig. 15.15).

Also, certain characteristic or pathognomonic features may be present in specific long bone areas: at the elbows, dislocations or fusions may occur; fibula overgrowth; the chevron and reverse chevron deformity in the distal femur and proximal tibia – achondroplasia; short or long femoral necks; accordion femurs – osteogenesis imperfecta type II; French telephone receiver femurs – thanatophoric dysplasia; key-shaped proximal femurs – Desbuquois dysplasia (Fig. 15.16).

At the hips one may recognize coxa vara, coxa valga or frank dislocations. At the knees genu valga or vara, a windswept deformity (combination of both) or dislocation

may also be found. The patella should be analyzed for absence, hypoplasia, dislocation, fragmentation and even enlargement.

Generalized intraosseous bone lesions may occur in certain skeletal dysplasias. They include osteopoikilosis, melorrheostosis, osteopathia striata, fibrous lucencies (whorls), popcorn calcifications and spurs. Even exostoses and enchondromas are very important.

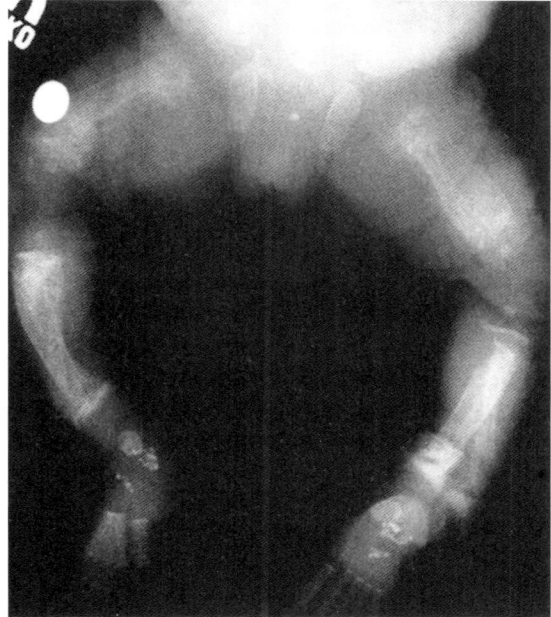

Figure 15.15 Mucolipidosis type II (I cell disease), newborn: radiograph of lower extremities demonstrating characteristic periosteal cloaking and stippled ossification centers.

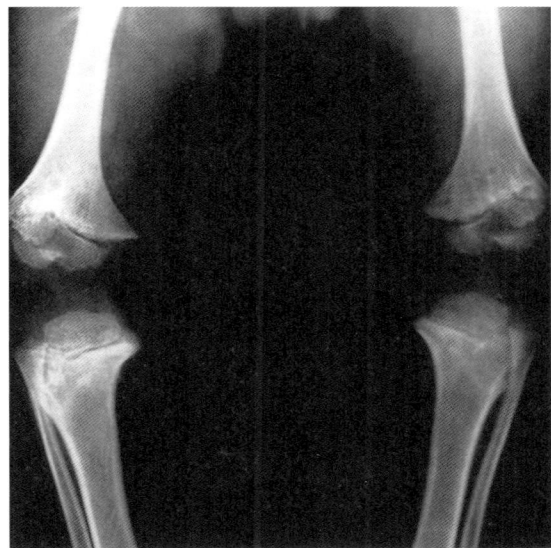

Figure 15.16 Achondroplasia: knee films demonstrating a modified 'chevron' deformity of the distal femurs and proximal fibular overgrowth.

CONCLUSIONS

The preceding pages have been a trip through the skeletal dysplasias using the radiologic assessment as the road map. This assessment must be put together with the other clinical findings to come up with a correct, specific diagnosis whenever possible for accurate genetic counseling and medical management. This can be performed by referring to Chapter 17 in this book and a variety of other texts, including several in the field of genetics.[1] Problem cases should be referred to the International Skeletal Dysplasia Registry or other skeletal dysplasia experts around the world. In the field of the skeletal dysplasias, it is most important to remember the adage, 'If it doesn't fit, don't force it'. An incorrect diagnosis will lead to incorrect genetic counseling and the failure of adequate management.

REFERENCES

1   Taybi H, Lachman RS. *Radiology of Syndromes, Metabolic Disorders and Skeletal Dysplasias*, 4th edn. Saint Louis: Mosby, 1996.
2   Lachman RS. Neurologic abnormalities in the skeletal dysplasias: A clinical and radiological perspective. *Am J Med Genet* 1997; **69**: 33–43.
3   Sorge G, Ruggieri M, Lachman RS. Spondyloperipheral dysplasia. *Am J Med Genet* 1995; **59**: 139–42.
4   Shohat M, Lachman RS, Gruber HE, Rimoin DL. Brachyolmia: radiographic and genetic evidence of heterogeneity. *Am J Med Genet* 1989; **33**: 209–19.
5   Shohat M, Rimoin DL, Gruber HE, Lachman RS. Perinatal lethal hypophosphatasia: clinical, radiologic and morphologic findings. *Pediatr Radiol* 1991; **21**: 421–7.
6   Mortier GR, Rimoin DL, Lachman RS. The scapula as a window to the diagnosis of the skeletal dysplasias. *Pediatr Radiol* 1997; **27**: 447–51.

FURTHER READING

Beighton P, ed. *McKusick's Heritable Disorders of Connective Tissue*, 5th edn. Chicago: Yearbook Medical Publishers, 1992.
Emery AEH, Rimoin DL, eds. *The Principles and Practice of Medical Genetics*, 3rd edn. Edinburgh: Churchill Livingstone, 1996.
Taybi H, Lachman RS. *Radiology of Syndromes, Metabolic Disorders and Skeletal Dysplasias*, 4th edn. Saint Louis: Mosby, 1996.

16

Psychological assessment

MELISSA COLSMAN, DAVID E SANDBERG

INTRODUCTION

Strategies for the clinical management of short children and adolescents have shifted from the guiding principle of 'hormone-replacement,' to the treatment of slow growth and 'short stature.' This move is evidenced by a disassociation between diagnosis and treatment. At present, the majority of youths receiving biosynthetic growth hormone (rhGH) are growth hormone (GH) sufficient.[1] Justification for the targeting of short stature for treatment hinges on patients', parents', and clinicians' understanding of the liabilities of being markedly short, as a youth and as an adult. For this reason, the clinical evaluation of the patient requires consideration of psychological and social contextual variables to ensure that medical intervention is warranted, likely to benefit the patient now or in the future, and that anticipated benefits outweigh any medical or psychological risks.

The focus of this chapter is on psychological assessment of children with short stature. It begins with case presentations designed to illustrate common medical management challenges. This is followed by a discussion of stereotypes and assumptions regarding the social, educational, and psychological sequelae of short stature that are thought to affect the quality of life (QOL) of the individual and, in turn, inform treatment decisions. Finally, a conceptual model guiding psychological assessment will be presented along with one example of that model put into practice.

CASES AND CLINICAL MANAGEMENT CONSIDERATIONS

Case 1

A 13-year-old boy growing steadily at the 5th percentile for height (−1.65 height SD, htSD) was referred to pediatric endocrinology by his primary care pediatrician for an evaluation of growth. The referral was initiated at the parents' insistence. Both parents are of average height: the mother is 163 cm (−0.1 htSD) and father is 177 cm (0.0 htSD). The mid-parental target height for this boy is 176.5 ± 10 cm (0.0 htSD). There is a paternal history of constitutional growth delay. The boy and his parents state they wish he was taller. He complains that he gets teased because of his height, cannot play sports very well, and has few friends. Given his height falling within the normal range, healthy growth velocity and slightly delayed bone age, the pediatric endocrinologist decided there was no indication for medical treatment; however, the parents are seeking help for a problem they define as 'medical' in nature.

Case 2

An 11-year-old boy below the 1st percentile for height (<−2.25 htSD) was referred by his pediatrician for an evaluation of growth. Mother's height is 154 cm (-1.7 htSD) and father's height is 164 cm (-2.0 htSD). The mid-parental target height for this boy is 165.5 ± 10 cm (-1.7 htSD). Predicted adult height based on bone age places this boy within the lower end of the range for target height (158 cm). Results of stimulation testing suggest that he is not GH-deficient (GHD). A comprehensive assessment, including history, physical examination, and laboratory tests, reveals this boy to be physically healthy. He is diagnosed with familial/genetic short stature. He complains about being teased at school and his parents report that his grades are poor.

Case 3

A 12-year-old girl below the 1st percentile for height (<-2.25 htSD) was referred by her pediatrician for an evaluation of growth. Both parents are short: the mother's height is 153 cm (-1.8 htSD) and father's height is 165 cm (-1.8 htSD). The mid-parental target height for their daughter is 152.5 ± 9 cm (-1.9 htSD) and her predicted height (as for Case 2) falls at the lower end of the range for target height. Results of stimulation testing indicate she is not GHD; a comprehensive assessment shows that she is physically healthy. The patient is diagnosed as having familial/genetic short stature. She presents as happy and well-adjusted.

Case 4

A 10-year-old girl growing at the 5th percentile for height (-1.65 htSD), was referred by her primary medical doctor for an evaluation of unexplained short stature. Both parents are tall: mother's height is 172 cm (1.4 htSD) and father's height is 186 cm (1.4 htSD). Her mid-parental target height is 172.5 ± 9 cm (1.5 htSD). Results of the evaluation indicated her karyotype is 45,XO/46,XX (i.e., Turner syndrome mosaic). The patient exhibits other physical features associated with Turner syndrome (TS), specifically, a narrow, high-arched palate and crowded teeth, cubitus valgus, and low posterior hairline. She has also been diagnosed with repeated otits media that has contributed to significant hearing loss. Neuropsychological testing provides evidence of a nonverbal learning disorder.[2] Both the child and her parents report 'she's doing pretty well.'

Considerations in clinical management

In Case 1, a pediatric endocrinologist would likely resist treatment with rhGH, instead referring the youth and his parents to a mental health professional to address his difficulties in social relationships. Inherent in this course of action is the potential dissatisfaction that the patient and parents may experience stemming from their belief that their

search for 'help' has been misunderstood, particularly because they attribute the son's difficulties to a 'medical condition,' i.e., short stature. However, the teasing and feelings of exclusion this child experiences, and the value that both he and his parents ascribe to stature, may be misattributed. In other words, there is the possibility that the boy's difficulties with peer relations are attributable to additional or other factors. The family may resist referral to a psychologist because of the implication that psychological, rather than medical, factors predominate. The family has been informed that their son does not qualify for treatment as it is 'not medically necessary'. However, the parents are not deterred and state they are willing to pay out-of-pocket.

Cases 2 and 3 are included, in part, due to the recent (2003) approval of rhGH for the treatment of idiopathic short stature (ISS) by the U.S. Food and Drug Administration (FDA).[3] In Case 2, the boy has difficulties at school (poor grades and is teased); in Case 3, the girl does not. In both, we must consider the risks and benefits of treating a condition through an invasive, chronic, and expensive intervention when there is no evidence that the treatment ameliorates an underlying disease state. This prompts the question: what are the explicit and implicit assumptions guiding the clinical care of these children?

Although there exists a broad consensus to provide rhGH therapy to girls with TS,[2] Case 4 was introduced to examine underlying assumptions. Prior to the introduction of rhGH, girls with TS were not treated because of the limited availability of cadaveric GH. Assuming the diagnosis was made early, girls with TS would return to the pediatric endocrinology clinic only when it was considered time to initiate puberty through sex hormone replacement. Since the approval by the FDA in 1997 of rhGH treatment for TS, pediatric endocrinologists have been involved in regular care of these girls from an earlier age than ever before. It has long been recognized that girls and women with TS often experience difficulties in social relationships, academic, and cognitive functioning.[4,5] They also exhibit chronic medical problems, some of which can further impact on QOL (for example, repeated otitis media with associated sensorineural hearing loss).[6] The lack of spontaneous puberty and infertility represent additional major developmental challenges for these girls and women. Might the intense focus on enhanced linear growth contribute to the belief among families (and clinicians) that improved growth is a strong predictor of QOL outcomes, possibly more critical than the other challenges these girls face? What is the evidence in support of this belief?

All four cases raise questions as to why it is that short stature has increasingly become a target for medical intervention. With the possible exceptions of GHD[7] and Prader–Willi syndrome (PWS),[8,9] for which metabolic benefits of rhGH have been ascribed, the primary rationale for treatment has traditionally rested on the assumption that short stature constitutes a physical disability, and otherwise serves as a significant psychosocial burden for the individual.[10]

Furthermore, treatment is predicated on the belief that rhGH-induced increases in height will improve QOL. The abundance of rhGH, and uncertainty regarding the diagnosis of GHD,[11] contribute to controversy regarding who should receive treatment. Allen and Fost infer from the growing number of conditions for which rhGH is prescribed that 'the cause of short stature is not morally relevant in deciding who is entitled to treatment.'[1] These authors proposed that rhGH therapy is indicated when a *disability* in adaptation attributable to short stature is identified (rather than by virtue of a medical diagnosis), and that treatment should be aimed at correcting this disability through treatment up to the point that an adult height within the 'normal range' is attained, i.e., the 5th percentile.

An additional question raised by these cases concerns the potential role of the pediatric endocrinology team in the assessment of the psychosocial aspects of children's slow growth. Because of their vast clinical experience in caring for such patients, these healthcare professionals will be very familiar with the predictable and, in individual cases, burdensome social challenges that these children face. Concluding that the particular child is not an appropriate candidate for rhGH therapy does not necessarily imply that other interventions are also unnecessary. In this context, consider Case 1. The American Academy of Pediatrics mandates that pediatricians take a leading role in addressing a wide range of medical conditions and developmental tasks, as well as coordinating care between medical and nonmedical specialists.[12] Although the pediatric endocrinologist is the specialist to whom patients are referred by primary care pediatricians, they are also the healthcare professionals with the most clinical experience in recognizing the psychosocial sequelae of short stature. For this reason, the pediatric endocrinology clinic is an ideal venue for providing comprehensive services – even if the needs are not entirely medical. The process of making recommendations for psychological care in the context of a medical evaluation is delicate. How can the findings and recommendations from such a comprehensive evaluation (e.g., for psychoeducational counseling) be provided in a manner that increases the likelihood families will follow through?[13]

With an evaluation that focuses *exclusively* on anthropometric and medical variables, the pediatric endocrinologist is limited to determining whether the patient is either physically 'healthy,' and therefore in no need of medical services, or that the patient has a medically treatable condition. This restricted decision tree constrains options and gives rise to ironic situations in which clinicians find themselves recommending rhGH treatment to a short, but well adjusted youth, while not providing treatment to youths who are a little taller (though still relatively short), but functioning poorly, *and* this situation is demonstrably related to the growth failure. By combining the psychological assessment with the medical evaluation in the endocrine clinic, additional opportunities for intervention become possible.

STEREOTYPES AND ASSUMPTIONS ABOUT THOSE WITH SHORT STATURE

Attitudes toward short stature and its treatment that are held by the child, parent, and clinician are informed by implicit beliefs about this physical characteristic and its psychosocial sequelae. Given that these beliefs can influence treatment decisions, it is imperative to examine putative links between short stature and psychosocial adaptation. One salient factor pertains to stereotypes held about those with short stature. A review of the specific stereotypes and assumptions implicit in the QOL rationale for rhGH therapy, as well as the clinical and epidemiologic data supporting them, may serve to inform clinical management decisions.

Stereotypes

Stereotyping refers to a process in which identical characteristics are assigned to all individuals within a group, regardless of the actual variation among group members. Negative stereotypes regarding experiences and characteristics of individuals with short stature are plentiful and exemplars in the research literature can be classified as follows: accompanying psychological characteristics, differential treatment by others, social relationships, and education/occupation.

Accompanying psychological characteristics

Children's and adults' beliefs about height demonstrate a bias toward the notion that 'taller is better.' In one study, elementary school children ascribed a positive valence to the word *short*, but then assigned significantly less favorable adjectives to short silhouettes than to either tall or average-sized silhouettes of children.[14]

In a study of college undergraduates, participants were provided with a written description of a hypothetical 24-year-old man or woman that included the individual's height in feet and inches.[15] The height descriptions provided to the students corresponded to either a short, average, or tall stature. The short man was rated less positively than the men of tall or average height on measures of personal adjustment, masculinity, and athletic orientation. The short woman was rated as less masculine than women of tall or average height; differences were not found with regard to personal adjustment, femininity, or athletic orientation. In a semantic differential task, in which research participants are asked to rate an object or concept (e.g., short man) on a series of bipolar evaluative dimensions (e.g., mature = 1 to immature = 7), male undergraduates rated 'short men' as significantly *less* mature, uninhibited, positive, secure, masculine, active, complete, successful, optimistic, dominant, capable, confident, and outgoing than men of tall or average height.[16] Similarly, female undergraduates rated short men as *more* immature, inhibited, negative, insecure, conforming, feminine, passive, and incomplete and as *less* successful and capable, but also as less pessimistic and withdrawn.[16] Using a variation of this paradigm, Gacsaly and Borges[17] asked college undergraduates to select which of six hypothetical males was mostly likely to represent each of 24 character traits. The six target stimuli represented not only two height conditions (short and tall) but also different body types (endomorph – heavy rounded body or fat; mesomorph – muscular; and ectomorph – light body build with little muscle mass). The combination of physical characteristics yielded results that contrasted with those of Martel and Biller[16] in which information about the hypothetical other was restricted to height. This study failed to detect differences in character trait attributions based on height alone. Instead, significant differences were found for height–body build combinations: the short endomorph figure was judged most likely to be an alcoholic and the short ectomorph was seen as more intelligent and helpful to others; no differences were found for the short and tall mesomorphs.

In summary, studies that focus on the physical characteristic of height suggest that individuals with short stature are viewed more negatively than others. Related to this phenomenon is the finding that youths and adults of both genders would prefer to be taller.[18–20]

Differential treatment by others

The words we use to describe everyday phenomena carry connotations that influence our thoughts about these traits.[21] Some argue that individuals with short stature experience disadvantages in the way they are treated due to stature-related societal perceptions.[22] When mothers of preschool children were shown photographs of one boy and one girl described as either 'short,' 'average,' or 'tall' and asked how long they would send the child to his or her room as punishment for pushing and hitting a baby that lived next door, the mothers assigned similar punishments for the male preschooler regardless of height status but assigned less severe punishment to the short girl than to her tall and average counterparts.[23]

'Personal space' (i.e., the area around a person's body into which others may not intrude without arousing discomfort) has been used as a proxy of respect. In two studies investigating the relationship between height and personal space, results were mixed. In both, college undergraduates were instructed to walk toward either a short or tall confederate (an individual who participates in the study under the direction of the investigator, but is presented as being a volunteer subject like the subjects themselves) and stop once they felt uncomfortable. In one study, participants stopped further away from the tall confederate than from the short.[24] In the second study, male participants were given additional information that 'the other person has been instructed to defend his territory and we would like to see to

what extent he will go to defend his area.'[25] When asked to rate the confederate as either nonaggressive or aggressive, weak or strong, or muscular or nonmuscular, students rated the tall confederate as more aggressive than the short one; however, there was no difference in measured physical proximity.

Social relationships

Research on the effects of height on social relationships focuses on heterosexual dating and partner selection. Findings support the conventional notion that taller is better in dating relationships, and this appears particularly true for males,[15,26–28] but less so for females.[15,28] In one study, female undergraduates were shown photographs of nine men varying in height (three short, three average, and three tall) and were asked to rate the men on several scales.[27] Shorter men were rated as less attractive and desirable as potential dates than men of average or tall stature. In addition, women liked both short and tall men less than those of average height. In this same study, male undergraduates were shown the photographs and asked to make ratings, assuming a woman's perspective. There were no differences in estimated attractiveness to or desirability as dates to women; however, male participants rated short men as liked more than tall men. In another study, female and male undergraduates rated hypothetical short men as less socially and physically attractive than tall men, but as no different from men of average height; no differences in perceptions of hypothetical short, average, or tall women were detected.[15] In a different study, romantically involved and uninvolved college men rated shorter women as more attractive than taller women, whereas uninvolved women rated taller men as more attractive than shorter men.[28] Regarding the importance of height in partner selection, the man's height is a more important consideration for women than the reverse.[17,29]

Education and occupation

When asked to evaluate classmates' competence, preschool boys rated small boys as better at 'Art' than tall boys; girls rated tall boys as smarter than small boys; but girls' height did not correlate with ratings.[23] Mothers rated tall boys and girls as more competent than small boys in the majority of domains,[23] and had greater expectations for mastery and achievement from taller children.[30]

Several studies have examined the perceived association between stature and an individual's occupational prestige or social status. When college students attending different sections of a course were asked to estimate the height of their course director and that of a male visitor who was introduced as having one of five different academic ranks (e.g., fellow student or visiting scholar), height estimates for the course director remained stable across student groupings, whereas mean height estimates for the other man increased with academic rank.[31] In related paradigms in which the description of a hypothetical other person varied in terms of height, college students indicated that, for both men and women, individuals of tall and average height are expected to have a higher professional status than their short counterparts.[15] Finally, when participants were asked to estimate the height of men in ten specified occupations, their height estimates were correlated with the prestige they associated with each profession.[32]

In view of the findings on stereotyped beliefs, it is understandable that parents of children with short stature, as well as healthcare professionals who treat these children, may be concerned about the child's psychosocial and educational adaptation. Even if the stereotypes represent gross overgeneralizations, the social consensus regarding the stigma associated with short stature becomes a reality unto itself. One way in which stereotyped beliefs and attitudes affect care is in how they shape our assumptions about those with short stature and the role of rhGH treatment.

Assumption 1: Individuals with short stature experience chronic psychosocial stress

Early studies showed that short stature was associated with teasing and juvenilization (i.e., treating individuals as if they were younger due to a misperception of their chronologic age).[10] However, participation in these investigations was generally restricted to patients with complex medical conditions and little attention was directed toward bias introduced by subject selection factors.[33] Thus, it is questionable to assume these findings are generalizable to the larger population of children with short stature currently seen by endocrinologists.

Two more recent clinic-based studies found that the majority of youths (approximately 60–70%) referred to pediatric endocrinologists for a growth evaluation, experienced teasing or juvenilization.[34,35] Contrary to expectations, the child's relative height (range: -3.1 to -0.2 htSD) was *not* significantly related to children's or parents' reports of stature-related psychosocial stressors.[35] Results of these clinical studies corroborate anecdotal reports that short stature elicits predictable social responses during childhood and adolescence, and conform to stereotypes that individuals with short stature are perceived and treated negatively. Missing from these clinic-based reports is an assessment of the degree to which teasing or juvenilization are associated with psychological dysfunction. Banter among friends that makes reference to the individual's height would not be expected to have the same long-term consequences as more pernicious teasing or bullying of any type. To date, published reports in this area have not taken the *quality* of such experiences into account by weighting self- or parental reports of such potentially stressful events by the degree to which they are perceived as distressing.

Assumption 2: Individuals with short stature exhibit clinically significant problems of psychosocial adaptation

A short youth was referred for endocrine evaluation. A commonly held assumption is that patients with short stature exhibit higher rates of clinically significant behavioral or emotional problems than those of average height in the general population.[10] Implicit in this belief is the expectation that the prevalence of psychiatric problems is significantly higher among patients with short stature than it is for the general population (estimated from epidemiological studies to be approximately 12%).[36,37] However, this does not appear to be the case when selection biases in participant recruitment are minimized. For example, self-reported self-esteem scale scores for short youths referred for evaluation of short stature were *higher* (i.e., more positive) than questionnaire norms despite reports that the majority of these individuals experienced teasing and juvenilization.[35] The same was true for behavior disturbances: patients reported significantly fewer problems than questionnaire norms, and parental reports indicated that patients were indistinguishable from the norms in terms of behavioral and emotional functioning.[35] Similar findings were reported by a European randomized clinical trial of the QOL benefits of rhGH therapy in children with ISS ($n = 36$; 5–12 years old; mean of -2.95 and -2.70 htSD for treatment and control groups, respectively).[38] Except in the area of 'social functioning,' scores before initiating treatment fell within normative ranges on self-esteem and health-related QOL measures.

In another clinic-based study of patients referred for an evaluation of short stature, by self-report, adolescent boys with short stature exhibited no more behavior problems than the community norms as measured by an extensively used problem checklist.[39] The girls reported significantly *fewer* problems than the norms. By parental report, girls with short stature were indistinguishable from the norms. In contrast, the boys were perceived as exhibiting significantly more behavior problems than the norms, but showed fewer problems than a psychiatric-referred comparison group. Interestingly, relatively taller children received *higher* problem scores (i.e., indicating more problems).[39]

In contrast, other studies reported significantly more behavioral and emotional problems among children with short stature relative to norms as measured by both self- and parent- report.[40,41] Unfortunately, key details essential to gauge the representativeness of the samples were not provided, e.g., the total number of eligible patients and the method of targeting participants for behavioral studies. These and other methodological concerns are discussed more fully elsewhere.[42] Studies featuring clinically representative samples have shown behavioral adjustment to be comparable to population-based norms[35,39] and classmates.[43]

Several studies have demonstrated that *perceived* height may differ substantially from actual *measured* height.[44–51] For example, when using the Silhouette Apperception Technique, Grew and colleagues[47] found that height overestimation was very common in families with a child with short stature due to hypopituitarism. A similar tendency to overestimate the short child's height has been demonstrated in other clinic-based samples[46,48,50] and in a community sample of adolescent boys.[52] The suggestion has been made that this phenomenon might serve the adaptive coping function of 'denial' of certain physical facts, awareness of which might generate emotional distress for the individual.[46,47,52] Support for this notion has come from studies demonstrating that self-perceptions of height are more strongly predictive of personality characteristics such as dominance (Ackerman and Herman's study as cited in Roberts et al.[53]) or self-esteem,[49] as well as psychosocial adaptation and satisfaction with stature than is measured height.[48]

Short youths in the general population

Although rarely articulated, it follows that short youths who are not referred for a medical evaluation are similarly at risk for psychosocial adaptation problems. In the prospective, longitudinal Wessex Growth Study, in which the sample is comprised of short but otherwise healthy children from the general population, no evidence of serious psychosocial or academic disadvantage was found.[54–57] The Wessex study is unique in that the sample is comprised of short (below the 3rd percentile) but otherwise healthy children from the general population.[58] Children with known organic disease were excluded, the age range lay within a tight band, a wide range of socioeconomic classes was represented, and the study incorporated case-matched (classmate) controls of average stature (10th to 90th percentile). Psychometric testing was largely based on well-validated and standardized tests. Although mean IQ significantly differed between the short and control groups, this was of no clinical import, as height explained only 2% of the variance in IQ, a finding that emphasizes the need to look beyond p values in statistical tests and consider effect size.[59] The Wessex data indicate that socioeconomic factors, rather than stature, best predict psychosocial and academic outcomes.[55] (Comparable findings for IQ have been reported for a national probability sample in the US.[60])

As others have found using self-report measures,[61] the children in the Wessex short stature group would have preferred to be taller, and they also reported more bullying than their taller peers.[19] Neither the desire for physical change nor bullying, however, had a measurable effect on school performance or self-esteem.[54,55] These findings suggest that stigmatized individuals are able to call on self-protective cognitive mechanisms that allow self-esteem to remain intact.[39]

In a recent study using a novel research design, the influence of height on students' ($n = 956$; grades 6 to 12; approximately 11 to 18 years old) psychosocial adaptation was assessed using peer informants.[62] Statistically significant relationships were not detected between height and measures of friendship, popularity, or most aspects of reputation among peers, despite substantial statistical power.

Findings did not vary by participant gender, peer- or self-report, whether data from the entire sample were used, or when subgroups of very short (≤ -2.25 htSD; 1st percentile) or very tall students ($\geq +2.25$ htSD; 99th percentile) students were contrasted with average height (25th to 75th percentile for norms) classmates. In the lower grades, classmates perceived shorter students as younger than their chronological age. However, this perception was not meaningfully related to measures of social acceptance or other aspects of reputation among peers. The authors concluded that extremes of stature in the general population – either short or tall – have minimal detectable influence on peer perceptions of social behavior, friendship, or acceptance.[62] Overall, it appears that the assumption that children with short stature have clinically significant problems of social and psychological adaptation is not supported. However, one might wonder about how their short stature may affect psychosocial adaptation in adulthood.

Short adults in the general population

A cohort study of 18-year-old Swedish conscripts ($n = 32\,887$) examined the association between men's stature and intellectual performance, psychological functioning, and other health concerns.[63] After excluding from data analyses cases with health conditions (e.g., asthma, congenital malformations, and mental retardation) that have a known association with height, investigators found that short men (≤ -2 htSD) scored more poorly than taller men in assessments of intellectual functioning, psychological functioning during mental stress, and suitability for leadership positions. However, despite attempting to control for health conditions that may have effects on both stature and psychological functioning, difficulties in interpretation remain: the study did not control for background variables such as socioeconomic status (SES), nor more subtle conditions that could lead to decreases in both stature and functioning, for example, premature birth.

The relationship between height and marriage rates varies by study. In the National Child Development Study (NCDS), a longitudinal study of British citizens, the probability of being married was 7% lower for short men (≤ 9th percentile) and 5% lower for tall women (≥ 90th percentile) than for adults of average height (20th to 79th percentiles), when statistically controlling for social class, education, health, race, and region of residence.[64] Contrasting findings derive from the US National Longitudinal Survey of Youth (NLSY), a study featuring a comparable research design. Although short men exhibited lower rates of first marriage than those of average height, this effect disappeared once family-of-origin variables (parental education, poverty status, and region of the country) were taken into account; no consistent relationship was found between women's height and marriage rates.[65,66]

Vågerö and Modin[67] used data from the Uppsala Birth Cohort (a lifelong follow-up study of individuals born between 1915 and 1929) to explore one path by which height may be related to marriage rates. They found that men with a birth weight for gestational age in the lowest fifth for this cohort were less likely to marry than those who were heavier. No such relationship was detected for women. Although analyses did not control for adult height, the investigators speculated that prenatal risk factors for growth retardation (such as maternal alcohol consumption, maternal tobacco use, or exposure to other toxic agents) may affect facial appearance; this may lead to subtle disadvantages, such as a reduced likelihood of marriage.

In the National Health and Nutrition Examination Survey (NHANES II, 1976–80), 20 325 men aged 20–65 years were physically examined and asked to complete questionnaires. Although a trend was found between taller stature and the likelihood of completing college, this relationship was not statistically significant.[68] Furthermore, taller men were not more likely to achieve higher professional status when in analyses that controlled for educational attainment.[68] In a study of job performance among male Navy recruits, height was not associated with ratings on standardized performance reviews.[69] In a study of women, supervisors rated tall (upper quartile), in-house applicants as more suitable as managers than short applicants.[70] In addition, a statistically significant difference in ratings was found on only one of 30 characteristics (after adjusting the p value for the number of statistical tests to protect against type I error): tall applicants were rated as being more able to think 'holistically' than short applicants. Within the nursing, business and administration, and skilled crafts professions, the participant's professional status accounted for 3% of the variance in height among female nurses, 3% of the variance among men in business and administration, and 4% of the variance among men in skilled trades after controlling for father's occupational status and subject's educational attainment.[71] In this same study, *perceptions* of social and professional success were also closely related to height; the author concluded that stereotypes contribute to a disproportionate rise to higher professional status among individuals with taller stature.[71] Of course, a causal hypothesis such as this cannot be tested through correlational research.

With regard to income, no consistent relationship was found in the NHANES II study between men's height and family income when the analysis controlled for age and education.[68] In contrast, Sargent and Blanchflower[72] detected a positive relationship between height at age 16 years and wages at age 23 years for men in the NCDS when the analysis statistically controlled for social class and measured intelligence. This study demonstrated that a difference of 10 cm in height was related to a 3% change in hourly wage, with taller individuals earning more. No relationship between height and income was found for women in the study. An analysis of more recently collected data from the NCDS longitudinal study[64] showed that men and women in the bottom 10% of the height distribution, as measured at age 33 years, earned 4.3% and 5.1% less income, respectively, than those in the average height group (20th to 79th percentiles).

Studies of the relationship between height and income often report that tall men and women earn more than their shorter colleagues.[64,68,72–74] However, when relevant background information (i.e., potentially confounding variables such as age, health, education and family of origin characteristics) are controlled for statistically, the relationship between height and income is attenuated.[68,74] A difficulty in interpreting this literature is that short stature might contribute to lower SES, and that by controlling for SES, its effect is obscured. In other words, the possibility exists that short stature contributes to downward socioeconomic mobility, perhaps due to social or psychological burdens associated with short stature. It also may be that a low SES, in which one lacks certain resources (e.g., good prenatal care, adequate healthcare or nutrition) may contribute to short stature.

Assumption 3: Height-related social stress results in significant problems of psychological adjustment

As both teasing[75,76] and psychological adaptation problems[37] are relatively common among children and adolescents, support for Assumption 3 should come from a demonstrated statistical link between stressful stature-related experiences and psychosocial dysfunction. In the one study that specifically addressed this issue, parental report of stature-related teasing statistically significantly predicted increased emotional problems.[34] The proportion of unique variance in problem scores attributable to teasing was approximately 2% and increased (to between 4% and 5%) when the frequency of teasing was taken into account. Juvenilization also contributed unique explanatory value, and summated with teasing as a negative influence on psychosocial adaptation.

To interpret the clinical significance of these effects, one must view them within the context of the mean level of behavior problems in this sample. As noted in Assumption 2, the psychological adaptation of short youths in this same clinic-referred cohort was comparable to community norms.[39] Thus, the possibility exists that stature-related stresses may contribute to variability in adaptation that falls within the 'normal range.'

Assumption 4: Increased growth velocity and height-induced by rhGH therapy result in improved quality of life

The final assumption underlying the 'increased height brings improved QOL' rationale for endocrine intervention relates to the anticipated psychological benefits of improved growth through rhGH therapy. Only three randomized controlled trials of GH treatment in ISS were designed to investigate psychological outcomes. We focus on ISS because the sole rational for rhGH treatment is acceleration of growth velocity during childhood and adolescence and increased adult height. In the case of other conditions for which rhGH is approved (e.g., GHD and PWS), metabolic benefits are posited in addition to increased growth.[7,8] Changes in QOL subsequent to rhGH could then be the consequence of either the metabolic benefits or taller stature.

In the Wessex Growth Study, 15 children were treated with rhGH beginning at the age of 7–8 years.[77] These children were compared to untreated short control participants and children of average height (10th to 90th percentiles) at recruitment, after 3 years, and after 5 years. Study participants were 12–13 years of age at the time of the 5-year follow-up. Only the treated group showed a significant height increase (htSD score changed from −2.44 to −1.21 over 5 years). The behavioral results were uncomplicated: across all behavioral measures, no significant differences were seen between treated and untreated short children or peers of average height at recruitment, after 3 years, or after 5 years of treatment.

In a more recent study,[38] 36 prepubertal children with ISS (5–12 years old) were randomly assigned to treatment or control groups. The children, their parents, and the treating physician answered health-related QOL and self-esteem questionnaires before initiating therapy and after 1 and 2 years of rhGH treatment. As noted in the discussion of Assumption 1, psychosocial adaptation and self-esteem of these children were comparable to norms for the general population at baseline (although see Assumption 1 for exception). After 2 years of rhGH therapy, the relative height of the treated group increased from −2.95 to −1.85 htSD, whereas that of the untreated control group remained essentially unchanged (−2.70 to −2.50 htSD). Despite significant increases in relative height, neither parents nor children reported an associated improvement in the child's health-related QOL. In some cases, treated children reported a *worse* health-related QOL or self-esteem than the untreated control group. In contrast, the *treating pediatricians* reported better perceived psychological functioning in the treatment group (compared with the control group) after 2 years of rhGH therapy. It is troubling that the clinician, rather than the child or parents, associated the lack of rhGH treatment in the control group with greater distress. The treating pediatrician's perception can, therefore, jeopardize established psychological mechanisms promoting adaptive coping.

A survey showed that 56% of physicians believed that height impairs emotional well-being in children whose height is below the 3rd percentile and 32% believed that QOL can be improved by increasing height.[78] As reviewed earlier, research supports neither belief. As such, parents can be reassured that short children are indistinguishable from children of average height in terms of global psychosocial adaptation. Additionally, shorter adults are difficult to distinguish from their taller peers. Problems that might be evident are not necessarily attributable to short stature, as in cases in which short stature is a single feature of a complex syndrome (e.g., TS).[79]

The third randomized controlled study of the psychological effects of rhGH on children with ISS added a placebo-treated control group.[50] In the above two studies, any

observed changes could have been attributed to a placebo effect. Placebo effects are particularly common and strong in research where the measured outcome is subjective and continuous as in the sorts of studies reviewed here.[80]

In the study by Ross et al.,[50] 59 prepubertal children (78% male; mean age 12.4 years at recruitment) diagnosed with ISS completed the Self-Perception Profile[81,82] and the Silhouette Apperception Technique,[47] and a parent completed the Child Behavior Checklist[83] at recruitment and at yearly intervals over 4 years of treatment with either rhGH or placebo. At recruitment, both groups' scores on all Self-Perception Profile and Child Behavior Checklist scales were indistinguishable from each other and from normative data. There was, however, a significant correlation between height and parental report of child internalizing (i.e., emotional) problems, such that *taller* children exhibited greater problems. (This counter-intuitive finding has previously been reported[39] and may be related to a bias in the referral of mildly short youths with behavioral or emotional problems to pediatric endocrinologists.) Self-perceptions of height, as measured by the Silhouette Apperception Technique, did not differentiate the groups, both of which overestimated their measured height. Subsequent assessments did not reveal statistically significant differences between treatment and control groups on the Self-Perception Profile and scores on the Child Behavior Checklist remained within the normative range.

In addition to these randomized controlled investigations, there is one notable report in which the QOL of 24 young adults who had been diagnosed with ISS and treated with rhGH in childhood was compared with a group of 65 former patients with the same diagnosis who had not been treated.[20] These latter patients participated in a retrospective study of the spontaneous growth of children with ISS. Thus no random assignment to groups was made and only the treated group was followed prospectively. At the time of the follow-up assessment, the mean adult height attained by both groups was approximately the same (−2.3 ± 0.9 htSD). The mean height gain of the treatment group (based on the predicted adult height before initiation of treatment) was 3.3 ± 5.6 cm (range: −9.9 to 13.4 cm). The level of educational attainment was comparable in the two groups, but the *treated* patients had a romantic partner *less* often than participants in the control group, even after adjustments were made for age and gender. Neither of two well-standardized health-related QOL measures revealed differences between the treatment and control groups, or between results for a combined group of ISS patients and age-specific norms for the questionnaires. Despite their relative short stature, the vast majority of participants in the treatment group (92%) and control group (86%) expressed satisfaction with their adult height. Even so, 58% and 62% of the treatment and control groups, respectively, wished to be taller. However, when faced with a hypothetical scenario designed to assess the strength of this desire, only 22% indicated they would take a medication to be taller if it were associated with a shorter life ('time trade-off' paradigm). In a second hypothetical situation, surgery to achieve taller stature was considered.

In this circumstance, only 11% indicated they would consider an operation if there were a risk of dying as a result of the procedure ('standard gamble' paradigm). Despite the limited gain in height (3.3 ± 5.6 cm), satisfaction with rhGH therapy was high. This surprising finding is likely related to the overestimation of adult height gained through treatment. Former patients and parents attributed 12 (±8) cm and 13 (±7) cm of additional height, respectively, to rhGH treatment.[20]

Although individuals who have received treatment may still want to be taller, they are likely to be satisfied with the decision for rhGH therapy because of the misattribution of *all* growth subsequent to treatment initiation to the benefits of rhGH.[20] This observation lessens concerns that variability in the results produced by rhGH may result in disappointment, a potential psychological side effect of treatment. Consequently, it is unlikely that former patients will complain of the unrealized benefit of rhGH treatment. Although this report suggests that most rhGH-treated patients are satisfied with treatment results regardless of its objective efficacy, a psychological downside to the treatment may yet exist. If perceived height is more closely related to psychosocial adaptation than is measured height, then a therapeutic approach concerned only with the outcome variable of measured height may result in unexpected (and possibly negative) psychological outcomes. rhGH therapy is a treatment involving daily subcutaneous injections, typically over the course of several years. The treatment itself may therefore highlight in youths' minds a sense of being different from others[84] and undo the adaptive aspects of misperceptions of height by either patients themselves or their parents. Although additional studies of this topic using rigorous research designs are required, no compelling evidence yet exists to suggest that rhGH therapy is associated with changes in behavior during childhood, adolescence, or young adulthood.

This review of the clinical research literature on psychosocial adaptation of individuals with short stature, and assumptions implicit in the recommendation for rhGH treatment, are based upon group data. It represents a summary of findings in the aggregate, which differs from the clinical setting where clinicians work with individual patients and their families. Therefore, while this review indicates that children with short stature, on average, are doing well, there is nothing in this literature that discounts the distress an individual may encounter as a function of his or her markedly short stature. For an individual child, height may interfere with healthy psychological development. As such, a comprehensive psychological assessment is warranted as a part of the evaluation.

PSYCHOLOGICAL EVALUATION

Conceptual model

The clinical management of short stature implies a number of assumptions about psychosocial stressors and risks of psychological problems in this patient group. Noeker and Haverkamp[85] developed a useful conceptual framework to guide the psychological assessment of youths with short stature that can be used to inform clinical management decisions. Three hierarchical levels of assessment are identified: stress exposure due to short stature (Level I), quality of adaptive coping responses (Level II), and occurrence of psychopathology (Level III).

Level I assessment includes evaluating stressful situations typically associated with short stature. These include stigmatization, juvenilization, and other stressors associated with complex medical conditions such as chronic renal failure, TS, or PWS. Level II concerns the individual's ability to mount effective coping responses. Factors that might intensify negative reactions to short stature are those that tax the individual's capacity to compensate; for example, low SES, poor academic performance related to a learning disability, or family discord. Conversely, protective factors, such as an easy-going temperament or strong family and peer support, can effectively buffer the individual against the sequelae of stature-related stresses. Finally, Level III involves assessing the patient's behavioral and emotional functioning, and identifying clinically significant impairment in family, peer, or educational functioning.

Clinical management is facilitated by a thorough psychosocial evaluation designed to delineate specific stressors experienced by the child, the pattern of coping, and psychosocial adaptation. Because of the salience of short stature and its potential to serve as a lightning rod that diverts attention from other stressors, clinicians must be watchful of misattributions by the child, parents, or others (including oneself). This influence may direct attention away from prescribing psychosocial interventions for maladaptive coping. This evaluation serves to assess individual characteristics (e.g., intelligence, temperament) and social-ecologic factors (e.g., degree of stress in the child's environment, salience of height to the family, social support from peers) that could moderate the influence of height on psychosocial adaptation. Finally, identifying adaptive coping strategies as an alternative (or adjunct) to rhGH therapy is an additional goal. Gathering such detailed information is prudent in view of the clinical evidence showing that the adult height of formerly treated GH-sufficient individuals often remains substantially below average.[86]

Model in practice: The psychosocial screening project

In light of older clinical reports suggesting an increased risk that children and adolescents with short stature show increased problems of academic and psychosocial adjustment,[10] patients referred for a growth evaluation at our institution routinely receive a psychosocial assessment. The *Psychosocial Screening Project* (PSP) refers to a clinical service provided to all new patients with short stature receiving a growth evaluation. The purpose of the PSP is to identify and provide psychosocial services to individuals who are currently experiencing difficulties and to provide anticipatory guidance to families where the child or adolescent is currently adapting well.

At the time of their initial visit to the pediatric endocrinology clinic, an accompanying parent of all patients 2 years and older, referred with a chief complaint of short stature, completes paper-and-pencil questionnaires selected to characterize the child's psychosocial profile. Children 8 years and older complete parallel self-assessment forms. The assessment protocol (30–40 min in duration) is completed during waiting intervals between physician examinations or while waiting for blood tests or a bone-age X-ray, and as such it does not require 'extra' time in clinic to complete. Feedback from the evaluation and any indicated recommendations from a doctoral level pediatric psychologist are provided to the family by telephone two weeks after the endocrine clinic visit. A summary of the psychosocial screening report is filed in the patient's endocrine chart.

Questionnaires used include the *Child Behavior Checklist*,[83] *Youth Self Report*,[87] *Self-Perception Profile*,[81,82] an *Educational Background Questionnaire*,[88] and a questionnaire pertaining to *Issues Related to Growth Problem and Height*.[34] This combination of generic and short stature-specific assessment tools was selected to characterize the general psychological, social, and educational adaptation of patients as well as negative experiences attributed to short stature.

This behavioral assessment can enhance clinical care by providing clinicians (physicians and mental health professionals) with important information that might otherwise go unreported. For patients whose questionnaire findings demonstrate positive adaptation, the PSP serves a preventive function. At the time of the initial visit, all families receive booklets about both the physical[89,90] and psychological aspects[91] of slow growth and short stature. The latter booklet discusses common psychosocial sequelae of short stature and provides strategies to counter these at home and in public.[91]

The services provided through the PSP extend beyond the initial assessment and treatment recommendations. Families have the option of receiving psychoeducational counseling or other interventions from the two pediatric psychologists attending the endocrine clinics. Follow-up visits to the endocrine clinic provide the opportunity to update patients' psychosocial status, whether or not any medical intervention is indicated. Finally, the PSP includes the services of an educational/vocational counselor who facilitates enrollment in various socialization experiences (e.g., organized after-school sports or interest-based programs, internships, and summer jobs) to support the development of age-appropriate social skills that counter the tendency of others to minimize expectations for the markedly short youth.

PSP applied to the four cases

The PSP is a comprehensive evaluation that provides information on psychosocial adaptation at each of the three levels recommended by Noeker and Haverkamp.[85] As a

screening evaluation, any recommendations based upon positive findings are considered provisional pending further evaluation. Likely PSP findings and recommendations for the four patients described earlier in this chapter are discussed below.

CASE 1

Both the child and his parents reported difficulties in psychosocial adjustment which they believe are related to the boy's height. Parent report on the *Child Behavior Checklist* indicated that the patient participates in fewer peer-oriented activities and experiences more internalizing behavior (i.e., problems of anxiety, depression, or withdrawn behavior) than are typically reported by parents of boys his age. He scored in the average range for all school subjects, and his parents reported he receives no special services at school. His self-report, on the *Youth Self-Report*, was comparable to his parents'. Self-perceptions of domain-specific competencies (per the *Self-Perception Profile*), fell in the low (i.e., negative) range for social acceptance, athletic competence, physical appearance, romantic appeal, close friends, and global self-worth, but in the positive range for scholastic competence, job competence, and behavioral conduct. On the *Issues Related to Growth Problem and Height*, he stated he is teased by his peers, who call him a combination of stature- and non-stature-related names (e.g., 'shorty' and 'dummy') and reported that he is 'very dissatisfied' with his height. In addition to wishing he could be taller, he also expressed the desire to be more muscular. He believes that his short stature is the major factor in why he is not chosen by his peers for sports teams. He reports that he reacts to the teasing by withdrawing; his parents, in turn, react with frustration and anger over the child's circumstances. Other than his expressed interest in sports, from which he frequently withdraws, he socializes little with his peers and plays video games alone at home.

Based on the combined medical and psychological evaluation, it is apparent that although both the child and his parents are dissatisfied with his height, and attribute many of his difficulties with peers to his stature, rhGH treatment is not an indicated treatment. Instead, recommendations include further assessment as to why he suspends his involvement in sports and other peer-based activities in favor of spending time alone. Based on the psychosocial screen, several factors may account for social withdrawal; for example, being teased, parental reaction to the teasing, or this youth's negative perception of his athletic competence. Further exploration of these may reveal that the parents' angry and frustrated reactions to hearing their son is teased and/or their attempts to be supportive may inadvertently reinforce their child's belief that his short stature is preventing him from joining in and enjoying the company of his peers. Another possibility may be that he is depressed – his withdrawal from others and elevated score on the *internalizing* scale of the *Child Behavior Checklist* indicate this is another area to evaluate more closely.

Psychoeducational counseling is indicated to disabuse the boy (and his parents) of unrealistic expectations that they have about the auxologic benefits of rhGH in GH-sufficient youth.[86] They would also be reassured, based on the empirical literature reviewed above, that short stature need not limit the range of interests, experiences, or accomplishments. To address the experience of being teased, consideration would be given to enrolling this youth in a cognitive behavioral psychotherapy group designed to enhance coping to the predictable psychosocial stresses associated with short stature,[92] i.e., bolster Level II adaptation according to Noeker and Haverkamp's model.[85]

The screening evaluation also revealed that this child may be dissatisfied with delayed pubertal development (i.e., complaints about lack of muscle strength) compared to others his age. An alternative to rhGH may be to consider testosterone treatment (see Stein et al.[93]).

CASE 2

Results of the *Child Behavior Checklist* indicated that this boy participates in few peer-oriented activities, and is doing below-average work at school. The parents noted his teacher reports he is easily distracted and does not consistently complete his homework. He is not receiving any special services at school to address these difficulties. His parents wonder if additional help might be appropriate. On the *Issues Related to Growth Problem and Height*, both the child and his parents complain about teasing and juvenilization. He added that others make remarks about his height and talk to him as if he were 7 or 8 years old, and of most concern to him is that his peers pick him up off the ground at school because he is 'so small.' On the *Self-Perception Profile*, the patient scored in the negative range on measures of scholastic competence, social acceptance, and close friendships.

The psychosocial screening evaluation highlights the teasing and juvenilization faced by this child, as well as academic difficulties. The basis for these problems is likely multi-determined: it may be that the teasing and juvenilization interfere with his ability to concentrate on his school work. Alternatively, it may be that his academic difficulties arise from an as-yet undiagnosed problem such as an attention deficit hyperactivity disorder (ADHD), the symptoms of which (i.e., distractibility, failure to sustain attention in tasks or play, difficulty waiting for his turn, etc.) provide a basis for teasing and juvenilization.[94] Further assessment of these difficulties is advised, as is psychoeducational counseling to address the teasing and juvenilization. The counseling could take the form of coaching on how to deal with taunts and forming a plan of action, likely involving adult intervention, for when other children attempt to pick him up off the ground.

CASE 3

Neither the child nor her parents reported any difficulties in psychosocial or educational areas, per the *Child Behavior Checklist*, *Youth Self-Report*, and *Educational Background Questionnaire*. Her parents reported that she enjoys dancing and gymnastics, is doing well academically, and has several close friends. On the *Issues Related to Growth Problem and Height*, both she and her parents noted that, while she looks approximately 2 years younger than her chronological age, this does not bother her or worry her parents since she behaves age-appropriately. She also stated that she is not particularly concerned about her height and scored in the positive range for all domains of the *Self-Perception Profile*.

Results of the psychosocial screening show that this child has positive adaptation in all areas: she encounters little teasing or juvenilization (Level I), is doing well in school, has reliable friendships, a supportive family environment (Level II), and does not experience any significant emotional or behavioral difficulties (Level III). An inherent psychological risk in recommending rhGH based on the diagnosis of ISS would be the implication that there is something 'wrong' with this child that requires chronic treatment.

CASE 4

The parents of this girl reported no difficulties of an internalizing or externalizing nature, per the *Child Behavior Checklist*; though they noted she is receiving failing grades for maths. She receives special accommodation at school which addresses her hearing loss and learning disorder. According to the *Issues Related to Growth Problem and Height*, her parents indicated they were 'somewhat satisfied' with their daughter's height, though curious why she was shorter than her younger sister. They also noted that although she is eager to join in with peers, she is not sought out by them. They commented that she engages in activities more suitable for younger children – for example, the clothes she wears and music she listens to are more appropriate for 7 or 8-year-old children. While this does not bother her, her parents are growing increasingly concerned that social and emotional problems will emerge as she grows older.

For this child, the psychosocial screening highlighted some differences between the child's and parents' perceptions. While all agreed that 'she's doing pretty well,' her parents had some concerns about her future development. With the parents' authorization, the pediatric psychologist from the endocrine clinic contacted the school psychologist who had conducted the educational evaluation. Information was provided regarding the neurocognitive features of TS as well as recommended remediation strategies.[95] With regard to delayed social maturity and social skills deficits, a recommendation was made to have this girl participate in a social skills group for pre-teens and to enroll in organized peer-group activities based upon her interests. Finally, the family was encouraged to contact the Turner Syndrome Society of the United States where they could find family-to-family support.

CONCLUSIONS

As illustrated both by these four cases and the research literature reviewed, there exist certain predictable psychosocial experiences associated with short stature. While not universal, these experiences (e.g., teasing or juvenilization) are very real and can place a child at risk for problems of psychosocial or educational adaptation. In cases where the short stature is associated with a medical condition, these place additional burdens on the child and family. Consider, for example, TS and children born small for gestational age in which neurocognitive deficits are found; PWS with associated mental retardation and behavioral disturbances; GHD and other pituitary hormone deficits in which spontaneous puberty (or lack thereof), infertility, and neurocognitive deficits may be involved.

Also consider that many children with GH-sufficient short stature remain shorter than same-aged peers even with treatment.[86] Pediatric endocrinologists and other healthcare professionals can be instrumental in countering negative stereotypes attributed to short stature as well as allaying parental concerns which are unfounded and which may be interpreted by the child as evidence that there is something 'wrong' with them. In addition, unfounded beliefs that short stature is strongly associated with negative experiences can result in parents attributing problems of a varied nature to the child's stature even when other factors are more directly responsible.

Additionally, in light of findings from studies using the Silhouette Apperception Test, it may be wise to consider how procedures in clinic (e.g., repeated height measurements), although necessary, potentially reduce the coping benefit of denial. Multiple studies suggest that denial of one's short stature may be an adaptive quality and that veridical perceptions in this context may be maladaptive.[46–48,52] Evidence of 'depressive realism,' the idea that a depressed person's judgments about him- or herself are more accurate than those of non-depressed individuals, is readily observable in experimental studies[96] (also see Ackerman and DeRubeis[97] for a review).

A patient's (and parents') reported satisfaction with rhGH treatment can serve as a powerful incentive for clinicians to continue prescribing the treatment in the face of empirical evidence demonstrating variable and generally modest effects on adult height. As reported in one study, high satisfaction with rhGH therapy can exist in the absence of appreciable benefits in growth.[20] The likelihood that rhGH treatment (for GH-sufficient short stature) is acting as a placebo with regard to subjective QOL outcomes is a distinct possibility.[80]

The possibility of unforeseen risks in treating children with pharmacologic doses of rhGH[98] is particularly salient to parents who report their main concern about rhGH treatment pertains to risks.[99] Clinicians should be aware that parents may evaluate factors for and against rhGH therapy for their children very differently from physicians.[99,100] Factors that parents consider (in order of descending importance)

include risk of long-term side-effects, out-of-pocket costs, the child's attitude toward wanting rhGH therapy, the likelihood of a height increase, the magnitude of the height increase, and the route of rhGH administration.[99] Given the importance of these factors to families, it is prudent to gear interactions toward addressing these priorities. To this list, we would add the importance of making explicit the assumptions that the child and family (and physician) hold concerning the liabilities of short stature and the expected benefits of rhGH therapy.

In conclusion, the preceding analysis suggests that a combined medical and psychosocial clinical management approach may result in substantial benefits to the patient with SS. Barriers to implementing an interdisciplinary approach are daunting however. The impetus for change will come from clinical trials demonstrating that an integrated approach yields enhanced short- and long-term quality of life benefits over either medical or psychological approaches alone.

KEY LEARNING POINTS

- Short stature has increasingly become a target for medical intervention.
- A rationale for rhGH treatment rests on the assumption that short stature constitutes a physical disability and otherwise serves as a significant psychosocial burden for the individual.
- There are predictable negative psychosocial experiences associated with short stature. While not universally encountered, they can place a child at risk for psychosocial or educational adaptation problems.
- The pediatric endocrine clinic is an ideal venue to conduct a comprehensive medical and psychosocial evaluation.
- Short stature can serve as a lightning rod that diverts attention from other stressors that are more directly responsible for adjustment difficulties.
- Components of the psychosocial assessment include: evaluating short stature as a psychosocial stressor, identifying psychological coping response quality (including risk and protective factors), and assessing behavioral and emotional functioning (including the presence of impaired family, social, or educational function).
- Incorporating a psychosocial assessment component within the medical evaluation increases the range of intervention options available to the clinician.
- Clinical trials demonstrating that an integrated medical and psychosocial approach yields enhanced short- and long-term quality of life benefits are badly needed.

REFERENCES

● = Seminal primary article
◆ = Key review paper

● 1 Allen DB, Fost N. hGH for short stature: ethical issues raised by expanded access. *J Pediatr* 2004; **144**: 648–52.

2 Sybert VP, McCauley E. Turner's Syndrome. *New Engl J Med* 2004; **351**: 1227–38.

3 U.S. Food and Drug Administration. FDA Talk Paper: FDA approves Humatrope for short stature. 7-25-2003. http://www.fda.gov/bbs/topics/ANSWERS/2003/ANS01242.html (accessed 1 January 2005).

4 Rovet JF. *The Cognitive and Neuropsychological Characteristics of Females with Turner Syndrome.* Boulder, CO: Westview, 1990.

5 Temple CM, Carney RA, Mullarkey S. Frontal lobe function and executive skills in children with Turner's syndrome. *Dev Neuropsychol* 1996; **12**: 343–63.

6 Hultcrantz M, Sylven L, Borg E. Ear and hearing problems in 44 middle-aged women with Turner's syndrome. *Hearing Res* 1994; **76**: 127–32.

7 Vance ML, Mauras N. Growth hormone therapy in adults and children. *New Engl J Med* 1999; **341**: 1206–16.

8 Carrel AL, Moerchen V, Myers SE, *et al.* Growth hormone improves mobility and body composition in infants and toddlers with Prader–Willi syndrome. *J Pediatr* 2004; **145**: 744–9.

9 Cassidy SB. Prader–Willi syndrome in the new millennium. *Endocrinologist* 2001; **10(Suppl 1)**: 1S–73S.

◆ 10 Meyer-Bahlburg HFL. Short stature: Psychological issues. In: Lifshitz F, ed. *Pediatric Endocrinology.* New York: Marcel Dekker, 1990: 173–96.

11 Rosenfeld RG. Is growth hormone deficiency a viable diagnosis? *J Clin Endocrinol Metab* 1997; **82**: 349–51.

12 Committee on Pediatric Workforce. Scope of practice issues in the delivery of pediatric health care. *Pediatrics* 2003; **111**: 426–35.

13 Drotar D. Consultation and collaboration in pediatric inpatient settings. In: Drotar D, ed. *Consulting with Pediatricians: Psychological Perspectives.* New York: Plenum Press, 1995: 49–63.

14 Clopper R, Mazur T, Ellis AM, Michael P. Height and children's stereotypes. In: Stabler B, Underwood LE, eds. *Growth, Stature, and Adaptation.* Chapel Hill, NC: University of North Carolina at Chapel Hill, 1994: 7–18.

15 Jackson LA, Ervin KS. Height stereotypes of women and men: The liabilities of shortness for both sexes. *J Soc Psychol* 1992; **132**: 433–45.

16 Martel LF, Biller H. *Stature and Stigma: the Biopsychosocial Development of Short Males.* Lexington, MA: Lexington Books, 1987.

17 Gacsaly SA, Borges CA. The male physique and behavioral expectancies. *J Psychol* 1979; **101**: 97–102.

18 Arkoff A, Weaver HB. Body image and body dissatisfaction in Japanese-Americans. *J Soc Psychol* 1966; **68**: 323–30.

● 19 Voss LD, Mulligan J. Bullying in school: are short pupils at risk? Questionnaire study in a cohort. *BMJ* 2000; **320**: 612–3.

● 20 Rekers-Momberg LT, Busschbach JJ, Massa GG, *et al.* Quality of life of young adults with idiopathic short stature: effect of growth hormone treatment. *Acta Paediatr* 1998; **87**: 865–70.

21 Hensley WE, Angoli M. Message valence, familiarity, sex, and personality effects on the perceptual distortion of height. *J Psychol* 1981; **104**: 149–56.

22 Underwood LE. The social cost of being short: Societal perceptions and biases. *Acta Paediatr Suppl* 1991; **377**: 3–8.

23 Eisenberg N, Roth K, Bryniarski KA, Murray E. Sex differences in the relationship of height to children's actual and attributed social and cognitive competencies. *Sex Roles* 1984; **11**: 719–34.

24 Hartnett JJ, Bailey KG, Hartley CS. Body height, position, and sex as determinants of personal space. *J Psychol* 1974; **87**: 129–36.

25 Bailey KG, Caffrey JV, Hartnett JJ. Body size as implied threat: Effects on personal space and person perception. *Percept Mot Skills* 1976; **43**: 223–30.

26 Beigel HG. Body height in mate selection. *J Soc Psychol* 1954; **39**: 257–68.

27 Graziano W, Brothen T, Berscheid E. Height and attraction: Do men and women see eye-to-eye? *J Pers* 1978; **46**: 128–45.

28 Hensley WE. Height as a basis for interpersonal attraction. *Adolescence* 1994; **29**: 469–74.

29 Pierce CA. Body height and romantic attraction: A meta-analytic test of the male-taller norm. *Soc Behav Personal* 1996; **24**: 143–50.

30 Brackbill Y, Nevill DD. Parental expectations of achievement as affected by children's height. *Merrill–Palmer Q* 1981; **27**: 429–41.

31 Wilson PR. Perceptual distortion of height as a function of ascribed academic status. *J Soc Psychol* 1968; **74**: 97–102.

32 Lechelt EC. Occupational affiliation and ratings of physical height and personal esteem. *Psychol Rep* 1975; **36**: 943–6.

◆ 33 Sandberg DE. Short stature: Intellectual and behavioral aspects. In: Lifshitz F, ed. *Pediatric Endocrinology*, 3rd edn. New York, NY: Marcel Dekker, 1996: 149–62.

● 34 Sandberg DE, Michael P. Psychosocial stresses related to short stature: does their presence imply psychiatric dysfunction? In: Drotar D, ed. *Assessing Pediatric Health-Related Quality of Life and Functional Status: Implications for Research.* Mahwah, NJ: Lawrence Erlbaum Associates, 1998: 287–312.

● 35 Zimet GD, Cutler M, Litvene M, *et al.* Psychological adjustment of children evaluated for short stature: a preliminary report. *J Dev Behav Pediatr* 1995; **16**: 264–70.

36 Gould MS, Wunsch-Hitzig R, Dohrenwend B. Estimating the prevalence of childhood psychopathology. A critical review. *J Am Acad Child Psychiatry* 1981; **20**: 462–76.

37 Shaffer D, Fisher P, Dulcan MK, *et al.* The NIMH Diagnostic Interview Schedule for Children Version 2.3

(DISC-2.3): description, acceptability, prevalence rates, and performance in the MECA Study. Methods for the Epidemiology of Child and Adolescent Mental Disorders Study. *J Am Acad Child Adolesc Psychiatry* 1996; **35**: 865–77.

- 38 Theunissen NC, Kamp GA, Koopman HM, *et al.* Quality of life and self-esteem in children treated for idiopathic short stature. *J Pediatr* 2002; **140**: 507–15.

- 39 Sandberg DE, Brook AE, Campos SP. Short stature: a psychosocial burden requiring growth hormone therapy? *Pediatrics* 1994; **94**: 832–40.

- 40 Stabler B, Clopper RR, Siegel PT, *et al.* Academic achievement and psychological adjustment in short children. The National Cooperative Growth Study. *J Dev Behav Pediatr* 1994; **15**: 1–6.

- 41 Steinhausen HC, Dorr HG, Kannenberg R, Malin Z. The behavior profile of children and adolescents with short stature. *J Dev Behav Pediatr* 2000; **21**: 423–8.

- 42 Sandberg DE, Kranzler J, Bukowski WM, Rosenbloom AL. Psychosocial aspects of short stature and growth hormone therapy. *J Pediatr* 1999; **135**: 133–4.

- 43 Gilmour J, Skuse D. Short stature – the role of intelligence in psychosocial adjustment. *Arch Dis Child* 1996; **75**: 25–31.

44 Davis H, Gergen PJ. Self-described weight status of Mexican–American adolescents. *J Adolesc Health* 1994; **15**: 407–9.

45 Dowdney L, Woodward L, Pickles A, Skuse D. The Body Image Perception and Attitude Scale for children: Reliability in growth retarded and community comparison subjects. *Int J Methods Psychiatr Res* 1995; **5**: 29–40.

46 Erling A, Wiklund I, Albertsson-Wikland K. Prepubertal children with short stature have a different perception of their well-being and stature than their parents. *Qual Life Res* 1994; **3**: 425–9.

47 Grew RS, Stabler B, Williams RW, Underwood LE. Facilitating patient understanding in the treatment of growth delay. *Clin Pediatr* 1983; **22**: 685–90.

- 48 Hunt L, Hazen RA, Sandberg DE. Perceived versus measured height. Which is the stronger predictor of psychosocial functioning? *Horm Res* 2000; **53**: 129–38.

49 Prieto AG, Robbins MC. Perceptions of height and self-esteem. *Percept Motor Skills* 1975; **40**: 395–8.

- 50 Ross JL, Sandberg DE, Rose SR, *et al.* Psychological adaptation in children with idiopathic short stature treated with growth hormone or placebo. *J Clin Endocrinol Metab* 2004; **89**: 4873–8.

51 Tienboon P, Wahlqvist ML, Rutishauser IH. Self-reported weight and height in adolescents and their parents. *J Adolesc Health* 1992; **13**: 528–32.

52 Stabler B, Whitt JK, Moreault DM, *et al.* Social judgments by children of short stature. *Psychol Rep* 1980; **46**: 743–6.

53 Roberts JV, Herman CP. The psychology of height: an empirical review. In: Herman PC, Zanna MP, Higgins ET, eds. *Physical Appearance, Stigma, and Social Behavior: The Ontario Symposium.* Hillsdale, NJ: Lawrence Erlbaum Associates, 1986: 113–40.

- 54 Voss LD, Mulligan J. The short 'normal' child in school: self-esteem, behavior and attainment before puberty (The Wessex Growth Study). In: Stabler B, Underwood LE, eds. *Growth, Stature and Adaptation.* Chapel Hill, NC: University of North Carolina at Chapel Hill Press, 1994: 47–64.

- 55 Downie AB, Mulligan J, Stratford RJ, *et al.* Are short normal children at a disadvantage? The Wessex growth study. *BMJ* 1997; **314**: 97–100.

56 Voss LD. Short but normal. *Arch Dis Child* 1999; **81**: 370–1.

- 57 Ulph F, Betts P, Mulligan J, Stratford RJ. Personality functioning: the influence of stature. *Arch Dis Child* 2004; **89**: 17–21.

- 58 Voss LD, Walker J, Lunt H, *et al.* The Wessex Growth Study: first report. *Acta Paediatr Scand Suppl* 1989; **349**: 65–72.

- ◆ 59 Sandberg DE. Should short children who are not deficient in growth hormone be treated? *West J Med* 2000; **172**: 186–9.

60 Wilson DM, Hammer LD, Duncan PM, *et al.* Growth and intellectual development. *Pediatrics* 1986; **78**: 646–50.

61 Crowne EC, Shalet SM, Wallace WH, *et al.* Final height in boys with untreated constitutional delay in growth and puberty. *Arch Dis Child* 1990; **65**: 1109–12.

- 62 Sandberg DE, Bukowski WM, Fung CM, Noll RB. Height and social adjustment: Are extremes a cause for concern and action? *Pediatrics* 2004; **114**: 744–50.

- 63 Tuvemo T, Jonsson B, Persson I. Intellectual and physical performance and morbidity in relation to height in a cohort of 18-year-old Swedish conscripts. *Horm Res* 1999; **52**: 186–91.

64 Harper B. Beauty, stature and the labour market: A British cohort study. *Oxf Bull Econ Stat* 2000; **62**: 771–800.

65 Fu H, Goldman N. Incorporating health into models of marriage choice: Demographic and sociological perspectives. *J Marriage Fam* 1996; **58**: 740–58.

66 Fu H, Goldman N. The association between health-related behaviours and the risk of divorce in the USA. *J Biosoc Sci* 2000; **32**: 63–88.

- 67 Vågerö D, Modin B. Prenatal growth, subsequent marital status, and mortality: longitudinal study. *BMJ* 2002; **324**: 398.

- 68 Ekwo E, Gosselink C, Roizen N, Brazdziunas D. The effect of height on family income. *Am J Hum Biol* 1991; **3**: 181–8.

69 Gunderson EK. Body size, self-evaluation, and military effectiveness. *J Pers Soc Psychol* 1965; **2**: 902–6.

70 Lindeman M, Sundvik L. Impact of height on assessments of Finnish female job applicants' managerial abilities. *J Soc Psychol* 1994; **134**: 169–74.

- 71 Schumacher A. On the significance of stature in human society. *J Hum Evol* 1982; **11**: 697–701.

- 72 Sargent JD, Blanchflower DG. Obesity and stature in adolescence and earnings in young adulthood. Analysis of a British birth cohort. *Arch Pediatr Adolesc Med* 1994; **148**: 681–7.

73 Persico N, Postlewaite RJ, Silverman D. The effect of adolescent experience on labor market outcomes: The case of height. *J Polit Econ* 2004; **112**: 1019–53.

● 74 Judge TA, Cable DM. The effect of physical height on workplace success and income: preliminary test of a theoretical model. *J Appl Psychol* 2004; **89**: 428–41.

75 Keltner D, Capps L, Kring AM, *et al.* Just teasing: a conceptual analysis and empirical review. *Psychol Bull* 2001; **127**: 229–48.

76 Warm TR. The role of teasing in development and vice versa. *J Dev Behav Pediatr* 1997; **18**: 97–101.

● 77 Downie AB, Mulligan J, McCaughey ES, *et al.* Psychological response to growth hormone treatment in short normal children. *Arch Dis Child* 1996; **75**: 32–5.

● 78 Cuttler L, Silvers JB, Singh J, *et al.* Short stature and growth hormone therapy. A national study of physician recommendation patterns. *JAMA* 1996; **276**: 531–7.

79 Skuse DH, James RS, Bishop DV, *et al.* Evidence from Turner's syndrome of an imprinted X-linked locus affecting cognitive function. *Nature* 1997; **387**: 705–8.

80 Hrobjartsson A, Gotzsche PC. Is the placebo powerless? An analysis of clinical trials comparing placebo with no treatment. *New Engl J Med* 2001; **344**: 1594–602.

81 Harter S. *Manual for the Self-perception Profile for Children*. Denver, CO: University of Denver, 1985.

82 Harter S. *Manual for the Self-perception Profile for Adolescents*. Denver, CO: University of Denver, 1988.

83 Achenbach T. *Manual for the Child Behavior Checklist/4-18 and 1991 Profile*. Burlington, VT: University of Vermont Department of Psychiatry, 1991.

● 84 Lantos J, Siegler M, Cuttler L. Ethical issues in growth hormone therapy. *JAMA* 1989; **261**: 1020–4.

● 85 Noeker M, Haverkamp F. Adjustment in conditions with short stature: a conceptual framework. *J Pediatr Endocrinol Metab* 2000; **13**: 1585–94.

● 86 Finkelstein BS, Imperiale TF, Speroff T, *et al.* Effect of growth hormone therapy on height in children with idiopathic short stature: a meta-analysis. *Arch Pediatr Adolesc Med* 2002; **156**: 230–40.

87 Achenbach T. *Manual for the Youth Self Report and 1991 Profile*. Burlington, VT: University of Vermont, Department of Psychiatry, 1991.

88 Sandberg DE. *Educational Background Questionnaire*. Unpublished questionnaire, 1991.

89 Rieser P, Underwood LE. *Growing children: A parent's guide*. 4th So. San Francisco, CA: Genentech, Inc., 2002.

90 Eli Lilly and Co. *Ready, Set, Grow*. Indianapolis, IN: Eli Lilly and Co., 2002.

◆ 91 Rieser PA, Meyer-Bahlburg HFL. *Short & OK*. Falls Church, VA: Human Growth Foundation, 1991.

92 Eminson DM, Powell RP, Hollis S. Cognitive behavioral interventions with short statured boys: a pilot study. In: Stabler B, Underwood LE, eds. *Growth, Stature, and Adaptation*. Chapel Hill, NC: The University of North Carolina at Chapel Hill, 1994: 135–50.

93 Stein MT, Frasier SD, Stabler B. Parent requests growth hormone for child with idiopathic short stature. *Pediatrics* 2004; **114**: 1478–82.

94 Mrug S, Hoza B, Gerdes AC. Children with attention-deficit/hyperactivity disorder: peer relationships and peer-oriented interventions. *New Direct Child Adolesc Dev* 2001; **91**: 51–77.

95 Rovet JF. The psychoeducational characteristics of children with Turner syndrome. *J Learn Disab* 1993; **26**: 333–41.

96 Alloy LB, Abramson LY. Judgment of contingency in depressed and nondepressed students: Sadder but wiser? *J Exp Psychol: Gen* 1979; **108**: 441–85.

97 Ackermann R, DeRubeis RJ. Is depressive realism real? *Clin Psychol Rev* 1991; **11**: 565–84.

98 Slyper A. The safety and effectiveness of human growth hormone using pharmacological dosing. *Med Hypotheses* 1995; **45**: 523–8.

● 99 Finkelstein BS, Singh J, Silvers JB, *et al.* Patient attitudes and preferences regarding treatment: GH therapy for childhood short stature. *Horm Res* 1999; **51(Suppl 1)**: 67–72.

● 100 Singh J, Cuttler L, Shin M, *et al.* Medical decision-making and the patient: understanding preference patterns for growth hormone therapy using conjoint analysis. *Med Care* 1998; **36(Suppl 8)**: AS31–AS45.

PART 3

CHRONIC PEDIATRIC DISORDERS AND MANAGEMENT OF THE ASSOCIATED GROWTH DISTURBANCE

17

Short stature syndromes

GEERT R MORTIER, JOHN M GRAHAM JR, DAVID L RIMOIN

INTRODUCTION

Height is a measurable physiological quantity that approximates a Gaussian distribution in the normal population. This wide range of human stature is present not only within but also between various populations. The height of an individual is the culmination of an interaction between many genes (the genotype) and various environmental factors such as nutritional status and hormonal milieu. 'Short stature' is therefore a relative term and related to a person's ethnic, familial and nutritional background. The cut-off demarcating short stature has been variously defined as the lowest 5%,[1] 3%[2] or even 0.4%[3] values on growth curves for a clearly defined population at a given time in history. Traditionally, short stature is defined as a height that lies 2 standard deviations below the mean for age compared with sex-specific and ethnic-matched standards based on an appropriate healthy population. Allowances must be made for parental height, nutritional status, and sexual maturity before the diagnosis of pathologic short stature can be made. Familial short stature and constitutional growth delay are considered physiological variants of normal stature. In this chapter we will discuss the most common genetic conditions with short stature as a major feature.

DIAGNOSTIC WORK-UP OF SHORT STATURE

The presence of numerous disorders with short stature makes a specific diagnosis challenging. Nevertheless, a correct diagnosis is important because each condition has a different prognosis and may have preventable complications or predictable responses to treatments. In the case of a genetic condition, only a specific diagnosis will allow accurate genetic counseling.

The diagnostic work-up starts with a careful history and analysis of the pedigree. Knowledge of birth length and postnatal growth data are essential to determine whether the growth deficiency was of prenatal or postnatal onset. The possibility of a congenital infection or other teratogenic exposure during pregnancy should be solicited in cases of fetal growth deficiency (Tables 17.1 and 17.2). Fetal alcohol syndrome is the most frequent teratogenic disorder presenting with intrauterine growth deficiency that persists postnatally with microcephaly and distinctive facial features (thin smooth upper lip with short palpebral fissures). The history should also focus on the postnatal course with special attention to environmental insults, congenital anomalies, the psychomotor development and musculoskeletal complaints. Proportionate short stature in association with mental retardation and other congenital anomalies may suggest a recognizable syndrome, teratogenic disorder or chromosomal abnormality, whereas a patient with disproportionate short stature with or without complaints of joint pain and waddling gait may suggest a chondrodysplasia. During family history, the stature of at least first degree relatives should be noted and the possibility of a heritable condition considered when other family members are short-statured. The possibility of consanguinity should also be ascertained.

The first step in the clinical evaluation is to measure height, weight and head circumference of the patient. It is important to assess whether the body habitus is proportionate or disproportionate. This is usually apparent on casual examination but in more subtle conditions may require measurement of sitting height, upper/lower segment ratio and arm span. Children with disproportionate

Table 17.1 Etiology of fetal growth restriction

Factors that influence fetal growth	Conditions associated with fetal growth restriction
Maternal factors – maternal size – maternal nutritional status – maternal disease – maternal infections – maternal exposure	– women who were born 'small for gestational age' – women with unusual dietary restrictions – chronic diseases: autoimmune, kidney, lungs, heart – AIDS, CMV, rubella – drugs of abuse: alcohol, tobacco, cocaine (Table 17.2) – medications: anticonvulsants, anticoagulants, folic acid antagonists (Table 17.2) – other teratogenic exposures
Uteroplacental factors – uterine size – uterine anomalies – uteroplacental circulation – multiple fetuses – confined placental mosaicism	– small uterus – septate uterus – decidual vasculopathy causing maternal hypertension – twin pregnancies – placental tissue trisomic for chromosome 16
Fetal factors – chromosomal aberrations – single gene defects	– see Table 17.3 – see the section 'Monogenic disorders with short stature'

Table 17.2 Teratogenic (non-genetic) syndromes with short stature

Teratogenic syndrome	Key features
Alcohol embryopathy	Irritability in infancy; hyperactivity in childhood; mild to moderate mental retardation; microcephaly; short palpebral fissures; short nose; thin smooth upper lip
Hydantoin embryopathy	Learning disabilities, cleft lip/palate; small nose; distal phalangeal (and nail) hypoplasia
Valproate embryopathy	Mental retardation; small nose; metopic ridge; distal phalangeal (and nail) hypoplasia; neural tube defects; genital anomalies
Warfarin embryopathy	Mental retardation (30%); hypoplastic nose; choanal stenosis; epiphyseal stippling; brachydactyly
Folate antagonist (aminopterin, methotrexate) embryopathy	Normal to low IQ; craniosynostosis; hypertelorism; micrognathia; brachy- and syndactyly; neural tube defects

short stature usually have a skeletal dysplasia, while those with proportionate short stature may have a more generalized disorder (i.e., endocrine disorder, malformation syndrome, chronic disease with malnutrition or malabsorption, psychosocial deprivation). Physical examination should also include a careful evaluation of all body parts, with special attention to dysmorphic features and the presence of minor and major congenital anomalies.

SHORT STATURE SYNDROMES

Many genetic conditions and multiple congenital anomaly syndromes present with short stature as a major manifestation of the disorder.[4] With respect to etiology, they can be divided into chromosomal disorders, monogenic disorders (due to a single gene defect) and syndromes of unknown etiology. In the last decade, the genetic defect has been unraveled for an increasing number of monogenic syndromes.

CHROMOSOMAL DISORDERS WITH SHORT STATURE

Abnormalities of chromosomes may be either numerical or structural. Aneuploidy refers to an abnormal chromosome number due to an extra or missing chromosome. Most aneuploidies for the autosomes will result in a miscarriage early on in pregnancy. There are only a few exceptions: trisomy 21 (Down syndrome), trisomy 13 (Patau syndrome) and trisomy 18 (Edwards syndrome) can give rise to a liveborn baby, usually with multiple congenital anomalies. Full monosomy for an autosome in all somatic cells is not compatible with life (and will therefore also result in early miscarriages).

Numerical chromosome aberrations

DOWN SYNDROME

Down syndrome or trisomy 21, is by far the most common and best known of the chromosome disorders and is the single most common genetic cause of moderate mental retardation.[5] At birth, neonates with Down syndrome show mild growth retardation with a slightly smaller placenta.[6] Growth velocity in infancy is near-normal, but after the first year it falls, so that by 3 years of age, height approaches −3 SD. Final adult height average is 151 cm for males and 141 cm for females. Growth charts for children with Down syndrome are available.[7,8]

EDWARDS SYNDROME AND PATAU SYNDROME

Intrauterine growth retardation is common in Edwards syndrome (trisomy 18) and Patau syndrome (trisomy 13), although normal growth parameters at birth can be observed.[9] In both conditions multiple congenital anomalies, including congenital heart disease, renal anomalies and structural defects of the brain and the eye, are frequently present. Cleft lip/palate (especially median cleft lip), holoprosencephaly, scalp defects and polydactyly are the more distinguishing features of trisomy 13. Most infants die within months after birth. In survivors, profound physical and mental retardation is inevitable.[10]

TURNER SYNDROME

Turner syndrome, or monosomy X, is a common chromosomal abnormality associated with short stature. Affected females have gonadal dysgenesis in association with variable physical anomalies including webbed neck, low posterior hairline, broad chest with widely spaced nipples, short (fourth) metacarpals and dysplastic nails. There is an increased frequency of renal and cardiovascular anomalies (especially coarctation of the aorta).[11] In full-term infants with Turner syndrome, the mean birth weight is between the 25th and 50th centiles for normal females and the mean birth length is at the 5th centile for the normal female population.[12] Children are usually referred for short stature around the age of 5–10 years, when growth failure becomes apparent, or around pubertal age because of lack of growth spurt and delayed puberty. Growth hormone treatment has become standard in this group of patients. Gain in final adult height is variable (from no gain to as much as 9.7 cm) and seems to depend on age at start, duration of therapy, and dosage of recombinant human growth hormone.[12]

Structural chromosome aberrations

Various structural anomalies of the chromosomes have been described over the years.[13] Many of them are rare and patient-unique while others are more common and known as particular syndromes. Short stature and mental retardation are frequently observed in patients with unbalanced structural autosomal aberrations. This suggests that genes controlling growth and brain function are numerous and dispersed throughout the entire human genome. Extremely short stature, as is found in many monogenic skeletal dysplasias, is not characteristic for chromosome aberrations.

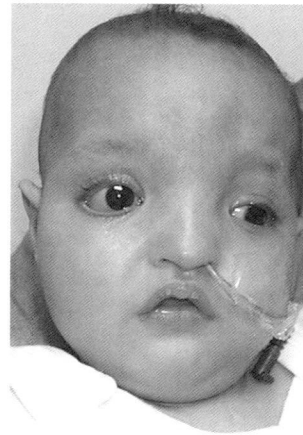

Figure 17.1 Infant with Wolf–Hirschhorn syndrome. Note the high forehead, prominent glabella, broad nasal root and hypertelorism (Greek helmet). Please see Plate 2.

If extreme dwarfism is found in a patient with a chromosome abnormality, other causes such as growth hormone deficiency should be considered.[13] We will discuss here the most frequent structurally abnormal chromosome conditions with short stature as an important feature.

WOLF–HIRSCHHORN SYNDROME

Wolf–Hirschhorn syndrome is caused by a deletion on the distal part of the short arm of chromosome 4. The most common breakpoint is probably 4p15.[13] The critical region for development of this disorder is located within chromosome band 4p16.3.[14] The syndrome is characterized by a marked growth retardation of prenatal onset and usually severe mental retardation. Mean weight, length, and head circumference of full-term newborns are 2000 g, 44.4 cm and 29 cm, respectively.[13] Patients with this deletion syndrome have a distinctive face (Fig. 17.1). The high forehead with prominent glabella, hypertelorism and broad nose resembles a Greek helmet. Congenital malformations are very common and may be found in almost every organ, particularly in the brain, heart, eye and kidney.[15,16] As with most microdeletion syndromes, the severity of the phenotype correlates to some extent with the size of the microdeletion.[17]

CRI-DU-CHAT SYNDROME

Partial deletion of the short arm of chromosome 5 results in the cri-du-chat syndrome. The name of this syndrome refers to the distinctive cry of affected infants, which at resembles the mewing of a cat. The critical region for the phenotype is located on band 5p15, a region containing the telomerase reverse transcriptase gene.[18] Microcephaly with a round face, hypotonia and congenital heart defects are common features of the syndrome.[4] Mental retardation is usually severe.[19] Low birth weight and slow growth are frequently observed in patients with cri-du-chat syndrome. The microcephaly is more obvious than the short stature.[20]

Table 17.3 Most common chromosomal disorders with short stature

Disorder	Chromosomal defect	Key clinical features
Down syndrome	Trisomy 21 (95%) Robertsonian translocation (5%)	Hypotonia, excess skin on back of neck, flat facial profile, upslanted palpebral fissures, small ears, single palmar crease, endocardial cushion defects
Patau syndrome	Trisomy 13 (80%) Robertsonian translocation (20%)	Holoprosencephaly, scalp defects, cleft lip/palate, polydactyly
Edwards syndrome	Trisomy 18 (80%) Translocation (20%)	Short sternum, clenched fingers, rocker-bottom feet, congenital heart disease
Turner syndrome	Monosomy X or 45,X (50%) Mosaicism or structural defects of the X chromosome (50%)	Gonadal dysgenesis, coarctation of the aorta, webbed neck, short fourth metacarpal
Wolf–Hirschhorn syndrome	Del (4) (pter → p15)	Greek helmet facies, iris coloboma, cleft lip/palate, sacral dimple, hypospadias
Cri-du-chat syndrome	Del (5) (pter → p15)	Mewing cry, microcephaly, heart defect
WAGR syndrome	Del (11p13)	Wilms' tumor, aniridia, ambiguous genitalia, ptosis
Prader–Willi syndrome	Del (15) (q11 → q13)pat	Neonatal hypotonia, small genitalia, obesity, hypogonadism, small hands/feet,
Del (13q) syndrome	Del (13) (q13 → q31)	Microcephaly, retinoblastoma, genital anomalies, absent thumbs
Del (18p) syndrome	Del (18) (pter → p11.2 to q11)	Holoprosencephaly, microcephaly, large ears, webbed neck
Del (18q) syndrome	Del (18) (q21 → qter)	Stenotic ear canals, IgA deficiency, sensorineural hearing loss, hypospadias, heart defects

WAGR SYNDROME

The WAGR syndrome refers to the association of Wilms' tumor, aniridia, genito-urinary malformations and mental retardation. It is due to an interstitial deletion on the short arm of chromosome 11 (band 11p13), involving the genes for aniridia (PAX6) and Wilms' tumor (WT1). This contiguous gene deletion syndrome is characterized by mild prenatal and more significant postnatal growth retardation in about 50% of the affected children.[4,13] Microcephaly usually becomes apparent after birth. Obesity has been reported in several cases.[21]

PRADER–WILLI SYNDROME

Prader–Willi syndrome can be the result of a small interstitial deletion on the paternally derived chromosome 15 (band 15q11.2). Less common causes for this syndrome are maternal uniparental disomy for chromosome 15, abnormalities of imprinting and structural rearrangements involving the region 15q11q13 on chromosome 15.[22] This syndrome demonstrates the relevance of genetic imprinting in the pathogenesis of human disease. Prader–Willi syndrome is characterized by severe muscular hypotonia and feeding problems in infancy, hyperphagia resulting in obesity in early childhood, hypogonadism and short stature. Patients have mild to moderate mental retardation and characteristic facial features including almond shaped eyes, narrow bitemporal diameter, upslanting palpebral fissures and strabismus. Approximately 90–95% of patients with Prader–Willi syndrome have short stature, usually related to growth hormone deficiency.[23] Growth hormone stimulation testing has become standard for patients with Prader–Willi syndrome. Recent studies have shown that growth hormone therapy improves linear growth, final height, physical strength and agility in Prader–Willi syndrome patients.[24] However, sudden deaths in markedly obese, growth hormone-treated patients, suggest a need for further sleep apnea studies should also be considered for such patients.[25, 26]

LESS COMMON CHROMOSOMAL DELETIONS SYNDROMES

Growth retardation is frequently observed in other less common chromosomal deletion syndromes, including the del(13q) syndrome (prenatal onset), the del(18p) syndrome (postnatal onset – growth hormone deficiency reported) and the del(18q) syndrome (pre- and postnatal onset – growth hormone deficiency reported).[4] Key clinical findings of these syndromes are listed in Table 17.3.

MONOGENIC DISORDERS WITH SHORT STATURE

Monogenic disorders are defined as genetic conditions that can be caused by a mutation in a single gene. The identification of genetic defects for this group of disorders has been progressing at a rapid rate over the past decade. These new insights have shown that a variety of mutations in one gene can result in a broad phenotypic spectrum, sometimes including different clinical entities, that were previously defined as separate conditions (allelic heterogeneity). On the other hand, it also has become clear that one disorder can be caused by mutations in different genes (locus heterogeneity), which complicates the molecular genetic analysis for confirmation of the diagnosis.

Similar to the group of chromosomal disorders, many monogenic conditions are characterized by short stature, either of prenatal or postnatal onset.[4] We will focus on the most frequent disorders. A list of all monogenic conditions with links to various databases can be found on the world wide web (Online Mendelian Inheritance In Man – URL: http://www.ncbi.nlm.nih.gov/entrez/query.fcgi?db= OMIM).

Monogenic syndromes with disproportionate short stature

Children with disproportionate short stature usually have a skeletal dysplasia. Depending on which parts of the skeleton are mainly affected, chondrodysplasias will either result in short-limb dwarfism or short-trunk dwarfism.[27] Achondroplasia, pseudoachondroplasia, cartilage hair hypoplasia and Schmid metaphyseal dysplasia represent the most common forms of short-limb dwarfism. The type I collagenopathies (various forms of osteogenesis imperfecta) and type II collagenopathies (in particular, spondyloepiphyseal dysplasia congenita and Kniest dysplasia) can be considered as the most frequent causes of short-trunk dwarfism. It should be emphasized that patients with osteogenesis imperfecta can also have short limbs or even normal body proportions. These entities will not be discussed here in detail since they are the subject of another chapter in this book (Chapter 19). We will discuss only a few short stature syndromes with brachydactyly as the major manifestation of skeletal involvement.

AARSKOG SYNDROME

Aarskog syndrome, or faciogenital dysplasia, is probably a genetically heterogeneous condition characterized by a distinct craniofacial dysmorphism, brachydactyly, and urogenital abnormalities. It was originally considered to represent an X-linked condition but subsequently some families with an autosomal dominant inheritance were reported.[28,29] The gene (*FGD1*) responsible for the X-linked form has been

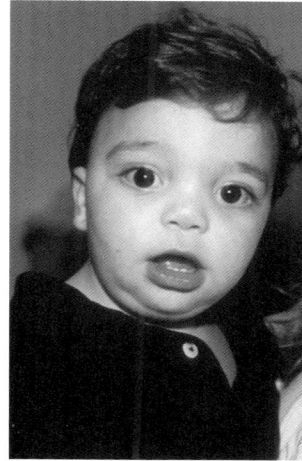

Figure 17.2 Boy with Aarskog syndrome. Typical facial features include hypertelorism, short nose with anteverted nares and long philtrum. Please see Plate 3.

identified.[30] The *FGD1* gene encodes a guanine nucleotide exchange factor for members of the Rho/Rac family of small GTP-binding proteins. The craniofacial phenotype of affected patients (usually boys) is characterized by hypertelorism, down-slanting palpebral fissures, small nose with anteverted nares and long philtrum (Fig. 17.2). Ptosis of the upper eyelids is observed in about 50% of the cases.[31] Frequent urogenital anomalies include cryptorchidism, shawl or overriding scrotum and inguinal herniae. The short stature in Aarskog syndrome is mild but disproportionate, mainly due to acromelic shortening of the limbs. The hands are short and broad with brachydactyly, interdigital webbing and laxity of finger joints. Patients usually have normal intelligence. Mutations in *FGD1* have been established in only a minority of patients.[32] This may be explained by the genetic heterogeneity of the disorder and the overlapping clinical features with other syndromes, in particular Noonan syndrome and Robinow syndrome.

ROBINOW SYNDROME

Brachydactyly in association with hypertelorism is also found in Robinow syndrome. Both autosomal recessive and autosomal dominant inheritance have been described in this condition. The gene (*ROR2*) for the autosomal recessive form has been identified.[33,34] *ROR2* codes for a receptor tyrosine kinase. Children with Robinow syndrome have a distinct face, sometimes compared with a fetal face because of the laterally displaced eyes (hypertelorism) and short upturned nose. Other characteristic orofacial features include broad forehead, prominent eyes (due to deficiency of the lower eyelid), midfacial hypoplasia, tented upper lip with tethering in the center (sometimes exposing the incisors and upper gum), ankyloglossia, crowded teeth and gum hypertrophy.[35] Genital abnormalities may be noted after birth. They can range from small penis or clitoris and labia minora to ambiguous genitalia. Sometimes these genital anomalies are associated with malformations of the renal tract. Around 15% of the published cases are reported with a congenital heart defect, most frequently pulmonary stenosis or atresia.[35] Short stature is most pronounced in the autosomal recessive forms. It is disproportionate because of acromesomelic involvement of the limbs (especially short forearms) and vertebral segmentation defects of the spine. Brachydactyly with shortening of the distal phalanges is frequently observed. Radiographs may show symphalangism, carpal fusion and splitting of the distal phalanges. The segmentation defects of vertebrae and ribs may resemble those found in spondylothoracic and spondylocostal dysostosis. Intelligence is usually normal but developmental delay occurs in 10–15% of cases.[35]

ALBRIGHT HEREDITARY OSTEODYSTROPHY

Brachydactyly in association with short stature is also a feature of Albright hereditary osteodystrophy (AHO). AHO is an autosomal dominant disorder characterized by one or more of the following clinical features: short stature, brachydactyly, subcutaneous calcifications, obesity and mental retardation.[4] The condition is caused by loss-of-function mutations in the gene (GNAS1) coding for the α-subunit of the G_s protein.[36] G proteins are heterotrimeric guanine nucleotide-binding proteins that transmit signals from cell-surface receptors (G protein-coupled receptors) to effectors that generate intracellular signals altering cell function (G protein-coupled signal transduction).[37] The severity of the AHO phenotype is variable and some patients with GNAS1 mutations have few or no symptoms.[38] Interestingly, patients who inherited the GNAS1 mutation from their mother also develop resistance to various hormones (parathyroid hormone [PTH], thyroid stimulating hormone [TSH], luteinizing hormone [LH], and follicle stimulating hormone [FSH]), a condition referred to as pseudohypoparathyroidism type 1a. In contrast, patients who inherit the same mutation from their father develop only AHO, a condition referred to as pseudopseudohypoparathyroidism. This observation is explained by a tissue-specific (paternal) imprinting of the GNAS1 gene. Although the gene is biallelically expressed in most tissues (including red blood cells), it is expressed primarily from the maternal allele in various hormonal target tissues such as the renal proximal tubule, thyroid and pituitary gland.[39] Therefore, loss-of-function mutations in the active maternal allele will not only result in AHO but also in resistance to various hormones including PTH, whereas mutations in the paternal allele will only cause AHO without affecting hormone signaling. In pseudohypoparathyroidism type 1b, only resistance to PTH (and mild resistance to TSH in some cases) is present without signs of AHO. This is due to an imprinting defect of the GNAS1 gene with silencing of the maternal allele, affecting mainly the renal proximal tubules.[40] Short stature in AHO is usually of postnatal onset.[41] Obesity is present in about 65% of adolescents but usually less pronounced in cases of pseudopseudohypoparathyroidism.[41] The face

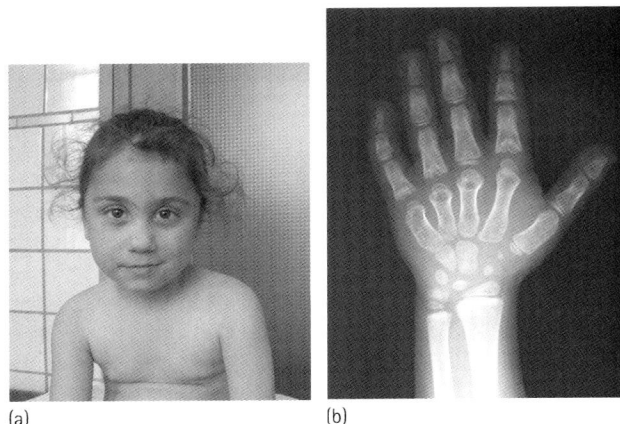

(a)   (b)

Figure 17.3 (a) Girl with Albright hereditary osteodystrophy due to a mutation in the GNAS1 gene. (b) Hand radiograph shows shortening of the metacarpals (especially III to V) and phalanges with cone-shaped epiphyses. Note the subcutaneous calcification in the carpal region below the distal ulnar epiphysis. Please see Plate 4.

in AHO is characteristically round with full cheeks, low nasal bridge and mild hypertelorism. Short fourth and fifth metacarpals are a useful diagnostic sign (absent knuckles) that becomes apparent when the patient makes a fist. The distal phalanx of the thumb is often small, manifested by a short and broad nail. Subcutaneous calcifications can be found in the scalp and the extremities, in particular the periarticular regions of hands and feet (Fig. 17.3). Short fourth and fifth metacarpals in association with mental retardation, can also be found in patients with a terminal deletion on the long arm of chromosome 2 (2q37). Therefore, chromosome studies (fluorescence in situ hybridizaiton [FISH] analysis) should be performed in patients with an AHO-like phenotype and normal activity of the α-subunit of the G_s protein in red blood cells and/or normal results after GNAS1 mutation screening.[42] Type E brachydactyly represents the mildest end of this clinical spectrum with short fourth and fifth metacarpals and mild short stature. This autosomal dominant condition is one of the most common causes of mild short stature that segregates within families.

ACRODYSOSTOSIS

Acrodysostosis should not be confused with AHO. Both conditions show varying degrees of metacarpal and phalangeal shortening with cone-shaped epiphyses on hand radiographs. However, endocrine abnormalities are not found in acrodysostosis. In addition, normal activity of the α-subunit of the G_s protein has been documented in several cases.[43,44] Acrodysostosis has in common with AHO the short stature, brachydactyly and mental retardation but differs from it by the presence of nasal hypoplasia, midface deficiency and varying degrees of hearing loss. In addition, spinal stenosis seems to be common in acrodysostosis but not in AHO.[44]

Monogenic syndromes with proportionate short stature of prenatal onset

These monogenic disorders present at birth with proportionate short stature as a result of a more generalized growth failure of prenatal onset. They should be differentiated from other causes of fetal growth restriction (Table 17.1).

DISORDERS WITH INCREASED CANCER RISK

Growth retardation and an increased risk for cancer are common features of the so-called DNA repair disorders. These conditions are caused by a monogenic defect in one of the DNA repair pathways. In some of them, this DNA repair defect is reflected by cytogenetic analysis showing an increased number of chromosome breakages. The skin, mucosae, and immune system are also frequently affected in these disorders.

Bloom syndrome

Bloom syndrome is an autosomal recessive disorder caused by a mutation in the BLM gene. The gene product, RECQ protein-like 3, belongs to the RecQ family of DNA helicases.[45] RecQ helicases are important for the maintenance of genome integrity. The condition is quite rare (less than one case per million) but frequent in the Ashkenazi Jewish population where the incidence is 1 in 10 000. The principal clinical features of this syndrome are prenatal and postnatal growth retardation, sensitivity to sunlight, reduced fertility (especially in males), decreased serum immunoglobulins and an increased risk of cancer.[46] Typical is the telangiectatic rash in sun-exposed areas, particularly on the cheeks, resembling to some extent lupus erythematosus because of the butterfly distribution across the nose (Fig. 17.4a). Hyperpigmented spots with café-au-lait color can also be observed (Fig. 17.4b). Birth weight is usually less than 2300 g at term. Mean birth length is 44 cm. Final height attainment rarely exceeds 145 cm in males and 130 cm in females.[4] Intelligence is normal. The major complication is the substantially increased risk for malignancies. Affected individuals are predisposed to the development of most cancer types, a feature that is apparently unique amongst familial cancer syndromes. The mean age of cancer diagnosis is about 24 years.[47,48] Cells from patients with Bloom syndrome show an increased frequency of chromosomal breaks but the hallmark feature, which is used for diagnostic purposes, is the approximately 10-fold elevation in the rate of sister chromatid exchanges (SCE).[49] SCEs arise from crossing over of chromatid arms during homologous recombination, a ubiquitous process that exists to repair DNA double-stranded breaks and damaged replication forks. The cytogenetic test for SCE is a simple and reliable screening test for confirmation of the diagnosis. Molecular testing is also available and important for prenatal diagnosis in subsequent pregnancies. Bloom syndrome should be differentiated from other conditions with sunlight sensitivity such as Rothmund–Thomson syndrome, xeroderma pigmentosum and Cockayne syndrome.

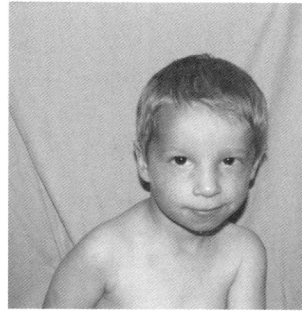

(a)

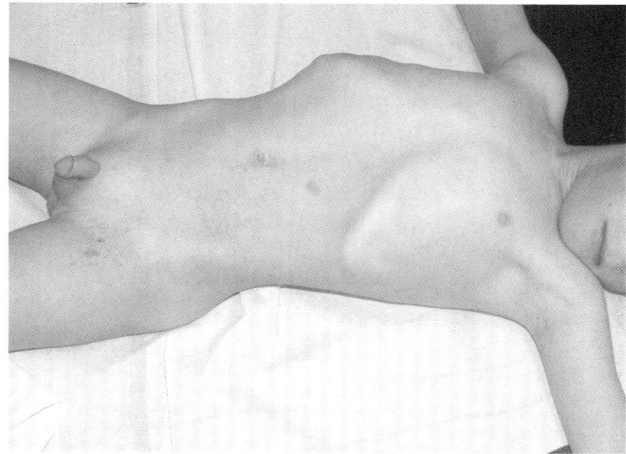

(b)

Figure 17.4 Boy with Bloom syndrome showing (a) the telangiectatic rash on the cheeks and (b) hyperpigmented spots on the abdomen and in the left groin.

However, in the former two conditions stature is normal and in the latter disorder, growth retardation only becomes evident during the second year of life (see the section 'Disorders with premature aging' on p. 274. Please see Plate 5.).

Fanconi anemia

Pre- and postnatal growth retardation are also features of Fanconi anemia, another DNA-repair disorder. This condition shows autosomal recessive inheritance and is characterized by congenital abnormalities and a predisposition to bone marrow failure and malignancies.[50] Fanconi anemia is a genetically heterogeneous disorder. Nine genetic subtypes have been described, most of which have been connected to distinct disease genes.[51] To date, 11 different genes have been identified which complicates the molecular genetic testing for diagnostic purposes. Cells from Fanconi anemia patients are hypersensitive to chromosomal breakage by cross-linking agents such as diepoxybutane (DEB) and mitomycin C (MMC). This trait has been exploited to assess the diagnosis by means of cytogenetic analysis, both in prenatal and postnatal situations. Increased rates of spontaneous chromosomal breakage may be seen in other chromosomal breakage syndromes (Bloom syndrome, ataxia–telangiectasia) but it is the increased breakage and formation of radicals in response to DEB/MMC that distinguish Fanconi anemia from these other syndromes. Patients with Fanconi anemia can have a wide variety of clinical abnormalities. The disorder is associated with altered growth both *in utero* and after birth. Low birth weight is common and the median height lies around the 5th centile.[50] Deficiency of growth hormone and thyroid hormone may contribute to the growth failure.[52] The most common and typical skeletal abnormalities are the radial ray defects such as hypoplasia of the thumbs and radius (rarely polydactyly can be present). Microphthalmia, conductive hearing loss, microcephaly and developmental delay are also frequent features. Urogenital abnormalities are present in about one third of the patients.[50] Less common abnormalities include atresia along the gastrointestinal tract (esophageal, duodenal, jejunal, anal), congenital heart defects and structural abnormalities of the central nervous system. Affected subjects often have areas of increased or decreased skin pigmentation. Up to one-third of the cases do not have any obvious congenital abnormalities. In these instances the diagnosis is made because of the hematological abnormalities, another key manifestation of the disorder. Fanconi anemia is the most common type of inherited bone marrow failure. At birth, the blood count is usually normal and macrocytosis is often the only detected abnormality, followed by thrombocytopenia and neutropenia. Pancytopenia typically presents between the ages of 5 and 10 years.[53] By age 40–48 years, the estimated cumulative incidence of bone marrow failure is 90%. There is an increased risk of acute myeloid leukemia and certain solid tumors, notably hepatic tumors and squamous cell carcinomas.[54] Fanconi anemia should be differentiated from other genetic conditions with hematological abnormalities (Diamond–Blackfan anemia) and radial ray defects (Table 17.4).

DISORDERS WITH MENTAL RETARDATION AND MICROCEPHALY

Intrauterine growth retardation, microcephaly and mental retardation are features of de Lange syndrome, Seckel syndrome and Dubowitz syndrome.

de Lange syndrome

de Lange syndrome (also called Brachmann–de Lange syndrome and Cornelia de Lange syndrome) is an autosomal dominant condition characterized by pre- and postnatal growth retardation and severe mental retardation. Recently, heterozygous mutations in genes coding for cohesin regulators and cohesin structural components have been identified in individuals with de Lange syndrome. The cohesin proteins compose an evolutionarily conserved complex of proteins that are important for chromosome cohesion and segregation of sister chromatids. Mutations in the *NIPBL* gene (on chromosome 5p13) are responsible for about 50% of cases with de Lange syndrome.[55,56] *NIPBL* is the vertebrate homolog of the yeast sister chromatid cohesion 2 (Scc2) protein and is a regulator of cohesin loading and unloading. Mutations in the genes *SMC1A* and *SMC3*, which each code for a subunit of the cohesin heterodimer, contribute to 5% of individuals with de Lange syndrome and result in a milder phenotype.[57,58] de Lange syndrome is a multisystem disorder affecting the eye, heart, limbs, and the gastrointestinal and urogenital tracts.[59,60] Ocular anomalies, including myopia, ptosis, and nystagmus, are present in 57% of the patients. Approximately 15% of the affected individuals have a congenital heart defect. The limb anomalies range from small hands and feet with clinodactyly of the fifth fingers, to severe phocomelia, usually involving the upper limb. Radiographs of the hands show a characteristic

Table 17.4 Common genetic disorders with radial ray defects

Disorder	Inheritance	Gene	Short stature	Key distinguishing features
Baller–Gerold syndrome	AR	RECQL4	yes	Craniosynostosis; anal atresia
Fanconi anemia	AR	Many genes [51]	yes	Pancytopenia; abnormal skin pigmentation; various congenital malformations
Holt–Oram syndrome	AD	TBX5	no	Atrial or ventricular septal defect
Nager acrofacial dysostosis	Usually sporadic	unknown	yes	Coloboma of the lower eyelid; hypoplasia of the zygomata and maxilla, cleft palate, severe micrognathia, hearing loss
RAPADILINO syndrome	AR	RECQL4	yes	Absent or hypoplastic patellae; diarrhea; joint dislocations; cleft palate
TAR syndrome	AR	unknown	yes	Thrombocytopenia, preservation of thumbs
Townes–Brock syndrome	AD	SALL1	no	Microtia; hearing loss; anal atresia
VATER association	Usually sporadic	unknown	yes	Vertebral defects; anal atresia, tracheoesophageal fistula, cardiac defects, renal anomalies

metacarpophalangeal profile with shortening of the first metacarpal and short middle phalanges of fourth and fifth fingers.[61] The kidneys are often hypoplastic, dysplastic or cystic and various structural and functional gastrointestinal abnormalities have been reported. Feeding problems and gastroesophageal reflux are common features in infancy. The typical craniofacial dysmorphism consists of microcephaly, low hairline, synophrys, long eyelashes, small nose with anteverted nostrils, small ears, thin upper lip, and widely spaced teeth (Fig. 17.5). Micrognathia is common and sometimes a mental spur can be palpated. Also quite typical are the cutis marmorata and generalized hirsutism. Growth retardation is an almost universal finding and typically has a prenatal onset. The degree of intrauterine growth retardation seems to correlate with the severity of the phenotype. Both height and weight usually remain far below the third centile for age.[62] The mental retardation is often severe with a mean IQ of 53 and many children have self-injurious behavior.[63] Important for the differential diagnosis and genetic counseling, is the observation that patients with a duplication of the long arm of chromosome 3 (band 3q26) can have overlapping phenotypic features with the de Lange syndrome.[64]

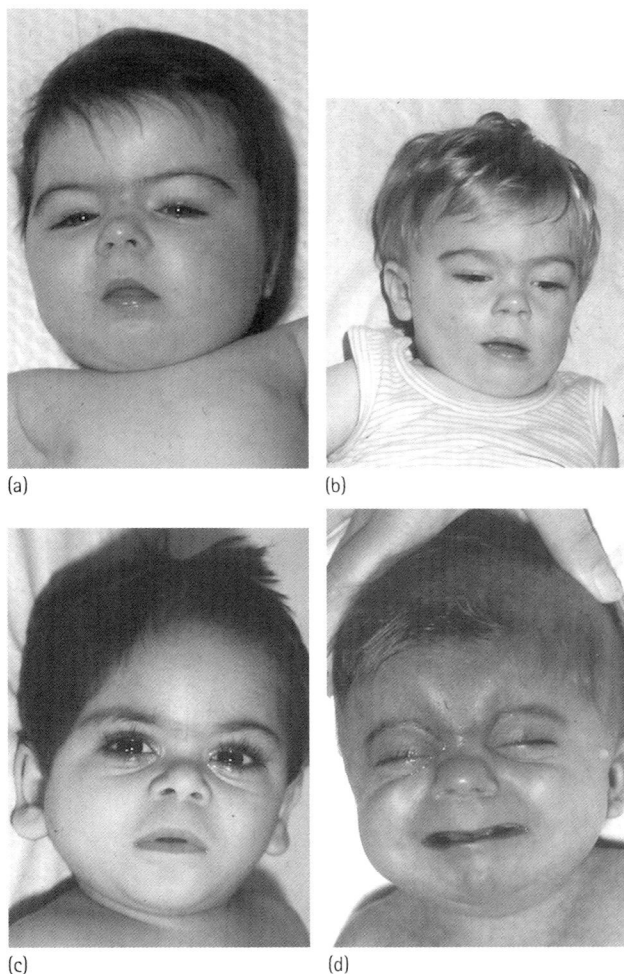

(a) (b)

(c) (d)

Figure 17.5 Typical facial features of the Brachmann–de Lange syndrome in four unrelated children. (Courtesy of J. Leroy). Please see Plate 6.

Seckel syndrome

Seckel syndrome is an autosomal recessive condition characterized by marked intrauterine and postnatal growth retardation, microcephaly and mental retardation. Patients with Seckel syndrome have a distinct face with receding forehead, relatively large eyes, large beak-like nose, and micrognathia, giving the face a 'bird-like' appearance. Craniosynostosis due to poor brain growth has been documented in approximately 50% of the cases.[4] Seckel syndrome is a genetically heterogeneous condition. At least three different loci have been identified.[65–67] Recently, O'Driscoll et al. identified ATR as the gene mutated at the first defined locus on 3q22.1–q24.[68] The ATR gene encodes for the ataxia–telangiectasia and Rad3-related protein. This protein functions in cell-cycle checkpoint and DNA repair pathways which may explain the chromosome instability sometimes observed in cells from Seckel syndrome patients.[69] Mean birth weight of affected newborns at term is approximately 1540 g (range, 1000–2055 g). Postnatal growth deficiency is on average 7 SD below the mean (range −5.1 to −13.5 SD). All patients are mentally retarded, with half having an IQ below 50.[4] Seckel syndrome should be differentiated from microcephalic osteodysplastic primordial dwarfism (MOPD), where the growth retardation is more severe and skeletal dysplastic changes are present (Table 17.5).[70,71]

Dubowitz syndrome

Dubowitz syndrome is an autosomal recessive condition with variable expression, probably due to genetic heterogeneity. The main features of the disorder are intrauterine growth retardation, proportionate short stature, microcephaly and a distinct facies.[72] Intrauterine growth retardation with average birth weight of 2.413 g for males and 2.221 g for females is noted in 68% of the affected newborns. Head circumference at birth averages 31 cm.[73] The face is characterized by a high sloping forehead, broad nasal bridge, telecanthus, flat supraorbital ridges with arched and laterally sparse eyebrows, ptosis of the eyelids (often asymmetrical), small palpebral fissures, low-set ears, and micrognathia (Fig. 17.6). Facial asymmetry can be observed and, more importantly, 60% of the affected infants have an eczematous skin eruption in the face, usually from birth on.[73] Sparse or thin hair and eczema are the most common ectodermal manifestations of the disease. Infancy is usually complicated by poor feeding, frequent vomiting, and diarrhea. The degree of microcephaly does not correlate with the mental retardation, which is usually mild. Most children are hyperactive, shy, hate crowds, and like music.[73] Submucous cleft palate and velopharyngeal insufficiency have been reported.[72,74] Also characteristic is the high-pitched voice. Immunodeficiency, anemia, and malignancies (leukemia, lymphoma) have been associated with the disorder.

DISORDERS WITH NORMAL HEAD CIRCUMFERENCE

Short stature and low weight at birth in association with a normal for age (and therefore disproportionately large) head size is a feature of several conditions discussed in this session.

Table 17.5 Major distinguishing features between Seckel syndrome and the two types of microcephalic osteodysplastic primordial dwarfism (MOPD)

	Seckel syndrome	MOPD type 1/3 *	MOPD type 2
Intrauterine growth retardation	++ (birth weight at term less than 2100 g)	+++	+++(birth weight at term less than 1500 g and length less than 40 cm)
Postnatal growth retardation	++	+++	+++(adult height less than 110 cm); progressively disproportionate
Microcephaly	Present at birth	Present at birth	At birth proportionate for body size, later on true microcephalic
Precocious puberty	Not reported	Not reported	Often seen
Neuronal migration anomalies	Can be present	Can be present	Not documented
Hair	Normal	Sparse	Sparse
Skin	No anomalies reported	Dry	Progressive appearance of areas of increased pigmentation
Facial features			
Forehead	Receding at birth	Receding at birth	Normal at birth
Ears	Relatively large	Relatively normal	Simple; missing lobule
Intelligence	Severe mental retardation	Severe mental retardation	Normal intelligence or mild to moderate menal retardation
Skeleton	No bone dysplasia	Bone dysplasia: foreshortened vertebral bodies; short iliac wings; short and squared metacarpals and phalanges	Bone dysplasia: foreshortened vertebral bodies; high and narrow iliac wings; gracile and overtubulated bones; coxa vara, capital femoral epiphysiolysis; V-shaped distal femoral metaphyses and triangular distal femur epiphyses; ivory epiphyses in hands; hypoplastic distal phalanges

*There is evidence that MOPD type 1 and type 3 are variant expressions of the same entity

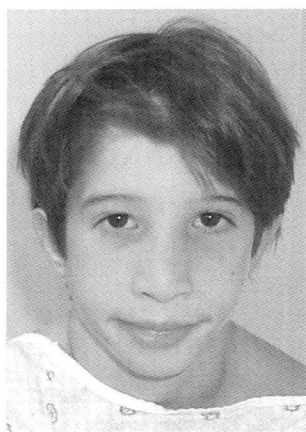

Figure 17.6 Patient with Dubowitz syndrome. A mild ptosis of the right upper eyelid is present. Please see Plate 7.

Russell–Silver syndrome

Russell–Silver syndrome (RSS) is characterized by pre- and postnatal growth retardation resulting in a proportionate short stature with normal head circumference (Fig. 17.7).[75] For full-term babies at birth, mean weight is 1940 g for boys and 1897 g for girls. Mean length of full-term babies at birth is 43.1 cm in both sexes.[76] The head circumference is usually appropriate for gestation, giving the skull a 'pseudohydro-cephalic' appearance. The average adult height of males is 151 cm and that of females is 139 cm.[76,77] Hypoglycemia is a well-known complication in the neonatal period. The typical facial phenotype consists of a broad and prominent forehead with small triangular face and small, narrow chin. Additional features that can be diagnostically helpful are limb length asymmetry, significant clinodactyly of the fifth fingers and the presence of café-au-lait spots. In contrast to conditions with hemihypertrophy, RSS patients do not seem to have a significantly increased risk for malignancies. Developmental delay and learning disabilities seem to occur with increased frequency in RSS.[78] Gastrointestinal problems, including failure to thrive, gastroesophageal reflux and food aversion, are common in individuals with RSS.[79] RSS is most likely a genetically heterogeneous condition.[80] In about 10% of

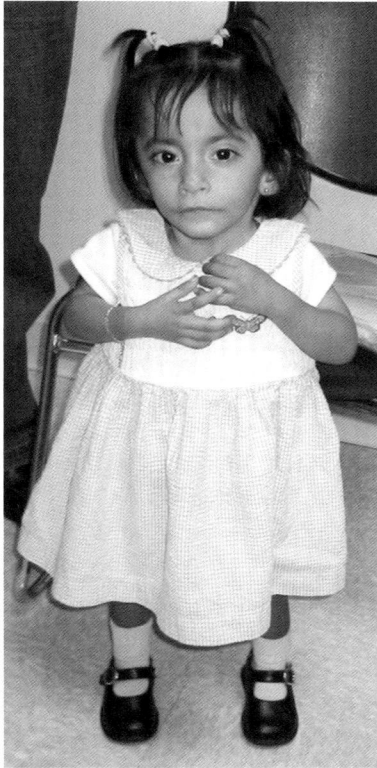

Figure 17.7   Girl with the Russell–Silver syndrome. Please see Plate 8.

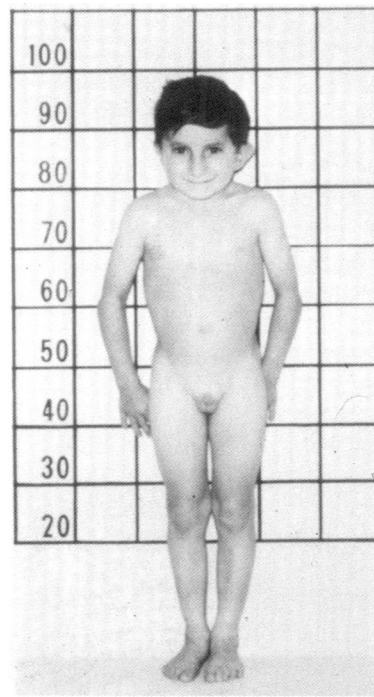

Figure 17.8   Boy with the Floating Harbor syndrome as originally reported from the Harbor General Hospital in Torrance. (From *Smith's Recognizable Patterns of Human Malformation*, Jones, KL(ed.), Saunders).

the patients, uniparental (maternal) disomy for chromosome 7 has been documented.[81] There is evidence that the paternally imprinted *GRB10* gene, mapped to chromosome 7p11.2–p12, is responsible for the growth disturbance in these patients. *GRB10* codes for the growth factor receptor-bound protein 10, a member of the family of adaptor proteins that mediate interactions between disparate proteins. Disruption of the imprinted homolog *Grb10* in mice results in overgrowth, suggesting that this maternally expressed gene suppresses growth in both humans and mice.[82] Rearrangements of chromosome 17 (17q25) have also been observed in RSS patients.[83] In this chromosomal region genes coding for growth factor receptor-bound proteins (*GRB2;GRB7*) and genes coding for components of the growth hormone gene cluster (*GH; CSH1;CSH2*) have been localized. Deletion of the *CSH1* gene has been documented in two cases of RSS but subsequently ruled out in a panel of 106 RSS patients.[80] Most cases of RSS are sporadic. However, recurrence in sibs and vertical transmission in families have been reported.[84,85]

3-M syndrome

Russell–Silver syndrome should not be confused with the 3-M syndrome, an autosomal recessive condition also characterized by intrauterine growth retardation and relatively large head. However, patients with the 3-M syndrome have a different facial phenotype (frontal bossing, full eyebrows, hypoplastic midface, pointed and prominent chin,

upturned nose and full lips), do not show limb length asymmetry and have mild skeletal dysplastic changes on radiographs.[86–88] The long tubular bones are usually slender and the vertebral bodies high and foreshortened in patients with 3-M syndrome. The same radiographic abnormalities are also found in dolichospondylic dysplasia.[89]

Floating Harbor syndrome

Floating Harbor syndrome is a rare condition characterized by proportionate short stature, usually of prenatal onset, with normal head circumference.[4] The name is derived from one patient seen at Boston Floating Hospital[90] and another being reported from Harbor General Hospital in Torrance (Fig. 17.8).[91] The etiology of the syndrome is still unknown and most of the reported cases (approximately 20 patients) have been sporadic.[4] Recognition of the facial dysmorphism is important for the diagnosis. Characteristic facial features include prominent eyes in infancy that become deep-set with age, long eyelashes, posteriorly rotated ears, typical nose, short philtrum, and wide mouth with thin lips. The nose has a broad bridge and broad tip with wide columella in early infancy. In later childhood the nose is more prominent, but the nasal bridge and tip become smaller, and hypoplasia of the alae nasi becomes more pronounced.[92,93] At least 50% of the reported cases are small for gestational age at birth with normal head circumference.[4] Short stature in childhood and adolescence is variable and can range from normal to a height of less than 6 standard deviations below the mean.[94,95] Several reports have emphasized its particular association with delayed development of expressive speech. Nasal speech and high-pitched voice have been noted.[95]

Mulibrey nanism

Mulibrey nanism is an autosomal recessive condition, first described in Finland and characterized by severe growth failure of prenatal onset and multiple organ manifestations.[96] The term 'mulibrey' refers to the *mu*scle, *li*ver, *br*ain and *ey*e involvement. The disorder occurs worldwide but is more common in the Finnish population.[97] Mulibrey nanism is caused by mutations in the *TRIM37* gene.[98,99] The *TRIM37* gene encodes a novel zinc finger protein of unknown function, located in the peroxisomes.[100] In a series of 85 patients, 95% were small for gestational age.[97] Birth length standard deviation score (SDS) was on average −3.1 (range, −6.4 to 0.7) and mean birth weight SDS was −2.8 (range, −4.0 to 0.5). The head circumference is usually normal for age and therefore relatively macrocephalic in comparison with the rest of the body. Feeding problems and failure to thrive are common in the newborn period and during infancy.[97] Episodes of respiratory failure, induced by an infection, occurred in 25% of the infants. Psychomotor development is normal or slightly delayed (due to muscular hypotonia) in the majority of cases. Children have a slender but short habitus with a relatively scaphocephalic skull and triangular face, characterized by broad and prominent forehead, hypertelorism and low nasal bridge. Features or complications that may suggest the diagnosis are (1) restrictive cardiomyopathy or constrictive pericarditis, sometimes resulting in congestive heart failure and hepatomegaly; (2) characteristic ocular findings including yellow dots in the midperiphery of the fundus or other retinal abnormalities;[101] and (3) a low and shallow (J shaped) sella turcica and fibrous dysplasia, usually in the lower limbs.

SHORT syndrome

SHORT syndrome is an acronym referring to the association of *s*hort stature, *h*yperextensibility of joints and/or inguinal *h*ernia, *o*cular depression, *R*ieger anomaly and delayed eruption of *t*eeth. About 70% of the affected newborns have intrauterine growth retardation with normal head circumference.[102] During infancy, babies usually have poor weight gain despite good appetite and this, together with a lipodystrophy that becomes more apparent with age, gives the affected individuals a dystrophic and progeroid appearance. The lipodystrophy is due to lack of subcutaneous fat, predominantly in the face, chest and upper extremities (relatively sparing the legs). Although lipodystrophy is not mentioned in the mnemonic term SHORT, some authors believe that this feature is more important for the syndrome than the short stature.[102] The face is triangular with a prominent forehead, deep-set eyes, midface hypoplasia, thin alae nasi and small chin. The most typical ocular malformation is Rieger anomaly. Sometimes this is apparent

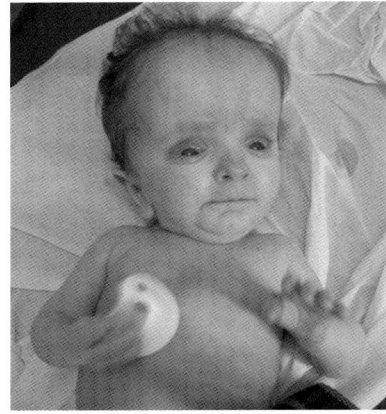

Figure 17.9   Infant with Wiedemann–Rautenstrauch syndrome. The skull is relatively large with high and prominent forehead, sparse hair and prominent veins. Please see Plate 9.

soon after birth because of congenital glaucoma or absence of the iris stroma. In most cases, however, a pediatric ophthalmologist needs to look carefully for this malformation in order to establish the diagnosis. Nearly all patients have delayed dental eruption. In addition, the teeth can be small or show enamel hypoplasia. Dental prosthesis because of early-onset dental caries is not unusual. Intelligence is usually normal to slightly subnormal. Delayed bone age, large epiphyses and gracile tubular bones have been reported as radiographic manifestations of the disorder.[103] The genetic defect is not known but autosomal dominant inheritance has been postulated.[102]

Wiedemann–Rautenstrauch syndrome

Deficiency of subcutaneous fat in association with intrauterine growth retardation are also features of the Wiedemann–Rautenstrauch syndrome (WRS). This neonatal progeroid syndrome is a rare autosomal recessive disorder. The genetic defect is not yet known. All affected children have intrauterine growth retardation with subsequent failure to thrive and short stature.[104] The head circumference is usually within normal limits for age. The generalized lack of subcutaneous fat, low birth weight, relatively large head with sparse hair, prominent scalp veins and large fontanelles give these infants a progeroid appearance at birth (Fig. 17.9). The face is rather tiny and triangular in contrast to the large cranial size. This disproportion between cranium and face becomes more apparent with age. The presence of natal teeth is a useful diagnostic feature distinguishing this condition from other progeroid syndromes. The hands and feet are rather large with long fingers and toes. A large penis has been observed in several cases.[105] Interestingly, in other conditions with generalized lipoatrophy (leprechaunism, Berardinelli–Seip syndrome) patients frequently have phallic enlargement. Children with WRS often suffer from feeding difficulties and respiratory tract infections. Insulin resistance, abnormalities of lipid metabolism and dysfunction of the hypothalamic–pituitary pathway have been reported in WRS.[105] The condition is usually lethal by the

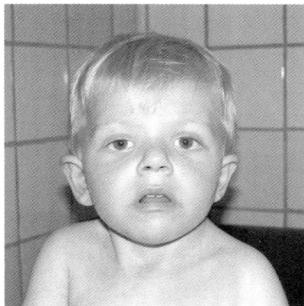

Figure 17.10 Typical facial features in a boy with Noonan syndrome: hypertelorism with downslanting palpebral fissures, low-set ears with thickened helix and clearly outlined philtrum. Please see Plate 10.

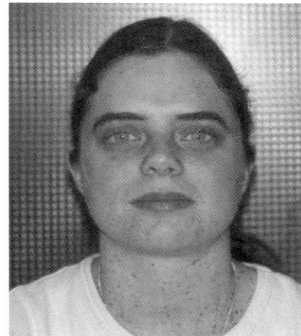

Figure 17.11 Woman with LEOPARD syndrome showing light-colored irides and multiple lentigines in face and neck. Please see Plate 11.

age of 7 months. However, on rare occasions, patients have survived into their teens.[105] Mental retardation is a variable manifestation of WRS.

Monogenic syndromes with proportionate short stature of postnatal onset

DISORDERS WITH MENTAL RETARDATION AND NORMAL HEAD CIRCUMFERENCE

Noonan syndrome and related disorders

Noonan syndrome is probably the most common monogenic condition characterized by proportionate short stature of postnatal onset. The disorder shows autosomal dominant inheritance. Heterozygous mutations in at least three genes involved in the RAS pathway have been identified. In more than 50% of cases with Noonan syndrome, mutations are found in either the *PTPN11* or *KRAS* genes.[106] These mutations result in an increased *RAS*-mitogen-activated protein kinase (*MAPK*) signaling. In about 15–20% of individuals with Noonan syndrome, gain-of-function mutations in *SOS1* are present.[107] The *SOS1* gene codes for a RAS-specific guanine nucleotide exchange factor. Cardinal features of the syndrome include short stature, congenital heart defect, broad and webbed neck, chest deformity (pectus carinatum superiorly and pectus excavatum inferiorly), developmental delay of variable degree, cryptorchidism, and characteristic facies. The distinct face is most striking during infancy and middle childhood but often subtle in adulthood.[108] Key facial features are hypertelorism with downslanting palpebral fissures, light-colored irides, low-set and posteriorly rotated ears with a thickened helix, and a deeply grooved philtrum (Fig. 17.10). Hair may be wispy in the toddler and often curly or wooly in the older child and adolescent.[109] Pulmonary valve stenosis is the most common congenital heart defect. Hypertrophic cardiomyopathy is found in 20–30% of the patients. About one-third of the patients have a coagulation defect, presenting as either severe surgical hemorrhage, clinically mild bruising or as a laboratory

abnormality with no clinical consequences. Thrombocytopenia, platelet dysfunction or coagulation factor defects may be responsible for the hemorrhagic diathesis.[109] Lymphatic abnormalities may cause general or localized lymphoedema. Dorsal limb lymphoedema is commonly found after birth and usually disappears during childhood. Varying degrees of edema or hydrops can be found on ultrasound during intrauterine life. Length at birth is usually normal. Mean prepubertal growth follows the third centile for height and weight. Onset of puberty is usually delayed and the pubertal growth spurt often reduced. However, study of growth data around puberty suggests a catch-up in late adolescence.[110] Mean adult height is 162.5 cm in males and 152.7 cm in females.[111] Females manifest normal fertility whereas reduced fertility in males may occur. Several studies have reported the results of growth hormone treatment in Noonan syndrome. Although these reports seem to confirm an increase in medium-term height velocity, the effect on final height is not yet well established.[109,112,113] Most school-age children perform well in a normal educational setting, but 10–15% require special education.[114] Mild mental retardation is seen in up to one-third of the affected individuals and tends to correlate with the severity of feeding problems during early childhood.

Since the identification of the *PTPN11* gene, it has become clear that Noonan syndrome and LEOPARD syndrome are allelic conditions.[115] The presence of sensorineural hearing loss and multiple lentigines distinguishes LEOPARD syndrome from Noonan syndrome (Fig. 17.11). Cardiofaciocutaneous syndrome (CFCS) also shows overlapping features with Noonan syndrome because of similar cardiac and lymphatic findings. However, CFCS differs from Noonan syndrome by the more severe mental retardation, more coarse facial features and more pronounced skin abnormalities (Fig. 17.12). CFCS is caused by mutations in *BRAF* (over 50% of cases) with some patients demonstrating mutations in *MEK1*, *MEK2* or *KRAS*.[116] Costello syndrome is a third disorder in this group of related syndromes caused by mutations in the *RAS-MAPK* pathway. Costello syndrome is characterized by mental retardation, hypertrophic cardiomyopathy and/or rhythm disturbances, pulmonary stenosis,

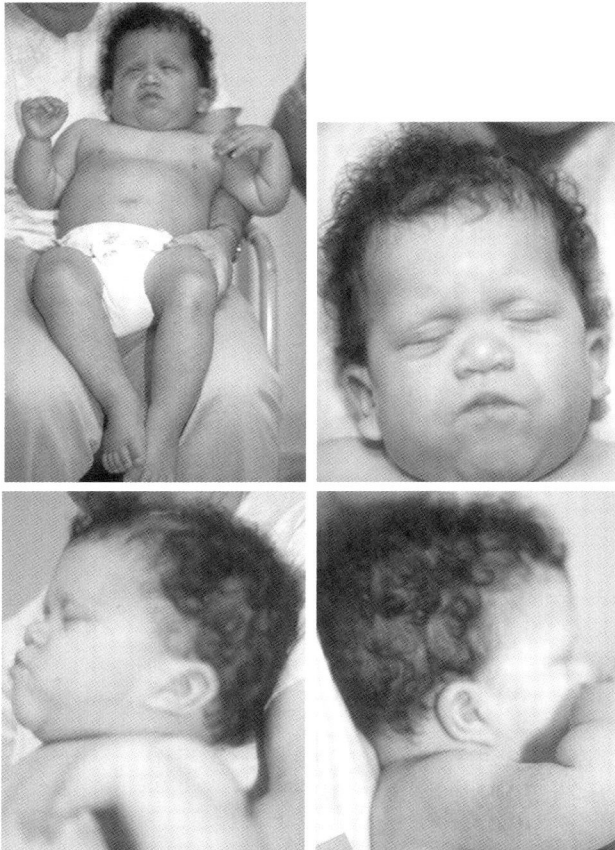

Figure 17.12   Coarse facial features in a child with the cardiofaciocutaneous syndrome due to a mutation in *BRAF*. Please see Plate 12.

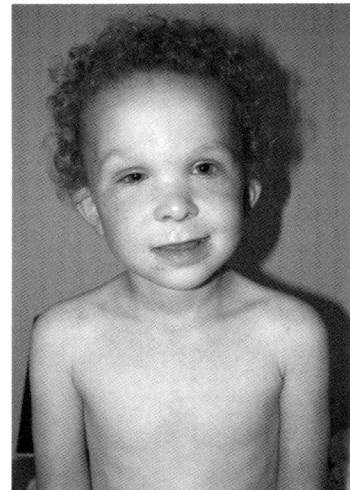

(a)

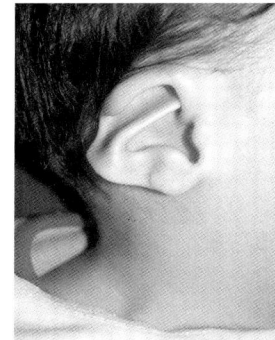

(b)

Figure 17.13   (a) Girl with CHARGE syndrome. Note the facial asymmetry due to paresis of the right facial nerve. (b) Typical shape of the external ear in CHARGE syndrome. Please see Plate 13.

short stature, coarse facial features, peri-mucosal papillomata developing during childhood, musculoskeletal abnormalities, and tumor predisposition (predominantly rhabdomyosarcoma, neuroblastoma, and bladder carcinoma). Prenatal presentation is characterized by overgrowth, edema and polyhydramnios, and Costello syndrome is caused most commonly by a specific activating point mutation in *HRAS* in over 85% of cases.[116]

CHARGE syndrome

The CHARGE syndrome, first described by Bryan Hall[117] and Helen Hittner[118] in 1979, is a multiple congenital anomaly syndrome characterized by craniofacial malformations, postnatal growth retardation and developmental delay. Heart defects, esophageal atresia, and/or cleft lip/palate and renal malformations are well-known components of this condition. The syndrome was given the acronym CHARGE referring to the common manifestations such as *c*oloboma, *h*eart defect, *a*tresia choanae, *r*etarded growth and development, *g*enital hypoplasia, and *e*ar anomalies/deafness. The disorder was initially considered to represent an association but as more patients were reported, the

condition became accepted as a recognizable syndrome. Early studies emphasized the presence of choanal atresia or ocular colobomata as key diagnostic features. However, over time, it became clear that the ear anomalies with the characteristic temporal bone morphology (absence of semicircular canals), as well as the cranial nerve dysfunction were also important for establishing the diagnosis (Fig. 17.13). These features are now considered as major diagnostic criteria (Table 17.6).[119,120] The diagnosis of CHARGE syndrome is unquestionable when an individual meets either four major criteria or three major and three minor criteria. In neonates and infants the diagnosis needs to be considered when one or two major and several minor manifestations are present. The majority of patients with CHARGE syndrome have appropriate birth measurements but over 70% of them develop postnatal growth retardation.[121] Feeding problems in infancy with failure to thrive are due to pharyngeal incoordination and gastroesophageal reflux. Deficiency of growth hormone has been seen in a few patients, and most have hypothalamic hypogonadism.[122] Recently, a microdeletion on chromosome

Table 17.6 Diagnostic criteria for CHARGE syndrome

Diagnostic criteria	Clinical features
Major criterion	
– Coloboma	– coloboma of iris, retina, choroid; microphthalmia
– Choanal stenosis/atresia	– bony or membranous choanal stenosis or atresia
– Characteristic ear abnormalities	– lop or cup shaped external ear; hypoplasia/agenesis of semicircular canals; ossicular defects of middle ear
– Cranial nerve dysfunction	– anosmia (I); facial palsy (usually asymmetric) (VII); hearing loss and defective vestibular function (VIII); dysphagia (IX/X)
Minor criterion	
– Genital hypoplasia	– cryptorchidism, small penis; hypoplastic labia; delayed or incomplete pubertal development
– Developmental delay	– hypotonia, mental retardation
– Cardiac defects	– usually conotruncal defects
– Growth failure	– short stature
– Orofacial clefting	– cleft lip/palate
– Tracheoesophageal defects	– tracheoesophageal fistula

8q12 has been identified in a few patients with CHARGE syndrome and heterozygous mutations in the *CHD7* gene have been found in another subset of patients.[123] The *CHD7* gene is localized within the microdeletion interval on 8q12 and belongs to the family of chromodomain helicase DNA-binding (*CHD*) genes that play a pivotal role in early embryonic development.

KBG syndrome

The KBG syndrome is a rather rare, autosomal dominant condition characterized by mild mental retardation, short stature and facial dysmorphism.[124] The disorder was first described in 1975 in seven patients from three unrelated families.[125] The name of the syndrome was derived from the first letters of the surnames of each family. Characteristic facial features include round face, bushy eyebrows with synophrys, long palpebral fissures, thin lips, and protruding ears. An important distinguishing feature of the syndrome is the macrodontia with wide upper central incisors and prominent, supernumerary mamelons (some as many as five) on the incisal edges.[126] Costovertebral abnormalities, including cervical ribs, block vertebrae and spina bifida occulta are also quite common in this condition and may therefore be helpful for making the diagnosis.[127]

DISORDERS WITH MENTAL RETARDATION AND SMALL HEAD CIRCUMFERENCE

Rubinstein–Taybi syndrome

Rubinstein–Taybi syndrome (RTS) is an autosomal dominant condition. It is caused by either a microdeletion on chromosome 16p13 (in about 10% of the cases) or by a heterozygous mutation in the *CREBBP* gene (which is located in the microdeletion interval on 16p13).[128] The *CREBBP* gene codes for a nuclear protein (CREB-binding protein) that participates as a coactivator in cAMP-regulated gene expression.[129] Affected individuals have mental retardation with the most severe delay in expressive speech. Microcephaly is present in less than 50% of the patients and is usually of postnatal onset.[130] Length and weight are normal at birth but rapidly fall off in the first months of life. The lack of pubertal growth spurt further contributes to the short stature which is seen in these patients.[131] Individuals with RTS have a distinct face with down-slanting palpebral fissures, strabismus, beaked nose with the columella extending below the alae, and micrognathia. Grimacing or unusual smile have been observed frequently. The broad thumbs and great toes in association with the characteristic nose are cardinal features of the disorder (Fig. 17.14). Angulation deformities of the thumbs and halluces, usually caused by abnormally formed proximal phalanges, occur in about one third of the cases.[4] Common congenital anomalies include congenital heart defects (24–38%)[132] and renal abnormalities (52%).[133] Refractive errors, strabismus, coloboma, and lacrimal duct obstructions are more frequently observed than in the general population.[133–135] A significant number of boys have incomplete or delayed descent of the testes. Feeding problems are common during infancy. Orthopedic complications include dislocation of the radial head and patella, avascular necrosis or slipping of the capital femoral epiphysis and scoliosis.[133–135] Recently, medical guidelines for management of individuals with RTS have been published.[136]

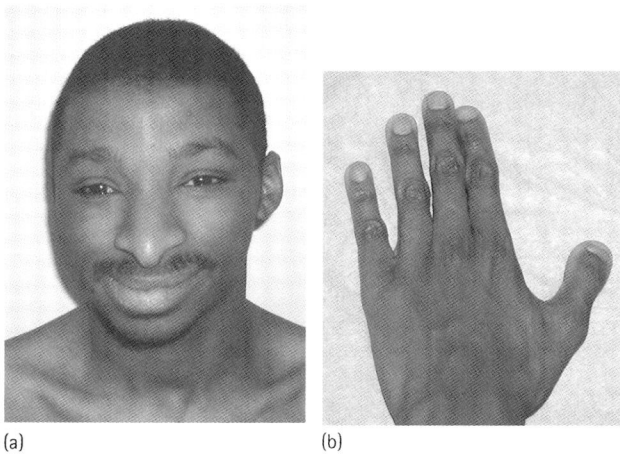

Figure 17.14 Boy with Rubinstein–Taybi syndrome. Note (a) the typical nose with the columella extending below the alae and (b) broad thumb. Please see Plate 14.

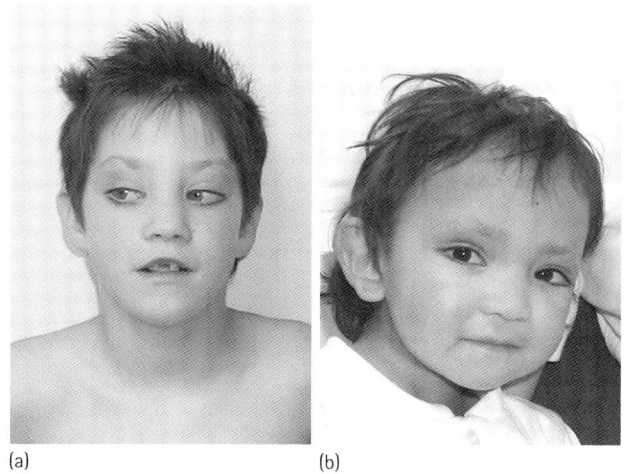

Figure 17.15 Two unrelated patients with Kabuki syndrome. Typical are the arched eyebrows, long palpebral fissures and eyelashes, and eversion of the lateral part of the lower eyelids. Please see Plate 15.

Briefly, physicians taking care of this group of patients should be aware of: (1) the easy collapsibility of the laryngeal walls that may complicate intubation procedures; (2) the higher likelihood to form keloids and hypertrophic scars after surgery; and (3) the increased risk of benign and malignant tumors such as leukemia and lymphoma.

Kabuki syndrome

Kabuki syndrome was described simultaneously by two Japanese groups as a syndrome with mental retardation, postnatal growth retardation, and a distinct face reminiscent of the make-up used in the Kabuki theatre.[137,138] Since the genetic defect is not yet known, the diagnosis of Kabuki syndrome is made on a clinical basis. Diagnostic criteria have not been published. Most affected individuals have a recognizable facial dysmorphism with the periorbital characteristics being most specific (Fig. 17.15).[139] The eyebrows are placed relatively high on the forehead and give the impression of being pulled up at their middle ('arched eyebrows'). The lateral third of the eyebrows is usually sparse or notched. The eyelashes are long and the palpebral fissures elongated, sometimes extending beyond the conjunctiva. The upper eyelids appear thick and are therefore often described as ptotic or droopy. The lateral part of the lower eyelids tends to be everted. The sclerae can have a bluish appearance. Other common orofacial features are tethered nasal tip, cleft lip/palate, prominent lower lip with pits or a midline depression, fissured tongue, and preauricular dimples, pits or fistulas. Growth retardation is usually of postnatal origin. Microcephaly is documented in about 25% of patients.[4] A mild to moderate global developmental delay is usually present. Feeding problems are common in infancy and may be due to various factors including hypotonia and congenital heart defects. Left-sided obstructive malformations and atrial and ventricular septal defects are the most frequently observed heart anomalies.[139] Development of areolar fullness in infancy has been reported in about 20% of the girls.[139] Persistence of fetal finger pads is characteristic but not pathognomonic for the disorder. The occurrence of lax joints, hernias and hyperextensible skin suggests connective tissue involvement. There is some evidence for abnormalities of the immune system, reflected by increased rates of infections, but no increased risk of cancer has been recognized so far.

DISORDERS WITH PREMATURE AGING

Premature aging in association with proportionate short stature of postnatal onset are features of the Cockayne syndrome and the Hutchinson–Gilford progeria syndrome.

Cockayne syndrome

Cockayne syndrome (CS) is a rare genetic disorder with autosomal recessive inheritance due to a defect in nucleotide excision repair (DNA repair disorder). It is characterized by growth failure and progressive multisystem failure.[140] In the classic form (Cockayne syndrome type I), prenatal growth is normal and growth failure becomes evident in the first two years. Gradually, all anthropometric measurements fall far below the fifth percentile. Usually, weight is more affected than height, which causes a cachectic phenotype ('cachectic dwarfism'). Reduced amounts of subcutaneous fat in the face, the sunken eyes (enophthalmia) and the beaked nose give the patients a typical, 'birdlike' facial appearance (Fig. 17.16). Progressive impairment of vision, hearing, and central and peripheral nervous system function lead to severe disability. Progressive neurologic dysfunction is manifested initially by developmental delay followed by progressive motor, behavioral and intellectual deterioration with evidence of leukodystrophy on brain MRI.[141] In addition,

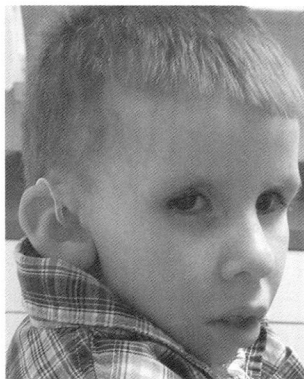

Figure 17.16 Characteristic facial features in a boy with Cockayne syndrome. Please see Plate 16.

demyelinating peripheral neuropathy may be present. Many patients have structural eye abnormalities, such as cataracts, ciliary body defects and pigmentary degeneration of the retina.[142] Dental caries are also common. Another characteristic feature of the condition is cutaneous photosensitivity with or without thin or dry skin and hair. The immune system is not affected and there is no increased risk of skin cancer. Cockayne syndrome is a progressive disorder with reduced life expectancy. Death usually occurs in the first or second decade. The diagnosis is usually made on a clinical basis. Cellular tests to document the DNA repair defect are highly specialized analyses and only available on a research basic. The most consistent findings in fibroblasts of patients with CS are marked sensitivity to UV radiation, deficient recovery of RNA synthesis after UV damage and impaired repair of actively transcribed genes.[143,144] Two genes are known to be associated with Cockayne syndrome. Both gene products appear to be involved in transcription-coupled DNA repair. About 80% of the patients (complementation group B) have a mutation in the *ERCC6* gene, whereas the remaining patients (complementation group A) carry a mutation in the *CKN1* gene.[145] Mutations in *ERCC6* have also been found in patients with the severe, congenital form of Cockayne syndrome (Cockayne syndrome type II – also known as cerebro-oculo-facial syndrome and Pena–Shokeir type II syndrome).[146] In this severe form, growth failure, cataracts, and joint contractures are already present at birth and little or no neurological development is observed postnatally. Children typically die by age 7 years.

Hutchinson–Gilford progeria syndrome

Premature aging is also a key feature of Hutchinson–Gilford progeria syndrome (HGPS), a rare autosomal dominant condition with an estimated incidence of 1 in 4 million.[147] Children with this condition generally appear normal at birth but by the age of 1 or 2 years begin to display the effects of accelerated aging.[148] As these children grow up, the disorder causes them to age about a decade for every year of their life. Key features of the disorder are widespread lack of subcutaneous fat, resulting in wrinkled skin, proportionate short stature with decreased weight for height, balding with loss of eyebrows and eyelashes, and failure to complete secondary sexual development. The prominent scalp veins, prominent eyes, beaked nose, delayed dental eruption and micrognathia accentuate the aged looking appearance of these patients. Intelligence is not affected by the disorder. On average, death occurs at the age of 13. Progressive atherosclerosis of the coronary and cerebrovascular arteries is the most common fatal complication of the disorder.[149] Recently, in a series of patients with HGPS, heterozygous mutations have been identified in the *LMNA* gene.[150,151] This gene codes for lamin-A, a structural protein of the nuclear lamina. The nuclear lamina is a protein-containing layer attached to the inner nuclear membrane. Interestingly, at least ten other human diseases have been shown to result from mutations in the *LMNA* gene: the autosomal recessive and dominant forms of Emery–Dreifuss muscular dystrophy type 2, an autosomal dominant form of dilated cardiomyopathy, autosomal dominant partial lipodystrophy (Dunnigan type), autosomal dominant limb-girdle muscular dystrophy type 1B, autosomal recessive axonal neuropathy (Charcot–Marie–Tooth disease type 2B1), mandibuloacral dysplasia and atypical forms of Werner syndrome (see OMIM, #150330).[152] These observations nicely illustrate how mutations in one particular gene can cause a spectrum of phenotypes.

CONCLUSION

The child with short stature usually poses a diagnostic challenge to the pediatric endocrinologist and clinical geneticist. Numerous disorders are known with growth failure as an important feature. For the differential diagnosis, it is important to distinguish between prenatal and postnatal onset of short stature. When the onset of growth deficiency is prenatal, one must differentiate between the numerous forms of intrauterine growth retardation. This is a very heterogeneous group of disorders with multiple causes ranging from placental insufficiency, to teratogenic exposure, to specific genetic and chromosomal syndromes. The clinical evaluation and analysis of dysmorphic features present in each case often permits reaching a conclusive diagnosis. In certain syndromes, diagnosis can be supported by specific laboratory studies. As genes for such syndromes become known and clinical molecular testing becomes available, mutation analysis may become more feasible, but such testing seldom demonstrates mutations in 100% of cases. For families with a known mutation demonstrated in a research laboratory, this mutation can be confirmed in a clinical molecular laboratory and used for clinical purposes. For syndromes of unknown etiology, new techniques such as molecular karyotyping by array comparative genomic hybridization (array-CGH), are promising tools to unravel the genetic defect in the very near future.

KEY LEARNING POINTS

- The diagnosis of a short stature syndrome mainly relies upon a careful and detailed evaluation of the patient with special attention to the presence of dysmorphic features and congenital anomalies.
- It is essential for diagnostic purposes to determine if the growth failure is of prenatal or postnatal onset.
- Children with disproportionate short stature usually have a skeletal dysplasia.
- A chromosomal abnormality should always be excluded in children with proportionate short stature, mental retardation and various congenital abnormalities, certainly if the association of anomalies does not seem to fit into a recognizable syndrome.
- Children with proportionate short stature and abnormalities of skin, mucosae or immune system may have a DNA-repair disorder.
- Measurement of the head circumference is important in the differential diagnosis of intrauterine growth retardation.

REFERENCES

● = Seminal primary article
◆ = Key review paper
* = First formal publication of a management guideline

- ● 1 Tanner JM, Davies PS. Clinical longitudinal standards for height and height velocity for North American children. *J Pediatr* 1985; **107**: 317–29.
- ● 2 Tanner JM, Whitehouse RH. Clinical longitudinal standards for height, weight, height velocity, weight velocity, and stages of puberty. *Arch Dis Child* 1976; **51**: 170–9.
- ● 3 Freeman JV, Cole TJ, Chinn S, *et al.* Cross sectional stature and weight reference curves for the UK, 1990. *Arch Dis Child* 1995; **73**: 17–24.
- ◆ 4 Gorlin RJ, Cohen MM, Hennekam RCM (eds). *Syndromes of the Head and Neck.* Oxford: University Press, 2001.
- ● 5 Cooley WC, Graham JM. Down syndrome – an update and review for the primary pediatrician. *Clin Pediatr* 1991; **30**: 233–53.
- ● 6 Clementi M, Calzolari E, Turolla L, *et al.* Neonatal growth patterns in a population of consecutively born Down syndrome children. *Am J Med Genet* 1990; **7(Suppl)**: 71–4.
- ● 7 Cronk C, Crocker AC, Pueschel SM, *et al.* Growth charts for children with Down syndrome: 1 month to 18 years of age. *Pediatrics* 1988; **81**: 102–10.
- ● 8 Toledo C, Alembik Y, Aguirre JA, Stoll C. Growth curves of children with Down syndrome. *Ann Genet* 1999; **42**: 81–90.
- ● 9 Baty BJ, Blackburn BL, Carey JC. Natural history of trisomy 18 and trisomy 13: Growth, physical assessment, medical histories, survival, and recurrence risk. *Am J Med Genet* 1994; **49**: 175–88.
- ● 10 Tolmie JL. Down syndrome and other autosomal trisomies. In: Rimoin DL, Connor JM, Pyeritz RE, Korf BR (eds). *Emery and Rimoin's Principles and Practice of Medical Genetics.* London: Churchill Livingstone, 2002: 1129–83.
- ● 11 Allanson JE, Graham GE. Sex chromosome abnormalities. In: Rimoin DL, Connor JM, Pyeritz RE, Korf BR, eds. *Emery and Rimoin's Principles and Practice of Medical Genetics.* London: Churchill Livingstone, 2002: 1184–201.
- * 12 Sybert VP. Turner syndrome. In: Cassidy SB, Allanson JE, eds. *Management of Genetic Syndromes.* New York: Wiley-Liss, 2001: 459–84.
- ◆ 13 Schinzel A, ed. *Catalogue of Unbalanced Chromosome Aberrations in Man.* Berlin: De Gruyter, 2001.
- ● 14 Zollino M, Lecce R, Fischetto R, *et al.* Mapping the Wolf–Hirschhorn syndrome phenotype outside the currently accepted WHS critical region and defining a new critical region, WHSCR-2. *Am J Hum Genet* 2003; **72**: 590–7.
- ● 15 Zollino M, Di Stefano C, Zampino G, *et al.* Genotype–phenotype correlations and clinical diagnostic criteria in Wolf–Hirschhorn syndrome. *Am J Med Genet* 2000; **94**: 254–61.
- ● 16 Wieczorek D, Krause M, Majewski F, *et al.* Effect of the size of the deletion and clinical manifestations in Hirschhorn syndrome: analysis of 13 patients with a de novo deletion. *Eur J Hum Genet* 2000; **8**: 519–26.
- ● 17 Van Buggenhout G, Melotte C, Dutta B, *et al.* Mild Wolf–Hirschhorn syndrome: micro-array CGH analysis of atypical 4p16.3 deletions enables refinement of the genotype–phenotype map. *J Med Genet* 2004; **41**: 691–8.
- ● 18 Zhang A, Zheng C, Hou M, *et al.* Deletion of the telomerase reverse transcriptase gene and haploinsufficiency of telomere maintenance in Cri du chat syndrome. *Am J Hum Genet* 2003; **72**: 940–8.
- ● 19 Mainardi PC, Perfumo C, Cali A, *et al.* Clinical and molecular characterization of 80 patients with 5p deletion: genotype–phenotype correlation. *J Med Genet* 2001; **38**: 151–8.
- ● 20 Marinescu RC, Mainardi PC, Collins MR, *et al.* Growth charts for cri-du-chat syndrome: an international collaborative study. *Am J Med Genet* 2000; **94**: 153–62.
- ● 21 Gul D, Ogur G, Tunca Y, Ozcan O. Third case of WAGR syndrome with severe obesity and constitutional deletion of chromosome (11)(p12p14). *Am J Med Genet* 2002; **107**: 70–1.
- ● 22 Spinner NB, Emanuel BS. Deletions and other structural abnormalities of the autosomes. In: Rimoin DL, Connor JM, Pyeritz RE, Korf BR, eds. *Emery and Rimoin's Principles and Practice of Medical Genetics.* London: Churchill Livingstone, 2002: 1202–36.
- ● 23 Cassidy SB. Prader–Willi syndrome. In: Cassidy SB, Allanson JE, eds. *Management of Genetic Syndromes.* New York: Wiley-Liss, 2001: 301–22.

∗ 24 Eiholzer U, Whitman BY. A comprehensive team approach to the management of patients with Prader–Willi syndrome. *J Pediatr Endocrinol Metab* 2004; **17**: 1153–75.

● 25 Allen DB, Carrel AL. Growth hormone therapy for Prader–Willi syndrome: a critical appraisal. *J Pediatr Endocrinol Metab* 2004; **17(Suppl 4)**: 1297–306.

◆ 26 Dattani M, Preece M. Growth hormone deficiency and related disorders: insights into causation, diagnosis, and treatment. *Lancet* 2004: **363**: 1977–87.

● 27 Mortier GR. The diagnosis of skeletal dysplasias: a multidisciplinary approach. *Eur J Radiol* 2001: **40**: 161–7.

● 28 Grier RE, Farrington FH, Kendig R, Mamunes P. Autosomal dominant inheritance of the Aarskog syndrome. *Am J Med Genet* 1983: **15**: 39–46.

● 29 van de Vooren MJ, Niermeijer MF, Hoogeboom JM. The Aarskog syndrome in a large family suggestive for autosomal dominant inheritance. *Clin Genet* 1983: **24**: 439–45.

● 30 Pasteris NG, Cadle A, Logie LJ, *et al.* Isolation and characterization of the faciogenital dysplasia (Aarskog–Scott syndrome) gene: a putative Rho/Rac guanine nucleotide exchange factor. *Cell* 1994: **79**: 669–78.

● 31 Porteous MEM, Goudie DR. Aarskog syndrome. In: Donnai D, Winter RM, eds. *Congenital Malformation Syndromes.* London: Chapman & Hall Medical, 1995: 106–11.

● 32 Orrico A, Galli L, Cavaliere ML, *et al.* Phenotypic and molecular characterization of the Aarskog–Scott syndrome: a survey of the clinical variability in light of FGD1 mutation analysis in 46 patients. *Eur J Hum Genet* 2004; **12**: 16–23.

● 33 Afzal AR, Rajab A, Fenske C, *et al.* Autosomal recessive Robinow syndrome is allelic to dominant brachydactyly type B and caused by loss of function mutations in ROR2. *Nat Genet* 2000; **25**: 419–22.

● 34 van Bokhoven H, Celli J, Kayserili H, *et al.* Mutation of the gene encoding the ROR2 tyrosine kinase causes autosomal recessive Robinow syndrome. *Nat Genet* 2000; **25**: 423–6.

● 35 Patton MA, Afzal AR. Robinow syndrome. *J Med Genet* 2002; **39**: 305–10.

● 36 Weinstein LS, Gejman PV, Friedman E, *et al.* Mutations of the G$_s$ α-subunit gene in Albright hereditary osteodystrophy detected by denaturing gradient gel electrophoresis. *Proc Natl Acad Sci USA* 1990; **87**: 8287–90.

◆ 37 Spiegel AM, Weinstein LS. Inherited diseases involving G proteins and G protein-coupled receptors. *Annu Rev Med* 2004; **55**: 27–39.

● 38 Miric A, Vechio JD, Levine MA. Heterogeneous mutations in the gene encoding the α-subunit of the stimulatory G protein of adenyl cyclase in Albright hereditary osteodystrophy. *J Clin Endocrinol Metab USA* 1993; **76**: 1560–8.

● 39 Germain-Lee EL, Ding C-L, Deng Z, *et al.* Paternal imprinting of Gαs in the human thyroid as the basis of TSH resistance in pseudohypoparathyroidism type 1a. *Biochem Biophys Res Commun* 2002; **296**: 67–72.

● 40 Weinstein LS, Liu J, Sakamoto A, *et al.* Minireview: GNAS: normal and abnormal functions. *Endocrinology* 2004; **145**: 5459–64.

● 41 Fitch N. Albright hereditary osteodystrophy. A review. *Am J Med Genet* 1982; **11**: 11–29.

● 42 Wilson LC, Leverton K, Oude Luttikhuis ME, *et al.* Brachydactyly and mental retardation: an Albright hereditary osteodystrophy-like syndrome localized to 2q37. *Am J Hum Genet* 1995; **56**: 400–7.

● 43 Wilson LC, Oude Luttikhuis ME, Baraitser M, *et al.* Normal erythrocyte membrane Gs-alpha bioactivity in two unrelated patients with acrodysostosis. *J Med Genet* 1997; **34**: 133–6.

● 44 Graham JM, Krakow D, Tolo VT, *et al.* Radiographic findings and Gs-alpha bioactivity studies and mutation screening in acrodysostosis indicate a different etiology from pseudohypoparathyroidism. *Pediatr Radiol* 2001; **31**: 2–9.

● 45 Ellis NA, Groden J, Ye TZ, *et al.* The Bloom syndrome gene product is homologous to RecQ helicases. *Cell* 1995; **83**: 655–66.

● 46 German J. Bloom syndrome: a Mendelian prototype of somatic mutational disease. *Medicine* 1993; **72**: 393–406.

● 47 German J. Bloom syndrome: the first 100 cancers gene. *Cancer Genet Cytogenet* 1997; **93**: 100–6.

● 48 Hickson ID. RecQ helicases: caretakers of the genome. *Nat Rev Cancer* 2003; **3**: 169–78.

● 49 Chaganti RS, Schonberg S, German J. A manyfold increase in sister chromatid exchanges in Bloom syndrome lymphocytes. *Proc Natl Acad Sci USA* 1974; **71**: 4508–12.

● 50 Tischkowitz MD, Hodgson SV. Fanconi anaemia. *J Med Genet* 2003; **40**: 1–10.

● 51 Levitus M, Rooimans MA, Steltenpool J, *et al.* Heterogeneity in Fanconi anemia: evidence for 2 new genetic subtypes. *Blood* 2004; **103**: 2498–503.

● 52 Wajnrajch MP, Gertner JM, Huma Z, *et al.* Evaluation of growth and hormonal status in patients referred to the International Fanconi Anemia Registry. *Pediatrics* 2001; **107**: 744–54.

● 53 Butturini A, Gale RP, Verlander PC, *et al.* Hematologic abnormalities in Fanconi anemia: an International Fanconi Anemia Registry study. *Blood* 1994; **84**: 1650–5.

● 54 Alter BP. Cancer in Fanconi anemia, 1927–2001. *Cancer* 2003; **97**: 425–40.

● 55 Krantz ID, McCallum J, DeScipio C, *et al.* Cornelia de Lange syndrome is caused by mutations in NIPBL, the human homolog of *Drosophila melanogaster* Nipped-B. *Nat Genet* 2004; **36**: 631–5.

● 56 Tonkin ET, Wang TJ, Lisgo S, *et al.* NIPBL, encoding a homolog of fungal Scc2-type sister chromatid cohesion proteins and fly Nipped-B, is mutated in Cornelia de Lange syndrome. *Nat Genet* 2004; **36**: 636–41.

● 57 Musio A, Selicorni A, Focarelli ML, *et al.* X-linked Cornelia de Lange syndrome owing to SMC1L1 mutations. *Nat Genet* 2006; **38**: 528–30.

● 58   Deardorff MA, Kaur M, Yaeger D, *et al*. Mutations in cohesin complex members SMC3 and SMC1A cause a mild variant of Cornelia de Lange syndrome with predominant mental retardation. *Am J Hum Genet* 2007; **80**: 485–94.

● 59   Jackson L, Kline AD, Barr MA, Koch S. de Lange syndrome: a clinical review of 310 individuals. *Am J Med Genet* 1993; **47**: 940–6.

● 60   Ireland M, Donnai D, Burn J. Brachmann–de Lange syndrome. Delineation of the clinical phenotype. *Am J Med Genet* 1993; **47**: 959–64.

● 61   Butler MG, Dahir GA, Gale DD, Meaney FJ. Metacarpo-phalangeal pattern profile analysis in Brachmann–de Lange syndrome. *Am J Med Genet* 1993; **47**: 1003–5.

● 62   Kline AD, Barr M, Jackson LG. Growth manifestations in the Brachmann–de Lange syndrome. *Am J Med Genet* 1993; **47**: 1042–9.

● 63   Kline AD, Stanley C, Belevich J, *et al*. Developmental data on individuals with the Brachmann–de Lange syndrome. *Am J Med Genet* 1993; **47**: 1053–8.

● 64   Holder SE, Grimsley LM, Palmer RW, *et al*. Partial trisomy 3q causing mild Cornelia de Lange phenotype. *J Med Genet* 1994; **31**: 150–2.

● 65   Goodship J, Gill H, Carter J, *et al*. Autozygosity mapping of a Seckel syndrome locus to chromosome 3q22.1-q24. *Am J Hum Genet* 2000; **67**: 498–503.

● 66   Børglum AD, Balslev T, Haagerup A, *et al*. A new locus for Seckel syndrome on chromosome 18p11.31-q11.2. *Eur J Hum Genet* 2001; **9**: 753–57.

● 67   Kilinç MO, Ninis VN, Ugur SA, *et al*. Is the novel SCKL3 at 14q23 the predominant Seckel locus. *Eur J Hum Genet* 2003; **11**: 851–57.

● 68   O'Driscoll M, Ruiz-Perez VL, Woods CG, *et al*. A splicing mutation affecting expression of ataxia-telangiectasia and Rad3-related protein (ATR) results in Seckel syndrome. *Nat Genet* 2003; **33**: 497–501.

● 69   Casper AM, Durkin SG, Arlt MF, Glover TW. Chromosomal instability at common fragile sites in Seckel syndrome. *Am J Hum Genet* 2004; **75**: 654–60.

◆ 70   Spranger JW, Brill PW, Poznanski A, eds. *Bone Dysplasias: An Atlas of Genetic Disorders of Skeletal Development*. Oxford: University Press, 2002.

● 71   Hall JG, Flora C, Scott CI, *et al*. Majewski osteodysplastic primordial dwarfism type II: natural history and clinical findings. *Am J Med Genet* 2004; **130A**: 55–72.

● 72   Winter RM. Dubowitz syndrome. In: Donnai D, Winter RM, eds. *Congenital Malformation Syndromes*. London: Chapman & Hall Medical, 1995: 133–6.

● 73   Tsukahara M, Opitz JM. Dubowitz syndrome: review of 141 cases including 36 previously unreported patients. *Am J Med Genet* 1996; **63**: 277–89.

● 74   Hansen KE, Kirkpatrick SJ, Laxova R. Dubowitz syndrome: long-term follow-up of an original patient. *Am J Med Genet* 1995; **55**: 161–4.

● 75   Price SM, Stanhope R, Garrett C, *et al*. The spectrum of Silver–Russell syndrome: a clinical and molecular genetic study and new diagnostic criteria. *J Med Genet* 1999; **36**: 837–42.

● 76   Wollmann HA, Kirchner T, Enders H, *et al*. Growth and symptoms in Silver–Russell syndrome: review on the basis of 386 patients. *Eur J Pediatr* 1995; **154**: 958–68.

● 77   Saal HM, Pagon RA, Pepin MG. Reevaluation of Russell–Silver syndrome. *J Pediatr* 1985; **107**: 733–7.

● 78   Lai KY, Skuse D, Stanhope R, Hindmarsh P. Cognitive abilities associated with the Silver–Russell syndrome. *Arch Dis Child* 1994; **71**: 490–6.

● 79   Anderson J, Viskochil D, O'Gorman M, Gonzales C. Gastrointestinal complications of Russell–Silver syndrome: a pilot study. *Am J Med Genet* 2002; **113**: 15–9.

● 80   Hitchins MP, Stanier P, Preece MA, Moore GE. Silver–Russell syndrome: a dissection of the genetic aetiology and candidate chromosomal regions. *J Med Genet* 2001; **38**: 810–9.

● 81   Kotzot D, Balmer D, Baumer A, *et al*. Maternal uniparental disomy 7 – review and further delineation of the phenotype. *Eur J Pediatr* 2000; **159**: 247–56.

● 82   Charalambous M, Smith FM, Bennett WR, *et al*. Disruption of the imprinted Grb10 gene leads to disproportionate overgrowth by an Igf2-independent mechanism. *Proc Natl Acad Sci USA* 2003; **100**: 8292–7.

● 83   Midro AT, Debek K, Sawicka A, *et al*. Second observation of Silver–Russell syndrome in a carrier of a reciprocal translocation with one breakpoint at site 17q25. *Clin Genet* 1993; **44**: 53–5.

● 84   Escobar V, Gleiser S, Weaver DD. Phenotypic and genetic analysis of the Silver–Russell syndrome. *Clin Genet* 1978; **13**: 278–88.

● 85   Duncan PA, Hall JG, Shapiro LR, Vibert BK. Three-generation dominant transmission of the Silver–Russell syndrome. *Am J Med Genet* 1990; **35**: 245–50.

● 86   Hennekam RC, Bijlsma JB, Spranger J. Further delineation of the 3-M syndrome with review of the literature. *Am J Med Genet* 1987; **28**: 195–209.

● 87   Flannery DB. 3-M syndrome. *Am J Med Genet* 1989; **32**: 252–4.

● 88   van der Wal G, Otten BJ, Brunner HG, van der Burgt I. 3-M syndrome: description of six new patients with review of the literature. *Clin Dysmorphol* 2001; **10**: 241–52.

● 89   Elliott AM, Graham JM, Curry CJ, *et al*. Spectrum of dolichospondylic dysplasia: two new patients with distinctive findings. *Am J Med Genet* 2002; **113**: 351–61.

● 90   Pelletier G, Feingold M. Case report 1. In: Bergsma D, ed. *Syndrome Identification*, Vol 1. New York: White Plains, National Foundation – March of Dimes, 1973: 8–9.

● 91   Leisti J, Hollister DW, Rimoin DL. Case report 2. In: Bergsma D, ed. *Syndrome Identification*, Vol 2. New York: White Plains, National Foundation – March of Dimes, 1974: 305.

● 92   Houlston RS, Collins AL, Dennis NR, Temple IK. Further observation on the Floating–Harbor syndrome. *Clin Dysmorphol* 1994; **3**: 143–9.

● 93   Wieczorek D, Wüsthof A, Harms E, Meinecke P. Floating–Harbor syndrome in two unrelated girls: mild short stature in one patient and effective growth hormone therapy in the other. *Am J Med Genet* 2001; **104**: 47–52.

● 94   Patton MA, Hurst J, Donnai D, *et al*. Floating–Harbor syndrome. *J Med Genet* 1991; **28**: 201–4.

● 95   Ala-Mello S, Peippo M. The first Finnish patient with the Floating–Harbor syndrome: follow-up of eight years. *Am J Med Genet* 2004; **130A**: 317–9.

● 96   Perheentupa J, Autio S, Leisti S, *et al*. Mulibrey nanism, an autosomal recessive syndrome with pericardial constriction. *Lancet* 1973; **2**: 351–5.

● 97   Karlberg N, Jalanko H, Perheentupa J, Lipsanen-Nyman M. Mulibrey nanism: clinical features and diagnostic criteria. *J Med Genet* 2004; **41**: 92–8.

● 98   Avela K, Lipsanen-Nyman M, Idänheimo N, *et al*. Gene encoding a new RING-B-box-Coiled-coil protein is mutated in mulibrey nanism. *Nat Genet* 2000; **25**: 298–301.

● 99   Hamalainen RH, Avela K, Lambert JA, *et al*. Novel mutations in the TRIM37 gene in mulibrey nanism. *Hum Mutat* 2004; **23**: 522.

● 100   Kallijärvi J, Avela K, Lipsanen-Nyman M, *et al*. The TRIM37 gene encodes a peroxisomal RING-B-Box-Coiled-Coil protein: classification of mulibrey nanism as a new peroxisomal disorder. *Am J Hum Genet* 2002; **70**: 1215–28.

● 101   Raitta C, Perheentupa J. Mulibrey nanism: an inherited dysmorphic syndrome with characteristic ocular findings. *Acta Ophthalmol Suppl* 1974; **123**: 162–71.

● 102   Koenig R, Brendel L, Fuchs S. SHORT syndrome. *Clin Dysmorphol* 2003; **12**: 45–49.

● 103   Haan E, Morris L. SHORT syndrome: distinctive radiographic features. *Clin Dysmorphol* 1998; **7**: 103–7.

● 104   Toriello HV. Wiedemann-Rautenstrauch syndrome. In: Donnai D, Winter RM, eds. *Congenital Malformation Syndromes*. London: Chapman & Hall Medical, 1995: 137–40.

● 105   Pivnick EK, Angle B, Kaufman RA, *et al*. Neonatal progeroid (Wiedemann–Rautenstrauch) syndrome: report of five new cases and review. *Am J Med Genet* 2000; **90**: 131–40.

● 106   Tartaglia M, Mehler EL, Goldberg R, *et al*. Mutations in PTPN11, encoding the protein tyrosine phosphatase SHP-2, cause Noonan syndrome. *Nat Genet* 2001; **29**: 465–8.

● 107   Roberts AE, Araki T, Swanson KD, et al. Germline gain-of-function mutations in SOS1 cause Noonan syndrome. *Nat Genet* 2007; **39**: 70–4.

● 108   Allanson JE, Hall JG, Hughes HE, *et al*. Noonan syndrome: the changing phenotype. *Am J Med Genet* 1985; **21**: 507–14.

∗ 109   Allanson JE. Noonan syndrome. In: Cassidy SB, Allanson JE, eds. *Management of Genetic Syndromes*. New York: Wiley-Liss, 2001: 253–68.

● 110   Noonan JA, Raaijmakers R, Hall BD. Adult height in Noonan syndrome. *Am J Med Genet* 2003; **123**: 68–71.

● 111   Witt DR, Keena BA, Hall JG, Allanson JE. Growth curves for height in Noonan syndrome. *Clin Genet* 1986; **30**: 150–3.

● 112   Kirk JM, Betts PR, Butler GE, *et al*. Short stature in Noonan syndrome: response to growth hormone therapy. *Arch Dis Child* 2001; **84**: 440–3.

● 113   Noordam C, van der Burgt I, Sengers RC, *et al*. Growth hormone treatment in children with Noonan syndrome: four year results of a partially controlled trial. *Acta Paediatr* 2001; **90**: 889–94.

● 114   van der Burgt I, Thoonen G, Roosenboom N, *et al*. Patterns of cognitive functioning in school-aged children with Noonan syndrome associated with variability in phenotypic expression. *J Pediatr* 1999; **135**: 707–13.

● 115   Keren B, Hadchouel A, Saba S, *et al*. PTPN11 mutations in patients with LEOPARD syndrome: French multicentric experience. *J Med Genet* 2004; **41**: e117.

● 116   Gelb BD, Tartaglia M. Noonan syndrome and related disorders: dysregulated RAS-mitogen activated protein kihase signal transduction. *Human Molec Genet* 2006; **15**: R220–6.

● 117   Hall BD. Choanal atresia and associated multiple anomalies. *J Pediatr* 1979; **95**: 395–8.

● 118   Hittner HM, Hirsch NJ, Kreh GM, Rudolph AJ. Colobomatous microphthalmia, heart disease, hearing loss and mental retardation: a syndrome. *J Pediatr Ophthalmol Strabismus* 1979; **16**: 122–8.

● 119   Amiel J, Attie-Bitach T, Marianowski R, *et al*. Temporal bone anomaly proposed as a major criteria for diagnosis of CHARGE syndrome. *Am J Med Genet* 2001; **99**: 124–7.

● 120   Graham JM Jr. Editorial comment: A recognizable syndrome within CHARGE association: Hall–Hittner syndrome. *Am J Med Genet* 2001; **99**: 120–3.

∗ 121   Oley CA. CHARGE association. In: Cassidy SB, Allanson JE, eds. *Management of Genetic Syndromes*. New York: Wiley-Liss, 2001: 71–84.

● 122   Tellier AL, Cormier-Daire V, Abadle V, *et al*. CHARGE syndrome: report of 47 cases and review. *Am J Med Genet* 1998; **76**: 402–9.

● 123   Vissers LE, van Ravenswaaij CM, Admiraal R, *et al*. Mutations in a new member of the chromodomain gene family cause CHARGE syndrome. *Nature Genet* 2004; **36**: 955–7.

● 124   Smithson SF, Thompson EM, McKinnon AG, *et al*. The KBG syndrome. *Clin Dysmorphol* 2000; **9**: 87–91.

● 125   Herrmann J, Pallister PD, Tiddy W, *et al*. The KBG syndrome – a syndrome of short stature, characteristic facies, mental retardation, macrodontia and skeletal anomalies. *BDOAS* 1975; **11**: 7–18.

● 126   Dowling PA, Fleming P, Gorlin RJ, *et al*. The KBG syndrome, characteristic dental findings: a case report. *Int J Paediatr Dent* 2001; **11**: 131–4.

● 127   Tekin M, Kavaz A, Berberoglu M, *et al*. The KBG syndrome: confirmation of autosomal dominant inheritance and further delineation of the phenotype. *Am J Med Genet* 2004; **130A**: 284–7.

● 128   Petrij F, Dauwerse HG, Blough RI, *et al*. Diagnostic analysis of the Rubinstein–Taybi syndrome: five cosmids should be used for microdeletion detection and low number of protein truncating mutations. *J Med Genet* 2000; **37**: 168–76.

● 129 Petrij F, Giles RH, Dauwerse HG, *et al.* Rubinstein–Taybi syndrome caused by mutations in the transcriptional co-activator CBP. *Nature* 1995; **376**: 348–51.

● 130 Allanson JE. Microcephaly in Rubinstein–Taybi syndrome. *Am J Med Genet* 1993; **46**: 244–6.

● 131 Stevens CA, Hennekam RCM, Blackburn BL. Growth in the Rubinstein–Taybi syndrome. *Am J Med Genet* 1990; **37(Suppl 6)**: 51–55.

● 132 Stevens C, Bhakta M. Cardiac abnormalities in the Rubinstein–Taybi syndrome. *Am J Med Genet* 1995; **59d**: 346–8.

● 133 Rubinstein J. Broad thumb-hallux (Rubinstein–Taybi) syndrome 1957–1988. *Am J Med Genet* 1990; **37(Suppl 6)**: 3–16.

● 134 Hennekam RCM, Van Den Boogaard MJ, Sibbles BJ, Van Spijker HG. Rubinstein–Taybi syndrome in the Netherlands. *Am J Med Genet* 1990; **37(Suppl 6)**: 17–29.

● 135 Stevens CA, Carey JC, Blackburn BL. Rubinstein–Taybi syndrome: a natural history study. *Am J Med Genet* 1990; **37(Suppl 6)**: 30–7.

∗ 136 Wiley S, Swayne S, Rubinstein JH, *et al.* Rubinstein–Taybi syndrome medical guidelines. *Am J Med Genet* 2003; **119A**: 101–10.

● 137 Kuroki Y, Suzuki Y, Chyo H, *et al.* A new malformation syndrome of long palpebral fissures, large ears, depressed nasal tip and skeletal anomalies associated with postnatal dwarfism and mental retardation. *J Pediatr* 1981; **99**: 570–3.

● 138 Niikawa N, Matsuura N, Fukushima, *et al.* Kabuki make-up syndrome: a syndrome of mental retardation, unusual facies, large and protruding ears, and postnatal growth deficiency. *J Pediatr* 1981; **99**: 565–9.

● 139 Armstrong L, El Moneim AA, Aleck K, *et al.* Further delineation of Kabuki syndrome in 48 well-defined new individuals. *Am J Med Genet* 2004; **132A**: 265–72.

● 140 Nance MA, Berry SA. Cockayne syndrome: review of 140 cases. *Am J Med Genet* 1992; **42**: 68–84.

● 141 Boltshauser E, Yalcinkaya C, Wichmann W, *et al.* MRI in Cockayne syndrome type I. *Neuroradiology* 1989; **31**: 276–7.

● 142 Dollfus H, Porto F, Caussade P, *et al.* Ocular manifestations in the inherited DNA repair disorders. *Surv Ophthalmol* 2003; **48**: 107–22.

● 143 Mayne LV, Lehmann AR. Failure of RNA synthesis to recover after UV-irradiation: an early defect in cells from individuals with Cockayne syndrome and xeroderma pigmentosa. *Cancer Res* 1982; **42**: 1473–8.

● 144 Van Gool AJ, Citterio E, Rademakers S, *et al.* The Cockayne syndrome B protein, involved in transcription-coupled DNA repair, resides in an RNA polymerase II-containing complex. *EMBO J* 1997; **16**: 5955–65.

● 145 Rapin I, Lindenbaum Y, Dickson DW, *et al.* Cockayne syndrome and xeroderma pigmentosum. *Neurology* 2000; **55**: 1442–9.

● 146 Meira LB, Graham JM Jr, Greenberg CR, *et al.* Manitoba aboriginal kindred with original cerebro-oculo-facio-skeletal syndrome has a mutation in the Cockayne syndrome group B gene. *Am J Hum Genet* 2000; **66**: 1221–8.

● 147 Brown WT. Progeria: a human disease model of accelerated ageing. *Am J Clin Nutr* 1992; **55**: 1222S–4S.

● 148 Pollex RL, Hegele RA. Hutchinson–Gilford progeria syndrome. *Clin Genet* 2004; **66**: 375–81.

● 149 Baker PB, Baba N, Boesel CP. Cardiovascular abnormalities in progeria. Case report and review of the literature. *Arch Pathol Lab Med* 1981; **105**: 384–6.

● 150 De Sandre-Giovannoli A, Bernard R, Cau P, *et al.* Lamin A truncation in Hutchinson-Gilford progeria. *Science* 2003; **300**: 2055.

● 151 Eriksson M, Brown WT, Gordon LB, *et al.* Recurrent de novo point mutations in lamin A cause Hutchinson–Gilford progeria syndrome. *Nature* 2003; **423**: 293–8.

∗ 152 Worman HJ. Nuclear envelope proteins and human disease. In: Evans DE, Hutchinson CJ, Bryant JA, eds. *The Nuclear Envelope.* New York: BIOS Scientific Publishers, 2004: 41–56.

18

Genetic and dysmorphic syndromes with increased stature

MICHAEL A PATTON, NAZNEEN RAHMAN

INTRODUCTION

In most cultures increased stature is less rarely perceived to be a problem than short stature. However, it may become socially unacceptable or it may be associated with other medical problems and will therefore present to the growth clinic. The initial approach to tall stature is similar to that used for short stature. It is important to assess the child's height against standard growth charts and to decide whether the child has normal body proportions or not. There will be a number of children with proportionate tall stature whose growth falls into the upper centiles of the normal distribution and some of these may be predicted from analysis of parental heights.

Where disproportionate growth occurs it is more likely that there is an underlying genetic syndrome. These are considered later. In most cases the genes and molecular pathology have not yet been fully elucidated, but for some syndromes fascinating insights into the control of local growth factors have been identified, and the border between overgrowth and malignant growth can be seen to be a fine dividing line.

There are various approaches to the classification of syndromes with tall stature[1] and some overlap with syndromes where there is local overgrowth without tall stature. In this chapter the disorders are considered in three groups:

1. Tall stature as a result of normal variation
2. Tall stature of pre-natal onset
3. Tall stature of post-natal onset

There is a more general discussion of the genetic control of growth and the medical and surgical management of tall stature elsewhere in this book (see Chapters 4, 46 and 47).

TALL STATURE AS A RESULT OF NORMAL VARIATION

It is obviously of great importance to decide first whether a child's excessive growth falls within the normal range or not, and to do this requires some understanding of the genetic determinants of height. Birth weight and birth length are largely determined by intrauterine factors and are not very good predictors of final adult height. One way of determining the genetic contribution to this is to study the correlation between monozygotic (MZ) twins and dizygotic (DZ) twins. In the former case the twins share the genetic information and should, in theory, have a correlation of 1.0 for genetic traits. In the latter case, they share only 50 percent of the genetic material in common and should have a correlation of 0.5 for genetic traits. At birth MZ twins are actually less alike than DZ twins. This initial discordance may reflect the fact that there was unequal division of the ovum or zygote or may be the result of unequal blood supply from the placenta or because one twin is being more compressed *in utero*. However, the position changes and by 4 years of age the correlation in height is 0.94 in MZ twins and 0.6 in DZ twins.[2]

Adult height shows a normal gaussian distribution in the population. This has been taken to indicate that there

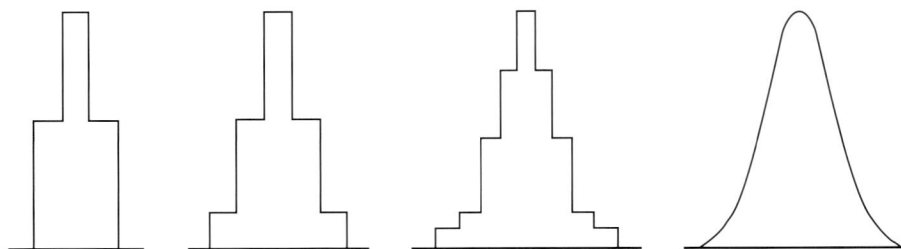

Figure 18.1   The additive effect of genes in polygenic inheritance will lead to a normal distribution.

are many genes and also many environmental factors that determine final height. The way in which many genes may have an additive effect to produce a normal distribution is illustrated in Fig. 18.1. It can be seen from this that the effect of even a relatively small number of genes will produce a normal distribution curve and it is not possible to calculate the number of genes that might be involved. However, in other areas where polygenic inheritance was proposed and in which the genes are being identified, it appears that there may be only a small number of major genes involved. It is, therefore, possible that the same may apply in determining height.

With the polygenic inheritance of stature, the effect of having a tall parent is corrected to some extent because only half the genes are inherited from the tall parent and the other half come from the other parent. This means that a child with one tall parent will tend to have a final height closer to the mean. However, the polygenic model assumes random or non-assortive mating. This is not always the case especially at either end of the height distribution, i.e., tall women may seek out tall men and vice versa. Here the additive effects may produce an exceptionally tall child whose height draws medical attention and the possibility of disorders such as Marfan syndrome may be raised.

A study of correlation of adult height between parent and child shows that the correlations are broadly similar between father and son (0.54), mother and daughter (0.47), father and daughter (0.52) and mother and son (0.53).[3] These figures are close to the theoretical correlation of 0.5. This fits with the polygenic model where all genes are of equal effect and none is dominant over the others. In clinical practice when a full pedigree with the heights of all relatives is recorded, it may occasionally be noted that the tall stature appears to be inherited predominantly from one side of the family. These unusual families may be explained by statistical variation, but could be of value in further genetic research to identify genes controlling final height.

In addition to assessing the genetic influence on final height, it may be important in the clinic to assess the genetic influence on the tempo of development. There is relatively little information about this other than in connection to the age of menarche. A significant part of the variation in this is genetic as the sister–sister correlation and mother–daughter correlation are both around 0.4. It is likely that skeletal maturity, as manifest by bone age or dental eruption, is also genetically determined. Better understanding of these correlations would be helpful in assessing the tall child who may reach puberty earlier than his or her peers.

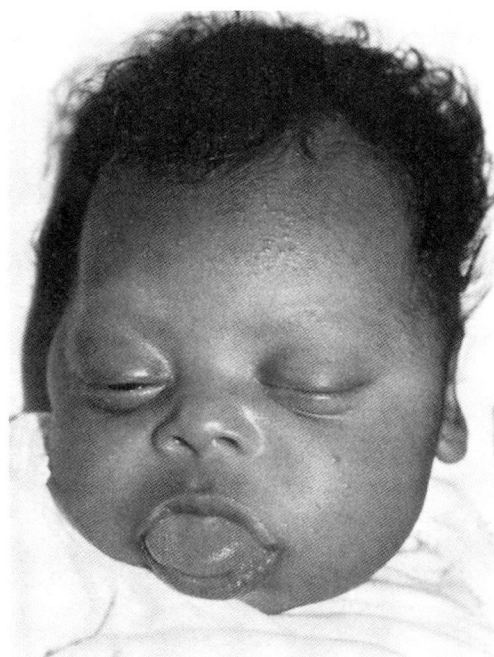

Figure 18.2   The macroglossia in Beckwith–Wiedemann syndrome can be striking in the neonatal period.

TALL STATURE WITH PRE-NATAL ONSET

Beckwith–Wiedemann syndrome

Beckwith–Wiedemann syndrome (MIM 130650) is characterized by pre-natal and post-natal overgrowth, macroglassia and anterior abdominal wall defects that range from mild umbilical hernia to exomphalos (Fig. 18.2). Additional features that are variably present include organomegaly, neonatal hypoglycemia, hemihypertrophy and urogenital abnormalities. Intelligence is usually normal but developmental delay is sometimes present, particularly if hypoglycemia occurs in the neonatal period. Creases on the anterior surface of the ear lobe and pits over the posterior surface of the pinna may be helpful in making the diagnosis. The syndrome affects approximately 1 in 14 000 births.[4]

Increased fetal growth is usually noted in the last trimester and may be accompanied by polyhydramnios, a large placenta and preterm delivery. The birth weight and birth length are usually increased, although occasionally the increased growth may not start until after birth. Growth velocity and bone age are advanced in the first 4–6 years of life, after which they may return to normal. Final height tends to be at the upper end of the normal range.[5]

Approximately 5 percent of children with Beckwith–Wiedemann syndrome develop embryonal tumors. Wilms' tumor occurs most frequently, but hepatoblastoma, adrenal carcinoma, rhabdomyosarcoma and pancreatoblastoma may also occur.[6] Over 90 percent of tumors develop by 7 years. The risk of tumors is greater in cases with hemihypertrophy and may differ according to the underlying cause.[7] There is controversy about the benefits of screening, but 3 monthly abdominal ultrasounds for at least 7 years are generally recommended.

The genetic basis of Beckwith–Wiedemann syndrome is complex and involves altered function of several closely linked genes in an imprinted region on chromosome 11p15.5.[8] Imprinting is an epigenetic modification that allows gene expression to be altered according to the parent-of-origin. Imprinted genes implicated in Beckwith–Wiedemann syndrome include the paternally expressed *IGF2* and *KCNQ1OT1* (*LIT1*) genes and the maternally expressed *H19*, *CDKNIC* (*P57KIP2*) and *KCNQ1* genes. There are three major subgroups of Beckwith–Wiedemann syndrome: chromosomal (2 percent, usually duplications of 11p15), familial (15 percent, of which 40 percent are due to *CDKNIC* mutations) and sporadic (83 percent). Sporadic Beckwith–Wiedemann cases can be further subdivided according to the underlying molecular pathology. Approximately 5 percent are due to *CDKNIC* mutations and 10–20 percent are due to uniparental disomy. Up to 60 percent of sporadic cases are due to epigenetic modifications known as epimutations that affect two separate imprinting centers. The second imprinting center is located in intron 10 of the *KCNQ1* gene and is known as KvDMR1. Loss of methylation at KvDMR1 is seen in up to 50 percent of sporadic Beckwith–Wiedemann cases and is the commonest known cause of the syndrome.[9]

Simpson–Golabi–Behmel syndrome

Simpson–Golabi–Behmel syndrome (MIM 312870) is an X-linked recessive condition characterized by pre-natal and post-natal overgrowth, dysmorphic features and a spectrum of congenital malformations that show some overlap with Beckwith–Wiedemann syndrome. Overgrowth is of pre-natal onset and continues post-natally. Birth length, birth weight and head circumference of affected males are usually well above the 97th centile and adult height can exceed 2 m, although height is variable.[10]

There is a characteristically coarse facial appearance with large protruding jaw, widened nasal bridge, central cleft of the lower lip and dental irregularity (Fig. 18.3). A very wide range of other malformations has been reported, including congenital heart disease, heart arrythmias, postaxial polydactyly, hypoplastic nails, accessory nipples, pectus excavatum, rib/vertebral anomalies, submucous cleft palate, umbilical hernia, hypospadias, cryptorchidism, and cystic

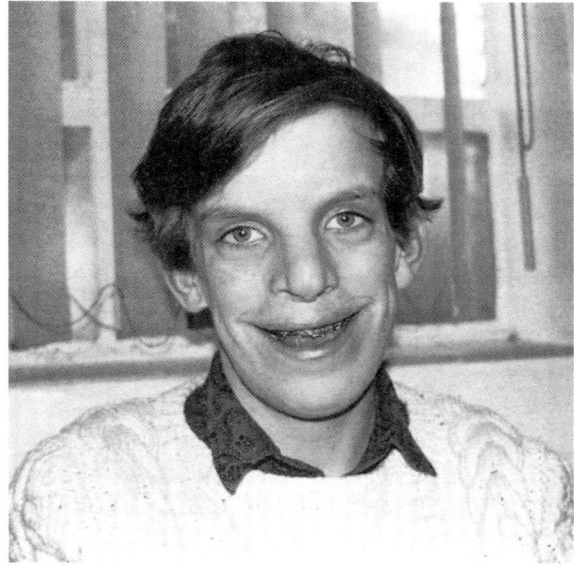

Figure 18.3 This boy has Simpson–Golabi–Behmel syndrome. Note the large jaw, wide mouth, dental problems and central cleft in the lower lip.

dysplasia of the kidneys.[10] The risk of embryonal tumors is similar to that of Beckwith–Wiedemann syndrome, but the condition is much less common. It is, however, sometimes associated with early mortality, which may be the result of cardiac arrhythmias.[11]

The Simpson–Golabi–Behmel syndrome is due to deletions or inactivating mutations in the glypican-3 gene (*GPC3*).[12] GPC3 is a cell surface proteoglycan implicated in regulating cell proliferation and apoptosis by modulating cellular responses to growth factors.[13] It was initially proposed that GPC3 acts as a growth suppressor by forming a complex with IGF2 that down-regulates IGF2 activity.[12] However, mouse models of Simpson–Golabi–Behmel syndrome demonstrate that overgrowth is largely IGF2 independent and suggest that the major GPC3 binding factor is not IGF2. Nevertheless, it is possible that the phenotypic overlap between Beckwith–Wiedemann syndrome and Simpson–Golabi–Behmel syndrome may result from downstream convergence of independent signaling pathways in which IGF2 and GPC3 participate.[14] A second locus associated with a more severe form of the disorder (MIM 300209) was mapped to Xp22 in a single family, but the causative gene has not been identified.[15]

Perlman syndrome

Perlman syndrome (MIM 267000) is an autosomal recessive condition characterized by pre-natal overgrowth, bilateral nephroblastomatosis, Wilms tumor, high mortality and characteristic facial features including a full round face and deeply set eyes. Originally reported by Perlman[16] in 1973, fifteen cases from six different families have been reported.[17] There is phenotypic overlap with both Beckwith–Wiedemann

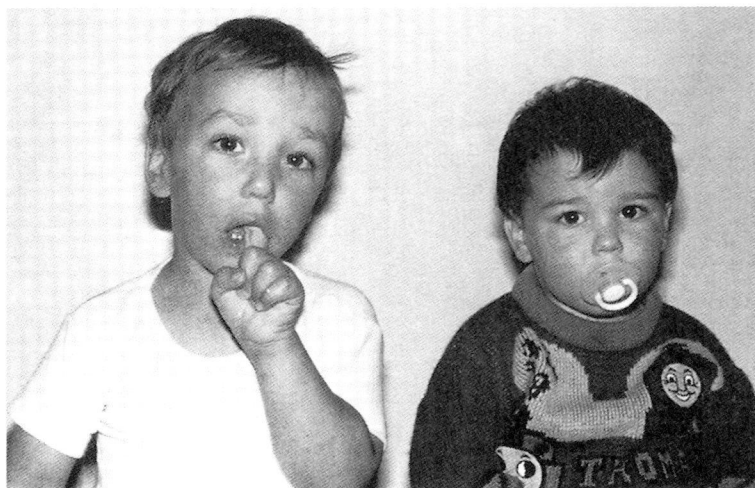

Figure 18.4 This illustrates the discrepancy in size and facial features in twin boys in which the brother on the left has Sotos syndrome and the other does not.

syndrome and Simpson–Golabi–Behmel syndrome, but the underlying molecular cause is unknown.

Sotos syndrome

Sotos et al.[18] described five children with excessively rapid growth, large heads and some developmental delay (MIM 117550). They used the term 'cerebral gigantism' to describe the condition but the eponymous 'Sotos syndrome' is generally used. Although there are overlapping features seen in a number of overgrowth syndromes, the phenotype was clearly defined in a series of 79 patients.[19] Affected children have increased length and increased head circumference at birth (both usually >97th centile). The length is greater in proportion than the weight, and both the height and head circumference tend to remain above the 97th centile during childhood, although final height is not necessarily increased. There is a recognizable facies (Fig. 18.4) with a large broad forehead and sparse hair over the frontoparietal region together with a prominent jaw and downslanting palpebral fissures.

Almost all children with Sotos syndrome have some developmental delay but this is very variable ranging from mild intellectual impairment in individuals that lead independent lives and have families of their own, to severe developmental and behavioral problems in individuals that require constant care. The majority of children have mild to moderate intellectual impairment. Advanced bone age, cardiac and genitourinary anomalies, neonatal jaundice, neonatal hypotonia, seizures and scoliosis are all fairly common in Sotos syndrome. A wide variety of tumors have been reported, but most of these were in unsubstantiated cases. In a review of >250 Sotos cases the overall incidence of tumors was very low and only neuroblastoma and sacrococcygeal teratomas occurred at increased frequency compared to the general population. However, the absolute risk of these tumors was low and the teratomas generally had a benign course.[20]

In 2002, Kurotaki et al.[21] reported a Sotos syndrome case with a de novo translocation t(5,8)(q35;q24.1) that bisected the NSD1 (nuclear receptor-binding SET domain containing protein) gene on chromosome 5q35.3 and identified microdeletions encompassing NSD1 and intragenic NSD1 mutations in several Sotos syndrome cases.[21] NSD1 is a histone methyltransferase implicated in transcriptional regulation and is believed to act as both a positive and negative regulator of transcription depending on the cellular context.[22]

Several other groups have confirmed that NSD1 alterations cause Sotos syndrome. In all populations examined outside Japan NSD1 mutations are the principal cause of Sotos syndrome accounting for >80 percent of typical Sotos syndrome cases.[23,24] Microdeletions account for approximately 10 percent of non-Japanese cases. It is likely that the remaining Sotos cases are due to undetected NSD1 abnormalities and there is no evidence of heterogeneity. Almost all cases are due to new mutations occurring in the child with Sotos syndrome and the recurrence risk of unaffected parents is extremely low. However, the offspring risk for Sotos syndrome cases that go on to have children is 50 percent.[20]

Weaver syndrome

In 1974, Weaver et al.[25] reported a syndrome of persistent overgrowth of pre-natal onset, accelerated osseous maturation, distinctive craniofacial appearance, developmental delay, widened distal long bones and camptodactyly (MIM 277590). There is overlap with Sotos syndrome, but classic Weaver syndrome cases can be distinguished by more pronounced hypertelorism, a small but prominent chin, which appears almost 'stuck on' and the presence of camptodactyly and prominent fetal pads on the finger tips (Fig. 18.5). Some cases with overlapping Sotos/Weaver phenotype have NSD1 mutations, but no classic Weaver syndrome case has been attributed to this gene and a separate, currently unknown

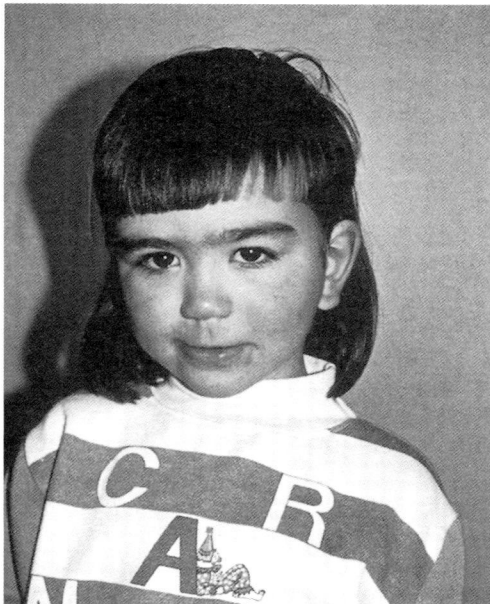

(a)

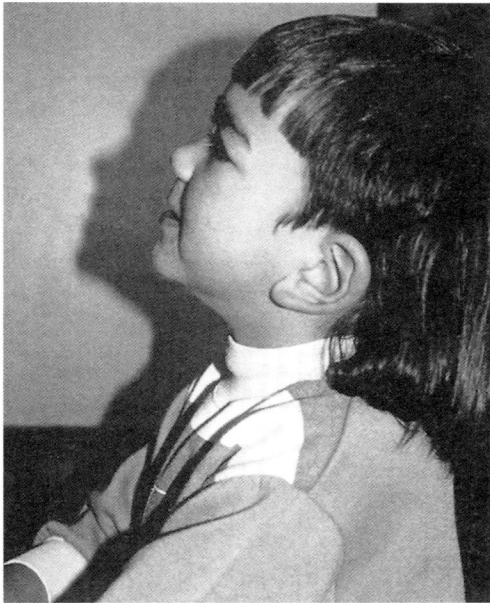

(b)

Figure 18.5 This girl has Weaver syndrome. She is large for her chronological age and has large ears and a small pointed chin.

cause, is likely to be responsible for this syndrome.[23] Most cases are sporadic.

Marshall–Smith syndrome

Infants with this syndrome (MIM 602535) have increased length and bone age at birth, but tend to be underweight. The facial features include prominent forehead, prominent eyes with shallow orbits, and a flat upturned nose, which may be associated with choanal atresia. Weight gain is poor and respiratory problems are common. Developmental delay is the rule and death in the first 2 years of life has been reported in most patients.[26]

The hand radiograph shows a characteristic pattern with thickened proximal and middle phalanges in the second to fifth digits, with small hypoplastic distal phalanges. Bone histology is also abnormal and it has been suggested that this may represent more than precocious bone maturation.[27] All cases of Marshall–Smith syndrome have been sporadic and the etiology is unknown.

Nevo syndrome

Nevo and colleagues[28] described three cases of 'cerebral gigantism' in a large consanguineous Israeli family (MIM 601451). They had increased birth length, generalized hypotonia and some advancement of the bone age. They did not have increased head circumferences or the facial features seen in Sotos syndrome. Another difference from Sotos syndrome was the presence of contractures and edema of the hands with spindle-shaped fingers and wrist drop. To date, seven children from five families have been reported.[29] Inheritance is autosomal recessive and Nevo syndrome is clearly distinct from Sotos syndrome. The cause is unknown.

Bannayan–Riley–Ruvalcaba syndrome

This autosomal dominant overgrowth syndrome (MIM 153480) includes macrocephaly, vascular malformations, lipomas, hamartomous polyps, and pigmented macules on the shaft of the penis and was initially described independently by three groups: Bannayan–Zonana, Riley– Smith and Ruvalcaba–Myre; Cohen[30] recognized that all had been describing the same disorder from slightly different standpoints. Birth weight is usually in excess of 4 kg and the birth length is above the 97th centile. The increased length only remains in the first few years of life and the final height is usually not increased. There is no increased bone age. However, the head circumference is increased at birth and remains increased throughout life. Developmental delay, speech defects, and hypotonia are frequent. In the bowel, polyps in the terminal ileum or colon may be associated with rectal bleeding or intussusception.

Approximately 50–60 percent of cases have inactivating mutations in *PTEN*.[31] This gene also causes Cowden syndrome (MIM 158350), a complex disorder including malignant and benign (hamartomatous) lesions affecting derivatives of all three germ layers.[32] Cowden syndrome is associated with increased risks of breast cancer, thyroid cancer and endometrial cancer. Although Bannayan–Riley– Ruvalcaba syndrome has not traditionally been associated with these cancers, the identification of germline *PTEN* mutations identical to those present in Cowden syndrome has led to cancer screening in affected adults with this condition.

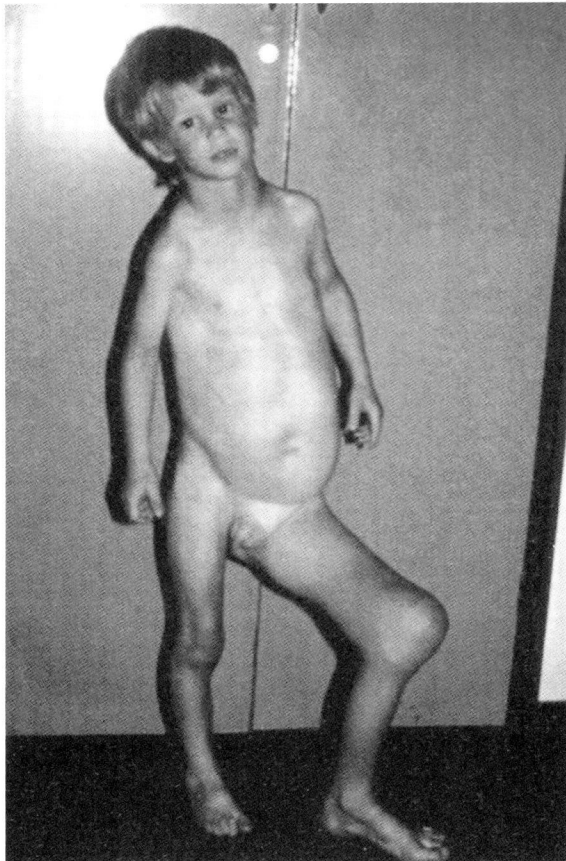

Figure 18.6 This boy had an initial diagnosis of Klippel–Trenauney–Weber syndrome, but was subsequently recognized as having Proteus syndrome. The leg discrepancy here was so great that amputation was ultimately required.

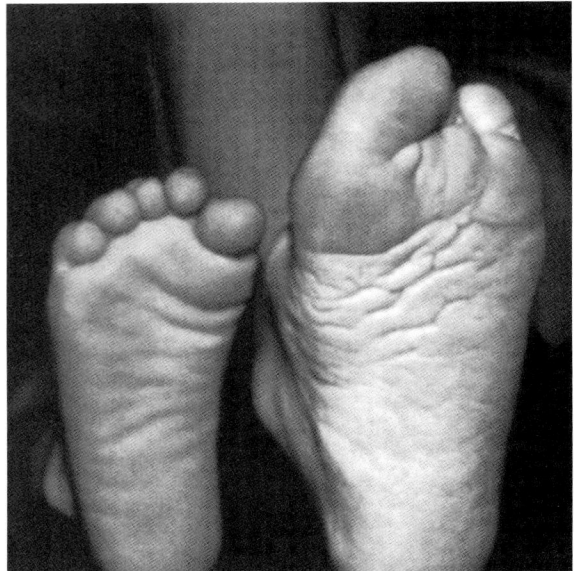

Figure 18.7 The deep verrucous skin on the soles of the feet is a characteristic sign of Proteus syndrome.

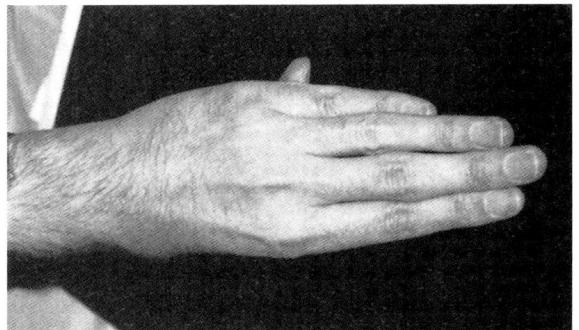

Figure 18.8 The Steinberg or thumb sign may be a feature of Marfan syndrome.

PTEN has also been implicated in some cases of Proteus syndrome (MIM 176920).[33] Although this condition is not associated with tall stature it can include progressive overgrowth of multiple tissues. The great majority of classic cases are not due to *PTEN* and the predominant cause(s) is unknown (Figs 18.6 and 18.7).

TALL STATURE SYNDROMES WITH POST-NATAL ONSET

Marfan syndrome

This autosomal dominant disorder (MIM 154700) was first described in 1896 by Antoinie Marfan[34] and it has been suggested that both Abraham Lincoln and Paginini were affected by this condition. It is one of the best known causes of tall stature and occurs in two per 10 000 births.

It is characterized by a height around or above the 97th centile with long limbs. It is usually said that the arm span is greater than the height, but this is not a very reliable diagnostic sign because a considerable proportion of the taller members of the population also have a greater arm span.[35] It is therefore better to take an arm span 8 cm greater than the height because this is found in only 5 percent of the normal tall population, but is seen in patients with Marfan syndrome. Similarly the presence of arachnodactyly with the Steinberg sign (deviation of the flexed thumb past the ulnar border of the hand) (Fig. 18.8) is suggestive, but not diagnostic, of Marfan syndrome, because it may also occur in the taller members of the general public. To make a diagnosis of Marfan syndrome as opposed to tall stature, where there is no family history of Marfan syndrome, it is important to have at least one characteristic sign in either the heart or the eyes.[36] The other skeletal features are kyphoscoliosis, joint laxity, pectus excavatum, pes planus, and a high arched palate with dental overcrowding.

Myopia is frequent and often appears early in childhood, and should therefore be screened for. Later, lens dislocation is frequent (Fig. 18.9). If the lens dislocates into the anterior chamber acute glaucoma may develop. Occasionally retinal detachment can occur.

The main cause of death in Marfan syndrome is as a result of aortic dissection. This occurs after the ascending aorta has

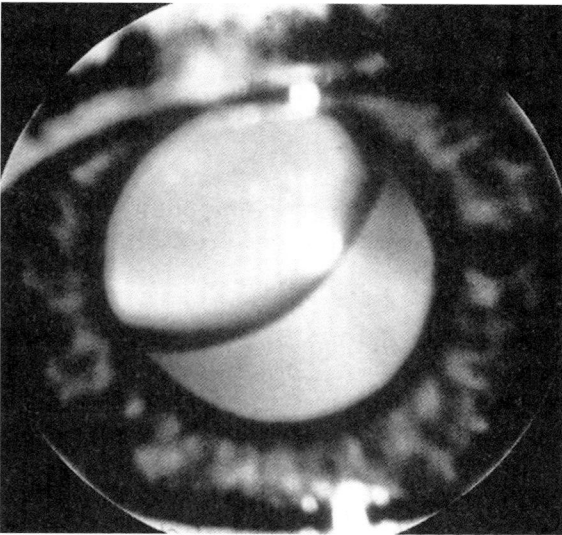

Figure 18.9   Lens dislocation may be a feature of Marfan syndrome.

become dilated, and it is important to use echocardiography to screen the aortic root diameter regularly. If it reaches 5 cm or more, a surgical correction using the Bentall procedure should be carried out.[37] This approach has improved the survival for patients with Marfan syndrome, although there is still a somewhat reduced lifespan especially for males.[38] Beta blockers are often prescribed to try to delay the aortic widening, but they often cause sleep disturbances and excessive lethargy when used in children. In children aortic problems are rare, but there may be mitral valve prolapse and this may go on to mitral valve regurgitation in adult life. Aortic valve regurgitation also frequently occurs.

Other systems are involved in Marfan syndrome. Pneumothorax occurs when there is rupture of lung bullae. Obstructive sleep apnea occurs frequently and is often overlooked because it is usually seen in obese rather than tall thin individuals and the tiredness may be attributed to cardiac problems.[39] Striae are frequently seen and are particularly characteristic over the lumbar spine, where they appear at right angles to the vertical growth in the spine at the onset of puberty. Hernias are also common. In the spine there may be protrusion of the dura seen on computed tomography and this may be associated with nerve root symptoms.

Inheritance is autosomal dominant with about one-third of cases arising as new mutations. The disorder was mapped by chromosome rearrangements and linkage studies to chromosome 15, and subsequently the disease was found to be caused by abnormalities in the fibrillin 1 gene (*FBN1*). This gene is large (110 kb) and has 56 exons. It has an epidermal growth factor (EGF)-like domain at the N-terminal end and cysteine-coding residues at a number of posts within the gene, which are responsible for the disulfide cross-binding sites in the protein. Most mutations that have been identified are point mutations in the cysteine-coding sequences, and in the very severe neonatal forms there have been mutations in the EGF-like domains (exons 24–32). Mutations

act by exerting a dominant negative effect, i.e., mutant fibrillin monomers act by disrupting the packing of the protein and hence the function of the microfibrils. Unfortunately, diagnostic testing is still complex as the majority of mutations are novel and require extensive sequence of the *FBN1* gene. The situation is further complicated by genetic heterogeneity. A similar phenotype (MIM 154705) without ocular complications.[40] has been mapped to chromosome 3p25 and identified to be due to mutations in TGF beta receptor 2 (TGFBR2).[41] There is another fibrillin gene (*FBN2*) located on chromosome 5 that causes the more severe skeletal complications seen in congenital contractural arachnodactyly or Beal's syndrome. Marfanoid features with craniosynostosis, craniofacial abnormalities, contractures and abdominal herniae have been described as Sprintzen–Goldberg syndrome (MIM 182212). Some cases of the Sphrintzen–Goldberg syndrome have been confirmed as having fibrillin 1 mutations.[42]

Abnormalities in fibrillin explain the pathophysiology of Marfan syndrome.[43] The ascending aorta, suspensory ligament of the lens and the periosteum all have large amounts of fibrillin and abnormalities in the protein will weaken these structures. In the periosteum, the weakness reduces the normal control of the growth in the long bones leading to excessive height.

A footnote should be made about the severe neonatal forms of Marfan syndrome that have been reported.[44] These have a considerably increased birth length and usually die from cardiac complications in the neonatal period.

Congenital contractural arachnodactyly (Beal syndrome)

This autosomal dominant disorder (MIM 121050) closely resembles Marfan syndrome but has, in addition, multiple joint contractures, severe kyphoscoliosis and large 'crumpled' ears. They may have similar cardiac complications. The disorder has been found to result from abnormalities in fibrillin 2 on chromosome 5q23–31.

Multiple endocrine neoplasia type 2B

In type 2b multiple endocrine neoplasia syndrome (MIM 162300) there is a combination of phaeochromocytoma, medullary thyroid carcinoma and mucosal neuroma (Fig. 18.10). In many of these patients there is also a marfanoid habitus with increased stature. This may be associated with some scoliosis and muscle wasting, but not with cardiac involvement. There is also ganglioneuromatosis in the bowel which may lead to a variety of gastrointestinal symptoms such as constipation, diarrhoea or feeding difficulties. The molecular abnormality has recently been identified as a mutation in the receptor tyrosine kinase gene *RET* on chromosome 10. It is also intriguing to note that different mutations in this gene can cause familial medullary thyroid

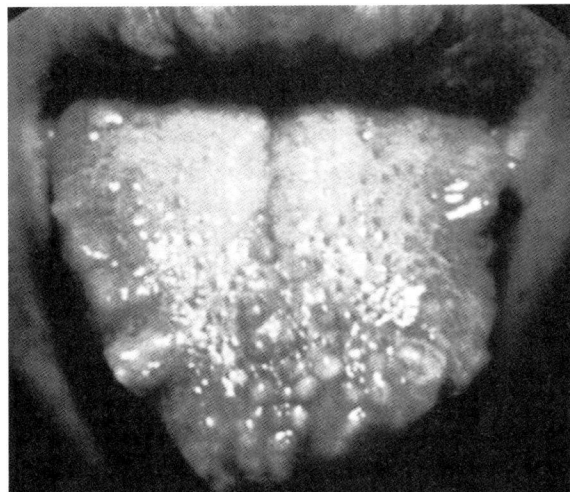

Figure 18.10 The presence of multiple neuromas on the edge of the tongue is characteristic of multiple endocrine neoplasia.

carcinoma, multiple endocrine neoplasia type 2a and more recently mutations in the same gene have been reported in some cases of Hirschsprung's disease.[45]

Other 'marfanoid' syndromes

The recognition of the tall thin habitus in Marfan syndrome has led to the use of the term 'marfanoid' habitus, and it has been found in a number of other rare disorders some of which also have mental handicap. These are listed in Table 18.1.

TALL STATURE ASSOCIATED WITH CHROMOSOMAL DISORDERS

Most chromosome disorders are usually seen with intrauterine growth retardation and short stature, however some of the sex chromosome aneuploidies may present with tall stature. In Klinefelter syndrome (47,XXY), tall stature may be the presentation before puberty and before the hypogonadism is apparent. The final height in prospective studies of Klinefelter syndrome has not been completely determined, but these boys tend to be taller than their sibs and on a higher centile than their parents.[51] In males with 46,XYY there are usually no physical stigmata but once again they may present when investigations for tall stature are being carried out. Boys with XYY have increased growth velocity towards puberty and attain a final height of 188.1 cm.[52]

Patients with fragile X syndrome have large heads, long ears and, after puberty, large testes. They may also have a height above average although within the wider range of normal.[53]

Sclerosteosis

This skeletal dysplasia (MIM 269500) causes increasing bone sclerosis and with that increasing height. The adult height in males is 178–207 cm and the adult female height is 168–190 cm.[54] There is also a great deal of thickening of the facial bones with frontal prominence and prognathism. Ultimately there may be cranial nerve compression and pressure on the medulla oblongata from the thickening around the calvarium and foramen magnum.

Sclerosteosis is found more commonly among the Afrikaner population in South Africa and is autosomal recessive. It has been found to be caused by a novel gene *SOST*, which regulates bone homeostasis and is located on chromosome 17q12–21.[55]

Beradinelli's lipodystrophy (congenital generalized lipodystrophy)

This disorder causes increased bone age and proportionate tall stature, but with premature puberty there may be a reduction in final height. It is also associated with diabetes mellitus and increased skin pigmentation including acanthosis nigricans, and patients frequently have a rather muscular appearance because of the loss of subcutaneous fat.

The disorder is autosomal recessive, and is due to the *BSCL1* gene on chromosome 9 (MIM 608594) or the *BSCL2* gene (seipin) on chromosome 11 (MIM 269700).[56] There may be further heterogeneity in this syndrome.[57] Pituitary tumors have also been associated with acanthosis nigricans and may be a cause of tall stature.[58]

Table 18.1 Marfanoid syndromes

Syndrome	Inheritance	Features	Reference
Lujan	XR	Marfanoid habitus, mental handicap, abnormal speech	Lujan[46]
Houlston	AR	Marfanoid habitus, mental handicap, microcephaly, glomerulonephritis, leukemia	Houlston et al.[47]
Fragoso	AR	Marfanoid habitus, mental handicap, coarse peculiar facies, underdeveloped muscles	Fragoso and Cantu[48]
Saul	?XR	Marfanoid habitus, mental handicap seizures, ectopic, pupils	Saul and Stevenson[49]
Tamminga	??	Marfanoid habitus, congenital contractures, leukodystrophy	Tamminga et al.[50]

XR, X-linked recessive; AR, autosomal recessive; ??, unknown.

It is seen from this review there is much to be learnt from the genetic disorders causing overgrowth through finding their causative genes and learning more about the underlying molecular mechanism leading to the overgrowth.

REFERENCES

1   Cohen MM. A comprehensive and critical assessment of overgrowth and overgrowth syndromes. *Adv Hum Genet* 1993; **18**: 181–303.

2   Wilson RS. Concordance in physical growth for monozygotic and dizygotic twins. *Ann Hum Biol* 1976; **3**: 1–10.

3   Susanne C. Genetics and environmental influence on morphological characteristics. *Ann Hum Biol* 1975; **2**: 279–88.

4   Elliott ML, Maher ER. Syndrome of the month: Beckwith–Wiedemann syndrome. *J Med Genet* 1994; **31**: 560–4.

5   Sippel WG, Partsch CJ, Wiedemann HR. Growth, bone maturation and pubertal development in children with the EMG syndrome. *Clin Genet* 1989; **35**: 20–8.

6   DeBaun MR, Tucker MA. Risk of cancer during the first four years of life in children from the Beckwith–Wiedemann Syndrome Registry. *J Pediatr* 1998; **132**: 398–400.

7   DeBaun MR, Niemitz EL, McNeil DE, *et al.* Epigenetic alterations of H19 and LIT1 distinguish patients with Beckwith–Wiedemann syndrome with cancer and birth defects. *Am J Hum Genet* 2002; **70**: 604–11.

8   Weksberg R, Smith AC, Squire JA, Sadowski P. Beckwith–Wiedemann syndrome demonstrates a role for epigenetic control of normal development. *Hum Mol Genet* 2003; **12**: R61–8.

9   Diaz-Meyer N, Day CD, Khatod K, *et al.* Silencing of CDKN1C (p57KIP2) is associated with hypomethylation at KvDMR1 in Beckwith–Wiedemann syndrome. *J Med Genet* 2003; **40**: 797–801.

10 Neri G, Gurrieri F, Zanni G, Lin A. Clinical and molecular aspects of the Simpson–Golabi–Behmel syndrome. *Am J Med Genet* 1998; **79**: 279–83.

11 Lin AE, Neri G, Hughes-Benzie R, Weksberg R. Cardiac anomalies in the Simpson–Golabi–Behmel syndrome. *Am J Med Genet* 1999; **83**: 378–81.

12 Pilia G, Hughes-Benzie RM, MacKenzie A, *et al.* Mutations in GPC3, a glypican gene, cause the Simpson Golabi Behmel overgrowth syndrome. *Nat Genet* 1996; **12**: 241–7.

13 Gonzales AD, Kaya M, Shi W, *et al.* GPC3, a plypican encoded by a gene that is mutated in the Simpson–Golabi–Behmel overgrowth syndrome, induces apoptosis in a cell-specific manner. *J Cell Biol* 1998; **141**: 1407–14.

14 Chiao E, Fisher P, Crisponi L, *et al.* Overgrowth of a mouse model of the Simpson–Golabi–Behmel syndrome is independent of IGF signaling. *Dev Biol* 2001; **243**: 185–206.

15 Brzustowicz LM, Farrell S, Khan MB, Weksberg R. Mapping of a new SGBS locus to chromosome Xp22 in a family with a severe form of Simpson–Golabi–Behmel syndrome. *Am J Hum Genet* 1999; **65**: 779–83.

16 Perlman M, Goldberg GM, Bar-Ziv J. Renal hamartomas and nephroblastomas with fetal gigantism: a familial syndrome. *J Pediatr* 1973; **83**: 414–18.

17 Henneveld HT, van Lingen RA, Hamel BCJ, *et al.* Perlman syndrome: Four additional cases. *Am J Med Genet* 1999; **86**: 439–46.

18 Sotos JF, Dodge PR, Muirhead D, *et al.* Cerebral gigantism in childhood. *New Engl J Med* 1964; **271**: 109–16.

19 Cole TRP, Hughes HE. Sotos syndrome: a study of the diagnostic criteria and natural history. *J Med Genet* 1994; **31**: 20–32.

20 Tatton-Brown K, Rahman N. Clinical features of NSD1-positive Sotos syndrome. *Clin Dysmorphol* 2004; **13**: 199–204.

21 Kurotaki N, Imaizumi K, Harada N, *et al.* Haploinsufficiency of NSD1 causes Sotos syndrome. *Nat Genet* 2002; **30**: 365–6.

22 Huang N, vom Baur E, Garnier JM, *et al.* Two distinct nuclear receptor interaction domains in NSD1, a novel SET protein that exhibits characteristics of both corepressors and coactivators. *EMBO J* 1998; **17**: 3398–412.

23 Douglas J, Hanks S, Temple IK, *et al.* NSD1 mutations are the major cause of Sotos syndrome and occur in some cases of Weaver syndrome but are rare in other overgrowth phenotypes. *Am J Hum Genet* 2003; **72**: 132–43.

24 Rio M, Clech L, Amiel J, *et al.* Spectrum of NSD1 mutations in Sotos and Weaver syndromes. *J Med Genet* 2003; **40**: 436–40.

25 Weaver DD, Graham CB, Thomas IT, Smith DW. A new overgrowth syndrome with accelerated skeletal maturation, unusual facies and camptodactyly. *J Pediatr* 1974; **84**: 547–52.

26 Marshall R, Graham C, Scott C, Smith D. Syndrome of accelerated skeletal maturation and relative failure to thrive: a newly recognised clinical growth disorder. *J Pediatr* 1971; **78**: 95–101.

27 Eich GF, Silver MM, Weksberg R, *et al.* Marshall–Smith syndrome: New radiographic, clinical and pathologic observations. *Radiology* 1991; **181**: 183–8.

28 Nevo S, Zelter M, Benderly A, Levy J. Evidence for autosomal recessive inheritance in cerebral gigantism. *J Med Genet* 1974; **11**: 158–65.

29 Dumic M, Vukelic D, Plavsic V, *et al.* Nevo syndrome. *Am J Med Genet* 1998; **76**: 67–70.

30 Cohen MM. Bannayan–Riley–Ruvalcaba syndrome: renaming three formerly recognized syndromes as one etiological entity [Letter]. *Am J Med Genet* 1990; **35**: 291.

31 Marsh DJ, Kum JB, Lunetta KL, *et al.* PTEN mutation spectrum and genotype-phenotype correlations in Bannayan–Riley–Ruvulcaba syndrome suggest a single entity with Cowden syndrome. *Hum Mol Genet* 1999; **8**: 1461–72.

32 Pilarski R, Eng C. Will the real Cowden syndrome please stand up? Expanding mutational and clinical spectra of the PTEN hamartoma tumor syndrome. *J Med Genet* 2004; **41**: 323–6.

33 Zhou XP, Hampel H, Thiele H, *et al.* Association of germline mutation in the PTEN tumor suppressor gene and a subset of Proteus and Proteus-like syndromes. *Lancet* 2001; **358**: 210–1.

34 Marfan AB. Un cas de deformation congenitale des quatre members plus prononcee aux extremités caracterisee par allongement des os avec un certain degre d'amincissement. *Bulletin et Memories de la Société Medicine Hôpitaux Paris* 1896; **13**: 200–6.

35 Schott GD. The extent of man from Vitruvius to Marfan. *Lancet* 1992; **340**: 1518–20.

36 Beighton P, de Paepe A, Danks D, *et al.* International nosology of heritable disorders of connective tissue. *Am J Med Genet* 1988; **29**: 581–94.

37 Gott VL, Pyeritz RE, Macgovern GJ, *et al.* Surgical treatment of aneurysms of the ascending aorta in the Marfan syndrome. *New Engl J Med* 1986; **314**: 1070–4.

38 Gray JR, Davies SJ. Marfan syndrome. *J Med Genet* 1996; **33**: 403–8.

39 Cistulli PA, Sullivan CE. Sleep apnea in Marfan's syndrome: increased upper airway collapsibility during sleep. *Chest* 1995; **108**: 631–5.

40 Boileau C, Jondeau G, Babron MC, *et al.* Autosomal dominant Marfan-like connective tissue disorder with aortic dilation and skeletal anomalies not linked to the fibrillin genes. *Am J Hum Genet* 1993; **53**: 46–54.

41 Mizuguchi T, Collod-Beroud G, Akiyama T, *et al.* Heterozygous TGFBR2 mutations in Marfan syndrome. *Nat Genet* 2004; **36**: 855–60.

42 Sood S, Eldadah ZA, Krause WL, *et al.* Mutation in fibrillin 1 and the Marfanoid-craniosynostosis (Sphrintzen–Goldberg) syndrome. *Nat Genet* 1996; **12**: 209–11.

43 Robinson PN, Godfrey M. The molecular genetics of Marfan syndrome and related microfibrillopathies. *J Med Genet* 2000; **37**: 9–25.

44 Buntinx IM, Willems PJ, Spitaels SE, *et al.* Neonatal Marfan syndrome with congenital arachnodactyly, flexion contractures, and severe cardiac valve insufficiency. *J Med Genet* 1991; **28**: 267–73.

45 Van Heyningen V. One gene–four syndromes. *Nature* 1994; **367**: 319–20.

46 Lujan JE. A form of X linked mental retardation with marfanoid habitus. *Am J Med Genet* 1984; **17**: 311–22.

47 Houlston RS, Iraggori S, Murday V, *et al.* Microcephaly, focal segmental glomerulonephritis and marfanoid habitus in two sibs. *Clin Dysmorphol* 1992; **1**: 111–13.

48 Fragoso R, Cantu JM. A new psychomotor retardation syndrome with peculiar facies and marfanoid habitas. *Clin Genet* 1984; **25**: 187–90.

49 Saul RA, Stevenson RE. Ectopic pupils, marfanoid habitus and mental retardation in two siblings. *Proc Greenwood Genet Cent* 1982; **1**: 14–15.

50 Tamminga P, Jennekens FGI, Barth PG. An infant with marfanoid phenotype and congenital contractures associated with ocular and cardiovascular anomalies, cerebral white matter hypoplasia and spinal axonopathy. *Eur J Paediatr* 1985; **143**: 228–31.

51 Ratcliffe S, Murray L, Teague P. Edinburgh study of growth and development of children with sex chromosomes. *Birth Defects: Original Articles Series* 1986; **22**: 73–118.

52 Ratcliffe SG, Pan H, McKie M. Growth during puberty in the XYY boy. *Ann Hum Biol* 1992; **19**: 579–87.

53 Sutherland GR, Hecht F. *Fragile Sites on Human Chromosomes.* Oxford: Oxford University Press, 1985.

54 Hamersma H, Gardner J, Beighton P. The natural history of sclerosteosis. *Clin Genet* 2003; **63**: 192–7.

55 Brunkow ME, Gardner JC, Van Ness J, *et al.* Bone dysplasia sclerosteosis results from loss of the SOST gene product, a novel cystine knot-containing protein. *Am J Hum Genet* 2001; **68**: 577–89.

56 Van Maldergem L, Magre J, Khallouf TE, *et al.* Genotype-phenotype relationships in Berardinelli–Seip congenital lipodystrophy. *J Med Genet* 2002; **39**: 722–33.

57 Rajab A, Heathcote K, Joshi S, *et al.* Heterogeneity for congenital generalized lipodystrophy in seventeen patients from Oman. *Am J Med Genet* 2002; **110**: 219–25.

58 Brown J, Winklemann RK, Randall RV. Acanthosis nigricans and pituitary tumours. *JAMA* 1966; **198**: 619–23.

19

Skeletal dysplasias

LARS HAGENÄS

INTRODUCTION

Skeletal dysplasias comprise a wide and heterogeneous group of disorders that have a generalized defect in skeletal development as a common trait. Linear growth and body proportion are also usually disturbed resulting in disproportionate short stature. However, the degree of severity may vary from the lethal entities or those conferring profoundly short stature to those going with mostly unaltered stature but with early onset osteoarthrosis. Altogether, more than 100 well described entities can be considered belonging to the skeletal dysplasias. An international classification system, last updated in 2001,[1] aims at grouping related entities based on molecular background or radiological/clinical similarities.

Even if the single skeletal dysplasia is rare or, often, extremely rare, together they occur with an estimated incidence of one to two cases per 4000 to 5000 births. Lethal skeletal dysplasias are estimated to occur with a frequency of 0.95 per 10 000 deliveries and of those, thanatophoric dysplasia and achondrogenesis account for about 60 percent. The four most common severe skeletal dysplasias are thanatophoric dysplasia, achondroplasia, osteogenesis imperfecta, and achondrogenesis. Examples of common mild skeletal dysplasias (which are usually diagnosed later in childhood) are hypochondroplasia and Leri–Weill dyschondrosteosis. The definition of what is to belong to the category of skeletal dysplasias is not clear, however. For example, Turner and Down syndromes may be regarded as belonging to the skeletal dysplasias since they confer skeletal changes together with disproportionate short stature.

CLASSIFICATION AND GENETICS OF SKELETAL DYSPLASIAS

Historically, skeletal dysplasias have been classified into short-trunk or short-limb categories. The further classification has previously to a large extent rested on the presence of radiological changes in epiphyses, metaphyses and vertebrae or combinations thereof. Thus, a certain disorder can be classified as, for example, predominantly metaphyseal, or epiphyseal, or in cases where vertebrae are also affected, as for example spondyloepiphyseal or spondyloepimetaphyseal. Spondyloepimetaphyseal dysplasia is typical in pseudoachondroplasia, for example. Emphasis on a whole-skeleton radiological survey has thus been a general rule for arriving at the diagnosis. It is also important to know that skeletal changes may be age-specific and that repeated radiological surveys can be useful for arriving at a diagnosis.

The last decade has shown a diverse genetic background of the skeletal dysplasias even if the causes of most entities are still not known. Some of the known backgrounds are: a change in amount or quality of connective tissue elements (e.g., different collagen types); a defect sulfate transporter; a constitutively increased or decreased receptor activity (e.g., fibroblast growth factor receptor-3 (FGFR3) and parathyroid hormone receptor (PTHR)); a defect of mitochondrial RNA-processing endo-ribonuclease (RMRP). Table 19.1 lists some of the known genetically elucidated skeletal dysplasias.

Many of the mutations have a dominant influence. This seems logical when, for example, an abnormal connective tissue element that is incorporated in the extracellular matrix may destroy its overall structure and function or when a constitutively activated receptor over-rides the function of the normal receptor. Sometimes, when a known dominant skeletal dysplasia seems to be transmitted in a recessive way in a family, it could be explained by germ line mosaicism in one of the parents.

CLINICAL EVALUATION OF THE SHORT CHILD WITH SUSPECTED SKELETAL DYSPLASIA

A significant portion of individuals with obvious skeletal dysplasia will not been given a specific diagnosis. This is due to the wide range of entities, each of which is usually rare or very rare, and that a single clinician cannot gain sufficient experience of the rarer entities. Furthermore, there may be a considerable variability in the phenotype of a disorder in addition to the lack of known genetic background for most entities.

The skeletal dysplasias will usually confer a disproportionate short stature in contrast to growth disorders caused by endocrinological, cardiac, renal or inflammatory disorders, which result in proportionate short stature. The trunk–leg relation can conveniently be evaluated by measuring sitting height and calculating its percentage of total height. Figure 19.1 gives the normal age variation and population distribution of this measure. Arm span measurement is valuable since normally, arm span is equal to height at least from the age of 6 years. The arms normally reach the middle of the thigh. Clinical observation of the patient can reveal if a short arm span is mostly due to a rhizomelic (proximal segment) or mesomelic (middle segment) shortening.

The same evaluation should be done for the lower limbs when sitting height percentage of total height exceeds +2 SDS meaning that the legs are significantly short in relation to the trunk. The size of hands and feet are important to note. Are the thumbs normally 'inserted'? Is there a metacarpal sign, i.e., when the fourth metacarpal is short leaving an absent knuckle? A short first metacarpal will give a more proximal 'insertion' of the thumb ('hitchhiker's thumb').

Furthermore, head circumference should be compared with that of the parents. A more comprehensive list of relevant items is found in Table 19.2. Blood levels of calcium, phosphorus, and alkaline phosphatase are, with a few exceptions, normal in the skeletal dysplasias.

DEVELOPMENT OF HEIGHT AND BODY PROPORTION IN SKELETAL DYSPLASIAS

Knowledge about growth pattern is missing for most of the entities even if information exists on birth size and final height for a few skeletal dysplasias. In particular, information on pubertal growth is lacking.

For some of the more common entities, information on, for example, final adult height is available but the sample is rarely systematic or large enough to obtain a convincing estimate of the variation around the mean. Furthermore, collecting auxological data is complicated by the phenotypic variability that often exists both within and between families, for a genetically defined skeletal dysplasia as well as genetic heterogeneity for other skeletal dysplasias.

Birth size

Intrauterine growth is compromised in certain skeletal dysplasias; for example, in diastrophic dysplasia or cartilage hair hypoplasia with a mean birth length of about −3 SDS. In other disorders that result in an extreme adult short stature, birth length will be more or less normal. Such examples are achondroplasia and pseudoachondroplasia.

Growth in infancy

The infancy growth period is compromised in many skeletal dysplasias, resulting in a rapid fall in the relative position on the growth curve (Fig. 19.2, page 296). The initial growth velocity may sometimes be normal; in achondroplasia, for example, the initial length position at birth is often maintained until 2–4 months of age before an abrupt decrease in growth velocity causes a decrease on the growth curve. In other skeletal dysplasias the fall in SDS position may be seen already from birth. A peculiar exception is found in pseudoachondroplasia where normal growth often is observed during the whole first year of life before a continuous, dramatic decrease in height position starts.

Childhood growth

From available growth data it seems that the relative height position is maintained during the childhood growth period in many skeletal dysplasias including achondroplasia and cartilage hair dysplasia. As mentioned, children with pseudoachondroplasia are an exception with their continuous fall in relative height position also during childhood growth.

Table 19.1 Genetic defects and molecular mechanisms in certain skeletal dysplasias

Skeletal dysplasia group (Ho)mozygous; (L)ethal Dominant diseases that seem to occur in a recessive way in a family may be caused by parental germ cell mosaicism	Gene/chromosomal location/ (D)ominant; (R)ecessive	Gene product function and molecular mechanisms
FGFR3 Thanatophoric dysplasia (L) Achondroplasia Hypochondroplasia	*FGFR3*/4p/D (fibroblast growth factor receptor-3)	Constitutive FGFR3 activation leading to inhibition of chondrocyte proliferation and differentiation and rhizomelic disproportionate short stature
SHOX Turner syndrome Leri-Weill dyschondrosteosis Langer mesomelic dysplasia (Ho)	*SHOX*/Xp and Yp/pseudoautosomal-D (short stature homeobox-containing gene)	Haploinsufficiency or total loss of the SHOX (homeobox) transcription factor leading to mesomelic disproportionate short stature
Type I collagen Osteogenesis imperfecta (OI) type I–IV	*COL1A1*/17q/D *COL1A2*/7q/D (collagen I alpha-1 and -2 chains)	Defective procollagen I compromise formation of mature homofibrils causing a more or less continuous spectrum of clinical severity. Type II OI is usually lethal
Type II collagen Achondrogenesis type 2 (L) Hypochondrogenesis (often L) Kniest dysplasia SEDC (spondyloepiphyseal dysplasia congenita) SEMD Strudwick Stickler syndrome type-1 Familial osteoarthrosis	*COL2A1*/12q/D (collagen type II alpha-1 chain)	Disturbed assembly and structure of type II collagen causes defect differentiation and growth of axial and juxta-axial skeleton. Type II collagen is also called cartilage collagen and is produced as a major collagen from proliferative chondrocytes in the growth plate

Type IX collagen
Multiple epiphyseal dysplasia
    type-6 (EDM6 – *COL9A1*)
    type-2 (EDM2 – *COL9A2*)
    type-3 (EDM3 – *COL9A3*)
	COL9A1/6q/D
	COL9A2/1p/D
	COL9A3/20q/D
	(collagen type IX alpha-1 to -3 chains)
		Type IX collagen is a heterotrimer of alpha-1, alpha-2, and alpha-3 chains. It is a cartilage-specific fibril-associated collagen. It is produced as a minor collagen from proliferative chondrocytes in the growth plate

Type X collagen Metaphyseal dysplasia Schmid type	*COL10A1*/6q/D (collagen type X alpha-1 chain)	Type X collagen is produced by hypertrophic chondrocytes in the epiphyseal growth plate
Type XI collagen Stickler syndrome type-2 (*COL11A1*) and type-3 (non-ocular form, *COL11A2*) Marshall syndrome (*COL11A1*)	*COL11A1*/1p/D *COL11A2*/6p/D (collagen type XI alpha-1 and -2 chains)	Type XI collagen 'decorates' type II collagen fibrils. It is produced as a minor collagen from proliferative chondrocytes in the growth plate and is also a structural component in the eye. Stickler type-2 (and type-1) is associated with ocular changes (myopia and risk of retinal detachment)
COMP Pseudoachondroplasia Multiple epiphyseal dysplasia type-1 (EDM1)	*COMP*/19p/D (cartilage oligomeric protein)	COMP is a homopentameric protein necessary for assembly of cartilage matrix. Mutated COMP may be retained in chondrocyte endoplasmatic reticulum causing premature cell death
RNAse MRP-RNA Cartilage hair hypoplasia (metaphyseal chondrodysplasia, McKusick type)	*RMRP*/9p/R (mitochondrial RNA-processing endoribonuclease)	RMRP is a nuclear gene product that is imported into mitochondria. Mutations confer metaphyseal dysplasia, immunological defects and anemia

(Continued)

Table 19.1 (Continued)

Skeletal dysplasia group (Ho)mozygous; (L)ethal Dominant diseases that seem to occur in a recessive way in a family may be caused by parental germ cell mosaicism	Gene/chromosomal location/ (D)ominant; (R)ecessive	Gene product function and molecular mechanisms
DTDST (SLC26A2) Achondrogenesis type 1B (L) Atelosteogenesis type 2 (L) Diastrophic dysplasia Multiple epiphyseal dysplasia type-4 (EDM4)	DTDST(SLC26A2)/5q/R (diastrophic dysplasia sulphate transporter); solute carrier family 26-sulfate transporter)	Defective sulfate transporter confer undersulfated proteoglycans in extracellular matrix leading to distorted joint formation; scoliosis and short stature
Matrilin-3 Multiple epiphyseal dysplasia type-5 (EDM5)	MATN3/2p/D (matrilin-3)	Defective matrilin-3 disturbs formation of cartilage matrix. Matrilin-3 is an oligomeric protein present in the cartilage extracellular matrix
PTH/PTHrP-receptor Metaphyseal dysplasia Jansen type Blomstrand dysplasia (L)	PTHR/3p/D,R (parathyroid hormone receptor)	Constitutively activating (dominant) mutations of parathyroid hormone receptor in Jansen dysplasia cause delayed terminal differentiation of chondrocytes with a chaotic process of ossification in metaphyseal areas. Inactivating (recessive) mutations in Blomstrand cause advanced skeletal maturation and generalized osteosclerosis
CDMP1 Acromesomelic dysplasia Grebe and Hunter–Thompson types Brachydactyly type C	CDMP1/20q/R (cartilage-derived morphogenetic protein-1)	CDMP1 initiates chondrogenic differentiation of mesenchymal stem cells. The loss of function mutations confer a phenotypic spectrum ranging from brachydactyly C in heterozygotes to the severe Grebe-type chondrodysplasia in the homozygous affected and seems to be due to CDMP1 gradient effects during pattern formation
NPRB Acromesomelic dysplasia Maroteaux type	NPRB/9p/R (natriuretic peptide receptor B gene)	NPRB is the homodimeric transmembrane natriuretic peptide receptor B
GNAS1 Pseudohypoparathyreoidism type 1a (PHP-1a) McCune Albright syndrome (fibrous dysplasia)	GNAS1/20q/D (stimulatory Gs alpha protein of adenylate cyclase)	Heterozygous inactivating mutations in exons of GNAS encoding the alpha subunit of the stimulatory Gs-alpha confer PHP-1a including Albright hereditary osteodystrophy, (AHO). Activating dominant mutations (always somatic mosaicism) cause polyostotic fibrous dysplasia of the bone in McCune–Albright syndrome
Cathepsin K Pyknodysostosis	Cathepsin K/1q/R	Cathepsin K is a cysteine lysosomal protease that is highly expressed in osteoclasts
Sedlin Spondyloepiphyseal dysplasia tarda	SEDL/Xp/XR	Sedlin is an endoplasmatic reticulum protein with a putative role in Golgi transport
SOX9 Campomelic dysplasia (often L)	SOX9/17q/D [SRY (sex reversal Y-chromosome) -related HMG-box 9 gene]	SOX9 is a transcription factor responsible for regulation of chondrocyte lineage and also for COL2A1. The latter may explain certain phenotypic similarities to SEDC, Stickler and Kniest dysplasia. The majority of karyotypic males show partial or complete sex reversal
TRPS1/EXT1 Tricho-rhino-phalangeal syndrome type-1 and -3 Tricho-rhino-phalangeal syndrome type-2 (Langer-Giedion syndrome)	TRPS1/8q/D (TRP type 1 and 3) (trichorhinophalangeal syndrome-1 gene) EXT1/8q/D (TRP type 2) (exostosin-1)	TRPS1 is a zinc finger protein functioning as a putative transcription factor. TRP type 2 is a contiguous gene syndrome involving loss of functional copies of the TRPS1 and EXT1 genes
CBFA1 Cleidocranial dysplasia	CBFA1/6p/D	The gene encodes the core binding (transcription) factor A1

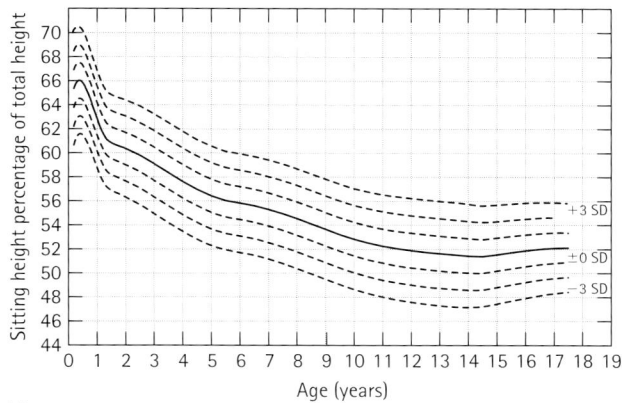
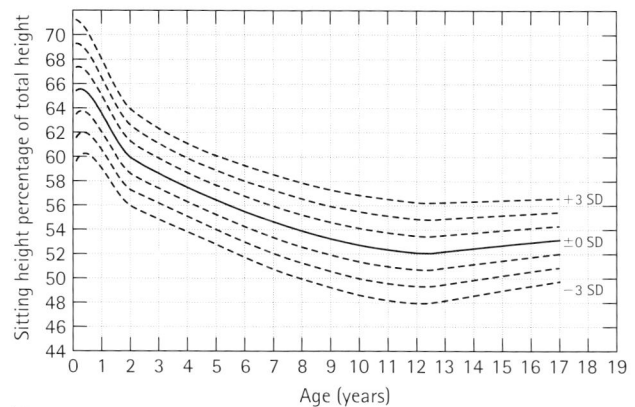

(a) Boys

(b) Girls

Figure 19.1   Relative sitting height (i.e., sitting height as a percentage of total height) development for normal boys and girls. Mean and ± 1,2,3 SD. Data from Gerver.[3]

Table 19.2   Clinical findings and historical details to consider when handling a patient with suspected skeletal dysplasia

Head, respiratory function, vision

Head circumference (expressed as SDS): comparison with other family member.

Face: decreased or increased vertical dimension of middle face; facial muscle hypotonia; ptosis; retrognathia; underdeveloped maxilla

Ears: low set position; anatomy of the earlobes; swelling or deformation of the pinnae. Otitis media; conductive or sensineuronal hearing impairment

Mouth: high arched palate, cleft palate, bifid uvula, congruency of the bite (malocclusion), pharynx narrowness; snoring; apneic episodes; sleeping position.

Vision: myopia; cataract; retinal detachment.

Arms and hands

Arm length: arms should normally reach middle thigh; reaching shorter or longer. Rhizomelia or mesomelia. Extension defect in elbows; cubitus valgus; Madelung deformity of the wrist and forearm. Muscle mass of the arms; muscle strength.

Hands: short hands (acromelia); only short metacarpals; metacarpal sign; trident finger configuration; hitchhiker's thumb (more proximal insertion than normal due to short first metacarpal bone); loose finger or wrist joints; telescoping fingers; swollen joints; joint restrictions; pain or stiffness.

Legs and walking

Disproportionate short legs; mesomelic or rhizomelic shortening. Varus or valgus deformity of femur and tibia.

Feet: short, or short and broad.

Joint pain or stiffness; swollen joints.

Muscle mass; muscle strength.

Increased or decreased patellar or achilles reflexes in relation to muscle tone.

Age for sitting and walking.

Leg pain, weakness or fatigability after exercise ('spinal claudication' is a sign of spinal stenosis).

Trunk and neck

Narrow thorax; compromised respiratory capacity; truncal hypotonia; pectus excavatum or carinatum; kypho-/scoliosis; cervical kyphosis, thoracolumbar kyphosis; lumbar lordosis

Lumbar pain or fatigability (sign of spinal claudiation).

Short or long trunk (measure sitting height and evaluate sitting height as a percentage of standing height); short neck.

Neck: search for signs of cervical spine instability; C1–C2 sublocation/dislocation may be present secondary to hypoplastic dens axis and/or abnormally lax ligament fixation of dens or between C1–C2. Head flexion or extension may in those cases cause pain or neurological symptoms due to displacement of bony parts of C2 into the medulla.

Growth history

Birth weight; birth length.

Height SDS development during first and second year? Presence of catch-up growth? Duration of catch-up.

Height SDS at 2, 3, 4 years of age. Is height SDS stabilizing during pre-pubertal years. Further loss in height SDS during puberty until final height.

Head circumference SDS.

Body proportion expressed as 'relative sitting height' (i.e., sitting height as a percentage of total height) expressed in SDS for age and sex (SH percent SDS).

Change in SH percent during childhood growth or during puberty.

Weight development; BMI may not be useful due to body disproportion. Waist circumference may be a better indicator of overweight.

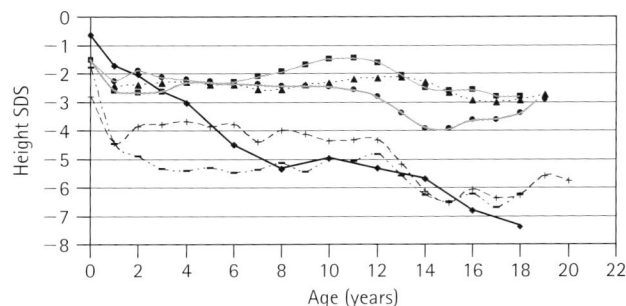

Figure 19.2 Development of average height SDS with age for certain skeletal dysplasias and syndromes. Typical for many entities is a compromised linear growth during infancy but constant relative height position during childhood growth. Pubertal growth is often compromised resulting in a further loss of height position on the curve. Achondroplasia (bars), 146 girls (from Hertel et al.[112]); diastrophic dysplasia (crosses), 68 girls (from Mäkitie and Kaitila[99]); Turner syndrome (circles), n = 598 (from Rongen-Westerlaken et al.[113]); Noonan syndrome (triangles), 55 girls (from Ranke et al.[114]); Down syndrome (squares), 151 girls (from Myrelid et al.[115]); pseudoachondroplasia (diamonds), 61 boys and girls (from Horton et al.[70]). Normal height standard is that of Karlberg.[116]

Pubertal growth

Timing of puberty is probably normal for most skeletal dysplasias. It is usually believed that pubertal growth may be compromised in some of the disorders, such as Leri–Weill dyschondrosteosis and hypochondroplasia. This could then result in a loss in height position of about 1.5 SDS or more during puberty.

Adult height

Adult height varies enormously in different skeletal dysplasias; in some entities a height well below 100 cm is not unusual whereas in other dysplasias total height may be only marginally compromised but with presence of body disproportion. Phenotypic variability, also regarding height, may be considerable for many skeletal dysplasias, even within an affected family. This also includes body disproportion. Knowledge of adult height and its variability awaits exploration for most skeletal dysplasias.

Weight development

Individuals with skeletal dysplasia may be prone to develop obesity due to restrictions in physical activity imposed by muscular hypotonia, arthrosis and other orthopedic problems. Weight for height indices as well as the BMI measure will be influenced by a significant body disproportion making comparison with population based standards impossible. The individual's waist circumference development may be easier to evaluate in relation to normal population standard.

Development of body proportions

TRUNK–LEG RELATIONSHIP

The trunk–leg relationship could easily be evaluated by routinely measuring sitting height and calculate 'relative sitting height'; i.e., sitting height as a percentage of total length or height ('SH percent'). Normally the young child has short extremities that grow proportionally faster than the trunk until the start of puberty. This will result in a continuous decrease in relative sitting height until the start of puberty when the trend reverses due to the sex steroid induced growth spurt of the spine. Figure 19.1 shows the normal pace of relative sitting height for girls and boys with mean and ± 3 SD from a normal Dutch population. Body proportion is partly dependent on height and, for short children, it has been suggested that the normal relative sitting height range extends to about +2.5 SDS.[2] Many syndromes with short stature will show deviant body proportions due to short extremities or a short trunk. In certain entities with a compromised growth capacity of the legs the relative trunk–leg disproportion is maintained (i.e., a constant relative sitting height SDS) from early childhood until at least the start of puberty when, depending on the skeletal dysplasia, amplification or improvement of the disproportion may be seen.

In skeletal dysplasias with abnormal growth capacity of the spine a continuous worsening in body proportions may be seen. Systematic data on development of trunk–leg ratio are missing in the literature however.

Except for the short-leg skeletal dysplasias some other syndromes will also confer disproportionate short legs. In Down syndrome patients the mean relative sitting height (SH percent) is about +3 SDS and in Turner syndrome about +2 SDS which could be compared with hypochondroplasia at +3 to +4 SDS; Leri–Weill dyschondrosteosis at +3 SDS and achondroplasia at about +10 SDS. Figure 19.3 shows height and other body measurements and proportions for achondroplasia, hypochondroplasia and Leri–Weill dyschondrosteosis.

ARM SPAN

Arm span normally equals height from the age of 6–7 years.[3] At younger ages, arm span is distinctly shorter. In certain skeletal dysplasias arm span is typically shortened in relation to height, e.g., in Leri–Weill dyschondrosteosis. In some skeletal dysplasias, the measurement of arm span can be hard to evaluate due to increasing extension defects of the elbow.

HEAD CIRCUMFERENCE

Head circumference is typically increased in achondroplasia at a mean of about +3 SDS of the normal. In some skeletal dysplasias head circumference is comparable with the normal mean but disproportionately large compared to height. Head circumference development mirrors growth of the brain and is not expected to be affected by the genetic–molecular mechanisms responsible for certain skeletal dysplasias.

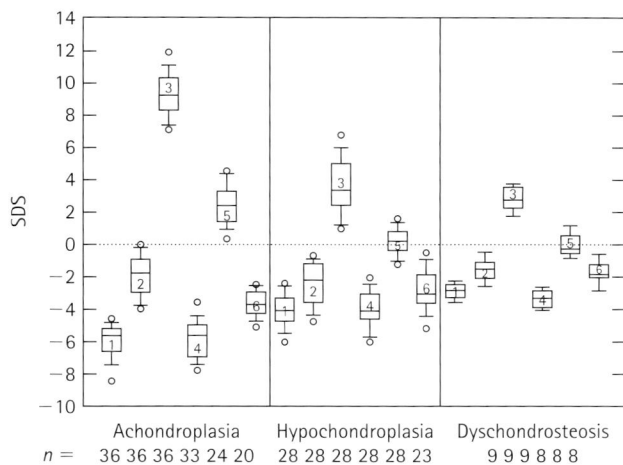

Figure 19.3   Height and body proportions in achondroplasia, hypochondroplasia and Leri—Weill dyschondrosteosis. Data are given for (1–6): height, absolute sitting height, relative sitting height (i.e., sitting height percentage of total height), arm span, head circumference and foot length. The number of measured subjects for each item is indicated in the figure. Data are given as SDS according to the standards of Gerver[3] (for arm span, absolute and relative sitting height and foot length) and of Karlberg for height.[116] The box plot denotes 5th, 10th, 25th, 50th, 75th, 90th, and 95th centiles.

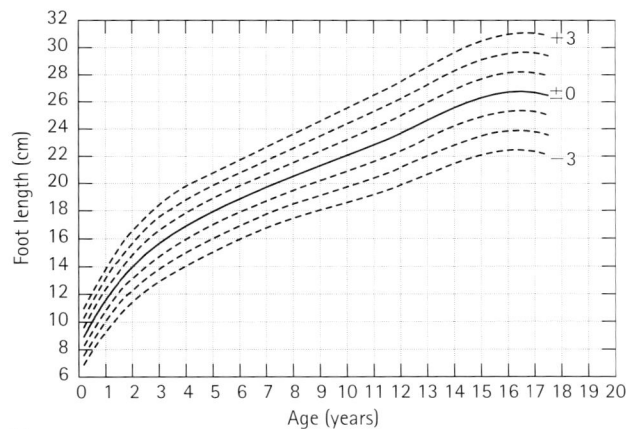

(a) Boys

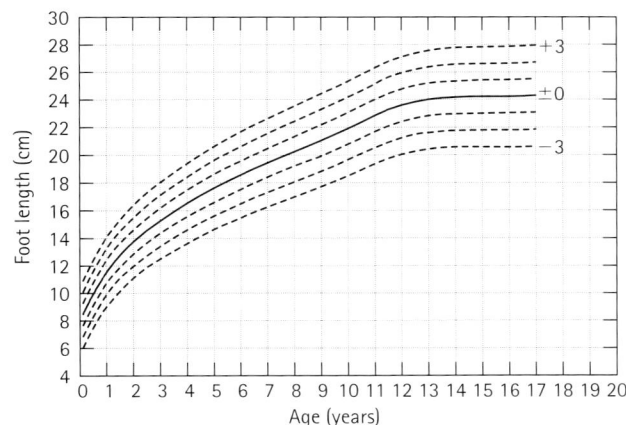

(b) Girls

Figure 19.4   Development of foot length in normal boys and girls. Mean ±3 SDS. Data from the Dutch population standard of Gerver.[3]

Comparison with head circumference of unaffected members of the family is then relevant.

FOOT LENGTH

Foot length can easily be measured and compared using a simple device commonly found in shoe shops. Comparison with normal population standards[3] (Fig. 19.4) can reveal varying degrees of growth restriction compared with total or sitting height. Feet (and hands) are particularly small in e.g. achondroplasia and acromesomelic dysplasia even if the former diagnosis shows considerable variability in foot length. On the other side of the spectrum spondyloepiphyseal dysplasia congenita shows most involvement of the trunk and juxtatrunkal skeleton with little abnormality of hands and feet.

ORTHOPEDIC, NEUROLOGICAL AND OTHER MEDICAL PROBLEMS

Many skeletal dysplasias confer significant complications that may be orthopedic or neurological or often both. Bone stability is typically not affected even if chronic immobilization and under-usage of muscle can cause osteopenia. The rare exceptions to a normal bone structure include osteogenesis imperfecta, osteopetrosis, and pyknodysostosis which give increased risk for fractures. On the other hand, in many of the skeletal dysplasias, skeletal and joint deformities contribute to a significant physical handicap. Extreme short stature and gross trunk–leg disproportion often compound these medical problems.

Muscle function

In many skeletal dysplasias motor development is, for unknown reasons, delayed (e.g., in achondroplasia) or permanently impaired (e.g., in pseudoachondroplasia or in spondyloepiphyseal dysplasia congenita). In achondroplasia this could be associated with spinal compression whereas in other diagnoses a defective connective tissue could be the cause of affected muscle function. On the other side of the spectrum, increased muscular function is often observed in Leri—Weill dyschondrosteosis and in hypochondroplasia-like mild skeletal dysplasias.

The spine

Development of kyphosis or kyphoscoliosis, which may be progressive, is found in some of the type II collagenopathies and in most individuals with diastrophic dysplasia. In achondroplasia a transient thoracolumbar kyphosis is commonly seen during infancy, usually disappearing when the child begins walking and is then replaced by a lumbar lordosis. A pronounced truncal muscular hypotonia may possibly increase the risk for a permanent and progressing thoracolumbar kyphosis.

The cervical medulla is potentially at risk in some of the common skeletal dysplasias. A threat to its neural integrity comes from a narrow foramen magnum or a reduced spinal canal diameter; both findings are common in achondroplasia. Likewise, an atlantoaxial instability due to underdeveloped dens axis and/or atlantoaxial ligament laxity as found in the type II collagenopathies (except for Stickler syndrome), osteogenesis imperfecta, cartilage hair hypoplasia or in pseudoachondroplasia can predispose to traumatic injury to the medulla.[4,5]

In diastrophic dysplasia kyphosis of the cervical spine can become pronounced and may occur together with atlantoaxial subluxation, also potentially causing cervical cord compression. These conditions also predispose to a risk in anaesthesia and intubation. Prospective, repeated radiological evaluation of provoked (flexion/extension) projections of atlantoaxial integrity is therefore essential in diagnoses at risk. Symptoms pointing to cervical neurological involvement should actively and prospectively be sought for and include lack of motor coordination (clumsiness), increased difficulties in walking, neck pain, and limited neck mobility, neurogenic bladder, spasticity, and lower limb hyperreflexia. Even in clinically unaffected cases magnetic resonance imaging (MRI) occasionally shows edema and gliosis of the cervicomedullary cord.

Joint function

Ligament laxity together with defect articular cartilage predispose to premature arthrosis with stiffness and pain that may be already evident in childhood. This is found in pseudoachondroplasia and in Stickler syndrome. On the contrary, contractures may dominate causing joint luxation or subluxation as is common in diastrophic dysplasia. Dysplastic formation of femoral head and/or acetabulum is found in achondroplasia and spondyloepiphyseal dysplasia congenita (SEDC), in the latter diagnosis sometimes causing hip luxation. Coxa vara, i.e., hips set at a wrong angle towards the body ('shepherd's hook') is found in SEDC, and contributes to a waddling gait.

Foot and hand deformities

Development of pes equinovarus may be dependent on delayed motor development and is found in diastrophic dysplasia and in Kniest dysplasia. Abnormal insertion of the thumb, hitchhiker's thumb, depends on a particularly short first metacarpal and is seen in diastrophic dysplasia.

Vision and hearing problems

Myopia and/or risk of retinal detachment are prevalent in some of the type II collagenopathies. Hearing defects due to sensorineural and/or conductive causes are common in Kniest dysplasia or osteogenesis imperfecta. Recurrent otitis media is a typical cause of hearing defect in achondroplasia.

Intelligence and other cognitive functions are generally fully normal in most skeletal dysplasias.

EFFECT OF GROWTH HORMONE TREATMENT, AND BONE–LENGTHENING ON HEIGHT AND BODY PROPORTION

Reported experience of growth hormone (GH) treatment in short children with skeletal dysplasia is sparse and often limited to short treatment periods. Knowledge of its effect on pubertal growth and adult height is generally lacking. Formal studies are almost all confined to achondroplasia as the most common entity. First year treatment response is typically a 2–3 cm increase in growth velocity in pre-pubertal achondroplastic children with a total gain over three to four pre-pubertal treatment years of about 1 SDS. For most other skeletal dysplasias knowledge, even from short term trials, is insufficient. Genetic heterogeneity and/or phenotypic variability for many of the diagnostic entities will perhaps also confound future results on short- and long-term trials with GH. This would be relevant for the fairly prevalent syndromes of hypochondroplasia and dyschondrosteosis.

The potential gain in final height from GH treatment can also be compared with that accomplished by surgical bone lengthening. According to one compilation from lengthening of 261 femora and tibia the average gain for femur was 11 cm (range, 3.5–17 cm) and 9 cm for tibia (range, 3–15.6 cm). The average total time for treatment of the tibia was 268 days (range, 110–497 days).[6]

Comparison with short term effect on statural growth in other syndromes

It is interesting to compare responses to GH treatment in different skeletal dysplasias with those in individuals with other non-GH-deficient conditions such as Turner syndrome or Noonan syndrome, or even in the poorly defined group of children with idiopathic short stature.

A placebo-controlled study of 232 Turner subjects report an increase in first year growth velocity of less than 3 cm compared with that of the controls.[7] In selected cases, using more extreme doses of GH growth velocity can be considerably increased. Thus, a study using roughly 0.1 mg kg^{-1} day^{-1} in a cohort of 40 girls with Turner syndrome reports a 6 cm first year increase in growth velocity (see Chapter 35). However, increases in IGF-I levels often become excessive during such high-dose therapy. In Noonan syndrome, increases in growth velocity of 2.4–3.5 cm year^{-1} during the first year of GH treatment are reported.[8,9] In children with idiopathic short stature, a large meta-analysis shows an estimated first year increase in growth velocity of 3.3 cm for 214 children in uncontrolled studies and 2.9 cm for 229 children in controlled trials. The mean estimated first-year gain in height for the children in the controlled studies was 0.6 SDS.[10]

Effect on body proportions

The knowledge of the effect of GH treatment on body proportion in different skeletal dysplasias is limited. At least during the pre-pubertal growth period, treatment does not seem to influence the degree of disproportion very much in achondroplasia, hypochondroplasia or Leri–Weill dyschondrosteosis. In this context it should be noted that short individuals with GH deficiency have normal relative sitting height as seen in Prader–Willi syndrome and in other GH deficient individuals. There is, furthermore, no correlation between degree of GH sufficiency and relative sitting height and GH treatment will not change body proportions in GHD or ISS children or in children with hypochondroplasia or in girls with Turner syndrome.[11]

PROFESSIONAL TEAM FOR DIAGNOSIS, HANDLING AND PROSPECTIVE SURVEILLANCE OF PATIENTS WITH SKELETAL DYSPLASIAS

Since the prevalence of skeletal dysplasias is low, but variability of auxological, orthopedic, ophthalmologic and other neurological problems are great, it is necessary to have a team of specialists seeing the majority of the patients at a referral clinic in order to acquire the necessary knowledge to handle the problems, both with respect to establishing a diagnosis and potential medical complications. Especially important are specialists in pediatric neurology, orthopedic surgery, neurosurgery, and neuroradiology. An early correct diagnosis is important for surveillance of possible medical complications. A correct diagnosis is also necessary for correct genetic counseling of the family.

ACHONDROPLASIA

Achondroplasia is the commonest of the severe skeletal dysplasias with an incidence of about one per 25 000 newborns. Its typical features usually suggest the diagnosis already at birth or at least during the first year of life when growth is faltering and body disproportion becomes more visible. Due to a range of medical complications that accompany achondroplasia it is necessary to have a good knowledge of the special anatomy with resulting possible neurological and other problems that may already be present from infancy.

Genetics and molecular mechanisms

Achondroplasia is the result of a heterozygous mutation of a single base in the transmembrane region of the *FGFR3* gene (fibroblast growth factor receptor 3). This nucleotide is one of the most mutable in the human genome and the mutation seems to be of exclusive paternal origin in new cases which account for about 80 percent of all cases. The mutation has complete penetrance and fairly constant phenotypic expression, at least regarding linear growth.

FGFR3 normally functions as an important negative regulator of chondrocyte proliferation and differentiation in the growth plate. Mutations of *FGFR3* which are associated with skeletal dysplasias (in order of increasing severity: hypochondroplasia, achondroplasia, SADDAN, and thanatophoric dysplasia) seem to induce ligand-independent activation and/or increased stability of the activated receptor prolonging its intracellular signalling. Increased *FGFR3* activity then induces premature termination of the proliferative cycle of the chondrocyte, which restricts linear growth.[12–14]

In achondroplasia, growth plates in the extremities are affected to a greater extent than those of the vertebrae resulting in short limbed skeletal dysplasia while trunk length is usually affected only to a minor degree. Homozygous achondroplasia is usually lethal in the newborn period due to underdevelopment of the thorax and compressed neural structures due to narrowing of the foramina in the skull base. Prenatal diagnosis is easily made by DNA analysis when suspicion of achondroplasia occurs from the finding of short femora on ultrasound examination, from about the 24th week of gestation.

Clinical traits

Achondroplasia is usually easily recognizable at birth because of a large head, sometimes with frontal bossing, in combination with short arms and legs. Although length at birth is within the normal range, extreme shortness develops during the first year of life, largely depending on deficient growth of the lower extremities, in particular the femora. In contrast, growth of the trunk is diminished to a lesser extent. Also the arms, especially the humeri, are extremely short and achondroplasia is therefore classified as a rhizomelic form of short limb skeletal dysplasia (from Greek *rhiza* meaning root).

Hands (as well as feet) are short with short metacarpals and phalanges; they are often described as 'trident hands' and with inability to approximate, in extension, the sides of distal fingers. Extension and rotation of the elbow joint are often limited. Ligament laxity is frequent and is noticeable in the large joints.

The head is larger than normal; i.e., there is absolute macrocephaly caused by a larger than normal brain in combination with slightly increased ventricular and extracerebral liquor space. The midface is usually hypoplastic including a depressed nasal bridge, which contrasts with prominent bossing of the frontal area. Secondary to the hypoplastic midface, airways are narrow causing increased airway resistance. A typically narrow thorax, may contribute to an increased respiratory load.

During infancy, it is common to see thoracolumbar kyphosis, which disappears when the child starts to walk. From this time a marked lumbar lordosis usually develops.

Growth and development of body proportions

Fetal growth is affected to a limited extent with birth length corresponding to about −1.5 SDS. Length development is

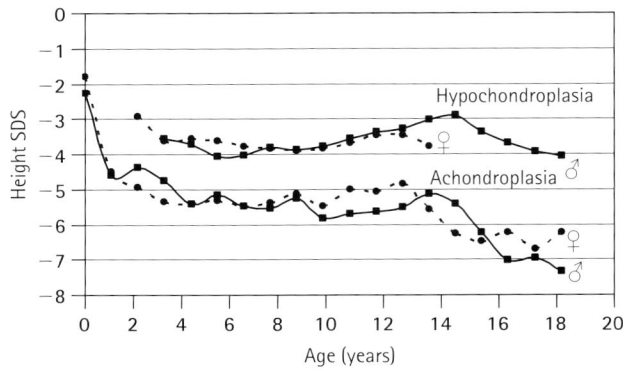

Figure 19.5 Height development for boys and girls with achondroplasia and hypochondroplasia. Data for hypochondroplasia: 56 boys and 28 girls (from Appan et al.[29]). Data for achondroplasia: 97 boys and 146 girls (from Hertel et al.[117]). Normal height standard is that of Karlberg.[116]

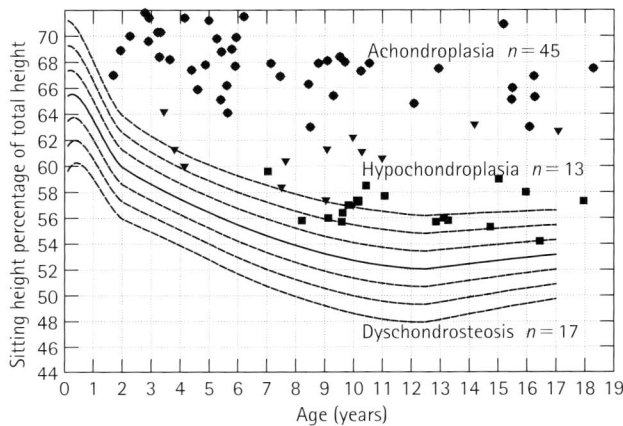

Figure 19.7 Absolute sitting height in 36 boys with achondroplasia plotted on the Dutch standard of Gerver.[3] (Neumeyer L, Hagenäs L, unpublished data.)

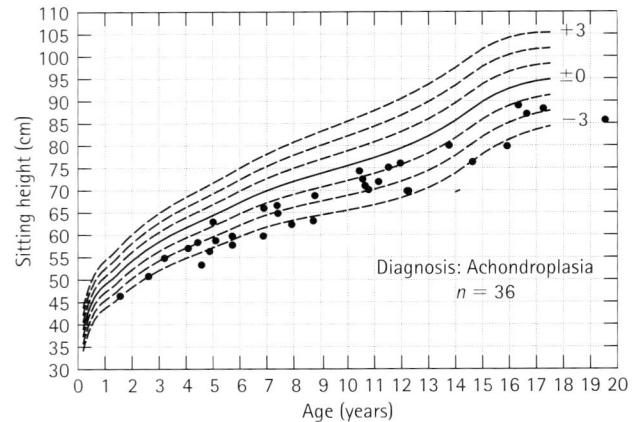

Figure 19.6 Relative sitting height (i.e., sitting height as a percentage of total height) in children with achondroplasia (diamonds), hypochondroplasia (triangles) and Leri–Weill dyschondrosteosis (squares) plotted on a Dutch standard with mean and ± 3SD.[3] There is almost no overlap between achondroplasia and hypochondroplasia (Neumeyer L, Hagenäs L, unpublished data.)

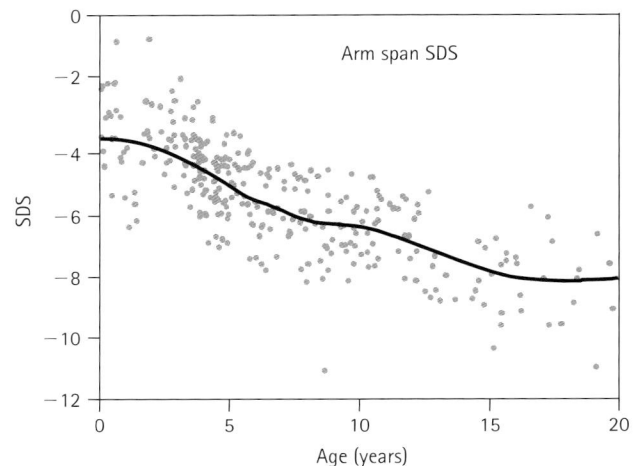

Figure 19.8 Arm span development in achondroplasia expressed as SDS using the normal Dutch standard of Gerver.[3] The continuous deterioration in arm span growth is partly dependent on increasing extension defect in the elbow. Semilongitudinal unpublished data.[112]

often fairly normal during the first few months of life; sometimes the relative length positioning is maintained for the first half year. Growth velocity then suddenly drops with a continuous fall on the growth curve to about −5.5 SDS at 2 years of age. This position is thereafter approximately maintained during childhood with a further fall in relative height during puberty due to a diminished pubertal component of growth resulting in adult height being about −6 to −7 SDS. Figure 19.5 shows the development of height SDS with age for boys and girls with achondroplasia.

The normally rapid growth of the extremities during early childhood is much impaired and development body proportions do not follow the normal growth pattern. Relative sitting height corresponds typically to about +10 SDS (Fig. 19.6). The pronounced shortness in achon-

droplasia is therefore dependent on a marked reduction in leg length whereas trunk length, as approximated by sitting height, is normal at all ages and may, not uncommonly, be above the mean for normal children (Fig. 19.7). The mean sitting height in achondroplasia is about −1.5 SDS of normal. Growth of the arms is impaired resulting in an extreme reduction of arm span (Fig. 19.8). Contributing to this is the extension defect of the elbow which often worsens with age.

Growth charts for children with achondroplasia have been produced by Horton et al. giving standards for height, growth velocity, head circumference and lengths for upper and lower body segments.[15] The height standards are based on mixed cross-sectional and longitudinal measurements of 189 boys and 214 girls.

ADULT HEIGHT

In a survey published by Murdoch *et al.* the mean height at 16 years or older was 131.6 cm for 51 boys (SD 5.6 cm) and 123.5 cm for 55 girls (SD 6.0 cm).[16] This corresponds to −6.8 SDS for boys and −6.4 SDS for girls, according to the standard of Tanner *et al.* The sex difference in height in this study was therefore 8.1 cm. No correlation was found between final height and parental height.

In the compilation of growth data for North American achondroplastic subjects, Horton *et al.* found that the mean adult height for men was 132 cm (±2 SD, 118–145 cm) and 125 cm for women (±2 SD, 112–136 cm) resulting in a sex difference of 7 cm[15]. Wynne-Davies *et al.* reported adult heights of 132.2 ±1.6 cm for men and 123.9 ±1.06 cm for women.[17]

Final height in Japanese achondroplastic individuals was reported to be 128.9 cm (SD 8.7 cm) for men and 124.0 (SD 4.8 cm) for women resulting in a sex difference of 4.9 cm.[18] When compared with Japanese growth standards final height corresponds to −7.3 SDS for men and −6.6 SDS for women.

WEIGHT DEVELOPMENT

Obesity is reported to be prevalent in individuals with achondroplasia. Due to the grossly disturbed body proportions, it is not possible, however, to use standard criteria for BMI or other weight for height indices when evaluating the weight situation. BMI values have been reported for 175 males and 262 females with achondroplasia.[19] The author's own results have shown a mean BMI at birth which corresponds to about ±0 SDS, increasing to about +1 SDS at 6 and 12 months of age, to +2.5 SDS at 24 months and to +3 SDS at 3 years of age ($n = 29$, unpublished data).

HEAD CIRCUMFERENCE

The available head circumference standard for achondroplasia is that of Horton *et al.*[15] plotted on the normal reference of Nellhaus.[20] At birth, head circumference is only slightly increased − about +1.5 SDS − but during the first few months of life, an increased rate of growth is typically observed and, at 6 months of age, the mean head circumference is about +2 SDS. If these data are plotted on a conventional head circumference reference, they could be mistaken as indicating hydrocephalic development. Therefore, the use of syndrome specific head circumference reference is strongly encouraged.

The mean head size for a child with achondroplasia is thus often clearly above the +2 SDS limit, for girls and boys respectively, over most of childhood. At 18 years of age, mean head circumference for females with achondroplasia is +2 SDS of the normal, but for males, it is almost +3 SDS. Thus, individuals with achondroplasia may have an absolute macrocephaly at all ages.

Medical complications

COGNITIVE FUNCTIONS

As for the majority of skeletal dysplasias, achondroplasia is associated with completely normal intelligence although speech delay and/or articulation problems may be present and motor milestones generally are delayed. Any sign of developmental delay affecting cognitive function should, however, be investigated immediately since CNS dysfunction as well as hydrocephalus may occur due to impaired liquor circulation that usually is independent of on aqueduct stenosis. In one large patient review as many as 11 percent of 198 individuals had received shunts due to either neurological/developmental or head circumference acceleration causes.[21]

NEUROLOGICAL DEVELOPMENT AND COMPLICATIONS

Gross motor development is delayed with a median age for walking of 17 months. Weakness in the trunk muscles similarly delays the child's sitting on its own. The delay in walking is a consequence of the combination of decreased muscular tone, ligament laxity − hyperextensibility of the knees is particularly common − and difficulties in supporting the large head. The foramen magnum is usually and the cervical spinal canal is often narrow, potentially contributing to late motor development through compression of the medulla. Increased reflexes in the legs are an indication of medullar compression. Neuroradiological investigation of the medulla in the foramen magnum and spinal canal is then often indicated to detect cases where surgical widening of the skeletal structures is necessary. Leg pain, parasthesias, and weakness with limitations in walking due to spinal stenosis is frequent in adults with achondroplasia but can also be present during childhood.

Due to potential compression of the spinal medulla, special considerations should be made in case of anesthesia, avoiding prolonged extreme positions of the head–neck. It is to be noted that non-traumatic cervical cord infarction has been reported during childhood.[22] Underdevelopment of the dens axis or atlantoaxial instability that occurs in type II collagen disorders is not typically present in achondroplasia, however. Functional medullary compression may be revealed by a compromised conductivity of nerve transmission or muscle excitability when tested using by electromyography, electroneurography or visual evoked responses.

RESPIRATORY PROBLEMS

Sleep problems are prevalent in the youngest children due to a narrow anatomy in the upper pharynx, especially when enlarged tonsils and adenoids contribute to the upper airway obstruction. The child then usually snores during sleep, sometimes with apneic episodes and with the head in a maximally extended position. If sleep apnea occurs, ventilation studies are obligatory in order to detect decreased oxygenation or carbon dioxide retention during sleep. Tonsil- and adenoidectomy may be helpful to relieve obstructive problems. At times, medullar compression from a narrow foramen magnum and/or cervical spine contributes to life-threatening apneic episodes due to brainstem dysfunction.[23]

Otitis media and conductive hearing loss are frequent findings in achondroplasia, often requiring ventilation tubes.

ORTHOPEDIC PROBLEMS

A thoracolumbar kyphosis is typically present during infancy, disappearing when the child starts to walk. In cases of its persistence, radiological investigation of the spinal canal is required. The sometimes very short and broad feet may require orthopedic shoes. Development of varus deformity of the lower legs during early or mid-childhood is common, also dependent on malalignment of the knee joint due to ligament laxity, and may require tibial osteotomy when malalignment of the ankle joint becomes pronounced. Extension defects in the elbows are usual and tend to increase with age depending on posterior bowing of the distal humerus.[24]

HYPOCHONDROPLASIA

Hypochondroplasia, as described in 1913 by Ravenna,[25] was long considered to be a mild form or allelic variant of achondroplasia ('achondroplasia tarda'). In contrast to achondroplasia, hypochondroplasia is usually diagnosed later in childhood due to mild body disproportion and variable short stature. The most severe cases may be hard to distinguish from achondroplasia, both clinically and radiologically, whereas the mildest cases may only show mild short stature with discrete body disproportion. It is, however, clear that hypochondroplasia is a heterogeneous diagnosis with mixed genetic background.

Genetics and molecular mechanisms

In 1995, it was confirmed that achondroplasia and hypochondroplasia are due to mutations of the same gene and are thus allelic disorders.[26,27] Whereas in achondroplasia, a single base is mutated altering the structure in the transmembrane region of *FGFR3*, hypochondroplasia is associated with different *FGFR3* mutations, mostly in the intracellular tyrosine kinase I region of the receptor. The mutations are, as in achondroplasia, thought to give increased activity of the receptor, thus mediating growth restriction at the epiphyseal growth plate. However, in a significant number of individuals with a clinical and radiological diagnosis of hypochondroplasia, *FGFR3* mutations cannot be found. Segregation analysis furthermore excludes *FGFR3* in some families.[28] The prevalence of hypochondroplasia is not established, but the disorder is not uncommon and may be more prevalent than achondroplasia. The trait is inherited in an autosomally dominant pattern with probably fairly constant expression.

Many of the cases are, as in achondroplasia, *de novo* mutations. It is not known whether these, as in achondroplasia, are of exclusive paternal origin.

Clinical traits

At birth, the clinical appearance is normal and discrete traits including lumbar lordosis, disproportionate short legs with mild varus deformity of tibia may become obvious later in childhood. Arm span is slightly reduced as compared to height. Hands may show brachydactyly. Facial features are normal and head circumference is typically at or just above normal mean. An absolute macrocephaly is thus not common. Although the spinal canal typically narrows in a caudal direction, skeletal dimensions are as a rule not sufficiently compromised to cause spinal stenosis or medullar compression from a narrow foramen magnum. The radiological hand-profile is typical for hypochondroplasia and could be helpful in establishing or refuting the diagnosis.

From a clinical point of view, the diagnosis contains considerate phenotypic variability and will probably, in the future, be sub-divided into several etiologies. In particular, it is often confused with Leri–Weill dyschondrosteosis which is a mesomelic (i.e., the middle segment of the limb is most affected) short limb skeletal dysplasia contrary to hypochondroplasia which is a rhizomelic (the proximal segment most affected) disorder.

Mild forms of hypochondroplasia may be hard to separate from idiopathic short stature only on clinical grounds and evaluation of body proportions, including the trunk–leg relation, may be decisive for considering the diagnosis. Measurement of sitting height and calculation of relative sitting height is helpful together with evaluation of a possible mesomelic or rhizomelic situation for leg and arm.

Growth and development of body proportions

Due to the diagnostic heterogeneity, height data are infrequent and depend on the diagnostic criteria used. Fetal growth is often marginally affected corresponding to about -1 to -1.5 SDS and short stature at -3 to -4 SDS develops during the first few years of life. The author's own experience from a small series of cases shows a mean height at 6 months of age corresponding to -2.4 SDS falling to -3.3 SDS at 12 months and to -4 SDS at 4 years of age. The position on the growth curve is probably then constant during the pre-pubertal years (Fig. 19.5). Puberty starts at normal age but pubertal growth is thought to be compromised resulting in a further reduction of final height.[29] Sufficient data for evaluation of pubertal growth are, however, not available.

Being a rhizomelic skeletal dysplasia, body disproportion in hypochondroplasia is generally not appreciated during childhood. Measurement of sitting height (measured in recumbent position for the youngest children) can reveal a relative increase in sitting height often corresponding to +3 SDS or more during early childhood. The trunk/leg disproportion becomes somewhat more pronounced with increasing age but clinically, the disproportion may be appreciated only after puberty. Head size is in the normal range at birth and subsequently follows the normal mean.

ADULT HEIGHT

Adult height is reported as 145–165 cm for males and 133–151 cm for females for cases using rather loose diagnostic criteria[29].

Medical complications

Genu varus deformity may develop during childhood and may require surgical correction. Lumbar lordosis is common but generally not as severe as in achondroplasia. Neurological complications from a narrow foramen magnum or spinal canal are not typical in hypochondroplasia.

LERI–WEILL DYSCHONDROSTEOSIS

The skeletal dysplasia (Leri–Weill) dyschondrosteosis (LWD) was described in 1929 by Leri and Weill.[30] They described a heritable trait characterized by mesomelic disproportional short stature together with a Madelung deformity of the wrist. The syndrome is characterized by a considerable intra- as well as inter-familial variability in phenotype with regard to stature and body disproportion. The prevalence of LWD is not known but estimates up to 1:2000 have been suggested.[31] It would then be one of the most common of the skeletal dysplasias but, due to discrete symptoms including moderate influence on stature, the condition is probably often overlooked.

Genetics and molecular mechanisms

In 1998, it was discovered that the genetic background to LWD was heterozygous mutations causing haploinsufficiency of the *SHOX* (short stature homeobox) gene. The *SHOX* gene is located in the major pseudoautosomal region (PAR1) on the short arms of the X and Y chromosomes.[32,33] Genes in this region escape X-chromosomal inactivation and the inheritance of LWD is then pseudoautosomal dominant or sex chromosome dominant. Due to the greatly increased rate of cross-over that occurs in PAR1 during meiosis,[34] a mutation residing on the X chromosome in an affected father could easily be transmitted via the Y chromosome to his son.

Altogether, about 60–80 percent of individuals with a clinical and radiological diagnosis of LWD have *SHOX*

mutations; most are large deletions. There seems to be no major phenotypic difference between those with or without demonstrable mutations.[35]

A homozygous *SHOX* mutation results in Langer mesomelic dysplasia, which is a severe mesomelic skeletal dysplasia with more pronounced short stature, hypoplasia or aplasia of the ulna and fibula, thickened and curved radius and tibia.

Clinical features

Apart from the presence of Madelung deformity, most prevalent in postpubertal females, mild short stature with body disproportion due to short legs is characteristic for LWD. The relative sitting height often corresponds to about +3 SDS in LWD and is a relevant screening measure. The body disproportion is evident also in the very young child and the SH percent SDS is probably constant during most of childhood. During puberty SH percent SDS may deteriorate further due to insufficient pubertal growth of the legs. Systematic longitudinal data of pubertal growth is, however, missing in LWD. Increased muscle mass and function is furthermore present in individuals with LWD.

There is a distinct sex difference in the expression in the Madelung deformity with females more often developing a clinically severe form that may require surgery. Furthermore, some authors report that height is more affected in females, which may further contribute to a bias of ascertainment that there are more females with LWD. It should be noted that idiopathic Madelung deformity without concomitant short stature and LWD is described as a separate syndrome.[36]

Medical complications

The Madelung deformity of the wrist usually develops slowly during childhood; only discernible on a radiograph at the beginning, but from puberty becoming clinically obvious. It is characterized by growth disturbance of the distal radial physis resulting in a progressive volar and ulnar tilted distal radial articular surface due to premature fusion of the ulnar portion of radial epiphysis. This will result in the radiological triangularization of the epiphysis with the radius becoming shortened and curved, both in ulnar and dorsal directions. The interosseus space between the radius and ulna is widened with the longitudinal level of the radius translated in the volar direction relative to the ulna. The carpal bones usually attain a wedged configuration, slipping down between radius and ulna.

Clinically, a volar subluxation of the hand and wrist, and a dorsally prominent distal ulna develops. Patients often experience increasing deformity and pain with limitation in movements especially supination and dorsiflexion. Pronation and flexion are usually normal. Although there is a distinct female preponderance in the prevalence of clinically expressed Madelung deformity, radiological signs are found in a majority of males with LWD.

Linear growth and development of body proportions

As with other clinical traits in LWD, influence on statural growth is variable and often moderate. Height SDS between −1.0 to −3.0 is typical, but a height that is near or even above average for age is probably not rare.[37]

There exist few reports on body height and proportions in the literature. These contain mostly data from probands with the Madelung deformity and may thus be biased. However, stature seems not to be associated with the presence of Madelung deformity.

Birth length is reduced indicating that fetal growth is affected. Thus, Munns et al. describes that, compared to unaffected siblings, birth length was 2.1 SDS shorter and that this difference was maintained during childhood.[38] Other authors confirm that height-SDS is unchanged during childhood.[31] Pubertal growth is repeatedly described as being deficient[37,39] (Fig. 19.9) but data on the consistency of this feature are missing. Deficient pubertal growth could to a certain extent be dependent on limited tibial growth, increasing the degree of mesomelia and body disproportion after puberty. It is not known whether the variability in height deficit is also reflected by a corresponding influence on the magnitude of pubertal growth.

However, other, mostly cross-sectional, studies find no difference between height SDS during childhood and at final height[40] or compared to affected parents.[31] The difference in height SDS compared to unaffected siblings is furthermore reported to be unchanged between childhood and at final height.[38]

Body proportions are most often deviant in LWD; an investigation of 28 probands showed a mean stature of

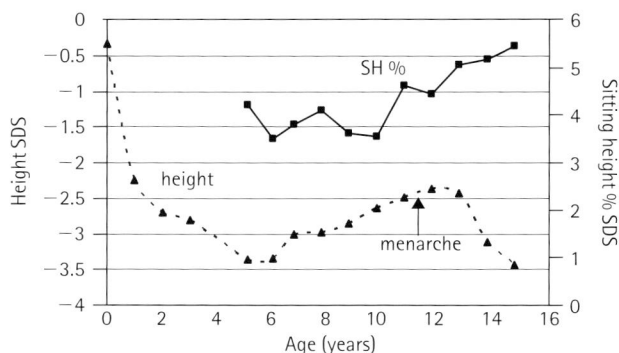

Figure 19.9 Growth curve as represented in SDS for a Japanese girl with Leri–Weill dyschondrosteosis. Height SDS is temporarily improved during pubertal years but final height position is similar to height SDS during mid-childhood. Body proportion measured as sitting height percent of total height deteriorates significantly during puberty due to better growth in the spine than in the legs (data from Fukami et al[37]). Normal height standard is that of Karlberg[116] and sitting height of Gerver.[3]

−2.1 SDS (range, −4.0 to +0.3 SDS). Relative sitting height (SH percent) was at a mean of +3.3 SDS (range, −0.3 to +6.4) and arm span at a mean of −3.5 SDS (range, −5.4 to −0.7).[41] See also Fig. 19.6 for distribution of relative sitting height.

SHOX mutations in idiopathic short stature

It has been reported that *SHOX* mutations are present at a low frequency in individuals with idiopathic short stature.[42–44] Auxological or radiological data to exclude LWD was not presented, however. A further investigation detected *SHOX* haploinsufficiency in three probands out of 140 short children.[45] In all three, skeletal and body proportion stigmata were consistent with the diagnosis in LWD. It is probable that individuals identified as having idiopathic short stature but with *SHOX* mutations, in fact, have LWD.

Leri–Weill dyschondrosteosis versus Turner syndrome and the influence of estrogen

Of interest as to the cause of the skeletal trait in LWD is that the prevalence of Madelung deformity in Turner syndrome is only 2 percent despite both conditions having haploinsufficiency of the *SHOX* gene.[46,47] This low frequency has been suggested to be due to estrogen deficiency. However, the number of girls with Turner syndrome that experience any extent of spontaneous puberty is substantial and as many as 10 percent with a 45,X cell line have menstruations.[48] Furthermore, in Turner syndrome, the length of the ulna is reduced compared to that of the radius,[47] i.e., the reverse of the situation in LWD. Radiological hand profile analysis gives similar patterns in Turner syndrome and LWD but still allows for 84 percent segregation between the entities.[49,50] The craniofacial features that are correlated to Turner syndrome, e.g., micrognathia, high arched palate and short neck are not as common in LWD.[51]

It is also to be noted that final height of untreated girls with Turner syndrome is not different for those with or without spontaneous puberty. The reduction of pubertal growth observed in both LWD and Turner syndrome may rather be caused by an inherent growth defect of the growth plate than by the influence of estrogens. The distinct sex difference in phenotype seen in LWD with regard to, at least, Madelung deformity remains to be investigated.

Effect of growth hormone therapy in Leri–Weill syndrome

Binder describes GH treatment in five children with LWD and *SHOX* mutations.[31] During a mean of 3.4 years of treatment (range, 1.5–9.8 years), the mean change in height SDS was 0.82 (SD 0.34). Thuestad report GH treatment of five children with LWD with a first year mean increase of growth velocity by 4.1 cm year^{-1}. At least three of the patients were, however, pubertal.[52]

The KIGS database show for 39 children with a given diagnosis of LWD a first year GH treatment change in height SDS of 0.47 (10th to 90th percentile, 0.32–0.76).[11]

MULTIPLE EPIPHYSEAL DYSPLASIA

Multiple epiphyseal dysplasia (MED) was described in more detail in 1947 by Thomas Fairbank.[53] It is a heterogeneous skeletal dysplasia, at present divided into six genetically distinct forms (EDM1-6). MED is characterized by mild short stature and childhood onset progressive osteoarthrosis, with bilateral pain and stiffness of weight bearing joints. On radiological investigation a more or less generalized involvement of all epiphyses is seen, with delayed and irregular ossification centers but with little abnormality of metaphyses or with spinal changes. MED is a common skeletal dysplasia with estimated prevalence of up to 1 per 10 000.[54]

Genetics and molecular mechanisms

MED is associated with dominant mutations in some of at least five genes: cartilage oligomeric protein (COMP; EDM1); the three type IX collagen genes (COL9A1-3; EDM6; EDM2; EDM3) and matrillin 3 (MTN3; EDM5). Furthermore, an autosomally recessive form of MED is linked to mutations in a sulfate transporter gene (DTDST or SLC26A2; EDM4).[54] Thus six variants, EDM1-6, exist in the MED spectrum of skeletal dysplasia. Still, fewer than half of cases with MED can presently be linked to any of these known genes.[55–57]

MED was formerly divided into the Fairbank type which was severe with involvement of almost all of the epiphyseal centers, and Ribbing type which was mild with epiphyseal ossification delay and dysplastic epiphysis primarily confined to the hips. However, it is now clear that all degrees of severity exist, and that both Ribbing and Fairbank types can result from mutations in the same genes.

The quality of the cartilage and linear growth may be differently affected in the various MED types. Thus both a COMP and a COL9A3 mutation giving a dominant arthropathy without affecting stature is described.[58,59]

Clinical traits

MED typically presents in early childhood with painful and stiff lower extremities. Hips and knees are most often affected in a symmetrical fashion and gait will be waddling.

The radiological abnormalities are most prominent in the hips, knees, wrists, and ankles. Growth of lower extremities is often disturbed with development of coxa vara, genu valgum or varum (or a combination; 'windswept deformity') and tibiotalar slant. Slipped epiphyses can be a complication of coxa vara. Perthe's disease, affecting a single joint, may be mistaken for MED if a general skeletal survey is not performed but many patients with MED present with bilateral Perthe's disease. In early adulthood the articular surfaces of the joints may be flattened, dysplastic and osteoarthrotic requiring athroplasty. Deficient linear growth may parallel the orthopedic problems. Furthermore, hands and feet may be short and stubby.

A distinct intra- as well as interfamilial clinical variability exists, from mild MED manifesting with pain and stiffness in the joints to more severe symptoms including marked short stature, ligamentous laxity and deformity of lower extremities.

As for the genetic diagnosis it has been suggested that MED patients with COMP mutations have the most severe changes in the hip joints with a progressive disease leading to early-onset hip osteoarthrosis, whereas patients with collagen IX mutations are more severely affected in the knee-joints with relative hip sparing.[60] COMP protein is normally present in the general circulation and levels are shown to be decreased in individuals with pseudoachondroplasia and MED depending on COMP mutations.[61]

The presence of pes equinovarus together with generalized epiphyseal involvement is common in the recessive DTDST-associated form of MED (EDM4).

Linear growth and body proportions

Stature in MED is often mildly affected and frequently normal. Systematic investigations for height and body proportion in MED are, however, largely lacking. Spranger reports adult height varying from 145 to 170 cm.[62] The correlation between radiological signs and stature is weak.[63] Six Japanese individuals with MED and COMP mutations were reported to have a median height of −2.0 SDS with the range −6.7 to −1.0 SDS.[64] In a study from Canada only ten of 25 individuals with the diagnosis of MED had a stature below the 3rd centile (corresponding to approximately below −2 SDS).[56] Figure 19.10 shows height SDS development in a girl with EDM1.

PSEUDOACHONDROPLASIA

Pseudoachondroplasia (PSACH) was described as a separate disorder by Maroteaux and Lamy in 1959.[65] It is a frequent severe skeletal dysplasia with profoundly short stature, childhood-onset joint laxity and severe arthrosis of weight-bearing joints. Radiological investigation shows epiphyseal as well as metaphyseal changes of the tubular bones and platyspondyly of the spine. The spectrum of clinical severity in PSACH also includes mildly affected cases. Appearance at birth is normal, also in severe cases, and growth failure together with orthopedic problems is usually not recognized until the second year of life. PSACH

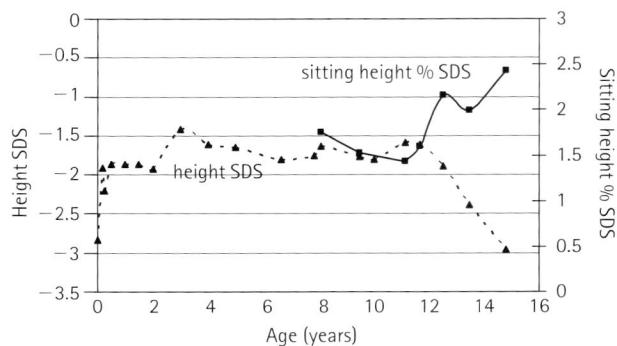

Figure 19.10 Growth curve as represented in SDS for height and body proportion in a girl with multiple epiphyseal dysplasia dependent on a *COMP* mutation (EDM1). The height SDS position is maintained during childhood but deteriorates during puberty due to deficient pubertal growth. The sitting height percentage of total height increases steeply during this period showing that growth of the spine is not as compromised as growth of the legs. At 15 years she is fully pubertal and has completed linear growth. Normal height standard is that of Karlberg[116] and sitting height of Gerver.[3]

is one of the more frequent skeletal dysplasias with an estimated prevalence of 1:30 000.

Genetics and molecular mechanisms

Pseudoachondroplasia is almost exclusively dependent on heterozygous mutations in the *COMP* (cartilage oligomeric protein) gene.[66–68] The majority of the cases with PSACH are associated with new mutations. Gonadal mosaicism can explain reports of affected successive children of unaffected parents. PSACH and certain types of MED (EDM1) are allelic disorders, representing a clinical spectrum with some phenotypical overlap.

The mutant COMP molecule has been shown to accumulate within the endoplasmatic reticulum of chondrocytes, presumably leading to decreased cellular viability with premature apoptosis and reduced linear growth capacity of the affected individual.

Clinical traits

The skull, face, and general appearance at birth are normal and growth disturbance as well as orthopedic problems will be obvious from the second year of life. Walking is delayed and abnormal hip involvement with small and irregular epiphyses leads to a waddling gait.

In the older child deformities of the lower limbs often develop, ranging from genu varum to genu valgum, to a windswept deformity (i.e., a combination of varum and valgum deformities). For example, surgical correction of bowlegs was performed in 70 percent of 61 cases with PSACH.[69] Ligamentous laxity, especially of the knees and ankles, joint stiffness and pain contribute to the orthopedic

problems. Uneven growth of epiphyses and metaphyses can lead to joint incongruity. The hands become broad with short metacarpals. The short fingers will have hyperlax joints that can be pulled out in a telescoping fashion. Arms are disproportionately short with incomplete extension at the elbows and ulnar deviations of the wrists.

Height development and body proportions

A severe short-limb stature develops during childhood but, in contrast to achondroplasia, trunk length is affected almost as much as leg length. Birth length is normal with a reported median of 50 cm for 47 individuals.[69] The postnatal growth pattern in PSACH is unusual because growth velocity can continue to be normal until about 1 year of age. The relative position on the growth curve thereafter starts a rapid and continuous decline reaching a severely compromised adult height. There seems to be poor correlation between stature and orthopedic complications.[69]

A growth curve for PSACH has been constructed by Horton *et al.* from data in 61 individuals (sexes combined).[70] Mean birth length was 49.4 cm with a SD of 2.0 cm indicating a perfectly normal intrauterine growth. At 2 years of age the position corresponds to about −2 SDS. Height position between 2 and 10 years of age decreases by 3 SDS and a further 2.4 SDS between 10 and 18 years of age. Mean adult height (at 18 years of age) of 30 individuals was 118.8 cm but with a SD of 12.2 cm.

Reports of adult height in other populations also exist. Nine, mostly adult, Korean individuals with PSACH and *COMP* mutations have been reported to have an average height at 17 years or older of 116.3 cm ($n = 6$) or a median height of −8.3 SDS with the range −13.8 to −3.5 SDS,[71] and another cohort of six adult Korean individuals had a mean height of 116 cm.[72] Seven Japanese individuals with PSACH and *COMP* mutations were reported to have a median height of −5.6 SDS with the range −12.2 to −1.6 SDS.[73] McKeand reports a median adult height in Caucasians of 116.6 cm for women and 120 cm for men.[69] Figure 19.11 shows development of growth and body proportion in a girl with PSACH.

THE TYPE II AND TYPE XI COLLAGENOPATHIES

Mutations in the *COL2A1*, *COL11A1* and *COL11A2* genes account for collagenopathies types II and XI. The members in this group of dominant skeletal dysplasias with overlapping traits are, in roughly decreasing degree of severity, the two lethal conditions achondrogenesis II and hypochondrogenesis, Kniest dysplasia, the severe spondyloepimetaphyseal dysplasia type Strudwick, spondyloepiphyseal dysplasia congenita of varying severity, the often mild Stickler artroophthalmopathy, and the autosomally dominant spondyloarthropathy.

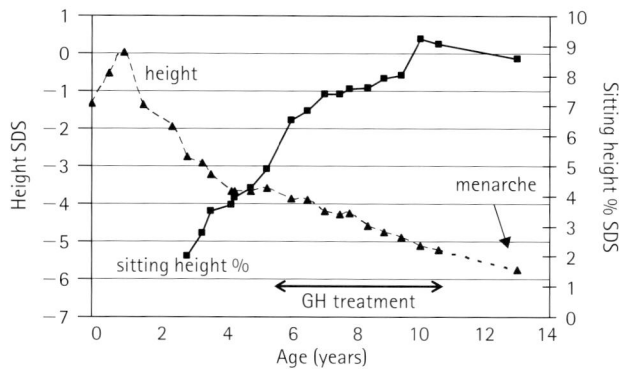

Figure 19.11 Growth curve as represented in SDS for height and body proportion in a girl with pseudoachondroplasia. Note a continuous decline in height SDS after 1 year of age. A trial with growth hormone as indicated, escalating to about 0.1 mg kg^{-1} day^{-1}, did not seem to alter the decreasing trend in height position. Body proportion measured as 'relative sitting height'; i.e., sitting height as a percentage of total height show a continuous increase dependent on abnormal growth of the legs. Normal height standard is that of Karlberg[116] and sitting height of Gerver.[3]

Type II collagen is a fibril-forming protein consisting of homotrimers of COL2A1 polypeptide chains twisted together to form a helical molecule. Important for the function is that every third amino acid is glycine. Mutations as well as deletions and premature stop codons can impair tertiary structure and assembly of the polypeptide chains into fibrils. Type XI collagen helps to maintain the spacing and diameter of type II collagen fibrils. Altogether, the type II and type XI collagenopathies have been estimated to occur in about one in 10 000.

SPONDYLOEPIPHYSEAL DYSPLASIA CONGENITA

Spondyloepiphyseal dysplasia congenita (SEDC) is a short trunk, skeletal dysplasia. It affects the development of the epiphyses and gives a retarded ossification, especially of the axial skeleton. It was named in 1966 by Spranger and Wiedemann, describing an entity with primary involvement of the vertebrae and proximal epiphyses of the limbs.[74] The incidence of SEDC is not known but estimations of one in about 100 000 have been given.

Genetics and molecular mechanisms

The genetic background of SEDC is mostly sporadic, heterozygous mutations, of the alpha chain of the collagen II gene (*COL2A1*) on chromosome 12. The mutation compromises the amount and quality of triple-stranded, helical, type II collagen, which is an extracellular matrix protein found in large amount in cartilage, the vitreous body of the eye, the inner ear, and in the nucleus pulposus of the intervertebral discs.

Clinical traits

At birth, more or less discrete clinical signs are present. These include diminished length, especially due to a short trunk, a flat face with a tendency towards wide set eyes and shallow orbits, a broad or barrel-shaped chest with increased anteroposterior diameter. Radiological investigation in infancy reveals delayed ossification of the skeleton with absence of ossification centers in, for example, the pubic bones and knee epiphyses. Vertebrae are typically ovoid in childhood but later become flattened, so-called platyspondyly.

The subsequent development shows a wide variability between affected individuals regarding linear growth and skeletal/orthopedic problems. It is common to encounter spinal deformities, including lumbar lordosis and/or scoliosis. Due to the short neck, the head may appear to rest more or less directly on the shoulders. Progressive coxa vara commonly develops as well as premature osteoarthrosis of the hips. Muscular hypotonia is present during infancy and walking is delayed. Gait will then be waddling due to a combination of coxa vara, muscular hypotonia, lumbar lordosis and the abnormalities of the hip joints including poorly formed femoral heads. The epiphyseal developmental defects are predominantly present in the spine and juxtatruncal epiphyses leaving the more distal bones less affected. Hands and feet are thus typically normal sized and with outstretched fingers. Severe cases of SEDC showing significant metaphyseal changes are usually classified as spondyloepimetaphyseal dysplasia type Strudwick. It has been suggested that this entity should be included in the SEDC diagnosis.[75]

Linear growth and body disproportion

A growth curve for SEDC is available, constructed from cross-sectional data of 62 individuals but combined for the sexes.[70] Mean birth length is 42 cm corresponding to about −6 SDS with a SD of 2.7 cm implicating a much-compromised intrauterine growth. Linear growth is very poor during the first year of life, but will from about 2 years of age follow about −5 SDS. Pubertal growth is scanty. Adult height is 115.5 cm corresponding to −8.9 SDS for males and −7.8 SDS for women. SD for adult height is 14.9 cm indicating much variability among individuals with SEDC for adult height. A range for adult height of 85 to 145 cm is reported.[76]

SEDC confers a general deficit in growth but the trunk is shorter than the extremities, which show a rhizomelic shortening. Hands and feet appear, on the contrary, little affected and head circumference is normal. Wynne-Davies and Hall suggested that individuals with SEDC and different degrees of coxa vara also had different degrees of height development.[77] In their survey, those with mild coxa vara fell just below −2 SDS in height, whereas those with severe coxa vara had a severely compromised adult height of 90–120 cm.

KNIEST DYSPLASIA

Kniest dysplasia, also known as metatropic dysplasia type II, was described in 1952 by Wilhelm Kniest.[78] It is a short trunk, short stature syndrome associated with enlarged joints and progressive increasing joint problems as well as abnormal vision and hearing. As for other members of the type II collagen disease group there is an overlap with other entities, especially SEDC.

Genetics

Kniest dysplasia is an autosomally dominant disorder dependent on mutations of *COL2A1* gene; most are small deletions giving shortened type II collagen fibers. The incidence of Kniest dysplasia is poorly known but estimations of fewer than one case per million have been given.

Clinical traits

Prenatal growth is affected with short limbs at birth and disproportional growth from the second trimester. The newborn furthermore has a flat round face with low nasal bridge. Shallow orbitae may be present making the eyes appear protruding. Cleft palate is present in 50 percent of individuals with Kniest. Clubfoot can be present. The joints are typically enlarged at birth and a radiologic survey shows large broad metaphyses and deformed large epiphyses.

Eye problems are present in about in 50 percent including myopia, retinal detachment, cataracts, and rarely congenital glaucoma. Hearing problems are often present (in 40 percent) and can be caused by a combination of a sensorineural defect and conduction deafness secondary to otitis media. Due to the platyspondyly and kyphoscoliosis, the trunk appears short in later childhood and the neck appears very short. Atlantoaxial instability is common due to odontoid hypoplasia.

Linear growth

The growth pattern is not reported in Kniest dysplasia. Average adult height in Kniest syndrome is reported to range between 100 and 140 cm corresponding to between −11 and −5 SDS for males and between −10 and −3.7 SDS for females. Figure 19.12 gives development of height and body proportion in a girl with Kniest dysplasia.

STICKLER SYNDROME

Stickler syndrome, or hereditary arthro-ophthalmopathy, is an autosomal disorder dependent on mutations in either type II or type XI collagen. The entity was described by Stickler *et al.* as being a condition characterized by among

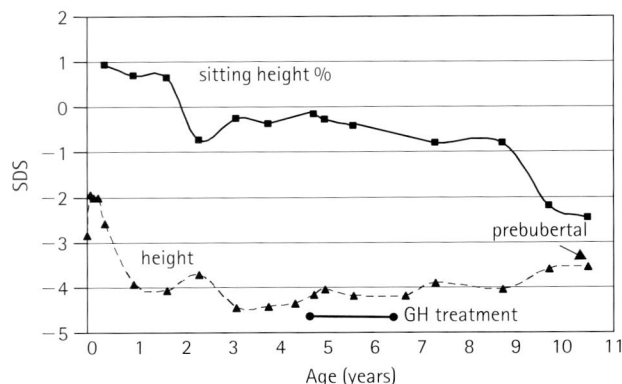

Figure 19.12 Growth curve in SDS for height and body proportions in a girl with Kniest dysplasia. A short trial of growth hormone therapy is shown. It was abandoned because of poor height gain. At 10 years she is still pre-pubertal. Note the periods with a decline in sitting height percentage of total height, dependent on deficient growth of the trunk. Normal height standard is that of Karlberg[116] and sitting height of Gerver.[3]

other midface hypoplasia, ocular manifestations, and joint hypermobility.[79] Marshall syndrome that is caused by mutations in type XI collagen is an allelic variant of or even regarded to be included in the Stickler syndrome diagnosis. The incidence of Stickler syndrome is estimated to be one out of 7500.

Genetics and molecular mechanisms

The majority of individuals have autosomal dominant mutations in *COL2A1* but mutations in *COL11A1* and *COL11A2* are also reported. In families without eye involvement *COL11A2* mutations have been described.[80]

Clinical traits

The midface is typically flat due to underdevelopment of the maxilla and nasal bridge. This trait usually diminishes with increasing age. A retro- or micrognathia is common and approximately 25 percent have cleft palate, often as part of a Pierre–Robin sequence. An isolated bifid uvula may be found. It is estimated that about 35 percent of children with Pierre–Robin sequence have Stickler syndrome.[81]

Myopia, usually severe but non-progressive, is a common problem found in Stickler syndrome. Cataract that is congenital or early onset, vitreous anomalies and retinal detachment also occur. A sensineuronal, progressive, high-frequency hearing loss is another major clinical finding.

Thoracolumbar spinal abnormalities or back pain are nearly uniformly observed and scoliosis is present in one-third but rarely needs corrective treatment.[82] Hip anomalies are common and manifest as slipped capital femoral epiphysis or Legg–Perthes-like disease.[83] The variability in phenotype of Stickler syndrome can be extensive indicating that this dominant trait can go unrecognized within a family until a child with Pierre–Robin sequence is born or a family member develops a cataract or has retinal detachment at a young age.[84]

Linear growth

Affected individuals are reported to have somewhat compromised height as compared to siblings but published systematic data on growth pattern including pubertal growth, are not available.

SPONDYLOEPIPHYSEAL DYSPLASIA TARDA

Spondyloepiphyseal dysplasia tarda (SEDT) is a skeletal dysplasia with late clinical onset. Individuals with SEDT appear normal at birth and show clinical signs of growth retardation, spinal and hip involvement from late childhood or during puberty.

Genetics and molecular mechanisms

SEDT is genetically heterogeneous. Most cases are X-linked recessive meaning that only males are affected. This form of SEDT is called SEDL and depends on mutations of the gene *SEDLIN* coding for a small, ubiquitously expressed, intracellular protein with unknown function.[85] An affected father with SEDL will thus contribute the mutated gene to none of the sons but to half of his daughters who, in turn, will be unaffected carriers. Autosomally recessive forms of SEDT with unclear genetic background also exist.

The incidence of SEDT is not known. In the UK, out of all skeletal dysplasia cases registered at the orthopedic clinics >9 percent were SEDT, with 22 percent being the X-linked recessive form.[86]

Clinical traits

Both clinical and radiological status is normal during infancy and the first years of life. Achievement of motor milestones is normal; i.e., no muscular weakness exists.

The initial clinical presentation occurs typically in late childhood with vague but progressive back and hip pain and numbness. There is a considerable variability in clinical expression but development of osteoarthrosis is common. The radiological changes may mimic Perthe's disease. A platyspondyly develops early resulting in deficient growth of the trunk. At times kyphoscoliosis is apparent during the pubertal years. Atlantoaxial instability, due to a hypoplastic odontoid process, may be present warranting radiological and clinical supervision.

Linear growth and body proportions

Growth restriction mostly affects the spine giving disproportionate short stature. The often mild shortening of the trunk is typical and can be quantified through measurement of sitting height. Subnormal growth probably starts first during late childhood. Adult height is reported below 150 cm (-4.3 SDS for males)[86] or ranging between 125 and 157 cm.[76]

An investigation of 11 mutational positive SEDL males showed an adult height range from 137 to 160 cm (-6.3 to -2.8 SDS) with an excess of arm span length over total height of 4.5 to 21.1 cm; median 16 cm.[87] The X-linked form of SEDT is reported to give a more pronounced short trunk condition compared to the autosomal forms.[88]

OSTEOGENESIS IMPERFECTA

Osteogenesis imperfecta (OI) is a heterogeneous, mostly autosomally dominant, skeletal dysplasia giving a defect of bone mass and stability with increased fracture rate. The prevalence has been estimated to about one in 5000 to 10 000.[89] The mildest variants do not affect linear growth whereas the severely affected individuals die *in utero* or have strongly affected development of the long bones with extreme short stature and major skeletal deformities.

Genetics and molecular mechanisms

OI is a mostly autosomally dominant disease that generally is caused by mutations in either of the two type I collagen genes *COL1A1-2* on chromosomes 17 and 7, respectively. The collagen type I molecule is a triple helix consisting of two COL1A1 chains and one COL1A2 chain. Cases of OI not linked to these loci also exist.[90] Missense mutations involving glycine codons in the central helix forming domain are typical in OI but genotype–phenotype correlation is often unpredictable.

The *COL1A1-2* mutations often compromise the triple-helix formation of type I collagen which disturb collagen fibril formation. The defect and/or insufficient matrix formation from the osteoblasts will cause abnormally low mineralized bone tissue as well as a deficiency in the amount of bone tissue. The result will be osteomalacia with a brittle bone structure.

Clinical traits

Except for diminished bone mass with increased fracture rates clinical findings may include blue or greyish-white sclera, skin hyperlaxity, joint hypermobility and decreased muscular tone. Dentinogenesis imperfecta, most evident in the primary teeth, is a variable finding in OI. The face often becomes small and triangular. Development of hearing loss is common in all variants of OI. At 40 years of age it occurs in about 40 percent of cases with type I OI.

Due to wide variability, OI is classified into groups of clinical severity. The commonly used classification was suggested by Sillence in 1979 and comprises four groups: types I–IV.[91]

Type I OI is the mildest, mostly non-deforming with little or no involvement of height. Vertebral fractures are typical and can, except for a short trunk condition, also lead to mild scoliosis. Fracture rates usually decrease after puberty. Sclera is usually blue. Dentinogenesis imperfecta may or may not be present.

Type II OI is severe and lethal *in utero* or during the perinatal period due to severely brittle bone with multiple fractures.

Type III OI is progressively deforming with a major influence on height. At birth the child typically shows frontal and temporal bossing of the skull and short, deformed fracture-prone extremities. During childhood development of deformed limbs, compressed vertebral bodies and severe kyphoscoliosis is common. The face will usually become short and triangular. Dentinogenesis imperfecta is common. Fractures heal with normal speed but occurrence of extensive callous formations and pseudarthroses are common. Prophylactic intramedullary rodding of the long bones in the lower extremities is a routine orthopedic procedure in these cases to prevent fractures and deformities.

Type IV OI is intermediate in clinical severity comprising cases that are not easily categorized in groups I–III. Symptoms in the type IV group sometimes present at birth but often later in childhood. Dentinogenesis imperfecta may or may not be present. The sclera is white after the age of 2 years. There is a marked intra- as well as interfamilial variability in the expression. Linear growth is moderately affected. Fractures often heal with extensive callus.

A further sub-classification of certain forms in the variable type IV group into types V, VI, and VII OI has been suggested according to radiological and genetic associations.[92]

Growth development and body proportion

Depending on the clinical type of OI, height and body disproportion can be vastly different. Height data are reported from a Dutch population of 49 children with OI with a mean (SD) age of 11.3 (3.8) years.[89] None of the children had been treated with bisphosphonate. Those with OI type I had a mean height of −1.8 (1.1; range, −3.8 to 0.9) SDS; those with OI type III −8.4 (1.8; range, −11.1 to −4.7) SDS and those with OI type IV −3.4 (1.6; range, −5.8 to −0.9) SDS. Body proportion as sitting height SDS showed means of −3.5, −7.7, and −4.7 for the respective groups type I, III, and IV. This suggests that even the least affected in the type I group are disproportional due to short trunk.

Another large cohort of children and adolescents with OI has been reported from Montreal.[93] Those with type I disease had a mean height SDS of −1.8 (n = 31; range, −4.0 to 0.9); those with type III had a mean height SDS of

−6.8 (n = 47; range, −12.4 to −3.0), and those with type IV −3.4 (n = 47; range, −9.0 to 1.1).

Treatment with bisphosphonate, physiotherapy, and intramedullary rodding: Effects on bone pain, fracture rate, and linear growth

Treatment of skeletal pain and bone turnover using bisphosphonate has been used in uncontrolled clinical trials in the last decade.[92,94] Bisphosphonate is incorporated into the inorganic bone tissue and seems to inhibit both osteoclast and osteoblast activity. This will then diminish an increased bone turnover in OI. The treatment also induces a transient decrease in serum calcium, which increases PTH secretion potentially stimulating osteoblast function. At present it is unclear whether bisphosphonate treatment will decrease development of skeletal deformities or scoliosis.[92] A large retrospective study of height development during 1 or 4 years of bisphosphonate treatment did show a minor height SDS improvement after 1 year of treatment only in type III OI (n = 42) (delta mean, 0.3; SD 0.8) but after 4 years only in type IV group (delta mean, 0.4; SD 0.7).[93] It is also to be noted that in children with polyostotic fibrous dysplasia (a localized bone abnormality associated with McCune–Albright syndrome) treated with bisphosphonate for 1–3 years, no significant effect on height development was observed.[95]

Treatment with growth hormone

Short trials with growth hormone treatment have been performed in OI. A report of treating types III and IV OI in 26 children with the GH dose 0.1–0.2 IU kg^{-1} day^{-1} on 6 days per week, showed that 14 of the children were 'responders' to GH treatment increasing their growth rate by at least 50 percent compared to baseline. The treatment growth rate for the responders was 6.4 (SD 2.0) cm year^{-1} compared with 4.0 (SD 1.7) cm for the non-responders during the first year of treatment. The average increase in height velocity was 3.3 cm ranging from 1.0 to 8.0 cm. S-IGF-I was almost tripled at 12 months of treatment compared to baseline. The responders had higher baseline values of carboxyterminal propeptide of collagen type I, suggesting that they had a higher capacity for collagen production. Most of the responders had OI type IV with moderate bone fragility and most of the non-responders had type III with severe bone fragility.[96]

DIASTROPHIC DYSPLASIA

Diastrophic dysplasia (DD) was named in 1960 by Lamy and Maroteaux who described it as a separate entity.[97] It is a short limb, short stature, skeletal dysplasia with generalized spine and joint involvement. Growth retardation as well as distortions of joints is usually already present at birth. In the past the condition was often named arthrogryposis multiplex congenita.

Genetics and molecular mechanisms

Recessive mutations in a sulfate transporter gene (*DTDST*) were recognized in 1994 as the background for DD.[98] Diastrophic dysplasia is particularly common in the Finnish population, where a founder *DTDST* mutation is present in about 1 percent of the population with more than 180 diagnosed cases of DD and an incidence of about 1:30 000.[99]

Recessive mutations in the *DTDST* gene also cause the mild skeletal dysplasia multiple epiphyseal dysplasia (EDM4) as well as the lethal conditions atelosteogenesis type 2 and achondrogenesis type 1B. Generally, there seems to be a correlation between the degree of loss of function of this membrane bound ion transporter and the phenotype.[100]

Clinical traits

Typical deformities seen in most individuals with DD are foot deformities, often pes equinovarus, and a short first metacarpal leading to a marked abducted position of the thumb – 'hitchhiker's thumb'. The fingers are short and broad with ulnar deviation.

Another typical sign in DD, occurring in the majority (85 percent) of cases, is acute cystic swelling of the pinnae of the ears starting during the first days or weeks of life. Facial features that are often present consist of a prominent cheek, circumoral fullness, and narrow nasal bridge. The cartilage of the larynx and trachea may be soft producing clinical signs of laryngomalacia. The cry may be hoarse.

Spine deformities and progressive articular degeneration and development of joint contractures with subluxation or dislocations are present. Scoliosis or kyphoscoliosis is reported to be present in the majority of cases[101] and considered to be progressive in 13 percent. Lumbar lordosis is usually present from early childhood and can be pronounced. Mechanistically it is associated to the hip contracture.

The development and growth of the cervical spine is commonly affected with spina bifida occulta (in average over three to four vertebrae) in 80 percent of cases, and childhood kyphosis that most often resolves spontaneously. The resolution of the cervical kyphosis coincides with the development of upright position and walking similarly with the case of thoracolumbar kyphosis seen in the achondroplastic child.[102] The spinal canal is narrow but neurological signs from a compromised medulla is, however, not very common.[103]

A uniform development of progressive deformities and contractures of the joints are the rule. Flexion contractures of knee and hip joints can severely compromise posture.

Hip joint dysplasia (occurring in 70 percent) with or without dislocation (occurring in 20 percent) as well as a general joint stiffness, early arthrosis and foot deformities produces difficulty in walking and the occasional need of a wheelchair.[103] Motor milestones are delayed and the average child sits unsupported at 8 months of age and walks at 24 months.[104]

Linear growth and body proportions

DD confers a short limb, short stature condition and compromised growth is evident at birth. Mäkitie[99] reported growth characteristics from 121 Finnish cases; thus derived from a homogeneous genetic background also for the DTDST-mutation[105] (Fig. 19.13).

Birth length was at a median of − 3.2 SDS (range, −8.1 to −0.6) for boys and − 3.0 SDS (range, −7.5 to −1.3) for girls. Birth head circumference was for boys and girls 0.7 and 0.1 SDS, respectively. During the first 2 years of life the position on the growth curve decreased by about 1 SDS and then remained more or less stable during most of childhood until puberty.

Pubertal growth was deficient with a median decrease in relative height of about 2 SDS (range, 0.1–4.6) for boys and 2.9 SDS (range, 1.4–4.1) in girls between 10 years of age and adulthood.

Median adult height for this Finnish DD population was 135.7 cm (−7.2 SDS; range, 114.0–158.3 cm) for men, and 129.0 cm (−6.7 SDS; range, 98.0–143.0 cm) for women. The variability of growth failure within the same sibship was considerable. The presence of contractures in hips and knees as well as scoliosis further reduces compromised growth.

Previous published studies from other populations have given mean adult statures of 112 cm (both sexes combined).[106] A growth reference for DD, combined for the sexes, is also published by Horton from data of 38 male and 34 female individuals. It gives a mean adult height of 118.3 cm (SD 12.0 cm; n = 18).[70]

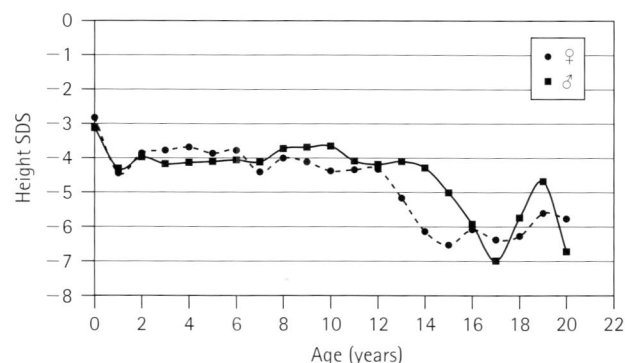

Figure 19.13   Height SDS development in boys (circles) and girls (squares) with diastrophic dysplasia. Mixed longitudinal and cross-sectional data from 53 boys and 68 girls applied on the normal population standard of Karlberg.[116] Data from Makitie and Kaitila.[99]

CARTILAGE HAIR HYPOPLASIA

Cartilage hair hypoplasia (CHH), synonyms McKusick-CHH or metaphyseal dysplasia McKusick type is a short limb skeletal dysplasia with extreme adult shortness. The diagnosis can be considered in cases with a combination of short limb metaphyseal skeletal dysplasia and generalized laxity of joint ligaments and sparse body hair. Other symptoms include deficiencies of the immune system and mild macrocytic anemia that mostly is transient during childhood, but occasionally is severe and persistent.[107]

There is a high degree of intrafamilial variability with regard to the combinations of symptoms. Cases with minimal extra-skeletal involvement may be misdiagnosed as Schmid type metaphyseal dysplasia.

Genetics and molecular mechanisms

The molecular basis of CHH is mutations in the mitochondrial RNA-processing endoribonuclease (RMRP). The disorder is prevalent in the Finnish population with about 150 registered individuals and an estimated incidence of 1:23 000 corresponding to a carrier frequency of about one in 76.[108] It is even more common among the religious isolates; the Old Order Amish in the US with an incidence of 1.5 in 1000 births. The disease occurs, however, sporadically in all populations.

Clinical traits

The short limb growth retardation is already obvious at birth. All segments of the limbs are proportionally shortened. Hands are short and broad with short fingernails. The hair, including the eyebrows and eyelashes, is most often fine, sparse, slow growing and depigmented. Cases with normal hair are also described. Ligament laxity is typical including hypermobility of wrists, fingers, and feet.

Other features include extension defect of the elbow, increased lumbar lordosis, scoliosis, genu varum, and narrow thorax with flaring of lower rib cage. Head circumference and face are normal.

Except for the metaphyseal dysplasia, platyspondyly, long fibula in relation to tibia, bow legs, narrowing of interpedicular distances in caudal direction, and occasional odontoid hypoplasia are important skeletal signs and features.

The immune defect occurring at high prevalence in CHH is linked to T-cell dysfunction but many cases have B-cell defects as well. Signs of a more general hematopoietic impairment are often present with defects in all myeloid lineages; erythroid, granulocyte–macrophages and megakaryocytes. The immune defect causes susceptibility to opportunistic infections, principally varicella, which could be life threatening.[109]

Probably due to the immune defect, the prevalence of malignancies, especially non-Hodgkin's lymphoma and leukemia, is also increased. Impaired spermatogenesis is

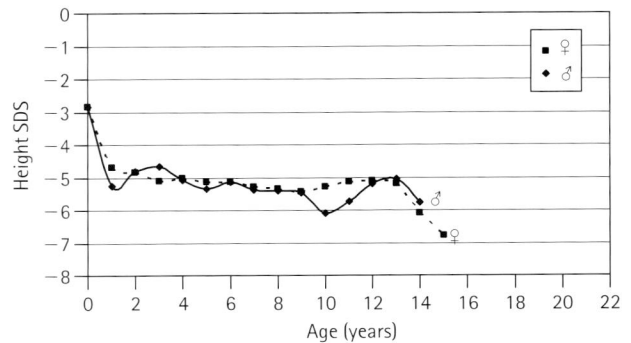

Figure 19.14 Height SDS development in boys (diamonds) and girls (squares) with cartilage hair hypoplasia. Mixed longitudinal and cross-sectional data from 44 males and 56 females (from Makitie et al.[110]) applied to the normal population standard of Karlberg.[116]

another feature of the generalized defect in cell proliferation; giving a low sperm count and abnormal sperm morphology. The prevalence of Hirschsprung's disease is increased (7 percent in the Finnish CHH population) and is associated with more severe forms of CHH.

Growth and development of body proportions

Growth curves for CHH are available based on 107 Finnish individuals (Fig. 19.14). Mean length at birth was −2.9 SDS for boys and −3.0 SDS for girls. Mean birth weight was −0.8 and −0.9 SDS for boys and girls respectively. Pre-term birth as well as breech presentation was over-represented.[110]

Growth velocity during the first year of life is severely subnormal, with a gain of only 8–9 cm, resulting in a length corresponding to about −5 SDS before 2 years of age. This relative height position is then maintained until 6 years of age, with a further reduction to −6 SDS before puberty.

Timing of puberty seems to be normal, but pubertal growth is weak, resulting in further loss of relative height. The sex difference in height is 2.5 cm or less during most of childhood, with boys being taller than girls.

All segments of upper and lower limbs are shortened and the short trunk is still disproportionately long compared to the legs. Sitting height, expressed as percentage of total height is increased. This measure corresponds to about + 3 SDS in the younger children with CHH, up to the age of six and then increases further to adulthood. The shortest individuals have the greatest disproportions in that respect. The mean difference between arm span and height is normal at all ages, suggesting that growth failure is more severe in the lower limbs.

HEAD CIRCUMFERENCE

At birth, head circumference corresponds to −0.2 SDS for boys and −0.5 SDS for girls, decreasing to about −1.0 SDS at two years of age. Adult head circumference is −0.9 SDS (range, −3.8 to +2.0 SDS).

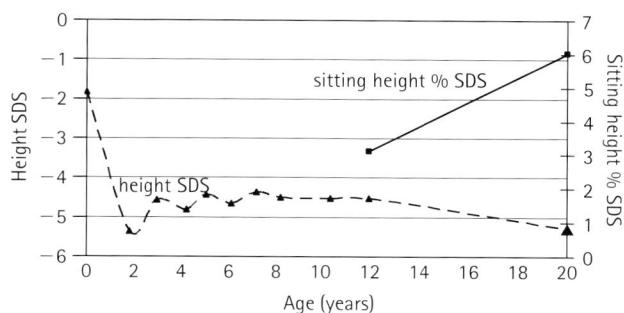

Figure 19.15 Growth curve in SDS for height and body proportion in a girl with cartilage hair hypoplasia. Pubertal development was average. Normal height standard is that of Karlberg[116] and sitting height of Gerver.[3]

ADULT HEIGHT

In the Finnish study, mean final height was 131.1 for males and 122.5 cm for females corresponding to −7.9 SDS for both sexes. The range of adult height was 111–149 cm for males and 104–137 cm for females. The sex difference in mean height was thus 8.6 cm. There was no correlation between final height and target height. Adult height for Amish individuals with CHH is reported to be within the range of 107–147 cm.[111] Figure 19.15 gives height and proportion development in a girl with CHH.

KEY LEARNING POINTS

- Evaluate sitting height percentage of total height in all short children compared to normal standard. A disproportionate short stature with relative sitting height above +2.5 SDS suggests a skeletal dysplasia or a syndrome. Growth failure due to hormonal, nutritional or psychosocial causes does not usually have body disproportions.
- Make a detailed evaluation of phenotypic skeletal and other morphologic traits in the patient and the family (see Table 19.2).
- Draw a family tree and include data on height and body proportion as well as other physical features.
- Consider the growth pattern of patient and family members. Any suspicion of deficient pubertal growth in fully grown family members?
- Evaluate possible signs of a generalized connective tissue abnormality (including hearing, vision, decreased muscle function).
- It is necessary to follow children with skeletal dysplasias in dedicated clinical centers to accumulate the necessary experience in diagnosing and prospective clinical management.
- It is advisable to follow patients with diagnoses at risk for cervical spine instability with repeated radiological and clinical evaluations.
- It is advisable to see patients with skeletal and/or joint problems together with a pediatric orthopedic surgeon and a pediatric neurologist.

REFERENCES

● = seminal primary article
◆ = key review article
∗ = management guidelines

∗   1   Hall CM. International nosology and classification of constitutional disorders of bone. *Am J Med Genet* 2002; **113**: 65–77.

●   2   Fredriks AM, van Buuren S, van Heel W, *et al.* Nation-wide age references for sitting height, leg length and sitting height/height ratio and their diagnostic value for disproportionate growth disorders. *Arch Dis Child* 2005.

●   3   Gerver WJM, de Bruin R. *Paediatric Morphometrics.* Utrecht: Wetenschappelijke uitgeverij Bunge, 1996.

∗   4   Lachman RS. The cervical spine in the skeletal dysplasias and associated disorders. *Pediatr Radiol* 1997; **27**: 402–8.

∗   5   Lachman RS. Neurologic abnormalities in the skeletal dysplasias: a clinical and radiological perspective. *Am J Med Genet* 1997; **69**: 33–43.

●   6   Noonan KJ, Leyes M, Forriol F, Canadell J. Distraction osteogenesis of the lower extremity with use of monolateral external fixation. A study of two hundred and sixty-one femora and tibiae. *J Bone Joint Surg Am* 1998; **80**: 793–806.

7   Quigley CA, Crowe BJ, Anglin DG, Chipman JJ. Growth hormone and low dose estrogen in Turner syndrome: results of a United States multi-center trial to near-final height. *J Clin Endocrinol Metab* 2002; **87**: 2033–41.

8   MacFarlane CE, Brown DC, Johnston LB, *et al.* Growth hormone therapy and growth in children with Noonan's syndrome: results of 3 years' follow-up. *J Clin Endocrinol Metab* 2001; **86**: 1953–6.

9   Kirk JM, Betts PR, Butler GE, *et al.* Group tU. Short stature in Noonan syndrome: response to growth hormone therapy. *Arch Dis Child* 2001; **84**: 440–3.

∗   10   Finkelstein BS, Imperiale TF, Speroff T, *et al.* Effect of growth hormone therapy on height in children with idiopathic short stature: a meta-analysis. *Arch Pediatr Adolesc Med* 2002; **156**: 230–40.

11   KIGS, Pfizer International Growth Database.

12   Cho JY, Guo C, Torello M, *et al.* Defective lysosomal targeting of activated fibroblast growth factor receptor 3 in achondroplasia. *Proc Natl Acad Sci USA* 2004; **101**: 609–14.

13   Lievens PM, Mutinelli C, Baynes D, Liboi E. The kinase activity of fibroblast growth factor receptor 3 with activation loop mutations affects receptor trafficking and signaling. *J Biol Chem* 2004; **279**: 43254–60.

14   Legeai-Mallet L, Benoist-Lasselin C, Munnich A, Bonaventure J. Overexpression of FGFR3, Stat1, Stat5 and p21Cip1 correlates with phenotypic severity and defective chondrocyte differentiation in FGFR3-related chondrodysplasias. *Bone* 2004; **34**: 26–36.

∗   15   Horton WA, Rotter JI, Rimoin DL, *et al.* Standard growth curves for achondroplasia. *J Pediatr* 1978; **93**: 435–8.

16   Murdoch JL, Walker BA, Hall JG, *et al.* Achondroplasia–a genetic and statistical survey. *Ann Hum Genet* 1970; **33**: 227–44.

17 Wynne-Davies R, Walsh WK, Gormley J. Achondroplasia and hypochondroplasia. Clinical variation and spinal stenosis. *J Bone Joint Surg Br* 1981; **63B**: 508–15.

18 Tachibana K, Suwa S, Nishiyama S, *et al.* Growth of patients with achondroplasia (in Japanese). *Shounikashinryo* (*J Pediatr Pract*) 1997; **60**: 1363–9.

19 Hecht JT, Hood OJ, Schwartz RJ, *et al.* Obesity in achondroplasia. *Am J Med Genet* 1988; **31**: 597–602.

20 Nellhaus G. Head circumference from birth to eighteen years. Practical composite international and interracial graphs. *Pediatrics* 1968; **41**: 106–14.

* 21 Hunter AG, Bankier A, Rogers JG, *et al.* Medical complications of achondroplasia: a multicentre patient review. *J Med Genet* 1998; **35**: 705–12.

22 Wieting JM, Krach LE. Spinal cord injury rehabilitation in a pediatric achondroplastic patient: case report. *Arch Phys Med Rehabil* 1994; **75**: 106–8.

23 Tasker RC, Dundas I, Laverty A, *et al.* Distinct patterns of respiratory difficulty in young children with achondroplasia: a clinical, sleep, and lung function study. *Arch Dis Child* 1998; **79**: 99–108.

24 Kitoh H, Kitakoji T, Kurita K, *et al.* Deformities of the elbow in achondroplasia. *J Bone Joint Surg Br* 2002; **84**: 680–3.

25 Ravenna F. Achondroplassia et chondrohypoplasie. Contribution clinique. *Nouvelle iconographie de la Salpêtrière* 1913; **26**: 157–84.

26 Bellus GA, McIntosh I, Smith EA, *et al.* A recurrent mutation in the tyrosine kinase domain of fibroblast growth factor receptor 3 causes hypochondroplasia. *Nat Genet* 1995; **10**: 357–9.

27 Shiang R, Thompson LM, Zhu YZ, *et al.* Mutations in the transmembrane domain of FGFR3 cause the most common genetic form of dwarfism, achondroplasia. *Cell* 1994; **78**: 335–42.

28 Grigelioniene G, Eklof O, Ivarsson SA, *et al.* Mutations in short stature homeobox containing gene (SHOX) in dyschondrosteosis but not in hypochondroplasia. *Hum Genet* 2000; **107**: 145–9.

29 Appan S, Laurent S, Chapman M, *et al.* Growth and growth hormone therapy in hypochondroplasia. *Acta Paediatr Scand* 1990; **79**: 796–803.

30 Leri A, Weill J. Une affection congenitale et symetrique du development osseux: la dyschondrosteose. *Bull Mem Soc Med Hop Paris* 1929; **53**: 1491–4.

31 Binder G, Renz A, Martinez A, *et al.* SHOX haploinsufficiency and Leri-Weill dyschondrosteosis: prevalence and growth failure in relation to mutation, sex, and degree of wrist deformity. *J Clin Endocrinol Metab* 2004; **89**: 4403–8.

32 Belin V, Cusin V, Viot G, *et al.* SHOX mutations in dyschondrosteosis (Leri-Weill syndrome). *Nat Genet* 1998; **19**: 67–9.

33 Shears DJ, Vassal HJ, Goodman FR, *et al.* Mutation and deletion of the pseudoautosomal gene SHOX cause Leri-Weill dyschondrosteosis. *Nat Genet* 1998; **19**: 70–3.

34 Lien S, Szyda J, Schechinger B, *et al.* Evidence for heterogeneity in recombination in the human pseudoautosomal region: high resolution analysis by sperm typing and radiation-hybrid mapping. *Am J Hum Genet* 2000; **66**: 557–66.

35 Schiller S, Spranger S, Schechinger B, *et al.* Phenotypic variation and genetic heterogeneity in Leri–Weill syndrome. *Eur J Hum Genet* 2000; **8**: 54–62.

36 Plafki C, Luetke A, Willburger RE, *et al.* Bilateral Madelung's deformity without signs of dyschondrosteosis within five generations in a European family – case report and review of the literature. *Arch Orthop Trauma Surg* 2000; **120**: 114–7.

37 Fukami M, Matsuo N, Hasegawa T, *et al.* Longitudinal auxological study in a female with SHOX (short stature homeobox containing gene) haploinsufficiency and normal ovarian function. *Eur J Endocrinol* 2003; **149**: 337–41.

38 Munns CF, Glass IA, Flanagan S, *et al.* Familial growth and skeletal features associated with SHOX haploinsufficiency. *J Pediatr Endocrinol Metab* 2003; **16**: 987–96.

39 Kosho T, Muroya K, Nagai T, *et al.* Skeletal features and growth patterns in 14 patients with haploinsufficiency of SHOX: implications for the development of Turner syndrome. *J Clin Endocrinol Metab* 1999; **84**: 4613–21.

40 Ross JL, Scott C Jr, Marttila P, *et al.* Phenotypes associated with SHOX deficiency. *J Clin Endocrinol Metab* 2001; **86**: 5674–80.

41 Grigelioniene G, Schoumans J, Neumeyer L, *et al.* Analysis of short stature homeobox-containing gene (SHOX) and auxological phenotype in dyschondrosteosis and isolated Madelung deformity. *Hum Genet* 2001; **109**: 551–8.

42 Rao E, Weiss B, Fukami M, *et al.* Pseudoautosomal deletions encompassing a novel homeobox gene cause growth failure in idiopathic short stature and Turner syndrome. *Nat Genet* 1997; **16**: 54–63.

43 Rappold GA, Fukami M, Niesler B, *et al.* Deletions of the homeobox gene SHOX (short stature homeobox) are an important cause of growth failure in children with short stature. *J Clin Endocrinol Metab* 2002; **87**: 1402–6.

44 Stuppia L, Calabrese G, Gatta V, *et al.* SHOX mutations detected by FISH and direct sequencing in patients with short stature. *J Med Genet* 2003; **40**: E11.

45 Binder G, Ranke MB, Martin DD. Auxology is a valuable instrument for the clinical diagnosis of SHOX haploinsufficiency in school-age children with unexplained short stature. *J Clin Endocrinol Metab* 2003; **88**: 4891–6.

46 Binder G, Fritsch H, Schweizer R, Ranke MB. Radiological signs of Leri–Weill dyschondrosteosis in Turner syndrome. *Horm Res* 2001; **55**: 71–6.

47 Tauber M, Lounis N, Coulet J, *et al.* Wrist anomalies in Turner syndrome compared with Leri–Weill dyschondrosteosis: a new feature in Turner syndrome. *Eur J Pediatr* 2004; **163**: 475–81.

♦ 48 Layman LC. Human gene mutations causing infertility. *J Med Genet* 2002; **39**: 153–61.

49 Laurencikas E, Söderman E, Davenport M, *et al.* Metacarpophalangeal pattern profile analysis as a tool for early diagnosis of Turner syndrome. *Acta Radiol* 2005.

50 Laurencikas E, Soderman E, Grigelioniene G, et al. Metacarpophalangeal pattern profile analysis in Leri–Weill dyschondrosteosis. Acta Radiol 2005; 46: 200–7.

51 Kosho T, Muroya K, Nagai T, et al. Skeletal features and growth patterns in 14 patients with haploinsufficiency of SHOX: implications for the development of Turner syndrome. J Clin Endocrinol Metab 1999; 84: 4613–21.

52 Thuestad IJ, Ivarsson SA, Nilsson KO, Wattsgard C. Growth hormone treatment in Leri–Weill syndrome. J Pediatr Endocrinol Metab 1996; 9: 201–4.

53 Fairbank T. Dysplasia epiphysialis multiplex. Proc R Soc Med (Ortho Sec) 1947: 39: 315–7.

54 Briggs MD, Chapman KL. Pseudoachondroplasia and multiple epiphyseal dysplasia: mutation review, molecular interactions, and genotype to phenotype correlations. Hum Mutat 2002; 19: 465–78.

55 Unger S, Hecht JT. Pseudoachondroplasia and multiple epiphyseal dysplasia: New etiologic developments. Am J Med Genet 2001; 106: 244–50.

56 Jakkula E, Makitie O, Czarny-Ratacjzak M, et al. Mutations in the known genes are not the major cause of MED; distinctive phenotypic entities among patients with no identified mutations. Eur J Hum Genet 2005; 13: 292–301.

57 Lachman RS, Krakow D, Cohn DH, Rimoin DL. MED, COMP, multilayered and NEIN: an overview of multiple epiphyseal dysplasia. Pediatr Radiol 2004; Oct 21 [Epub ahead of print]

58 Kawaji H, Nishimura G, Watanabe S, et al. Autosomal dominant precocious osteoarthropathy due to a mutation of the cartilage oligomeric matrix protein (COMP) gene: further expansion of the phenotypic variations of COMP defects. Skeletal Radiol 2002; 31: 730–7.

59 Nakashima E, Kitoh H, Maeda K, et al. Novel COL9A3 mutation in a family with multiple epiphyseal dysplasia. Am J Med Genet A 2005; 132A: 181–4.

60 Unger SL, Briggs MD, Holden P, et al. Multiple epiphyseal dysplasia: radiographic abnormalities correlated with genotype. Pediatr Radiol 2001; 31: 10–8.

61 Mabuchi A, Momohara S, Ohashi H, et al. Circulating COMP is decreased in pseudoachondroplasia and multiple epiphyseal dysplasia patients carrying COMP mutations. Am J Med Genet 2004; 129A: 35–8.

62 Spranger J. The epiphyseal dysplasias. Clin Orthop 1976; 114: 46–60.

63 Haga N, Nakamura K, Takikawa K, et al. Stature and severity in multiple epiphyseal dysplasia. J Pediatr Orthop 1998; 18: 394–7.

64 Mabuchi A, Momohara S, Ohashi H, et al. Circulating COMP is decreased in pseudoachondroplasia and multiple epiphyseal dysplasia patients carrying COMP mutations. Am J Med Genet 2004; 129A: 35–8.

65 Maroteaux P, Lamy M. Les formes pseudoachondroplastiques des dysplasies spondylo-epiphysaires. Presse Med 1959; 67: 383–6.

66 Briggs MD, Hoffman SM, King LM, et al. Pseudoachondroplasia and multiple epiphyseal dysplasia due to mutations in the cartilage oligomeric matrix protein gene. Nat Genet 1995; 10: 330–6.

67 Hecht JT, Nelson LD, Crowder E, et al. Mutations in exon 17B of cartilage oligomeric matrix protein (COMP) cause pseudoachondroplasia. Nat Genet 1995; 10: 325–9.

68 Spranger JW, Zabel B, Kennedy J, et al. A disorder resembling pseudoachondroplasia but without COMP mutation. Am J Med Genet A 2005; 132A: 20–4.

69 McKeand J, Rotta J, Hecht JT. Natural history study of pseudoachondroplasia. Am J Med Genet 1996; 63: 406–10.

* 70 Horton WA, Hall JG, Scott CI, et al. Growth curves for height for diastrophic dysplasia, spondyloepiphyseal dysplasia congenita, and pseudoachondroplasia. Am J Dis Child 1982; 136: 316–9.

71 Song HR, Lee KS, Li QW, et al. Identification of cartilage oligomeric matrix protein (COMP) gene mutations in patients with pseudoachondroplasia and multiple epiphyseal dysplasia. J Hum Genet 2003; 48: 222–5.

72 Song HR, Li QW, Oh CW, et al. Mesomelic dwarfism in pseudoachondroplasia. J Pediatr Orthop B 2004; 13: 340–4.

73 Mabuchi A, Manabe N, Haga N, et al. Novel types of COMP mutations and genotype-phenotype association in pseudoachondroplasia and multiple epiphyseal dysplasia. Hum Genet 2003; 112: 84–90.

74 Spranger J, Wiedemann HR. Dysplasia spondyloepiphysaria congenita. Acta Paediatr Helv 1966; 21: 598.

♦ 75 Spranger J, Winterpacht A, Zabel B. The type II collagenopathies: a spectrum of chondrodysplasias. Eur J Pediatr 1994; 153: 56–65.

* 76 Spranger JW, Brill PW, Poznanski A. Bone Dysplasias. An Atlas of Genetic Disorders of Skeletal Development, 2nd edn. Oxford: Oxford University Press; 2002.

77 Wynne-Davies R, Hall C. Two clinical variants of spondylo-epiphysial dysplasia congenita. J Bone Joint Surg Br 1982; 64: 435–41.

78 Kniest W. Zur abgrenzung der dysostosis encondralis von der chondrodystrophie. Z Kinderheilkunde 1952; 760: 633–40.

79 Stickler GB, Belau PG, Farell FJ, et al. Hereditary progressive arthro-ophthalmopathy. Mayo Clin Proc 1965; 40: 433–55.

80 Sirko-Osadsa DA, Murray MA, Scott JA, et al. Stickler syndrome without eye involvement is caused by mutations in COL11A2, the gene encoding the alpha2(XI) chain of type XI collagen. J Pediatr 1998; 132: 368–71.

81 van den Elzen AP, Semmekrot BA, Bongers EM, et al. Diagnosis and treatment of the Pierre Robin sequence: results of a retrospective clinical study and review of the literature. Eur J Pediatr 2001; 160: 47–53.

82 Rose PS, Ahn NU, Levy HP, et al. Thoracolumbar spinal abnormalities in Stickler syndrome. Spine 2001; 26: 403–9.

83 Rose PS, Ahn NU, Levy HP, et al. The hip in Stickler syndrome. J Pediatr Orthop 2001; 21: 657–63.

84 Liberfarb RM, Levy HP, Rose PS, et al. The Stickler syndrome: genotype/phenotype correlation in 10 families with Stickler syndrome resulting from seven mutations in the type II collagen gene locus COL2A1. Genet Med 2003; 5: 21–7.

85 Gedeon AK, Colley A, Jamieson R, et al. Identification of the gene (SEDL) causing X-linked spondyloepiphyseal dysplasia tarda. Nat Genet 1999; 22: 400–4.

86 Wynne-Davies R, Gormley J. The prevalence of skeletal dysplasias. An estimate of their minimum frequency and the number of patients requiring orthopaedic care. J Bone Joint Surg Br 1985; 67: 133–7.

87 Gedeon AK, Tiller GE, Le Merrer M, et al. The molecular basis of X-linked spondyloepiphyseal dysplasia tarda. Am J Hum Genet 2001; 68: 1386–97.

88 Iceton JA, Horne G. Spondylo-epiphyseal dysplasia tarda. The X-linked variety in three brothers. J Bone Joint Surg Br 1986; 68: 616–9.

89 Engelbert RH, Uiterwaal CS, Gerver WJ, et al. Osteogenesis imperfecta in childhood: impairment and disability. A prospective study with 4-year follow-up. Arch Phys Med Rehabil 2004; 85: 772–8.

90 Roughley PJ, Rauch F, Glorieux FH. Osteogenesis imperfecta – clinical and molecular diversity. Eur Cell Mater 2003; 5: 41–7.

* 91 Sillence DO, Senn A, Danks DM. Genetic heterogeneity in osteogenesis imperfecta. J Med Genet 1979; 16: 101–16.

◆ 92 Rauch F, Glorieux FH. Osteogenesis imperfecta. Lancet 2004; 363: 1377–85.

93 Zeitlin L, Rauch F, Plotkin H, Glorieux FH. Height and weight development during four years of therapy with cyclical intravenous pamidronate in children and adolescents with osteogenesis imperfecta types I, III, and IV. Pediatrics 2003; 111: 1030–6.

94 Astrom E, Soderhall S. Beneficial effect of long term intravenous bisphosphonate treatment of osteogenesis imperfecta. Arch Dis Child 2002; 86: 356–64.

95 Plotkin H, Rauch F, Zeitlin L, et al. Effect of pamidronate treatment in children with polyostotic fibrous dysplasia of bone. J Clin Endocrinol Metab 2003; 88: 4569–75.

96 Marini JC, Hopkins E, Glorieux FH, et al. Positive linear growth and bone responses to growth hormone treatment in children with types III and IV osteogenesis imperfecta: high predictive value of the carboxyterminal propeptide of type I procollagen. J Bone Miner Res 2003; 18: 237–43.

97 Lamy M, Maroteaux P. Le nanisme diastrophique. Presse Med 1960; 68: 1977–80.

98 Hastbacka J, de la Chapelle A, Mahtani MM, et al. The diastrophic dysplasia gene encodes a novel sulfate transporter: positional cloning by fine-structure linkage disequilibrium mapping. Cell 1994; 78: 1073–87.

* 99 Makitie O, Kaitila I. Growth in diastrophic dysplasia. J Pediatr 1997; 130: 641–6.

100 Karniski LP. Functional expression and cellular distribution of diastrophic dysplasia sulfate transporter (DTDST) gene mutations in HEK cells. Hum Mol Genet 2004; 13: 2165–71.

* 101 Remes V, Poussa M, Peltonen J. Scoliosis in patients with diastrophic dysplasia: a new classification. Spine 2001; 26: 1689–97.

* 102 Remes VM, Marttinen EJ, Poussa MS, et al. Cervical spine in patients with diastrophic dysplasia – radiographic findings in 122 patients. Pediatr Radiol 2002; 32: 621–8.

103 Remes V, Poussa M, Lonnqvist T, et al. Walking ability in patients with diastrophic dysplasia: a clinical, electrophysiological, treadmill, and MRI analysis. J Pediatr Orthop 2004; 24: 546–51.

* 104 Crockett MM, Carten MF, Hurko O, Sponseller PD. Motor milestones in children with diastrophic dysplasia. J Pediatr Orthop 2000; 20: 437–41.

105 Hastbacka J, Kerrebrock A, Mokkala K, et al. Identification of the Finnish founder mutation for diastrophic dysplasia (DTD). Eur J Hum Genet 1999; 7: 664–70.

106 Walker BA, Scott CI, Hall JG, et al. Diastrophic dwarfism. Medicine (Baltimore) 1972; 51: 41–5.

107 Williams MS, Ettinger RS, Hermanns P, et al. The natural history of severe anemia in cartilage-hair hypoplasia. Am J Med Genet 2005; 138:66–7.

108 Makitie O. Cartilage-hair hypoplasia in Finland: epidemiological and genetic aspects of 107 patients. J Med Genet 1992; 29: 652–5.

* 109 Makitie O, Kaitila I. Cartilage-hair hypoplasia – clinical manifestations in 108 Finnish patients. Eur J Pediatr 1993; 152: 211–7.

* 110 Makitie O, Kaitila I, Perheentupa J, Kaitila I. Growth in cartilage-hair hypoplasia. Ped Res 1992; 31: 176–80.

111 Mckusick VA, Eldridge R, Hostetler JA, et al. Dwarfism in the Amish II. Cartilage-hair hypoplasia. Bull Johns Hopkins Hosp 1965; 116: 285–326.

112 Hertel TH, Neumeyer L, Kaitila I, et al. Unpublished data.

113 Rongen-Westerlaken C, Corel L, van den Broeck J, et al. Reference values for height, height velocity and weight in Turner's syndrome. Acta Paediatr 1997; 86: 937–42.

114 Ranke MB, Heidemann P, Knupfer C, et al. Noonan syndrome: growth and clinical manifestations in 144 cases. Eur J Pediatr 1988; 148: 220–7.

115 Myrelid A, Gustafsson J, Ollars B, Anneren G. Growth charts for Down's syndrome from birth to 18 years of age. Arch Dis Child 2002; 87: 97–103.

116 Karlberg P, Taranger J, Engstrom I, et al. I. Physical growth from birth to 16 years and longitudinal outcome of the study during the same age period. Acta Paediatr Scand Suppl 1976; 258: 7–76.

117 Hertel TH, Neumeyer L, Kaitila I, et al. Unpublished data.

20

Respiratory disorders

JENNIFER A BATCH, RISTAN M GREER

EVIDENCE SCORING OF THERAPY

* Non-randomized controlled trials, cohort study, etc.
** One or more well designed randomized controlled trials
*** Systematic review or meta-analysis

INTRODUCTION

The impact on growth of chronic respiratory disease has always been a matter of great concern to the affected children, their parents and their medical advisers. When bronchiectasis was a common condition in children, one of its characteristic features was growth retardation. Fortunately, except when it is associated with cystic fibrosis, bronchiectasis is a rare problem in most developed countries.

It has been recognized for many years that children with very troublesome asthma are often stunted in growth and delayed in pubertal development. With the availability of effective prophylactic drugs, these complications of asthma are much less common, but regrettably inappropriate use of the corticosteroid-based prophylactic drugs rather than the asthma itself may now cause growth suppression, at least in the short term. Serious chronic lung infection, inadequate energy intake and incomplete control of malabsorption all contribute to the impaired growth, which remains a problem for many children and adolescents with cystic fibrosis. Some children with bronchopulmonary dysplasia (BPD) complicating neonatal respiratory distress syndrome remain below normal in their growth but it is difficult to separate out the contributions of the chronic lung disease and hypoxia from the effects of prematurity. Other chronic lung disease as a cause of growth suppression is rare. The major problem is that many of these uncommon disorders such as pulmonary fibrosis and obliterative bronchiolitis are treated with moderate-to-high dose oral corticosteroid therapy. This makes it difficult to determine the relative contributions to the growth impairment of the disease and the therapy.

Numerous congenital lung formations exist, which can lead to chronic pulmonary insufficiency and mimic the finding of premature infants with BPD. Among the most common and severe is congenital diaphragmatic hernia (CDH). This condition has an incidence of between 1 in 2000 and 1 in 10 000 live births. There are few follow-up data on these infants. However, studies have shown that there are persisting developmental abnormalities and severe nutritional problems in these infants.

This chapter deals with the three major respiratory conditions causing growth disturbance in childhood and adolescence: asthma, cystic fibrosis, and bronchopulmonary dysplasia.

ASTHMA

Asthma is the most common chronic medical condition occurring in childhood. It has long been thought that asthma can be associated with impaired growth, with the first report in 1868 by Salter who stated 'if the asthma has come on young, he is generally below the average height. Some asthmatics however. . . have nothing whatever the matter with their appearance and would be taken for perfectly healthy people'.[1] One of the earliest reports on asthma and growth was from Cohen,[2] who wrote of the importance of recording height, weight and physical maturity in assessing the progress of children with allergic disorders, including asthma. In milder cases, they found normal increments in height with poor weight gain but, as the constitutional symptoms progressed, stunting of growth and finally delayed maturation occurred. In the 1960s, Spock[3] compared the height of children attending an asthma clinic with a group of normal children without asthma. He found no difference between the heights of the two groups. In an extension of this study he did, however, find differences in the heights of steroid and nonsteroid treated asthmatic children, suggesting that asthma itself had little effect on growth, but that asthma treatment, particularly steroid treatment may affect growth.

Effects of asthma on growth, puberty, and final height

Chronic disease such as asthma is often regarded as a cause of growth failure, with growth suppressant effects independent of treatment. The causes of this perceived growth failure remain poorly defined, but growth-suppressing influences of endogenous cytokines and glucocorticoids produced in response to illness and inflammation may be responsible.

The Childhood Asthma Management Program study of 1041 children aged 5–12 years,[4] showed that mild–moderate persistent asthma of 4–7 years duration does not in itself produce an adverse effect on linear growth. Significant disease related growth suppression occurs only when asthma is persistent and of at least moderate severity. Furthermore, studies have also demonstrated that any apparent growth failure is due to delayed puberty. Hauspie et al.[5] showed that asthmatic boys had delayed puberty compared to control Dutch and English reference values, with a resultant delay in attaining peak height velocity of 1.3 years. The effect of asthma on delaying puberty has also been demonstrated in studies by Martin et al.[6] and Balfour-Lynn.[7]

Recent large studies of young people in the armed forces have provided data indicating that adult height in those with asthma is essentially normal. Shohat et al.[8] reported on approximately 92 000 17-year-old military conscripts, and found no difference between the asthmatic and nonasthmatic group. A Swedish study of approximately 173 000 military conscripts demonstrated a small but significant difference between asthmatics and normal controls, with a negative correlation between height and asthma severity. They were also able to demonstrate that despite a 40-fold increased use of inhaled corticosteroids between sub-cohorts in 1983 and 1996, there was a decrease in the growth difference between asthmatics and controls during that time period.[9]

Effects of asthma treatment

EFFECTS OF ORAL STEROIDS ON GROWTH

Corticosteroids are potent inhibitors of linear growth, with growth effects including blunting of pulsatile growth hormone release, down-regulation of growth hormone receptor expression, inhibition of insulin-like growth factor-I bioactivity and osteoblast activity, and suppression of collagen synthesis and adrenal androgen production.

Growth retardation in chronic asthma may be compounded by treatment with oral steroids in a dose and duration-dependent manner,[10] although it may be difficult to separate the different components contributing to growth failure. In a longitudinal study where disease severity was graded, oral steroids did have a significant effect on growth delay in comparison to those with the same grade of asthma severity but not treated with steroids.[6] Growth attenuation with oral steroids is dependent on the dose, the duration of therapy and frequency of administration. A dose of prednisolone as low as 2.5 mg day^{-1} has been reported to suppress short-term linear growth over 5 weeks.[11] In other longer-term studies, daily doses of less than or equal to 3 mg m^{-2} or less have been reported not to inhibit growth.[12] Doses approximately double this may be safe for alternate-day therapy. Treatment for periods of 1 week or two or three occasions a year will not affect growth, but more frequent administration of oral steroids for short time periods may slow growth velocity.[6]

EFFECTS OF INHALED CORTICOSTEROIDS

As oral steroid treatment could be associated with growth retardation in asthmatic children, the introduction of inhaled corticosteroids (ICS) in the early 1970s was welcomed by doctors and families alike. In contrast to the growth suppressant effects of oral steroids, ICS were initially thought to be effective with negligible side effects.

The first report of an adverse effect of ICS on growth occurred in 1988, when a study by Littlewood et al.[13] showed a significant negative impact on the height standard deviation score at the onset of commencement of regular beclamethasone dipropionate (BDP). The effects of inhaled corticosteroids on growth has been an area of intense research activity. All of the currently available ICS have been shown to cause a dose dependent growth suppression. The effects of ICS on growth have been summarized by several authors in terms of short ($\leq$3 months), medium (>3 months but not final height) and long-term growth studies (growth over many years $\pm$final height) (reviewed in Pedersen[14] and Randell et al.[15]).

Short–term growth

Short-term studies have utilized knemometry, an extremely accurate means of measuring lower leg growth. Early studies by Wolthers and Pedersen[16] using budesonide (BUD) in doses of 200–400 μg day^{-1} showed no significant effect on lower leg growth for 2 weeks, but a significant decrease in growth while receiving BUD 800 µg day^{-1}. Similar studies have been performed for BDP and fluticasone propionate (FP). BDP results in decreased short-term growth at a dose of 400–800 µg day^{-1}, while FP has no growth effects at a dose of 200 µg day^{-1} (reviewed in Doull[17]). Despite short-term studies suggesting an effect of various ICS on lower leg growth, knemometry and measurement of lower leg growth is a very poor correlate of statural growth and cannot be extrapolated to the longer term.

Growth in the medium term

A meta-analysis of studies on BDP calculated that at a dose of 400 µg day^{-1} of BDP that growth decreased by 1.5 cm per year.[18***] Younger, prepubertal children appear more sensitive to the growth suppressive effects of ICS (reviewed in Doull[17]). Medium-term studies of FP 200 µg day^{-1} showed growth suppression, while there appears to be more growth suppression with BDP 400 µg day^{-1} than FP 200 µg day^{-1} (reviewed in Doull[17]). Doull comments that 'the magnitude of reported growth suppression in medium term growth studies of ICS, flies in the face of clinical observations', and that medium-term studies give conflicting results on the duration of the growth effect, ranging from short lived to persisting for the duration of the study.

Long–term growth and final height

The Childhood Asthma Management Program (CAMP) Research Group has published a 4–6 year follow-up period showing that the effects of inhaled corticosteroids on growth are relatively short lived.[4**] The study compared the use of BUD, nedocromil or placebo. In the first year, the BUD group grew 1.1 cm less than the placebo group, however growth over the 4.3 year mean follow-up time was similar in both groups. There was also no significant change in bone age or bone density between any of the groups in the mean 4.3 year follow-up.

Agertoft and Pedersen[19] have reported the growth of a cohort of 300 asthmatic children (budesonide treated versus untreated and sibling controls) over a 14 year period. They showed that growth decreased after commencing budesonide and remained suppressed for 2 years, after which time the growth was no different from controls. Compared to predicted adult final height, there was no significant difference in attained adult height between those who received BUD, asthmatic controls or the sibling controls.

Safety of inhaled corticosteroids in young children

Most studies of the safety and efficacy of ICS have been done in prepubertal children. A study of 625 young children (1–3 years of age), which compared 1 year safety and efficacy of FP (100 µg twice daily) with that of sodium cromoglycate was reviewed by Allen.[20] There was no significant difference in mean adjusted growth rates between the two groups, with growth comparisons being independent of age, gender or previous steroid use.

EFFECTS OF INHALED CORTICOSTEROIDS ON ADRENAL FUNCTION

Adrenal suppression from inhaled corticosteroids may occur, and may contribute to growth failure. Adrenal suppression has been demonstrated by reduced overnight adrenal secretion, a delayed rise from the nocturnal cortisol nadir and low early morning cortisols that are possible with doses of inhaled corticosteroids as low as 400 mg per day.[21]

Symptomatic adrenal insufficiency resulting from ICS use is rare, but has been reported (reviewed in Allen[20]). Todd et al.[22] reported on 28 children who met diagnostic criteria for adrenal crisis, 23 of whom had symptomatic hypoglycaemia. All had been treated with 500–200 µg day^{-1} of ICS, with 90 percent receiving FP. Allen[20] notes that close inspection of cases of adrenal suppression with ICS reveal the following common characteristics: treatment with FP far in excess of recommended dosage for children; lack of follow-up visits to assess disease control and reduce dose of ICS; and provision of care by general practitioners in the absence of subspecialty consultations. Allen concludes that acute adrenal insufficiency after discontinuation of moderate-dose ICS therapy is rare, and children receiving low to moderate doses of ICS (e.g., <400 µg day^{-1} of BDP or ≤200 µg day^{-1} of FP or BUD) do not require routine monitoring of the hypothalamic pituitary axis (HPA) unless there is evidence of growth suppression.[20]

Randall et al.[15] point out that clinical indicators of systemic effects of ICS such as poor growth or Cushingoid features are not always present in children with documented biochemical adrenal insufficiency secondary to ICS. Allen[20] suggests that children with severe asthma requiring consistent high dose ICS, or who are receiving topical corticosteroids by additional routes (e.g., dermal for atopic eczema or intranasal for allergic rhinitis) are at increased risk for clinically significant HPA axis suppression. Morning cortisol levels should be monitored periodically in these children, and if low levels are detected, then consideration should be given to further adrenal axis testing. Considerable debate exists whether a standard or low dose adrenocorticotrophin (ACTH) test, is the better method for determining the adequacy of the adrenal response.

EFFECTS OF INHALED CORTICOSTEROIDS ON BONE DENSITY

Corticosteroids can potentially adversely affect bone metabolism in a number of ways. Bone resorption may be increased by uncoupling the balance between osteoblast and osteoclast activity. Increases in urinary calcium losses may occur, coupled with inhibition of vitamin D-mediated intestinal calcium absorption. These changes may result in total body calcium deficiency and secondary hyperparathyroidism. Bone accretion and attainment of peak bone mass normally parallels linear growth with rapid increases occurring during puberty. Inhibition of bone metabolism by ICS in childhood and adolescence could thus theoretically result in significant reduction in peak bone mass, and increased fracture risk.

A meta-analysis of the effect of inhaled steroids on bone density in adults[23]*** concluded that inhaled steroids for the treatment of asthma can be considered safe with respect to their effect on bone loss. A recently published study has examined the use of ICS and fracture risk in children and adolescents. Schlienger et al.[24] performed a population based nested case control analysis using data from the United Kingdom-based General Practice Research Database (GPRD). Within a base population of 273 456 individuals aged 5–79 years, they identified children and adolescents (5–17 years) with a fracture diagnosis and up to six control subjects per case matched to cases on age, gender, general practice attended, calendar time and years of history in the GPRD. They compared use of inhaled steroids before the index date between fracture cases and control patients and found that current exposure to inhaled steroids did not reveal a substantially altered fracture risk compared with nonusers, even in individuals with current longer term exposure. They concluded that exposure to inhaled corticosteroids does not materially increase the fracture risk in children or adolescents compared with non-exposed individuals. Allen[20] has reviewed the cross sectional and prospective studies of the effects of ICS on bone mineral density (BMD), and conclude that moderate dose ICS is not associated with significant changes in BMD, but more studies of high doses and of therapy in adolescence are needed to further address this issue.

Prevention and treatment of growth problems in asthma

Prevention of growth disturbance in asthma requires good control of the asthmatic process, whether by nonsteroidal or even steroidal medications. Unless the asthma is well controlled, growth may be impaired by the asthma itself. If oral steroid therapy is required it should be given as the smallest possible dose, preferably as an alternate-day medication. If inhaled corticosteroids are necessary, the smallest possible dose needed to control the asthma should be administered, with the use of devices such as spacers to minimize oral deposition and absorption. Doull[17] suggests that for most children this will be the equivalent of BDP $200\,\mu g\,day^{-1}$, where side effects are extremely unlikely. He suggests that all children receiving $400\,\mu g\,day^{-1}$ or more should have their height measured every six months, preferably by the same person using the same equipment. A small short-term decrement in height velocity may be seen, but more striking and prolonged decreases in height velocity are of greater concern, with recent reports highlighting significant and often symptomatic adrenal suppression in children receiving ICS, particularly FP. Doull observed that many of the children had associated growth suppression preceding the demonstration of adrenal suppression.[17] Although the majority of cases were receiving doses of ICS

well, above the recommended dose, some appeared to be receiving more conventional doses. Thus Doull suggests that it is prudent to recommend that any child who requires more that $400\,\mu g\,day^{-1}$ BDP equivalent to control their asthma should have the diagnosis and treatment reassessed. Any child receiving ICS with striking or prolonged decrease in height velocity should have an urgent assessment of adrenal function.[17]

In the face of steroid-treated asthma and growth failure, growth hormone (GH) treatment has been advocated by some groups with some short-term improvements in growth velocity. However, persistence of disease activity and high glucocorticoid doses (i.e., prednisone $>0.35\,mg$ $kg^{-1}\,day^{-1}$) appear to interfere with GH responsiveness.[25] Delayed puberty associated with asthma should be treated with the appropriate sex steroid, usually testosterone esters given intramuscularly for boys and oral ethinylestradiol in girls. Used appropriately, these therapies will have the dual benefit of growth enhancement and induction of secondary sexual characteristics without limitation of final height.

CYSTIC FIBROSIS

Since the earliest descriptions by Dorothy Anderson[26] of universally poor survival in cystic fibrosis (CF) the median survival in most developed countries is now into the third decade. In the United States, median survival has improved from 14 years in 1969 to 32 years in 2000.[27] The pattern of survival is similar in most countries with continuing improvement.[28] Females have shorter life expectancy than males by about 5 years.[29,30] CF is an autosomal recessive genetic disease caused by mutations in the gene encoding for the cystic fibrosis transmembrane conductance regulator (CFTR) on chromosome 7, where the defective protein prevents or reduces epithelial cell chloride secretion. Approximately 70 percent of patients carry the most common Δ F5087 mutation, although over 1300 mutations have now been identified. The CF phenotype ranges from 'classical CF' characterized by severe disease manifest in infancy or childhood, with progressive pulmonary impairment and pancreatic insufficiency, through to very mild disease with atypical presentation, frequently in adulthood.

The growth, pubertal development and final height of individuals with CF have assumed greater importance in recent years as a result of the optimism regarding longevity and the swing towards improving quality of life and self-esteem. Growth can be used as a marker of overall stability and well-being in CF, with decline in weight and growth retardation often heralding a spiralling decline in respiratory status. Failure to maintain body weight is a predictor of mortality risk for those aged over 17 years, a weight for height of less than 70 percent of the ideal has been associated with a mortality rate of more that 50 percent within 2 years.[31]

Factors adversely affecting growth in cystic fibrosis

PANCREATIC INSUFFICIENCY AND INTESTINAL MALABSORPTION

Eighty-five to ninety percent of people with CF have pancreatic insufficiency, which is frequently present at diagnosis, but may also develop during the first year of life.[32] Pancreatic sufficiency is associated with milder mutations and improved prognosis. Liver disease is common with an estimated prevalence of up to 37 percent. CF is also associated with bile salt malabsorption.[33,34*]

INFECTION AND INFLAMMATION

CF is associated with increased levels of circulating inflammatory cytokines and chronic inflammation, which occurs early in infancy, as does colonization with pulmonary pathogens.[35] Acquisition of *Pseudomonas aeruginosa* occurs eventually in most patients, associated with an accelerated rate of decline in pulmonary function.[36]

ENERGY IMBALANCE

Resting energy expenditure is reportedly increased in CF by 7–35 percent above that of non-CF subjects, exacerbating potential energy imbalance due to reduced energy availability associated with malabsorption, inappetance and gastrointestinal complications.[33*] Resting energy expenditure appears additionally increased in females with CF.[37,38]

PULMONARY FUNCTION AND NUTRITIONAL MANAGEMENT

Improved growth, nutritional status and pulmonary function are associated with improved outcome.[39***] The relationship between nutritional status and pulmonary function is still poorly understood. Nutritional status and pulmonary function are strongly associated; nutritional status may be an independent prognostic factor for survival in its own right. Corey *et al.* in their landmark paper compared survival in 534 Toronto patients (mean age 15.2 ± 8.3 years, range 1 month to 43 years) with 499 Boston patients (mean age 15.9 ± 9.6 years). The median age of survival of 30 years in Toronto was significantly higher than that of 21 years in Boston. The two groups had similar age-specific pulmonary function. Boston patients were significantly shorter than Toronto patients, and Toronto male patients maintained significantly better weight. These nutritional differences were associated with differing nutritional policies between the two clinics, where the Toronto clinic advocated a high fat, high calorie diet with aggressive pancreatic enzyme replacement, whereas the Boston clinic advocated a low fat, high calorie diet, with a lower dose of enzyme replacement.[40]

Growth in infancy

Growth failure and malnutrition are hallmarks of infants with CF diagnosed on clinical signs. Cross-sectional data from clinical studies and patient registries show that infants with CF under 1 year of age have mean weight and height consistently below the 50th percentile, varying from around the 15th to the 40th centile. Patient registry data indicate a consistent trend to catch-up growth after diagnosis, following initiation of therapy.[27,41] The Wisconsin neonatal screening trial of 650 341 newborns, conducted through 1985–91, compared growth in a group of 77 infants diagnosed with CF by screening with a control group of 81 infants conventionally diagnosed on clinical signs. Anthropometric indices of nutritional status (length/height, weight, head circumference) were significantly higher at diagnosis of CF in the screened group compared with the unscreened group. The growth differential between the two groups remained during 13 years of follow-up, providing evidence that infants and children with early malnutrition do not experience complete catch up growth.[42]

Wang *et al.*, in an analysis of patient registry data of 3625 CF infants and children diagnosed between 1982 and 1990, found that in infants with early asymptomatic diagnosis (median age at diagnosis 3.6 weeks) only 18 percent were at or below the 5th percentile for weight and 10 percent at or below the 5th percentile for height. In contrast, of children having later symptomatic diagnosis (median age 25 weeks), 48 percent were at or below the 5th percentile for weight and 42 percent at or below the 5th centile for height.[43]

Growth in childhood and adolescence

Although survival in childhood and adolescence in patients with CF has improved over the last decade,[28] studies examining secular trends in height and weight for age have shown few changes. Laursen *et al.* compared nutritional parameters in 270 patients between 1960 and 1990, finding height increased in only 1 of 12 age groups.[44] McNaughton *et al.* found similar results, in comparing 97 patients attending an Australian clinic in 1986 to 227 patients in 1996, where the 1996 males had lower weight for age and weight for height z-score than 1986 males, and 1996 females had lower height and weight for age z-scores than 1986 females.[45] These findings may be explained by the presence of patients with more severe disease in recent cohorts, who would not have survived in earlier years. Cross-sectional patient registry data show that children reach their 'best' weight and height for age percentile between 1 and 5–8 years of age, approaching the population norm

(50th percentile), but tend to deteriorate thereafter, with mean weight and height percentiles varying from the 15th to 40th percentiles across studies.[27,41]

Pubertal development

Historically, pubertal delay is common in CF,[33,34*] and recent studies suggest that it remains likely in modern cohorts. Arrigo et al., in a study of 25 girls with CF, found a menarcheal delay of approximately 1 year compared with their mothers; this delay was not related to genotype, disease severity, or glucose tolerance. The only factors which affected menarcheal age were maternal menarcheal age and nutritional status, where age at menarche was negatively correlated with body mass index percentile.[46] Aswani et al. undertook a retrospective review of peak height velocity in 30 CF subjects (16 male). Peak height velocity was significantly later in both genders compared with Tanner and Whitehouse standards, with boys reaching peak height velocity at 14.6 years and girls reaching peak height velocity at 12.6 years. Mean peak height velocity was lower in both genders (7.7 cm year^{-1} in boys and 6.4 cm year^{-1} in girls), but final heights did not differ significantly from UK normative data. Fifty-two percent of subjects attained or exceeded the mid-parental centile.[47]

Cystic fibrosis related diabetes

Cystic fibrosis related diabetes (CFRD) or glucose intolerance is associated with poor growth, delayed progression of puberty, failure to gain or maintain weight despite nutritional intervention, and deterioration in pulmonary function.[48*] It is characterized by reduced insulin secretion, insulinopenia and loss of beta cell mass secondary to pancreatic disease. Yung et al. found, in formal glucose tolerance tests, that CF subjects with normal glucose tolerance, as well as those with impaired glucose tolerance or those who had CFRD, had lower maximal insulin secretion and higher area under the plasma glucose concentration curve than normal controls.[49] Frequency of impaired glucose tolerance and diabetes increases with age in CF. Moran et al. found a CFRD prevalence of 9 percent, 26 percent, 35 percent and 43 percent, a glucose intolerance prevalence of 34 percent, 38 percent, 42 percent and 27 percent, and normal glucose tolerance of 57 percent, 36 percent, 23 percent, and 30 percent respectively, in patient age groups of 5–9, 10–19, 20–29, and 30+ years.[50] Microvascular complications occur with CFRD with reported prevalence of retinopathy 5–16 percent, nephropathy 3–16 percent, and neuropathy 5–21 percent. The risk of macrovascular complications appears small, but may need re-evaluation with increased survival of patients with CFRD.[48*]

DIAGNOSIS OF CYSTIC FIBROSIS RELATED DIABETES

Diagnostic criteria for CFRD include four glucose tolerance categories, based on the results of an oral glucose tolerance test with 1.75 g kg^{-1} (maximum 75 g):

- Normal glucose tolerance (fasting plasma glucose <7.0 mmol L^{-1}, 2 h plasma glucose <7.8 mmol L^{-1})
- Impaired glucose tolerance (fasting plasma glucose <7.0 mmol L^{-1}, 2 h plasma glucose 7.8–11.1 mol L^{-1})
- CFRD without fasting hyperglycemia (fasting plasma glucose <7.0 mmol L^{-1}, 2 h plasma glucose $\geq$ 11.1 mmol L^{-1})
- CFRD with fasting hyperglycemia (fasting plasma glucose = 7.0 mmol L^{-1}, oral glucose tolerance test not necessary)

HbA$_1$c is a poor screening tool for diabetes or impaired glucose tolerance in CF, as those with diabetes may have normal HbA$_1$c. CFRD may be chronic or intermittent, associated with stress due to infection, nutritional interventions, or glucocorticoid treatment of pulmonary disease. Women with CF are at high risk for gestational diabetes.[48*]

MANAGEMENT OF CYSTIC FIBROSIS RELATED DIABETES

Goals of treatment of CFRD with fasting hyperglycemia include maintenance of nutritional status, including normal growth and development; control of hyperglycemia and avoidance of diabetic complications, avoidance of severe hypoglycemia, and promotion of optimal psychological status. Insulin is the standard medical treatment, and the use of oral anti-diabetic agents is currently unproven both in terms of safety and efficacy. CFRD patients may require only low doses of insulin, but the dose should be tailored to interventions such as nocturnal gastrostomy or nasogastric feedings. Patients with intermittent CFRD require corresponding intermittent insulin therapy.[48*]

A trial of insulin therapy may be considered in patients with CFRD without fasting hyperglycemia, particularly in the setting of poor growth, delayed pubertal progression, or otherwise unexplained decline in pulmonary function. Patients with impaired glucose tolerance should be monitored closely for the development of clinical symptoms.

Acquisition of peak bone mass in cystic fibrosis

Bone density is reduced in adults with CF.[51] Several studies have found reduced bone density in adolescents while findings in children are more variable. Low bone density and bone mineral content in growing children and adolescents may be associated with small bone size and short stature, which should be carefully considered in clinical evaluation of bone density in patients with CF.[52–54] Bone metabolism is perturbed in CF, associated from adolescence with high bone resorption, low bone accretion, inflammatory cytokines, and abnormalities of vitamin D metabolism.[55]

Prevention of growth failure and delayed puberty

Care of the patient with CF is optimally carried out in a team environment which includes the support of the respiratory physician, nurse, physiotherapist, dietician, appropriate social support, and other specialist care as needed. Patients with CF should have normal growth. The aims of nutritional management are to:

- Achieve normal growth, including genetic potential for height, which is an important indicator of global nutritional sufficiency, and adequate weight for height, which is of clinical importance for the individual.
- Achieve normal bone mass.
- Achieve age appropriate pubertal development.

Achievement of normal growth is accomplished by:

- Monitoring growth and nutrition
- Utilizing strategies for preventing undernutrition
- Utilizing specific interventions for patients with nutritional failure.

MONITORING GROWTH

Special attention should be focused on growth and nutrition at three critical times: (1) the first 12 months after the diagnosis of CF; (2) birth to 12 months for infants diagnosed pre-natally or at birth, until normal growth patterns are established; (3) the peripubertal growth period (girls 9 to 16 and boys 12 to 18 years of age). Accurate, sequential measurements of head circumference, length/height and weight, using current reference data, are essential to the care of children with CF. Growth indices should be measured every 3 months at routine clinic visits. If BMI (body mass index, weight/height^2) is calculated, percentile charts should be used for interpretation, as BMI is not constant through childhood[34]), but in children and adolescents the use of BMI has shown no advantage over height and weight for documenting malnutrition.[33*]

Pubertal development should be assessed at least annually. In children 8 years or older, bone mass should be assessed using bone densitometry if any of the following risk criteria are present: candidate for organ transplantation, post-organ transplantation, end-stage lung disease, fracture associated with low-impact activity, chronic use of

corticosteroids, delayed pubertal development or nutritional failure. Serum calcium, phosphate, parathyroid hormone and vitamin D should be measured and the dietary intake of calcium and vitamin D assessed.[34]

PREVENTING MALNUTRITION

Optimal management of pulmonary disease is important. Treatment of acute and chronic lung infection has been shown to result in an increase in body weight.[33]

Pancreatic enzyme replacement therapy should be started as soon as pancreatic insufficiency is identified either on clinical signs (malodorous, frequent greasy stools) or tests such as 72 h fecal fat balance or duodenal intubation and stimulation. The European Consensus recommended a maximum lipase dose of 10 000 units daily, and the Cystic Fibrosis Foundation Consensus that the lipase dose should be restricted to 2500 U kg^{-1} per meal or less than 4000 U g^{-1} of fat per day, to avoid the risk of fibrosing colonopathy.[33,34*] Patients should be recommended a balanced, high energy diet with 35–40 percent of calories as fat (higher than recommended for the general population). Fat soluble vitamin (A, D, E and K) supplementation is recommended for most patients. Minerals should be supplemented based on the results of nutritional surveillance, and salt supplemented in conditions of high sweat loss, particularly in infants.[33,34*]

NUTRITIONAL INTERVENTION

Nutritional intervention should be based on behavioral and dietary evaluation, and consideration of co-morbidities including gastro-esophageal reflux, distal intestinal obstructive syndrome, and symptoms such as anorexia, bloating or nausea as well as diabetes, liver disease, and other complications. Specific interventions include the use of nutritional supplements, which may include standard calorically dense formulas or elemental or semi-elemental formulas. These may be used in conjunction with enteral feedings (nasogastric, orogastric, gastrostomy or jejunostomy) if required.[33,34*]

Insulin therapy should be considered on a case-by-case basis. Anabolic agents such as growth hormone and megestrol acetate have shown some benefit in the setting of randomized controlled trials, but present data does not show that the benefits outweigh the risks.[34]

BRONCHOPULMONARY DYSPLASIA

Bronchopulmonary dysplasia (BPD) was first described in 1967 as a syndrome of chronic lung disease in infants born pre-term who had been treated for respiratory distress syndrome with supplemental oxygen and mechanical ventilation.[56] Bronchopulmonary dysplasia continues to be an important consequence of prematurity and respiratory distress syndrome despite the use of surfactant therapy. It has become the most common form of chronic lung disease in the USA with about 7000 cases occurring each year.[57] Despite the frequent occurrence of BPD, relatively little has been published regarding the long-term prognosis for survivors with BPD, especially in the area of growth.

Factors contributing to growth failure in bronchopulmonary dysplasia

POOR EARLY NUTRITION

De Regnier[58] studied infants for the first 6 weeks post-term and found that growth failure occurred early in the post-natal period (weeks 2–4). Persistently poor growth in the first post-natal month was characteristic only on the infants who were developing BPD and was not reversed by full enteral feeding. These data support the idea that early growth failure contributes to long term problems in infants with bronchopulmonary dysplasia.

INCREASED ENERGY EXPENDITURE

Weinstein and Oh[59] measured the oxygen consumption of eight infants with BPD and seven matched controls. They found that the mean resting oxygen consumption for the BPD infants was higher than for the control infants and was paralleled by an increased respiratory rate in the BPD group, suggesting that an overall increase in respiratory effort was responsible for the increased oxygen consumption in infants with BPD. Kurzner[60] also found that the need for additional nutritional input in BPD infants persists through the first year of life.

IMPAIRED USE OF METABOLIC FUELS

Yunis and Oh[61] compared carbon dioxide production and energy expenditure in BPD and control patients under basal states and during glucose infusions. BPD infants increased O_2 consumption, CO_2 production and energy expenditure by roughly 20 percent yet controls had no change, indicating that the BPD group had impaired metabolism of glucose.

MEDICATIONS USED TO PREVENT OR TREAT BRONCHOPULMONARY DYSPLASIA

In 1972, Liggins and Howie[62] demonstrated that pre-natal corticosteroid therapy reduced the incidence of respiratory distress syndrome (RDS). Since then, 18 randomized controlled trails have been performed to demonstrate the benefits of pre-natal corticosteroid treatment in reducing neonatal mortality, intraventricular hemorrhage and

surfactant use in addition to the incidence of RDS and later bronchopulmonary dysplasia.[63]*** There have been concerns, however, regarding the potential adverse effects of repeated doses of pre-natal corticosteroids on fetal growth and development. Repeat courses of pre-natal steroids reduce birth weight by about 9 percent and head circumference by approximately 4 percent, without additional benefits for mortality or respiratory outcomes (reviewed in Halliday[64]).

Post-natally, medications used to treat bronchopulmonary dysplasia may also affect growth. The most important of these are corticosteroids. Short- and long-term steroid administration is a common feature of management of infants with BPD. Gibson[65] reported that knee–ankle growth, which is usually approximately 0.5 mm day^{-1} in premature infants, was reduced to zero after 9 days of dexamethasone therapy, and did not return to predicted values until 30 days after treatment was stopped.

Leitch et al.[66] showed that although as expected, growth rate was severely impaired in infants with BPD during dexamethasone treatment compared to non-treatment phases, this difference could not be related to differences in energy expenditure or energy intake. This finding suggests that dexamethasone alters the composition of weight gain by increasing fat and decreasing protein accretion relative to growth when dexamethasone is not administered.

Halliday[64] has reviewed outcomes based on meta-analyses when post-natal steroids are given at three post-natal age periods: early (<96 h), moderately early (7–14 days) and delayed (>3 weeks). Potential adverse effects of early steroid treatment include hyperglycemia and growth failure. Long-term adverse effects of post-natal steroids including adverse neurological outcomes are the subject of intense research activity. Yeh et al.[67] recently reported the outcomes in school age children who had participated in a double blind, placebo controlled trail of early post-natal dexamethasone therapy for the prevention of chronic lung disease of prematurity. They found that the dexamethasone treated group were significantly shorter than the controls and had a significantly smaller head circumference, and also had a range of other adverse neurodevelopmental outcomes compared to controls.

Short–term growth studies in bronchopulmonary dysplasia

Poor growth in early childhood is well described in infants with BPD, with most studies reporting relatively short follow-up periods, some as short as 12 months after hospital discharge. Yu et al.[68] found that the weight of 37 percent of infants with BPD was less than the 10th centile at 2 years of age, height was at the 10th to the 25th centile and head circumference was at the 50th centile. Markestad and Fitzhardinge,[69] in their follow-up of BPD infants to 2 years, demonstrated a similar growth outcome.

Longer term growth studies in bronchopulmonary dysplasia

Most longer-term follow-up studies of infants with BPD have tended to focus mainly on the respiratory or the neurodevelopmental outcome, and have generally concluded that early growth impairment in BPD infants persists into late childhood, adolescence and early adulthood.[70] Two more detailed growth analyses of follow-up of BPD infants suggest, however, a better long-term growth outcome for infants with BPD.[71,72] They reported an 8-year follow-up of three groups of neonates with differing severity of bronchopulmonary dysplasia and matched comparison groups, and found no major growth discrepancies between the BPD groups or between the matched control groups. Vrlenich et al.[71] performed a follow-up study of 406 infants including 95 with BPD and 311 without BPD. Significant differences were noted with regard to weight and head circumference at school age, but no difference in height was found. It was thought that the differences in growth of BPD and control children previously observed may be related to factors such as low birth weight and gestational age rather than to negative growth effects of BPD itself. Korhonen et al.[73] have evaluated whether 7-year-old very low birth weight (VLBW) survivors with and without BPD have similar growth patterns and adrenal androgen (AA) secretion. They found that at 7 years of age, VLBW children are shorter and tend to have higher AA levels than term controls, but VLBW children with and without BPD do not differ from each other in growth or AA status. Those born SGA have higher AA levels compared to non SGA cases. They conclude that the consequences of these findings to final height and to later metabolic and vascular health remain to be determined.

Prevention of growth problems in bronchopulmonary dysplasia

From a review of the studies presented above, it appears that BPD can certainly be accompanied by growth failure particularly in the first 2–3 post-natal years. However the longer-term growth outcome of these children is perhaps better than first thought. Increased attention should be aimed at prevention or amelioration of bronchopulmonary dysplasia. As adequate growth has been demonstrated in infants with BPD who have appropriate nutrition and adequate levels of home oxygen therapy, efforts to optimize this type of therapy should be part of the routine BPD management. Thus a general approach to prevention of growth failure in BPD includes ensuring adequate oxygenation, increasing nutrient intake, and monitoring growth and biochemical indices of malnutrition. A multidisciplinary clinic approach has been suggested as beneficial in the management of infants with BPD.

CONCLUSIONS

It is quite clear that chronic respiratory illness in childhood may have a significant negative effect on growth during childhood and adolescence. The outlook for growth and pubertal development in asthma may well improve as newer therapies with fewer side effects are developed and asthma control improves. Likewise the long-term outlook for children with bronchopulmonary dysplasia will most probably continue to improve as more effective treatments become available and greater emphasis is placed on early nutritional rehabilitation. The growth prognosis in cystic fibrosis may remain somewhat limited by the disease severity of cystic fibrosis, in terms of both pancreatic malabsorption and respiratory compromise. The challenge for thoracic physicians and endocrinologists remains to work together to optimize the growth and pubertal development of all children and adolescents with chronic respiratory disease.

KEY LEARNING POINTS

- Recent studies have provided evidence that asthma itself does not significantly affect final height outcome.
- Asthmatic children receiving conventional doses of ICS (400 µg of BDP equivalent) will attain their target height, and will have heights similar to non-asthmatic controls.
- Symptomatic adrenal insufficiency resulting from ICS is rare, but may occur, particularly if the ICS dose is in excess of the recommended dose for children.
- Growth as near normal as possible and good nutritional status are essential for good outcome and survival in cystic fibrosis.
- CF is a complex multi-system disease best managed in the setting of multi-disciplinary team care.
- Critical life stages which warrant special growth and nutritional surveillance are the periods after diagnosis and in the peri-pubertal years.
- Bronchopulmonary dysplasia is associated with short term growth impairment, which may be exacerbated by the use of post-natal steroids.
- Growth problems in bronchopulmonary dysplasia may be minimized by ensuring that infants have optimal nutrition, and adequate levels of home oxygen therapy.

REFERENCES

● = Seminal primary article

◆ = Key review paper

1 Salter H. *On Asthma: Its Pathology and Treatment*, 2nd edn. London: Churchill, 1868.

2   Cohen M, Weller R, Cohen S. Anthropometry in children. Progress in allergic children shown by increments in height, weight and maturity. *Am J Dis Child* 1940; **60**: 1058–66.

3   Spock A. Growth patterns in 200 children with bronchial asthma. *Ann Allergy* 1965; **23**: 608–15.

4   The Childhood Asthma Management Program Research Group. Long term effects of budesonide or nedocromil in children with asthma. *N Engl J Med* 2000; 343: 1054–63.

● 5   Hauspie R, Susanne C, Alexander F. Maturational delay and temporal growth retardation in asthmatic boys. *J Allergy Clin Immunol* 1977; **59**: 200–6.

6   Martin AJ, Landau LI, Phelan PD. The effect of growth on childhood asthma. *Acta Paed Scand* 1981; **70**: 683–8.

7   Balfour-Lynn L. Growth and childhood asthma. *Arch Dis Child* 1986; **61**: 1049–55.

● 8   Shohat M, Shohat T, Kedem R, *et al*. Childhood asthma ands growth outcome. *Arch Dis Child* 1987; **62**: 63–5.

9   Norjavaara E, Gerhardsson D, Verdier M, *et al*. Reduced height in Swedish men with asthma at the age of conscription for military service. *J Pediatr* 2000; **137**: 25–9.

● 10   Chang K, Miklich D, Barwise G, Chai H, Miles-Lawrence R. Linear growth of chronic asthmatic children: the effects of disease and various forms of steroid therapy. *Clin Allergy* 1982; **12**: 369–78.

11   Wolthers OD, Pedersen S. Short term growth in asthmatic children during treatment with prednisolone. *BMJ* 1990; **301**: 145–8.

12   Kerrebjin K, de Kroon J. Effect on height of corticosteroid therapy in asthmatic children. *Arch Dis Child* 1968; **43**: 556–61.

● 13   Littlewood JM, Johnson AW, Edwards PA, *et al*. Growth retardation in asthmatic children treated with inhaled beclamethasone dipropionate. *Lancet* 1988; **i**: 115–6.

◆ 14   Pedersen S. Long-term outcomes in paediatric asthma. *Allergy* 2002; **57(Suppl 74)**: 58–74.

◆ 15   Randell TL, Dohnaghue KC, Ambler GR, *et al*. Safety of the newer inhaled corticosteroids in childhood asthma. *Pediatr Drugs* 2003; **5**: 481–504.

16   Wolthers OD, Pedersen S. Controlled study of linear growth in asthmatic children during treatment with inhaled glucocorticosteroids. *Pediatrics* 1992; **89**: 839–42.

◆ 17   Doull IJM. The effect of asthma and its treatment on growth. *Arch Dis Child* 2004; **89**: 60–3.

18   Sharek PJ, Bergman DA. The effect of inhaled steroids on the linear growth of children with asthma: a metanalysis. *Pediatrics* 2000; **106**: 2034–44.

19   Agertoft L, Pedersen S. Effect of long term treatment with inhaled budesonide on adult height in children with asthma. *N Engl J Med* 2000; **343**: 1064–9.

◆ 20   Allen DB. Systemic effects of inhaled corticosteroids in children. *Curr Opin Pediatr* 2004; **16**: 440–4.

21   Law CM, Marchant JL, Honour J, *et al*. Nocturnal adrenal suppression in asthmatic children taking inhaled beclmethasone dipropionate. *Lancet* 1986; **i**: 942–4.

22   Todd GR, Acerini CL, Ross-Russell R, *et al*. Survey of adrenal crisis associated with inhaled corticosteroids in the United Kingdom. *Arch Dis Child* 2002; **87**: 457–61.

23   Sharma P, Malhotra S, Pandhi P, Kumar N. Effect of inhaled steroids on bone mineral density: a meta-analysis. *J Clin Pharmacol* 2003; **43**: 193–7.

24   Schlienger RG, Jick SS, Meier CR. Inhaled corticosteroids and the risk of fractures in children and adolescents. *Pediatrics* 2004; **114**: 469–73.

25   Rivkees S, Danon M, Herrin J. Prednisone dose limitation of growth hormone treatment of steroid induced growth failure. *J Pediatr* 1994; **125**: 322–5.

● 26   Andersen DH. Cystic fibrosis of the pancreas and its relation to celiac disease. A clinical and pathological study. *Am J Dis Child* 1938; **56**: 344–99.

27   Cystic Fibrosis Foundation Patient Registry, Annual Report. Bethesda, Maryland, 2002.

◆ 28   Lewis P. The epidemiology of cystic fibrosis. In: Hodson M, Gedded D, eds. *Cystic Fibrosis*, 2nd edn. London: Arnold, 2000.

● 29   Rosenfeld M, Davis R, FitzSimmons S, *et al*. Gender gap in cystic fibrosis mortality. *Am J Epidemiol* 1996; **145**: 794–803.

● 30   Davis P. The gender gap in cystic fibrosis survival. *J Gender Spec Med* 1999; **2**: 47–51.

31   Kerem E, Reisman J, Corey M, *et al*. Prediction of mortality in patients with cystic fibrosis. *N Engl J Med* 1992; **326**: 1187–91.

32   Couper R, Corey M, Moore D, *et al*. Decline of exocrine pancreatic function in cystic fibrosis patients with pancreatic insufficiency. *Pediatr Res* 1992; **32**: 179–82.

◆ 33   Sinaasappel M, Stern M, Littlewood JM, *et al*. Nutrition in patients with cystic fibrosis: a European consensus. *J Cyst Fibros* 2002; **1**: 51–75.

◆ 34   Borowitz D, Baker RD, Stallings V. Consensus report on nutrition for pediatric patients with cystic fibrosis. *J Pediatr Gastroenterol Nutr* 2002; **35**: 246–59.

35   Armstrong D, Grimwood K, Carzino R, *et al*. Lower respiratory infection and inflammation in infants with newly diagnosed cystic fibrosis. *BMJ* 1995; **310**: 1571–2.

36   Kosorok MR, Zeng L, West SEH, *et al*. Acceleration of lung disease in children with cystic fibrosis after *Pseudomonas aeruginosa* colonisation. *Pediatr Pulmonol* 2001; **32**: 277–87.

37   Allen JR, McCauley J, Selby A, *et al*. Differences in resting energy expenditure between male and female children with cystic fibrosis. *J Pediatr* 2003; **1**: 15–19.

38   Zemel BS, Kawchak DA, Cnaan A, *et al*. Prospective evaluation of resting energy expenditure, nutritional status, pulmonary function, and genotype in children with cystic fibrosis. *Pediatr Res* 1996; **40**: 578–86.

39   Navarro J, Rainisio M, Harms HK, *et al*. Factors associated with poor pulmonary function: cross-sectional analysis of data from the ERCF. European Epidemiologic Registry of Cystic Fibrosis. *Eur Respir J* 2001; **18**: 298–305.

● 40   Corey M, McLaughlin F, Williams M, Levison H. A comparison of survival, growth and pulmonary function in patients with cystic fibrosis in Boston and Toronto. *J Clin Epidemiol* 1988; **41**: 583–91.

41 Australasian Cystic Fibrosis Data Registry, Annual Data Report. Sydney: Cystic Fibrosis Australia, 1999.

42 Farrell PM, Kosorok MR, Rock MJ, *et al.* Early diagnosis of cystic fibrosis through neonatal screening prevents severe malnutrition and improves long-term growth. Wisconsin Cystic Fibrosis Neonatal Screening Study Group. *Pediatrics* 2001; **107**: 1–13.

43 Wang S, O'Leary L, FitzSimmons S, Khoury M. The impact of early cystic fibrosis diagnosis on pulmonary function in children. *J Paediatr* 2002; **141**: 804–10.

44 Laursen EM, Koch C, Petersen JH, Muller J. Secular changes in anthropometric data in cystic fibrosis patients. *Acta Paediatr* 1999; **88**: 169–74.

45 McNaughton S, Stormont D, Shepherd R, *et al.* Growth failure in cystic fibrosis. *J Paediatr Child Health* 1999; **35**: 86–92.

46 Arrigo T, De Luca F, Lucanto C, *et al.* Nutritional, glycometabolic and genetic factors affecting menarcheal age in cystic fibrosis. *Diabetes Nutr Metab* 2004; **17**: 114–9.

47 Aswani N, Taylor CJ, McGaw J, *et al.* Pubertal growth and development in cystic fibrosis: a retrospective review. *Acta Paediatr* 2003; **92**: 1029–32.

◆ 48 Moran A, Hardin D, Rodman D, *et al.* Diagnosis, screening and management of cystic fibrosis related diabetes mellitus: a consensus conference report. *Diabetes Res Clin Pract* 1999; **45**: 61–73.

49 Yung B, Noormohamed FH, Kemp M, *et al.* Cystic fibrosis-related diabetes: the role of peripheral insulin resistance and beta-cell dysfunction. *Diabet Med* 2002; **19**: 221–6.

50 Moran A, Doherty L, Wang X, Thomas W. Abnormal glucose metabolism in cystic fibrosis. *J Pediatr* 1998; **133**: 10–7.

● 51 Haworth CS, Selby PL, Webb AK, *et al.* Low bone mineral density in adults with cystic fibrosis. *Thorax* 1999; **54**: 961–7.

52 Laursen EM, Molgaard C, Michaelsen KF, *et al.* Bone mineral status in 134 patients with cystic fibrosis. *Arch Dis Child* 1999; **81**: 235–40.

53 Hardin DS, Arumugam R, Seilheimer DK, *et al.* Normal bone mineral density in cystic fibrosis. *Arch Dis Child* 2001; **84**: 363–8.

54 Buntain HM, Greer RM, Schluter P, *et al.* Bone mineral density in Australian children, adolescents and adults in cystic fibrosis: a controlled cross sectional study. *Thorax* 2003; **59**: 149–55.

55 Greer RM, Buntain HM, Potter JM, *et al.* Abnormalities of the PTH-vitamin D axis and bone turnover markers in children, adolescents and adults with cystic fibrosis: comparison with healthy controls. *Osteoporos Int* 2003; **14**: 404–11.

● 56 Northway W, Rosan R, Porter D. Pulmonary disease following respirator therapy of hyaline-membrane disease: bronchopulmonary dysplasia. *N Engl J Med* 1967; **276**: 357–68.

57 Farrell PM, Palta M. Bronchopulmonary dysplasia. In: Farrell PM, Taussig LM, eds. *Bronchopulmonary Dysplasia and Isolated Chronic Respiratory Disorders.* Columbus, OH: Ross Laboratories, 1986.

58 de Regnier RA, Guilbert T, Mills MMG. Growth failure and altered body composition are established by one month of age in infants with bronchopulmonary dysplasia. *J Nutr* 1996; **126**: 168–75.

59 Weinstein M, Oh W. Oxygen consumption in infants with bronchopulmonary dysplasia. *J Pediatr* 1981; **99**: 958–61.

60 Kurzner S, Garg M, Bautista D, *et al.* Growth failure in infants with bronchopulmonary dysplasia: nutrition and elevated resting metabolic expenditure. *Pediatrics* 1988; **81**: 379–84.

61 Yunis K, Oh W. Effects of intravenous glucose loading on oxygen consumption, carbon monoxide production and resting energy expenditure in infants with BPD. *J Pediatr* 1989; **115**: 127–32.

◆ 62 Liggins GC, Howie RN. A controlled trial of antepartum glucocorticoid treatment for the prevention of respiratory distress syndrome in premature infants. *Pediatrics* 1972; **50**: 512–23.

63 Crowley P, editor. *Prophylactic Corticosteroids for Preterm Delivery.* Cochrane Review. 4th edn. Oxford, 2001.

◆ 64 Halliday HL. Use of steroids in the perinatal period. *Paediatr Respir Rev* 2004; **5(Suppl A)**: S321–7.

65 Gibson AT, Pearse RG, Wales JK. Growth retardation after dexamethasone administration: assessment by knemometry. *Arch Dis Child* 1993; **69**: 505–9.

66 Leitch CA, Ahlrichs J, Karn C, Denne SC. Energy re-expenditure and energy intake during dexamethasone therapy for chronic lung disease. *Pediatr Res* 1999; **46**: 109–13.

67 Yeh TF, Lin YJ, Hung CL, *et al.* Outcomes at school age after postnatal dexamethasone therapy for lung disease of prematurity. *N Engl J Med* 2004; **350**: 1304–13.

68 Yu V, Orgill A, Lim S, *et al.* Growth and development of very low birthweight infants recovering from bronchopulmonary dysplasia. *Arch Dis Child* 1983; **58**: 791–4.

69 Markestad T, Fitzhardinge P. Growth and development in children recovering from bronchopulmonary dysplasia. *J Pediatr* 1981; **98**: 597–602.

70 Vohr B, Coll C, Lobato D, *et al.* Neurodevelopmental and medical status of low birth weight survivors of bronchopulmonary dysplasia 10–12 years of age. *Dev Med Child Neurol* 1991; **33**: 690–7.

71 Vrlenich L, Bozynski M, Shyr Y, *et al.* The effect of bronchopulmonary dysplasia on growth at school age. *Pediatrics* 1995; **95**: 855–9.

72 Robertson C, Etshes P, Goldson E, Kyle J. Eight year school performance, neurodevelopmental and growth outcome of neonates with bronchopulmonary dysplasia: a comparative study. *Pediatrics* 1992; **89**: 365–72.

73 Korhonen P, Hyodynmaa E, Lenko H-L, Tammela O. Growth and adrenal androgen status at 7 years in very low birth weight survivors with and without bronchopulmonary dysplasia. *Arch Dis Child* 2004; **89**: 320–4.

21

Gastrointestinal disorders

R M BEATTIE, M O SAVAGE

INTRODUCTION

Impaired growth is a well recognized complication of gastrointestinal disorders and can be a presenting feature. The pathophysiology of the growth failure is usually related to a nutritional impairment or in some cases chronic inflammation. Nutritional impairment may occur as a consequence of reduced intake, increased requirements, hypermetabolism or a combination of these factors. The presentation of the nutritional impairment is usually as poor weight gain in infancy and poor weight gain associated with reduced height velocity in older children. The recognition of gut pathology as a potential cause of growth failure requires a sound knowledge base of the spectrum of gastrointestinal disorders, their prompt recognition and appropriate treatment with careful attention to the nutritional management of the underlying disease process in particular.

This chapter will focus on the gastrointestinal disorders which are relevant in the assessment of children with growth failure. These include primary gastrointestinal conditions such as celiac disease and Crohn's disease both of which can present with growth failure in the absence of any other symptoms or signs. It also includes the many gastrointestinal conditions (common and rare), which may

impact on intake in particular and exacerbate growth failure secondary to another primary pathology.

PATHOPHYSIOLOGY OF GROWTH FAILURE IN GASTROINTESTINAL DISEASE

Growth failure in children with gut disease (manifest as either faltering growth or short stature) is generally secondary to nutritional impairment and correction of the nutritional impairment is the key to successful management. It is important to bear in mind the following points:

- The role of nutrition in the pathophysiology of gastrointestinal disease. Nutrition is relevant in the assessment and management of most gut pathology.
- Energy expenditure. This comprises resting energy expenditure and physical activity level. At rest approximately 70 percent of energy expenditure is resting energy expenditure (basal metabolic rate).
- Energy balance. A positive energy balance implies that intake exceeds requirements and a negative energy balance that intake is less than requirements (including the need for growth). A negative energy balance implies an

energy deficit. In children with energy deficit growth is likely to be impaired.

- Nutritional impairment. In broad terms nutritional impairment can occur as a consequence of one or more of the following:
  - Reduced intake
  - Increased metabolic demands
  - Malabsorption/maldigestion

Many gastrointestinal conditions result in nutritional impairment either by poor intake, increased needs or increased losses or a complex interaction between all three. Cystic fibrosis is a good example with the potential for nutritional impairment occurring as a consequence of all three factors.

Faltering growth

This refers to failure to grow at an adequate rate. This occurs as a consequence of nutritional impairment. Faltering growth can occur as a consequence of serious underlying diseases e.g. cardiac disease, gut disease, neurological disease. More commonly it may occur as a result of non-organic factors, e.g., psychosocial deprivation. In children with non-organic failure to thrive gastrointestinal pathologies such as gastroesophageal reflux, constipation and pharyngeal incoordination may be factors in the overall picture.

GROWTH FAILURE IN MALNUTRITION

Inadequate calorie and protein intake is the most common cause of growth failure worldwide. Growth failure in early life (mostly manifest by poor weight gain) has a long-term impact on final adult height[1] and although more common in developing countries is a feature in developed countries as well.[1,2]

Marasmus refers to an overall deficiency of calories. Kwashiokor refers to inadequate protein intake. In both conditions vitamin and mineral deficiencies are apparent and there is significant overlap between the two pathologies.

Malnutrition is a common feature of chronic diseases. This results in disturbance of the insulin-type growth factor-I (IGF-I) system with low serum IGF-I returning to normal with improved nutrition. The malnutrition can be self induced and is seen in anorexia nervosa. The effect can be dramatic as reported by Pugliese et al. as fear of obesity: a cause of short stature and delayed puberty with dramatic fall-off in linear growth parallel to weight loss with impressive catch up once nutrition is restored although following a lag.[3]

Malnutrition can also occur in children with food allergy/intolerance on restricted diets, particularly if careful attention is not paid to micronutrient and nutrient intake. Gastrointestinal manifestations of food allergy are wide including cow's milk hypersensitivity (gastroesophageal reflux, infantile colic, constipation), enteropathy, enterocolitis, and proctocolitis.[4]

Specific conditions

Conditions associated with reduced intake include:

- Oropharyngeal incoordination, e.g., bulbar palsy, normal variant
- Dysmotility, e.g., secondary to esophagitis
- Congenital abnormalities, e.g., tracheoesophgeal fistula, web, malrotation
- Gastroesophageal reflux and gastroesophgeal reflux disease
- Esophagitis
- Achalasia
- Peptic ulcer disease
- Food allergy and intolerance/restricted diets
- Eating disorders

Oropharyngeal incoordination can occur as a variant of normal in otherwise healthy children. It is more commonly seen in children with neurodisability and can occur secondary to esophagitis.

Achalasia is a motor disorder which presents as a functional obstruction of the distal esophagus. It results in failure of relaxation of the lower esophageal sphincter and therefore failure of food propulsion thus creating dilation of the lower esophageal sphincter. It is a rare condition. Presenting features are age dependent but include dysphagia, regurgitation, and retrosternal pain. Weight loss can be a prominent feature particularly in younger children. Investigation includes barium radiology, endoscopy, and manometry. Treatment is generally surgical by either balloon dilatation or myotomy. As a potent cause of poor intake it is a potent cause of growth failure. Growth failure has been reported as a prominent feature at diagnosis with catch up post pneumatic dilatation in both infants[5] and older children.[6,7] The long-term outcome of surgery is good.[8]

GASTROESOPHAGEAL REFLUX AND ESOPHAGITIS

This is a common condition in childhood. It is a common cause of poor intake in infancy and, although less common, in older children. It can occur without vomiting.

Gastroesophageal reflux

Gastroesophageal reflux is the passage of gastric contents into the lower esophagus. It is a normal physiological phenomenon and is seen commonly in infancy. It is also seen in older children and adults particularly after meals and is secondary to transient relaxation of the lower esophageal sphincter not associated with swallowing.

Gastroesophageal reflux disease implies reflux with significant morbidity including failure to thrive, respiratory disease, and esophagitis or complications of esophagitis such as stricture. There is an increased prevalence in children with neurodisability.

Reflux esophagitis

Esophagitis implies acid or rarely alkali induced damage to the lower esophagus which can be painful. Crying and irritability may be symptoms of esophagitis in infants, similar to the adult complaint of heart burn and chest pain. There is much speculation about this. In an infant this may be difficult to distinguish from infantile colic. Children with esophagitis can develop a food aversion as a consequence of experiencing pain when they eat and food refusal can be the presenting feature.[9] This is likely to be a significant factor in the failure to thrive seen in some children with reflux.

Investigation of gastroesophageal reflux

Mild or functional reflux is common and rarely requires specific investigation. More severe cases require further investigation. Investigation of reflux is often invasive and not necessarily precise and needs careful planning. Evidence-based and cost effective algorithms are not available although guidelines produced by the North American Society of Pediatric Gastroenterology, Hepatology and Nutrition are useful.[10]

Specific tests include barium radiology, pH study, milk scanning, and upper gastrointestinal endoscopy. Barium radiology assesses the patient over only a short period. It will demonstrate reflux although is not particularly sensitive or specific. The pH study is considered by many to be the 'gold standard'. Its advantages are the ability to quantify reflux over a period of time and establish temporal relationships with atypical symptoms and events such as apnea. There is a standard protocol for the methodology and interpretation of pH studies.[11] Medication should be stopped prior to the procedure. A reflux episode occurs when the pH falls below 4. Most of the commercial software gives a printout of the whole recording period with data including time pH less 4 (percent), number of reflux episodes/24 h, number of reflux episodes greater than 30 min/24 h and the longest reflux episode. Interpretation requires review of the whole recording. The time pH less than 4 (percent) is quoted as the reflux index: 5–10 percent = mild reflux, 10–20 percent = moderate reflux which is usually controlled by medical therapy, 30 percent plus = severe and often requires surgical intervention. Indications for a pH study are:

- Children with simple reflux do not require pH study.
- Gastroesophageal reflux in whom there is diagnostic uncertainty, no response to treatment.
- If surgery is being considered.
- Children in whom doing the test will lead to a change in management.

- Suspicion of occult reflux.
- Unexplained or difficult to control respiratory disease.
- Unexplained apnea.

THE CHILD WITH NEURODISABILITY

Poor intake resulting in poor growth is a common phenomenon in children with neurodisability.[12] This can have a significant adverse effect in terms of general health, linear growth and cognitive function. Requirements are very variable in such children and are often difficult to achieve.[13] Nutritional difficulty can occur as a consequence difficulty feeding secondary to posture and seating, pharyngeal incoordination, primary aspiration secondary to bulbar weakness or severe gastroesophageal reflux.

In children in whom nutrition is poor and therefore likely to impact on growth, factors such as appropriate food, posture and seating are relevant. Hip dislocation needs to be considered. Therapeutic options include a change in feed volume or feed type (either increased calorie density or use of a pre-digested feed), nasogastric or gastrostomy tube feeding.

Gastrostomy tubes are increasingly used for children with neurodisability to improve nutritional status and reduce time taken over feeding. Long-term studies have shown that gastrostomy is an efficient and cost effective feeding method although there are complications including the development or exacerbation of pre-existing gastroesophageal reflux and 10–20 percent will require an anti-reflux procedure either at the time of gastrostomy insertion or subsequently.[14, 15]

HELICOBACTER PYLORI

Helicobacter pylori infects at least 50 percent of the world's population with a higher incidence in developing countries associated with poor socio-economic status and overcrowding. Most infections are asymptomatic. Persistent infection causes a chronic gastritis which may be asymptomatic. There is a strong relationship between *Helicobacter* infection and peptic ulceration. Transmission is feco-oral and familial clustering is common.

Symptomatic peptic ulceration is a potential cause of poor intake. There is controversy about the postulated association between *H. pylori* and short stature.[16,17] Potentially confounding variable such socio-economic status may contribute to both malnutrition and *H. pylori* colonization.

Non-invasive tests for *H. pylori* include serology (positive in active infection), urea breath tests and most recently fecal antigen. Endoscopy and biopsy remains the gold standard with rapid urea testing of biopsies taken from the stomach. Endoscopy is indicated in children with prominent epigastric symptoms including night pain.[18]

Treatment is indicated for gastritis or peptic ulceration. There are various regimes: the one most commonly used in children is omeprazole, amoxicillin and either clarithromycin or metronidazole for 1 week.[19] Outcome following treatment is variable.

CHRONIC DIARRHEA

This refers to diarrhea that has persisted for more than 2–3 weeks. Causes include:

- Enteropathy, e.g., celiac disease, cow's milk protein sensitive, post enteritis syndrome, giardiasis, auto-immune enteropathy, microvillous inclusion disease
- Carbohydrate intolerance
- Cystic fibrosis
- Short bowel syndrome
- Bacterial overgrowth
- Protein losing enteropathy
- Infections/immunodeficiency
- Inflammatory bowel disease

Enteropathies

This implies small bowel mucosal damage, which is detected by small bowel biopsy either via the endoscope or Crosby capsule. Celiac disease is the most common enteropathy in the developed world and will be discussed in detail below. It is important however particularly in the context of chronic diarrhea with poor weight gain to consider other potential causes of enteropathy.[20] Cow's milk, particularly in infancy, can induce an enteropathy with consequent poor weight gain secondary to malabsorption which resolves completely on milk exclusion using a cow's milk protein free milk as a substitute with the usual potential to tolerate a normal diet by the second or third birthday.[21] A post-enteritis syndrome with enteropathy responsive to milk exclusion can occur following enteric infection.[22] Children with immunodeficiency can develop an enteropathy secondary to chronic infection. Rarer causes include autoimmune enteropathy, Tufting enteropathy and congenital microvillous inclusion disease.[23] Such cases may be so severe, e.g., microvillous inclusion disease that total parenteral nutrition (TPN) is required to deliver nutrient intake.

The differential diagnosis of chronic diarrhea is as above. Clearly any child with chronic diarrhea has the potential either through reduced intake, malabsorption/maldigestion or increased losses to develop an energy deficit and can present with poor weight gain/impaired growth.

CELIAC DISEASE

Celiac disease (CD) is an immune-mediated enteropathy caused by a permanent sensitivity to gluten which is present in wheat, barley, and rye. The prevalence of symptomatic celiac disease is between 1:300 and 1:1000 (precise prevalence data are much debated). Prevalence in screened populations is between 1:100 and 1:300.[24] There are associations with HLA DQ2 and DQ8. There is an increased incidence in first-degree relatives (approximately 1:10). Intolerance is to

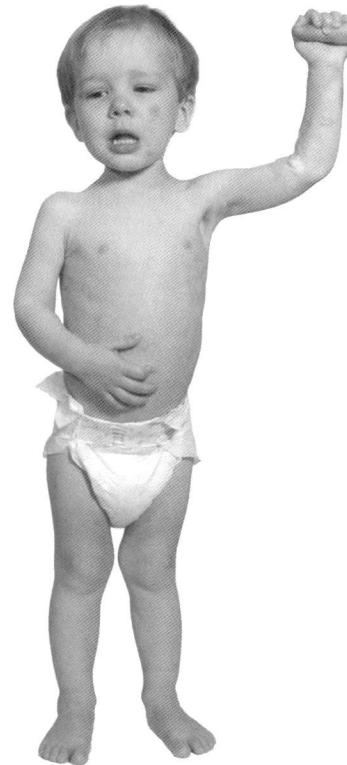

Figure 21.1 Child with celiac disease at presentation age 2 years. Note the misery, pallor, wasting and abdominal distension. Please see Plate 17.

gliadin in gluten which is present in wheat, rye, barley and oats (oat is probably not a primary pathogen but cross contaminated with the other grains during production).

Celiac disease presents after 6 months of age (i.e., after gluten has been introduced into the diet). The classical presentation is with irritability, weight loss, pallor, and abdominal distension (Fig. 21.1). Children can, however, present with a wide range of symptoms including diarrhea, abdominal pain, vomiting, constipation, anemia of unexplained origin, abdominal distension, and faltering growth, short stature and delayed puberty.

Atypical presentations with less-specific symptoms including recurrent abdominal pain are increasingly common and detected early with the advent of antibody screening.

Growth failure in celiac disease

Growth failure can be the first manifestation of the disease. Groll *et al.* reported 34 children with short stature (delayed bone age) of undetermined cause with no overt gastrointestinal symptoms who underwent jejunal biopsy to exclude celiac disease. Eight showed the characteristic enteropathy, seven of which showed a significant acceleration in both height and weight velocity on a gluten-free diet.[25] There have been numerous subsequent publications to confirm this observation. In a recently published evidence-based review addressing the question 'What is the prevalence of celiac disease in children with short stature with no other gastrointestinal symptoms?' Eleven papers were reviewed with pooled data which suggested an incidence of celiac disease of 1.7–8.3 percent in children in whom no preliminary work up to exclude endocrine causes of short stature and 18.6–59.1 percent in children in whom endocrine causes of short stature had been excluded. The wide variation in the range is likely to reflect referral patterns, definition of short stature and patient selection for the individual reports. Nevertheless the clear message from the review and papers that contributed to it is that children with short stature should be evaluated for celiac disease and that the diagnostic yield of investigation is high.[26]

Celiac disease must be considered in the differential diagnosis of unexplained short stature. Children with short stature should have celiac serology checked whether or not there are gut symptoms. Conditions with an increased prevalence of celiac disease include:

- Type 1 diabetes mellitus
- IgA deficiency
- Down syndrome
- Turner syndrome
- Williams syndrome
- First degree relatives of those with CD

Diagnosis

Measurement of IgA antibody to human recombinant tissue transglutaminase (TTG) and serum IgA is recommended for initial testing for CD.[27] IgA antibody to endomysium is observer-dependent and expensive. Antigliadin antibody tests are less accurate and not advised. It is important to exclude IgA deficiency as a cause of falsely negative serology. If CD is clinically suspected in children with IgA deficiency they should be referred for consideration of a small bowel biopsy.

It is crucial that children having CD testing are on a normal, gluten-containing diet prior to serological and histological diagnosis. All children with positive serology should have an endoscopy with multiple duodenal biopsies prior to starting a gluten-free diet. Children for whom there is a high clinical suspicion, e.g. faltering growth with chronic diarrhea should be referred for consideration of a biopsy even if their serology is negative as other enteropathies may be found.

Diagnosis now is based on a single biopsy showing characteristic histological findings of: partial or complete villous atrophy, crypt hyperplasia, and increased intraepithelial lymphocytes in the presence of positive serology.

The diagnosis is confirmed by complete symptom resolution on a strict gluten-free diet. Positive serology should revert to negative over time on a strict gluten-free diet. If there is no decline in anti-TTG after 6 months on a gluten-free diet compliance should be reviewed.

Gluten-free diet for life is the only effective treatment for CD. Children should all be seen by a pediatric dietician on a regular basis to help with compliance and assess the nutritional adequacy considering both calorie and micronutrient intake.

Catch-up growth during treatment of celiac disease

There is good evidence for improvement in nutritional status[28] with improved linear growth[29,30] in children with celiac disease on treatment. Improved nutrition is the driving force behind catch-up. Boersma et al. reported a series of 28 children with celiac disease who showed a malnutrition-like state of the somatrophic axis at diagnosis with rapid return to normal after institution of a gluten free diet.[31] There is a need for caution however in predicting the growth response to gluten exclusion in children with celiac disease presenting with short stature as highlighted by Gillis, who reported four children with failure of catch up following diagnosis who had familial short stature and stunting.[32]

PANCREATIC INSUFFICIENCY

Cystic fibrosis

This is covered in the respiratory section. Gastrointestinal problems are common, however. Pancreatic insufficiency is part of the pathophysiology in more than 90 percent. Pancreatic insufficiency can occur from other causes both congenital and acquired and these should be considered in children with pancreatic insufficiency not due to cystic fibrosis.

Schwachmann–Diamond syndrome

This is an autosomal recessive disorder. Incidence is 1:20 000 to 1:200 000. The main features are pancreatic insufficiency, neutropenia, and short stature. Other features include metaphyseal dysostosis, mild hepatic dysfunction, increased frequency of infections, and further hematological abnormalities (including thrombocytopenia and increased risk of malignancy).

INTESTINAL FAILURE

Intestinal failure is reduction of functional gut mass below that needed for digestion and absorption of nutrients and fluids required for maintenance and growth. There are three main groups of causes: short bowel syndrome, neuromuscular disease of the gastrointestinal tract (long segment Hirschprung's disease and chronic intestinal pseudo-obstruction), and congenital disease of the intestinal epithelium, e.g., microvillous inclusion disease (see earlier). In children with intestinal failure feeding has to be either exclusive TPN or a combination of enteral and parental feeding. This clearly has major implications in terms of growth in that it will only occur if adequate nutrients and micronutrients are delivered. This subject is well reviewed elsewhere.[33]

Short bowel syndrome

One of the commonest causes of intestinal failure is short bowel syndrome which is interesting to consider because of the bowel's potential to adapt, particularly in the preterm. This is defined as intestinal failure secondary to massive resection. Etiologies include:

- Neonatal – necrotizing enterocolitis, intestinal atresia, volvulus
- Older child – trauma, inflammatory bowel disease, vascular abnormalities

Factors that determine outcome include:

- Length of bowel resected, remaining bowel length (preterm bowel is likely to undergo further growth, bowel length increases by 100 percent in the 3rd trimester)
- Quality of bowel remaining – ischemic, distended, ileum has a greater potential to adapt than jejunum
- Presence of ileo-cecal valve – loss of ileo-cecal valve results in faster transit. Backflow (loss of the one-way valve) makes bacterial overgrowth more likely
- Presence or absence of colon with improved outcome if colon (which facilitates salt and water reabsorption) is still present
- Co-existent disease, e.g. enteropathy, is an adverse risk factor
- Presence of liver disease is an adverse risk factor

Management

There are three phases of intestinal adaptation: acute (TPN dependent, post-operative ileus), adaptive (increasing enteral nutrition can take months to years), and chronic. The priority is to maintain normal growth and development through adequate calorie, nutrient, and micronutrient intake during these phases. The early introduction of enteral feeds promotes intestinal adaptation and will improve subsequent feed tolerance. Less than 40 cm of small bowel is usually associated with the need for long-term nutritional support.

INFLAMMATORY BOWEL DISEASE

Growth failure is a common feature and a major problem in inflammatory bowel disease presenting in childhood and adolescence. Twenty five percent of cases of inflammatory bowel disease (IBD) presents in childhood, often in adolescence, and usually as Crohn's disease (CD) or ulcerative colitis (UC). The incidence of IBD in childhood is 5.2 per 100 000 and 58 percent of these have Crohn's disease.[34] Growth failure is well described and can be the presenting feature.[34] Colitis is defined as colonic inflammation and characteristic features include abdominal pain, tenesmus, bloody diarrhea and blood and mucous per rectum. Ten to fifteen percent of colitis is indeterminate which means the histology is consistent with inflammatory bowel disease but not characteristic of Crohn's disease or ulcerative colitis.

Crohn's disease is a chronic inflammatory disorder that can affect any part of the bowel, from mouth to anus. The most common sites are terminal ileum, ileo-colon, and colon. The typical pathological features are transmural inflammation and granuloma formation, which may be patchy.

Ulcerative colitis is an inflammatory disease limited to the colonic and rectal mucosa. The characteristic histology is mucosal and submucosal inflammation with goblet cell depletion, cryptitis, and crypt abscesses but no granulomas. The inflammatory change is usually diffuse rather than patchy.

Clinical features

Common presenting features of Crohn's disease include abdominal pain, diarrhea and weight loss. In ulcerative colitis this tends to be abdominal pain, diarrhea and blood per rectum with weight loss a less prominent feature. In the BPSU survey June 1998–99 of 739 children with inflammatory bowel disease at diagnosis, weight loss was a feature in 58 percent of Crohn's and 35 percent of ulcerative colitis at diagnosis with reduced mean weight and height SDS scores in both conditions, more prominent in Crohn's disease than ulcerative colitis.[35] Seidman reported in their experience of more than 50 cases per year over many years that 50 percent of children with Crohn's disease had growth failure and 90 percent were underweight at diagnosis.[36] Figure 21.2 shows height in (a) 72 boys and (b) 42 girls with Crohn's disease at referral to the pediatric inflammatory bowel disease clinic at St Bartholomew's Hospital, London.[37] Figure 21.3 shows a 14-year-old boy with Crohn's disease at presentation.

Investigations

Inflammatory bowel disease should be suspected if any of the presenting features are present. It is straightforward in

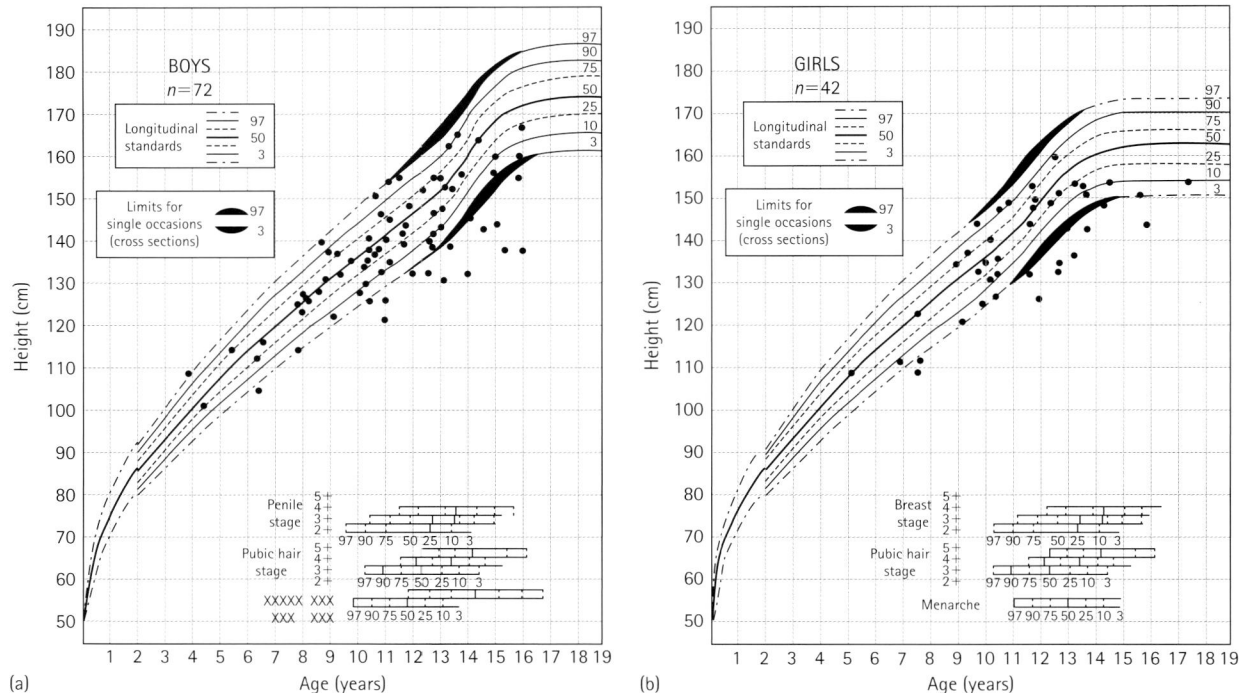

Figure 21.2 Height in (a) 72 boys and (b) 42 girls with Crohn's disease at referral to the pediatric inflammatory bowel disease clinic at St Bartholomew's Hospital, London. (From Brain and Savage.[37]) Copyright, 1994. With permission from Elsevier.

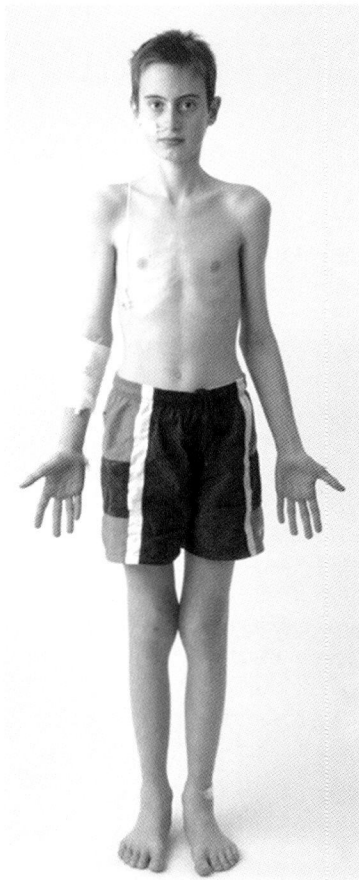

Figure 21.3 A 14-year-old boy with Crohn's disease at presentation. Note the pre-pubertal facies, pallor, reduced subcutaneous fat and poor muscle bulk. Please see Plate 18.

children with colitis symptoms to investigate further if stool cultures are negative. It is less clear in children with abdominal pain which in itself is common and then investigation should be considered in any child with systemic symptoms and/or abnormal physical signs which point to significant gastrointestinal pathology. The diagnosis should be considered in any child who presents with growth failure.

Basic screening investigations include stool culture to exclude infection, full blood count, basic biochemistry and inflammatory markers. Inflammatory markers are generally although not always raised in children with Crohn's disease at diagnosis.[38,39] Further investigation requires upper and lower gastrointestinal endoscopy and barium radiology.[40] It is important that the investigation is complete as if for example ileoscopy is not done then Crohn's confined just to the ileum can be missed.[41]

Pathogenesis of growth failure in inflammatory bowel disease

The mechanism of growth failure in Crohn's disease is likely to be multifactorial with malnutrition, active inflammatory and steroid therapy being likely contributory influences.

The growth failure is characterized by delayed skeletal maturation and delayed onset of puberty with a reasonable final adult height in most cases provided treatment is optimized particularly during the pubertal growth spurt[42,43] with continued growth into the late teens followed by delay in onset of puberty. Therapies that induce disease remission are associated with significant growth acceleration. This is seen most dramatically in children post surgical resection.[44–46]

Role of the IGF–I system in growth failure in Crohn's disease

Serum IGF-I is reduced in active Crohn's disease and improves with treatment.[47,48] The effect on the IGF-I axis predates any significant change in the nutritional state.[49]

These findings have suggested that the effect may not just be as a consequence of poor nutrition and there is increasing evidence for a cytokine effect by suppressing growth factors. C-reactive protein (CRP) as a marker of systemic disease activity in Crohn's disease is induced by interleukin 6 (IL-6). IL-6 expression is increased in Crohn's disease and circulating levels parallel disease activity.[49] IL-6 overexpression in transgenic mice results in growth faltering and reduced circulating IGF-I in the presence of normal growth hormone reversed by a neutralizing antibody to IL-6.[50]

In a rat model TNBS-induced (raised IL-6) granulomatous colitis also causes growth retardation. Compared with pair fed healthy controls growth impairment was more prominent despite similarly controlled intake.[51] Sawczenko et al. reported in rats with TBNS-induced colitis administration of IL-6 antibody restored linear growth and increased IGF-I but did not improve nutrient intake or reduce intestinal inflammation when compared with untreated disease controls.[52] Growth retardation at diagnosis (and high circulating CRP) was more common in children with the IL-6 GG genotype compared with the GC or CC genotypes.

The association between disease site and growth failure is not clear although data have suggested a link between jejunal involvement and short stature at diagnosis.[34] Wine, however, reported that in a series of 93 patients there was no association between disease site and growth failure, the predictor being disease severity. There was also no association between the recently discovered NOD2 gene which correlates with ileal disease and growth failure.[53]

Final adult height

There are few long-term studies of outcome in childhood inflammatory bowel disease. The recent advent of the much wider use of immunosuppressive agents and biologicals is not yet reflected in outcome studies. The impact of corticosteroids on growth is well known. Markowitz analyzed the records of 48 adults who had had IBD diagnosed in early adolescence and depending on the criteria used reported permanent growth failure in 19–35 percent with a positive correlation between corticosteroid use and permanent growth impairment.[54] One hundred and thirty-five patients from the Netherlands were reported in 2001, all of whom had had onset of Crohn's disease before puberty with reduced final adult height (although not when corrected for target height), with patients who had received cortico-steroids during puberty shorter than those who had not, i.e., the use of corticosteroids resulting in a reduced final adult height.[55]

The impact of corticosteroids on growth is well known. There are no studies comparing corticosteroids with other treatments with long term outcome on growth. There is, however, a pragmatic presumption that if corticosteroids can be avoided and alternative treatments used to induce a remission that would at least negate the potential impact of corticosteroid therapy on growth and/or minimize it.

Management of inflammatory bowel disease

GENERAL PRINCIPLES

Children and adolescents with inflammatory bowel disease should be managed in centers with expertise in the condition. This is best done as a clinical network with rapid access to diagnostic facilities, common protocols and ongoing support. The key priority is to control symptoms using the least toxic therapeutic regimens while maintaining normal growth, social and pubertal development.

Therapeutic options include enteral nutrition, corticosteroids, and immunosuppressive agents such as azathioprine, biological therapies, and surgery. Nutrition, either as enteral nutrition or supplemental nutrition is a key priority long term.

ENTERAL NUTRITION AS PRIMARY THERAPY IN CROHN'S DISEASE

In 1981 Kirschner reported seven children with moderately active Crohn's disease with significant growth retardation that responded well to aggressive nutritional supplementation with improved well being and an increase in height velocity.[56] In 1983 O'Morain reported 15 children treated for 4 weeks with elemental diet followed by 4 weeks of food reintroduction. During the study period all of the children improved with six patients crossing into a higher centile channel for weight and three for height.[57] By the middle of the 1980s elemental diet was widely used in the UK as primary therapy in children with Crohn's disease.

Sanderson compared the peptide-based, semi-elemental diet Flexical (Mead Johnson) with steroids in the treatment of children with small bowel disease and found equal efficacy in both groups but a better effect on long-term linear growth in the group treated with enteral nutrition. The diet was given for 6 weeks as sole therapy. At the end of the 6 week period food was reintroduced slowly, one new food every 2 days according to a strict protocol.[58] There have been numerous subsequent studies.

Since the 1990s, cheaper and more palatable polymeric (whole protein based) formulae have been used with equal efficacy. Fell[59] reported the successful use of the polymeric formula CT3211 (Nestlé) subsequently marketed as Modulen IBD. Seventy-nine percent achieved clinical remission (based on PCDAI). As with other cohorts of children treated with enteral nutrition, the response in terms of reduced symptoms, improved nutrition and reduction in serum inflammatory markers was dramatic. There have been subsequent published cohort studies.[49,60]

There have been numerous trials that suggest polymeric diets are as effective as elemental diets in adult patients and there has been a Cochrane review[61] with nine studies included comparing elemental diet ($n = 170$) with non-elemental diet ($n = 128$) with no significant difference in outcome.

DRUG THERAPY IN PEDIATRIC INFLAMMATORY BOWEL DISEASE

This subject is well reviewed elsewhere.[62–65] In addition to toxicity on growth there is evidence that bone health is impaired in Crohn's disease and that corticosteroid use is a factor.[66–68] It is essential to optimize calcium and vitamin intake whilst on steroids. A significant percentage, however, will relapse within the first 12 months whether enteral nutrition or steroids are used. Maintaining remission is therefore a major challenge and key to optimizing growth and pubertal development. Long-term immunosuppressive agents such as azathioprine or 6-mercaptopurine are frequently needed. More recently biologicals including infliximab (tumor necrosis monoclonal antibody therapy) has been used. Surgery is indicated for either acute complications, e.g., abscess or stricture or disease resistant to medical therapy particularly if resectable (i.e., not pan-enteric) and growth failure is present in the pre- or peri-pubertal patient.

MANAGEMENT OF GROWTH FAILURE IN PEDIATRIC INFLAMMATORY BOWEL DISEASE

Growth needs to be monitored at every clinic review with pubertal staging at least 6 monthly. This needs to be seen in the context of the mid-parental expected height centile. There needs to be a low threshold to re-investigate if there is impaired linear growth and to optimize therapy using steroid sparing strategies if possible.

Children often continue to grow into late adolescence and early adult life outside normal pediatric age range. Growth and pubertal development therefore continue as key priorities in late adolescence/early adult life. This is in the pediatric, transition and young adult clinic. It is important to be aware, in the young adult who is short and not yet through puberty, that there is a potential for catch-up growth.

Delayed growth and onset of puberty (looking younger than your colleagues) will have a significant negative impact on the child's psychosocial development and transition from early (dependent upon parents) to late adolescence (dependent on self) and thereby the transition to adulthood. The optimal management of growth equates to the optimal management of disease activity. Disease remission with treatment results in improved growth and nutritional status with a reasonable final adult height in most cases providing appropriate therapy is offered particularly during the mid-pubertal growth spurt. Other than the

studies looking at the outcome of surgical resection, very few studies have looked at growth as a primary outcome.

In the Cochrane review published on intervention for growth failure in childhood Crohn's disease, only three randomized controlled trials were identified with growth as the outcome. The two with interventions with a positive impact on growth were those of Sanderson[58] and Thomas.[48] Mention is made of cohort-based surgical outcome studies (with impressive catch-up growth post surgical resection) and cyclical enteral nutrition.[69]

In 1988 Belli et al. reported their experience with cyclical exclusive enteral nutrition which reduced disease activity and prednisolone usage in a cohort with Crohn's disease with improved linear growth.[70] Published in abstract form only but more fully reported in Seidman in a randomized controlled study (the maintenance phase of a larger trial) cyclical exclusive enteral nutrition resulted in fewer relapses and improved growth compared with alternate day low dose prednisolone.[71] In essence cyclical refers to 4 weeks on 8 weeks off exclusive enteral nutrition.

Borrelli reported 18 children with Crohn's disease all symptomatic with failure to respond to steroids and aza-thioprine treated with infliximab at 0, 2, and 6 weeks with positive results in terms of clinical response, reduced steroid use and improved linear growth over the 6 month follow-up period.[72]

GENERAL PRINCIPLES OF THE NUTRITIONAL MANAGEMENT OF GASTROINTESTINAL DISEASE

This is fundamental to the management of gastrointestinal disease and in particular the prevention of growth failure in children with gut disease:

1. Treat underlying pathology
2. Assess requirements and method of feeding
3. Increase calories by increasing calorie density and/or volume of feed
4. Consider change in feed regimen or feed type
5. Consider change in method of feeding, e.g., nasogastric tube, gastrostomy tube feeding

Enteral feeding

Enteral feeding strictly refers to enteral feed given directly into the gastrointestinal tract. For the purpose of this chapter, however, we have considered an enteral feed as a supplementary feed, i.e., not included foods normally taken by mouth and therefore refer principally to feeds given either by nasogastric or gastrostomy tube or in rare cases via a jejunostomy. Indications for enteral tube feeding are:

- Insufficient energy intake by mouth
- Wasting
- Stunting

KEY LEARNING POINTS

- Growth delay is a well recognized feature of gastrointestinal disease and can be the presenting feature.
- Nutritional impairment is the most common cause and can occur as a consequence of poor intake, increased losses or hypermetabolism.
- Children with growth failure should be screened for celiac disease and inflammatory bowel disease should be considered as part of the differential diagnosis.
- Management of growth failure secondary to gut disease requires treatment of the underlying condition and correction of nutritional impairment.
- Nutrition is therefore fundamental to the management and in particular the prevention of growth failure in children with gut disease.

REFERENCES

◆ = Key review paper

∗ = First formal publication of a management guideline

1 Liu Y, Albertsson-Wikland K, Karlberg J. Long term consequences of early growth retardation in Swedish children. *Pediatr Res* 2000; **47**: 475–85.

2 Shen T, Habicht JP, Chang Y. Effect of economic reforms on child growth in urban and rural areas of China. *N Engl J Med* 1996; **335**: 400–6.

3 Pugliese MT, Lifshitz F, Grad G, *et al*. Fear of obesity: A cause of short stature and delayed puberty. *N Engl J Med* 1983; **309**: 513–8.

◆ 4 Sichere SH. Clinical aspects of gastrointestinal food allergy in childhood. *Pediatrics* 2003; **111**: 1609–16.

5 Starinsky R, Berlovitz I, Mares AJ, *et al*. Infantile achalasia. *Pediatr Radiol* 1984; **14**: 113–5.

6 Schober E, Frisch H. Growth retardation and reduced growth hormone secretion in a boy with Achalasia. *Eur J Pediatr* 1995; **154**: 109–11.

7 Kocabas E, Tumgor G. Achalasia with growth retardation [Letter]. *Indian Pediatr* 2004; **41**: 745.

8 Morris-Stiff G, Khan R, Foster ME, Lari J. Long-term results of surgery for childhood achalasia. *Ann R Coll Surg Engl* 1997; **79**: 432–4.

9 Dellert SF, Hymans JF, Treem WR, *et al*. Feeding resistance and gastro-esophageal reflux in infancy. *J Pediatr Gastroenterol Nutr* 1993; **17**: 66–71.

∗ 10 Rudolph CD, Mazur LJ, Liptak GS. Guidelines for Evaluation and Treatment of Gastroesophageal Reflux in Infants and Children: Recommendations of the North American Society for Pediatric Gastroenterology and Nutrition. *J Pediatr Gastroenterol Nutr* 2001; **32(S2)**: 1–31.

∗ 11 Vandenplas Y, Belli D, Boige N, *et al*. A standardized protocol for the methodology of esophageal pH monitoring and interpretation of the data for the diagnosis of gastro-oesophageal reflux. ESPGHAN society statement. *J Pediatr Gastroenterol Nutr* 1992; **14**: 467–71.

12 Motion S, Northstone K, Emond A, *et al*. Early feeding problems in children with cerebral palsy: weight and neurodevelopmental outcomes. *Dev Med Child Neurol* 2002; **44**: 40–3.

13 Sullivan PB, Juszczak E, Lamberet BR, *et al*. Impact of feeding problems and nutritional intake and growth: Oxford Feeding Study II. *Dev Med Child Neurol* 2002; **44**: 461–7.

◆ 14 Sullivan PB. Gastrostomy feeding in the disabled child: when is an anti reflux procedure required? *Arch Dis Child* 1999; **81**: 463–4.

◆ 15 Sleigh G, Brocklehurst P. Gastrostomy feeding in cerebral palsy: a systemic review. 2004; **89**: 534–9.

16 Patel P, Mendall MA, Khulusis K, *et al*. *Helicobacter pylori* infection in childhood: risk factors and effects of growth. *BMJ* 1994; **309**: 1119–23.

◆ 17 Sood MR, Joshi S, Akobeng AK, *et al*. Growth in children with *Helicobacter pylori* infection and dyspepsia. *Arch Dis Child* 2005; **90**: 1025–8.

◆ 18 Campbell DI, Thomas JE. *Helicobacter pylori* infection in paediatric practice. *Arch Dis Child* 2005; **90**: ep25–30.

19 Gold BD, Colletti RB, Abbott M, *et al*. *Helicobacter pylori* infection in children: Recommendations for diagnosis and treatment. *J Pediatr Gastroenterol Nutr* 2000; **31**: 490–7.

20 Larcher VF, Shepherd R, Francis DEM, Harries JT. Protracted diarrhoea in infancy. Analysis of 82 cases with particular reference to diagnosis and management. *Arch Dis Child* 1977; **52**: 597–605.

21 Walker-Smith JA. Cow's milk protein intolerance: transient food intolerance of infancy. *Arch Dis Child* 1975; **50**: 347–51.

22 Walker-Smith JA. Cow's milk intolerance as a cause of postenteritis diarrhoea. *J Pediatr Gastroenterol Nutr* 1982; **1**: 163–75.

23 Phillips AD, Schmitz J. Familial microvillous atrophy: a clinico-pathological survey of 23 cases. *J Pediatr Gastroenterol Nutr* 1992; **14**: 380–96.

24 Csizmadia CGDS, Mearin ML, von Bloberg BM, *et al*. An iceberg of celiac disease in the Netherlands. *Lancet* 1999; **353**: 813–4.

25 Groll A, Candy DC, Preece MA, *et al*. Short stature as the primary manifestation of coeliac disease. *Lancet* 1980; **22**: 1097–9.

◆ 26 van Rijn JCW, Grote FK, Oostdijk W, Wit JM. Short stature and the probabililty of celiac disease, in the absence of gastrointestinal symptoms. *Arch Dis Child* 2004; **89**: 882–3.

∗ 27 Hill ID, Dirks MH, Liptak GS, *et al*. Guideline for the Diagnosis and Treatment of Celiac Disease in children: Recommendations of the North American Society for Pediatric Gastroenterology, Hepatology and Nutrition. *J Pediatr Gastroenterol Nutr* 2005: **40**: 1–19.

28 Rea F, Politi C, Di Toro A, *et al*. Restoration of body composition in celiac children after 1 year of

gluten-free diet. *J Pediatr Gastroenterol Nutr* 1996; **23**: 408–12.

29   Gemme G, Vignolo M, Naselli A, Garzia P. Linear growth and skeletal maturation in subjects with treated coeliac disease. *J Pediatr Gastroenterol Nutr* 1999; **29**: 339–42.

30   Patwari AK, Kapur G, Satyanarayana L, *et al.* Catch-up growth in children with late diagnosed coeliac disease. *Br J Nutr* 2005; **94**: 437–42.

31   Boersma B, Houwen RH, Blum WF, *et al.* Catch-up growth and endocrine changes in childhood celiac disease. Endocrine changes during catch up growth. *Horm Res* 2002; **58(Suppl 1)**: 57–65.

32   Gillis D, Shteyer E, Landau H, Granot E. Celiac disease and short stature – not always cause and effect. *J Pediatr Endocrinol Metab* 2001; **14**: 71–4.

◆ 33   Goulet O, Ruemmele F, Lacaille F, Colomb V. Irreversible intestinal failure. *J Pediatr Gastroenterol Nutr* 2004; **38**: 250–69.

34   Sawczenko A, Sandhu BK, Logan RF, *et al.* Prospective survey of childhood inflammatory bowel disease in the British Isles. *Lancet* 2001; **357**: 1093–4.

35   Sawczenko A, Sandhu BK. Presenting features of inflammatory bowel disease in Great Britain and Ireland. *Arch Dis Child* 2003; **88**: 995–1000.

36   Seidman E, Bagnell P, Griffiths AM, *et al.* Canadian Collaborative Pediatric Crohn's disease study: growth failure and nutritional deficiencies in pediatric patients with active Crohn's disease. *Gastroenterology* 1991; **100**: A29.

◆ 37   Brain CE, Savage MO. Growth and puberty in chronic inflammatory bowel disease. *Ballieres Clin Gastroenterol* 1994; **8**: 83–100.

38   Beattie RM, Walker-Smith JA, Murch SH. Indications for investigation of chronic gastrointestinal symptoms. *Arch Dis Child* 1995; **73**: 354–5.

39   Cabrera-Arreu JC, Davies P, Matek Z, Murphy MS. Performance of blood tests in diagnosis of inflammatory bowel disease in a specialist clinic. *Arch Dis Child* 2004; **89**: 69–71.

∗ 40   IBD Working Group of the European Society for Paediatric Gastroenterology, Hepatology and Nutrition (ESPGHAN). Inflammatory bowel disease in children and adolescents: recommendations for diagnosis – The Porto criteria. *J Pediatr Gastroenterol Nutr* 2005; **41**: 1–7.

41   Escher JC, Ten KF, Lichtenbelt K, *et al.* Value of rectosigmoidoscopy with biopsies for diagnosis of inflammatory bowel disease in children. *Inflamm Bowel Dis* 2002; **8**: 16–22.

42   Hildebrand H, Karlberg J, Kristiansson B. Longitudinal growth in children and adolescents with inflammatory bowel disease. *J Pediatr Gastroenterol Nutr* 1994; **18**: 165–73.

43   Ferguson A, Sedgewick DM. Juvenile onset inflammatory bowel disease: height and body mass index in adult life. *BMJ* 1994; **308**: 1259–63.

44   Lipson AB, Savage MO, Davies PS, *et al.* Acceleration of linear growth following intestinal resection for Crohn disease. *Eur J Pediatr* 1990; **149**: 687–90.

45   Davies G, Evans CM, Shand WS, Walker-Smith JA. Surgery for Crohn's disease in childhood: influence of site of disease and operative procedure on outcome. *Br J Surg* 1990; **77**: 891–4.

46   McLain BI, Davidson PM, Stkes KB, Beasley SW. Growth after gut resection for Crohn's disease. *Arch Dis Child* 1990; **65**: 760–7.

47   Beattie RM, Camacho-Hübner C, Wacharasindhu S, *et al.* Responsiveness of IGF-I and IGFBP-3 to therapeutic intervention in children and adolescents with Crohn's disease. *Clin Endocrinol* 1998; **49**: 483–9.

48   Thomas AG, Holly JM, Taylor F, Miller V. Insulin like growth factor-I, insulin like growth factor binding protein-1, and insulin in childhood Crohn's disease. *Gut* 1993; **34**: 944–7.

49   Bannerjee K, Camacho-Hübner C, Babinska, *et al.* Anti-inflammatory and growth stimulating effects precede nutritional restitution during enteral feeding in Crohn's disease. *J Pediatr Gastroenterol Nutr* 2004; **38**: 270–5.

50   De Benedetti F, Alzoni T, Moretta A, *et al.* Interleukin 6 causes growth impairment in transgenic mice through a decrease in insulin–like growth factor-I. A model for stunted growth in children with chronic inflammation. *J Clin Invest* 1997; **99**: 643–50.

51   Ballinger AB, Azzoz O, El-Haj T, *et al.* Growth failure occurs through a decrease in insulin-like growth factor 1 which is independent of undernutrition in a rat model of colitis. *Gut* 2000; **46**: 694–700.

52   Sawczenko A, Azzoz O, Paraszczuk J, *et al.* Intestinal inflammation-induced growth retardation acts through IL6 in rats and depends on the − 174 IL-6 G/C polymorphism in children. *Proc Nat Acad Sci* 2005; **102**: 13260–5.

53   Wine E, Reiff SS, Leshinsky-Silver E, *et al.* Pediatric Crohn's disease and growth retardation: the role of genotype, phenotype, and disease severity. *Pediatrics* 2004; **114**: 1281–6.

◆ 54   Markowitz J, Grancher K, Rosa J, *et al.* Growth failure in pediatric inflammatory bowel disease. *J Pediatr Gastroenterol Nutr* 1993; **16**: 373–80.

55   Alemzadeh N, Rekers-Mombarg LTM, Mearin ML, *et al.* Adult height in patients with early onset of Crohn's disease. *Gut* 2001; **51**: 26–9.

56   Kirschner BS, Klich JR, Kalman SS, *et al.* Reversal of growth retardation in Crohn's disease with therapy emphasizing oral nutritional restitution. *Gastroenterology* 1981; **80**: 10–5.

57   O'Morain C, Segal AM, Levi AJ, Valman HB. Elemental diet in acute Crohn's disease. *Arch Dis Child* 1983; **58**: 44–7.

58   Sanderson IR, Udeen S, Davies PS, *et al.* Remission induced by an elemental diet in small bowel Crohn's disease. *Arch Dis Child* 1987; **62**: 123–7.

59   Fell JM, Paintin M, Arnaud-Battandier F, *et al.* Mucosal healing and a fall in mucosal pro-inflammatory cytokine mRNA induced by a specific oral polymeric diet in paediatric Crohn's disease. *Aliment Pharmacol Ther* 2000; **14**: 281–9.

60   Afzal NA, Van Der Zaag-Loonen HJ, Arnaud-Battandier F, *et al.* Improvement in quality of life of children with acute

Crohn's disease does not parallel mucosal healing after treatment with exclusive enteral nutrition. *Aliment Pharmacol Ther* 2004; **20**: 167–72.

61 Zachos M, Tondeur M, Griffiths AM. Enteral nutritional therapy for inducing remission of Crohn's disease (Cochrane Review). *Cochrane Database Syst Rev* 2004.

∗ 62 Carter MJ, Lobo AJ, Travis SP, *et al.*, on behalf of the British Society of Gastroenterology. Guidelines for the management of inflammatory bowel disease in adults. *Gut* 2004; **53(Suppl V)**: 1–16.

◆ 63 Escher JC, Taminau JA, Nieuwenhuis EE, *et al.* Treatment of inflammatory bowel disease: best available evidence. *Inflamm Bowel Dis* 2003; **9**: 34–58.

◆ 64 Bremner AR, Beattie RM. Therapy of Crohn's disease in childhood. *Expert Opin Pharamacother* 2002; **3**: 809–25.

◆ 65 Bremner AR, Griffiths DM, Beattie RM. Therapy of ulcerative colitis in childhood. *Expert Opin Pharamacother* 2004; **5**: 37–53.

66 Boot AM, Bouquet J, Krenning EP, Muinck Keizer-Schrama SM. Bone mineral density and nutritional status in children with chronic inflammatory bowel disease. *Gut* 1998; **42**: 188–94.

67 Semeao EJ, Jawad AF, Stouffer NO, *et al.* Risk factors for low bone mineral density in children and young adults with Crohn's disease. *J Pediatr* 1999; **135**: 593–600.

68 Sylvester F. IBD and skeletal health: Children are not small adults. *Inflamm Bowel Dis* 2005; **11**: 1020–3.

69 Newby EA, Sawczenko A, Thomas AG, Wilson D. Interventions for growth failure in childhood Crohn's disease [Review]. *Cochrane Collab* 2005; Issue 3.

70 Belli D, Seidman EG, Bouthillier L, *et al.* Chronic intermittent elemental diet improves growth failure in children with Crohn's disease. *Gastroenterology* 1988; **94**: 603–10.

71 Seidman E. Nutritional therapy for Crohn's disease: Lessons from the Ste.-Justine Hospital experience. *Inflamm Bowel Dis* 1997; **3**: 49–53.

72 Borrelli O, Bascietto C, Viola F, *et al.* Infliximab heals intestinal inflammatory lesions and restores growth in children with Crohn's disease. *Dig Liver Dis* 2004; **36**: 342–7.

22

Renal disorders

ELKE WÜHL, FRANZ SCHAEFER

INTRODUCTION

Despite advances in the treatment of childhood-onset chronic renal failure (CRF), impairment of growth remains one of the major obstacles to successful rehabilitation. Final height is reduced below the third percentile in 30–50 percent of all patients who enter end-stage renal failure during childhood.[1–4] Although this has not been analyzed in depth, the incidence in permanent growth failure is assumed to be even higher in patients with onset of CRF in infancy. Chronic renal failure in childhood is not a homogeneous disease entity, but is the final common pathway of various renal abnormalities which may be congenital or acquired, manifest early or late in childhood, show rapid or slow progression and which may receive a variety of medications and renal replacement treatment modalities. The growth curve of a child with CRF may therefore be affected not only by renal dysfunction but by various co-morbid conditions and treatment-related effects. This review summarizes the present state of knowledge regarding the clinical manifestations, the underlying patho-physiological mechanisms and current management of growth failure in children with CRF.

CHRONIC RENAL FAILURE: CLINICAL PRESENTATION

The pattern of growth in children with congenital CRF is characterized by a rapidly increasing height deficit during the first 2 years of life, which is followed by a percentile-parallel growth pattern in the mid-childhood years. In the late pre-pubertal years, height velocity again decreases disproportionately. A late pubertal growth spurt of diminished amplitude eventually results in a decreased adult height.

Growth in infancy

Untreated CRF during early infancy is usually associated with severe growth retardation.[5–8] The mean loss in height in untreated patients is as high as 0.6 SD per month during the first year of life. A detailed analysis of the early infantile growth pattern observed in children with congenital CRF using the infancy–childhood–puberty model revealed that the 'infancy' growth phase, from intrauterine life to the second year of life, is affected in 50 percent of the patients.[9] Height standard deviation score (SDS), already reduced at birth, decreased further during the first three postnatal months, was normal between the 3rd and 9th month, and again decreased between the 10th and 12th month of life. The intrauterine period, the first three postnatal months and the period preceding the first birthday each contributed by about one-third to the overall reduction in height SDS observed in congenital CRF. The observed intrauterine growth retardation suggests that prenatal accumulation of certain circulating substances not cleared by the placenta in children with severe renal hypoplasia may compromise fetal growth. Conversely, intrauterine malnutrition could be the primary cause not only of fetal growth retardation but also of abnormal renal morphogenesis. With regard to early postnatal life, anorexia, water and electrolyte imbalances, recurrent vomiting, and catabolic responses to infections, metabolic acidosis, and secondary hyperparathyroidism are the main factors compromising growth. Appropriate early management can usually prevent severe stunting. Forced enteral feeding using nasogastric tubes, gastrostomies, and even fundoplication appears essential to prevent or reverse malnutrition.[10,11] Under optimal conditions it is possible to keep infants with CRF within 1–2 SD below the mean height for age.[11,12]

After a transient stabilization of growth rates, a further loss in relative height is commonly seen between 9 and 18 months of age. This period reflects the transition from the 'infancy' to the 'childhood' growth phase. An irregular onset or maintenance of the 'childhood' growth component was observed in 60 percent of the patients and resulted in a further decrease in mean standardized height by 0.7 SDS.[9] The reasons for this secondary deterioration of growth in infancy, which may occur despite adequate nutritional and medical supplementation, are poorly understood.

Growth during mid-childhood

In mid-childhood, patients with hypoplastic renal diseases usually grow along the percentiles attained around the end of infancy.[13] Patients who develop CRF after the second year of life exhibit a loss of relative height early in the course of disease and follow the growth percentile after stabilization of the disease process. The degree of renal dysfunction is the principal determinant of the variability in growth during this period. Spontaneous mid-childhood growth tends to be subnormal when glomerular filtration rate (GFR) is below $25 \, \text{mL} \, \text{min}^{-1} \, 1.73 \, \text{m}^{-2}$.[6,13–15]

A retrospective analysis of mid-childhood growth in patients with CRF showed a slightly lower annual growth rate in patients with GFR below $25 \, \text{mL} \, \text{min}^{-1} \, 1.73 \, \text{m}^{-2}$, accumulating a mean height difference of 6 cm between these subgroups at the age of 10 years (Fig. 22.1).[13] Given the heterogeneity of renal dysfunction and co-morbid conditions in this population, the observed variability of growth during the mid-childhood years was small, with height standard deviations averaging only 1.6 times those in healthy children. Growth rates during mid-childhood were most consistently correlated with the patients' average GFR, although only 10–15 percent of the variability in growth was actually accounted for by this parameter. The degree of anaemia, metabolic acidosis and malnutrition contributed only marginally to the annual growth rates.

The more or less percentile-parallel growth of uraemic children in mid-childhood has been interpreted as a 'normal' growth pattern that could be expected after a loss of growth potential in early infancy. Such readjustment of the growth channel is seen in children with cardiac diseases after surgery or in children with adrenal insufficiency overtreated

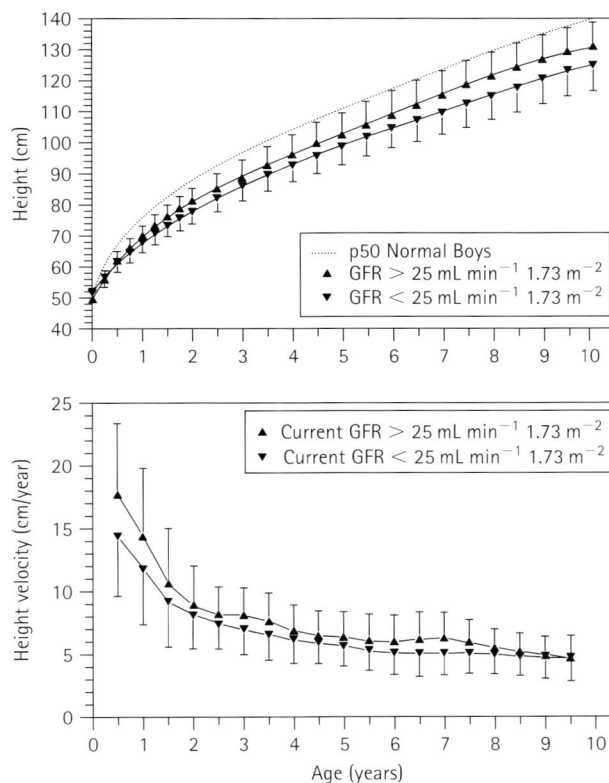

Figure 22.1 GFR-dependent growth pattern in children with chronic renal failure due to hypoplastic/dysplastic renal disorders. Approximately 100 children per age interval were evaluated. Upper panel: Mean ± SD of height in children with average GFR less or greater than $25 \, \text{mL} \, \text{min}^{-1} \, 1.73 \, \text{m}^{-2}$. Lower panel: Annual height velocity in children with current GFR greater or less than $25 \, \text{mL} \, \text{min}^{-1} \, 1.73 \, \text{m}^{-2}$ in the year of observation. (Adapted from Schaefer et al.,[13] with permission.)

in infancy.[16] However, the observation that complete catch-up growth, although not common, does occur in children in whom renal function is normalized by successful renal transplantation and glucocorticoid treatment can be withdrawn[17,18] suggests that catch-up growth is continuously suppressed in the uremic milieu. The percentile-parallel growth pattern during this period may therefore reflect a net balance between the growth-suppressive effect of uremia and the child's inherent tendency for catch-up growth.

Pubertal growth

The height gain achieved during the pubertal growth spurt is usually reduced.[19–22] In a longitudinal analysis of growth in 29 adolescents with various degrees of CRF, the growth spurt started with an average delay of 2.5 years.[22] The degree of the delay was correlated with the duration of CRF. Although an acceleration of growth during puberty occurred, the total pubertal height gain was reduced in both sexes to approximately 50 percent of normal late-maturing children. This reduction was due to a marked suppression of the late pre-spurt height velocity, a subnormal peak height velocity, and a shortening of the pubertal growth period by 1 year in boys and 1.5 years in girls. Notably, the prolonged pre-pubertal growth phase permitted the patients to grow up to an almost normal immediate pre-spurt height (-1 SDS in boys, $+0.1$ SDS in girls). Subsequently, relative height was lost during the pubertal growth spurt, ending up in an average relative height of -2.9 SDS in boys and -2.3 SDS in girls. This pattern of pubertal growth was recently confirmed in a control group of end-stage renal disease (ESRD) patients followed in the late 1990s who were not treated with recombinant GH.[23]

In pre-pubertal children with long-standing renal failure, bone maturation is retarded.[24–27] In dialysis patients, skeletal maturation is increasingly retarded before puberty and then accelerates dramatically. This observation and the fact that uremic boys respond to exogenous testosterone esters by an exaggerated increase in skeletal maturation,[27] suggests that the sensitivity of the growth plate to sex steroids is conserved. Because proliferation, i.e., growth, cannot keep pace with differentiation, bone maturation and growth potential may irreversibly be lost during puberty.

In contrast, in many transplant patients, an apparent standstill of bone maturation is observed, even when the patient is growing and puberty is progressing. This phenomenon is thought to be related to direct interference of corticosteroids with the differentiation of the growth plate. Despite the delayed bone age, late growth is usually not observed.[3,22,28] In fact, the successive stages of the pubertal growth spurt seem to occur at increasingly earlier bone ages than would be assumed in a normal population.[22]

Final height

A crucial question in the rehabilitation of children with chronic renal disease relates to the degree of compromise of final height. Of the patients with childhood-onset (ESRD) in the EDTA Registry, 50 percent achieved adult heights below the 3rd percentile. Children with continued dialysis until adulthood reached a lower mean final height than children who received a renal transplant.[1,3,4,29–32] Final height was more severely compromised in boys than in girls, reflecting the higher incidence of congenital nephropathies in boys. Final height is most compromised in patients with severe congenital renal disorders, among which nephropathic cystinosis leads to the most obvious growth retardation.[33] However, patients with acquired glomerular diseases usually exhibit a marked loss in height SDS in the early course of the disease, resulting in the need for growth-promoting treatment.

RENAL TRANSPLANTATION

Post-transplant growth and development has been studied most systematically in renal allograft recipients. While a wide variety of growth patterns after kidney transplantation has been reported by individual centers, ranging from progressive growth failure to almost complete catch-up growth,[19,20,34–46] most reports agree about the main determinants of post-transplant growth. These are the age and the degree of stunting at time of transplantation,[37,38,46–49] the level of allograft function and the modalities of glucocorticoid treatment.

The intense therapeutic attention to growth failure has resulted in improved growth in the pre-transplant phase. In the annual reports of the North American Pediatric Renal Transplant Registry (NAPRTCS),[50] mean standardized height at the time of first kidney transplantation has increased from -2.2 SDS in 1987 to -1.5 SDS in 1999.

The potential for post-transplant catch-up growth appears to be inversely related to age at transplantation. Excellent catch-up growth is observed in infants.[37,47–49,51] The critical age beyond which a significant improvement in height SDS was no longer observed was 2,[48] 6,[47,49] 7,[37] 10,[52] and 12 years[45] in different studies. Pubertal growth benefits least from renal transplantation. As in dialyzed patients, puberty and the pubertal growth spurt are delayed in renal allograft recipients by approximately 2 years. Although acceleration of height velocity occurs, total pubertal height gain is subnormal.[53] An inverse relationship between pubertal peak height velocity and cumulative glucocorticoid intake has been observed.[22,53]

In addition to the impact of age, the change in height following renal transplantation is correlated to the height at time of grafting.[51,54] Hence, the principle of catch-up growth 'by demand', i.e., the tendency of an organism to return to a pre-determined growth channel after removal of growth-inhibitory conditions, holds true for renal allograft recipients.

Post-transplant growth appears to be very sensitive to the function of the allograft. Whereas native kidney function only affects growth when glomerular filtration rate is reduced to less than 30 mL min^{-1} 1.73 m^{-2}, post-transplant growth velocity is significantly reduced at any GFR below 60 mL min^{-1} 1.73 m^{-2}.[36,47] Multivariate analyses have confirmed that the growth-suppressive effects of poor graft function is independent of glucocorticoid dosage.[42,45]

In view of the growth-suppressive endocrine and metabolic effects of glucocorticoids, this immunosuppressive medication plays a major role in post-transplant growth. Results from clinical trials using modified steroid administration, complete steroid withdrawal or even primary steroid avoidance have provided evidence that glucocorticoids affect catch-up growth in renal transplant recipients.[17,18,55] On the other hand, few studies found a consistent correlation between steroid dosage and the post-transplant change in standardized height.[22,34] The area under the serum methyl prednisolone concentration curve was superior to the administered glucocorticoid dose in predicting post-transplant growth rates.[56]

After more than three decades of pediatric renal transplantation, several thousand patients worldwide have achieved final adult height. This provides the opportunity to assess post-transplant catch-up growth, and to analyze the eventual impact of the modulatory factors mentioned above on the endpoint of longitudinal growth. Final height has been assessed in three single-center studies and one registry report.[53,54,57,58] Adult height was found below the normal range in 25–41 percent of all patients who developed end-stage renal disease and underwent kidney transplantation during childhood. In 237 children reported to the NAPRTCS registry who had received a graft at age ⩽12 years, final height SDS was identical to standardized height at the time of transplantation, indicating no overall catch-up growth.[58] As found for early post-transplant growth in the studies cited above, final height was inversely related to the age at transplantation, significant catch-up growth being limited to pre-pubertal patients. The most severely stunted patients exhibited the most marked post-transplant growth improvement, and renal graft function was an additional independent predictor of final height. The height attained at time of transplantation remained the most significant predictor of final height, illustrating the limited potential for post-transplant catch-up growth in the ESRD population. In addition, an average prednisone dosage in excess of $0.15\,\mathrm{mg\,kg^{-1}\,day^{-1}}$ was independently associated with a retarded final height in the NAPRTCS analysis.[58]

ETIOLOGY OF UNDERLYING RENAL DISEASE

The pathogenesis of impaired growth in CRF is complex and only partially understood. Although a particular cause can occasionally be found, a combination of several factors is generally responsible for growth impairment. Furthermore, the patient's age, the type, duration, and severity of renal disease, the treatment modality, and the patient's social environment all play important roles.

Congenital renal hypoplasia/dysplasia

A variety of kidney disorders may cause growth failure independent of the presence or absence of CRF. Congenital renal dysplasia or hypoplasia is the most common cause of end-stage renal failure during the first years of life. As discussed above, growth failure usually develops during the first year of life. In the care of these patients it is important to compensate for tubular electrolyte loss and acidosis. Pharmacological reno-protective therapy with renin–angiotensin system antagonists may slow down progression of renal failure and thereby have a positive long-term impact.

Glomerulonephritis

Progressive glomerular injury may appear as acute or chronic glomerulonephritis, or as nephrotic disease. Growth rates decline in patients with progressive glomerulonephritis as glomerular function deteriorates. Growth velocity is affected even in mild renal insufficiency.[14] In patients with nephrotic syndrome, proteinuria per se impairs growth, both in congenital nephrosis and resistant nephrotic syndrome that appears later in childhood.[59,60] The dose and duration of glucocorticoid treatment in nephrotic syndrome and the evolution of renal function are predominant factors affecting growth. Prolonged high-dose corticosteroid administration suppresses growth rates.[60–63] Final height was -0.22 SDS in a sample of 28 patients with childhood steroid-sensitive nephrotic syndrome.[62] In steroid-resistant nephrotic disease, focal–segmental glomerulosclerosis usually leads to progressive renal insufficiency and it is difficult to differentiate between the impact of proteinuria and decreasing GFR on statural growth. Congenital nephrotic syndrome usually is associated with severe stunting during the first months of life while GFR still is in the normal range but massive edema and proteinuria are present. Growth failure in these infants may be secondary to edema, recurrent infections, endocrine alterations due to losses of peptide and protein-bound hormones, and protein-calorie malnutrition. Bilateral nephrectomy, replacing proteinuria, edema and cachexia by ESRD, may be associated with improved growth.[64]

Tubulopathies and interstitial disorders

Primary tubular dysfunctions and interstitial disorders may lead to growth impairment. Patients with either proximal or distal renal tubular acidosis may present with growth failure during the first years of life.[65,66] Growth impairment may be due to tissue catabolism, volume depletion, electrolyte disorders and/or to malnutrition. Catch-up growth is observed after correction of acidosis with alkaline therapy in distal renal tubular acidosis (RTA).[65,67] Growth retardation occurs in about 50 percent of patients with nephrogenic diabetes insipidus. Maintaining water balance and treatment with indomethacin are associated with catch-up growth.[68] Bartter's syndrome and related disorders are characterized by failure to thrive.[69] Experimental potassium deficiency leads to growth failure[70,71] In patients with hyperprostaglandin E syndrome, indomethacin medication induces partial catch-up growth.[72] Complex disorders of proximal and distal tubular function, such as idiopathic Fanconi syndrome[73,74] or hereditary fructose intolerance may develop severe growth failure. In these cases, only partial catch-up growth is possible even with rigorous electrolyte supplementation.[65,67,69,72] Severe growth failure may also develop in children with cystinosis or oxalosis and occurs even with optimal substitution of tubular losses, due to the generalized deposition of cystine crystals which result in local growth plate and hypothalamopituitary dysfunction and hypothyroidism. In a survey by the EDTA only 13 of 106 cystinotic patients on renal replacement therapy who were between 8 to 21 years had a height above the third centile.[75] Treatment with cysteamine or phosphocysteamine appears to slow the rate of deterioration of GFR and to improve growth rates.[76–78] Recombinant GH was effective in stimulating growth independently of renal function and cysteamine treatment.[33]

In patients with chronic or recurrent interstitial disease, minor growth retardation may develop. Persistent or recurrent urinary tract infections may cause growth impairment by tubular dysfunction, by the catabolic effect of chronic disease, and/or progressive renal insufficiency. Growth rates may increase after medical and/or surgical intervention.[79–81] In patients with vesicoureteric reflux, moderate growth retardation has been demonstrated.[82] Whereas previous reports noted a growth spurt after successful antireflux surgery,[80,81] multiple regression analysis in 54 patients with obstructive urinary tract malformations suggested a positive relationship between the increase in relative height and the duration of antibiotic treatment, but no independent effect of surgical intervention.[83] Severe growth failure was observed in patients with posterior urethral valves.[84]

PROTEIN–ENERGY MALNUTRITION

One of the cardinal abnormalities associated with CRF is a loss of appetite. Energy intake is inversely related to the degree of renal failure,[85] and is correlated with growth rates if it is less than 80 percent of recommended dietary allowances.[86] However, further augmentation of energy intake above this level results in obesity rather than in a further stimulation of growth.[86,87] Height SDS is correlated with body cell mass and serum transferrin or albumin in infants, emphasizing the importance of malnutrition for growth failure in this age group.[5,88,89] In later childhood, food intake is usually low when related to the patient's age, but normal when adjusted for body mass.[90,91] The same is true for the body protein content of children with CRF and short stature, which is adequate for height but not for age.[92]

At any given protein intake, the conversion of dietary to body protein is less efficient in uremic compared with pair-fed control animals.[93] Resistance to the anabolic effects of insulin and IGF-I and increased protein breakdown by activation of proteolytic pathways may contribute to poor growth. In contrast to deficient calorie intake, protein malnutrition is infrequently seen in children with CRF.[90,91] In a prospective study deliberately limiting protein intake to the safe levels of the WHO (e.g., 0.8–1.1 $g\,kg^{-1}\,day^{-1}$) but ensuring adequate calorie intake, no impairment of weight gain and length gain was seen over 3 years.[94]

METABOLIC ACIDOSIS

Once the reduction of GFR exceeds 50 percent, the kidney's ability to excrete ammonia is increasingly compromised. The severity of the acidosis is aggravated by nutritional protein and acid load, catabolism and altered electrolyte balance. Metabolic acidosis is associated with increased glucocorticoid production and increased protein degradation by activating branched chain ketoacid catabolism and the ubiquitin–proteasome pathway.[95–97] In young children with CRF, the degree of protein wasting is tightly correlated with serum bicarbonate levels.[98] Moreover, metabolic acidosis has profound suppressive effects on the somatotropic hormone axis by downregulating GH secretion,[99] GH receptor and IGF-I gene expression[100] and serum IGF-I levels.[101] Hence acidosis per se causes a state of GH insensitivity.

DISTURBANCES OF WATER AND ELECTROLYTE METABOLISM

Many congenital renal diseases lead to a loss of electrolytes and a reduced ability of the kidney to concentrate urine. Polyuria, an expression of the reduced ability of the kidney to concentrate the urine, is seen in patients with Fanconi's syndrome and in nephronophthisis, but also in hypoplastic kidney disease.

It is not possible to independently assess the extent to which water and electrolyte disturbances contribute to growth retardation in individual patients with CRF. In rats, sodium deficiency decreases protein synthesis and growth, which is only partially reversible by sodium repletion.[102,103] Part of the effects usually attributed to sodium deficiency are actually caused by concomitant depletion of chloride, which per se, if removed selectively from a sodium-replete diet, causes growth retardation and diminished muscle protein synthesis.[104]

ANEMIA

Children with CRF develop increasing anemia as a result of erythropoietin (EPO) deficiency. Theoretically, anemia may interfere with growth via various mechanisms such as poor appetite, intercurrent infections, cardiac complications and poor oxygenation of the cartilage cells in the growth plate.

RENAL OSTEODYSTROPHY

Renal osteodystrophy was originally considered to be important in the development of renal growth retardation. This issue is, however, viewed differently today. Although gross skeletal deformities can contribute to growth retardation, renal osteodystrophy is not inevitably paralleled by alterations in epiphyseal growth of the long bones. Metaphyseal changes are often detected radiologically in patients with relatively good growth rates. In such cases, osteopathy may be unmasked by rapid growth.[105] Growth is only arrested completely when secondary hyper-parathyroidism results in severe destruction of metaphyseal bone architecture and epiphyseal slipping.[106]

ENDOCRINE DISORDERS IN UREMIA

Distinct abnormalities of the somatotrophic and gonadotrophic hormone axes have been identified which corroborate the view that growth failure in uremia may be interpreted as a syndrome of multiple endocrine resistance.

Somatotrophic hormone axis

Fasting GH concentrations are variably elevated in uremic children and adults[107,108] The kidney is a major site of GH degradation.[109] In patients with endstage renal failure, the metabolic clearance rate of GH is reduced by approximately 50 percent.[110,111] Deconvolution analyses of GH plasma concentration profiles revealed that the increase in plasma GH concentrations is mainly due to an increased plasma half-life of the hormone, whereas the actual pituitary GH secretion rate varied between patients and studies. GH secretion rate was high-normal in pre-pubertal children with ESRD and increased in adult patients on hemodialysis, possibly as a result of attenuated bioactive IGF-I feedback on the hypothalamo-pituitary unit.[112,113] In pubertal patients with advanced CRF reduced GH secretion rates were observed, indicating an altered sensitivity of the somatotropic hormone axis to the stimulatory effect of sex steroids during this stage of development.[114]

The variability of plasma GH levels in CRF may in part be due to associated conditions such as acidosis and malnutrition, which independently affect GH secretion. Metabolic acidosis suppresses GH release both in rodents and humans.[99]

Dysregulation of GH secretion may be related to abnormalities of central neuroendocrine control mechanisms. Evidence for this is provided by several hypothalamo-pituitary function tests.[107,115-119] However, the altered metabolic clearance rates of GH as well as of the provocative agents in renal failure[120] make a clinical interpretation of such tests virtually impossible.

Growth failure despite elevated circulating GH concentrations suggests a state of GH resistance in children with CRF. Indeed, GH-induced hepatic IGF-I synthesis is markedly reduced in rats with CRF.[121,122] This GH insensitivity may in part be due to deficient GH receptor expression, although this is controversial. In humans serum levels of GH binding protein were decreased in some, but normal in other studies.[111,123-126] Another mechanism accounting for the resistance to GH in uremia is provided by a marked post-receptor GH signaling defect recently observed in livers of chronically uremic rats.[122]

As most metabolic effects of GH are mediated by IGF-I, GH insensitivity in uremia may also be due to IGF resistance. Indeed, numerous studies in the rat as well as in humans have documented marked IGF-I resistance in CRF.[127-130]

The effect of GH on longitudinal growth is partially mediated by stimulating the production of somatomedins, the two most important of which are the insulin-like growth

factors (IGF) I and II. Serum IGF-I and IGF-II levels in children with preterminal CRF are in the normal range, whereas in end-stage renal disease mean age-related serum IGF-I levels are slightly decreased and IGF-II levels moderately elevated.[131] Hence, total immunoreactive IGF levels in CRF serum are normal. In contrast, IGF bioactivity is markedly reduced. Similarly, the level of free IGF-I is reduced by 50 percent in relation to the degree of renal dysfunction.[132] This finding is one of the key abnormalities of the GH/IGF axis in children with CRF.

The discrepancy between low IGF-I activity by bioassay and normal or elevated insulin-like growth factor by radioimmunossay or radioreceptor assay suggests the presence of circulating somatomedin inhibitors in uremia. An early study suggested the presence of a low-molecular weight IGF inhibitor (approx. 1 kDa).[133]

The most likely explanation for the inhibition of IGF-I action in uremia has emerged from the identification of six insulin-like growth factor-binding proteins (IGFBP-1 to -6). In children with CRF, the serum concentrations of IGFBP-1, IGFBP-2, IGFBP-4 and IGFBP-6 are increased in a manner inversely related to glomerular filtration rate.[131,134-139] Experimental evidence suggests that the increase of IGFBP-1 and IGFBP-2 is not only due to reduced renal metabolic clearance but also to increased hepatic synthesis.[140] An important question is whether the imbalance between normal total IGF and the excess of unsaturated IGFBPs contributes to growth failure in children with CRF. Serum levels of IGFBP-1, IGFBP-2 and IGFBP-4 correlate inversely with standardized height in CRF children.[131,139,141] In uremic rats the effect of IGF-I and various IGF-I analogs on protein turnover was suppressed.[127] The observation that the inhibitory effect of IGF-I and its analogs were affected to a similar degree indicates that the resistance arises because of a defect at a cellular level and not because of changes in the IGFBP levels. The pattern of elevated GH, normal total IGF and markedly elevated plasma IGFBP concentrations in uremia has interesting implications with respect to the estimated IGF production rate. In a functioning homeostatic system, the diminished free IGF-I levels would be expected to stimulate IGF production in order to restore the steady-state between bound and unbound hormone at a higher level. In uremia, however, total IGF concentrations are normal rather than increased. Kinetic modeling suggests that the metabolic half-life of IGFs is elevated, and the IGF production rate is decreased 10- to 100-fold in uremia.[142] Taken together, the markedly deficient IGF-I synthesis and the modest elevation of plasma GH levels strongly support the notion of a multi-level homeostatic failure of the GH–IGF-I system.

During puberty, GH secretion physiologically increases three-fold compared with the pre-pubertal level driven by the rise in circulating sex steroid levels. In CRF, the pubertal increase of GH secretion is absent.[114] The observed lack of a correlation between serum testosterone levels and GH secretion rates indicates an altered sensitivity of the somatotrophic hormone axis to the stimulatory effects of sex steroids in the pubertal period.[22]

Glucocorticoids and the GH–IGF hormone axis

Following renal transplantation, the glucocorticoids interfere with the GH–IGF-I axis on various levels. Although short-term glucocorticoid administration stimulates GH release,[143,144] high-dose, long-term glucocorticoid treatment tends to suppress GH secretion in pediatric renal allograft recipients, mainly by a reduction of amplitudes of the GH secretory bursts.[145,146] The physiological increase of GH burst amplitudes during puberty is blunted, and the normal correlation between sex steroid plasma levels and GH secretion rate is absent.[146] GH release after insulin-induced hypoglycemia is inadequate.[145] The insufficiency of spontaneous and stimulated GH secretion in post-transplant patients is most likely explained by a glucocorticoid-induced enhancement of hypothalamic somatostatin release.[147] On the target tissue level, glucocorticoids suppress GH receptor and IGF-I gene transcription.[148,149] Nevertheless, basal IGF-I plasma levels in renal transplant recipients are in the normal range.[20,150,151] Whereas circulating immunoreactive IGF-I concentrations are not consistently reduced, IGF bioactivity is markedly diminished in patients on glucocorticoid treatment.[150,152] This may be due to the induction of IGF inhibitors of 12–20 kDa molecular weight and/or to increased serum IGFBP-3 levels.[150,152] Moreover, increased IGFBP-2 concentrations are found in patients with Cushing's syndrome[153] which may act as a IGF-I inhibitor in patients receiving chronic glucocorticoid treatment.

Glucocorticoids also interfere with chondrocyte growth and enchondral bone formation in various ways. They inhibit sulfate incorporation into cartilage matrix as well as mineralization and formation of new bone.[154] In cultured epiphyseal chondrocytes, dexamethasone decreases DNA synthesis and cell proliferation, GH receptor expression and paracrine IGF-I secretion.[155]

Gonadotrophic hormone axis

The endocrine profile of pre-pubertal or peripubertal patients with CRF is characterized by increased gonadotrophin (LH and FSH) and low–normal sex steroid concentrations.[156] This constellation has been interpreted as a state of compensated hypergonadotrophic hypogonadism. Indeed, human chorionic gonadotrophin (HCG) stimulation studies revealed impaired testicular responsiveness even in prepubertal children with CRF, with hyporesponsiveness being most severe in end-stage CRF patients.[157] Recently, the presence of a circulating substance acting as an endogenous LH inhibitor in uremic serum has been demonstrated.[158]

The degree of hypergonadotrophism typically seen in CRF is usually inadequate for the degree of hypogonadism, suggesting an additional defect of hypophyseal gonadotrophin secretion. Moreover, the rise in nocturnal pulsatile gonadotrophin secretion heralding the imminent onset of puberty, is delayed in CRF patients by about 2 years.[159] Deconvolution analysis of nocturnal LH concentration profiles revealed, both in humans[160] and in rats[161] that the elevation of basal plasma LH concentrations is the result of diminished renal clearance rate of the hormone. The subnormal pituitary gonadotrophin secretion has been demonstrated in vitro and in vivo to be caused by a diminished release of gonadotrophin-releasing hormone (GnRH) into the hypophyseal portal circulation.[162,163] The spectrum of LH isoforms secreted from the pituitary is shifted towards less bioactive alkaline isoforms in children and adults with CRF.[164–166]

TREATMENT OF UREMIC GROWTH FAILURE

Conservative treatment

Adequate nutrition is the most important prerequisite for infantile growth. Growth rates in this period are correlated with energy intake.[86] Consequently, nasogastric tube, gastrostomy or even fundoplication is an essential component in the management of infantile CRF.[10,11,167] In later childhood, adequate nutrition is permissive for growth; however, catch-up growth cannot be obtained by dietary manipulations alone. Metabolic acidosis should be treated systematically, and water and electrolyte losses must be consequently compensated.[12,168,169]

Dialysis and transplantation

DIALYSIS

The institution of dialysis usually does not improve growth in uremic children. Several studies found mean annual losses of 0.4–0.8 SD standardized height.[170–172] As with hemodialysis, catch-up growth is not commonly observed in children on peritoneal dialysis. Whereas early experience suggested continued significant losses of standardized height on CAPD/CCPD,[8,173–175] more recent studies suggest percentile-parallel growth patterns or slight losses of less than 0.5 SD per year.[176,177] Even catch-up growth could be achieved in children on daily hemodiafiltration regimen[178] or with enhanced nutrition and clearance.[179] Residual renal function is a more important predictor of growth on PD than dialytic clearance.[177] In addition, a high peritoneal transporter state predicted poor growth (−0.5 SD per year) in a prospective study of 51 children followed for 18 months.[176] It is currently believed that apart from causing increased dialytic protein losses, the high transporter status may be an indicator of microinflammation, a putative cause of GH resistance in uremia.

RENAL TRANSPLANTATION

Only successful renal transplantation is able to restore the conditions for normal growth. However, growth rates after transplantation vary widely, from further deterioration of height SDS to complete catch-up growth.[19,20,37,39–42,51,57,180,181] Whereas pubertal patients tend to lose relative height following transplantation,[46] a potential for post-transplant catch-up growth exists in patients younger than 6 years.[36,51,54,180] Infant allograft recipients typically exhibit excellent spontaneous growth rates, with a relative height gain of 1.5 SD within 2–7 years.[37,51,182] Apart from the inverse relationship with age, the degree of growth retardation positively predicts post-transplant growth rate.[47,51,54,180,181,183] Furthermore, post-transplant growth critically depends on graft function.[31,47,51,54,58,180,181,183] A marked deceleration in post-transplant growth is observed when GFR is below 60 mL min^{-1} 1.73 m^{-2}.[21] The daily dose as well as the cumulative dose of corticosteroids seem to be inversely related to the post-transplant growth rate.[22,34,56] Alternate-day corticosteroid administration improved growth by 0.25–0.5 SD of height per year.[40,45] The most impressive catch-up growth has been observed in patients in whom steroids could be completely withdrawn[17,39,43,184,185] with an improvement of 0.6 to 0.8 SD during the first post-transplant year. Ellis *et al.* found a cumulative height increment by 1.5 SD within 3 years in children less than 5 years of age with tacrolimus monotherapy, and apparent catch-up growth even in pubertal patients.[184] The results of steroid withdrawal studies should be interpreted with caution since usually only patients with low risk for rejection with good allograft function were included. The advent of several potent new immunosuppressive agents in recent years may allow complete withdrawal of steroids in pediatric renal transplantation.[185,186] The risk of rejection and loss of renal function by steroid withdrawal, historically rated as 40–50 percent,[39,187,188] may have diminished considerably with the new immunosuppressive protocols.

HORMONE TREATMENT

Vitamin D analogs

Whereas treatment with vitamin D and 1,25(OH)$_2$D$_3$ improves growth in uremic rats,[189] an equivalent therapeutic success has not been achieved in children with CRF. Treatment with 5000 to 10 000 IU vitamin D$_3$ per day did not affect growth in dialyzed children.[190] An early optimistic report in four patients receiving 1,25(OH)$_2$D$_3$[191] could not be validated in the long term.[192] The extent to which secondary hyperparathyroidism contributes to growth impairment is unclear. Parathyroid hormone (PTH) is an anabolic hormone and an intrinsic growth factor, stimulating mitosis in osteoprogenitor cells and growth plate chondrocytes and up-regulates the vitamin D receptor.[193,194] Intermittent PTH administration stimulates the skeletal growth of normal and uremic rats.[195] However, resistance to the effect of PTH is observed in uremia, characterized by reduced cAMP production in growth plate chondrocytes.[193]

A low bone turnover state induced by relatively low PTH levels may contribute to growth impairment.[196] At the other end of the spectrum, excessive secretion of PTH can lead to the destruction of growth plate architecture,[197] epiphyseal displacement[106] and metaphyseal fractures.[198]

Erythropoietin

Whereas short-term stimulatory effects of recombinant erythropoietin were observed in single patients,[199] no persistent growth improvement was observed in prospective trials.[159] Although the correction of anemia by erythropoietin resulted in well-being and sometimes in stimulation of appetite,[200] no systematic improvement of growth was observed. In a European multicenter study, 29 children with dialysis treatment were treated with erythropoietin to achieve a target hemoglobin of 10 g L^{-1}. Height SDS, which declined during the year before the start of erythropoietin treatment, further declined during several years of erythropoietin treatment.[159]

Growth hormone

The GH resistance observed in uremia and during glucocorticoid treatment, and the experimental proof that GH resistance can be overcome by supraphysiological doses of exogenous GH[201] have provided a rationale for treating children with CRF and after renal transplantation with recombinant human growth hormone (rGH). Administration of rGH increases IGF-I production to a greater degree than IGFBP concentrations, thereby raising the availability of free IGF-I at the tissue level.[126]

rGH TREATMENT IN PREDIALYSIS AND DIALYSIS CHILDREN

In pre-pubertal children, numerous studies including two double-blind placebo-controlled trials rGH demonstrated that rGH induces a nearly two-fold increase in height velocity during the first treatment year, with a diminishing but still significant effect on growth rate during the second year.[203–209] Although the maximal height increment occurs in the first three treatment years, standardized height continues to increase slightly during extended treatment. After 5–6 years of rGH administration, mean height SDS had increased from −2.6 at baseline to −0.7 in a North American study,[209] from −3.4 to −1.9 in German children[208] and from −3 to −0.5 in Dutch patients.[210] The remarkable pre-pubertal growth acceleration was not associated with a disproportionate advancement of bone age, resulting in a remarkable increase in predicted adult height at the end of the pre-pubertal phase.[208] Pre-pubertal children on dialysis respond less well to rGH than children with CRF on conservative treatment (Fig. 22.2).[208,211] Children on chronic peritoneal dialysis do not respond differently to rGH than

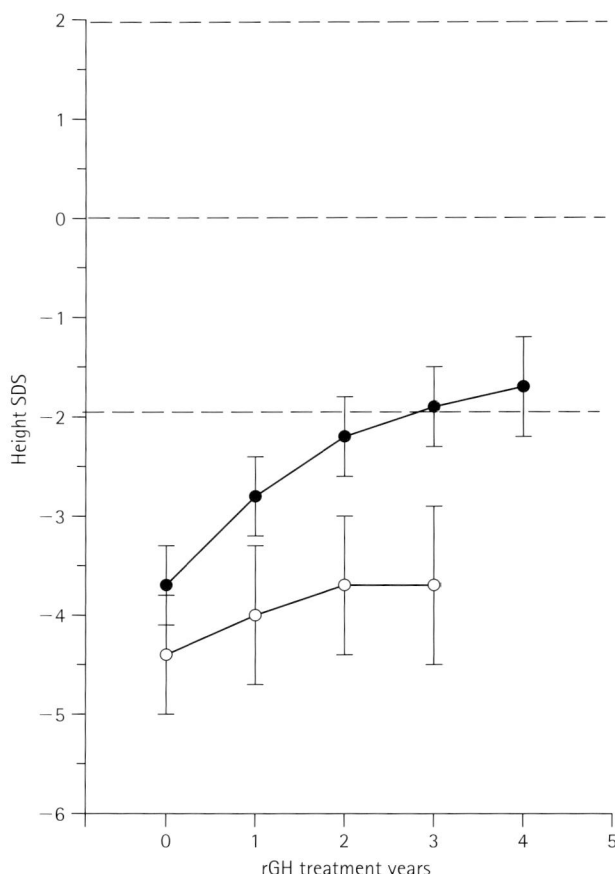

Figure 22.2 Superior efficacy of recombinant growth hormone (rGH) treatment in children with pre-endstage chronic renal failure (CRF) (●, $n = 19$) compared to children on dialysis (○, $n = 6$). (Adapted from Haffner et al.,[208] with permission.)

hemodialysis patients.[212] In pre-pubertal children with nephropathic cystinosis, GH increased height by 1.6 SDS within 3 treatment years.[33]

POST-TRANSPLANTATION TREATMENT

In pre-pubertal renal allograft patients, in whom alternate-day corticosteroid treatment does not induce catch-up growth and discontinuation of corticosteroid medication is not considered an option for safety reasons, a therapeutic trial with GH may be considered. Several studies have demonstrated a growth promoting effect of GH in pre-pubertal children with renal allografts over average treatment periods of 1 to 3 years.[151,213–219]

USE OF GROWTH HORMONE IN PUBERTY

A systematic analysis of rGH treatment efficacy in pubertal children is difficult due to methodological problems.[219] These include delayed puberty with a lack of appropriate growth reference data, potential effects of rGH on the onset and duration of the pubertal growth spurt, and frequent changes in treatment modalities with variable relative

efficacy of rGH. In addition, rGH is usually discontinued at the time of transplantation but is sometimes reinstituted if the growth rate remains low, introducing large variability in the duration of rGH treatment during puberty.

Haffner et al. followed 38 children with CRF in whom rGH was initiated at pre-pubertal age until they reached adult height.[23] Since rGH was stopped at the time of transplantation, the patients received rGH during 50 percent of the pubertal observation time. Fifty children, matched for age and degree of CRF, who did not receive rGH because their height was normal, served as controls. The children receiving rGH showed sustained catch-up growth, whereas the control children developed progressive growth failure (Fig. 22.3). Dissection of the pre-pubertal and the pubertal growth phases disclosed that the additional height gain relative to the control group was almost entirely limited to the pre-pubertal period, whereas pubertal height gain was insignificantly greater in the rGH treated patients than in the controls. Hokken-Koelega et al. demonstrated that allograft recipients may respond very well to rGH even in late puberty,[206] with an almost three-fold greater 2-year height gain compared to untreated historical controls.[221]

Neither in the German study nor in the Dutch cohort[210] advanced onset of puberty were observed, although a subtle acceleration of bone maturation and a slight shortening of the pubertal growth spurt was noted by Haffner et al.[23]

Adult height

In the German multicenter study, the mean adult height of 38 children who received rGH for a mean of 5.3 years was −1.6 SDS, with two-thirds of patients ending up at a height above the 3rd percentile.[23] The patients gained 1.4 SD when compared to their standardized height at baseline. Conversely, mean height SDS decreased in the untreated control group from −1.5 to −2.1 SDS at attainment of adult height. Figures in the same range were reported from several other trials.[210,215,217,222–224] Of course, the variability of final height outcomes is large. Cumulative height gain appears to be positively affected by the height deficit at the start of rGH and the total duration of rGH administration,[23] negatively by the cumulative duration of periods spent on dialysis. Growth was positively associated with the initial target-height deficit and the duration of rGH therapy and negatively associated with the percentage of the observation period spent on dialysis.[23,210] The relative height attained at transplantation seems to be maintained to final height.[223,225]

General treatment strategies

The response to rGH is positively influenced by the residual GFR, target height, the initial target height deficit and the duration of GH treatment, and negatively by the age at start of treatment.[220] A curvilinear dose–response relationship

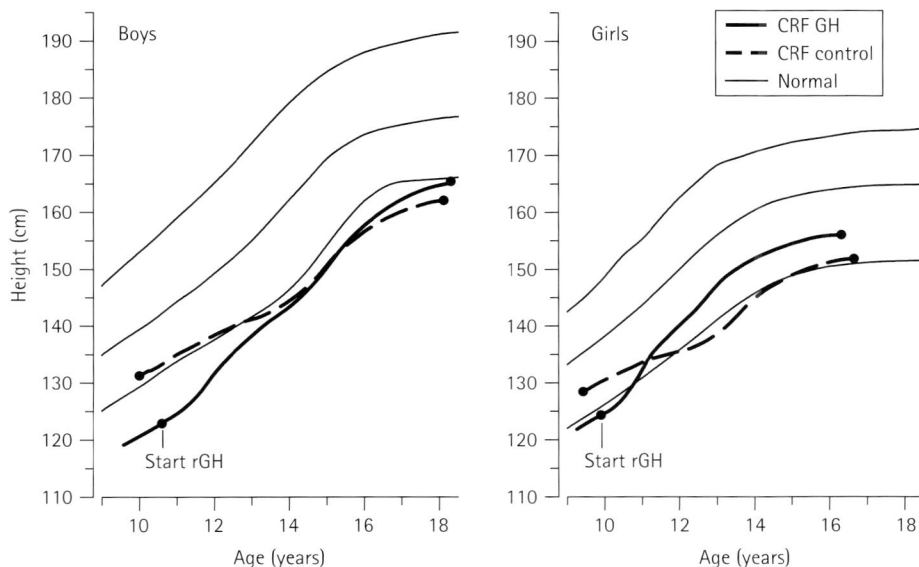

Figure 22.3 Favorable effect of long-term rGH treatment on final adult height in children with CRF. Synchronized mean growth curves during GH treatment for 38 children (32 boys and 6 girls) with CRF, compared with 50 control children with CRF not treated with GH. Normal values are indicated by the 3rd, 50th, and 97th percentiles. The circles indicate the time of the first observation (the start of GH treatment in the treated children) and the end of the pubertal growth spurt. (Adapted from Haffner et al.,[23] with permission.)

appears to exist. Although a dosage of $4 \, \text{IU} \, \text{m}^{-2} \, \text{day}^{-1}$ was more efficient than $2 \, \text{IU} \, \text{m}^{-2} \, \text{day}^{-1}$ in a double-blind trial,[226] no further improvement of the growth response was observed with $8 \, \text{IU} \, \text{m}^{-2} \, \text{day}^{-1}$, at least in a pubertal cohort.[221] Daily dosing is more efficacious than three applications per week.[227] Discontinuation of GH treatment will result in loss of height SDS in 75 percent of children with CRF on conservative treatment,[228] whereas catch-down growth seems to be uncommon when rGH is discontinued due to renal transplantation.[223,228]

Since the absolute growth response to rGH (in centimeters height gain per year) is independent of age but the reference range increases with age,[208] GH treatment should be started as early as possible in the course of renal disease. A fixed daily dose of $1.4 \, \text{mg} \, \text{m}^{-2} \, \text{day}^{-1}$ should be used and should be continued when the patient becomes dialysis-dependent. If GH is initiated in a small child already on dialysis, transplantation should not be postponed for the sake of approved GH treatment, since the efficacy of rGH in dialysis patients is limited and short-lasting. Treatment should be stopped at the time of renal transplantation to observe the spontaneous evolution of growth. If no or insufficient catch-up growth occurs within 12 months, glucocorticoid withdrawal is the first option. If unsuccessful, rGH reinstitution should be considered. Treatment decisions should be made without delay to save growth potential. The question of rGH continuation through puberty is still controversial. The pubertal growth spurt occurs independent of concomitant rGH treatment, rendering any judgment about treatment efficacy exceedingly difficult. Controlled prospective study results are not available. Hence, the decision to continue or re-start rGH in puberty must be made on an individual basis, taking into account the

degree of growth retardation, the residual growth potential and the expected therapeutic compliance of the adolescent.

It is also an issue of current consideration whether in patients with imminent or early puberty skeletal maturation should be delayed by pharmacological intervention by GnRH analogs or aromatase inhibitors to prolong the prepubertal growth phase for GH treatment.

Adverse effects of growth hormone treatment

Given its remarkable efficacy, GH treatment causes surprisingly few side effects in children with CRF.

DIABETES MELLITUS

Concern was raised initially that prolonged GH treatment might provoke diabetes mellitus, because patients with CRF already show impaired glucose tolerance due to peripheral insulin resistance. However, not a single case of irreversible diabetes mellitus has been observed in children with CRF.[229,230]

EPIPHYSEAL SLIPPING

Epiphyseal slipping[231,232] and femoral head necrosis[233] have been reported as rare events during treatment with rGH. Whether these complications were caused or intensified by rGH is unclear, since both complications are noted with increased incidence in children with CRF without GH treatment.[197,198] An aggravation of secondary hyperparathyroidism has been reported rarely.[234,235] This seems not to be due to a direct stimulation of the parathyroid gland by GH, but represent an indirect effect of small decreases of ionized calcium as a consequence of GH-stimulated bone apposition or an increase in serum phosphate concentration secondary to improved appetite. Furthermore, a pre-existing renal osteodystrophy may be unmasked by an increased growth rate and may become radiographically apparent.[105]

RENAL FUNCTION

Concern has also been raised that GH may cause glomerular hyperfiltration and accelerated deterioration of renal function. However, the physiologic acute increase of GFR induced by GH in healthy subjects is obliterated in patients with CRF.[236] Long-term observations for up to 8 years showed no acceleration of renal failure progression in predialytic patients with CRF due to cystinosis,[237] other renal disorders[23,207,209] and in renal allograft recipients.[23]

ALLOGRAFT REJECTION

Since GH is an immunomodulatory substance,[238,239] allograft rejection might be triggered by rGH administration in post-transplant patients. However, several controlled trials provided evidence that an increased risk of rejection is limited to high-risk patients with more than one acute rejection episode prior to start of GH treatment.[215,217,240,241]

MALIGNANCY

Contrary to previous concerns,[242] an extended survey of thousands of patients failed to disclose any significant relationship between GH treatment and malignancy.[243–245] Recent reports on renal cell carcinoma developing in two patients 9 and 11 years post-transplant who had received GH, a case of leukemia in an 18-year-old GH-treated patient with a failing transplant[243] and a report of premalignant tubuloepithelial changes in a pediatric renal allograft[246] raise the suspicion that tumor risk may be selectively increased by GH in post-transplant children receiving long-term immunosuppression.

RETENTION OF SODIUM AND WATER

GH induces an IGF-I-mediated increase in distal tubular sodium reabsorption and up-regulates the renin–angiotensin system.[247,248] As a consequence, a transient, usually mild retention of sodium and water occurs during the first few days of treatment. In this context, benign intracranial hypertension has been reported as a rare adverse effect of GH treated patients with various underlying diseases. In CRF, the the risk for this complication is increased tenfold.[249,250] A recent survey noted signs or symptoms of intracranial hypertension in 15 out of 1670 patients with renal disease receiving GH (0.9 percent).[251] All but two patients were symptomatic; the symptoms generally abated when GH therapy was discontinued, but two patients had persistent blindness. At least four of these patients had recurrence of intracranial hypertension after reinitiation of GH therapy. Intracranial hypertension manifested within a median of 13 weeks of treatment. We therefore recommend that a baseline fundoscopy is performed and that the dose is gradually increased from 50 to 100 percent of the maintenance dose within 4 weeks. Headache, vomiting and other clinical signs of increased intracranial hypertension make careful clinical investigation, including fundoscopy, essential.

REFERENCES

1 Chantler C, Broyer M, Donckerwolcke RA, et al. Growth and rehabilitation of long-term survivors of treatment for end-stage renal failure in childhood. Proc Eur Dial Transplant Assoc 1981; 18: 329–39.

2 Rizzoni G, Broyer M, Guest G, et al. Growth retardation in children with chronic renal disease: scope of the problem. Am J Kidney Dis 1986; 7: 256–61.

3 van Diemen-Steenvoorde R, Donckerwolcke RA, Brackel H, et al. Growth and sexual maturation in children after kidney transplantation. J Pediatr 1987; 110: 351–6.

4 Schaefer F, Gilli G, Schärer K. Pubertal growth and final height in chronic renal failure. In: Schärer K, ed. Growth and Endocrine Changes in Children and Adolescents with Chronic Renal Failure: Pediatric and Adolescent Endocrinology, vol. 22. Basel: Karger, 1989: 59–69.

5 Jones RWA, Rigden SP, Barratt TM, Chantler C. The effects of chronic renal failure in infancy on growth, nutritional status and body composition. Pediatr Res 1982; 16: 784–91.

6 Kleinknecht C, Broyer M, Huot D, et al. Growth and development of nondialyzed children with chronic renal failure. Kidney Int 1983; 24:40–7.

7 Rizzoni G, Basso T, Setari M. Growth in children with chronic renal failure on conservative treatment. Kidney Int 1984; 26: 52–8.

8 Warady BA, Kriley MA, Lovell H, et al. Growth and development of infants with end-stage renal disease receiving long-term peritoneal dialysis. J Pediatr 1988; 112: 714–9.

9 Karlberg J, Schaefer F, Hennicke M, et al. Early age-dependent growth impairment in chronic renal failure. European Study Group for Nutritional Treatment of Chronic Renal Failure in Childhood. Pediatr Nephrol 1996; 10: 283–7.

10 Ramage IJ, Geary DF, Harvey E, et al. Efficacy of gastrostomy feeding in infants and older children receiving chronic peritoneal dialysis. Perit Dial Int 1999; 19: 231–6.

11 Kari JA, Gonzalez C, Lederman SE, et al. Outcome and growth of infants with severe chronic renal failure. Kidney Int 2000; 57: 1681–7.

12 Van Dyck M, Bilem N, Proesmans W. Conservative treatment for chronic renal failure from birth: a 3-year follow-up study. Pediatr Nephrol 1999; 13: 865–9.

13 Schaefer F, Wingen AM, Hennicke M, *et al.* Growth charts for prepubertal children with chronic renal failure due to congenital renal disorders. European Study Group for Nutritional Treatment of Chronic Renal Failure in Childhood. *Pediatr Nephrol* 1996; **10**: 288–93.

14 Hodson EM, Shaw PF, Evans RA, *et al.* Growth retardation and renal osteodystrophy in children with chronic renal failure. *J Pediatr* 1983; **103**: 735–40.

15 Polito C, Greco L, Totino SF, *et al.* Statural growth of children with chronic renal failure on conservative treatment. *Acta Paediatr Scand* 1987; **76**: 97–102.

16 Rappaport R, Bouthreuil E, Marti-Henneberg C, Basmaciogoul-Lari A. Linear growth rate, bone maturation and growth hormone secretion in prepubertal children with congenital adrenal hyperplasia. *Acta Paediatr Scand* 1973; **62**: 513–9.

17 Klare B, Strom TM, Hahn H, *et al.* Remarkable long-term prognosis and excellent growth in kidney-transplant children under cyclosporine monotherapy. *Transplant Proc* 1991; **23**: 1013–7.

18 Hamiwka LA, Burns A, Bell L. Prednisone withdrawal in pediatric kidney transplant recipients on tacrolimus-based immunosuppression: Four-year data. *Pediatr Transplant* 2006; **10**: 337–44.

19 Offner G, Hoyer PF, Jüppner H, *et al.* Somatic growth after kidney transplantation. *Am J Dis Child* 1987; **141**: 541–6.

20 Rees L, Greene SA, Adlard P, *et al.* Growth and endocrine function after renal transplantation. *Arch Dis Child* 1988; **63**: 1326–32.

21 Broyer M, Guest G. Growth after kidney transplantation – a single centre experience. In: Schärer K, ed. *Growth and Endocrine Changes in Children and Adolescents with Chronic Renal Failure. Pediatric and Adolescent Endocrinology*, vol. 20. Basel: Karger, 1989: 36–45.

22 Schaefer F, Seidel C, Binding A, *et al.* Pubertal growth in chronic renal failure. *Pediatr Res* 1990; **28**: 5–10.

23 Haffner D, Schaefer F, Nissel R, *et al.* Effect of growth hormone treatment on adult height of children with chronic renal failure. *N Engl J Med* 2000; **343**: 923–30.

24 Schärer K and study group on pubertal development in chronic renal failure. Growth and development of children with chronic renal failure. *Acta Paediatr Scand Suppl* 1990; **366**: 90–2.

25 Betts PR, White RHR. Growth potential and skeletal maturity in children with chronic renal insufficiency. *Nephron* 1976; **16**: 325–32.

26 Cundall DB, Brocklebank JT, Buckler JMH. Which bone age in chronic renal insufficiency and end-stage renal disease? *Pediatr Nephrol* 1988; **2**: 200–4.

27 van Steenbergen MW, Wit JM, Donckerwolcke RAMG. Testosterone esters advance skeletal maturation more than growth in short boys with chronic renal failure and delayed puberty. *Eur J Pediatr* 1991; **150**: 676–780.

28 Grushkin CM, Fine RN. Growth in children following renal transplantation. *Am J Dis Child* 1973; **125**: 514–6.

29 Rizzoni G, Broyer M, Brunner FP, *et al.* Combined report on regular hemodialysis and transplantation in Europe, 1985. *Proc Eur Dial Transplant Assoc* 1986; **23**: 55–83.

30 Gilli G, Mehls O, Schärer K. Final height of children with chronic renal failure. *Proc Eur Dial Transplant Assoc* 1984; **21**: 830–6.

31 Fennell RS, III, Love JT, Carter RL, *et al.* Statistical analysis of statural growth following kidney transplantation. *Eur J Pediatr* 1986; **145**: 377–9.

32 Hokken-Koelega AC, Van Zaal MA, van Bergen W, *et al.* Final height and its predictive factors after renal transplantation in childhood. *Pediatr Res* 1994; **36**: 323–8.

33 Wühl E, Haffner D, Offner G, *et al.* Long-term treatment with growth hormone in short children with nephropathic cystinosis. *J Pediatr* 2001; **138**: 880–7.

34 DeShazo CV, Simmons RL, Berstein SM, *et al.* Results of renal transplantation in 100 children. *Surgery* 1974; **76**: 461–3.

35 Potter DE, Holliday MA, Wilson SJ, Salvatierra JO. Alternate day steroids in children after renal transplantation. *Transplant Proc* 1975; **7**: 79.

36 Pennisi AJ, Costin G, Phillips LS, *et al.* Linear growth in long-term renal allograft recipients. *Clin Nephrol* 1977; **8**: 415–21.

37 Ingelfinger JR, Grupe WE, Harmon WE, *et al.* Growth acceleration following renal transplantation in children less than 7 years of age. *Pediatrics* 1981; **68**: 255–9.

38 Bosque M, Munian A, Bewick M, *et al.* Growth after renal transplants. *Arch Dis Child* 1983; **58**: 110–4.

39 Reisman L, Lieberman KV, Burrows L, Schanzer H. Follow-up of cyclosporine-treated pediatric renal allograft recipients after cessation of prednisone. *Transplantation* 1990; **49**: 76–80.

40 Broyer M, Guest G, Gagnadoux M-F. Growth rate in children receiving alternate-day corticosteroid treatment after kidney transplantation. *J Pediatr* 1992; **120**: 721–5.

41 Kaiser BA, Polinsky MS, Palmer JA, *et al.* Growth after conversion to alternate-day corticosteroids in children with renal transplants: a single-center study. *Pediatr Nephrol* 1994; **8**: 320–5.

42 Hokken-Koelega AC, Van Zaal MA, de Ridder MA, *et al.* Growth after renal transplantation in prepubertal children: impact of various treatment modalities. *Pediatr Res* 1994; **35**: 367–71.

43 Chao SM, Jones CL, Powell HR, *et al.* Triple immunosuppression with subsequent prednisolone withdrawal: 6 years' experience in paediatric renal allograft recipients. *Pediatr Nephrol* 1994; **8**: 62–9.

44 Ellis D. Clinical use of tacrolimus (FK-506) in infants and children with renal transplants. *Pediatr Nephrol* 1995; **9**: 487–94.

45 Jabs K, Sullivan EK, Avner ED, Harmon WE. Alternate-day steroid dosing improves growth without affecting graft survival or long-term graft function. A report of the North American Pediatric Renal Transplant Cooperative Study. *Transplantation* 1996; **61**: 31–6.

46 Tejani A, Cortes L, Sullivan EK. A longitudinal study of the natural history of growth post-transplantation. *Kidney Int* 1996; **53**: 103–8.

47 Tejani A, Fine R, Alexander S, et al. Factors predictive of sustained growth in children after renal transplantation. The North American Pediatric Renal Transplant Cooperative Study. J Pediatr 1993; 122: 397–402.

48 Helling TS, Nelson PW, Reed L, et al. A seven year experience with kidney transplantation for pediatric end stage renal disease. Mo Med 1994; 91: 33–7.

49 Kohaut EC, Tejani A. The 1994 annual report of the North American Pediatric Renal Transplant Cooperative Study. Pediatr Nephrol 1996; 10: 422–34.

50 North American Pediatric Renal Transplant Cooperative Study (NAPRTCS). 2001 Annual Report. Rockville, MD: Emms Corporation; 2001.

51 Qvist E, Marttinen E, Rönnholm K, et al. Growth after renal transplantation in infancy or early childhood. Pediatr Nephrol 2002; 17: 438–43.

52 Fine RN, Stablein D. Long-term use of recombinant human growth hormone in pediatric allograft recipients: a report of the NAPRTCS Transplant Registry. Pediatr Nephrol 2005; 20: 404–8.

53 Nissel R, Brazda I, Feneberg R, et al. Effect of renal transplantation in childhood on longitudinal growth and adult height. Kidney Int 2004; 66: 792–800.

54 Englund MS, Tyden G, Wikstad I, Berg UB. Growth impairment at renal transplantation – A determinant of growth and final height. Pediatr Transplant 2003; 7: 192–9.

55 Höcker B, John U, Plank C, et al. Successful withdrawal of steroids in pediatric renal transplant recipients receiving cyclosporine A and mycophenolate mofetil treatment: results after four years. Transplantation 2004; 78: 228–34.

56 Sarna S, Hoppu K, Neuvonen PJ, et al. Methylprednisolone exposure, rather than dose, predicts adrenal suppression and growth inhibition in children with liver and renal transplantation. J Clin Endocrinol Metab 1997; 82: 75–7.

57 Rodriguez-Soriano J, Vallo A, Quintela MJ, et al. Predictors of final adult height after renal transplantation during childhood: a single-center study. Nephron 2000; 86: 266–73.

58 Fine RN, Ho M, Tejani A. The contribution of renal transplantation to final adult height: a report of the North American Pediatric Renal Transplant Cooperative Study (NAPRTCS). Pediatr Nephrol 2001; 16: 951–6.

59 Polito C, la Manna A, Olivieri AN, di Toro R. Proteinuria and statural growth. Child Urol Nephrol 1988; 9: 286–9.

60 Schärer K, Essigmann HC, Schaefer F. Body growth of children with steroid-resistant nephrotic syndrome. Pediatr Nephrol 1999; 13: 828–34.

61 Lam CN, Arneil GC. Long-term dwarfing effects of corticosteroid treatment for childhood nephrosis. Arch Dis Child 1968; 43: 589–94.

62 Foote KD, Brocklebank JT, Meadow SR. Height attainment in children with steroid-responsive nephrotic syndrome. Lancet 1985; 2: 917–9.

63 Rees L, Greene SA, Adlard P, et al. Growth and endocrine function in steroid sensitive nephrotic syndrome. Arch Dis Child 1988; 63: 484–90.

64 Holtta TM, Ronnholm KA, Jalanko H, et al. Peritoneal dialysis in children under 5 years of age. Perit Dial Int 1997; 17: 573–80.

65 Nash MA, Torrado AD, Greifer I, et al. Renal tubular acidosis in infants and children. J Pediatr 1972; 80: 738–48.

66 Tsuru N, Chan JCM. Growth failure in children with metabolic alkalosis and with metabolic acidosis. Nephron 1987; 45: 182–5.

67 Morris RC, Sebastian AC. Renal tubular acidosis and Fanconi syndrome. In: Stanbury JB, Wyngaarden JB, Frederickson DS, eds. The Metabolic Basis of Inherited Disease, 3rd ed. New York: McGraw-Hill, 1983: 1808.

68 Niaudet P, Dechaux M, Trivin C. Nephrogenic diabetes insipidus. Clinical and pathophysiological aspects. Adv Nephrol 1983; 13: 247–60.

69 Simopoulos AP. Growth characteristics in patients with Bartter's syndrome. Nephron 1979; 23: 130–5.

70 Taymans JM, Wintmolders C, Riele TE, et al. Detailed localization of regulator of G protein signaling 2 messenger ribonucleic acid and protein in the rat brain. Neuroscience 2002; 114: 39–53.

71 Bergwitz C, Abou-Samra AB, Hesch RD, Jüppner H. Rapid desensitisation of parathyroid hormone dependent adenylate cyclase in perfused human osteosarcoma cells (SaOS-2). Biochim Biophys Acta 1994; 1222: 447–56.

72 Seidel C, Timmermanns G, Seyberth H, Schärer K. Body growth in hyperprostaglandin E syndrome (HPGS) treated by indomethacin. Pediatr Nephrol 1992; 6: C108.

73 Haffner D, Weinfurth A, Seidel C, et al. Body growth in primary de Toni-Debre-Fanconi syndrome. Pediatr Nephrol 1997; 11: 40–5.

74 Haffner D, Weinfurth A, Manz F, et al. Long-term outcome of paediatric patients with hereditary tubular disorders. Nephron 1999; 83: 250–60.

75 Ehrich JHH. Combined Report on Regular Dialysis and Transplantation in Europe Part III: Renal Replacement Therapy in Children. Presentation at the XXIX Congress of European Renal Association – The European Dialysis and Transplant Association, Paris, 28 June to 1 July 1992.

76 da Silva VA, Zurbrügg RP, Lavanchy P, et al. Long-term treatment of infantile nephropathic cystinosis with cysteamine. N Engl J Med 1985; 313: 1460–3.

77 Gahl WA, Reed GF, Thoene JG, et al. Cysteamine therapy for children with nephropathic cystinosis. N Engl J Med 1987; 316: 971–7.

78 van't Hoff WG, Gretz N. The treatment of cystinosis with cysteamine and phosphocysteamine in the United Kingdom and Eire. Pediatr Nephrol 1995; 9: 685–9.

79 Smellie JM, Preece MA, Paton AM. Normal somatic growth in children receiving low-dose prophylactic co-trimoxazole. Eur J Pediatr 1983; 140: 301–4.

80 Merrell RW, Mowad JJ. Increased physical growth after successful antireflux operation. J Urol 1979; 122: 523–7.

81 Sutton R, Atwell JD. Physical growth velocity during conservative treatment and following subsequent surgical treatment for primary vesicoureteric reflux. Br J Urol 1989; 63: 245–50.

82 Polito C, la Manna A, Capacchione A, *et al.* Height and weight in children with vesicoureteral reflux and renal scarring. *Pediatr Nephrol* 1996; **10**: 564–7.

83 Seidel C, Schaefer F, Schärer K. Body growth in urinary tract malformation. *Pediatr Nephrol* 1993; **7**: 151–5.

84 Drozdz D, Drozdz M, Gretz N, *et al.* Progression to end-stage renal disease in children with posterior urethral valves. *Pediatr Nephrol* 1998; **12**: 630–6.

85 Norman LJ, Coleman JE, Macdonald IA, *et al.* Nutrition and growth in relation to severity of renal disease in children. *Pediatr Nephrol* 2000; **15**: 259–65.

86 Arnold WC, Danford D, Holliday MA. Effects of calorie supplementation on growth in uremia. *Kidney Int* 1983; **24**: 205–9.

87 Betts PR, Magrath G, White RHR. Role of dietary energy supplementation in growth of children with chronic renal insufficiency. *Br Med J* 1977; **1**: 416–8.

88 Lucas LM, Kumar KL, Smith DL. Gynecomastia: a worrisome problem for the patient. *Postgrad Med* 1987; **82**: 73–81.

89 Jones RWA, Dalton RN, Turner C, *et al.* Oral essential aminoacid and ketoacid supplements in children with chronic renal failure. *Kidney Int* 1983; **24**: 95–103.

90 Orejas G, Santos F, Malaga S, *et al.* Nutritional status of children with moderate chronic renal failure. *Pediatr Nephrol* 1995; **9**: 52–6.

91 Foreman JW, Abitbol CL, Trachtman H, *et al.* Nutritional intake in children with renal insufficiency: a report of the Growth Failure in Children with Renal Diseases Study. *J Am Coll Nutr* 1996; **15**: 579–85.

92 Baur LA, Knight JF, Crawford BA, *et al.* Total body nitrogen in children with chronic renal failure and short stature. *Eur J Clin Nutr* 1994; **48**: 433–41.

93 Mehls O, Ritz E, Gilli G, *et al.* Nitrogen metabolism and growth in experimental uremia. *Int J Pediatr Nephrol* 1980; **1**: 34–41.

94 Wingen AM, Fabian-Bach C, Schaefer F, Mehls O. Randomised multicentre study of a low-protein diet on the progression of chronic renal failure in children. European Study Group of Nutritional Treatment of Chronic Renal Failure in Childhood. *Lancet* 1997; **349**: 1117–23.

95 May RC, Kelly RA, Mitch WE. Metabolic acidosis stimulates protein degradation in rat muscle by a glucocorticoid-dependent mechanism. *J Clin Invest* 1986; **77**: 614–21.

96 May RC, Hara Y, Kelly RA, *et al.* Branched-chain amino acid metabolism in rat muscle: abnormal regulation in acidosis. *Am J Physiol* 1987; **252**: E712–18.

97 Bailey JL, Wang X, England BK, *et al.* The acidosis of chronic renal failure activates muscle proteolysis in rats by augmenting transcription of genes encoding proteins of the ATP-dependent ubiquitin-proteasome pathway. *J Clin Invest* 1996; **97**: 1447–53.

98 Boirie Y, Broyer M, Gagnadoux MF, *et al.* Alterations of protein metabolism by metabolic acidosis in children with chronic renal failure. *Kidney Int* 2000; **58**: 236–41.

99 Challa A, Krieg RJ Jr, Thabet MA, *et al.* Metabolic acidosis inhibits growth hormone secretion in rats: mechanism of growth retardation. *Am J Physiol* 1993; **265**: E547–53.

100 Challa A, Chan W, Krieg RJ Jr, *et al.* Effect of metabolic acidosis on the expression of insulin-like growth factor and growth hormone receptor. *Kidney Int* 1993; **44**: 1224–7.

101 Brüngger M, Hulter HN, Krapf R. Effect of chronic metabolic acidosis on the growth hormone/IGF1 endocrine axis: new cause of growth hormone insensitivity in humans. *Kidney Int* 1997; **51**: 216–21.

102 Wassner SJ. Altered growth and protein turnover in rats fed sodium-deficient diets. *Pediatr Res* 1989; **26**: 608–13.

103 Wassner SJ. The effect of sodium repletion on growth and protein turnover in sodium-depleted rats. *Pediatr Nephrol* 1991; **5**: 501–4.

104 Heinly MM, Wassner SJ. The effect of isolated chloride depletion on growth and protein turnover in young rats. *Pediatr Nephrol* 1994; **8**: 555–60.

105 Mehls O, Salusky IB. Recent advances and controversies in childhood renal osteodystrophy. *Pediatr Nephrol* 1987; **1**: 212–23.

106 Mehls O, Ritz E, Krempien B, *et al.* Slipped epiphyses in renal osteodystrophy. *Arch Dis Child* 1975; **50**: 545–54.

107 Ramirez G, O'Neill WM, Bloomer A, Jubiz W. Abnormalities in the regulation of growth hormone in chronic renal failure. *Arch Intern Med* 1978; **138**: 267–71.

108 Davidson MB, Fisher MB, Dabir-Vaziri N, Schaffer M. Effect of protein intake and dialysis on the abnormal growth hormone, glucose, and insulin homeostasis in uremia. *Metabolism* 1976; **25**: 455–64.

109 Johnson V, Maack T. Renal extraction, filtration, absorption, and catabolism of growth hormone. *Am J Physiol* 1977; **233**: F185–96.

110 Haffner D, Schaefer F, Girard J, *et al.* Metabolic clearance of recombinant human growth hormone in health and chronic renal failure. *J Clin Invest* 1994; **93**: 1163–71.

111 Schaefer F, Baumann G, Haffner D, *et al.* Multifactorial control of the elimination kinetics of unbound (free) growth hormone (GH) in the human: regulation by age, adiposity, renal function, and steady state concentrations of GH in plasma. *J Clin Endocrinol Metab* 1996; **81**: 22–31.

112 Tönshoff B, Veldhuis JD, Heinrich U, Mehls O. Deconvolution analysis of spontaneous nocturnal growth hormone secretion in prepubertal children with chronic renal failure. *Pediatr Res* 1995; **37**: 86–93.

113 Veldhuis JD, Iranmanesh A, Wilkowski MJ, Samojlik E. Neuroendocrine alterations in the somatotropic and lactotropic axes in uremic men. *Eur J Endocrinol* 1994; **131**: 489–98.

114 Schaefer F, Veldhuis J, Stanhope R, *et al.* Alterations in growth hormone secretion and clearance in peripubertal boys with chronic renal failure and after renal transplantation. *J Clin Endocrinol Metab* 1994; **78**: 1298–306.

115 Bessarione D, Perfumo F, Giusti M, *et al.* Growth hormone response to growth hormone-releasing hormone in normal and uraemic children: comparison with hypoglycemia following insulin administration. *Acta Endocrinol (Copenh)* 1987; **114**: 5–11.

116 Giordano C, De Santo NG, Carella C, et al. TSH response to TRH in hemodialysis and CAPD patients. Int J Artif Organs 1984; 7: 7–10.

117 Alvestrand A, Mujagic M, Wajngot A, Efendic S. Glucose intolerance in uremic patients: the relative contributions of impaired beta-cell function and insulin resistance. Clin Nephrol 1989; 31: 175–83.

118 Marumo F, Sakai T, Sato S. Response of insulin, glucagon and growth hormone to arginine infusion in patients with chronic renal failure. Nephron 1979; 24: 81–4.

119 Rodger RSC, Dewar JH, Turner SJ, et al. Anterior pituitary dysfunction in patients with chronic renal failure treated by hemodialysis or continuous ambulatory peritoneal dialysis. Nephron 1986; 43: 169–72.

120 Duntas L, Wolf CF, Keck FS, Rosenthal J. Thyreotropin-releasing hormone: pharmacokinetic and pharmacodynamic properties in chronic renal failure. Clin Nephrol 1992; 38: 214–8.

121 Chan W, Valerie KC, Chan JCM. Expression of insulin-like growth factor-1 in uremic rats: Growth hormone resistance and nutritional intake. Kidney Int 1993; 43: 790–5.

122 Schaefer F, Chen Y, Tsao T, et al. Impaired JAK-STAT signal transduction contributes to growth hormone resistance in chronic uremia. J Clin Invest 2001; 108: 467–75.

123 Baumann G, Shaw MA, Amburn K. Regulation of plasma growth hormone-binding proteins in health and disease. Metabolism 1989; 38: 683–9.

124 Postel-Vinay MC, Tar A, Crosnier H, et al. Plasma growth-hormone binding is low in uremic children. Pediatr Nephrol 1991; 5: 545–7.

125 Tönshoff B, Cronin MJ, Reichert M. Reduced concentration of serum growth hormone (GH)-binding protein in children with chronic renal failure: correlation with GH insensitivity. J Clin Endocrinol Metab 1997; 82: 1007–13.

126 Powell DR, Liu F, Baker BK, et al. Modulation of growth factors by growth hormone in children with chronic renal failure. The Southwest Pediatric Nephrology Study Group. Kidney Int 1997; 51: 1970–9.

127 Ding H, Gao XL, Hirschberg R, et al. Impaired actions of insulin-like growth factor 1 on protein synthesis and degradation in skeletal muscle of rats with chronic renal failure. Evidence for a postreceptor defect. J Clin Invest 1996; 97: 1064–75.

128 Phillips LS, Kopple JD. Circulating somatomedin activity and sulfate levels in adults with normal and impaired kidney function. Metabolism 1981; 30: 1091–5.

129 Fouque D. Insulin-like growth factor 1 resistance in chronic renal failure. Miner Electrolyte Metab 1995; 22: 133–7.

130 Fouque D, Peng SC, Kopple JD. Impaired metabolic response to recombinant insulin-like growth factor-1 in dialysis patients. Kidney Int 1995; 47: 876–83.

131 Tönshoff B, Blum WF, Wingen AM, Mehls O. Serum insulin-like growth factors (IGFs) and IGF binding proteins 1, 2 and 3 in children with chronic renal failure: relationship to height and glomerular filtration rate. J Clin Endocrinol Metab 1995; 80: 2684–91.

132 Frystyk J, Ivarsen P, Skjaerbaek C, et al. Serum-free insulin-like growth factor I correlates with clearance in patients with chronic renal failure. Kidney Int 1999; 56: 2076–84.

133 Phillips LS, Fusco AC, Unterman TG, del Greco F. Somatomedin inhibitor in uremia. J Clin Endocrinol Metab 1984; 59: 764–72.

134 Blum WF, Ranke MB, Kietzmann K, et al. Excess of IGF-binding proteins in chronic renal failure: evidence for relative GH resistance and inhibition of somatomedin activity. In: Drop SLS, Hintz RL, eds. Insulin-like Growth Factor Binding Proteins. Amsterdam: Elsevier, Science Publishers, 1989: 93–9.

135 Lee PD, Hintz RL, Sperry JB, et al. IGF binding proteins in growth-retarded children with chronic renal failure. Pediatr Res 1989; 26: 308–15.

136 Powell DR, Liu F, Baker B, et al. Insulin-like growth factor-binding protein-6 levels are elevated in serum of children with chronic renal failure: a report of the Southwest Pediatric Nephrology Study Group. J Clin Endocrinol Metab 1997; 82: 2978–84.

137 Powell DR, Durham SK, Brewer ED, et al. Effects of chronic renal failure and growth hormone on serum levels of insulin-like growth factor-binding protein-4 (IGFBP-4) and IGFBP-5 in children: A report of the Southwest Pediatric Nephrology Study Group. J Clin Endocrinol Metab 1999; 84: 596–601.

138 Powell DR, Liu F, Baker BK, et al. Effect of chronic renal failure and growth hormone therapy on the insulin-like growth factors and their binding proteins. Pediatr Nephrol 2000; 14: 579–83.

139 Ulinski T, Mohan S, Kiepe D, et al. Serum insulin-like growth factor binding protein (IGFBP)-4 and IGFBP-5 in children with chronic renal failure: Relationship to growth and glomerular filtration rate. Pediatr Nephrol 2000; 14: 589–97.

140 Tönshoff B, Powell DR, Zhao D, et al. Decreased hepatic insulin-like growth factor (IGF)-I and increased IGF binding protein-1 and -2 gene expression in experimental uremia. Endocrinology 1997; 138: 938–46.

141 Powell D, Liu F, Baker B, et al. Modulation of growth factors by growth hormone in children with chronic renal failure. Kidney Int 1997; 51: 1970–9.

142 Blum WF. Insulin-like growth factors (IGF) and IGF-binding proteins in chronic renal failure: evidence for reduced secretion of IGF. Acta Paediatr Scand 1991; 379(Suppl): 24–31.

143 Casanueva FF, Burguera B, Tome M. Depending on the time of administration, dexamethasone potentiates or blocks growth hormone-releasing hormone-induced growth hormone release in man. Neuroendocrinology 1990; 47: 46–9.

144 Veldhuis JD, Lizarralde G, Iranmanesh A. Divergent effects of short term glucocorticoid excess on the gonadotropic and somatotropic axes in normal men. J Clin Endocrinol Metab 1992; 74: 96–102.

145 Pennisi AJ, Costin G, Phillips LS, et al. Somatomedin and growth hormone studies. Am J Dis Child 1979; 133: 950–4.

146 Schaefer F, Hamill G, Stanhope R, *et al.* Pulsatile growth hormone secretion in peripubertal patients with chronic renal failure. *J Pediatr* 1991; **119**: 568–77.

147 Wehrenberg WB, Janowski BA, Piering AW. Glucocorticoids: Potent inhibitors and stimulators of growth hormone secretion. *Endocrinology* 1990; **126**: 3200–3.

148 Luo J, Murphy LJ. Dexamethasone inhibits growth hormone induction of insulin-like growth factor-I (IGF-I) messenger ribonucleic acid (mRNA) in hypophysectomized rats and reduces IGF-I mRNA abundance in the intact rat. *Endocrinology* 1989; **125**: 165–71.

149 Gabrielsson BG, Carmignac DF, Flavell DM, Robinson ICAF. Steroid regulation of growth hormone (GH) receptor and GH binding protein messenger ribonucleic acids in the rat. *Endocrinology* 1995; **133**: 2445–52.

150 Tönshoff B, Haffner D, Mehls O, *et al.* Efficacy and safety of growth hormone treatment in short children with renal allografts: three year experience. *Kidney Int* 1993; **44**: 199–207.

151 van Dop C, Jabs KL, Donohue PA, *et al.* Accelerated growth rates in children treated with growth hormone after renal transplantation. *J Pediatr* 1992; **120**: 244–50.

152 Unterman TG, Phillips LS. Glucocorticoid effects on somatomedins and somatomedin inhibitors. *J Clin Endocrinol Metab* 1985; **61**: 618–26.

153 Bang P, Degerblad M, Thoren M, *et al.* Insulin like growth factor (IGF) I and II and IGF binding protein (IGFBP) 1, 2 and 3 in serum from patients with Cushing's syndrome. *Acta Endocrinol* 1993; **128**: 397–404.

154 Silbermann M, Maor G. Mechanisms of glucocorticoid-induced growth retardation: impairment of cartilage mineralization. *Acta Anat (Basel)* 1978; **101**: 140–9.

155 Jux C, Leiber K, Hügel U, *et al.* Dexamethasone inhibits growth hormone (GH)-stimulated growth by suppression of local insulin-like growth factor (IGF)-I production and expression of GH- and IGF-I receptor in cultured rat chondrocytes. *Endocrinology* 1998; **139**: 3296–305.

156 Schaefer F, Mehls O. Endocrine, metabolic and growth disorders. In: Holliday MA, Barratt TM, Avner ED, eds. *Paediatric Nephrology*. Baltimore, MD.: Williams & Wilkins, 1994: 1241–86.

157 Schärer K, Broyer M, Vecsei P, *et al.* Damage to testicular function in chronic renal failure of children. *Proc Eur Dial Transplant Assoc* 1980; **17**: 725–9.

158 Dunkel L, Raivio T, Laine J, Holmberg C. Circulating luteinizing hormone receptor inhibitor(s) in boys with chronic renal failure. *Kidney Int* 1997; **51**: 777–84.

159 Schaefer F, André JL, Krug C, *et al.* Growth and skeletal maturation in dialysed children treated with recombinant human erythropoietin (rhEPO) – a multicenter study. *Pediatr Nephrol* 1991; **5**: 61.

160 Schaefer F, Veldhuis JD, Stanhope R, *et al.* Alterations in growth hormone secretion and clearance in peripubertal boys with chronic renal failure and after renal transplantation. *J Clin Endocrinol Metab* 1994; **78**: 1298–306.

161 Schaefer F, Daschner M, Veldhuis JD, *et al.* In vivo alterations in the gonadotropin-releasing hormone pulse generator and the secretion and clearance of luteinizing hormone in the castrate uremic rat. *Neuroendocrinology* 1994; **59**: 285–96.

162 Wibullaksanakul S, Handelsman DJ. Regulation of hypothalamic gonadotropin-releasing hormone secretion in experimental uremia: in vitro studies. *Neuroendocrinology* 1991; **54**: 353–8.

163 Schaefer F, Veldhuis JD, Bornemann T, *et al.* Dynamics of pituitary secretion and metabolic clearance of immunoreactive and bioactive LH in pubertal patients with chronic renal failure. *Pediatr Res* 1991; **29**: 85A.

164 Talbot JA, Rodger RSC, Robertson WR. Pulsatile bioactive luteinising hormone secretion in men with chronic renal failure and following renal transplantation. *Nephron* 1990; **56**: 66–72.

165 Schaefer F, Seidel C, Mitchell R, *et al.* Pulsatile immunoreactive and bioactive luteinizing hormone secretion in pubertal patients with chronic renal failure. *Pediatr Nephrol* 1991; **5**: 566–71.

166 Mitchell R, Bauerfeld C, Schaefer F, *et al.* Less acidic forms of luteinizing hormone are associated with lower testosterone secretion in men on hemodialysis treatment. *Clin Endocrinol* 1994; **41**: 65–73.

167 Strife CF, Quinlan M, Mears K, *et al.* Improved growth of three uremic children by nocturnal nasogastric feedings. *Am J Dis Child* 1986; **140**: 438–43.

168 Rodriguez-Soriano J, Arant BS, Brodehl J, Norman ME. Fluid and electrolyte imbalances in children with chronic renal failure. *Am J Kidney Dis* 1986; **7**: 268–9.

169 Parekh RS, Flynn JT, Smoyer WE, *et al.* Improved growth in young children with severe chronic renal insufficiency who use specified nutritional therapy. *J Am Soc Nephrol* 2001; **12**: 2418–26.

170 Trachtman H, Hackney P, Tejani A. Pediatric hemodialysis: A decade's (1974–1984) perspective. *Kidney Int* 1986; **30**: S15–22.

171 Fennell RS III, Orak JK, Hudson T, *et al.* Growth in children with various therapies for end-stage renal disease. *Am J Dis Child* 1984; **138**: 28–31.

172 Chantler C, Donckerwolcke RA, Brunner FP, *et al.* Combined Report on Regular Dialysis and Transplantation of Children in Europe 1976. In: *Dialysis Transplantation Nephrology*. vol.14. Tunbridge Wells: Pitman Medical Publications, 1977.

173 Potter DE, Luis ES, Wipfler JE, Portale AA. Comparison of continuous ambulatory peritoneal dialysis and hemodialysis in children. *Kidney Int* 1986; **30**: 11–14.

174 von Lilien T, Gilli G, Salusky IB. Growth in children undergoing continuous ambulatory or cycling peritoneal dialysis. In: Schärer K, ed. *Pediatric and Adolescent Endocrinology*, vol. 20. Basel: Karger, 1989; 27–35.

175 Fine RN, Mehls O. CAPD/CCPD in children: Four years' experience. *Kidney Int* 1986; **30**: S7–10.

176 Schaefer F, Klaus G, Mehls O, the Mideuropean Pediatric Peritoneal Dialysis Study Group. Peritoneal transport properties and dialysis dose affect growth and nutritional

status in children on chronic peritoneal dialysis. *J Am Soc Nephrol* 1999; **10**: 1786–92.

177 Chadha V, Blowey DL, Warady BA. Is growth a valid outcome measure of dialysis clearance in children undergoing peritoneal dialysis? *Perit Dial Int* 2001; **21**: S179–84.

178 Fischbach M, Terzic J, Laugel V, *et al.* Daily on-line hemodiafiltration: a pilot trial in children. *Nephrol Dial Transplant* 2004; **19**: 2360–7.

179 Tom A, McCauley L, Bell L, *et al.* Growth during maintenance hemodialysis: impact of enhanced nutrition and clearance. *J Pediatr* 1999; **134**: 464–71.

180 Fine RN. Growth post-renal transplantation in children: lessons from the North American Pediatric Renal Transplant Cooperative Study (NAPRTCS). *Pediatr Transplant* 1997; **1**: 85–9.

181 Ninik A, McTaggart SL, Gulati S, *et al.* Factors influencing growth and final height after renal transplantation. *Pediatr Transplant* 2002; **6**: 219–23.

182 So SKS, Chang P-N, Najaran JS, *et al.* Growth and development in infants after renal transplantation. *J Pediatr* 1987; **110**: 343–50.

183 Nissel R, Brazda I, Feneberg R, *et al.* Effect of renal transplantation in childhood on longitudinal growth and adult height. *Kidney Int* 2004; **66**: 792–800.

184 Ellis D. Growth and renal function after steroid-free tacrolimus-based immunosuppression in children with renal transplants. *Pediatr Nephrol* 2000; **14**: 689–94.

185 Motoyoma O, Hasagawa A, Ohara T, *et al.* A prospective trial of steroid cessation after renal transplantation in pediatric patients treated with cyclosporine and mizoribine. *Pediatr Transplant* 1997; **1**: 29–36.

186 Chakrabati P, Wong HY, Scantlebury VP, *et al.* Outcome after steroid withdrawal in pediatric renal transplant patients receiving tacrolimus-based immunosuppression. *Transplantation* 2000; **15**: 5–760.

187 Ingulli E, Sharma V, Singh A, *et al.* Steroid withdrawal, rejection and the mixed lymphocyte reaction in children after renal transplantation. *Kidney Int Suppl* 1993; **43**: S36–9.

188 Klaus G, Jeck N, Konrad M, *et al.* Risk of steroid withdrawal in pediatric renal transplant patients with suspected steroid toxicity. *Clin Nephrol* 2001; **56**: S37–42.

189 Mehls O, Ritz E, Gilli G, *et al.* Effect of vitamin D on growth in experimental uremia. *Am J Clin Nutr* 1978; **31**: 1927–31.

190 Mehls O, Ritz E, Gilli G, Heinrich U. Role of hormonal disturbances in uremic growth failure. *Contrib Nephrol* 1986; **50**: 119–29.

191 Chesney RW, Moorthy AV, Eisman JA, *et al.* Increased growth after long-term oral 1-alpha-25-vitamin D3 in childhood renal osteodystrophy. *N Engl J Med* 1978; **298**: 238–42.

192 Chesney RW, Moorthy AV, Eisman JA, Jax DK. Influence of oral 1,25-vitamin D in childhood renal osteodystrophy. *Contrib Nephrol* 1980; **18**: 55–71.

193 Kreusser W, Weinkauf R, Mehls O, Ritz E. Effect of parathyroid hormone, calcitonin and growth hormone on

cAMP content of growth cartilage in experimental uremia. *Eur J Clin Invest* 1982; **12**: 337–43.

194 Klaus G, von Eichel B, May T, *et al.* Synergistic effects of parathyroid hormone and 1,25- dihydroxyvitamin D3 on proliferation and vitamin D receptor expression of rat growth cartilage cells. *Endocrinology* 1994; **135**: 1307–15.

195 Schmitt CP, Hessing S, Oh J, *et al.* Intermittent administration of parathyroid hormone (1-37) improves growth and bone mineral density in uremic rats. *Kidney Int* 2000; **57**: 1484–92.

196 Kuizon BD, Goodman WG, Jüppner H, *et al.* Diminished linear growth during intermittent calcitriol therapy in children undergoing CCPD. *Kidney Int* 1998; **53**: 205–11.

197 Krempien B, Mehls O, Ritz E. Morphological studies on pathogenesis of epiphyseal slipping in uremic children. *Virchows Arch A* 1974; **362**: 129–43.

198 Mehls O, Ritz E, Oppermann HC, Guignard JP. Femoral head necrosis in uremic children without steroid treatment or transplantation. *J Pediatr* 1981; **6**: 926–9.

199 Seidel C, Schaefer F, Walther U, Schärer K. The application of knemometry in renal disease: preliminary observations. *Pediatr Nephrol* 1991; **5**: 467–71.

200 Huth MD. Structured abstracts for papers reporting clinical trials. *Ann Intern Med* 1987; **106**: 626–7.

201 Alexander SR. Pediatric uses of recombinant human erythropoietin: the outlook in 1991. *Am J Kidney Dis* 1991; **18(suppl 1)**: 42–53.

202 Mehls O, Ritz E, Hunziker EB, *et al.* Improvement of growth and food utilization by human recombinant growth hormone in uremia. *Kidney Int* 1988; **33**: 45–52.

203 Koch VH, Lippe BM, Nelson PA, *et al.* Accelerated growth after recombinant human growth hormone treatment of children with chronic renal failure. *J Pediatr* 1989; **115**: 365–71.

204 Rees L, Rigden SPA, Ward G, Preece MA. Treatment of short stature in renal disease with recombinant human growth hormone. *Arch Dis Child* 1990; **65**: 856–60.

205 Tönshoff B, Dietz M, Haffner D, *et al.* Effects of two years growth hormone treatment in short children with renal disease. *Acta Paediatr Scand* 1991; **379(Suppl)**: 33.

206 Hokken-Koelega AC, Stijnen T, de Muinck-Keizer-Schrama SM, *et al.* Placebo controlled, double blind, cross-over trials of growth hormone treatment in prepubertal children with chronic renal failure. *Lancet* 1991; **338**: 585–90.

207 Fine RN, Kohaut EC, Brown D, *et al.* Growth after recombinant human growth hormone treatment in children with chronic renal failure. *J Pediatr* 1993; **124**: 374–82.

208 Haffner D, Wühl E, Schaefer F, *et al.* Factors predictive of the short- and long-term efficacy of growth hormone treatment in prepubertal children with chronic renal failure. German Study Group for Growth Hormone Treatment in Children with Chronic Renal Failure. *J Am Soc Nephrol* 1998; **9**: 1899–907.

209 Fine RN, Kohaut E, Brown D, *et al.* Long-term treatment of growth retarded children with chronic renal insufficiency, with recombinant human growth hormone. *Kidney Int* 1996; **49**: 781–5.

210 Hokken-Koelega A, Mulder P, De Jong R, *et al.* Long-term effects of growth hormone treatment on growth and puberty in patients with chronic renal insufficiency. *Pediatr Nephrol* 2000; **14**: 701–6.

211 Wühl E, Haffner D, Nissel R, *et al.* Short dialyzed children respond less to growth hormone than patients prior to dialysis. German Study Group for Growth Hormone Treatment in Chronic Renal Failure. *Pediatr Nephrol* 1996; **10**: 294–8.

212 Schaefer F, Wühl E, Haffner D, *et al.* Stimulation of growth hormone in children undergoing peritoneal or hemodialysis treatment. *Adv Perit Dial* 1994; **10**: 321–6.

213 Johannson G, Janssens F, Proesmans W. Treatment with Genotropin in short children with chronic renal failure, either before active replacement therapy or with functioning renal transplants. An interim report on five European studies. *Acta Paediatr Scand* 1990; **370**: 36–42.

214 Fine RN, Yadin O, Nelson PA, *et al.* Recombinant human growth hormone treatment of children following renal transplantation. *Pediatr Nephrol* 1991; **5**: 147–51.

215 Hokken-Koelega AC, Stijnen T, de Jong RC, *et al.* A placebo-controlled, double-blind trial of growth hormone treatment in prepubertal children after renal transplant. *Kidney Int Suppl* 1996; **53**: S128–34.

216 Guest G, Berard E, Crosnier H, *et al.* Effects of growth hormone in short children after renal transplantation. *Pediatr Nephrol* 1998; **12**: 437–46.

217 Janssen F, Van Damme-Lombaerts R, Van Dyck M, *et al.* Impact of growth hormone treatment on a Belgian population of short children with renal allografts. *Pediatr Transplant* 1997; **1**: 190–6.

218 Fine RN, Stablein D, Cohen AH, *et al.* Recombinant human growth hormone post-renal transplantation in children: a randomized controlled study of the NAPRTCS. *Kidney Int* 2002; **62**: 688–96.

219 Fine RN, Stablein D. Long-term use of recombinant human growth hormone in pediatric allograft recipients: a report of the NAPRTCS Transplant Registry. *Pediatr Nephrol* 2005; **20**: 404–8.

220 Haffner D, Wühl E, Tönshoff B, Mehls O. Growth hormone treatment in short children: 5-year experience German Study Group for Growth Hormone Treatment in Chronic Renal Failure. *Nephrol Dial Transplant* 1994; **9**: 960–1.

221 Hokken-Koelega AC, Stijnen T, de Ridder MA, *et al.* Growth hormone treatment in growth-retarded adolescents after renal transplant. *Lancet* 1994; **343**: 1313–17.

222 Mehls O, Berg U, Broyer M, Rizzoni G. Chronic renal failure and growth hormone treatment: review of the literature and experience in KIGS. In: Ranke MB, Wilton P, eds. *Growth Hormone Therapy in KIGS – 10 Years Experience.* Heidelberg: Barth, 1999: 327–40.

223 Rees L, Ward G, Rigden SPA. Growth over 10 years following a 1-year trial of growth hormone therapy. *Pediatr Nephrol* 2000; **14**: 309–14.

224 Fine RN, Sullivan EK, Tejani A. The impact of recombinant human growth hormone treatment on final adult height. *Pediatr Nephrol* 2000; **14**: 679–81.

225 Fine RN, Sullivan EK, Kuntze J, *et al.* The impact of recombinant human growth hormone treatment during chronic renal insufficiency on renal transplant recipients. *J Pediatr* 2000; **136**: 376–82.

226 Hokken-Koelega AC, Stijnen T, de Jong MC, *et al.* Double blind trial comparing the effects of two doses of growth hormone in prepubertal patients with chronic renal insufficiency. *J Clin Endocrinol Metab* 1994; **79**: 1185–90.

227 Fine RN, Pyke-Grimm K, Nelson PA. Recombinant human growth hormone (rhGH) treatment in children with chronic renal failure (CRF): long-term (one to three years) outcome. *Pediatr Nephrol* 1991; **5**: 477–81.

228 Fine RN, Brown DF, Kuntze J, *et al.* Growth after discontinuation of recombinant human growth hormone therapy in children with chronic renal insufficiency. *J Pediatr* 1996; **129**: 883–91.

229 Filler G, Franke D, Amendt P, Ehrich JH. Reversible diabetes mellitus during growth hormone therapy in chronic renal failure. *Pediatr Nephrol* 1998; **12**: 405–7.

230 Stefanidis CP, Papathanassiou A, Michelis K, *et al.* Diabetes mellitus after therapy with recombinant human growth hormone. *Br J Clin Pract Suppl* 1996; **85**: 66–7.

231 Mehls O, Broyer M, on behalf of the European/Australian Study Group. Growth response to recombinant human growth hormone in short prepubertal children with chronic renal failure with or without dialysis. *Acta Paediatr Suppl* 1994; **399**: 81.

232 Watkins SL. Is severe renal osteodystrophy a contraindication for recombinant human growth hormone treatment? *Pediatr Nephrol* 1996; **10**: 351.

233 Boechat M, Winters W, Hogg R, *et al.* Avascular necrosis of the femoral head in children with chronic renal disease. *Radiology* 2001; **218**: 411–3.

234 Kaufman D. Growth hormone and renal osteodystrophy: a case report. *Pediatr Nephrol* 1998; **12**: 157–9.

235 Picca S, Cappa M, Rizzoni G. Hyperparathyroidism during growth hormone treatment: a role for puberty? *Pediatr Nephrol* 2000; **14**: 56–8.

236 Haffner D, Zacharewicz S, Mehls O, *et al.* The acute effect of growth hormone on GFR is obliterated in chronic renal failure. *Clin Nephrol* 1989; **32**: 266–9.

237 Wühl E, Haffner D, Gretz N, *et al.* Treatment with recombinant human growth hormone in short children with nephropathic cystinosis: no evidence for increased deterioration rate of renal function. *Pediatr Res* 1998; **43**: 484–8.

238 Auernhammer CJ, Strasburger CJ. Effects of growth hormone and insulin-like growth factor I on the immune system. *Eur J Endocrinol* 1995; **133**: 635–45.

239 Melk A, Daniel V, Mehls O, *et al.* Longitudinal analysis of T-helper cell phenotypes in renal-transplant recipients undergoing growth hormone therapy. *Transplantation* 2004; **78**: 1792–801.

240 Hokken-Koelega ACS, Stijnen T, de Jong RC, *et al.* A placebo-controlled double-blind trial of growth hormone treatment in prepubertal children with renal allografts. *Kidney Int* 1996; **49(Suppl)**: S128–34.

241 Maxwell H, Rees L, for the British Association for Paediatric Nephrology. Randomised controlled trial of recombinant human growth hormone in prepubertal and pubertal renal transplant recipients. *Arch Dis Child* 1998; **79**: 481–7.

242 Stahnke N, Zeisel HJ. Growth hormone therapy and leukaemia. *Eur J Pediatr* 1989; **148**: 591–6.

243 Tyden G, Wernersson A, Sandberg J, Berg U. Development of renal cell carcinoma in living donor kidney grafts. *Transplantation* 2000; **70**: 1650–6.

244 Boose AR, Pieters R, Delemarre-Van de Waal HA, Veerman AJ. Growth hormone therapy and leukemia. *Tijdschr Kindergeneeskd* 1992; 1.

245 Furlanetto R. Guidelines of the use of growth hormone in children with short stature. A report by the Drug and Therapeutics Committee of the Lawson Wilkins Pediatric Endocrine Society. *J Pediatr* 1995; **127**: 857.

246 Janssen F, Van Damme-Lombaerts R, Van Dyck M, *et al.* Impact of growth hormone treatment or a Belgian population of short children with renal allografts. *Pediatr Transplant* 1997; **1**: 190–6.

247 Lampit M, Nave T, Hochberg Z. Water and sodium retention during short-term administration of growth hormone to short normal children. *Horm Res* 1998; **50**: 83–8.

248 Hanukoglu A, Belutserkovsky O, Phillip M. Growth hormone activates renin-aldosterone system in children with idiopathic short stature and in a pseudohypoaldosteronism patient with a mutation in epithelial sodium channel alpha subunit. *J Steroid Biochem Mol Biol* 2001; **77**: 49–57.

249 Malozowski S, Tanner LA, Wysowski D, Fleming GA. Growth hormone, insulin-like growth factor I and benign intracranial hypertension. *N Engl J Med* 1993; **329**: 665–6.

250 Wingenfeld P, Schmidt B, Hoppe B, *et al.* Acute glaucoma and intracranial hypertension in a child on long-term peritoneal dialysis treated with growth hormone. *Pediatr Nephrol* 1995; **9**: 742–5.

251 Koller EA, Stadel BV, Malozowski SN. Papilledema in 15 renally compromised patients treated with growth hormone. *Pediatr Nephrol* 1997; **11**: 451–4.

23

Metabolic bone diseases: Disorders of calcium and phosphate metabolism

OLIVER FRICKE, ECKHARD SCHÖNAU

EVIDENCE SCORING OF THERAPY

   * Non-randomized controlled trials, cohort study etc.
  ** One or more well-designed randomized controlled trials
*** Systematic review or meta-analysis

INTRODUCTION

Calcium and phosphate are the main components of hydroxylapatite $[Ca_{10}(PO_4)_6(OH)_2]$. A deficiency of one of these components results in defective mineralization of the organic bone matrix, which is called osteomalacia in adulthood and rickets in childhood.[1] Rickets mainly affects the mineralization of the growth plate, whereas osteomalacia is characterized by decreased mineralization of cortical and trabecular bone. In general, rickets can be classified into two types: calcipenic and phosphopenic.[2] Calcipenic rickets result from calcium malabsorption, whereas phosphopenic rickets is usually caused by renal phosphate loss.

The regulation of calcium and phosphate metabolism under the leading regulatory hormones vitamin D and parathormone is shown in Fig. 23.1. Intestinal calcium absorption is mainly controlled by vitamin D. The cholesterol derivate 7-dehydrocholesterol is the origin of all premetabolites of vitamin D, which are synthesized in the dermis and epidermis under the influence of ultra-violet light. Vitamin D is stored in liver cells and hydroxylated to 25-(OH)-vitamin D, which is finally transformed to 1,25-(OH)$_2$-vitamin D by 1α-hydroxylase in the renal tubule cell. This last enzymatic step takes place under the control of the second regulatory hormone parathormone, which is synthesized in the parathyroid epithelia bodies. Moreover, the epithelia bodies are the sensors for calcium and phosphate. The decrease of the blood calcium concentration induces synthesis and excretion of parathormone, which activates vitamin D and increases the intestinal calcium absorption. Moreover, parathormone regulates the renal calcium excretion and the mobilization of calcium from hydroxylapatite. In addition to its synthesis, the vitamin D supply is dependent on the amount of nutritional vitamin D and the capacity of absorption of fatty nutritional components.

RICKETS CAUSED BY VITAMIN D DEFICIENCY

Pathophysiology

Even today, vitamin D deficiency is the most frequent cause of calcipenic rickets. Extremely vegetarian nutritional intake with avoidance of vitamin D supplementation in the first year of life might cause severe rickets.[3,4] Renal failure (renal osteopathy) and liver insufficiency are also frequent reasons for disturbances of the vitamin D metabolism. A secondary vitamin D deficiency is caused by gastrointestinal diseases, which are characterized by maldigestion and malabsorption. Because vitamin D controls the intestinal calcium absorption, vitamin D deficiency causes decreased intestinal calcium absorption, which induces hypocalcemia with secondary hyperparathyroidism resulting in increased urinary phosphate excretion

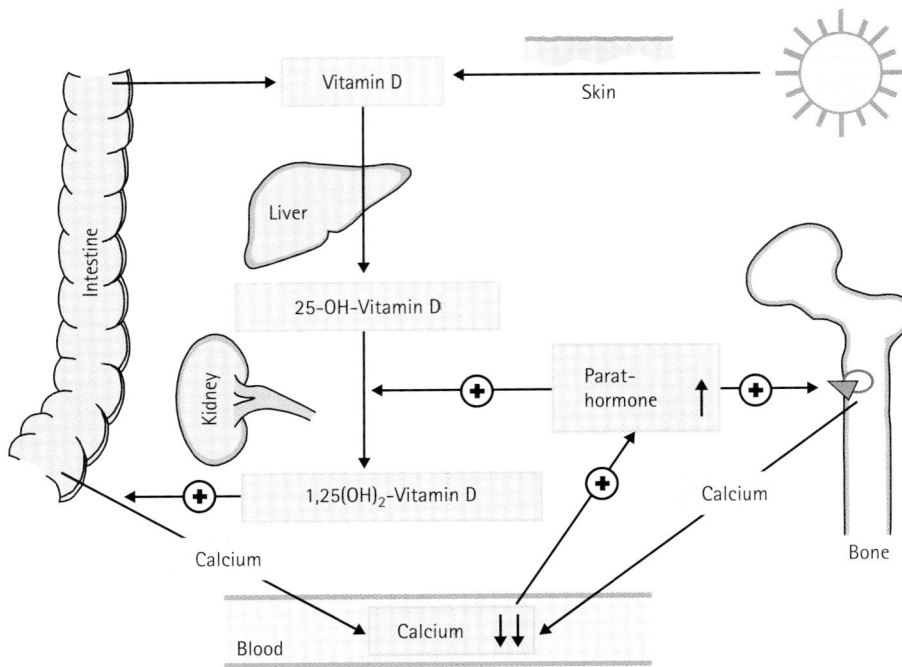

Figure 23.1 Vitamin D metabolism. Intestinal, liver and kidney diseases and imbalances of parathormone influence calcium and phosphate metabolism.

and hypophosphatemia. Diminished calcium and phosphate levels produce defective bone mineralization and the secondary hyperparathyroidism causes increased bone resorption.

Clinical features

Rickets is a clinical syndrome characterized by the failure of enchondral calcification of growth plates of long bones, which results in the deformation of the growth plate, reduction of longitudinal growth and the development of bone deformities. The disease is also associated with osteomalacia, which is a failure of mineralization of preformed osteoid on the trabecular and cortical bone surface. When the growth plates have fused and growth has ceased, only characteristics of ostemalacia are present.

The maturation of metaphyseal bone is also decreased resulting in insufficient biomechanical properties of the bone. Therefore, skeletal axes are bowed in bone areas of skeletal elements, which are under high biomechanical strain. This results in deformation, mainly affecting lower limbs developing genua vara or genua valga. These deformities are the reason for the early development of arthrosis in adulthood. Because calcium has a global role in human physiology, calcipenic rickets are combined with generalized disturbance of many organ functions (e.g.. muscle contraction, propagation of action potentials in neurons and muscle cells). Moreover, individuals affected with rickets have disturbances of dental mineralization, resulting in late dentition and dental enamel defects.

The most important clinical signs of rickets are summarized in Table 23.1. Transitions from cartilage tissue to bone

Table 23.1 Prevalence of symptoms and signs in children aged 18 months and older with radiological characteristics of rickets in Nigeria. (From: Pettifor JM. *Pediatric Bone*. Academic Press, 2003: p. 550).

	Characteristics	Prevalence (%) (*n* = 278)
Symptoms	Weakness	65
	Leg pain when walking	60
	Excessive falling	58
	Unable to walk	11
	Previous fracture	9
Signs	Enlarged costochondral junctions	77
	Enlarged wrists	75
	Genu varum	48
	Enlarged ankles	38
	Genu valgum	32
	Rib cage deformities	15
	Windswept deformities	14
	Open anterior fontanelle	12
	Dental enamel defects	11

(growth plates) are enlarged. Deformations of skeletal elements (e.g., rachitic saber shins, scoliosis) follow the mechanical strain as mentioned above. Typical signs of rickets in a 1½-year-old girl with vitamin D deficiency are shown in Fig. 23.2. The typical rachitic rosary can be noticed at the transition from cartilage tissue to bone of the thoracic skeleton. Moreover, the growth plates are enlarged at the wrists. In more severe cases, the blood calcium concentration decreases

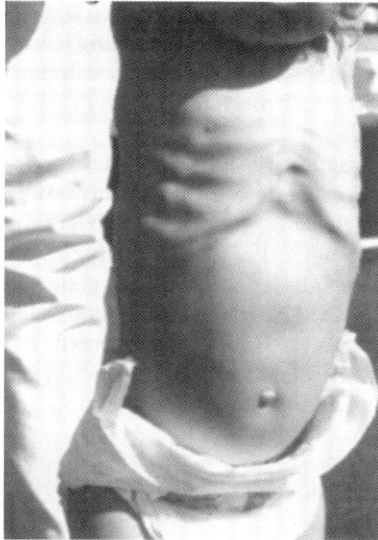

Figure 23.2 An 18-month-old girl with vitamin D deficiency. Costochondral enlargement of ribs form the rachitic rosary. Please see Plate 19.

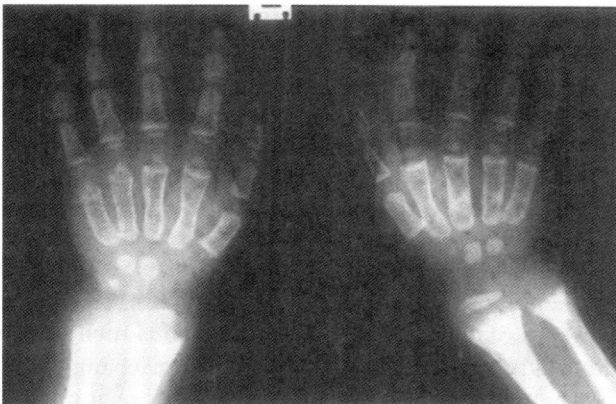

Figure 23.3 Radiographic characteristics of rickets caused by vitamin D deficiency in a 2-year-old child. The wrist shows marked widening of the growth plates at the distal radius and ulna. The distal metaphyses are splayed, cupped, and frayed. The trabecular structure of the metaphyses is coarsened and the cortices are ill defined.

resulting in neuromuscular dysfunction (tetany, muscular hypotonia, cerebral seizures), which can result in a delay of psychomotor development. Furthermore, severe calcipenia causes cardiac arrhythmia with a possible lethal outcome.

Diagnostic features

RADIOLOGY

The combination of typical clinical signs and radiological signs in X-rays of skeletal elements are main evidences of rickets. Characteristic enlarged distal radius and distal ulna in a 2-year-old child with rickets are shown in Fig. 23.3.

LABORATORY TESTS

Further evidence of rickets is shown by typical constellations of chemical parameters of calcium–phosphate metabolism (Fig. 23.4). Alkaline phosphatase is mainly synthesized by osteoblasts and is elevated due to an increased bone turnover. Decreased activity of alkaline phosphatase (AP) is rare and a sign of hypophosphatasia. The next diagnostic step focuses on the parathormone serum level. Vitamin D deficiency induces increased parathormone levels to mobilize calcium from the bone compartment. A normal parathormone concentration suggests the presence of phosphopenic rickets. When parathormone is increased, the final diagnostic step is the determination of vitamin D. When 25(OH)-vitamin D is inside the normal range and the active metabolite 1, 25-(OH)$_2$-vitamin D is decreased, an enzymatic deficiency in vitamin D synthesis can be suggested. In contrast, elevated levels suggest a vitamin D receptor defect.

Therapy

The supplementation of vitamin D (500 IE day^{-1}) over the first 12 months of life is the optimal prevention of rickets due to vitamin D deficiency. Therapy for rickets consists of the administration of high vitamin D doses (5000 IE/day) over 3–6 weeks, which should be followed by regular vitamin D supplementation in the first year of life *. The initial vitamin D therapy needs strict monitoring of the blood calcium level, because an elevated bone mineralization can induce decreased calcium levels with the complication of cardiac arrhythmia. This side effect can be prevented by the additive supplementation of calcium. Hypocalcemia with tetany is treated with intravenous calcium substitution *. Treatment with vitamin D and calcium normalizes chemical parameters (alkaline phosphatase) and clinical signs in 6–12 weeks. Deformities of skeletal elements normally disappear in the first year of therapy. The early diagnosis and the fast treatment of rickets can prevent the need for surgical corrections of skeletal deformities.

VITAMIN D-DEPENDENT RICKETS

Pathophysiology

Vitamin D-dependent rickets is divided into types I and II. Both types are transmitted in an autosomal recessive way and are rare. Type I is a deficiency of the activity of the renal 1α-hydroxylase.[5] Therefore, the synthesis of biological active 1,25-(OH)$_2$-vitamin D is reduced. Most individuals affected with type II derive from Arab families. Type II is characterized by a resistance to 1,25-(OH)$_2$-vitamin D.[6] Therefore, affected individuals often have supranormal 1,25-(OH)$_2$-vitamin D levels. The culture of dermal fibroblasts delivers the opportunity to detect defects of the vitamin D receptor or its intracellular signal pathway. These defects mainly affect

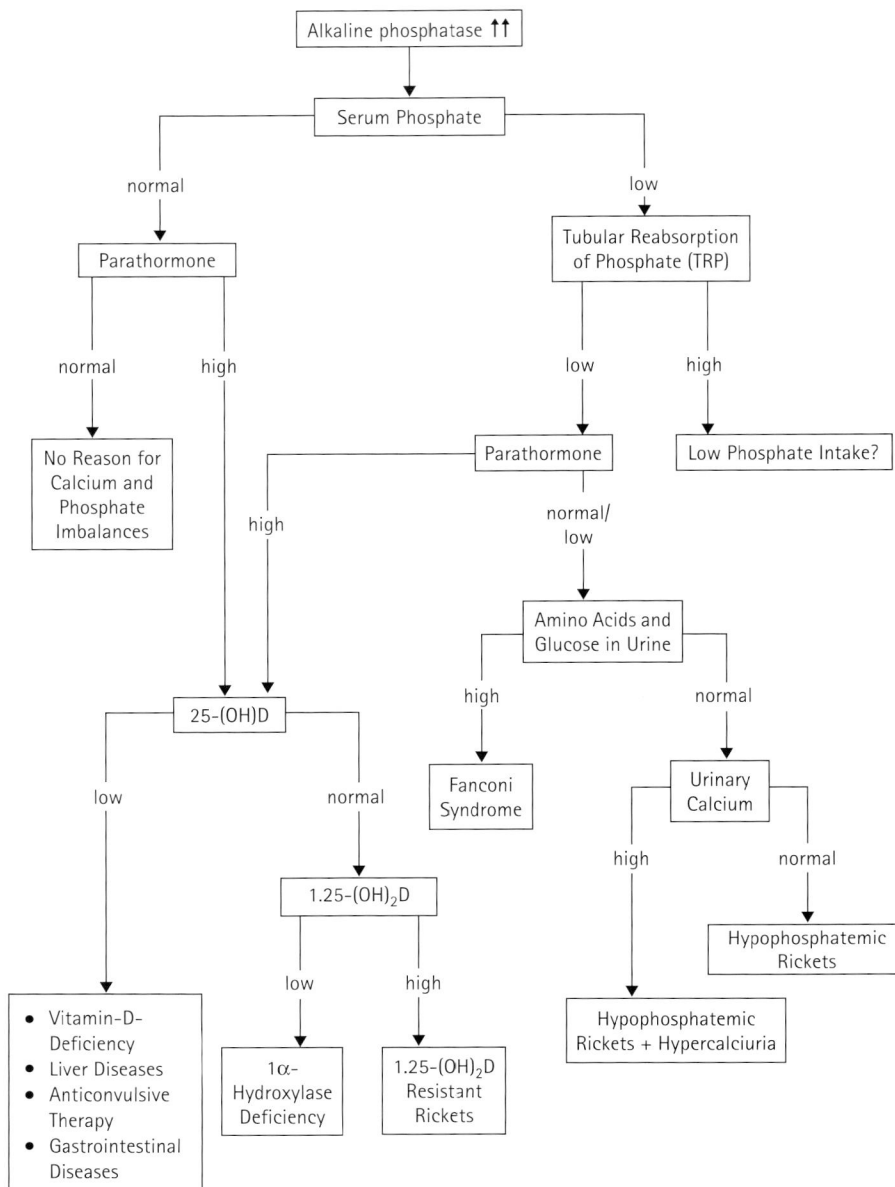

Figure 23.4 Flow chart for the diagnosis of rickets.

the intestinal calcium absorption. The biochemical pattern of vitamin D dependent rickets is heterogeneous. The definite diagnosis is obtained by proving the mutation of the receptor gene or a gene connected to the intracellular vitamin D signaling pathway.

Clinical features

The clinical pattern of vitamin D-dependent rickets is very similar to rickets caused by vitamin D deficiency. Type II is connected with the presence of a total alopecia in 50% of individuals. The time of manifestation of both type I and type II is mainly the second year of life.

Therapy

Type I is treated with a life-long substitution of the biologically active metabolite 1,25-(OH)$_2$-vitamin D (0.5–2 μg calcitriol day^{-1})*. The dose of vitamin D must be reduced to an individual amount of supplementation, which is necessary to optimize skeletal mineralization and to stabilize the blood calcium concentration. Parathormone is an important and useful parameter for the adjustment of the individual vitamin D dose.

The therapy of type II is more difficult than in type I. Because of the cellular resistance to vitamin D, extremely high doses of 1,25-(OH)$_2$-vitamin D (up to 50 μg day^{-1}) are needed for successful therapy*. When the oral administration of vitamin D cannot achieve sufficient vitamin D levels, oral or intravenous supplementation of calcium is necessary.

SECONDARY VITAMIN D DEFICIENCY

Renal diseases and renal osteodystrophy

DEFINITION AND PATHOGENESIS

Osteodystrophy is characterized by decreased growth rate and disturbances of bone turnover (remodeling) in childhood.[7,8] Renal failure affects the calcium–phosphate metabolism by decreased phosphate excretion, secondary hyperparathyroidism, decreased renal $1,25\text{-}(OH)_2$-synthesis and direct effects of uremia toxins.

CLINICAL FEATURES

Individuals with renal osteodystrophy show a reduced growth rate and deformities of the long skeletal bone tubes. X-ray signs of affected bones are related to radiological patterns of rickets, but bones affected with osteodystrophy have less enlarged growth plates in contrast to rickets. Moreover, disturbance of trabecular bone turnover (metaphyseal fibrosis) and subperiostal absorbed bone by hyperparathyroidism are classical signs of osteodystrophy. Hyperparathyroidism is caused by secondary hyperphosphatemia due to decreased renal phosphate excretion in the early renal failure.

THERAPY

The reduction of nutritional phosphate supply is the most important therapeutic issue for individuals with early renal failure*. When orally administered phosphate binding drugs are used, these preparations should not contain aluminum. Furthermore, the substitution of vitamin D under control of the parathormone level might be necessary, which can often be completed by oral calcium supplementation*. Parathormone levels should be adjusted in the upper part of the normal range, because suppressed parathormone inactivates bone metabolism. Parathormone is one of the most powerful anabolic hormones involved in bone metabolism.

GASTROINTESTINAL DISEASES

After intestinal absorption vitamin D is transported in chylomicrons through the lymphatic system to the blood circulation. Syndromes of intestinal malabsorption and of insufficient bile excretion followed by decreased intestinal absorption of fatty particles can cause vitamin D deficiency.[9] Therefore, diseases related to cholestasis and insufficient bile production might cause rickets (congenital liver cirrhosis, atresia of biliary channels, cystic fibrosis). Frequent monitoring of parathormone and alkaline phosphatase are important for the recognition of a additional need of vitamin D supplementation. Depending on the required supply, vitamin D is administered in combination with vitamins A, E and K in a high oral dose or by intramuscular injection in a time interval of 2–3 weeks.

Rickets associated with anticonvulsive medication

Children treated with anticonvulsive medication have a higher risk of developing rickets.[10] An increased vitamin D metabolism by liver cells is discussed to be responsible in a pathogenetic point of view.[11,12] Moreover, decreased motor activity and decreased sun exposure of handicapped children might present an additional reason for decreased bone mass (inactivity osteoporosis). The therapy is no different from the therapeutic approach to rickets caused by vitamin D deficiency. In addition, physical therapy might provide benefits for these children.

Osteopathy of the preterm infant

The combination of osteopenic and low mineralized bone is typical for this osteopathy, which can be recognized in preterm infants with an extremely low birth weight ($<1500\,g$ or <28 weeks).[13] Different factors contribute to this osteopathy:

- insufficient supply of calcium and phosphate
- long-term respiratory assistance
- drug treatment with diuretic agents (e.g., furosemide) and glucocorticoids

The daily requirement for calcium ($130\,mg\,kg^{-1}$) and phosphate ($70\,mg\,kg^{-1}$) for sufficient bone mineralization in the last trimester of pregnancy is higher than that provided by breast milk. Therefore, an additional supply of calcium and phosphate is needed for this high risk population to prevent the appearance of rickets. The prevention of rickets is completed by administering vitamin D. A typical side effect of these preventive issues might be the development of nephrocalcinosis in preterm infants. Therefore, monitoring of urinary calcium and phosphate excretion is necessary.[14] Mild defects of mineralization have a good prognosis in preterm infants and disappear in the first year of life. Severe defects of mineralization concern the skull development as well and can have effects on orbit development with later vision problems.

Hypophosphatasia

Alkaline phophatases are enzymes located in the cellular plasma membrane. How the alkaline phosphatase in osteoclasts contributes to bone mineralization is still unknown. When the activity of the alkaline phosphatase isoenzyme, located in liver, bone and cartilage tissue, is decreased for hereditary reasons, the mineralization of the bone matrix is disturbed.

CLINICAL FEATURES

Clinical signs and age of manifestation are highly variable. Rickets, like skeletal signs, is obvious and there is growth retardation as well. Emphasis should be put on the presence of a frayed metaphyseal area. Hypophosphatasia can be distinguished into three different types depending on age of manifestation.[15]

Infantile type

Clinical signs of severe mineralization defects, fractures and bone deformities are present at birth or develop in the first month of life. Affected children have a high risk of dying from secondary respiratory complications due to costal fractures and thorax instability. Moreover, those children suffer from growth retardation, preterm closure of skull sutures, cerebral seizures, hypercalcemia, and nephrocalcinosis.

Juvenile type

Typical signs are short stature, rickets and premature loss of deciduous teeth at the beginning of the second year of life.

Adult type

This type is the mildest type of hypophosphatasia. Typical clinical signs are bone pain, deformities of skeletal elements, and a generalized osteoporosis as well.

DIAGNOSTIC FEATURES

The first step is the determination of a reduced alkaline phosphatase in blood serum; the second step is the proof of gene mutation, which is related to hypophosphatasia. The interpretation of the alkaline phosphatase level should be interpreted on the background of the age dependent range of this enzyme. Furthermore, large quantities of urinary phosphoethanolamine are excreted and plasma inorganic pyrophosphate and pyridoxal-5-phosphate levels are elevated as a result of a lack of degradation in the absence of adequate alkaline phosphatase activity.

THERAPY

A causal therapy of hypophosphatasia is not available, but the clinical course of this condition may improve spontaneously as the child matures. Surgical procedures for the correction of skeletal deformities are possible and may improve the conditions of children affected with hypophosphatasia*. Supplementation with vitamin D is absolutely not indicated, because these children have an increased risk of developing nephrocalcinosis.

Phosphopenic rickets

PATHOPHYSIOLOGY

Phosphate is one of the main components of hydroxylapatite as mentioned above. Therefore, a phosphate deficiency causes defects of the bone mineralization. Hypophosphatemic rickets are characterized by the combination of low serum phosphate and increased phosphate excretion. The increased phosphate excretion can be solitary or related to a complex pathologic pattern of urinary excretion (glucose, amino acids, hydrogen carbonate). The most frequent type is the isolated increased renal-tubular phosphate excretion. The typical clinical feature is phosphate diabetes, which is also called X-linked familial hypophosphatemic rickets or hereditary hypophosphatemic vitamin D resistant rickets. A special type is the combination of hyperphosphaturia with hypercalcuria, which follows a still unknown hereditary trait.

EPIDEMIOLOGY

Hypophosphatemic rickets is the most frequent type of hereditary transmitted rickets and possesses a frequency of 1:20 000 to 1:25 000 in newborn infants. The hereditary transmission is X-chromosome-dominant.[16] The affected gene shows homology to the family of endopeptidases genes and is called PEX, or recently PHEX (phosphate regulating with homologies to endopeptidases on the X-chromosome).[17] Actually, fibroblast growth factor 23 (FGF-23) is discussed as the enzymatic target of PEX. FGF-23 induces phosphaturia and decreases the serum phosphate level.[18,19] Moreover, there seems to be a primary abnormality of osteoblasts leading to hypomineralized periosteolytic lesions.[20] The sporadic appearance of the adult type occurs infrequently. This type has to be clearly distinguished from the paraneoplastic type of phosphate diabetes, for which the tumor-induced secretion of a phosphate excretion regulating factor is discussed.

CLINICAL FEATURES

Hypophosphatemic rickets is typically recognized in the second year of life. Typical signs are short stature (body height below the third percentile) or a decreased growth rate (below the 25th percentile). Deformities of the lower limbs (genua vara) are the essential reason for short stature. Therefore, growth retardation progresses under the increasing biomechanical strain on the lower limbs in the second year of life. Precise assessment of body height can also detect a growth retardation in the first year of life. As phosphate diabetes mainly affects the growth of the legs – the major contributor to body size in early childhood – affected individuals present with disproportion between sitting height and leg length.[21]

During adolescence, when the trunk grows slightly faster than the legs, untreated individuals show no further growth retardation.[22] A relationship between the deficits of height and the degree of hypophosphatemia does not exist.[23] The final height of untreated or treated individuals is often shorter than 2–3 SD below the mean of unaffected adults.[21,24] Figure 23.5 shows a 2½-year-old girl with phosphate diabetes and genua vara. Genua valga are typical signs of phosphate diabetes in older children and adolescents.

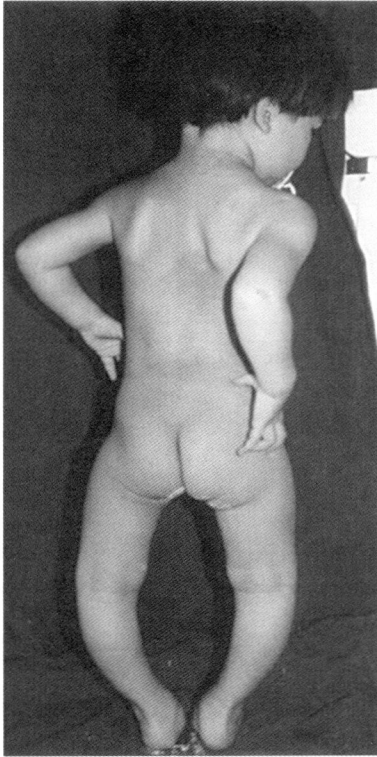

Figure 23.5 Extreme bowing of the femurs and tibias in a 2.5-year-old girl with hypophosphatemic rickets. Please see Plate 20.

Moreover, bone pain, wedge-shaped defects of the medial surface of the proximal tibia, fractures, and pseudo-fractures are typical signs of phosphate diabetes. The compression of the spinal channel and hearing loss are rarely described. Infants and children have a delayed dentition and change to adult teeth, sometimes connected with defects of the enamel of teeth. Adolescents and adults can be frequently affected with enamel defects. Untreated adults may have no symptoms or show calcifications of tendons, ligaments and joint capsules. When phosphopenic rickets are combined with hypercalcuria, nephrocalcinosis can appear.

DIAGNOSTIC FEATURES

Figure 23.4 displays the diagnostic approach when clinical signs indicate the presence of a bone disease with increased phosphate excretion. Phosphopenic rickets shows decreased renal phosphate absorption and decreased maximal tubular phosphate transportation capacity (TmP/GFR). TmP/GFR indicates the limit of tubular phosphate absorption. Below the TmP/GFR phosphate is completely absorbed from the urine. Hypophosphatemic rickets is characterized by elevated serum alkaline phosphatase activity. Levels of serum phosphate and calcium are in the normal range and normal parathormone levels are typical as well. The assessment of the urinary excretion of glucose, amino acids and hydrogen bicarbonate distinguishes between a generalized tubular defect of absorption (Fanconi syndrome) and the isolated

insufficiency of phosphate absorption. The assessment of urinary calcium excretion delivers the possibility to detect the type of phosphate diabetes connected with hypercalciuria. The detection of a mutation of the *PEX* gene might secure genetic proof of phosphopenic rickets.

THERAPY

Therapeutic issues are mainly focused on the supplementation of phosphate (50–70 mg elemental phosphorus kg^{-1} day^{-1})*. The distribution of the daily phosphate dose into five to six single doses is important. Moreover, the phosphate administration is combined with vitamin D (about 30 ng kg^{-1} calcitriol in two or three doses) to prevent a secondary hyperparathyroidism and to increase the intestinal phosphate absorption*. Phosphopenic rickets in combination with hypercalcuria can be additionally treated with hydrochlorothiazide, which increases the renal calcium absorption improving growth and fracture healing*.[24] The development of a nephrocalcinosis is an important side effect of the treatment of phosphopenic rickets, especially when vitamin D is administered. Therefore, the urinary calcium excretion has to be monitored and ultrasonographic controls of the kidneys help to detect nephrocalcinosis early.

Drug therapy should be continued up to adolescence when growth plates are closed. Bone pain is an indication to continue phosphate supplementation also during adulthood. The surgical correction of skeletal deformities might be necessary, even with sufficient drug treatment.[25,26] Sufficient treatment of phosphopenic rickets normalizes growth rate. Adjuvant growth hormone therapy can support catch-up growth as well.[27] Growth hormone treatment has to be monitored very carefully because growth hormone therapy can aggravate a pre-existent disproportionate stature by improving sitting height more than leg length.[28] The level of alkaline phosphatase should be in the higher normal range with adequate therapy.

Hypoparathyroidism

Hypoparathyroidism is characterized by insufficient parathormone (PTH) secretion resulting in hypocalcemia and hyperphosphatemia. Hypoparathyroidism may occur idiopathically or secondary to damage of the parathyroid glands by surgery, iron deposition in hemosiderosis, malignant infiltration or irradiation, as well as in hypomagnesemia. Transient neonatal hypoparathyroidism is more frequent than idiopathic persistent hypoparathyroidism, which can be distinguished into three different types:[2]

- sporadic or familial isolated hypoparathyroidism
- polyglandular autoimmune disease
- sporadic or familial hypoparathyroidism associated with further abnormalities

Sporadic or familial isolated hypoparathyroidism is autosomal dominant, autosomal recessive and X-linked recessive inherited and occurs as a solitary endocrine disorder.[2] Polyglandular autoimmune disease type I or autoimmune polyendocrinopathy–candidiasis–ectodermal dystrophy (APECED) is usually inherited as an autosomal recessive trait. Most patients develop candidiasis, hypoparathyroidism, and Addison's disease in the first decades of life.[29] Several syndromes and abnormalities may be related to sporadic or familial hypoparathyroidism (DiGeorge syndrome, Russel–Silver syndrome, Hallerman–Streiff syndrome, Dubowitz syndrome, Kearns–Sayre syndrome, sensorineural deafness, nephropathy, and lymphedema). Moreover, the association of hypoparathyroidism with severe growth retardation has been described in several children mainly from the Middle East. An autosomal recessive trait is suspected for those cases.[30–32] Mutations of the calcium sensing receptor gene increase the receptor's sensitivity to calcium, which induces life-long hypoparathyroidism and hypocalcemia with mild symptoms.[33]

Pseudohypoparathyroidism

Pseudohypoparathyroidism (PHP) is characterized by a resistance to biologically active parathormone.[2] The clinical feature may be heterogeneous, but most patients show a syndrome of hypocalcemia, hyperphosphatemia and secondary hyperparathyroidism. Biochemical parameters present the opportunity to distinguish between two different types of PHP.[34] Individuals affected with type I do not show any increased cyclic AMP (cAMP) in urine and plasma due to the high doses of PTH administered. Type II is characterized by a normal elevation of cAMP, but the urinary phosphate excretion is not increased due to PTH. Therefore, the defect is localized distal from cAMP formation in type II. PHP type I can be further classified into two subtypes. Type Ia is called Albright's hereditary osteodystrophy (AHO) and consists of the combination of short stature, round facies, short neck, obesity, subcutaneous calcification, and shortened metacarpals and metatarsals.

AHO without the presence of PHP is called pseudo-PHP and can be found in relatives of individuals affected with PHP type Ia. AHO is caused by mutations of the *GNAS1* gene (chromosome 20q13) encoding the alpha subunit of the G-protein coupling membrane receptor and adenylate cyclase. Therefore, individuals affected with type Ia show resistance to several hormones using G-coupled receptors for signal transduction (thyroid stimulating hormone, TSH; gonadotropins). Individuals suffering from AHO without PHP type Ia have also diminished Gs-α activity, but do not show any hormone resistance. Therefore, an additional factor is necessary for the development of hormone resistance, which may be related to genomic imprinting. This suggestion is emphasized by the result that PHP Ia appears in maternal transmission, whereas pseudo-PHP occurs in a paternal hereditary trait.[35] A causal therapy of PHP does not

exist. Hypothyroidism, delayed puberty, hypocalcemia, and hyperphosphatemia are symptomatically treated with thyroxine, sexual steroids, and vitamin D. In contrast to rickets, the supplementation of vitamin D does not influence the growth velocity. Obesity may be a problem, which has to be treated by dietary measures and physical activity.

Jansen–type metaphyseal dysplasia

Jansen-type metaphyseal dysplasia is a rare disorder that results from an activating PTH-receptor mutation.[36] This disorder is characterized by hypercalcemia and hypophosphatemia, as well as the abnormal formation of enchondral bone and severe growth delay. PTH serum levels are typically diminished.[37] Therapeutic issues are mainly focused on surgical correction of skeletal deformities. Solitary individuals were treated with bisphosphonates in an experimental therapeutic approach.

BONE DISEASES WITH INCREASED FRACTURE RATE: OSTEOPENIA AND OSTEOPOROSIS

Definition

Bone fractures appear under a highly increased mechanical strain in healthy individuals. Pathological fractures are fractures that happen under a normal biomechanical strain. Spontaneous fractures are pathological fractures without any recognizable mechanical strain. Pathological fractures occur in skeletal element, which consist of bone with a decreased capability to resist mechanical stress. This reduced bone stability can be localized to one or several skeletal elements, but it can also affect the complete skeleton (generalized osteoporosis) as well. Osteopenia can be called preclinical osteoporosis and indicates reduced bone mass without the occurrence of fractures. Osteoporosis is characterized by reduced bone mass in combination with bone fractures. Thereby, the reduced bone mass is the consequence of a lowered amount of organic bone matrix. In contrast to rickets, osteoporosis does not primarily develop due to deficits of bone mineralization. Osteoporosis is a disease of the organic components of the skeleton and is mainly caused by:

- reduced collagen synthesis or synthesis of pathologic collagen
- defect adaptation of the skeleton to its biomechanical environment (disease of the mechanostat, see Rauch and Schoenau[38])
- reduced mechanical stimulation (motor inactivity, muscle diseases)

Figure 23.6 illustrates the regulation of the skeleton. The most important examples for a disturbance of this feedback loop are indicated and are discussed in the following section.

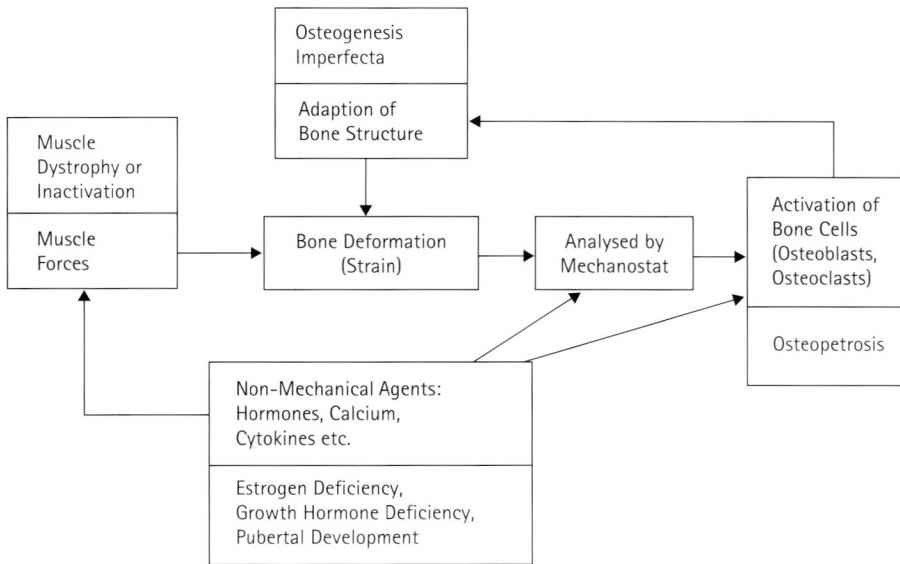

Figure 23.6 Mechanostat theory of muscle bone interaction and associated diseases.

An essential differential diagnosis to osteoporosis is child abuse (battered child syndrome). Battered child syndrome can be ruled out by recognizing typical additional signs (e.g., hematoma, retinal bleeding spots) and by the use of scintigraphic methods and X-rays of skeletal elements revealing fracture patterns which are not typical of osteoporosis.

Osteogenesis imperfecta

Phenotypes of osteogenesis imperfecta are heterogeneous. The most frequent reasons are point mutations of genes responsible for the expression of both chains of collagen I.[39] The hereditary transmission is autosomal dominant, less frequently recessive. Osteogenesis imperfecta possesses a frequency of 4:100 000 to 10:100 000.

CLINICAL FEATURES

Clinical features of osteogenesis imperfecta are highly variable and typically dominated by the occurrence of bone fractures. The range comprises association with intrauterine death, but manifestation of the disease in the middle age of life as well. Osteogenesis imperfecta is distinguished into four different types following genetic and clinical criteria described by Sillence *et al.* (Table 23.2).[40] In addition to this classification three further types (V–VII) are also described.[41,42]

Core symptoms of osteogenesis imperfecta are:

* frequent occurrence of bone fractures
* deformities of skeletal elements
* growth retardation

In addition, wormian bones are present in the skull and dentinogenesis imperfecta is described. There is a generalized decreased stability of connective tissue (ligaments, an

increased risk of bleeding, blue sclera, myopia, hernia, congenital heart disease, and hard of hearing or deafness) is characteristic.[40] Affected newborn infants may also be recognized by muscular hypotonia.

DIAGNOSTIC FEATURES

X-rays reveal an increased transparency of the skeleton due to osteopenia. Moreover, fresh and old fractures with normal callus, deformities of bone tubes and vertebra (kyphoscoliosis) and wormian bones can be recognized. The diagnosis follows clinical and radiological characteristics. Histology of bone tissue and molecular biology can be used to confirm the diagnosis in uncharacteristic cases.

THERAPY

The most important therapeutic issue is the early commencement of physiotherapy to increase muscular power. Long-bone tubes can be stabilized by telescope nails after bone fractures. Immobilization should be avoided because it leads to muscular hypotonia and is followed by additional inactivity osteoporosis, which deteriorates the physical conditions of the affected children. First results of clinical trials using bisphosphonates for the therapy of osteogenesis imperfecta revealed a benefit for treated individuals**.[43,44] Those drugs are inactivators of the osteoclastic function and may increase bone stability in children affected with osteogenesis imperfecta.

Osteopetrosis (Albers–Schoenberg disease)

PATHOPHYSIOLOGY

Osteopetrosis is characterized by four different types.[45] Milder forms are dominant inherited, the severer forms

Table 23.2 Phenotype classification of osteogenesis imperfecta according to Sillence et al.[40] (modified)

Type	Severity	Typical features	Genotype	Phenotype
I	Mild, non-deforming	Normal height or mild short stature; blue sclera; no dentinogenesis imperfecta	Premature stop codon in COL1A1	Quantitative collagen defect
II	Perinatal lethal	Fractures at birth +++; deformities +++; broad long bones; soft skull; dark sclera	Glycine substitutions in COL1A1 or COL1A2	Qualitative collagen defect
III	Severely deforming	Short +++; triangular face; scoliosis ++; grayish sclera; dentinogenesis imperfecta	Glycine substitutions in COL1A1 or COL1A2	Qualitative collagen defect
IV	Moderately deforming	Short ++; scoliosis +; grayish or white sclera; dentinogenesis imperfecta	Glycine substitutions in COL1A1 or COL1A2	Qualitative collagen defect
V	Moderate to severely deforming	Hyperplastic callus formation, calcified interosseous membrane	Unknown	
VI	Moderate to severely deforming	Osteoid thickness (histomorphometry) increased, mineralization defect	Unknown	
VII	Moderate to severely deforming	Short stature with rhizomelia	Unknown	

follow recessive inheritance. Osteopetrosis is a rare disease that is part of the family of sclerosing bony dysplasias. Estimates of the prevalence of this disease do not exist. Individuals with osteopetrosis have a normal count of osteoclasts, but they are functionally inactive. Therefore, remodeling is decreased, which implicates increased bone thickness (hyperostosis) and increased mineralization (osteosclerosis) as well. Because osteoclasts derive from cells with macrophagic function, monocyte function is also decreased in osteopetrosis resulting in an increased susceptibility for infectious diseases. Moreover, increasing bone thickness decreases the bone marrow cavity inducing anemia. Cranial nerves can be damaged in the skull perforating channels by compressing bone.[46]

DIAGNOSTIC FEATURES

Typical X-ray signs of osteopetrosis are the missing bone marrow cavity, enlargement and vertical metaphyseal stripes of long bone tubes and emphasized shape of vertebral bodies. The analysis of biochemical parameters reveals calcium and phosphate levels in the lower normal range in combination with elevated parathormone and vitamin D levels. Biochemical parameters of osteoblastic function (bone specific alkaline phosphatase and osteocalcin) are inside the normal range. Osteoclastic parameters such as the bone specific isoenzyme of acid phosphatase are decreased.

CLINICAL FEATURES

Osteopetrosis tarda is the most frequent type of osteopetrosis and is often detected by chance when X-rays are performed for different reasons. Symptoms might be an increased rate of bone fractures, anemia and dental erosions. Congenital or malign osteopetrosis are less frequent diseases. In addition to the symptoms already described for the osteopetrosis tarda, this type is characterized by hepatosplenomegalia, pancytopenia, enlarged lymph nodes, paralysis of cranial nerves (deafness, blindness), hydrocephalus internus, and an increased susceptibility for infectious diseases. Individuals affected with congenital osteopetrosis have a typical facies with macrocephalia, prominent forehead, hypertelorism, ptosis, and strabism. Intermedium and reno-cerebral types are rare diseases.

THERAPY

Mild manifestations of osteopetrosis are treated with transfusion, antibiotic therapy, and osteosynthesis in a symptomatic way. Severe cases are treated with early bone marrow transplantation in a curative approach.[47] The life span of the congenital type is lowered by the occurrence of secondary complications (anemia, infection).

Idiopathic juvenile osteoporosis

The etiology of idiopathic juvenile osteoporosis is still unknown. The recent discussion focuses on an increased bone turnover and a delayed skeletal adaptation to body height and body weight in individuals affected with idiopathic juvenile osteoporosis. Idiopathic juvenile osteoporosis is a rare disease.

CLINICAL FEATURES

The presence of idiopathic juvenile osteoporosis is described in children under 5 years in single cases, but the main age of manifestation is around the beginning puberty. Bone

Table 23.3 Differential diagnosis of osteoporosis in children and adolescents (From: Ward LM, Glorieux FH. *Pediatric Bone.* Academic Press, 2003: p. 405).

1. **Heritable Disorders of Connective Tissue**
   a. Osteogenesis Imperfecta
   b. Bruck Syndrome
   c. Osteoporosis Pseudoglioma Syndrome
   d. Ehlers–Danlos Syndrome
   e. Marfan Syndrome
   f. Homocystinuria

2. **Neuromuscular Disorders**
   a. Cerebral Palsy
   b. Duchenne Muscular Dystrophy
   c. Prolonged Immobilization

3. **Endocrine and Reproductive Disorders**
   a. Disorders of Puberty
   b. Turner Syndrome
   c. Growth Hormone Deficiency
   d. Hyperthyroidism
   e. Diabetes Mellitus
   f. Hyperprolactinemia
   g. Athletic Amenorrhea
   h. Glucocorticoid Excess

4. **Chronic Illness**
   a. Leukemia
   b. Rheumatologic Disorders
   c. Anorexia Nervosa
   d. Cystic Fibrosis
   e. Inflammatory Bowel Disease
   f. Other: primary biliary cirrhosis, cyanotic congenital heart disease, thalassemia, malabsorption syndrome, organ transplantation

5. **Inborn Errors of Metabolism**
   a. Lysinuric Protein Intolerance
   b. Glycogen Storage Disease
   c. Galactosemia
   d. Gaucher Disease

6. **Iatrogens**
   a. Glucocorticoids
   b. Methotrexate
   c. Cyclosporine
   d. Heparin
   e. Radiotherapy
   f. Medroxyprogesterone acetate
   g. GnRH agonists
   h. L-Thyroxine suppressive therapy

density normalizes and clinical signs disappear over a range of 3–4 years. Clinical symptoms are bone pain and fractures of vertebral bodies. The presence of fish-shaped vertebral bodies is very characteristic. Metaphyseal fractures of long bone tubes may also occur.

DIAGNOSTIC FEATURES

Table 23.3 displays the differential diagnosis, which has to be ruled out before the final diagnosis of idiopathic juvenile osteoporosis can be accepted. The clear separation from mild types of osteogenesis imperfecta can be difficult. Biochemical analyses of bone specific parameters do not reveal any pathological signs. The bone histology is characterized by a decreased rate of mineralization in the presence of normal bone absorption. Therefore, the histology indicates an imbalance of bone turnover with emphasis on bone resorption.

THERAPY

Therapeutic issues should be carefully considered, because spontaneous recovery is normal after puberty. Standardized therapies do not exist. Therapeutic approaches comprise bisphosphonates and vitamin D in combination with calcium and calcitonin*.

INACTIVITY OSTEOPOROSIS

Inactivity is the most frequent reason for osteoporosis in children and adolescents. Table 23.3 summarizes typical diseases that are linked with muscular inactivity and secondary osteoporosis. An insufficiently developed muscle system and lowered muscular tone are responsible for a decreased biomechanical stimulation of the skeletal system. Acute diseases induce a reduction of bone mass, chronic diseases mainly result in an insufficient gain of bone mass in childhood and adolescence.

KEY LEARNING POINTS

- Rickets can be distinguished into two types: calcipenic and phosphopenic. Calcipenic rickets results from calcium malabsorption, whereas phosphopenic rickets is usually caused by renal phosphate loss.
- Vitamin D-dependent rickets is divided into types I and II. Both types are transmitted in an autosomal recessive way. Type I is a deficiency of the activity of the renal 1α-hydroxylase. Type II is characterized by a resistance to 1,25-$(OH)_2$-vitamin D.

- Hypophosphatasia is characterized by a decreased activity of alkaline phosphatase isoenzymes and can be distinguished into three different types dependent on the age of manifestation: infantile, juvenile, and adult type.
- Hypophosphatemic rickets is characterized by the combination of low serum phosphate and increased phosphate excretion. The most frequent type is the isolated increased renal-tubular phosphate excretion.
- Hypoparathyroidism is characterized by insufficient PTH secretion resulting in hypocalcemia and hyperphosphatemia. Hypoparathyroidism may occur idiopathically or secondary to damage of the parathyroid glands by surgery, iron deposition in hemosiderosis, malignant infiltration or irradiation, as well as in hypomagnesemia.
- Osteopenia can be called preclinical osteoporosis and indicates reduced bone mass without the occurrence of fractures. Osteoporosis is characterized by reduced bone mass in combination with bone fractures.
- Phenotypes of osteogenesis imperfecta are heterogeneous and typically dominated by the occurrence of bone fractures. The range comprises affection with intrauterine death, but manifestation of the disease in the middle age of life as well.
- Inactivity is the most frequent reason for osteoporosis in children and adolescents. An insufficiently developed muscle system and lowered muscular tone are responsible for a decreased biomechanical stimulation of the skeletal system.

REFERENCES

● = Seminal primary article
◆ = Key review paper

◆ 1   Mankin HJ. Rickets, osteomalacia and renal osteodystrophy. Part I and II. *J Bone Joint Surg* 1974; **56**: 101–28, 352–86.

◆ 2   Kruse K. Disorders of calcium and bone metabolism. In: Brook CGD, ed. 3rd edn. Oxford: Blackwell, 1995: 735–78.

3   Pettifor JM. Nutritional rickets: deficiency of vitamin D, calcium, or both? *Am J Clin Nutr* 2004; **80(6 Suppl)**: 1725S–9S.

4   Greer FR. Issues in establishing vitamin D recommendations for infants and children. *Am J Clin Nutr* 2004; **80(6 Suppl)**: 1759S–62S.

● 5   Prader A, Illig R, Heierli, E. Eine besondere Form der primaeren Vitamin-D-resistant Rachitis mit Hypocalcaemie und autosomal-dominantem Erbgang. Die hereditaere Pseudo-Mangel-Rachitis. *Helvet Paediatr Acta* 1961; **16**: 452–68.

6   Liberman KA, Marx SJ. Vitamin D resistance. In: Weintraub BC, ed. *Molecular Endocrinology: Basic Concepts and Clinical Correlations*. New York: Raven Press, 1995: 425–44.

7   Martin KJ, Olgaard K, Coburn JW, *et al.* Bone Turnover Work Group. Diagnosis, assessment, and treatment of bone turnover abnormalities in renal osteodystrophy. *Am J Kidney Dis* 2004; **43**: 558–65.

8   Salusky IB, Kuizon BG, Juppner H. Special aspects of renal osteodystrophy in children. *Semin Nephrol* 2004; **24**: 69–77.

9   Sylvester FA. Bone abnormalities in gastrointestinal and hepatic disease. *Curr Opin Pediatr* 1999; **11**: 402–7.

10   Sheth RD. Bone health in pediatric epilepsy. *Epilepsy Behav* 2004; **5(Suppl 2)**:S30–5.

11   Rieger-Wettengl G, Tutlewski B, Stabrey A, *et al.* Analysis of the musculoskeletal system in children and adolescents receiving anticonvulsant monotherapy with valproic acid or carbamazepine. *Pediatrics* 2001; **108**: E107.

12   Liakakos D, Papadopoulos Z, Vlachos P, *et al.* Serum alkaline phosphatase and urinary hydroxyproline values in children receiving phenobarbital with and without vitamin D. *J Pediatr* 1975; **87**: 291–6.

13   Specker B. Nutrition influences bone development from infancy through toddler years. *J Nutr* 2004; **134**: 691S–5S.

14   Pohlandt F, Mihatsch WA. Reference values for urinary calcium and phosphorus to prevent osteopenia of prematurity. *Pediatr Nephrol* 2004; **19**: 1192–3.

15   Whyte MP. Hypophosphatasia. In: Scriver CR, Beandet AL, Sly WS, Valle D, eds. *The Metabolic and Molecular Basis of Inherited Diseases*, 7th edn. New York: McGraw-Hill, 1995: 4095–111.

16   Rasmussen H, Tenenhouse HS. Mendelian hypophosphatemias. In: Scriver CR, Becudet AL, Sly WS, Valle D, eds. *The Metabolic and Molecular Basis of Inherited Disease*, 7th edn. New York: McGraw-Hill, 1995: 3717–45.

17   Sabbagh Y, Jones AO, Tenenhouse HS. PHEXdb, a locus-specific database for mutations causing X-linked hypophosphatemia. *Hum Mutat* 2000; **16**: 1–6.

18   Blumsohn A. What have we learnt about the regulation of phosphate metabolism? *Curr Opin Nephrol Hypertens* 2004; **13**: 397–401.

● 19   White KE, Jonsson KB, Carn G, *et al.* The autosomal dominant hypophosphatemic rickets (ADHR) gene is a secreted polypeptide overexpressed by tumors that cause phosphate wasting. *J Clin Endocrinol Metab* 2001; **86**: 497–500.

● 20   Ecarot B, Glorieux FH, Desbarats M, *et al.* Defective bone formation by Hyp mouse bone cells transplanted into normal mice: evidence in favour of an intrinsic osteoblastic defect. *J Bone Miner Res* 1992; **7**: 215–20.

21   Steendijk R, Hauspie RC. The pattern of growth and growth retardation of patients with hypophosphatemic vitamin D-resistant rickets: a longitudinal study. *Eur J Pediatr* 1992; **151**: 422–7.

22   Steendijk R, Latham SC. Hypophosphatemic vitamin D-resistant rickets: an observation on height and serum inorganic phosphate in untreated cases. *Helvet Paediatr Acta* 1971; **26**: 179–84.

23 Glorieux FH, Marie PJ, Pettifor JM, Delvin EE. Bone response to phosphate salts, ergocalciferol and calcitriol in hypophosphataemic vitamin D-resistant rickets. *New Engl J Med* 1980; **303**: 1023–31.

24 Stickler GB. Familial hypophosphatemic vitamin D-resistant rickets: the neonatal period and infancy. *Acta Paediatr Scand* 1969; **58**: 213–9.

25 Rubinovitch M, Said SE, Glorieux FH, *et al*. Principles and results of corrective lower limb osteotomies for patients with vitamin D-resistant hypophosphataemic rickets. *Clin Orthop* 1988; **237**: 264–70.

26 Paley D. Problems, obstacles and complications of limb lengthening by the Ilizarov technique. *Clin Orthop* 1990; **250**: 81–104.

27 Wilson DM, Lee PDK, Morris AH. Growth hormone therapy in hypophosphatemic rickets. *Am J Dis Child* 1991; **145**: 1165–70.

28 Haffner D, Wuehl E, Blum WF, *et al*. Disproportionate growth following long-term growth hormone treatment in short children with X-linked hypophosphatemia. *Eur J Paediatr* 1995; **154**: 610–3.

29 Ahonen P, Myllaerniemi S, Silpilae J, Perheentupa J. Clinical variation of autoimmune polyendocrinopathy-candidiasis–ectodermal dystrophy (APECED) in a series of 68 patients. *New Engl J Med* 1990; **322**: 1829–36.

● 30 Richardson RJ, Kirk JMW. Short stature, mental retardation and hypoparathyroidism: a new syndrome. *Arch Dis Child* 1990; **65**: 1113–7.

31 Sanjad SA, Sakoti NA, Abu-Osba YK, *et al*. A new syndrome of congenital hypoparathyroidism, severe growth failure, and dysmorphic features. *Arch Dis Child* 1991; **66**: 193–6.

32 Hershkovitz E, Shalitin S, Levy J, *et al*. The new syndrome of congenital hypoparathyroidism associated with dysmorphism, growth retardation, and developmental delay – a report of six patients. *Isr J Med* 1995; **31**: 293–7.

◆ 33 Brown EM, MacLeod RJ. Extracellular calcium sensing and extracellular calcium signaling. *Physiol Rev* 2001; **81**: 239–97.

34 Levine MA, Germain-Lee E, Jan de Beur S. Genetic basis for resistance to parathyroid hormone. *Horm Res* 2003; **60(Suppl 3)**: 87–95.

35 Spiegel AM, Weinstein LS. Pseudohypoparathyroidism. In: Scriver CR, Beandet AL, Sly WS, Valle D, eds. *The Metabolic and Molecular Basis of Inherited Diseases*, 7th edn. New York: McGraw-Hill, 1995: 3073–89.

● 36 Schipani E, Kruse K, Jueppner H. A constitutively active mutant PTH-PTHrP receptor in Jansen-type metaphyseal chondrodysplasia. *Science* 1995; **268**: 98–100.

37 Kruse K, Schuetz C. Calcium metabolism in the Jansen type of metaphyseal dysplasia. *Eur J Paediatr* 1993; **152**: 912–5.

◆ 38 Rauch F, Schoenau E. The developing bone: slave or master of its cells and molecules? *Pediatr Res* 2001; **50**: 309–14.

● 39 Cole WG, Chow CW, Bateman JF, Silence DO. The phenotypic features of osteogenesis imperfecta resulting from a mutation of the carboxyl-terminal pro alpha 1 (I) propeptide that impairs the assembly of type I procollagen and formation of the extracellular matrix. *J Med Genet* 1996; **33**: 965–7.

40 Sillence D, Butler B, Latham M, Barlow K. Natural history of blue sclerae in osteogenesis imperfecta. *Am J Med Genet* 1993; **45**: 183–6.

● 41 Labuda M, Morissette J, Ward LM, *et al*. Osteogenesis imperfecta type VII maps to the short arm of chromosome 3. *Bone* 2002; **31**: 19–25.

42 Roughley PJ, Rauch F, Glorieux FH. Osteogenesis imperfecta – clinical and molecular diversity. *Eur Cell Mat J* 2003; **30**: 41–7.

◆ 43 Rauch F, Glorieux FH. Osteogenesis imperfecta. *Lancet* 2004; **363**: 1377–85.

● 44 Glorieux FH, Bishop NJ, Plotkin H, *et al*. Cyclic administration of pamidronate in children with severe osteogenesis imperfecta. *New Engl J Med* 1998; **339**: 947–52.

45 Stoker DJ. Osteopetrosis. *Semin Musculoskeletal Radiol* 2002; **6**: 299–305.

46 Stewart CG. Neurological aspects of osteopetrosis. *Neuropathol Appl Neurobiol* 2003; **29**: 87–97.

47 Peters C, Steward CG; National Marrow Donor Program; International Bone Marrow Transplant Registry; Working Party on Inborn Errors, European Bone Marrow Transplant Group. Hematopoietic cell transplantation for inherited metabolic diseases: an overview of outcomes and practice guidelines. *Bone Marrow Trans* 2003; **31**: 229–39.

24

Diabetes

DAVID B DUNGER, M LYNN AHMED

INTRODUCTION

In 1934 Mauriac described the case of a 10-year-old girl with poorly controlled type 1 insulin-dependent diabetes mellitus (TIDM) who had hepatomegaly, short stature, and excessive fat deposition on the shoulders and abdomen. She had recurrent ketoacidosis and puberty was delayed.[1] In those years, immediately after the introduction of insulin therapy, short stature was consistently reported in patients with TIDM[2,3] and clinical reports relating to the 'Mauriac syndrome' were still reasonably common in the 1950s. In 2001 Franzese and colleagues[4] reported a case of a 14-year-old girl with an 11-year history of type 1 diabetes mellitus. At diagnosis her height had been on the 95th centile and weight on the 50th centile. She was lost to follow-up for 5.5 years and presented again at 19 years with height on the 5th–10th centile and weight on the 10th–25th centile. She was Cushingoid, with hepatomegaly, a high AST, ALT and gamma-glutamyltransferase levels and was pre-pubertal. Intense insulin treatment $(1.6 \, U \, kg^{-1})$ and strict medical surveillance led to an improvement in her metabolic control, normalization of her biochemistry and resulted in catch-up growth indicating that deficient insulin replacement may have been the principal cause of the Mauriac syndrome.

In addition there have been a few studies reflecting the negative effect on longitudinal growth that may occur: Tattersall and Pyke[5] reported a mean difference of 2.5 inches in the final adult height and a 4–5 year difference in the age of menarche between identical twins with and without diabetes and reductions in the final height of children developing diabetes were reported even in apparently well-controlled subjects.[6–8]

Overall, however, the prognosis for growth of children with TIDM has gradually improved over the last five decades, reflecting the many advances in diabetic care. Most recent studies have suggested that final height is likely to be in the normal range for the majority of children with TIDM, although subtle abnormalities of growth, particularly during puberty, are still reported.[9] The study of the growth in TIDM remains an interesting area of research because it provides insights into the mechanisms whereby insulin and nutrition regulate growth and pubertal maturation. Furthermore studies on the growth of children, who later develop diabetes, may provide clues as to the complex interaction between the genetic predisposition and environmental influences that are central to the pathogenesis of TIDM.

GROWTH BEFORE TIDM DIAGNOSIS

Association between birth weight and the risk of developing diabetes has been found in some large population cohort studies. In 2001, Stene et al. reported on 1824 children with type 1 diabetes diagnosed between 1989 and 1998.[10] They found that the incidence of TIDM increased almost linearly with increasing birth weight over a wide range of birth weights. In 1988 a postal survey[11] of all newly diagnosed cases of TIDM in children under the age of 15 years was conducted in the United Kingdom. The results showed that children who subsequently developed diabetes were more likely to be heavier at birth compared to the national reference. Dahlquist *et al.* in a study of seven European centers compared 892 cases of TIDM with over 2000 controls and reported that low birth weight (<2500 g) and short birth length (<50 cm) were protective against TIDM.[12] In a Finnish study, Podar *et al.* reviewed 782 TIDM children and compared them to birth date and sex matched controls randomly selected from the Finnish national population register.[13] Boys with TIDM were longer and heavier at birth than controls while girls were just longer at birth.

Such associations between TIDM risk and size at birth could reflect subsequent postnatal weight gain. In a comprehensive review of nutritional risk factors and type 1 diabetes, Virtanen and Knip cite 20 references that have shown an association (before the diagnosis of TIDM) between increased infant weight gain and/or increased height and weight gains during childhood and greater risk of TIDM.[14] Height gain during infancy was also positively associated with risk in two studies[15,16] but not in another.[17]

The reports on weight gain during childhood are mixed, Blom *et al.*[18] and Bruining[17] found no relation to risk of developing TIDM, whereas in the EURODIAB study and a Finnish group[15,16] as well as a study of Swedish children over the first 2 years of life,[19] a positive association was observed.

Other studies have examined the growth of children before diagnosis of diabetes. Blom *et al.*[18] found rapid linear growth, but only in the boys who went on to develop diabetes, whereas Price and Burden[20] observed that both boys and girls with diabetes were taller at diagnosis. Both Finnish[16] and Dutch[17] children were observed to have a positive association between an increased height gain in childhood and the risk of subsequent TIDM. Bruining[17] also observed that both the children with TIDM and their siblings were taller than population controls. In both studies the parental heights of the control and TIDM children were similar. In contrast, one study by Leslie *et al.*[21] of 12 twin pairs observed a significant decrease in height velocity in the twin who subsequently developed diabetes. The growth nadir occurred at a mean of 1.2 (range 0.3–2.3) years before diagnosis.

It has been argued that variations in nutrition might predispose both to tall stature and to the development of diabetes. Obesity is related to tall stature during childhood and children destined to develop TIDM may weigh more during infancy.[22] Johansson *et al.*[19] retrospectively studied the growth, during the first years of life, in relation to the type of feeding in a group of 297 children who subsequently developed TIDM. They found that early weight gain was a risk factor for development of diabetes and argued that the lower weight gain in breast-fed babies might be a protective factor. A hypothesis put forward by Blom *et al.*[18] was that in the prediabetic phase there might be a tendency for hyperinsulinaemia that would accelerate growth.

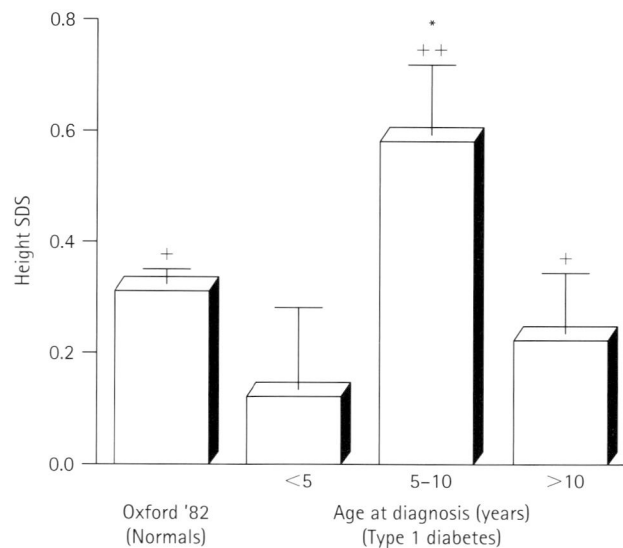

Figure 24.1 Height SD scores (from Tanner's data) at diagnosis of children with type 1 insulin-dependent diabetes mellitus (TIDM) and a representative sample of normal Oxford children. $+p < 0.05$ vs Tanner, $++p < 0.001$ vs Tanner, $*p < 0.05$ vs Oxford.

HEIGHT AT DIAGNOSIS

Several studies reported that children who developed TIDM were taller than controls at diagnosis,[6,23–28] whereas others refuted these observations.[5,7,29–31] It may be that this discrepancy is caused by the choice of control subjects. The choice of controls must reflect any secular trend in childhood growth that has occurred since many national growth references were first established.[32] This was exemplified in the study of Brown *et al.*,[33] who compared the height at diagnosis of 184 children with TIDM with the UK standards of Tanner *et al.*[34] The TIDM children were uniformly taller than controls. However, when the data were reanalyzed using contemporary controls, the authors found that only children diagnosed between the ages of 5 and 10 years were taller than controls (Fig. 24.1).

Controversy as to the height at diagnosis continues. Taller stature at diagnosis has been reported by several investigators.[18,20,35–39] Huang *et al.*[40] divided their Chinese cohort into pubertal and pre-pubertal subjects and found that only pubertal girls had a significantly elevated height SDS at diagnosis. Lebl *et al.*[41] in a review of 587 TIDM patients born in Vienna and Prague from 1962 to 1993 with a similar genetic background found the girls' mean height SDS at diagnosis to be $+0.74 \pm 1.46$, $p < 0.01$ and boys was $+0.15 \pm 1.1$, $p = 0.02$. Luna and colleagues[42] observed in a group of 83 newly diagnosed Spanish children that girls had a height SDS of $+0.40$ whereas the boys' height SDS was only $+0.08$. Thon *et al.*[43] and Cianfarani *et al.*[44] found those with diabetes to be of equal height at diagnosis to healthy controls.

Tall stature at diagnosis could be related to social class distribution, since it had been suggested that there was a bias towards the upper social classes in populations of children with TIDM.[26] However, Brown et al.[33] did not find any difference in social class distribution between control subjects and children with TIDM that would explain height differences in children diagnosed between the ages of 5 and 10 years.

The data presented by Brown et al.[33] were similar to those reported earlier by Songer and colleagues[27] from a large cohort of children in Pittsburgh, USA. Again, children diagnosed between the ages of 5 and 10 years were taller than national standards and the siblings of children with diabetes, who tested positive for islet cell antibodies, were also taller than those who tested negative. In this study, no direct association was found between height and HLA status. Barker et al.[45] have recently reported on the DAISY (Diabetes Auto-immunity Study in the Young) study. This is a prospective study to determine if earlier diagnosis in autoantibody children affects the clinical course after diagnosis (including any effect on growth). Both the high risk earlier diagnosed group and the community-diagnosed group had height SD scores at diagnosis that were greater than zero ($+0.12$ and $+0.41$, respectively).

Genetic heterogeneity may be responsible for the finding of the Pittsburgh (USA) group who compared their data with a comparable group of children with TIDM in Japan, and found striking differences in height at diagnosis.[46] More recently Ramachandran et al.[47] reported normal heights in children diagnosed in southern India.

There are also differences in height at diagnosis that relate to age at diagnosis. Heights of children under the age of 5 years reported by Brown et al.[33] were slightly smaller than control subjects and they tended to come from shorter families. Thus, the size at birth may be an important risk factor for the development of TIDM in children diagnosed before the age of 5 years. In contrast, subjects developing TIDM over the age of 10 years appear to have a normal height at diagnosis.[27,33]

GROWTH AFTER THE DIAGNOSIS OF TIDM

Most studies have reported a reduction in height SDS over the first 3 or 4 years after diagnosis.[26,33,35–38,40,43,48,49] However, one recent study reported normal pre-pubertal growth in a group of Belgium children with TIDM.[50] In the Oxford studies, Brown et al.[33] reported the greatest losses of height SDS, between diagnosis and the onset of puberty, in those children who were tallest at diagnosis, i.e., those diagnosed between the ages of 5 and 10 years. In those children the loss of height averaged 0.06 SDS per year. This loss of height could be considered as 'catch-down', although the mechanisms regulating growth in these children is still not clear, as discussed later. A recent study from Donaghue et al.[51] retrospectively compared the growth of children with TIDM stratified into two groups; one group was diagnosed between 1974 and 1990 and the second group between 1991 and 1995. Summarized from their data, Table 24.1 shows

Table 24.1 Height SDS from diagnosis of two cohorts of TIDM children

Ht SDS	Diagnosed 1974–90	Diagnosed 1991–95
At diagnosis	0.28 (1.01)	0.38 (0.99)
5 years follow-up	0.07 (0.99)	0.37 (0.94)
10 years follow-up	0.04 (0.87)	0.36 (0.89)

that the more recently diagnosed children do not lose height SDSs from diagnosis. This was ascribed to intensification of insulin treatment.

PUBERTAL GROWTH AND DEVELOPMENT

Delayed pubertal development was invariably reported in early studies of children with TIDM but this now appears to be less common,[26,28,33,52] although one study[50] revealed quite marked delay of puberty particularly in boys whereas another[48] demonstrated delayed puberty in the girls and not the boys. The Oxford puberty study of Ahmed et al.[36] reported no differences in the ages at the start of puberty between those children with TIDM and controls and no difference between the ages of menarche between the two (13.23 years compared to 13.00 years). Similarly no pubertal delay as evidenced by the age of menarche was observed in the Australian study of Donaghue et al.[51] reported to be 13 years in those girls diagnosed between 1974 and 1990 and 12.8 years in those diagnosed between 1991 and 1995.

There is a considerable consensus about the effects of diabetes on pubertal growth. Most investigators have noted that the pubertal growth spurt is blunted, particularly in girls with TIDM.[28,33,50] (Fig. 24.2). In many of the early studies the timing of peak height velocity was also delayed,[6,26] but recent data indicate that the timing and duration of the pubertal growth spurt are normal. Mean peak height velocity SDS ($\pm$SD) in the Oxford children was -1.09 ± 1.02 in the girls and -0.50 ± 1.14 in the boys.[33] Salardi et al.[28] reported that the poorest pubertal growth occurred in girls diagnosed just before the onset of puberty, whereas the Oxford data suggested that greatest loss of height during puberty was observed in those diagnosed under the age of 5 years.[33] Furthermore, there may be a sexual dimorphism as the study of pubertal growth by Ahmed et al.[36] observed that ages at peak height velocity were not different between subjects with TIDM and controls but that the girls (but not the boys) with TIDM had lower peak height velocities ($7.7 \pm 1.1 \, \mathrm{cm \, year^{-1}}$ compared to $8.4 \pm 0.9 \, \mathrm{cm \, year^{-1}}$).

FINAL HEIGHT IN TIDM

Despite the conflicting data in the literature about height at diagnosis and subsequent growth in TIDM, there is an overall impression that the outcome in terms of final height has

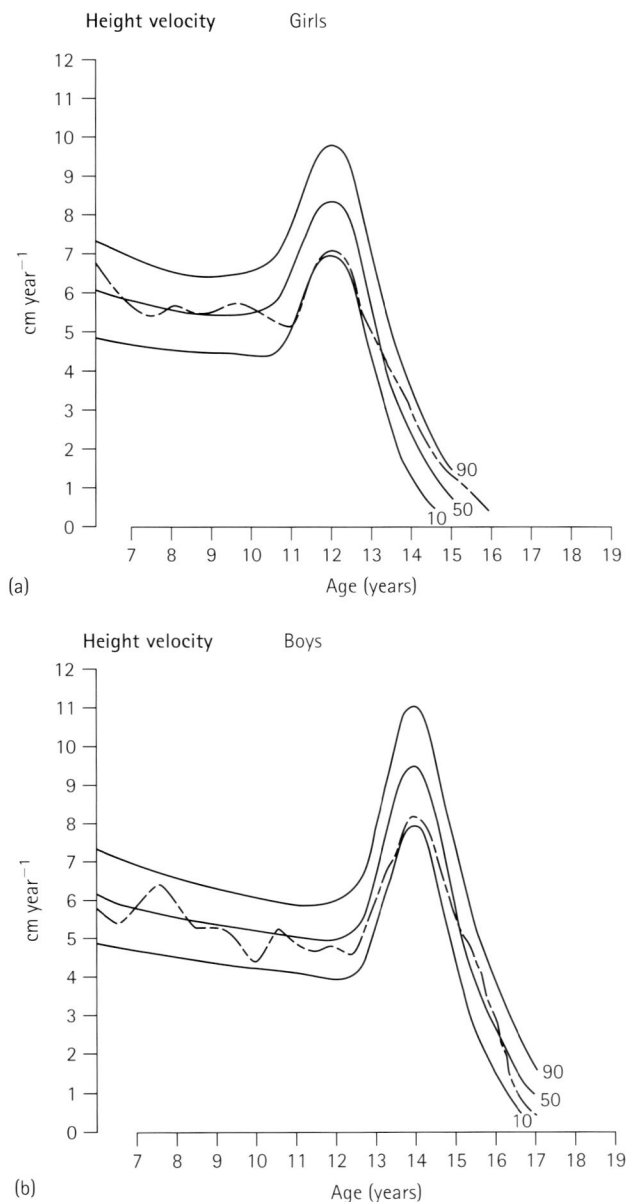

Figure 24.2 Mean height velocity during Puberty (---); (a) Girls and (b) Boys with TIDM. Data are compared to Tanner references and aligned with age at peak height velocity.

improved over the last 30 years. The final height data from the 80 children in the Oxford study did not differ significantly from the mid-parental height SDS;[33] nevertheless, the duration of diabetes was important, because those children diagnosed under the age of 5 years fared worse than this with a mean final height SDS of −0.74. However, as was pointed out earlier, in that study the children diagnosed under the age of 5 years tended to come from shorter families, and it is not therefore clear whether the poor outcome in terms of final height related to metabolic or genetic factors.[33] In a large study of children with TIDM and unaffected siblings, Holl et al.[37] concluded that longitudinal growth in diabetes may be temporarily reduced compared with unaffected siblings,

but this effect is small compared with genetic influences on height in any individual child. Even reported data about final height may be an underestimate because Heinz et al.[53] provided some evidence of continued growth, albeit at a very slow rate, right up until the age of 20 years. In a group of Chinese children, Huang et al. reported that height SDS was lost from diagnosis but final height was well within the normal range (girls −0.05 ± 0.86; boys, −0.13 ± 0.66).[40]

Conventional therapy, however, does not always guarantee optimal growth, especially in girls.[50] In the study by Ahmed et al., the girls were tall at diagnosis, but following their poor pubertal growth, the final height SD score (even when corrected for their mid-parental height) was significantly reduced in the girls but not the boys.[36] In all of the reported studies there is a very wide variation in growth rates but blunting of the pubertal growth spurt in girls, who have had a long duration of diabetes, may lead to considerable reductions in final height.[33] The Australian study from Kanumakala et al.[54] on children diagnosed pre-pubertally observed that boys and not girls had a decline in height SDS from diagnosis and their 'near final height' (age > 17.99) SD score loss from diagnosis was significant while the girls was not. Whereas Luna's (2004) Spanish children demonstrated a significant height loss in both sexes with a height SDS for the girls from 0.40 to 0.13 and in the boys from 0.08 to −1.02.[42] Thus conclusive data are still awaited but may be confounded by comparisons of different populations with varying glycemic control and insulin doses.

Weight gain in TIDM

Until recently the weight gain of children and adolescents with TIDM has been studied less often than stature. It has generally been observed that the range of body weights fell into the normal age-related distribution.[52] However, Thon et al.[43] in Germany demonstrated that, over the first 3 years from diagnosis, there was a greater increase in weight despite the relative reduction in length compared with controls. They also reported that the weight gain was not associated with accelerated skeletal maturation as reported in simple obesity. Pitukcheewanont et al.[55] noted a negative correlation between change in weight and height during puberty in TIDM.

In the study by Ahmed et al.,[56] BMI confirmed results from earlier studies that children with TIDM tended to gain more weight relative to height as they progressed through puberty.[37,43,55,57–59] In that study, body composition (assessed by skin folds) revealed that in the girls this increased BMI was largely due to an accumulation of fat mass and in the boys to a reduction in percent body fat. A summary of these changes (means ± SEM) in fat mass and percent body fat during puberty from that study is presented in Table 24.2.

Ingberg et al.[60] studying 18 post-menarcheal girls with TIDM, using dual-energy X-ray absorptiometry (DXA) and skin folds, also observed a higher body fat in the TIDM subjects and this was concentrated in the upper part of the body and associated with abdominal fat, insulin dose and

Table 24.2 Changes in fat mass and percent body fat in TIDM and control children

	TIDM	Controls	*p*
Fat mass (kg)			
Girls	10.7 ± 1.0	8.2 ± 0.4	0.04
Boys	3.5 ± 0.5	4.7 ± 0.8	0.2
Percent body fat			
Girls	8.1 ± 1.2	7.6 ± 1.1	0.8
Boys	−3.7 ± 0.8	−0.2 ± 1.0	0.008

HbA$_1$c. These observations of excessive weight gain may correspond to the introduction of intensified insulin therapy. Although this form of treatment may improve glycemic control, it does not necessarily reverse the blunting of the pubertal growth spurt. Furthermore, it can lead to excessive weight gain.[61,62] However, it may be that a recently introduced long acting insulin analogue that can be used to intensify insulin therapy and thus improve glycemic control does not inevitably lead to weight gain.[63]

Excessive weight gain can be associated with menstrual irregularity[64] and may be related to physiological, rather than psychological, factors. Yet excessive weight gain is frequently encountered in girls with TIDM during late adolescence.[60,65,66] Some studies indicate that, although adolescent girls may be more concerned than control subjects about weight and diet, and display features of disordered eating patterns, there is no definite evidence of an increased prevalence of overt eating disorders.[65,67] A recent Canadian study of 91 late teenage women with TIDM found that 29 percent had highly or moderately disordered eating behaviour.[68] Prospective studies of Bryden *et al.*,[67] however, suggest insulin omission may be common in adolescent girls in an attempt to control weight gain.

THE PATHOGENESIS OF GROWTH FAILURE IN TIDM

General considerations

The detection of slow growth in a child with TIDM may be the result of coincident thyroid or celiac disease. Autoimmune thyroiditis is very common in TIDM, thyroid microsomal antibodies being present in as many as 10.5 percent of all patients.[69] Frank hypothyroidism may develop in as many as 2.6–4.0 percent of patients and routine screening for thyroid disease in children with TIDM has been recommended.[70] Total thyroxine (T$_4$) and thyroxine-binding globulin (TBG) levels may be low in TIDM, and it is important to measure free thyroid hormones and thyroid-stimulating hormone (TSH) levels to establish the thyroid status.[69]

Celiac disease and TIDM are closely related and studies have suggested that the prevalence rates of celiac disease

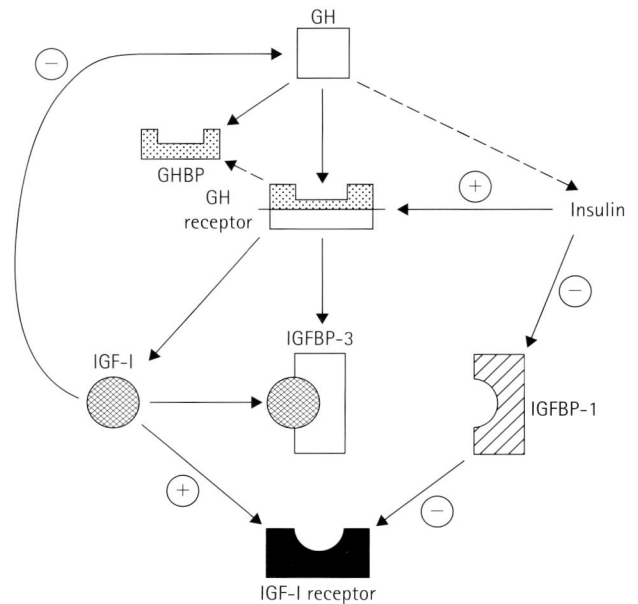

Figure 24.3 A schematic diagram of the GH/IGF-I axis and its relationship to insulin.

with TIDM may be 1–10 percent.[71–74] Many of these cases may be clinically asymptomatic or atypical in presentation and growth may not be affected. Nevertheless, appropriate screening tests using endomysial or antigliadin antibodies should be carried out in any child with TIDM who has growth retardation.[75] Amin *et al.*[76] recently showed that there was a recovery of their BMI SD score after 12 months on a gluten-free diet. Saadah *et al.*[77] also demonstrated a significant improvement in BMI and weight SD scores and also an increase in height SDS, although the latter did not reach statistical significance. It should also be remembered that there may also be coincident growth hormone (GH) or gonadotrophin deficiency and occasionally cases of Crohn's disease or other chronic diseases that affect growth will be encountered. These considerations apart, the pathogenesis of growth failure in TIDM appears to be closely linked to abnormalities of the growth hormone/insulin-like growth factor I (GH/IGF-I) axis and the regulation of that axis by insulin and nutrition.

The growth hormone/insulin–like growth factor–I axis

The GH/IGF-I axis is perturbed in TIDM (Fig. 24.3) and these disturbances can be attributed to portal insulin deficiency, down regulation of the hepatic growth hormone receptors and subsequent reduced circulating levels of IGF-I. Whereas spontaneous GH secretion is invariably increased in children and adolescents with TIDM[78,79] (Fig. 24.4) circulating levels of IGF-I are generally low or in the low–normal range.[80–82] It is likely that the poor pubertal growth seen in TIDM is related to the reduced levels of IGF-I[83] (Fig. 24.5). In a longitudinal study, Ahmed *et al.*[36]

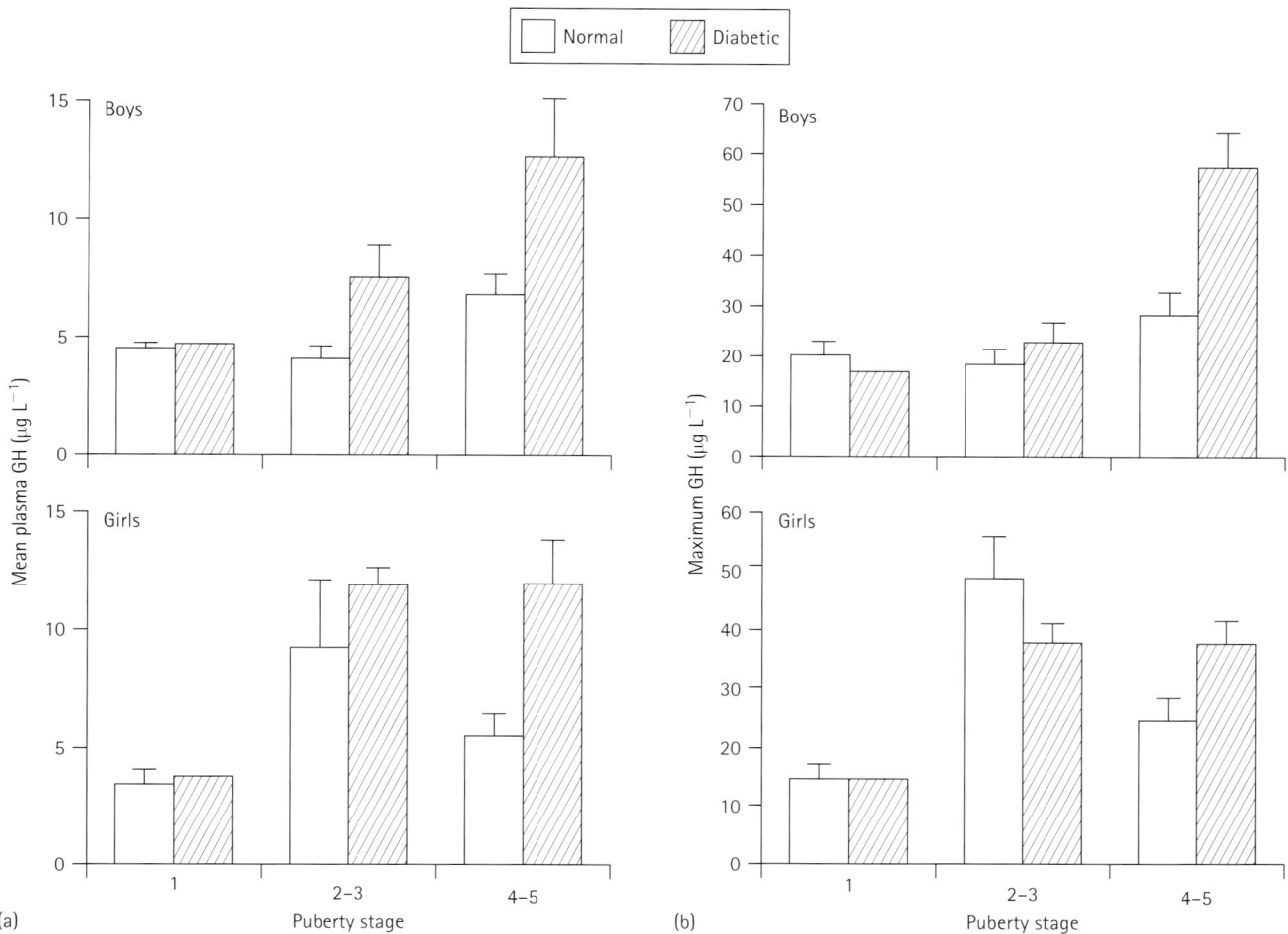

Figure 24.4   Mean ± SEM of growth hormone (GH) in TIDM and normal adolescents by sex and puberty stage. (a) Mean overnight GH concentration; (b) maximum GH concentration.

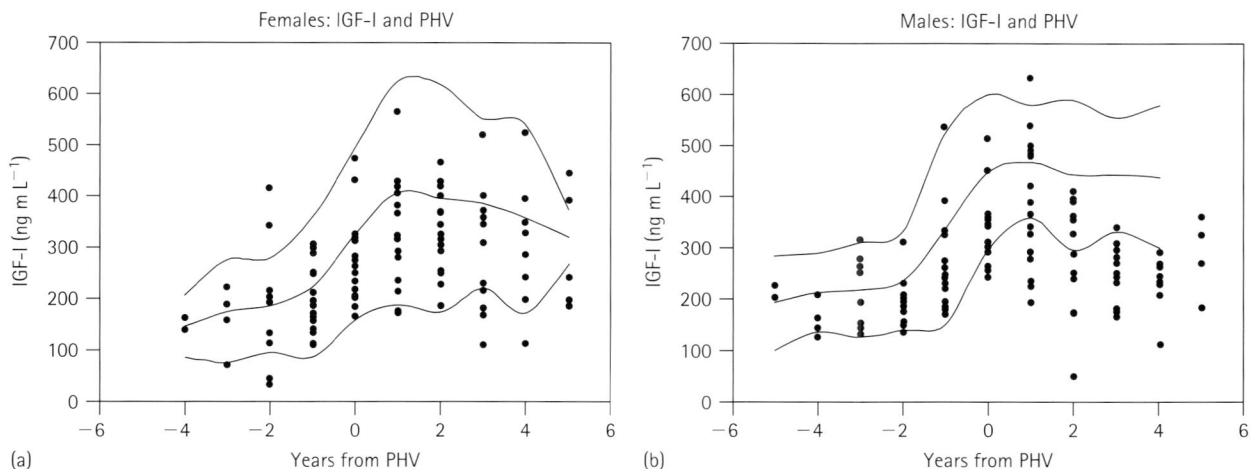

Figure 24.5   Levels of IGF-I in relation to years before and after peak height velocity (PHV) in (a) girls and (b) boys with TIDM. Curves are the mean and 95% CI for normal children.

observed low levels of IGF-I in TIDM subjects during puberty and also reported that IGF-I SD scores were lower in the boys despite reduced pubertal growth in the girls. Low IGF-I levels have been observed in both pre-pubertal[84] and pubertal subjects with TIDM[85] and levels of IGFBP-3 are

also low and fail to show the normal rise during puberty.[86] In contrast, levels of IGFBP-2 may be raised.[87]

A reduced IGF-I response to exogenous GH administration has been reported in children with TIDM[88] and there appears to be resistance to the effects of growth hormone at the level of the hepatic GH receptor. Some confirmation of this GH receptor resistance has come from studies of the circulating GH-binding protein (GHBP), which appears to be identical to the extracellular domain of the GH receptor and may reflect receptor numbers or function.[89] In adolescents with TIDM, GHBP levels are low compared with normal controls.[85,90–92] The development of GH resistance in TIDM is related to the relative insulin deficiency and occurs even in subjects on standard replacement therapy.

The role of insulin and nutrition in the regulation of the GH/IGF-I axis

Insulin has an important role in the regulation of the GH/IGF-I axis. *In vitro* studies suggest that insulin enhances hepatic IGF-I production, either by direct regulation of the GH receptor or by a permissive effect on post-GH receptor events.[93,94] In children with TIDM, levels of GHBP are closely related to insulin dose;[85,92,95] although GHBP levels are low in newly diagnosed patients an increase in levels is noted after 3 months of insulin therapy.[96] It follows that levels of circulating IGF-I are also closely related to total insulin dose in subjects with TIDM.[85,92,97]

Insulin also has a role in the regulation of IGF bioactivity through its effect on IGFBP-1.[98] Levels of IGFBP-1 vary inversely with levels of insulin and in most bioassay systems it appears to be an inhibitor of IGF bioactivity.[99,100] Thus high IGFBP-1 observed in children with TIDM during puberty may in part explain the reduced IGF bioactivity that has been observed.[82] Insulin may also have an important role in the regulation of IGFBP-3 protease activity[101] and thus regulate both the bioavailability and the bioactivity of IGF-I. Zachrisson et al.[102] in a study of boys in puberty observed elevated IGFBP-3 proteolysis in stage 3 compared to stage 5.

Intensified insulin therapy does not necessarily correct all of these abnormalities of IGF-I production. Once subjects are on therapy, it is the levels of insulin in the portal vein, rather than the systemic circulation, that determine IGF-I, IGFBP-1 and overall bioavailability of IGF-I in TIDM.[103] Even with intensified insulin therapy, portal levels of insulin may still be inadequate for normal generation of IGF-I and full correction of the GH/IGF-I axis.[9] Only direct portal administration of insulin will totally correct these abnormalities.[104]

Reduced portal insulin levels in children receiving standard therapy and the coexisting peripheral hyperinsulinism may also explain the excessive weight gain and menstrual abnormalities in TIDM.[64] Weight gain was an important complication observed after intensive insulin therapy in the diabetes complications and control trial in the USA, particularly during adolescence.[61] The relative imbalance between portal and systemic insulin with low levels of IGF-I may explain the correlation observed by Pitukcheewanont et al.[55] between excessive weight gain and insufficient increment in height.

Nutritional status is also an important regulator of GH receptor function and there are close correlations between

IGF-I levels and body mass index.[105] Restricted nutritional intake may have had a part to play in the pathogenesis of poor growth in the early days when strict carbohydrate restriction was recommended. Many of the children presenting with Mauriac syndrome had a very low energy intake and were thus maintained on a very small insulin dose. Correction of these problems was often enough to achieve catch-up growth (Fig. 24.6). These children had not only reduced circulating IGF-I levels, but also evidence suggesting resistance to the effects of IGF-I at a tissue level.[106]

IGF–I insufficiency as a cause of growth failure in TIDM

Although there is compelling evidence to attribute the growth problems in TIDM to abnormalities of IGF-I and its binding proteins, many observations are not explained by this simple analysis. Levels of IGF-I in TIDM are equally low in boys and girls during puberty (Fig. 24.5), yet blunting of the pubertal growth spurt is more marked in the girls (Fig. 24.2). This may reflect the observation that, in normal subjects, the pubertal growth spurt is more closely related to GH secretion in girls and to testosterone levels in boys.[107] Meyer and Kiess et al.[108] observed that in late puberty there is a higher level of both free and total testosterone in both boys and girls with TIDM. Levels of free testosterone may, if anything, be enhanced in boys because of low levels of sex hormone-binding globulin[109] and androgen levels may be the more important regulators of circulating IGF-I and IGFBP-3 levels in boys.[110]

Many recent studies that have examined the relationship between IGF-I levels and growth in TIDM have not allowed for these sex differences. Nevertheless, in very large studies, such as those carried out by Strasser-Vogel et al.,[111] although correlations were observed between IGF-I levels and growth in pre-pubertal children, these associations were lost during puberty. Ahmed et al.[36] have reported a detailed longitudinal analysis of growth in TIDM during puberty in both sexes. They were unable to detect any relationship between peak height velocity SDS and IGF-I SDS in patients with TIDM of either sex.

HbA₁c levels and growth in TIDM

The relationship between glycemic control, as judged by HbA$_1$c levels, and the growth of children with TIDM has proved difficult to define. Many studies have been unable to detect any relationship between HbA$_1$c and growth in these children with TIDM,[6,8,25,28,43,52,55] whereas another has reported a significant relationship between the two, most marked in the pre-pubertal years.[112] Methodological differences and, in particular, the retrospective cross-sectional design of many of these studies may explain the discrepancies. Two longitudinal studies identified a relationship between growth and HbA$_1$c: Gunczler et al.[113] were able to

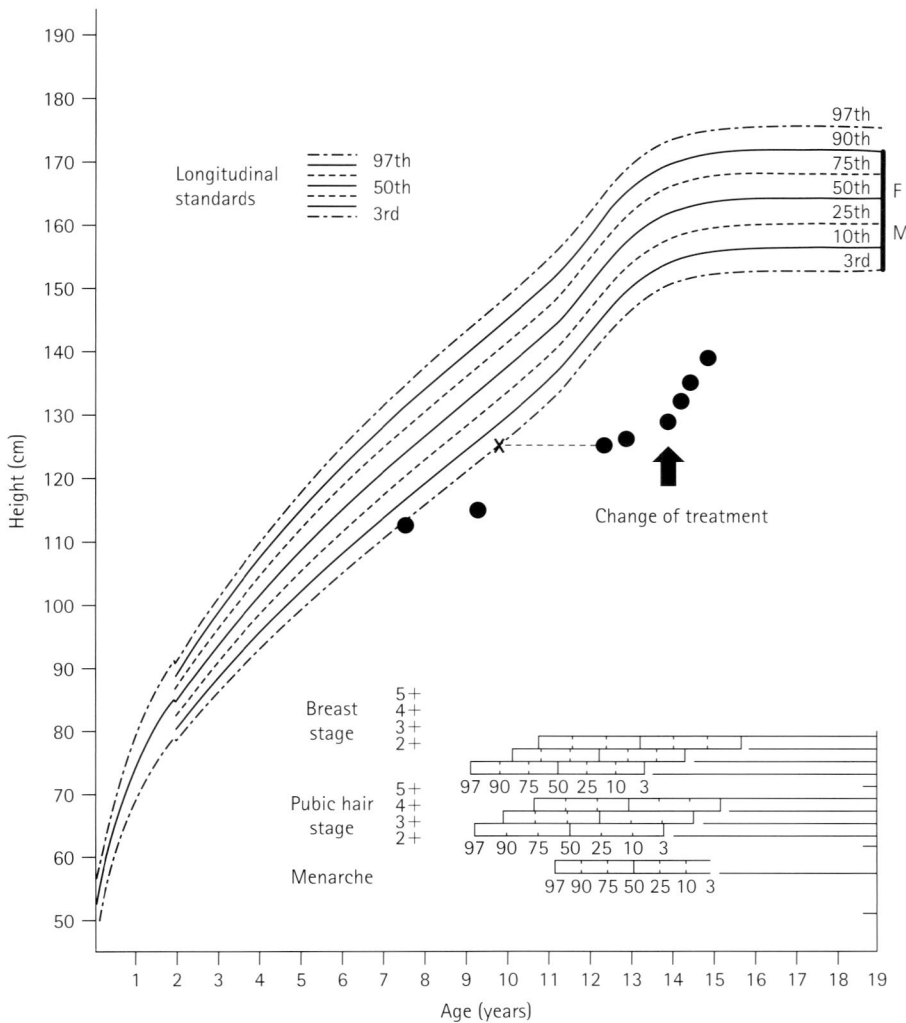

Figure 24.6 A child with Mauriac syndrome: response to treatment.

show that growth velocity over a five year period was significantly lower in children with higher HbA₁c levels and in their prospective studies, Ahmed et al.[36] demonstrated a clear negative relationship between peak height velocity SDS and HbA₁c (Fig. 24.7).

Levels of IGF-I and IGF bioactivity also show a weak correlation with HbA₁c,[97,111] although the relationship with insulin dose is stronger[85,92] (Fig. 24.8). Thus it remains difficult to resolve the conflicting data about the interrelationships of IGF-I, HbA₁c and growth in TIDM. Again these problems may in part relate to methodology, because measurements of IGF-I levels by radioimmunoassay may not accurately reflect free IGF-I levels and, more importantly, IGF bioavailability as a result of the complex interactions with the IGFBPs.[100] As our understanding of IGF-I/IGFBP interactions improves, these relationships may become clearer.

An alternative explanation is that poor glycemic control, as judged by HbA₁c, may have effects on bone metabolism, directly or indirectly through local paracrine changes in IGF-I and the IGFBPs. Bouillon et al.[114] reported decreased osteoblast function in children and reduced bone density has been reported in children[115,116] and osteoporosis in

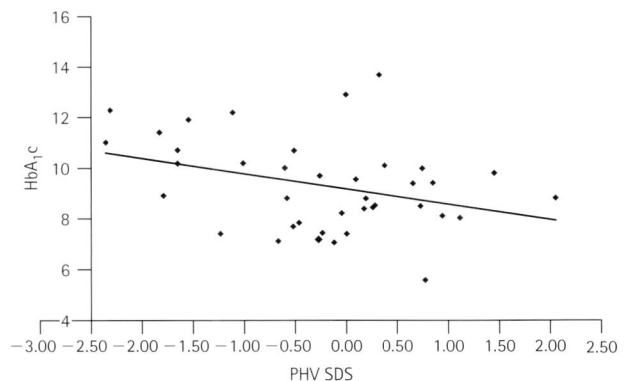

Figure 24.7 Relationship between PHV SDS and HbA₁c in TIDM children ($r = -0.35$, $p = 0.03$).

adults with TIDM.[117,118] However, a recent study by Ingberg using dual energy X-ray absorptiometry on 38 patients and age and sex matched controls found no difference in the bone mineral density between the two groups.[119] Bouillon et al.[114] concluded that any abnormalities in bone metabolism might be related to changes in IGF-I bioavailability, though other investigators have suggested that altered bone

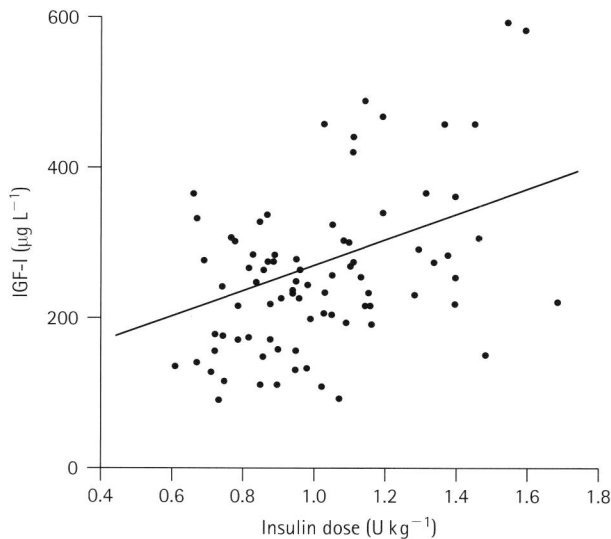

Figure 24.8 Relationship between IGF–I levels and insulin dose. From Clayton KI *et al.*[85]

density might be related to the persisting hypercalciuria which is frequently observed in TIDM.[120,121]

THE TREATMENT OF GROWTH DISORDERS IN TIDM

The detection of slow growth in patients with TIDM may indicate the development of coincident hypothyroidism or celiac disease[70,75] and in those cases appropriate treatment with thyroxine or a gluten-free diet will restore growth to normal. However, if these or other childhood diseases causing growth failure have been excluded, then slow growth is likely to be a direct result of diabetes and its treatment.

In children where growth velocity is impaired, treatment with growth hormone is clearly not an option, because the dose required would have to be high to overcome the GH resistance. This is likely to lead to deterioration in glycemic control with a possible increased risk for the development of diabetic microangiopathic complications.[122]

The close relationship of insulin dose, IGF–I and IGFBP-1 levels would indicate that intensified insulin therapy should improve growth velocity. The only study to examine this hypothesis directly was that reported by Rudolf *et al.*[123] Although those authors showed improved growth velocity with the introduction of continuous subcutaneous insulin delivery, many of the children were in early puberty and the changes might have related to the spontaneous pubertal growth spurt. Furthermore, intensive insulin therapy with multiple injection therapy or continuous subcutaneous insulin therapy may lead to excessive weight gain[61] and, as was stated earlier, may not correct all the abnormalities of the GH/IGF–I axis. Portal insulin delivery might be more appropriate in this respect, but it remains an experimental procedure.

Recombinant IGF–I could provide a logical method for improving the growth of children with TIDM,[124] and it

might bring the added benefit of improving insulin sensitivity by reducing excessive GH secretion.[125–127] A recent study by Saukkonen *et al.*[128] using a complex of IGF–I and IGFBP-3 on 15 young adults with TIDM resulted in increases in IGF–I and IGFBP-3 and reductions in overnight GH levels. However, it is yet to be determined whether increases in circulating IGF–I levels may have deleterious effects on the development of microvascular complications.[9] Several ongoing longitudinal studies should resolve these issues and determine whether recombinant IGF–I could have a place in the treatment of children with TIDM.

CONCLUSIONS

There can be no doubt that the prognosis in terms of growth of children with TIDM has improved considerably over the last 50 years, and relatively normal growth and the attainment of genetic height potential can be expected in most patients. Variations in heights at diagnosis and subsequent growth could relate to variations in glycemic control achieved in different centers or genetic differences in the populations studied. Nevertheless, blunting of the pubertal growth spurt and some loss of final height can still occur, particularly in girls with diabetes of long duration. These subtle growth abnormalities are closely related to changes in IGF–I and its binding proteins, but whereas these may be worse in children with poor glycemic control, the relationship between growth abnormalities and glycemic control is difficult to define. Although intensified insulin therapy may improve HbA$_1$c levels, it is yet to be proved whether this will prevent blunting of pubertal growth. The subcutaneous, rather than the portal, mode of administration of insulin may be critical in determining whether complete correction of the GH/IGF–I axis is achieved, and thus standard or intensified therapy may not completely correct growth abnormalities.

The peripheral hyperinsulinemia resulting from subcutaneous insulin delivery may explain excessive weight gain, despite poor statural growth, and this may be a limiting factor in attempts to achieve good compliance during adolescence. It is hopeful that newer analogs may be available that will intensify therapy without the concomitant weight gain. Recombinant IGF–I therapy might prove to be an appropriate alternative therapy for growth problems in TIDM but this has yet to be confirmed by long-term clinical trials, which must exclude any potential adverse effects on microangiopathic complications. Newer preparations of IGF–I complexed to its binding protein IGFBP-3 hold exciting possibilities of avoiding the adverse effects of IGF–I therapy.

Although the prognosis for growth in children with TIDM has improved, it will remain an area of intense interest, because it provides insights into the role of insulin in the regulation of growth and weight gain, and so serves as a model for our understanding of the regulation of growth in other nutritional disorders.

KEY LEARNING POINTS

- Children who develop type 1 diabetes (TIDM) tend to have higher birth weights than children who do not have TIDM.
- Early infant weight gain may be a risk factor in development of TIDM and this may explain the apparent protective effect of breast feeding (with its subsequent lower weight gain).
- Although controversy exists, tall stature at diagnosis is usually reported with a subsequent loss of height SDS although final height is generally within the expected familial range.
- A blunted pubertal growth spurt is observed especially in the girls and final height may be compromised in those girls with a long duration of TIDM.
- Increased BMI in girls with TIDM in later puberty was due to excess body fat compared to controls, whereas the boys with TIDM had a reduction in their percent body fat as they progressed through puberty.
- An imbalance in the GH/IGF-I axis exists with high levels of GH and low levels of IGF-I which result from low portal insulin levels with a relative peripheral hyperinsulinemia in TIDM that subcutaneous administration of insulin cannot prevent.
- New long acting analogues may address the problems of intensifying therapy and avoiding the concomitant weight gain.

REFERENCES

● = Seminal primary article
❋ = Key review paper

1 Mauriac P. Hepatomegalies de l'enfance avec troubles de la croissance et du metabolisme des glucides. *Paris Medecin* 1934; **2**: 525–8.
2 Joslin EP, Root HF, White P. The growth, development and prognosis of diabetic children. *JAMA* 1925; **85**: 420–2.
3 Wagner R, White P, Bogan I. Diabetic dwarfism. *Arch Dis Child* 1942; **63**: 667–727.
4 Franzese A, Iorio R, Buono P, *et al.* Mauriac syndrome still exists. *Diabetes Res Clin Pract* 2001; **54**: 219–21.
5 Tattersall RB, Pyke DA. Growth in diabetic children. Studies in identical twins. *Lancet* 1973; **2**: 1105–9.
6 Jivani SK, Rayner PH. Does control influence the growth of diabetic children? *Arch Dis Child* 1973; **48**: 109–15.
7 Petersen H, Korsgaard B, Deckert T, Nielsen E. Growth, body weight and insulin requirements in diabetic children. *Acta Paediatr Scand* 1978; **67**: 453–7.
8 Herber SM, Dunsmore IR. Does control affect growth in diabetes mellitus? *Acta Paediatr Scand* 1988; **77**: 303–5.
❋ 9 Dunger DB. Insulin and insulin-like growth factors in diabetes mellitus. *Arch Dis Child* 1995; **72**: 469–71.
10 Stene LC, Magnus P, Lie RT, *et al.* Birth weight and childhood onset type 1 diabetes: population based cohort study. *BMJ* 2001; **322**: 889–92.
11 Metcalfe MA, Baum JD. Family characteristics and insulin dependent diabetes. *Arch Dis Child* 1992; **67**: 731–6.
12 Dahlquist GG, Patterson C, Soltesz G. Perinatal risk factors for childhood type 1 diabetes in Europe. The EURODIAB Substudy 2 Study Group. *Diabetes Care* 1999; **22**: 1698–702.
13 Podar T, Onkamo P, Forsen T, *et al.* Neonatal anthropometric measurements and risk of childhood-onset type 1 diabetes. DiMe Study Group. *Diabetes Care* 1999; **22**: 2092–4.
❋ 14 Virtanen SM, Knip M. Nutritional risk predictors of beta cell autoimmunity and type 1 diabetes at a young age. *Am J Clin Nutr* 2003; **78**: 1053–67.
15 Group TESS. Rapid early growth is associated with increased risk of childhood type 1 diabetes in various European populations. *Diabetes Care* 2002; **25**: 1755–9.
16 Hypponen E, Virtanen SM, Kenward MG, *et al.* Obesity, increased linear growth, and risk of type 1 diabetes in children. *Diabetes Care* 2000; **23**: 1755–60.
17 Bruining GJ. Association between infant growth before onset of juvenile type-1 diabetes and autoantibodies to IA-2. Netherlands Kolibrie study group of childhood diabetes. *Lancet* 2000; **356**: 655–6.
18 Blom L, Persson LA, Dahlquist G. A high linear growth is associated with an increased risk of childhood diabetes mellitus. *Diabetologia* 1992; **35**: 528–33.
19 Johansson C, Samuelsson U, Ludvigsson J. A high weight gain early in life is associated with an increased risk of type 1 (insulin-dependent) diabetes mellitus. *Diabetologia* 1994; **37**: 91–4.
20 Price DE, Burden AC. Growth of children before onset of diabetes. *Diabetes Care* 1992; **15**: 1393–5.
21 Leslie RD, Lo S, Millward BA, *et al.* Decreased growth velocity before IDDM onset. *Diabetes* 1991; **40**: 211–6.
22 Baum JD, Ounsted M, Smith MA. Weight gain in infancy and subsequent development of diabetes mellitus in childhood [Letter]. *Lancet* 1975; **2**: 866.
23 Drayer NM. Height of diabetic children at onset of symptoms. *Arch Dis Child* 1974; **49**: 616–20.
24 Edelsten AD, Hughes IA, Oakes S, *et al.* Height and skeletal maturity in children with newly-diagnosed juvenile-onset diabetes. *Arch Dis Child* 1981; **56**: 40–4.
25 Hjelt K, Braendholt V, Kamper J, Vestermark S. Growth in children with diabetes mellitus. The significance of metabolic control, insulin requirements and genetic factors. *Dan Med Bull* 1983; **30**: 28–33.
26 Lee T, Stewart-Brown S, Wadsworth J, Savage D. Growth in children with diabetes. In: Borms J, ed. *Human Growth and Development*. New York: Plenum Press, 1984: 613–8.
27 Songer TJ, LaPorte RE, Tajima N, *et al.* Height at diagnosis of insulin dependent diabetes in patients and their

non-diabetic family members. *BMJ (Clin Res Ed)* 1986; **292**: 1419–22.

28 Salardi S, Tonioli S, Tassoni P, *et al.* Growth and growth factors in diabetes mellitus. *Arch Dis Child* 1987; **62**: 57–62.

29 Evans N, Robinson VP, Lister J. Growth and bone age of juvenile diabetics. *Arch Dis Child* 1972; **47**: 589–93.

30 Hoskins PJ, Leslie RD, Pyke DA. Height at diagnosis of diabetes in children: a study in identical twins. *BMJ (Clin Res Ed)* 1985; **290**: 278–80.

31 Emmerson AJ, Savage DC. Height at diagnos s in diabetes. *Eur J Pediatr* 1988; **147**: 319–20.

32 Chinn S, Price CE, Rona RJ. Need for new reference curves for height. *Arch Dis Child* 1989; **64**: 1545–53.

● 33 Brown M, Ahmed ML, Clayton KL, Dunger DB. Growth during childhood and final height in type 1 diabetes. *Diabet Med* 1994; **11**: 182–7.

34 Tanner JM, Whitehouse RH, Takaishi M. Standards from birth to maturity for height, weight, height velocity, and weight velocity: British children, 1965. I. *Arch Dis Child* 1966; **41**: 454–71.

35 Bognetti E, Riva MC, Bonfanti R, *et al.* Growth changes in children and adolescents with short-term diabetes. *Diabetes Care* 1998; **21**: 1226–9.

● 36 Ahmed ML, Connors MH, Drayer NM, *et al.* Pubertal growth in IDDM is determined by HbA1c levels, sex, and bone age. *Diabetes Care* 1998; **21**: 831–5.

37 Holl RW, Heinze E, Seifert M, *et al.* Longitudinal analysis of somatic development in paediatric patients with IDDM: genetic influences on height and weight. *Diabetologia* 1994; **37**: 925–9.

38 Holl RW, Grabert M, Heinze E, *et al.* Age at onset and long-term metabolic control affect height in type-1 diabetes mellitus. *Eur J Pediatr* 1998; **157**: 972–7.

39 Scheffer-Marinus PD, Links TP, Reitsma WD, Drayer NM. Increased height in diabetes mellitus corresponds to the predicted and the adult height. *Acta Paediatr* 1999; **88**: 384–8.

40 Huang CY, Lee YJ, Huang FY, *et al.* Final height of children with type 1 diabetes: the effects of age at diagnosis, metabolic control, and parental height. *Acta Paediatr Taiwan* 2001; **42**: 33–8.

41 Lebl J, Schober E, Zidek T, *et al.* Growth data in large series of 587 children and adolescents with type 1 diabetes mellitus. *Endocr Regul* 2003; **37**: 153–61.

42 Luna R, Fluiters E, Rodriguez I, Garcia-Mayor RV. Growth in Type 1 diabetic children. *Diabet Med* 2004; **21**: 1054–6.

43 Thon A, Heinze E, Feilen KD, *et al.* Development of height and weight in children with diabetes mellitus: report on two prospective multicentre studies, one cross-sectional, one longitudinal. *Eur J Pediatr* 1992; **151**: 258–62.

44 Cianfarani S, Bonfanti R, Bitti ML, *et al.* Growth and insulin-like growth factors (IGFs) in children with insulin-dependent diabetes mellitus at the onset of disease: evidence for normal growth, age dependency of the IGF system alterations, and presence of a small (approximately 18-kilodalton) IGF-binding protein-3 fragment in serum. *J Clin Endocrinol Metab* 2000; **85**: 4162–7.

45 Barker JM, Goehrig SH, Barriga K, *et al.* Clinical characteristics of children diagnosed with type 1 diabetes through intensive screening and follow-up. *Diabetes Care* 2004; **27**: 1399–404.

46 Anonymous. Height at onset of IDDM in high and low risk countries. Japan and Pittsburgh Childhood Diabetes Research Groups. *Diab Res Clin Prac* 1989; **6**: 173–6.

47 Ramachandran A, Snehalatha C, Joseph TA, *et al.* Height at onset of insulin-dependent diabetes in children in southern India. *Diabetes Res Clin Pract* 1994; **23**: 55–7.

48 Tillmann V, Adojaan B, Shor R, *et al.* Physical development in Estonian children with type 1 diabetes. *Diabet Med* 1996; **13**: 97–101.

49 Salerno M, Argenziano A, Di Maio S, *et al.* Pubertal growth, sexual maturation, and final height in children with IDDM. Effects of age at onset and metabolic control. *Diabetes Care* 1997; **20**: 721–4.

50 Du Caju MV, Rooman RP, op de Beeck L. Longitudinal data on growth and final height in diabetic children. *Pediatr Res* 1995; **38**: 607–11.

51 Donaghue KC, Kordonouri O, Chan A, Silink M. Secular trends in growth in diabetes: are we winning? *Arch Dis Child* 2003; **88**: 151–4.

52 Clarson C, Daneman D, Ehrlich RM. The relationship of metabolic control to growth and pubertal development in children with insulin-dependent diabetes. *Diabetes Res* 1985; **2**: 237–41.

53 Heinze HJ, Lowitt S, DeClue TJ, Malone JI. Blunting of the pubertal growth spurt with an extended period of linear growth through age 20 in subjects with type 1 diabetes mellitus. *Pediatr Res* 1993; **33**: 1134.

54 Kanumakala S, Dabadghao P, Carlin JB, *et al.* Linear growth and height outcomes in children with early onset type 1 diabetes mellitus – a 10-yr longitudinal study. *Pediatr Diabetes* 2002; **3**: 189–93.

55 Pitukcheewanont P, Alemzadeh R, Jacobs WR, *et al.* Does glycemic control affect growth velocity in children with insulin-dependent diabetes mellitus. *Acta Diabetol* 1995; **32**: 148–52.

56 Ahmed ML, Ong KK, Watts AP, *et al.* Elevated leptin levels are associated with excess gains in fat mass in girls, but not boys, with type 1 diabetes: longitudinal study during adolescence. *J Clin Endocrinol Metab* 2001; **86**: 1188–93.

57 Holl RW, Grabert M, Sorgo W, *et al.* Contributions of age, gender and insulin administration to weight gain in subjects with IDDM. *Diabetologia* 1998; **41**: 542–7.

58 Danne T, Kordonouri O, Enders I, Weber B. Factors influencing height and weight development in children with diabetes. Results of the Berlin Retinopathy Study. *Diabetes Care* 1997; **20**: 281–5.

59 Gregory JW, Wilson AC, Greene SA. Body fat and overweight among children and adolescents with diabetes mellitus. *Diabet Med* 1992; **9**: 344–8.

60 Ingberg CM, Sarnblad S, Palmer M, *et al.* Body composition in adolescent girls with type 1 diabetes. *Diabet Med* 2003; **20**: 1005–11.

61   Drash AL. The child, the adolescent, and the Diabetes Control and Complications Trial. *Diabetes Care* 1993; **16**: 1515–6.

62   Anonymous. Influence of intensive diabetes treatment on body weight and composition of adults in the Diabetes Control and Complications Trial. *Diabetes Care* 2001; **24**: 1711–21.

63   Fritsche A, Haring H. At last, a weight neutral insulin? *Int J Obes Relat Metab Disord* 2004; **28(Suppl 2)**: S41–6.

64   Adcock CJ, Perry LA, Lindsell DR, *et al*. Menstrual irregularities are more common in adolescents with type 1 diabetes: association with poor glycaemic control and weight gain. *Diabet Med* 1994; **11**: 465–70.

65   Peveler RC, Fairburn CG, Boller I, Dunger D. Eating disorders in adolescents with IDDM. A controlled study. *Diabetes Care* 1992; **15**: 1356–60.

66   Domargard A, Sarnblad S, Kroon M, *et al*. Increased prevalence of overweight in adolescent girls with type 1 diabetes mellitus. *Acta Paediatr* 1999; **88**: 1223–8.

67   Bryden KS, Neil A, Mayou RA, *et al*. Eating habits, body weight, and insulin misuse. A longitudinal study of teenagers and young adults with type 1 diabetes. *Diabetes Care* 1999; **22**: 1956–60.

68   Rydall AC, Rodin GM, Olmsted MP, *et al*. Disordered eating behavior and microvascular complications in young women with insulin-dependent diabetes mellitus. *N Engl J Med* 1997; **336**: 1849–54.

69   Connors MH, Dunger DB, Chapel H, *et al*. Diminished thyroxine-binding globulin in pubertal diabetic children. *Diabetes Care* 1996; **19**: 246–8.

70   McKenna MJ, Herskowitz R, Wolfsdorf JI. Screening for thyroid disease in children with IDDM. *Diabetes Care* 1990; **13**: 801–3.

71   Koletzko S, Burgin-Wolff A, Koletzko B, *et al*. Prevalence of coeliac disease in diabetic children and adolescents. A multicentre study. *Eur J Pediatr* 1988; **148**: 113–7.

72   Barera G, Bianchi C, Calisti L, *et al*. Screening of diabetic children for coeliac disease with antigliadin antibodies and HLA typing. *Arch Dis Child* 1991; **66**: 491–4.

73   Lorini R, Scaramuzza A, Vitali L, *et al*. Clinical aspects of coeliac disease in children with insulin-dependent diabetes mellitus. *J Pediatr Endocrinol Metab* 1996; **9(Suppl 1)**: 101–11.

74   Saukkonen T, Savilahti E, Reijonen H, *et al*. Coeliac disease: frequent occurrence after clinical onset of insulin-dependent diabetes mellitus. Childhood Diabetes in Finland Study Group. *Diabet Med* 1996; **13**: 464–70.

75   Rossi TM, Albini CH, Kumar V. Incidence of celiac disease identified by the presence of serum endomysial antibodies in children with chronic diarrhea, short stature, or insulin-dependent diabetes mellitus. *J Pediatr* 1993; **123**: 262–4.

76   Amin R, Murphy N, Edge J, *et al*. A longitudinal study of the effects of a gluten-free diet on glycemic control and weight gain in subjects with type 1 diabetes and celiac disease. *Diabetes Care* 2002; **25**: 1117–22.

77   Saadah OI, Zacharin M, O'Callaghan A, *et al*. Effect of gluten-free diet and adherence on growth and diabetic control in diabetics with coeliac disease. *Arch Dis Child* 2004; **89**: 871–6.

78   Edge JA, Dunger DB, Matthews DR, *et al*. Increased overnight growth hormone concentrations in diabetic compared with normal adolescents. *J Clin Endocrinol Metab* 1990; **71**: 1356–62.

79   Miller JD, Wright NM, Lester SE, *et al*. Spontaneous and stimulated growth hormone release in adolescents with type I diabetes mellitus: effects of metabolic control. *J Clin Endocrinol Metab* 1992; **75**: 1087–91.

80   Tamborlane WV, Hintz RL, Bergman M, *et al*. Insulin-infusion-pump treatment of diabetes: influence of improved metabolic control on plasma somatomedin levels. *N Engl J Med* 1981; **305**: 303–7.

81   Amiel SA, Sherwin RS, Hintz RL, *et al*. Effect of diabetes and its control on insulin-like growth factors in the young subject with type I diabetes. *Diabetes* 1984; **33**: 1175–9.

82   Taylor AM, Dunger DB, Grant DB, Preece MA. Somatomedin-C/IGF-I measured by radioimmunoassay and somatomedin bioactivity in adolescents with insulin dependent diabetes compared with puberty matched controls. *Diabetes Res* 1988; **9**: 177–81.

83   Dunger DB. Diabetes in puberty. *Arch Dis Child* 1992; **67**: 569–70.

84   Tapanainen P, Kaar ML, Leppaluoto J, *et al*. Normal stimulated growth hormone secretion but low peripheral levels of insulin-like growth factor I in prepubertal children with insulin-dependent diabetes mellitus. *Acta Paediatr* 1995; **84**: 646–50.

85   Clayton KL, Holly JM, Carlsson LM, *et al*. Loss of the normal relationships between growth hormone, growth hormone-binding protein and insulin-like growth factor-I in adolescents with insulin-dependent diabetes mellitus. *Clin Endocrinol (Oxf)* 1994; **41**: 517–24.

86   Batch JA, Baxter RC, Werther G. Abnormal regulation of insulin-like growth factor binding proteins in adolescents with insulin-dependent diabetes. *J Clin Endocrinol Metab* 1991; **73**: 964–8.

87   Knip M, Tapanainen P, Pekonen F, Blum WF. Insulin-like growth factor binding proteins in prepubertal children with insulin-dependent diabetes mellitus. *Eur J Endocrinol* 1995; **133**: 440–4.

88   Lanes R, Recker B, Fort P, Lifshitz F. Impaired somatomedin generation test in children with insulin-dependent diabetes mellitus. *Diabetes* 1985; **34**: 156–60.

89   Leung DW, Spencer SA, Cachianes G, *et al*. Growth hormone receptor and serum binding protein: purification, cloning and expression. *Nature* 1987; **330**: 537–43.

90   Menon RK, Arslanian S, May B, *et al*. Diminished growth hormone-binding protein in children with insulin-dependent diabetes mellitus. *J Clin Endocrinol Metab* 1992; **74**: 934–8.

91   Holl RW, Siegler B, Scherbaum WA, Heinze E. The serum growth hormone-binding protein is reduced in young

patients with insulin-dependent diabetes mellitus. *J Clin Endocrinol Metab* 1993; **76**: 165–7.

92   Massa G, Dooms L, Bouillon R, Vanderschueren-Lodeweyckx M. Serum levels of growth hormone-binding protein and insulin-like growth factor I in children and adolescents with type 1 (insulin-dependent) diabetes mellitus. *Diabetologia* 1993; **36**: 239–43.

93   Baxter RC, Bryson JM, Turtle JR. Somatogenic receptors of rat liver: regulation by insulin. *Endocrinology* 1980; **107**: 1176–81.

94   Maes M, Underwood LE, Ketelslegers JM. Low serum somatomedin-C in insulin-dependent diabetes: evidence for a postreceptor mechanism. *Endocrinology* 1986; **118**: 377–82.

95   Kratzsch J, Keliner K, Zilkens T, *et al*. Growth hormone-binding protein related immunoreactivity is regulated by the degree of insulinopenia in diabetes mellitus. *Clin Endocrinol (Oxf)* 1996; **44**: 673–8.

96   Arslanian SA, Menon RK, Gierl AP, *et al*. Insulin therapy increases low plasma growth hormone binding protein in children with new-onset type 1 diabetes. *Diabet Med* 1993; **10**: 833–8.

97   Rogers DG. Puberty and insulin-dependent diabetes mellitus. *Clin Pediatr (Phila)* 1992; **31**: 168–73.

98   Holly JM, Biddlecombe RA, Dunger DB, *et al*. Circadian variation of GH-independent IGF-binding protein in diabetes mellitus and its relationship to insulin. A new role for insulin? *Clin Endocrinol (Oxf)* 1988; **29**: 667–75.

99   Taylor AM, Dunger DB, Preece MA, *et al*. The growth hormone independent insulin-like growth factor-I binding protein BP-28 is associated with serum insulin-like growth factor-I inhibitory bioactivity in adolescent insulin-dependent diabetics. *Clin Endocrinol (Oxf)* 1990; **32**: 229–39.

100   Bereket A, Lang CH, Blethen SL, *et al*. Insulin treatment normalizes reduced free insulin-like growth factor-I concentrations in diabetic children. *Clin Endocrinol (Oxf)* 1996; **45**: 321–6.

101   Bereket A, Lang CH, Blethen SL, *et al*. Insulin-like growth factor binding protein-3 proteolysis in children with insulin-dependent diabetes mellitus: a possible role for insulin in the regulation of IGFBP-3 protease activity. *J Clin Endocrinol Metab* 1995; **80**: 2282–8.

102   Zachrisson I, Brismar K, Carlsson-Skwirut C, *et al*. Increased 24 h mean insulin-like growth factor binding protein-3 proteolytic activity in pubertal type 1 diabetic boys. *Growth Horm IGF Res* 2000; **10**: 324–31.

103   Brismar K, Fernqvist-Forbes E, Wahren J, Hall K. Effect of insulin on the hepatic production of insulin-like growth factor-binding protein-1 (IGFBP-1), IGFBP-3, and IGF-I in insulin-dependent diabetes. *J Clin Endocrinol Metab* 1994; **79**: 872–8.

104   Shishko PI, Kovalev PA, Goncharov VG, Zajarny IU. Comparison of peripheral and portal (via the umbilical vein) routes of insulin infusion in IDDM patients. *Diabetes* 1992; **41**: 1042–9.

105   Counts DR, Gwirtsman H, Carlsson LM, *et al*. The effect of anorexia nervosa and refeeding on growth hormone-binding protein, the insulin-like growth factors (IGFs), and the IGF-binding proteins. *J Clin Endocrinol Metab* 1992; **75**: 762–7.

106   Mauras N, Merimee T, Rogol AD. Function of the growth hormone-insulin-like growth factor I axis in the profoundly growth-retarded diabetic child: evidence for defective target organ responsiveness in the Mauriac syndrome. *Metabolism* 1991; **40**: 1106–11.

107   Merimee TJ, Russell B, Quinn S, Riley W. Hormone and receptor studies: relationship to linear growth in childhood and puberty. *J Clin Endocrinol Metab* 1991; **73**: 1031–7.

108   Meyer K, Deutscher J, Anil M, *et al*. Serum androgen levels in adolescents with type 1 diabetes: relationship to pubertal stage and metabolic control. *J Endocrinol Invest* 2000; **23**: 362–8.

109   Holly JM, Dunger DB, al-Othman SA, *et al*. Sex hormone binding globulin levels in adolescent subjects with diabetes mellitus. *Diabet Med* 1992; **9**: 371–4.

110   Crawford BA, Handelsman DJ. Androgens regulate circulating levels of insulin-like growth factor (IGF)-I and IGF binding protein-3 during puberty in male baboons. *J Clin Endocrinol Metab* 1996; **81**: 65–72.

111   Strasser-Vogel B, Blum WF, Past R, *et al*. Insulin-like growth factor (IGF)-I and -II and IGF-binding proteins-1, -2, and -3 in children and adolescents with diabetes mellitus: correlation with metabolic control and height attainment. *J Clin Endocrinol Metab* 1995; **80**: 1207–13.

112   Wise JE, Kolb EL, Sauder SE. Effect of glycemic control on growth velocity in children with IDDM. *Diabetes Care* 1992; **15**: 826–30.

113   Gunczler P, Lanes R, Esaa S, Paoli M. Effect of glycemic control on the growth velocity and several metabolic parameters of conventionally treated children with insulin dependent diabetes mellitus. *J Pediatr Endocrinol Metab* 1996; **9**: 569–75.

114   Bouillon R, Bex M, Van Herck E, *et al*. Influence of age, sex, and insulin on osteoblast function: osteoblast dysfunction in diabetes mellitus. *J Clin Endocrinol Metab* 1995; **80**: 1194–202.

115   Roe TF, Mora S, Costin G, *et al*. Vertebral bone density in insulin-dependent diabetic children. *Metabolism* 1991; **40**: 967–71.

116   Ponder SW, McCormick DP, Fawcett HD, *et al*. Bone mineral density of the lumbar vertebrae in children and adolescents with insulin-dependent diabetes mellitus. *J Pediatr* 1992; **120**: 541–5.

117   Saggese G, Bertelloni S, Baroncelli GI, *et al*. Bone demineralization and impaired mineral metabolism in insulin-dependent diabetes mellitus. A possible role of magnesium deficiency. *Helv Paediatr Acta* 1989; **43**: 405–14.

118   Shao AH, Wang FG, Hu YF, Zhang LM. Calcium metabolism and osteopathy in diabetes mellitus. *Contrib Nephrol* 1991; **90**: 212–6.

119 Ingberg CM, Palmer M, Aman J, *et al.* Body composition and bone mineral density in long-standing type 1 diabetes. *J Intern Med* 2004; **255**: 392–8.

120 Malone JI, Lowitt S, Duncan JA, *et al.* Hypercalciuria, hyperphosphaturia, and growth retardation in children with diabetes mellitus. *Pediatrics* 1986; **78**: 298–304.

121 Hough FS. Alterations of bone and mineral metabolism in diabetes mellitus. Part II. Clinical studies in 206 patients with type I diabetes mellitus. *S Afr Med J* 1987; **72**: 120–6.

122 Press M, Tamborlane WV, Sherwin RS. Importance of raised growth hormone levels in mediating the metabolic derangements of diabetes. *N Engl J Med* 1984; **310**: 810–5.

123 Rudolf MC, Sherwin RS, Markowitz R, *et al.* Effect of intensive insulin treatment on linear growth in the young diabetic patient. *J Pediatr* 1982; **101**: 333–9.

124 Dunger DB, Cheetham TD, Holly JM, Matthews DR. Does recombinant insulin-like growth factor I have a role in the treatment of insulin-dependent diabetes mellitus during adolescence? *Acta Paediatr Suppl* 1993; **388**: 49–53.

125 Acerini CL, Patton CM, Savage MO, *et al.* Randomised placebo-controlled trial of human recombinant insulin-like growth factor I plus intensive insulin therapy in adolescents with insulin-dependent diabetes mellitus. *Lancet* 1997; **350**: 1199–204.

126 Cheetham TD, Jones J, Taylor AM, *et al.* The effects of recombinant insulin-like growth factor I administration on growth hormone levels and insulin requirements in adolescents with type 1 (insulin-dependent) diabetes mellitus. *Diabetologia* 1993; **36**: 678–81.

127 Bach MA, Chin E, Bondy CA. The effects of subcutaneous insulin-like growth factor-I infusion in insulin-dependent diabetes mellitus. *J Clin Endocrinol Metab* 1994; **79**: 1040–5.

128 Saukkonen T, Amin R, Williams RM, *et al.* Dose-dependent effects of recombinant human insulin-like growth factor (IGF)-I/IGF binding protein-3 complex on overnight growth hormone secretion and insulin sensitivity in type 1 diabetes. *J Clin Endocrinol Metab* 2004; **89**: 4634–41.

25

Hemoglobinopathies

BEATRIX WONKE, VINCENZO DE SANCTIS

INTRODUCTION

The hemoglobinopathies (thalassemias and sickle-cell disease) are the most commonly inherited genetic disorders worldwide with some 240 000 infants born annually with major hemoglobinopathies and at least 190 million carriers worldwide. They are all inherited in a mendelian recessive manner so the person with the carrier or trait state is healthy.

The hemoglobinopathies have arisen as a result of mutations in and around the globin gene on chromosomes 16 and 11. These mutations have arisen and persisted within particular ethnic groups because of the selective advantage against *Plasmodium falciparum* malaria offered by the carrier state. The hemoglobinopathies are therefore not endemic to or found in the northern European population, but have come to this region with population migration. As a result there is hardly any large industrial town where patients with this disorder would not be present.

Patients with thalassemia and sickle-cell disease are now surviving into their fourth and fifth decades of life; however, many show problems with growth and sexual development in their adolescent years. In this chapter the clinical manifestations and management of growth in these patients are discussed.

THALASSEMIA

Pathophysiology

The basic genetic defect results in the destruction of the thalassemic red cells before the erythroblasts are well hemoglobinized; this is a consequence of the imbalance between the production of the α- and β-globin chains. This results in ineffective erythropoiesis leading to severe anemia, increased production of erythropoietin and expansion of the bone marrow by 15 to 30 times the normal. This marrow expansion results in distortion and fragility of the bone and an increased blood volume. The reticuloendothelial cells become congested by these abnormal red cells and consequently hepatosplenomegaly develops.

The growth and maturation of the thalassemic child are retarded and, in the absence of diagnosis and treatment, most die before the age of 5 years.[1] With the treatment now available, patients with thalassemia have a much improved prognosis. In a recently reported study by Cao *et al.*[2] the overall survival rate from birth was 97 percent at 10 years and 84 percent at 20 years.

Inheritance and genetic lesions

The inheritance is mendelian recessive and when two carriers (trait) mate there is a one in four chance in each pregnancy that the child will have thalassemia major. Thalassemia carriers can be identified by their low mean cell hemoglobin (MCH < 27 pg) and their raised hemoglobin A_2 (HbA$_2$ >3.5 percent). Once at-risk couples are identified, genetic counseling is given so as to allow the parents to make an informed decision regarding prenatal diagnosis. Safe and accurate diagnosis is possible in most cases before 10 weeks of gestation by chorionic villous sampling and gene mapping. Pre-natal diagnosis has led to a marked reduction in thalassemia in southern Europe and Cyprus (Fig. 25.1).

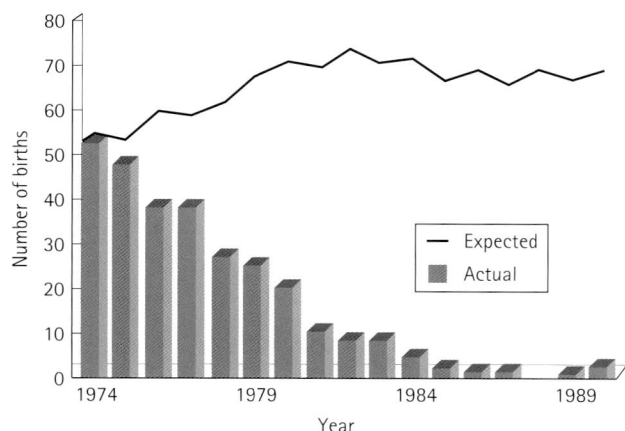

Figure 25.1   Annual incidence of thalassemia at birth since the introduction of prevention programs in Cyprus.

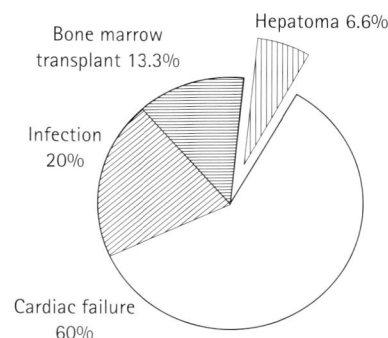

Figure 25.2   Causes of death in 15 thalassemia patients who died over the last two decades in the practices of one of the authors.[4]

Treatment

The recommended treatment for thalassemia is regular blood transfusions and chelation therapy, maintaining the overall mean hemoglobin level of about $12\,g\,dL^{-1}$. Pre-transfusion hemoglobin should be $9.5\,g\,dL^{-1}$ whereas post-transfusion hemoglobin should be a maximum of $14–15\,g\,dL^{-1}$. The aim is to transfuse $10–20\,mL\,kg^{-1}$ body weight of packed filtered red cells over a period of $2–3\,h$ throughout life. This ensures that erythroid marrow suppression preserves excellent health and normal development. The effectiveness of blood transfusion can be measured and frequency calculated from the rate of hemoglobin fall. In a splenectomized patient the fall is $1.0\,g\,dL^{-1}$ of hemoglobin a week, in a non-splenectomized patient it is $1.5\,g\,dL^{-1}$.

SIDE EFFECTS OF TRANSFUSION

Chronic transfusions may be associated with the following serious side effects:

- Allosensitization of clinically important antigens occurs in 25 percent of thalassemic patients receiving multiple transfusions. To avoid this complication, donor's red cells are matched closely with recipient red cells.
- Febrile transfusion reaction, cytomegalovirus infection and immunosuppression can be prevented by filtering the blood.
- Transfusion-associated viral infections (hepatitis B and C and HIV) are the most important problems in multiply transfused patients worldwide. In Europe and North America donors are now tested for these and the incidence is declining.
- Transfusion results in iron overload; if the iron is not chelated all patients die by the age of 20.[2] Cardiac iron overload causes heart failure and death (60 percent), greatly exceeding death from infections (15 percent) and liver disease (6 percent).[3]

Causes of death in some thalassemia patients are given in Fig. 25.2.

Complications of thalassemia major

Most of the complications are attributable to iron overload which may be the result of economic circumstances (expense of the chelation therapy), late onset of chelation therapy or poor compliance with the desferrioxamine treatment. Compliance is the major problem in Europe and North America. In iron overload, excess iron deposited in the tissues causes damage. Toxicity starts when the iron load in a particular tissue exceeds the tissue or blood-binding capacity of iron, and free non-transferrin iron appears.[5,6] The 'free iron' is a catalyst of the production of oxygen species that damage cells and peroxidize membrane lipids leading to cell destruction. Heart cells generate only small amounts of storage proteins and are therefore sensitive to 'free iron'-induced oxygen radicals. This leads to cardiomyopathy secondary to myocardial fibrosis and eventual cardiac failure and death.[7,8] Other organs sensitive to the 'free iron'-induced oxygen radicals are the endocrine glands, whereas the liver has a large capacity to produce proteins that bind the iron and store it in the form of ferritin and hemosiderin.

Influence of β-thalassemia on growth

Growth disturbances are a major clinical feature of patients with thalassemia. Although some patients show normal growth and development, many have growth retardation and failure of puberty.

FACTORS CONTRIBUTING TO GROWTH RETARDATION IN THALASSEMIA

- Chronic anemia
- Hypersplenism
- Endocrine disorders secondary to iron overload
- Chronic liver disease
- Desferrioxamine toxicity.

In a collaborative study of the Italian Paediatric Society,[10] short stature was present in over 20 percent of 3099 thalassemic patients. In chronic diseases, such as thalassemia, there is more than one factor that can cause growth retardation. Not all the factors are operative in every child at any one time, but many of them can be inter-related.

CHRONIC ANEMIA

The severity of the anemia depends on the type of the genetic mutation inherited by the child. In the most severe cases, the infant fails to thrive and requires transfusion before 2 years of age. In the late-onset type of thalassemia, the child may present after 2 years of age with growth impairment, lack of muscular tissue, giving the limbs a characteristic bony appearance, together with limited exercise tolerance. Hepatosplenomegaly and facial changes may also be present. Patients with thalassemia intermedia maintain a higher hemoglobin level ($>7\,g\,dL^{-1}$) which ensures normal growth in most cases. The beneficial effects of blood transfusion on growth and bone structure have been very well recognized since 1964. To ensure normal growth the mean pre-transfusional hemoglobin level should not be below $8.5–9\,g\,dL^{-1}$.[11] Well-transfused patients are physically indistinguishable from their normal peers: they show normal growth, are free of facial and skeletal deformities, and can perform strenuous exercise.

HYPERSPLENISM

Inadequate transfusion leads to massive hypersplenism caused by extramedullary erythropoiesis. A large spleen increases blood consumption, accelerates iron overload, worsens anemia and causes growth retardation. Splenectomy should be undertaken when the annual blood consumption is greater than $200\,mL\,kg^{-1}$ body weight. Before splenectomy meningococcal, pneumococcal and *Hemophilus influenzae b* vaccines should be given and penicillin prophylaxis is recommended for life afterwards. In patients with thalassemia intermedia after splenectomy, high platelet counts may cause thromboembolic complications. Low-dose soluble aspirin 75 mg daily or an antiplatelet-aggregating agent is recommended. In thalassemia intermedia folic acid deficiency may aggravate the severity of anemia and treatment with oral folic acid 5 mg daily is recommended.

Post-splenectomy, blood consumption declines and in late-onset thalassemia regular transfusions may stop, growth accelerates and the genetically determined height may be reached within 12 months.

EFFECTS OF NUTRITIONAL FACTORS

Undernutrition is an important cause of growth retardation in thalassemic children living in poor countries. Short stature is primarily caused by inadequate nutrient intake (zinc, folic acid, carotenoids and retinal binding proteins).[12]

IRON OVERLOAD

As the management of thalassemia has changed gradually over the years, some factors responsible for growth

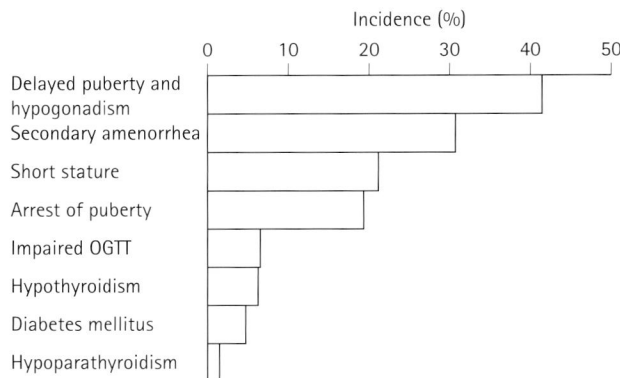

Figure 25.3   Incidence (percent) of growth retardation and endocrinopathies in 3099 thalassemia patients. OGTT, oral glucose tolerance test.

retardation, such as anemia or folic acid deficiency, are no longer important because they can be corrected by transfusions. Iron overload resulting from repeated blood transfusions is always present in thalassemia despite iron chelation therapy, and has been thought to be the cause of endocrine abnormalities. This is supported by histological studies of different endocrine glands. The incidence of growth retardation and endocrinopathies in a large multicenter study[10] is shown in Fig. 25.3.

SHORT STATURE

Thalassemic children of both sexes show reduced growth around the age of 10–11 years. This results in a final height which is below the predicted mid-parental height. The cause of this is not fully understood, but several mechanisms have been suggested. First, disorders of growth hormone (GH) secretion:

- Neurosecretory dysfunction
- Hypothalamic GHRH deficiency
- Pituitary GH deficiency
- Increased somatostatin activity

Second, disorders of post-GH secretion:

- Defective synthesis of insulin-like growth factors (IGFs) or damage to the site of IGF production
- Growth hormone resistance

The above factors are attributed to hypothalamic–pituitary damage by hemosiderosis and defective hepatic synthesis of IGF-I. Recently, De Luca *et al.*[13] reported that an increased somatostatin tone may be responsible for the low GH reserves in some patients.

The first author's group recommends that a careful assessment of growth is made at each follow-up visit from early childhood. Growth parameters should include linear height, sitting height and height velocity. All these parameters should be plotted on a growth chart in order to detect a variation of growth at an early stage (Fig. 25.4).

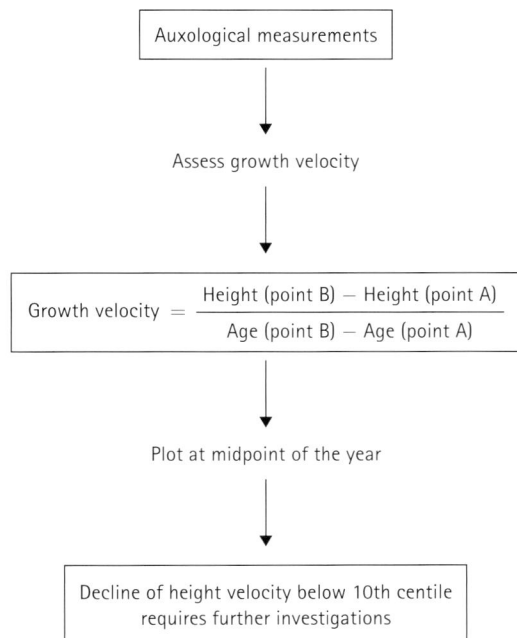

Figure 25.4   Flow chart for monitoring growth in thalassemia.

The investigation and treatment protocol in thalassemic patients with short stature and/or reduced growth velocity are shown in Table 25.1.

RECOMMENDED PROTOCOL FOR INVESTIGATION OF THALASSEMIC PATIENTS WITH GROWTH HORMONE INSUFFICIENCY

Selection criteria

1. Prepubertal and pubertal patients with potential for growth.
2. Short stature (less than 3rd centile) and/or reduced growth velocity (<10th centile for the bone age).
3. Priming with sex steroids is necessary in boys with a bone age of 10 years or greater. An intramuscular injection of testosterone ester (Sustanon) 100 mg is given 7 days before GH stimulation tests. Ethinyl estradiol 50 mg is given orally for 3 days before GH stimulation tests in girls aged 9 years or older. Girls whose bone age is less than 9 years and boys whose bone age is less than 10 years do not need priming. Desferrioxamine (Desferal) should be discontinued 7 days before priming and during the stimulation tests.
4. Significant GH insufficiency may be diagnosed by a reduced response of growth hormone to two provocative tests (GH peak <10 ng mL^{-1}).

Treatment

Recombinant human growth hormone (rhGH) is given subcutaneously and self-administered every evening for 6

Table 25.1   Protocol of investigation and treatment of thalassemia patients with short stature/slow growth

Investigations
> Auxological examination: standing and sitting height, arm length (from acromion) and pubertal staging (Tanner)
> Bone age (Tanner–Whitehouse)
> Assessment of GH secretion with conventional tests
> Thyroid function tests: TSH and free T4
> IGF-I and IGFBP-3 plasma assay (if available)
> Routine blood tests: full blood count and differential, liver function tests, calcium and phosphate, alkaline phosphatase, serum creatinine, electrolytes, serum ferritin and serum zinc
> Transglutaminase antibodies
> Urine analysis (protein, blood and glucose)

Treatment
> Recombinant human growth hormone is self-administered subcutaneously, every evening 6 days a week (Sunday excluded). Patient response can vary:
> *Responders*: growth velocity above 4 cm year^{-1} greater than the previous year
> *Partial responders*: growth velocity equal to 2–4 cm year^{-1} above the previous year
> *Non-responders*: growth velocity less than 2 cm year^{-1} above the previous year

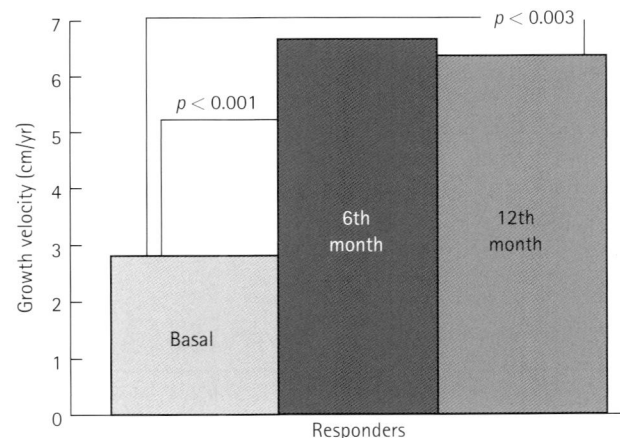

Figure 25.5   Growth velocity (cm year^{-1}) before and 6 months and 12 months after rhGH treatment.

days a week. The recommended rhGH dose is 0.6–0.8 IU kg^{-1} week^{-1} (divided into six doses).

It seems that the treatment gives positive results only in a small number of patients (Fig. 25.5) and the results are satisfactory mainly in the first year of treatment.[14]

Better results have been reported by Theodoridis *et al.*,[15] in 13 patients treated with rhGH (0.5 IU kg^{-1} week^{-1}) for 1.7–9 years. In these patients the final height, at the end of therapy, increased by 1 SD.

At present it is difficult to explain the suboptimal response to rhGH treatment observed in some thalassemic patients.

Table 25.2   Clinical features and grades of hypothyroidism

Hypothyroidism	Serum T_4	Serum FT_4	Serum TSH	TSH response to TRH
Pre-clinical	Normal	Normal	Marginally increased	Increased
Mild	Marginally low	Marginally low	Elevated	Exaggerated
Overt	Low	Low	Elevated	Exaggerated

Adapted from Evered et al.[17]

T_4, thyroxine; FT_4, free thyroxine; TSH, thyroid-stimulating hormone; TRH, thyrotrophin-releasing hormone.

The most likely hypothesis is a partial GH insensitivity[16] and/or a platyspondily of vertebral bodies.

HYPOTHYROIDISM

Hypothyroidism is observed in over 17 percent of iron-overloaded patients but it is rare in well-treated patients. In iron-overloaded patients with hypothyroidism, the thyroid glands contain large amounts of iron granules in the follicular epithelium and iron-laden macrophages can be seen in the interstitium. Fibrosis of the thyroid gland is moderate to marked. In mild-to-severe hypothyroidism, the following clinical features can be observed: decreased activity, dry skin, growth retardation, cardiac failure and pericardial effusion. The thyroid gland is normally not enlarged. Anti-thyroglobulin and antimicrosomal antibodies are not usually present. A summary of clinical and laboratory investigations is given in Table 25.2.[16] Treatment depends on the severity of organ failure. Replacement with L-thyroxine is recommended. Growth improves with treatment. Secondary hypothyroidism, caused by iron-mediated damage to the pituitary gland, occurs very rarely.

DELAYED PUBERTY AND HYPOGONADISM

Delayed puberty and hypogonadotrophic hypogonadism are the most common endocrine complications in patients with thalassemia (see Fig. 25.3). Transfusional hemosiderosis into the cells of the pituitary gonadotrophs which cause gonadotrophin deficiency is responsible for this endocrine dysfunction. The anterior pituitary gland is particularly sensitive to the free radicals caused by the oxidative stresses experienced, and exposure to this early in childhood results in pituitary damage. Histological examination of the gonads show minimal siderosis with occasional iron-containing macrophages in the ovaries and reduced numbers of primordial follicles. In the testes most of the iron is deposited in seminiferous tubules and the interstitial tissue and only a minimal amount in Leydig's cells. Clinically, patients are sexually infantile or have arrested puberty and markedly reduced growth velocity.

Treatment

The treatment of delayed or arrested puberty, and hypogonadotrophic hypogonadism depends on factors such as age, severity of iron overload, damage to the hypothalamic–pituitary–gonadal axis, chronic liver disease, and the presence of psychological problems resulting from hypogonadism. Collaboration between endocrinologists and other doctors is critical.

For girls, therapy may begin with the oral administration of ethinyl estradiol (2.5–5 μg daily) for 6 months, followed by hormonal reassessment. If spontaneous puberty does not occur within 6 months after stopping the treatment, oral estrogen is re-introduced with gradually increasing dosages (ethinyl estradiol from 5–10 μg daily) for another 12 months, If breakthrough uterine bleeding does not occur, then low estrogen–progesterone hormone replacement is the recommended treatment.

For delayed puberty in males, low dosages of intramuscular depot-testosterone esters (25 mg m^{-2}) are given monthly for 6 months. This is followed by hormonal reassessment. In patients with hypogonadotrophic hypogonadism, the therapy (50 mg m^{-2}) can be continued until the growth rates wane. The fully virilizing dose is 50–75 mg of depot-testosterone esters every 7–10 days administered intramuscularly. The same effects can be achieved with transdermal non-scrotal testosterone patches.

For pubertal arrest, the treatment consists of testosterone esters as for delayed puberty and hypogonadotrophic hypogonadism. The treatment of pubertal disorders is a complex issue due to the many associated complications; each patient has to be assessed individually.

DESFERRIOXAMINE TOXICITY

Maintenance transfusions preserve excellent health but, without treatment of iron overload, it leads to severe organ damage and eventually to cardiac death. At present the only available iron-chelating agent is desferrioxamine. The iron chelation therapy starts when serum ferritin (measure of iron overload) reaches 1000 mg L^{-1}. Desferrioxamine is given either subcutaneously, from a small portable syringe-driver pump infused over 8–12 h, at least 5–6 nights a

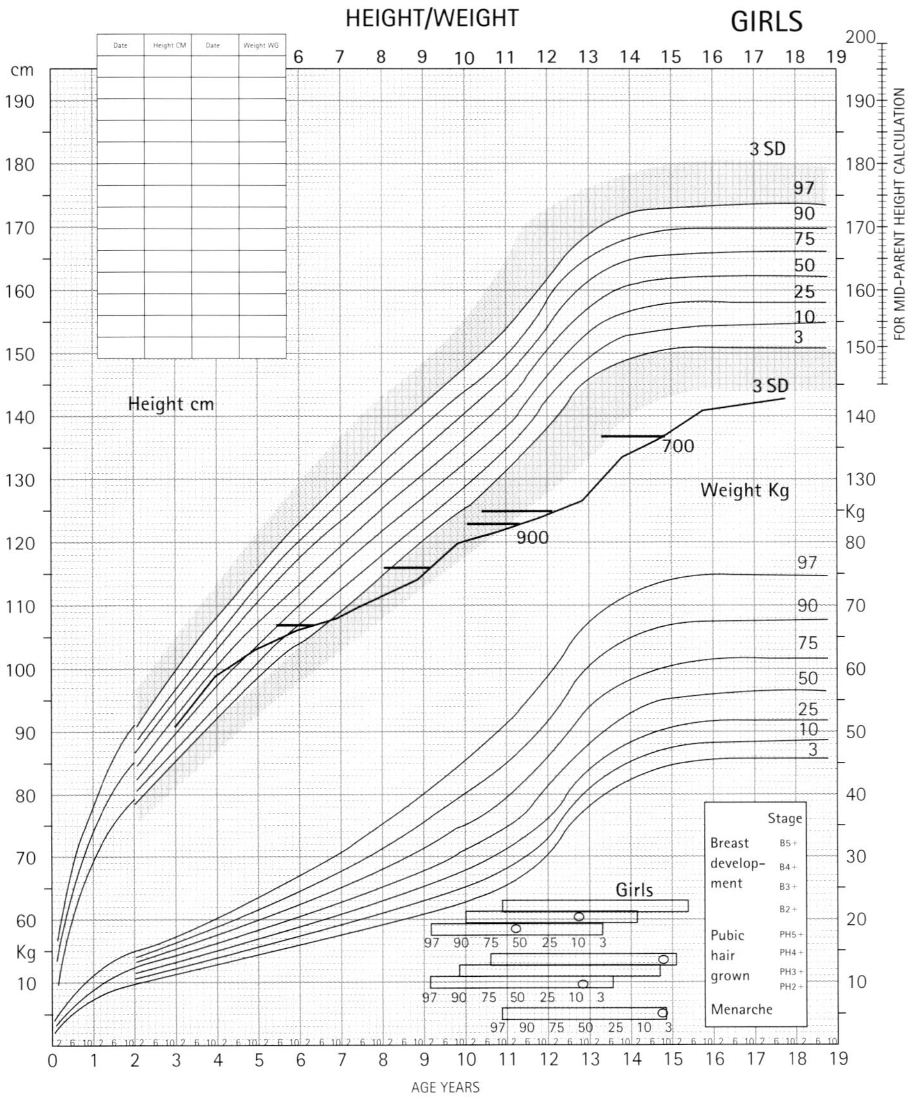

Figure 25.6 Growth curves in a patient with desferrioxamine toxicity. The numbers refer to serum ferritin (μg L^{-1}) levels.

week, or intravenously through an intravenous continuous delivery device. Desferrioxamine is a remarkably safe drug when given from early childhood and continued for life. However, ophthalmic complications and autotoxicity have been observed in patients receiving high doses of intravenous desferrioxamine.[18] The toxic effect of high doses of desferrioxamine on skeletal growth is still unresolved. It is known that desferrioxamine inhibits DNA synthesis, fibroblast proliferation and collagen formation, and possibly also causes zinc deficiency.

In well-treated and chelated patients with thalassemia three phases of growth have been observed:

1. Normal or subnormal growth velocity between birth and the first years of age
2. Decreased height velocity in peripubertal years of age
3. Reduced pubertal growth spurt

Patients who receive inappropriately high doses of desferrioxamine when the iron burden is minimal frequently complain of pain in the hips and lower back, and have difficulties in walking with growth arrest and reduction of growth velocity (Fig. 25.6). The body measurements are disproportionate: characteristically they have short trunks with discrepancy between the upper and lower segments (Fig. 25.7). Radiographic features include vertebral demineralization flatness of vertebral bodies (Fig. 25.8a) and pseudorickets-like lesions of the extremities (Fig. 25.8b, c).

Using microradiography and X-ray diffraction (XRD) of bone biopsies, we found in thalassemic subjects a reduced and irregular mineralization of the bone (compared with controls). Bone tissue microhardness was also significantly reduced. Nevertheless, bone apatite lattice was unaltered and no 'foreign' crystallographic phase was recorded by XRD.[19]

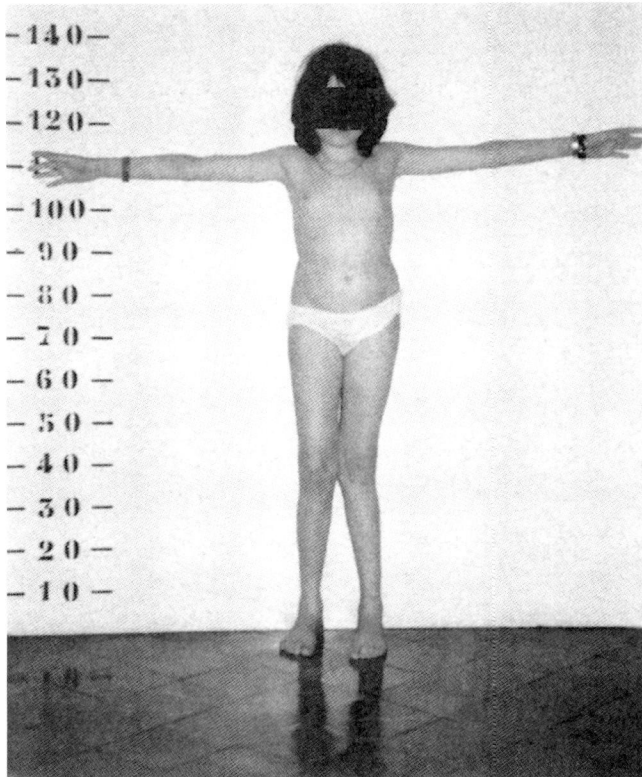

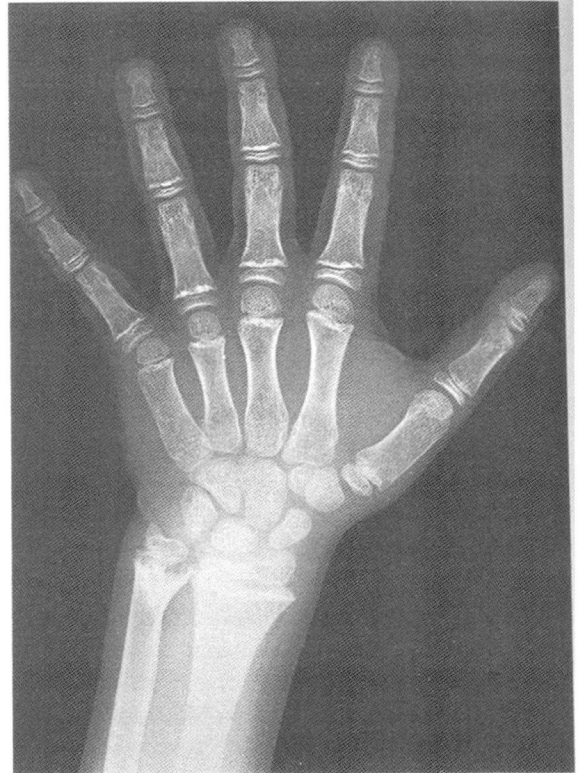

(b)

Figure 25.7 Disproportionate body segments resulting from desferrioxamine toxicity.

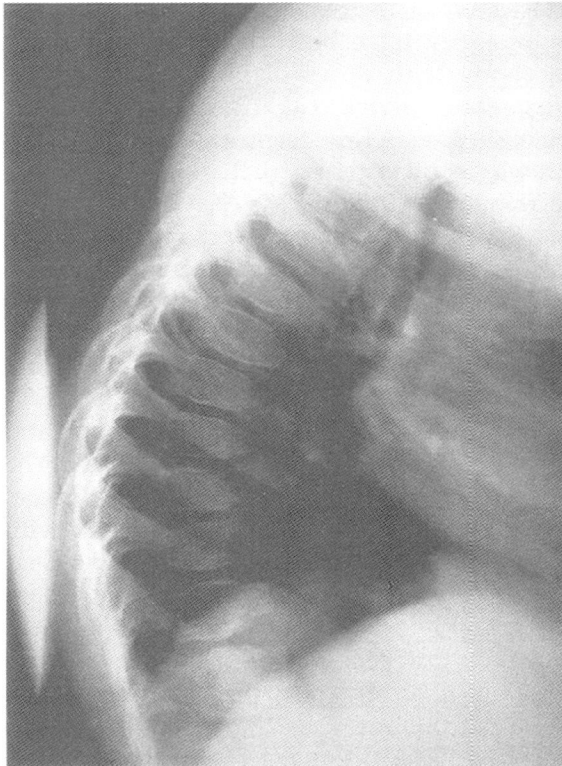

(a)

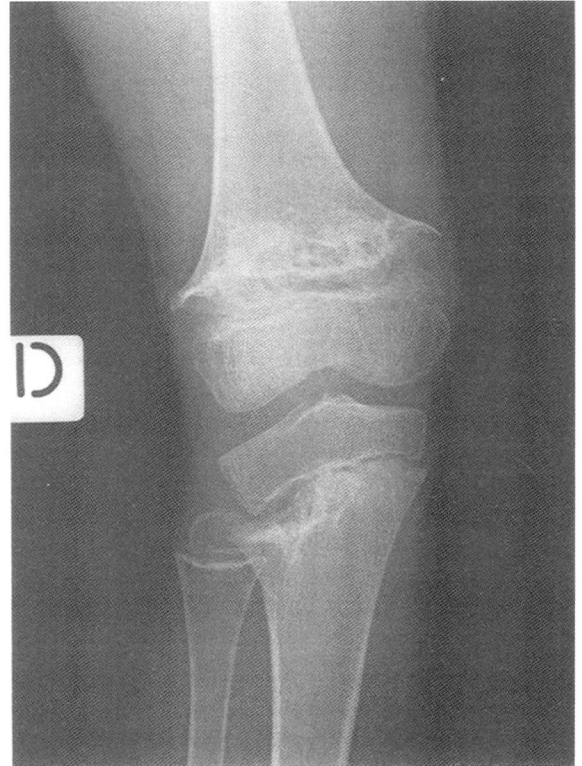

(c)

Figure 25.8 Marked platyspondylosis of the vertebrae (a) and rickets-like radiological lesions of the wrist (b) and knee (c) secondary to desferrioxamine toxicity.

Abnormal chondrocytes, alteration of cartilage staining pattern, irregular columnar cartilage, and lacunae in the cartilaginous tissue were revealed histologically. Osteoid thickness was either normal of slightly increased. Some bone trabeculae had microfractures and some had cartilaginous oases. In some cases, iron deposition was detectable by Perls' Prussian Blue staining.[20]

The serum ferritin levels in these patients are usually, but not invariably, below 1000–1500 mg L^{-1}. Growth hormone assessment in these patients is usually normal and the response to GH treatment is poor.

These results suggest that an ideal therapeutic regimen, which avoids the toxic effects of iron overload and of continuous subcutaneous chelation therapy has not yet been found, and therefore further studies and long-term observations on the effects of subcutaneous chelation therapy are needed before this intriguing puzzle is solved.

Desferrioxamine induced 'toxicity' can be prevented or avoided in the majority of patients by careful assessment of body iron burden and monitoring the desferrioxamine dose. An oral chelator (deferiprone) has been used successfully in one patient with osteochondrodystrophic lesions of long bones. However, the height velocity and severity of platyspondylosis did not improve during treatment indicating that some bone lesions are irreversible.[21,22]

SICKLE–CELL DISEASE

Sickle-cell disease (SCD) is the most common genetically inherited disorder worldwide. It is inherited in a mendelian recessive manner, so that people with the carrier state are generally healthy. Homozygous and confound heterozygous individuals have symptomatic disease. Four genotypes – sickle cell anemia (HbSS), sickle-hemoglobin cell disease (HbSC), and two types of sickle β-thalassemia (Sβ^+-thalassemia and Sβ°-thalassemia) – account for most SCD.[23] The clinical spectrum of homozygous SCD varies widely between patients. Factors contributing to this variability include α-thalassemia, persistence of high HbF levels, social circumstances and geographical variation. The disease is caused by a point mutation in the β-globin gene resulting in a substitution from adenine to thymine, which in turn results in substitution of the amino acid valine for glutamic acid at the sixth position of the β-globin chain. This results in β^s protein production which has a tendency to gel on deoxygenation. This liquid crystal distorts the red blood cells into their rigid sickle cell, leading to chronic hemolysis. The rigid cells aggregate in the microcirculation causing stasis and promoting hypoxia which leads to further sickling. The end result is vascular occlusion. Patients with sickle-cell disease suffer from anemia and sickling crises. Sickle-cell disease remains a major risk to health with high mortality and morbidity at all ages. In childhood the peak incidence of death is between 1 and 3 years of age, predominantly related to infection. In adolescents cerebrovascular accidents are the most common causes of death and, in adults, death is most often related to respiratory and renal conditions. With careful management the proportion of patients expected to survive to the age of 20 is 85 percent.[24]

Growth and development

The birth weight of babies with SCD is normal. Subsequently, a pattern of delayed growth emerges after 6 months of age, at the time that the levels of fetal hemoglobin (HbF) begin to decrease and clinical symptoms become apparent. By 2 years of age, the median height and weight percentiles fall below the 50th percentile, with the deficits increasing with age.[25,26]

Low weight is more pronounced than short stature[27] and is most evident in subjects older than 7 years of age.[28] By adulthood, both men and women acquired normal or near normal height, but their mean weights are still lower than those of control patients.[28]

Children with SS and Sβ° thalassemia are consistently smaller and less sexually developed than those with HbSC and HbSβ^+ thalassemia.

Height and weight growth reference curves for children and adolescents (0–18 years) with homozygous sickle cell disease in Kingston, Jamaica have been reported by Thomas et al.[29] Sexual development also is delayed in patients with SCD. This delay is found in both males and females[30] and follows the same patterns of other hemoglobinopathies.

As in any chronic disease menarcheal age in SCD is delayed by 1–2 years[31,32] and hypogonadism may occur in SS adults. Both chronic hemolysis and anemia may contribute to delayed growth and pubertal development.

Chronic hemolysis may lead to a state of high protein turnover and increased basal metabolic requirements.[33] Chronic anemia may result in cardiovascular stress with a state of high cardiac output and, possibly, increased energy expenditure.[34] Several reports have suggested increased requirements for zinc, folic acid, vitamins A, E, and B$_6$, riboflavin, but consistent correlations between deficiencies and growth retardation have not been established.[35]

Thyroid function and growth hormone secretion, usually, are normal.[26] However, Soliman et al.[36] observed defective GH release in 53 percent of prepubertal children with SCD resulting from a probable defect in GH secretion secondary to hypoxic–ischemic insults in the hypothalamus–pituitary area. All children had height-for-age below 2 SDS and were receiving regular blood transfusions to keep their hemoglobin concentrations above 9 g dL^{-1}. Therefore, it is possible that these children had GH deficiency secondary to pituitary iron overload.

Short stature and delayed puberty may be an indication for a through evaluation, including a dietary history, nutritional assessment and endocrinologic evaluation to identify impairment of growth hormone–insulin-like growth factor axis and/or gonadal function. Treatment of SCD is generally supportive or by transfusion, hydroxyurea or bone marrow transplant.[37]

KEY LEARNING POINTS

- The hemoglobinopathies (thalassemias and sickle-cell disease) are the most commonly inherited genetic disorders worldwide.
- The thalassemias present a spectrum of clinical features with a large degree of phenotypic heterogeneity. The clinical variability can usually be explained by the type of molecular defect inherited.
- The recommended treatment for thalassemia is regular blood transfusions and chelation therapy.
- Growth disturbances are a major clinical feature of patients with thalassemia.
- Most of the complications are attributable to iron overload which may be the result of economic circumstances (expense of the chelation therapy), late onset of chelation therapy or poor compliance with the desferrioxamine treatment.
- It is important that the physicians are aware that endocrine abnormalities may develop especially in patients with iron overload and poor compliance to treatment, particularly after the age of 10 years.
- Children with sickle cell anemia often have delayed growth and development, although the magnitude of this delay is variable.
- Multiple and complex mechanisms are likely to be involved in producing growth retardation in sickle cell anemia.

REFERENCES

● = Seminal primary article
◆ = Key review paper
✳ = First formal publication of a management guideline

1 Modell B, Berdoukas V. *The Clinical Approach to Thalassaemia*. London: Grune & Stratton, 1984.

◆ 2 Cao A, Galanello R, Rosatelli MC, *et al*. Clinical experience of management of thalassaemia: the Sardinia experience. *Semin Haematol* 1996; **33**: 66–75.

3 Zurlo MG, De Stefano P, Borgna-Pignatti C *et al*. Survival and causes of death in thalassaemia major. *Lancet* 1989; **2**: 27–30.

● 4 Modell B, Khan M, Darlison M. Survival in beta thalassaemia major in UK: data from the UK Thalassaemia Register. *Lancet* 2000; **355**: 205–52.

5 Brittenham GM, Farell DE, Harris JW, *et al*. Magnetic-susceptibility measurements of human iron stores. *New Engl J Med* 1982: **307**: 1671–5.

6 Kaltwasser JP, Goltchalke R, Schalke KP, *et al*. Non-invasive quantitation of liver iron-overload by magnetic resonance imaging. *Br J Haematol* 1990; **74**: 360–3.

7 Anderson LJ, Holden S, Davis B *et al*. Cardiovascular T_2 star (T_2^*) magnetic resonance for early diagnosis of myocardial iron overload. *Eur Heart J* 2001; **22**: 2171–9.

✳ 8 Anderson LJ, Wonke B, Prescott E *et al*. Comparison of effects of oral deferiprone and subcutaneous desferrioxamine on myocardial iron concentrations and ventricular function in beta-thalassaemia. *Lancet* 2002; **360**: 516–20.

✳ 9 Wonke B, Wright C, Hoffbrand AV. Combined therapy with deferiprone and desferrioxamine. *Br J Haematol* 1998; **103**: 361–4.

● 10 Italian Working Group on Endocrine Complications in Non-endocrine Diseases. Thalassaemia and endocrinopathies: multicenter study of 3092 patients. In: Andò S, Brancati C, eds. *Endocrine Disorders in Thalassaemia*. Berlin: Springer Verlag, 1995: **91**: 3.

✳ 11 De Sanctis V, Katz M, Vullo C, *et al*. Effect of different treatment regimes on linear growth and final height in b-thalassaemia major. *Clin Endocrinol* 1994; **40**: 791–8.

12 Fuchs GJ, Tienboon P, Linpisarn S, *et al*. Nutritional factors and thalassaemia major. *Arch Disease Child* 1996; **74**: 224–7.

13 De Luca G, Maggiolini M, Bria M, *et al*. GH secretion in thalassaemia patients with short stature. *Horm Res* 1995; **44**: 158–63.

14 Cavallo L, Acquafredda A, Zecchino C, *et al*. Recombinant growth hormone treatment in short patients with thalassaemia major: results after 24 and 36 months. *J Pediatr Endocrinol Metab* 2001; **14**: 1133–7.

15 Theodoridis C, Ladis V, Papatheodorou A, *et al*. Growth and management of short stature in thalassaemia major. *J Pediatr Endocrinol Metab* 1998; **11**: 835–44.

16 Zachmann M, Kempken B, De Sanctis V. Acute metabolic effects of human growth hormone on ^{15}N-nitrogen balance in patients with thalassaemia as compared to patients with other types of short stature. *J Pediatr Endocrinol Metab* 1998; **11**: 851–6.

● 17 Evered DC, Ormstron BJ, Smith PA, *et al*. Grades of hypothyroidism. *BMJ* 1973; **2**: 657–62.

18 Olivieri N, Buarcic R, Chew N, *et al*. Visual and auditory neurotoxicity in patients receiving subcutaneous desferrioxamine infusion. *New Engl J Med* 1986; **314**: 869–73.

19 De Sanctis V, Savarino L, Stea S, *et al*. Microstructural analysis of severe bone lesions in seven thalassaemic patients treated with desferrioxamine. *Calcif Tissue Int* 2000; **67**: 128–33.

20 De Sanctis V, Stea S, Savarino L, *et al*. Osteochondrodystrophic lesions in chelated thalassaemic patients: A histological analysis. *Calcif Tissue Int* 2000; **67**: 134–40.

✳ 21 Mangiagli A, De Sanctis V, Campisi S, *et al*. Treatment with deferiprone (L1) in a thalassaemic patient with bone lesions due to desferrioxamine. *J Pediatr Endocrinol Metab* 2000; **13**: 677–80.

◆ 22 De Sanctis V. Growth and puberty and its management in thalassaemia. *Horm Res* 2002; **58(Suppl 1)**: 72–9.

◆ 23 Committee on Genetics. Health supervision of children with sickle cell disease. *Pediatrics* 2002; **109**: 526–35.

24 Leikin SL, Gallagher D, Linney TR, *et al*. Mortality in children and adolescents with sickle cell disease. *Pediatrics* 1989; **84**: 500–8.

25 Glowry MF, Desai P, Ashcroft MT, et al. Height and weight of Jamaican children with homozygous sickle cell disease. Hum Biol 1977; 49: 429–36.

26 Oberfield SE, Wethers DL, Kirkland JL et al. Growth hormone response to growth hormone releasing factor in sickle cell disease. Am J Pediatr Haematol Oncol 1987; 9: 331–4.

27 Luban NL, Leikin SL, August GA. Growth and development in sickle-cell anemia: preliminary report. Am J Pediatr Hematol Oncol 1982; 4: 61–5.

◆ 28 Platt OS, Rosenstock W, Espleland MA. Influence of sickle hemoglobinopathies on growth and development. New Engl J Med 1984; 311: 7–12.

29 Thomas PW, Singhal A, Hemmings-Kelly M, Serjeant GR. Height and weight reference curves for homozygous sickle cell disease. Arch Dis Child 2000; 82: 204–8.

30 Serjeant G. Emerging understanding of sickle cell disease. Br J Haematol 2001; 112: 3–18.

31 Jimenez CT, Scott RB, Henry WL, et al. Studies in sickle cell anemia. The effects of homozygous sickle cell disease on the onset of menarche, pregnancy, fertility, pubescent changes and body growth in Negro subjects. Am J Disease Child 1996; 111: 497–504.

32 Balgir RS. Age at menarche and first conception in sickle cell haemoglobinopathy. Indian Pediatr 1994; 31: 827–32.

33 Heyman MB, Katz R, Hurst D, et al. Growth retardation in sickle-cell disease treated by nutritional support. Lancet 1985; 1: 903–6.

34 Barden EM, Zemel BS, Kawchak DA, et al. Total and resting energy expenditure in children with sickle-cell disease. J Pediatr 2000; 136: 73–9.

35 Gee BE, Platt OS. Growth and development. In: Embury SH, Hebbel RP, Mohandas N, Steinberg MH, Eds. Sickle-cell Disease: Basic Principles and Clinical Practice. New York: Raven Press, 1994: 589–97.

36 Soliman AT, El Banna N, Al Salmi I, et al. Growth hormone secretion and circulating insulin-like growth factor I (IGFI) and IGF binding protein-3 concentrations in children with sickle cell disease. Metabolism 1997; 46: 1241–5.

37 Raghavan M, Davies SC. The management of haemoglobinopathies. Curr Pediatr 2002; 12: 290–7.

26

Psychological disorders associated with short stature

DAVID SKUSE, JANE GILMOUR

PSYCHOSOCIAL CONSEQUENCES OF SHORT STATURE

To a substantial extent our physical appearance shapes our social interactions, in adulthood and especially in childhood. We can probably recognize from our own experience that characteristics such as body shape and size influence the way in which we respond to them.[1] Children are even more sensitive to such personal characteristics, especially when they perceive a peer as 'different' in some easily identifiable way. Factors such as obesity and physical attractiveness can influence social acceptance.[2-4] Children who suffer from obvious skin rashes, facial anomalies or orthopaedic conditions may experience teasing and exclusion from their peer group. Here we consider the case of short stature, which may at first sight appear less 'serious' a cause of psychological disturbance in childhood than an overt deformity, although pediatricians have assumed for years that it does have major significance for emotional and behavioral development.

Medical treatments for short stature are aimed primarily at reducing social handicap, although this aspect of the outcome is rarely explicitly evaluated. Although there is a considerable volume of literature on the benefits in terms of increased stature of growth hormone (GH) therapy, for example, in the case of Turner syndrome, there is increasing evidence that in particular, children with 'normal' short stature (who have no associated condition) in the community, have no major adjustment problems at all.[5] Practically no research has been done on whether the putative gain of a few centimetres is associated with better social adjustment. This is a difficult subject to evaluate because cause and effect are so closely

intertwined. Children who are rejected by their peers have poorer social skills than accepted children,[6,7] but because they are rejected they are likely to have less opportunity to develop such skills. Also, the benefits of treatment may differ at different ages. During the early years at school, children who appear much younger than their peer group because of their small stature may be regarded as 'babies' and given special attention for that reason. Such engagement may be pleasant enough in some respects, for example, being cast as the infant in games of 'mothers and fathers', but it is likely to be associated with limited opportunities for normal social development. As adolescence approaches children who appear small and physically immature may find themselves excluded from peer activities for which they are both emotionally and physically unprepared. However, these hypotheses remain largely untested. The impact of short stature on adjustment in adolescence is complicated by the interaction of two related influences: sexual maturity and height. Children who enter an early puberty (with a growth spurt that leads to relatively greater stature than their peer group for a period) may have fewer difficulties coping with an eventual stature that is lower than average than children who are sexually immature for several years, but whose eventual stature is within the average range.

The psychological adjustment of some children with short stature will be influenced by a number of factors in addition to their height. These include other evidence of deformity, facial appearance and the associated body habitus – especially obesity, which may be a cause of social stigmatization in childhood.[8,9] Individual differences such as intellectual ability[10] seem also to be influential. If the syndrome in question adversely affects intelligence, the child is likely to present more problems than if such ability is unaffected.[11] Anecdotal evidence also indicates that associated learning difficulties can be exacerbated by lower expectations of achievement in children whose physical appearance suggests that they are younger than they really are. In other words, there is a risk that children with persistent short stature such as those who were exceptionally small for gestational age (SGA),[12] will fail to achieve their potential because of this 'expectation effect'. It is at least theoretically possible that early treatment with GH therapy, starting well before the child enters school, may have indirect benefits by rendering the child of relatively normal stature by the time formal education begins. Even if their gain in height is not sustained throughout the school years, such children would not start with the double disadvantage of having potential learning difficulties and an immature physical appearance.

The psychological adjustment of children with exceptionally short stature is considered in three broad diagnostic clusters: the GH-deficiency syndromes, Turner syndrome and 'normal' short stature. In each case psychological development is reviewed in terms of: first, cognition, which encompasses both general intellectual functioning (measured by the IQ), and specific areas of cognitive functioning such as visual–motor or verbal skills; second, social behavior, encompassing both prosocial and anti-social behavior in relation to peers as well as adults; and third, the evidence for emotional adjustment and self-concept is considered, which includes self-worth or self-esteem, ambition for the future and self-image with respect to short stature itself.

HYPOPITUITARISM

Hypopituitarism is one of the most intensively studied of the growth-restricting conditions. When considering the intellectual abilities of these children distinctions have not always been drawn in the literature between the various etiologies of pituitary insufficiency, especially the potentially important distinction between isolated growth hormone deficiency (IGHD) and multiple pituitary hormone deficiencies (MPHD). For example, associated thyroid hormone deficiency may have an important part to play in influencing the clinical picture.[13] Earlier studies were inconsistent in their findings, some reporting no differences in average intelligence between the two groups[14,15] and others describing lower IQs in those with MPHD.[16] Visual–motor abilities may be specifically impaired[17] and a lower nonverbal than verbal IQ is often found according to Siegel and Hopwood.[18] More recent research[13] has not replicated the latter finding in either of two large groups of IGHD and MPHD patients aged 6–26 years. However, striking evidence was found of educational failure that was out of keeping with the measured intelligence of individuals with hypopituitarism. Such learning difficulties have also been described by others.[19–21] The etiology of relatively poor academic performance has never been properly elucidated, but

is likely to reflect a complex interaction of others' expectations, resultant self-esteem issues[22,23] and also perhaps associated problems of an essentially organic etiology such as deficient attention skills.

In terms of their social adjustment, children with hypopituitarism have the added handicap that their facial appearance tends to be rather immature. It is interesting that they are reported to perceive even average-sized children of their own age as in some way more 'grown up' than themselves[14] and feel less competent than younger siblings of normal stature. As a result of their immature appearance, they may evoke responses, especially from adults, that would be more appropriate for a child of their height rather than their age. Consequently, they may adopt an immature social role which is so powerful a stimulus to inappropriate adult responsiveness that even professionals, who have been intensively counseled about the undesirability of such behavior, find themselves engaging in it.[24]

Most studies of hypopituitary children report that they try to avoid conflict or confrontation.[25] Afraid of being physically hurt in situations over which, because of their size, they have relatively little control, they avoid activities such as sports in which body contact is an important ingredient. For some such children avoidance of conflicts that tend to occur at school may gradually generalize, so that conflict avoidance becomes a habitual style that dominates the child's personality. It can then become associated with difficulty handling frustration.[14]

Children with hypopituitarism are often said to be immature emotionally.[14,15,17,25] But, in general, samples have been small, highly selected and there has been a singular lack of normal comparison children of similar age and sex.[13] Accordingly, reports which state that self-concept tends to be poor, with a low self-esteem that is related to a failure to achieve goals and a sense of being subject to social discrimination, need to be considered with a degree of scepticism.[26] Furthermore, it is important to bear in mind that boys and girls can respond very differently to the potential handicap of exceptionally short stature. Boys are over-represented among clinic referrals in all studies. That said, boys do seem to be relatively more vulnerable to emotional and behavioral problems, especially in the elementary school age range.[26] Finally, as already emphasized, emotional adjustment to hypopituitarism will be influenced by the concomitant influence of the underlying condition upon sexual maturity in children nearing adolescence.[27] Strangely, this particular aspect of the syndrome has been studied relatively little to date. It is likely to be of great clinical relevance when decisions have to be made about whether to treat the sexual immaturity at the possible expense of final stature.

TURNER SYNDROME

Turner syndrome often presents with excessively short stature.[28] It is associated with specific cognitive and neuropsychological deficits, rather than a generalized retardation of intellectual functioning.[29] There is in general no impairment of verbal intelligence, but poor visuospatial organization leads to a relatively low Non-verbal Index score on intelligence tests.[30] The clinical phenotype of Turner syndrome may be associated with a wide variety of chromosomal anomalies; the genetic factors associated with this have yet to be clarified.[31] There is some evidence that those with a ring chromosome (about 30% of mosaics)[32] are more likely to have learning difficulties that will require special educational provision.[33,34]

In general, adjustment difficulties in Turner syndrome are not the result primarily of the short stature, which is often the main focus of early pediatric intervention if there are no other significant medical complications, but of the non-specific effect of haploinsufficiency of 'Turner genes' on brain development and functioning.[35] The clinical presentation of these associated motor, cognitive and social deficits occurs in quite distinct ways at different ages, with earlier manifesting disorders continuing to be of importance in their influence on day-to-day functioning right through to adolescence in some children.

Often the earliest problem encountered is a disorder of oral–motor skills, which results from a complex interaction of anatomical and functional abnormalities (such as a high arched palate and poor coordination of chewing and swallowing mechanisms). Resultant feeding difficulties are observed in up to 74 percent of affected girls.[36] This is increasingly recognized as a key aspect of the phenotype. For some girls, significant eating difficulties persist right through to early adulthood, reducing the motivation to try unfamiliar textures and occasionally manifesting in frankly anorexic behavior,[37] which may compound the growth deficiency.[38] By the time girls get to school age the most striking abnormality of behavior is an attention-deficit disorder with hyperactivity, manifesting in impulsivity, physical overactivity and poor concentration especially at school.[39,40] Despite verbal intelligence within the normal range, learning difficulties are common and are undoubtedly the result of quite subtle cognitive deficits which have yet to be fully explained.[41] For example, there is increasing evidence that dyscalculia may also be a characteristic part of the phenotype.[42] The authors' own research on over 200 girls with Turner syndrome recruited from a national survey has found that about half are likely to receive a statement of special educational needs by the time they leave school.[43] These cognitive difficulties seem to persist into adulthood.[44]

Social difficulties become most striking during adolescence,[40] because this is a period of development when there is need for a far more sophisticated style of social interaction than is required at elementary school. Many girls with Turner syndrome find it difficult to maintain friendships with peers, although they may have superficial relationships, especially with younger children. Group interactions usually present far more difficulty than one-to-one interactions, but this problem has little or nothing to do with short stature and probably little to do with sexual immaturity. The key disorder in forming and keeping social relationships with peers concerns a deficiency in social cognition which is an integral part of the Turner syndrome phenotype.[45] This problem is evident both in expressive[46] and receptive[47,48] social skill. Appropriate interventions for this difficulty, which makes it hard for most girls with the condition to interpret body language or the more subtle nuances of speech such as irony or sarcasm, are not well developed, but simply increasing height for age is likely to have little benefit. Effective treatments are more likely to take the form of social skills training similar to that used for children with high functioning autism, indeed the authors have presented evidence that a frank autistic-like picture is relatively common in Turner syndrome.[49] These primary social problems are likely to be exacerbated by functional speech and language difficulties that are common in affected girls.[50] Girls with the condition need more structure than average to encourage their participation in social interactions (e.g., organized games) because of the difficulty they often experience in understanding social cues. Simply providing treatment with growth hormone, in the hope that increased height will lead to better psychosocial functioning, is hard to support on the basis of the scientific evidence. Studies that have evaluated the psychological consequences of such treatment have not found convincing benefits in terms of self-concept, social interaction or behavioral adjustment.[51]

NORMAL SHORT STATURE

It is hard to draw firm conclusions from the findings of previous studies into the quality of life of children with normal short stature because of numerous methodological inadequacies. These include a lack of sample homogeneity and a lack of sensitivity of the measures of adjustment used. Research into the psychosocial adjustment of children with 'normal' short stature has relied largely on clinically referred samples and parental or teacher reports. It may be subject to bias for that reason, and the criticism has been trenchantly made that a very different clinical picture may emerge from the study of normal short children identified by screening the general population.[52,53]

We should, however, bear in mind that parental perceptions of stature are important in mediating psychosocial adjustment.[54] Indeed there is evidence that parental control is the key mediating factor in short children's social activity.[55] Children are often aware of their parents' views and parental dissatisfaction can lead to children's own dissatisfaction with their body image[56] and low self-esteem.[57] In cases of normal short stature, as in any other case, parents' and teachers' low expectations of academic abilities may evoke performance that is poor relative to ability. On the other hand, some families emphasize achievement in the scholastic field in order to compensate for the short child's difficulties in competing in physical activities.[20,58] The most comprehensive recent investigation of the cognitive abilities of children with normal short stature, identified in the general population of schoolchildren, found no evidence for impairment, once due allowance had been made for the fact that such children are over-represented among those of lower than average socioeconomic status.[59]

The authors' group[10,40] asked whether short normal children are excluded from their peer group. Are they at risk both of being teased and bullied, and of being treated within their peer group as 'the baby'? Could they internalize aggression, expecting to be teased and bullied? Is their predominant mode of behavior conflict avoidance?[60]

The authors' group investigated these matters using a combination of standardized instruments to measure the children's quality of life, such as measures of their self-perception, and they also obtained judgements from their teachers and parents, as well as their peers. Children were deliberately recruited from growth clinics at teaching hospitals because they were more likely to exhibit emotional and behavioral difficulties than a sample obtained by means of epidemiological screening[40] and it is believed that they were representative of the population of children who will be offered GH treatment. Cases were aged between 6 and 11 years, were all prepubertal with a height below −2 standard deviation score (SDS),[61] height velocity over the last year above −1.5 SDS and a bone age delayed not more than 2 years. No child was receiving any medical treatment for growth retardation. Comparison cases – children of normal stature – were chosen from each case child's class at school.

Measures of psychological adjustment were obtained by interviewing the children themselves and included self-concept in terms of global self-worth, social competence, athletic competence, behavioral competence, scholastic competence and physical appearance. Children reported the social support that they believed they received from teachers, classmates, friends and parents. The Body Image Perception and Attitude Scales for Children (BIPAS) were used,[62] which were developed by the authors' group to measure the child's satisfaction with their size and their shape (in terms of fatness and thinness).

A unique aspect of the design of the authors' investigation enabled them to compare the support that children perceive they are obtaining from their classmates with how they are actually seen by their peers. Sociometry was used to measure the extent to which the subjects were accepted by their peer group.[63] The exercise was carried out in school using standard techniques, the basis of which entailed giving questionnaires to the whole class which contained the case and comparison subjects; these questionnaires were filled out contemporaneously. All the children were asked to rate each other on specified behavioral characteristics.

Social competence was measured indirectly by asking the children how they would solve a series of hypothetical interpersonal problems, for example, 'Jill wants Pamela to be her friend. What can Jill do so that Pamela will be her friend?' The quantity and the quality of their responses could then be ascertained. Cognitive ability was measured using a standard scale of intelligence.[64]

Short children and their comparisons described themselves as being equally well supported by parents, classmates and friends, although short children reported having less support from their teachers. On the basis of the sociometric analyses similar proportions of cases and controls were rated as shy by their peers (5 percent vs 5 percent), disruptive (5 percent vs 9 percent) and liable to start fights (5 percent vs 9 percent), and a few were unable to take a teasing (5 percent vs 9 percent). Surprisingly, exceptionally short children were not perceived by their peers as being easy to push around (27 percent vs 18 percent), but they were regarded as being less trustworthy (18 percent vs 31 percent), although more cooperative than their normal stature peers (28 percent vs 18 percent). Fewer cases than control children were judged to be kind (5 percent vs 27 percent). None of these differences is statistically significant. Similar proportions of cases and controls were rated as popular by their peers (44 percent vs 40 percent) and there was a trend for more case than control children to be regarded as average (50 percent vs 25 percent). No case child was rejected (15 percent controls) or neglected (10 percent controls). There were no statistically significant differences between the groups. Children's height (in standard scores) was then correlated with the raw totals of nominations for 'easy to push around'. No trend was found for significance for either boys or girls in either of the study groups. In other words, there was no evidence that peers viewed very short children as easier to push around than average.

Children were assigned a score that summarizes their social impact on their classmates, the extent to which they are socially visible and their social preference – which refers to whether they are liked by their peers. Some interesting trends were observed. First, in neither group did these dimensions correlate significantly. In other words, to be socially preferred a child did not have to have a high impact on his or her classmates. Interestingly, for the case children only the raw number of nominations for 'being kind' was substantially different for boys than for girls ($p < 0.001$). For the case children only, higher social preference was significantly correlated with being less shy and with being more able to put up with teasing.

On our measure of social competence cases did not, on the whole, generate as many relevant solutions to the three interpersonal problems posed as the controls. Exploratory analyses showed that these figures were positively correlated with IQ in both the case groups, and when IQ was entered as a covariate in group comparisons differences in terms of social competence were not sustained. Case and control children were also similar in terms of social problem-solving style, as judged by the quality of their solutions.

There were no case and control group differences for any of the dimensions of self-perception or self-esteem. No main effect of sex and no interaction effects between sex and group status were found. On the BIPAS there were significant group differences in terms of perceived stature only. Only two of three case boys correctly chose the image corresponding to the shortest 20 percent as being their actual height, whereas five of six girls did so. A similar proportion of boys in the case group wanted, ideally, to be in the tallest 20 percent, and half the girls wished to be this tall. In contrast, within the control groups only one in three boys wished to be exceptionally tall, and two of nine girls. Thus, both boy and girl cases were dissatisfied with their stature, and most wanted not only to be taller but their aim was ideally to be much taller than average. This observation may have importance for their potential expectations of GH therapy, or other medical or surgical intervention designed to increase stature. A similar finding was reported by Erling et al.,[65] who assessed a Swedish population of children referred for investigation of short stature: in that study the children had unrealistically optimistic expectations of the potential benefits of treatment.

Despite the evidence from sociometry that short children were not much more likely than their peers to be perceived as easy to push around, for boys being short was associated with being teased and bullied. Responses recorded from boys during the administration of the BIPAS included: 'I don't like being a midget', 'My dad would like me to be taller, so I could pick back on him (the bully)' and 'My friends call me matchsticks – I don't like it'. The benefits to boys of being tall include 'You can stand up for yourself', 'Other kids won't pick on you' and 'You can be good at … football, basketball', etc. For girls the greatest ambition was to be slim as well as taller, although they certainly did not want to be 'skinny'. For example, one case girl commented 'I think I'm fat – my mum doesn't like me thinking I'm fat' and another said 'My dad says I'd be perfect if I was slimmer'. A comparison girl told us 'I hate wearing PE [physical education] kit – it's embarrassing', and another added 'When I wear shorts I sometimes feel my legs look fat'. We also asked the children to choose body images, in terms of stature and body shape, that represented what they thought their parents would ideally prefer them to be. These preferences were remarkably similar for the case and the control groups, girls and boys alike. Children thought, on the whole, that their parents would like them to look average. These data provide evidence that short children *perceive* that their parents are dissatisfied with their body height; a situation likely to impact negatively on a child's self-image over time. It remains to be seen if children are indeed accurately reporting parental preferences.

DISCUSSION

In ascertaining the psychological adjustment of exceptionally short children we should bear in mind the axiom 'size is relative and height generally has no meaning other than in comparison to others'.[66] The distinction between cognitive, social, and emotional development and self-concept is valuable for the purposes of discussion and research, but in the real world these variables are interrelated. For instance, emotional immaturity (fostered, perhaps, by others' perceptions) may lead to poor coping skills in social situations, resulting in frustration and a negative self-concept.

This, in turn, may be associated with diminished attention in the classroom and consequent learning problems.

Some themes are pertinent to the management of all the conditions that have been discussed. The term 'anticipatory guidance' has been coined[25] to indicate that many potentially serious conflicts and confusions may be avoided by creative and constructive forethought. Handling frustrating situations, for example, can be facilitated by teaching the child adaptive assertion or problem-solving techniques and these are a wise alternative to impulsive anger or withdrawal. Role-playing can be useful; the child can be helped to think out and rehearse assertive constructive responses. Group work may also be attempted, and parents may also benefit from groups, where opportunities exist for sharing experiences, obtaining emotional support and working out social management strategies.

Most (80 percent) of the short normal boys that the authors studied and all case girls were dissatisfied with their height, and all had of course been brought by their parents to a growth clinic. Not surprisingly, almost all reported their parents wanting them to be taller. Why had they been brought to medical attention? One hypothesis is that they were unhappy at school, that they were being neglected or rejected by their peers. Yet no evidence of this was found in the authors' unique direct measurements in the classroom. It has also been demonstrated that short children have social skills that are equivalent to those of their peers. This is important information because there is a strong association between social competence and acceptance in a peer group.[6] The authors also examined the possibility that short children may not solve interpersonal problems as well as their peers, but they found no evidence of this. Former reports describing social withdrawal[23] or aggression in children of short stature[67] were not replicated by the authors' data. The case children reported receiving comparable social support to children of normal height from peers, parents and friends, but they believed that they were receiving less support from teachers. This finding may be a true reflection of teachers' reactions to the children's underachievement at school.[40]

Short normal children did not appear to possess a negative self-concept, at least at this stage in development. The authors' sample was not lacking in confidence and self-esteem, in contrast to previous findings based on parental report.[57, 68] Yet they did accurately perceive their height relative to others, and they did want to change; indeed, they wanted to be taller than average! Evidently physical appearance caused short children dissatisfaction. Comparing stature and cognitive abilities as predictors of psychosocial adjustment, the authors' group found that IQ was a better predictor than height for self-concept and social competence.

Why, if their children appear well adjusted at this stage, did the parents of the case subjects bring their child for investigation at a growth clinic? Children who are exceptionally short are likely to have the same range of problems in peer relationships and in academic achievement as children of normal stature, assuming that there is no organic explanation for their growth failure which affects behavioral or cognitive function directly. It might reflect parent dissatisfaction with their child's body height or it may be that parents attribute any difficulties the child may have to his or her short stature. Although this hypothesis has yet to be tested directly, other research confirms the impression that parents of exceptionally short children regard those children as more maladjusted than is suggested by direct assessment of the children themselves.[65] The relevance of height to social adjustment may also become greater during adolescence. However, studies designed to investigate that possibility must find ways of dealing with the potentially confounding influence of sexual maturity, which may be more relevant for social acceptance and social skill acquisition than stature alone, and which will not be perfectly correlated with it. Whereas most studies on the adjustment of short children have focused on the prepubertal age group, there is some evidence that increasing age is associated with poorer self-esteem, and the expectation is that treatment benefits are likely to be seen maximally in adolescence.[69] However, to date there is little convincing evidence that GH treatment for children who are not GH deficient is going to be markedly beneficial to their quality of life.[70,71]

PSYCHOSOCIAL CAUSES OF SHORT STATURE

It is now widely accepted that an adverse family and social environment can retard children's physical development, but the mechanisms involved are puzzling. Evidence of an association between social deprivation and impaired physical growth has accumulated mainly from cross-sectional epidemiological studies. When growth failure occurs during infancy, it is usually described in terms of poor gain in weight (which is easier to measure accurately than length) and is known as 'failure to thrive'. Failure to thrive in the absence of physical disease or disability is termed 'non-organic'. Non-organic failure to thrive used to be considered as indicative of neglect, but it is not usually associated with frankly abusive or neglectful parenting. In most cases the etiology is unknown.[72] Recent evidence suggests, in developed countries, that the condition is often the outcome of a maladaptive interaction between specific child characteristics (failure to signal hunger unambiguously or oral–motor dysfunction) and specific parental characteristics, such as a failure to interpret feeding cues appropriately (S. Reilly et al., unpublished data).

If failure to thrive persists long enough it will eventually lead to stunting, in which height is low in relation to genetic potential (as assessed by mid-parental height). Adverse psychosocial circumstances can delay the rate of skeletal maturation by other mechanisms too. A few studies have suggested that boys are more vulnerable to the effects of psychosocial stress than girls.[73]

Height is normally distributed in the general population, but among schoolchildren in this country the distribution is 'spaced out' at the lower extremes of social class, so that elementary school-aged children of manual workers are about 2 cm shorter than those of non-manual workers at the 50th centile, but nearly 4 cm shorter at the 3rd centile.[74] Differences in height between children of the employed and unemployed have been found within each social class, but the effect is also greatest (up to 5 cm at school age) among the offspring of manual workers.[75]

Can we be more specific about the nature of the risks for impaired growth that are associated with low socioeconomic status? A cluster of factors seems to be important. They include single parenthood, overcrowding, low disposable income, paternal ill health, dependence on social welfare, and abuse of alcohol and drugs.[76] A number of studies have also found an association between the quality of maternal care, as assessed by health visitors, and children's stature.[77]

How do poor home conditions 'cause' short stature? Deprivation and stress are not synonymous, although there is a tendency for co-occurrence, especially among socio-economically disadvantaged families. Few attempts have been made to disentangle their influence. By far the greater part of the growth retardation in disadvantaged groups, relative to national norms, is evident by the time the child enters elementary school. Thereafter children from deprived or psychosocially stressed homes develop at much the same rate as those from more advantaged backgrounds, both in terms of height for age and in terms of bone age (skeletal maturation). Thus, the deficit seen at school age usually dates back to the preschool period. A number of lines of evidence converge to suggest that deprivation or stress during a 'sensitive period' of infancy is the crucial factor. In other words, a given insult that affects growth during this time in a child's life may have more severe and persistent impact than an equivalent insult during a later period of development.

Epidemiological surveys using longitudinal data have shown that many short children at school entry failed to thrive during infancy. However, neither in the developed nor in the developing world, where a similar association is found between stature and socioeconomic status, is 'growth faltering' (poor weight gain) during infancy a necessary condition for later stunting. It seems to be the result of a lag in the onset of the hormonally mediated 'childhood phase' of linear growth[78] but we do not know why. Further research in this area is needed. Surprisingly, indicators of adversity, such as exposure to infection or abnormal feeding patterns, do not seem to be necessary causal factors.

Growth trajectories are largely established within the first year or so of life when the infant is especially vulnerable to environmental insults, because the rate of growth is greater than at any other time, even puberty. Diminution in that normal velocity for a relatively brief time may have long-lasting consequences. If the child's growth trajectory diverges substantially and persistently from the population norm as a result of environmental adversity during this period, there is probably limited opportunity for full catch-up growth in later childhood, even if circumstances improve. How much catch-up growth is achieved depends on the degree to which biological maturation is delayed. If maturation is not delayed substantially, there will be less opportunity to catch up through a prolonged growth period. Some evidence suggests that accelerated growth rates are possible when deprived children are moved into a substantially more advantaged environment. Unfortunately, this may be at the expense of accelerated maturation, the consequence being an early puberty and short adult stature. The mechanism by which accelerated maturation occurs is unknown.

Over 30 years ago a condition was reported in which apparently idiopathic hypopituitarism[79,80] occurred in association with a variety of unusual behaviors, including hyperphagia (insatiable appetite) and polydipsia (insatiable thirst). Such growth failure, without organic etiology but with characteristic behavioral features, has subsequently been called 'psychosocial short stature'. Evidence is accumulating to suggest that affected children are genetically vulnerable to stress, and respond in an idiosyncratic way. It is typically, but not invariably, associated with emotional abuse. To avoid nosological confusion with other cases of stunting seen in association with psychosocial disadvantage, the term 'hyperphagic short stature' (HSS) is preferred.[81,82]

It used to be thought that food restriction was the cause of these children's obsession with eating. The condition has nothing to do with malnutrition, yet parents of hyperphagic children often go to extraordinary lengths to stop uncontrolled eating behavior at home. They lock food cupboards, refrigerators and freezers, and put alarms on kitchen doors. Phenotypically HSS children are very similar to those with the Prader–Willi syndrome,[83] which is caused by a small deletion on the paternal chromosome 15q11–13. Children with Prader–Willi syndrome are typically obese and hyperphagic; their parents usually attempt to restrict food intake by similar means. Strangely, although on average overweight for their height, HSS children are never obese. Perhaps this is in part because, in stark contrast to the lethargic Prader–Willi child, they are almost invariably hyperactive.[81]

The condition has other intriguing features too. Investigations of GH dynamics show that HSS children secrete very small quantities of growth hormone while living under conditions of high stress, typically at home, but they do not respond to therapy with exogenous growth hormone.[84] Yet if they are removed from the abusive parent or stressful home environment, for example, into hospital, there is a rapid and spontaneous increase in their endogenous GH output to above normal levels within a few weeks. If the reduction in stress can be sustained for a period of several months there will be catch-up growth of a degree that is often spectacular. This ceases rapidly if the child is once more returned to the stressful home environment. Other behaviors associated with the syndrome, including the hyperphagia, wax and wane in severity in parallel with the rate of linear growth.

Not all children whose growth is impaired in association with exposure to high levels of stress, usually intrafamilial in origin, respond with hyperphagia. But there is substantial evidence from the authors' own research that children who do show this form of response have a familial predisposition to do so which is almost certainly genetic in origin.[81] On the other hand, in the authors' study of growth failure in response to stress,[81] 74 percent of non-hyperphagic cases were found to be anorexic, with a low body mass index and normal GH responses to provocation tests. Perhaps humans have genetically mediated predispositions to respond to stress with an alteration in appetite that is dichotomous – either an increase in or a decrease in the desire for food. There is some intriguing research to back up this hypothesis. In a study by Willenbring et al.,[82] 44 percent of the sample of stressed adults experienced an increase in appetite and 48 percent experience a decrease. We speculate that the origins of some adult eating disorders may lie in such genetic predispositions.[83]

REFERENCES

1 Alley TR. Growth produced changes in body shape and size as determinants of perceived age and adult caregiving. *Child Dev* 1983; **54**: 241–8.

2 Byrnes DA. The physically unattractive child. *Childhood Educ* 1987; **64**: 80–5.

3 Banis HT, Varni JW, Wallander JL, et al. Psychological and social adjustment of obese children and their families. *Child Care Health Dev* 1988; **14**: 157–73.

4 Kennedy JH. Determinants of peer social status: contributions of physical appearance, reputation, and behaviour. *J Youth Adolesc* 1990; **19**: 233–4.

5 Voss L. Short stature. Does it matter? A review of the evidence. In: Eiholzer U, Haverkamp F, eds. *Growth, Stature and Psychosocial Well-being*. Hogrefe & Huber Publisher, 1999: 7–14.

6 Dodge KA, Asher SR, Parkhurst JT. Social life as a goal coordination task. *Child Dev* 1989; **63**: 1344–50.

7 Brochin HA, Wasik BH. Social problem solving among popular and unpopular children. *J Abnorm Child Psychol* 1992; **20**: 377–91.

8 Jarvie GJ, Lahey BB, Graziano W, Framer E. Childhood obesity and social stigma: what we know and what we don't know. *Dev Rev* 1983; **3**: 237–73.

9 Cohen R, Klesges RC, Summerville M, Meyers AW. A developmental analysis of the influence of body weight on the sociometry of children. *Addict Behav* 1989; **14**: 473–6.

10 Gilmour J, Skuse D. Short stature: the role of intelligence in psychosocial adjustment. *Arch Dis Child* 1996; **75**: 25–31.

11 Lai KC, Skuse D, Stanhope R, Hindmarsh P. Cognitive abilities associated with the Silver Russell syndrome. *Arch Dis Child* 1994; **71**: 490–6.

12 Smedler AC, Faxellus G, Bremme K, Lagerstrom M. Psychological development in children born with very low birthweight after severe intrauterine growth retardation: a

10-year follow-up study. *Acta Paediatr Scand* 1992; **81**: 197–203.

13 Frisch H, Hausler G, Lindenbauer S, Singer S. Psychological aspects in children and adolescents with hypopituitarism. *Acta Paediatr Scand* 1990; **79**: 644–51.

14 Rotnem D, Genel M, Hintz RL, Cohen DJ. Personality development in children with growth hormone deficiency. *J Am Acad Child Psychiatry* 1977; **16**: 412–26.

15 Steinhausen HC, Stahnke N. Negative impact of growth-hormone deficiency on psychological functioning in dwarfed children and adolescents. *Eur J Paediatr* 1977; **126**: 263.

16 Meyer-Bahlburg HFL, Feineman JA, MacGillivray MH, Aceto T Jr. Growth hormone deficiency, brain development and intelligence. *Am J Dis Child* 1978; **132**: 565–72.

17 Abbott D, Rotnem D, Genel M, Cohen DJ. Cognitive and emotional functioning in hypopituitary short-statured children. *Schizophr Bull* 1982; **8**: 310–9.

18 Siegel PT, Hopwood NJ. The relationship of academic achievement and the intellectual functioning and affective conditions of hypopituitary children. In: Stabler B, Underwood LE, eds. *Slow Grows the Child.* London: Lawrence Erlbaum, 1986: 57–71.

19 Rosenbloom AL, Smith DW, Loeb DG. Scholastic performance of short-statured children with hypopituitarism. *J Pediatr* 1969; **69**: 1131.

20 Holmes CS, Thompson RG, Hayford JT. Factors related to grade retention in children with short stature. *Child Care Health Dev* 1984; **10**: 159–210.

21 Stabler B, Clopper RR, Siegel P, *et al.* Academic achievement and psychological adjustment in short children. *J Dev Behav Pediatr* 1994; **15**: 1–6.

22 Pollitt E, Money J. Studies in the psychology of dwarfism. I. Intelligence quotient and school achievement. *J Paediatr* 1964; **64**: 415–21.

23 Money J, Pollitt E. Studies in the psychology of dwarfism II. Personality maturation and response to growth hormone treatment in hypopituitary dwarfs. *J Pediatr* 1966; **68**: 381–90.

24 Dorner S, Elton A. Short, taught and vulnerable. *Special Educ* 1973; **62**: 12–16.

25 Drotar D, Owens R, Gotthold J. Personality adjustment of children and adolescents with hypopituitarism. *Child Psychiatry Hum Dev* 1980; **11**: 59–66.

26 Sandberg DE, Brook AE, Campos SP. Short stature: a psychosocial burden requiring growth hormone therapy. *Pediatrics* 1994; **94**: 832–40.

27 Albanese A, Stanhope R. Investigation of delayed puberty. *Clin Endocrinol* 1995; **43**: 105–10.

28 Brook CGD. Turner syndrome. *Arch Dis Child* 1986; **61**: 305–9.

29 El Abd S, Turk J, Hill P. Psychological characteristics of Turner syndrome. *J Child Psychol Psychiatry* 1995; **36**: 1109–25.

30 Bender B, Puck M, Salbenblatt J, Robinson A. Cognitive development of unselected girls with complete and partial *X* monosomy. *Pediatrics* 1984; **73**: 175–82.

31 Ogata T, Matsuo N. Turner syndrome and female sex chromosome aberrations: deduction of the principal factors involved in the development of clinical features. *Hum Genet* 1995; **95**: 607–29.

32 Jacobs PA, Betts PR, Cockwell AE, *et al.* A cytogenetic and molecular reappraisal of a series of patients with Turner syndrome. *Ann Hum Genet* 1990; **54**: 209–23.

33 Dennis NR, Collins AL, Crolla JA, *et al.* Three patients with ring (*X*) chromosomes and a severe phenotype. *J Med Genet* 1993; **30**: 482–6.

34 Collins AL, Cockwell AE, Jacobs PA, Dennis NR. A comparison of the clinical and cytogenetic findings in nine patients with a ring (*X*) cell line and 16 45, *X* patients. *J Med Genet* 1994; **31**: 528–33.

35 Murphy DGM, DeCarli C, Daly E, *et al.* X-chromosome effects on female brain: a magnetic resonance imaging study of Turner's syndrome. *Lancet* 1993; **342**: 1197–200.

36 Starke M, Wikland K, Miller A. Parents' descriptions of development and problems associated with infants with Turner syndrome: a retrospective study. *J Paediatr Child Health* 2003; **39**, 293–8.

37 Skuse D. Feeding difficulties among infants and older children with Turner syndrome. In: Rovet J, ed. *Turner's Syndrome across the Life Span.* Toronto: University of Toronto Press, 1995: 17–26.

38 Sandberg DE, Smith MM, Fornari V, *et al.* Nutritional dwarfing: is it a consequence of disturbed psychosocial functioning? *Pediatrics* 1991; **88**: 926–33.

39 McCauley E, Ito J, Kay T. Psychosocial functioning in girls in Turner's syndrome and short stature: social skills, behavior problems and self-concept. *J Am Acad Child Psychiatry* 1986; **25**: 105–12.

40 Skuse D, Percy EL, Stevenson J. Psychosocial functioning in the Turner syndrome: a national survey. In: Stabler B, Underwood LE, eds. *Growth, Stature, and Adaptation.* Chapel Hill: University of North Carolina, 1994: 151–64.

41 Pennington BF, Heaton RK, Karzmark P, *et al.* The neuro-psychological phenotype in Turner syndrome. *Cortex* 1985; **21**: 391–404.

42 Bruandet M, Molko N, Cohen N, Stanislas D. A cognitive characterization of dyscalculia in Turner syndrome. *Neuropsychologia* 2004; **42**: 288–98.

43 Skuse D, James RS, Bishop DVM, *et al.* An imprinted X-linked locus affecting cognitive function: evidence from Turner syndrome. *Nature* 1997; **387**: 705–8.

44 Ross J, Stefanatos GA, Kushner H, *et al.* Persistent cognitive deficits in adult women with Turner syndrome. *Neurology* 2002; **58**: 218–25.

45 Skuse D, Cave S, O'Herlihy A, South R. Health related quality of life in Turner syndrome: perspectives on psychological adjustment in childhood. In: Drotar D, ed. *Assessing Pediatric Health-related Quality of Life and Functional Status: Implications for Research, Practice and Policy.* Philadelphia, PA: Lawrence Erlbaum, 1997: 315–28.

46 Lesniak-Karpiak K, Massocco M, Ross J. Behavioural assessment of social anxiety in females with Turner or fragile X . *J Autism Dev Disord* 2003; **33**: 55–67

47 Lawrence K, Kuntsi J, Coleman M, *et al.* Face and emotion recognition deficits in Turner Syndrome: A possible role for X-linked genes in amygdale development. *Neuropsychology* 2003; **17**: 39–49.

48 Lawrence K, Campbell R, Swettenham J, *et al.* Interpreting gaze in Turner syndrome: Impaired sensitivity to intentional and emotion, but preservation of social cuing. *Neuropsychologia* 2003; **41**: 894–905.

49 Cresswell C, Skuse D. Autism in association with Turner syndrome: Genetic implications for male vulnerability to pervasive developmental disorders. *Neurocase* 1999; **5**: 511–8

50 Van-Borsel J, Dhooge I, Verhoye K, *et al.* Communication problems in Turner syndrome. *J Commun Disord* 1999; **32**: 435–446.

51 Huisman J, Slijper FME, Sinnema G, *et al.* Psychosocial effects of two years of human growth hormone treatment in Turner syndrome. *Horm Res* 1993; **39(Suppl 2)**: 56–9.

52 Voss L. Short stature: does it matter? A review of the evidence. *J Med Screen* 1995; **2**: 130–2.

53 Downie AB, Mulligan J, Stratford RJ, *et al.* Are short normal children at a disadvantage? The Wessex Growth Study. *BMJ* 1997; **314**: 97–100.

54 Belfer M. *The Development and Sustenance of Self-esteem in Childhood.* New York: International Universities Press, 1983.

55 Caldwell L, Finkelstein J, Dermers B. Exploring the leisure behaviour patterns of youth with endocrionological disorders: Implications for therapeutic recreation. *Ther Recreat J* 2001; **35**: 236–49.

56 Pierce JW, Wardle J. Self-esteem, parental appraisal and body size in children. *J Child Psychol Psychiatry* 1993; **34**: 1125–36.

57 Stabler B. Growth hormone insufficiency during childhood has implications for later life. *Acta Paediatr Scand Suppl* 1991; **377**: 9–13.

58 Holmes CS, Hayford JT, Thompson RG. Parents' and teachers' differing views of short children's behaviour. *Child Care Health Dev* 1982; **8**: 3.

59 Voss LD, Mulligan J. The short normal child in school: self-esteem, behaviour and attainment before puberty (the Wessex growth study). In: Stabler B, Underwood LE, eds. *Growth, Stature, and Adaptation.* Chapel Hill: University of North Carolina; 1994: 47–64.

60 Young-Hyman D. Effects of short stature on social competence. In: Stabler B, Underwood L, eds. *Slow Grows the Child.* London: Lawrence Erlbaum, 1986: 22–45.

61 Tanner JM, Whitehouse RH. Clinical longitudinal standards for height, weight, height velocity, weight velocity, and stages of puberty. *Arch Dis Child* 1976; **51**: 170–9.

62 Dowdney L, Woodward L, Pickles A, Skuse D. The Body Image Perception and Attitude Scale for Children: reliability in growth retarded and community comparison subjects. *Int J Methods Psychiatr Res* 1995; **5**: 29–40.

63 Asher SR, Dodge KA. Identifying children who are rejected by their peers. *Dev Psychol* 1986; **22**: 444–9.

64 Wechsler D. *Wechsler Intelligence Scales for Children – Revised.* New York: Psychological Corporation; 1976.

65 Erling A, Wiklund I, Albertsson-Wikland K. Prepubertal children with short stature have a different perception of their well-being and stature than their parents. *Qual Life Res* 1994; **3**: 425–9.

66 Kelnar CJH. Pride and prejudice – stature in perspective. *Acta Paediatr Scand Suppl* 1990; **370**: 5–15.

67 Lee PDK, Rosenfeld RG. Psychosocial correlates of short stature and delayed puberty. *Paediatr Adolesc Endocrinol* 1987; **34**: 851–63.

68 Gordon M, Crouthamel C, Post EM, Richman RA. Psychosocial aspects of constitutional short stature: social competence, behavior problems, self-esteem and family functioning. *J Pediatr* 1982; **101**: 477–80.

69 Zimet GD, Cutler M, Litvene M, *et al.* Psychological adjustment of children evaluated for short stature: a preliminary report. *J Dev Behav Pediatr* 1995; **16**: 264–70.

70 Boulton TJC, Dunn SM, Quigley CA, *et al.* Perceptions of self and short stature: effects of two years of growth hormone treatment. *Acta Paediatr Scand Suppl* 1991; **377**: 20–7.

71 Pilpel D, Leiberman E, Zadik Z, Carel CA. Effect of growth hormone treatment on quality of life of short-stature children. *Horm Res* 1995; **44**: 1–5.

72 Skuse D. Epidemiological and definitional issues in failure to thrive. *Child Adolesc Psychiatr Clin North Am* 1993; **2**: 37–9.

73 Rudolf MC, Hochberg Z. Are boys more vulnerable to psychosocial growth retardation? *Dev Med Child Neurol* 1990; **32**: 1022–5.

74 Skuse D. Psychosocial adversity and impaired growth: in search of causal mechanisms. In: Williams P, Wilkinson G, Rawnsley K, eds. *The Scope of Epidemiological Psychiatry. Essays in honour of Michael Shepherd.* London: Routledge, 1989: 240–63.

75 Eveleth PB, Tanner JM. *Worldwide Variation in Human Growth*, 2nd edn. Cambridge: Cambridge University Press, 1990.

76 Wright CM, Aynsley-Green A, Tomlinson P, *et al.* A comparison of height, weight and head circumference of primary school children living in deprived and non-deprived circumstances. *Early Hum Dev* 1994; **31**: 157–62.

77 Parkin M. Epidemiology of growth failure. In: Wilkin TJ, ed. *Growth in Childhood.* London: Harwood Academic, 1989: 37–50.

78 Karlberg J. On the construction of the infancy-childhood–puberty growth standard. *Acta Paediatr Scand Suppl* 1989; **356**: 26–37.

79 Powell GF, Brasel JA, Raiti S, Blizzard RM. Emotional deprivation and growth retardation simulating idiopathic hypopituitarism: I. Clinical evaluation of the syndrome. *New Engl J Med* 1967; **276**: 1271–8.

80 Powell GF, Brasel JA, Raiti S, Blizzard RM. Emotional deprivation and growth retardation simulating idiopathic hypopituitarism: II. Endocrinologic evaluation of the syndrome. *New Engl J Med* 1967; **276**: 1279–83.

81 Skuse D, Albanese A, Stanhope R, *et al.* A new stress related syndrome of growth failure and hyperphagia in children, associated with reversibility of growth hormone insufficiency. *Lancet* 1996; **348**: 353–8.

82 Skuse D, Gilmour J, Stanhope R, *et al.* Stress-related growth failure. *Lancet* 1996; **348**: 1104–5.

83 Curfs LM, Fryns JP. Prader-Willi syndrome: a review with special attention to the cognitive and behavioural profile. *Birth Defects: Original Article Series*, 1992; **28**: 99–104.

84 Frasier SD, Rallinson ML. Growth retardation and emotional deprivation: relative resistance to treatment with human growth hormone. *J Pediatr* 1972; **80**: 603–9.

27

Etiology and management of growth failure in tropical and developing countries

PALANY RAGHUPATHY

CHILDREN'S GROWTH AS A DIAGNOSTIC TOOL AND AN INDICATOR OF HEALTH

Childhood growth has been repeatedly endorsed as a very sensitive and objective indicator of their health and nutritional status[1,2] and will serve as a tool for evaluation of the health programs and medical care projects in the community.[1] A change in growth rate is indeed a warning signal of ill-health, warranting the need for urgent intervention. Faltering growth may herald a chronic debilitating illness. As a corollary, good and steady growth in a child is very reassuring, denoting absence of any major illness and precludes the necessity for extensive investigation or active management as in the case of a child with maturational growth delay. Improved growth standards in children, following socioeconomic changes or the general health of the population, observed in regular periodic cross-sectional studies will be helpful in assessing the success of the national health programs in a given country.

Normal growth results from a complex interaction of genetic, racial, socioeconomic, nutritional, metabolic, and endocrine factors. By and large, growth potential is determined by polygenic inheritance, which is reflected in the heights of parents and relatives. The endocrine mechanisms involved are through the secretion of growth hormone (GH) by the pituitary which is in turn regulated by the GH-releasing hormone secreted by the hypothalamus and by certain GH-releasing peptides. Insulin-like growth factor (IGF-I) is released peripherally, or at active sites of bone growth. IGF-I circulates in the blood mainly bound to the binding protein IGFBP-3. While a new peptide hormone, ghrelin, produced by the stomach also stimulates GH release, somatostatin secreted by the hypothalamus inhibits GH secretion.

Intrauterine phase of growth is the most rapid in one's life. Size at birth, therefore, provides an estimate of the maternal and neonatal well-being. There is a gradual decline in growth rate after birth, reaching a steady rate of nearly 5 cm year^{-1} until puberty.[1] During this period, regular growth monitoring activity will evaluate the influence on growth in children by the country's public health and nutrition programs which usually cover health education, better nutrition, immunization and family planning. Such monitoring also helps in detection of undernourished children and those growing poorly, who may be given special care for treatment.

Plotting of growth after careful measurement helps in understanding whether the anthropometry is in the normal range for age and sex. Whether one set of international or local national standards from a representative sample of the population should be used continues to be a matter of debate. Nationally available Agarwal's charts are widely used in India.[3,4] Secular changes and improvement in nutritional status were observed in a recent study from Vellore.[5] However, it is generally agreed that the National Center of Health Statistics (NCHS) reference charts (2000) may be used.[6] It would also be more useful to determine if growth velocity of the children is in the normal range or whether deviating downwards following an illness or other disorder such as hypothyroidism or whether there is increased height velocity as in the case of precocious puberty. These clues obtained from growth curves would help greatly in planning appropriate treatment of the child. Improvement with treatment may also be demonstrated by catch-up growth.

LOW BIRTHWEIGHT AND LATER EFFECTS ON GROWTH

Maternal malnutrition before or during pregnancy leads to retarded fetal growth and consequently to the birth of an infant who is small for gestational age (SGA). The definition of SGA is given differently in various publications, including birth weight or length below the 10th percentile, 5th percentile, or 3rd percentile for gestational age, making it difficult to standardize incidence and prevalence data. A recommended definition is that used by Usher and McLean:[7] birth length and/or weight below an SD score (SDS) of -2 (i.e., less than 3rd percentile). Postnatal growth may be affected in these infants when catch-up growth (defined as a height velocity greater than normal after a period of growth inhibition) does not occur. Nearly 85% of SGA infants will show catch-up growth in the first 2 years of life. The others will be short during childhood and as adults. A seven-fold higher risk of being shorter has been reported in SGA subjects than those who were not SGA.[8] Lack of catch-up growth in a short child who was born SGA may be defined as a height that remains below -2 SD for age.

Persistent short stature is a long-term adverse outcome in an infant born SGA, along with the attendant psychosocial disadvantages. The other consequences encountered are adverse neurodevelopmental outcomes, increased insulin resistance, dyslipidemia and a metabolic syndrome (syndrome X) that consists of type 2 diabetes, hypertension, and obesity. In a large birth cohort (10 691 live births) studied at Vellore, India, wherein 2,218 young adults (mean age, 28 years) were followed up, diabetes was associated with low ponderal index at birth in men ($p = 0.02$) and low birthweight ($p = 0.02$) and short birth length ($p = 0.003$) in women. After adjustment for adult lifestyle factors, lower birthweight was associated with a higher prevalence of diabetes and impaired glucose tolerance (IGT) combined ($p = 0.02$) and higher 120-min glucose concentrations ($p = 0.003$). In the sexes combined, insulin resistance was positively related to birthweight ($p = 0.003$) (unpublished data).

Recent evidence from India also suggests that SGA is occurring with a greater frequency in developing countries. Excessive weight gain during adolescence in individuals whose weight was low at birth presents a particularly poor prognosis for the development of coronary heart disease in later life. Similarly current data from India do indicate that greater body mass index (BMI) in adolescence is associated with a greater risk of developing IGT in early adulthood.[9]

GROWTH MEASUREMENT IN ASSESSMENT OF NUTRITIONAL STATUS

Anthropometry

This is the most useful and practical tool in the assessment of the nutritional status of children. The two most common causes of impaired growth in children in developing countries are: inadequate energy intake mainly related to poverty and recurrent infections. Both these factors directly affect the size and rate of growth of an individual child. Although biochemical, immunological and other measures are available for assessing nutritional status, these are elaborate, expensive and not within the reach of a large majority.

The methods of population survey and data collection for obtaining anthropometric standards, are by no means simple to carry out. Access to the target population is required besides accurate portable equipment, specially trained personnel and uniformity of techniques used. Cross-sectional or longitudinal standards are available. The NCHS data[6] are cross-sectional data which are advocated for worldwide use. Tanner and Davies[10] constructed longitudinal growth charts which account for the pubertal changes during adolescence. These charts have been constructed from cross-sectional and longitudinal data.[10] They are based on the fact that children between the age of 2 years and the onset of puberty have a steady rate of growth. Any deviation from the normal velocity indicates ill-health and needs to be evaluated further.

In addition to these charts for assessing normal children, disease-specific growth charts for achondroplasia, Down syndrome, Turner syndrome etc. are now available.[11-13] The usefulness of these charts lies in the fact that any deviation from these centiles will denote the association of another underlying disease.

It is essential that the accuracy of the weighing and measuring equipment is maintained constantly in order to obtain clinically useful data.

Weight for age

Body weight is recorded to the nearest 10 g by using an electronic scale or a beam balance. The scales used should be periodically checked and recalibrated if necessary. In the clinic, the scale should be calibrated daily to maintain accuracy of the weight records. Weighing is usually done with the minimum of clothes (nude weight is ideal but impractical in most circumstances).

Height for age

Height measurements are taken using a Harpenden stadiometer (or with an inexpensive portable Microtoise height-measuring device) mounted appropriately. A hand-painted wooden vertical board mounted on the wall is often used but is very inaccurate. The child should be 'standing tall' and erect with the head held in the Frankfurt plane (the outer canthus of the eye and the external auditory meatus are in the same horizontal plane). The occiput, back, buttocks, and the backs of the heels should be touching the mounted wooden board of the stadiometer or the wall if Microtoise is used. Standing height is recorded in children aged over 2 years, whereas supine body length is measured in younger children. Accuracy in measurement is essential and is best done by a single individual with appropriate training and experience. This is necessary especially when height velocity is being assessed on chronic patients who are followed up regularly at periodic intervals. Such serial measurements are best obtained at the same time of the day because diurnal variation in standing height has been documented.[14]

Body length is determined by using an infantometer. This is essentially a horizontal board on which the infant is laid supine with the head held close to a vertical wooden board fixed at one end. A sliding wooden board at the other end is moved flush with the soles of the infant's feet and the body length is measured. Two people are needed to take this measurement accurately. While the assistant holds the head close to the headboard with the head in the Frankfurt plane, the examiner may hold the knees close together and in full extension.

Weight/height ratio

Weight for height is a good index for ascertaining the current health status of a child. It is also an indicator whether the child is 'wasted'. When combined with height for age, it will be most useful to monitor the nutritional status in surveillance programs. Height for age gives an indication of whether the child is 'stunted'. These terms 'wasting' and 'stunting' convey more meaning than 'acute' and 'chronic' malnutrition.

Skeletal maturation (bone age assessment)

Various ossification centers of the skeleton appear at different ages and follow a set pattern, so these data can also be used for comparison. Standard deviations have been worked out for various stages of skeletal development. An extensive skeletal survey is not required for bone age assessment. A radiograph of the left hand and wrist is commonly used and bone age assessed by comparing with the conventionally accepted standards of Greulich and Pyle.[15] Tanner et al.[16] and subsequently Tanner et al.[17] have developed a more elaborate scoring system for each bone in the hand and wrist. Both methods deal with data pertaining to normal children and cannot be readily applied to children with an endocrine disorder, skeletal dysplasias or other disorders.

Bayley and Pinneau[18] have devised the height prediction charts based on Greulich and Pyle data. These data too are quite accurate for predicting the heights of normal children.

Sex differences

All the growth parameters including skeletal maturation are different for the two sexes and different sets of charts are available for boys and girls. The differences are more pronounced during puberty and in attaining the final height.

Mid-upper arm circumference

This is measured using a (non-stretchable) fiberglass measuring tape. The length of the arm, from the acromial end of the clavicle to the tip of the olecranon process of the ulna, is recorded first and the midpoint is determined at half this distance. The midarm circumference is taken by passing the tape around the arm in that plane. It is recorded accurately to the nearest 0.1 cm without compressing the muscle mass of the arm.

This is a relatively age-independent method for quick assessment of the nutritional status and mass screening of children aged under 5 in the community. It does not give a precise diagnosis and at best, although useful for quick screening by community health workers, it is only a rough measure.

GROWTH DISORDERS

A child is considered short if his or her height is below the third percentile (roughly equivalent to height less than 2 standard deviations below the mean). Many of these children actually have normal growth velocity. These short children include those with familial short stature or constitutional delay in growth and maturation. When considering all children with short stature, only a few actually have a specific treatable diagnosis. Most of these are children with a slow growth velocity.

'Constitutional' growth delay

This terminology is applied by clinicians to different conditions. Delay in growth and onset of puberty are noted as a result of decreased GH secretion which is probably transient. The term 'maturational growth delay' is more appropriate for this condition, especially when there is a family history with one of the parents being affected. This is the most common cause of short stature and delayed puberty in adolescents.

However, most frequently, constitutional growth delay refers to 'normal variant short stature' in which the child's height centile deviates to the 5th centile or so around 2 years of age. Bone age is delayed. The estimated mature height is usually normal. The hormonal profile is entirely normal including the GH provocative test (with sex steroid priming in the peripubertal age group). If levels of IGF-I and IGFBP-3 in the serum are low and the GH response to provocative testing is poor even after sex steroid priming, further detailed investigation is warranted to rule out an intracranial pathology. Some children may be found to have familial short stature in addition to constitutional delay.

Familial (genetic) short stature

These children remain short throughout childhood and as adults. Many pathological conditions presenting with short stature have a genetic basis. This includes both endocrine and non-endocrine causes. GH insensitivity, genetic GH deficiency and pseudohypoparathyroidism are some examples of endocrine conditions presenting with familial short stature. The non-endocrine causes include many inborn errors of metabolism, skeletal dysplasias, chromosomal disorders and others.

Pathological short stature

This may be diagnosed when a child is of short stature and has a reduced height velocity, with significantly delayed bone age. Such a child usually presents with delayed puberty and the final height depends on the severity of the underlying clinical condition. This group includes nutritional, endocrine, chromosomal, skeletal and metabolic disorders, as well as chronic illnesses, intrauterine growth retardation (IUGR) and several birth defects. This group constituted 1.7% of general outpatient children seen at the Christian Medical College (CMC) Hospital, Vellore, India. As noted in other series, some children born with IUGR who failed to show catch-up growth presented with short stature.

CAUSES OF SHORT STATURE (VELLORE)

Most of the data in the literature on short stature refer only to the children who presented to a pediatric endocrinology or growth clinic for the specific complaint of poor growth. Children with Down syndrome, mucopolysaccharidosis, skeletal dysplasia, etc., and those seen in a specialty clinic for conditions such as malabsorption in a gastroenterology clinic or congenital heart disease in a cardiology clinic, may not reach the growth clinic at all. In other words, the data on short stature from a growth clinic often do not include, for example, all cases of Down syndrome, achondroplasia or even hypothyroidism that may also have the associated symptom of short stature. The true prevalence of short stature in the community is thus not evaluated. Hence a height survey of 21 712 children seen for various symptoms in a general pediatric outpatient clinic was carried out. The heights were recorded and plotted on the growth charts (Figs 27.1 and 27.2). Of this number, a total of 385 children (1.8%) were found to have short stature. Pathological causes of short stature were found in 367 cases (1.7%) and the causes were found to be as shown in Table 27.1; endocrine causes accounted for nearly one-third.

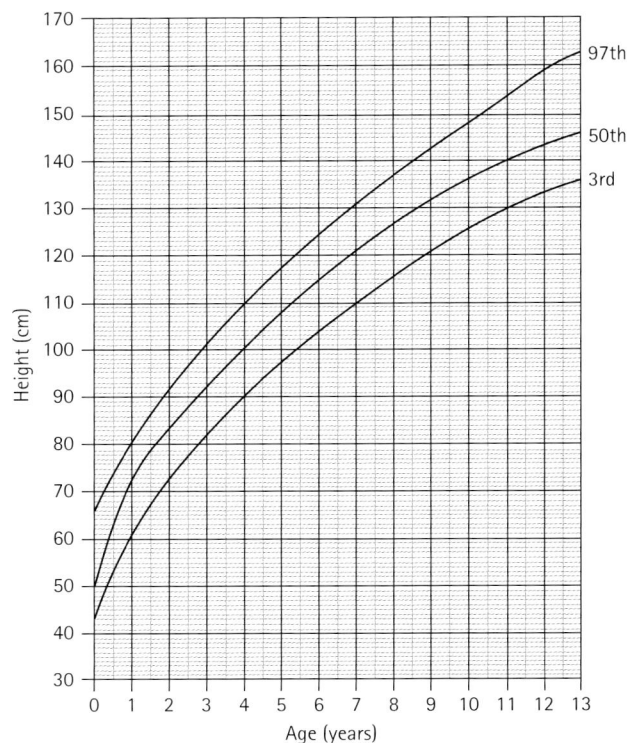

(a)

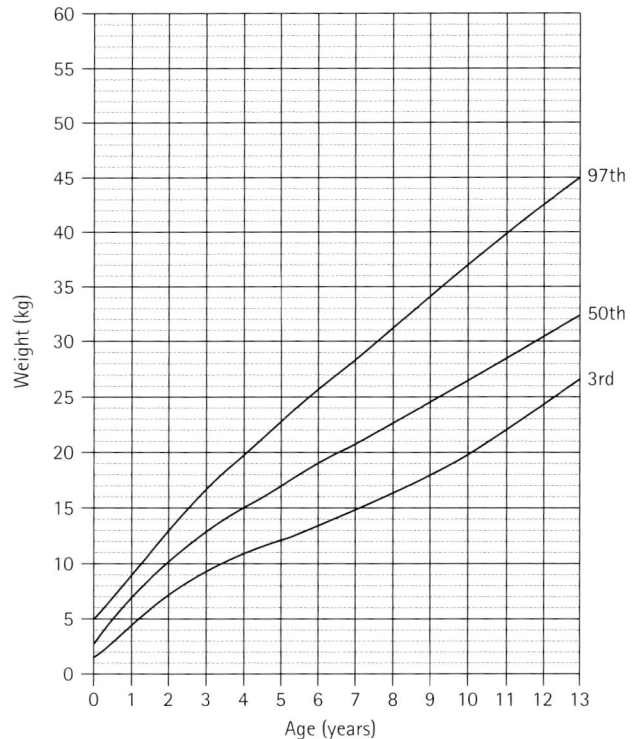

(b)

Figure 27.1 (a) Height centile chart and (b) weight centile chart for boys 1–12 years, resident in the Vellore District, Tamilnadu, India.

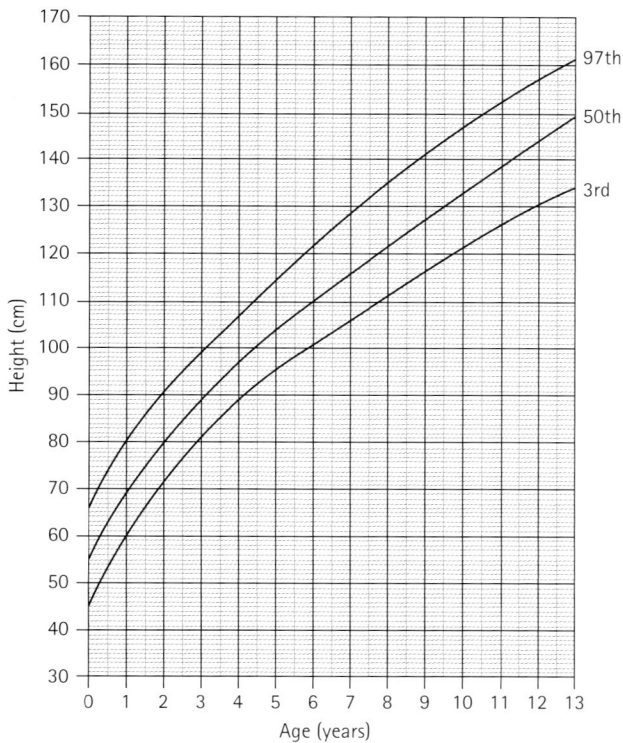

(a)

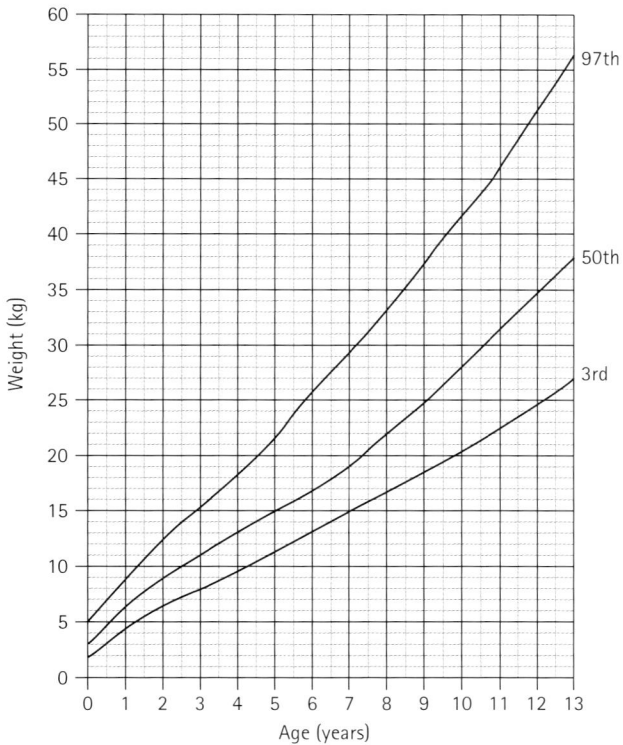

(b)

Figure 27.2 (a) Height centile chart and (b) weight centile chart for girls 1–12 years, resident in the Vellore District, Tamilnadu, India.

Table 27.1 Causes of short stature seen among children in the general pediatric outpatient clinic at CMC Hospital, Vellore

Causes	Number of children
Endocrine	128*
Genetic syndromes	22
Low birthweight	7
Cardiac	9
CNS	24
Hematological	59
Skeletal	13
Renal	17
Infections	14
Malignancy	2
Nutritional/gastrointestinal	34
Miscellaneous	56
Total	385

* Includes 18 cases of maturational (constitutional) growth delay.

Table 27.2 Cases of short stature registered in the pediatric endocrinology clinic at the CMC Hospital, Vellore (1986–97)

Causes	Number registered
Endocrine	347*
Genetic	15
Low birthweight	2
Cardiac	1
CNS	9
Hematological	7
Skeletal	10
Renal	4
Infections	2
Malignancy	1
Nutritional/gastrointestinal	10
Miscellaneous	3
Total	411

* Includes 84 cases of maturational (constitutional) growth delay and 263 cases of pathological causes of short stature.

Although the data presented in Table 27.1 are hospital-based, it still gives an idea of the problem of short stature in the community to an extent. The figures are different from those obtained from a general population in the West.[19] The cases of short stature registered over a 12-year period are shown in Table 27.2. In contrast to the figures in Table 27.1, endocrine causes constitute nearly 85% of cases. Among the 347 endocrine cases, pituitary causes make up 190 cases (56%), indicating the referral bias to a specialist clinic. The diagnosis of GH deficiency is based on clinical grounds in several cases, because these children were not investigated as a result of financial constraints both for investigation as well as subsequent therapy with GH at exorbitant costs.

INVESTIGATION OF CASES OF SHORT STATURE

In most developing countries like India, the investigation and treatment of a case of short stature are not deemed a priority in view of the heavy expenditure involved which may be afforded by only a few affluent families. If the parents cannot ultimately afford human growth hormone (hGH) therapy, one may have to consider the wisdom of detailed investigations at the cost of a considerable sum of money. Detailed history pertaining to the family height potential, maternal health status, birth size, growth pattern and chronic illnesses is important. Mid-parental height and estimated mature height will need to be calculated. Physical examination should include nutritional assessment, pubertal staging, body segment proportions and skeletal maturation. Simple screening tests such as complete blood count, erythrocyte sedimentation rate, renal, thyroid and liver function tests, venous blood gases, together with simultaneous measurement of urine pH, will help to rule out many treatable disorders utilizing much less expenditure. Girls with short stature will need to be investigated for Turner syndrome by karyotyping or at least a buccal smear. Radiological skeletal survey and certain biochemical estimations will be essential for diagnosing skeletal dysplasias and those of metabolic origin. Pituitary stimulation tests are mandatory for proving the diagnosis of GH deficiency. Insulin-induced hypoglycemia requires special expertise and should not be carried out in the ward without a blood glucose analyzer for immediate measurement of blood levels. The clonidine stimulation test has proved to be a highly useful test[20] – it eliminates the risks associated with the insulin-induced hypoglycemia test.

Random GH levels requested by many specialists with the intention of cost-saving are virtually useless and do not give any idea of the natural secretory potential of the pituitary. At best, it may be useful in ruling out the rare possibilities of GH insensitivity and biologically inactive GH secretion, presenting with normal or elevated levels of GH on random testing.

It has been argued that multiple blood samples collected for GH estimation during provocative pituitary stimulation tests are too expensive. However, this should be considered an essential expense to establish the diagnosis of GH deficiency on firm grounds instead of being 'penny wise' and must certainly be done before embarking on GH therapy which involves very much higher expenditure. Study of the neurosecretory abnormalities of GH secretion by multiple overnight blood sampling cannot be undertaken for cost considerations.

One way to reduce the cost of investigations will be to measure serum IGF-I and IGFBP-3 levels as a screening test. If IGFBP-3 is within the normal range for age, the possibility of non-GH-deficient short stature is more likely. IGFBP-3 is a technically simple assay, and is independent of age and nutritional status, but correlates strongly with GH secretion.

MANAGEMENT

The practical difficulties involved in management of growth disorders are many. With so many medical priorities in a developing country, growth defects cannot find a place in the list of conditions warranting therapy.

Health planners and even physicians, in general, are reluctant to recommend hGH therapy in deserving cases, as they are still quite skeptical about the results of treatment. Financial constraints limit the use of hGH therapy in deserving cases and, very often, therapy is started very late around the time of puberty as a desperate measure, when the short child suffers from peer pressures. It is natural to expect that the results of such therapy would be poor but are viewed by family physicians as failure of hGH to produce an appreciable response. Anti-GH antibodies are not found in these individuals. There are also some old discouraging reports which showed that one-half of boys and 85% of girls treated with GH do not achieve adult heights above the 3rd centile.[21] As a consequence, even families who can afford the therapy are dissuaded by family pediatricians from procuring therapy.

MATURATIONAL DELAY

In the presence of a strong family history of similarly affected members, the management consists mainly of ruling out other causes of delayed puberty and abnormal growth, with regular and periodic monitoring of height and adequate parental counseling. Height predictions using bone age assessment and the use of Bayley–Pinneau charts can be reassuring to parents. This is by far the most rewarding condition to treat, provided the diagnosis is confirmed beyond doubt, because the GH therapy required for treatment of the other conditions is not within the reach of a vast majority.

Unlike in the West, the aim of most of these children and their parents is for the child to achieve mid-parental height or even the height of one of the parents. If the short stature is the cause of severe psychological problems in the child, treatment with short-term sex steroid therapy at around the age of normal puberty has been advised.[22,23]

GROWTH HORMONE DEFICIENCY

Despite all the advances in easy availability of hGH, and a massive stride from the era of pituitary-derived hGH, therapy still remains the most frustrating area in pediatric endocrinology in developing countries, because of the enormity of expenditure involved. Most other endocrine disorders in children can be treated appropriately and adequately to a satisfactory extent, with funds raised from philanthropists and others for providing the relevant drugs. Provision of hGH therapy on similar lines is simply impossible, considering the long duration of expensive treatment.

One of the problems encountered is obesity in the children with GH deficiency. When obesity is noted before treatment, it is not improved with hGH therapy. It does worsen in many children who are found euthyroid. There appears to be no adequate explanation for this phenomenon.

OTHER ENDOCRINE DISORDERS CAUSING SHORT STATURE

In hypothyroidism, gonadotropin deficiency or gonadal insufficiency, appropriate replacement therapy is instituted to facilitate growth. In the case of hormone excess, e.g., hyperthyroidism, glucocorticoid excess, true precocious puberty, suppressive treatment or removal of a causative factor such as a tumor is performed. Nutritional and psychological rehabilitation is also provided when needed.

CHRONIC DISORDERS CAUSING SHORT STATURE

The primary disorder such as a chronic debilitating illness leading to growth failure in children needs to be treated first. hGH or IGF-I therapy may be quite useful in improving the final height attainment. If the child is receiving long term steroid therapy concurrently, the response may not be satisfactory. In a developing country, management ideals tend to be utopian because very often the parents are already at the end of their tether treating the initial chronic illness, e.g. chronic renal failure. Naturally, they will neither have the inclination nor the resources to consider hGH therapy.

The indications for hGH therapy have widened over the years[24] and good results have been demonstrated with the use of hGH alone or in combination with oxandrolone. hGH therapy is now used for Turner's syndrome,[25] chronic renal failure,[26] Prader–Willi syndrome,[27] and IUGR.[28] In India and the rest of the developing world, use of hGH for these conditions and several other new indications will probably not get the approval of health authorities in the near future, owing to the many pressing health problems faced by these nations.

SIDE EFFECTS OF GROWTH HORMONE THERAPY

Creutzfeld–Jacob disease was fortunately not seen in India as the pituitary-derived hGH was not available in the past and hence not used. Other side effects described in the literature have not been noticed, probably because very few cases have been treated on a long term basis.

In conclusion, any developing country will benefit from a national health policy and consensus guidelines on investigation and treatment of children with short stature.

REFERENCES

1 Gelander L. Children's growth: a health indicator and a diagnostic tool. *Acta Paediatr* 2006; **95**: 517–18.

2 Tanner JM. Growth as a monitor of nutritional status. *Porch Nutr Soc* 1976; **35**: 315–22.

3 Agarwal DK, Agarwal KN. Physical growth of affluent Indian children (birth to 6 years). *Indian Pediatr* 1994; **31**: 377–413.

4 Agarwal DK, Agarwal KN, Upadhyay SK, *et al.* Physical and sexual growth pattern of affluent Indian children for 5 to 18 years of age. *Indian Pediatr* 1992; **29**: 1203–68.

5 Gerver WJM, de Bruin R, Zwaga N, *et al.* Nutritional status in children based on anthropometric data. A description of an Indian population (Vellore). *Acta Med Auxolog* 2000; **32**: 93–103.

6 National Center of Health Statistics (NCHS) Reference Charts; www.cdc.gov/nchs (2000).

7 Usher R, McLean F. Intrauterine growth of live-born Caucasian infants at sea level: standards obtained from measurements in 7 dimensions of infants born between 25 and 44 weeks of gestation. *J Pediatr* 1969; **74**: 901–10.

8 Karlberg J, Albertsson-Wikland K. Growth in full-term small for gestational age infants: from birth to final height. *Pediatr Res* 1995; **38**: 733–9.

9 Bhargava SK, Sachdev HS, Fall CH, *et al.* Relation of serial changes in childhood body-mass index to impaired glucose tolerance in young adulthood. *N Engl J Med* 2004; **350**: 865–75.

10 Tanner JM, Davies SWD. Clinical longitudinal standards for height and height velocity for North American children. *J Pediatr* 1985; **107**: 317.

11 Horton WA, Rotter JI, Rimoin DL, *et al.* Standard growth curves for achondroplasia. *J Pediatr* 1978; **93**: 435.

12 Cronk C, Crocker AC, Pueschel SM, *et al.* Growth charts for children with Down syndrome: 1 month to 18 years of age. *Pediatrics* 1988; **81**: 102–10.

13 Lyon AL, Preece MA, Grant DB. Growth curve for girls with Turner syndrome. *Arch Dis Child* 1985; **60**: 932.

14 Whitehouse RH, Tanner JM, Healy MJR. Diurnal variation in stature and sitting height in 12–14 year old boys. *Ann Hum Biol* 1974; **1**: 103.

15 Greulich WW, Pyle SI. *Radiographic Atlas of Skeletal Development of the Hand and Wrist*, 2nd edn. Stanford, CA: Stanford University Press, 1959.

16 Tanner JM, Whitehouse RH, Marshall WA, *et al. Assessment of Skeletal Maturity and Prediction of Adult Height (TW2 Method)*, 2nd edn. London: Academic Press, 1983.

17 Tanner JM, Whitehouse RH, Cameron N, *et al. Assessment of Skeletal Maturity and Prediction of Adult Height (TW3 Method)*, 3rd edn. London: WB Saunders, 2001.

18 Bayley N, Pinneau S. Tables for predicting adult height from skeletal age: revised for use with the Greulich–Pyle hand standards. *J Pediatr* 1952; **40**: 423.

19 Lacey KA, Parkin JM. Causes of short stature. A community study of children in Newcastle-upon-Tyne. *Lancet* 1974; i: 42–5.

20 Fraser NC, Seth J, Brown S. Clonidine is a better test for growth hormone deficiency than insulin hypoglycaemia. *Arch Dis Child* 1983; **58**: 355–8.

21 Burns EC, Tanner JM, Preece MA, *et al.* Final height and pubertal development in 55 children with idiopathic growth hormone deficiency, treated for between 2 and 15 years with human growth hormone. *Eur J Paediatr* 1981; **137**: 155.

22 Rosenfeld RG, Northcraft GB, Hintz RL. A prospective, randomized trial of testosterone treatment of constitutional short stature in adolescent males. *Pediatrics* 1982; **69**: 681.

23 Richman RA, Kirsch LR. Testosterone treatment in adolescent boys with constitutional delay in growth and development. *New Engl J Med* 1988; **319**: 1563.

24 Lee PA, Kendig JW, Kerrigan JR. Persistent short stature, other potential outcomes, and the effect of growth hormone treatment in children who are born small for gestational age. *Pediatrics* 2003; **112**: 150–62.

25 Cave CB, Bryant J, Milne R. Recombinant growth hormone in children and adolescents with Turner syndrome (Cochrane Review). *The Cochrane Database of Systematic Reviews* (2003).

26 Vimalachandra D, Hodson EM, Willis NS, *et al.* Growth hormone for children with chronic kidney disease (Cochrane Review). *The Cochrane Database of Systematic Reviews* (2006).

27 Burman P, Ritzén ME, Lindgren AC. Endocrine dysfunction in Prader–Willi syndrome: A review with special reference to GH. *Endocr Rev* 2001; **22**: 787–99.

28 Cutfield WS, Lindberg A, Rapaport R, *et al.* Safety of growth hormone treatment in children born small for gestational age: The US Trial and KIGS analysis. *Horm Res* 2006; **65(Supp l3)**: 153–9.

ENDOCRINE CAUSES OF ABNORMAL GROWTH

28

Abnormalities of growth hormone secretion

FRANK B DIAMOND, BARRY B BERCU

BACKGROUND: PHYSIOLOGY OF NORMAL AND ABNORMAL GROWTH HORMONE SECRETION

The periodic pulsatile release of human growth hormone from the pituitary somatotroph reflects the organized integration of various stimulatory and inhibitory influences. GH secretion is augmented through the hypothalamic growth hormone releasing hormone (GHRH)/growth hormone releasing hormone receptor (GHRHR) unit and by the gut/brain-derived growth hormone secretagogue, ghrelin. GH release is inhibited by hypothalamic somatostatin, extra- and intra-pituitary feedback of insulin-like growth factor-1 (IGF-I), and GH suppressive effects of circulating metabolites such as glucose and free fatty acids. A panoply of neurotransmitters (adrenergic, cholinergic, histaminergic), neuropeptides (opioids, galanin, bombesin, melatonin, neuropeptide Y, substance P) and hormones (glucocorticoids, sex steroids, thyroid hormone, leptin) centrally modulate GHRH and somatostatin release. Somatostatin principally programs the episodic pulses of pituitary GH, while the GHRH/GHRHR regulates GH pulse amplitude. Analysis of GH secretion requires quantitative assessment of ultradian rhythms (episodic GH release over short intervals) and 24 h secretory patterns (circadian rhythms) in the context of a 'patterned orderliness' (approximate entropy).[1] Deconvolutional analyses calculate both GH secretory burst properties including amplitude, frequency and GH mass as well as half-life. Altered GH half-life is rare, but occurs in obese subjects and in individuals with severely impaired hepatic or renal function.[2]

A description of factors that regulate GH secretion appears in Table 28.1. Hypothalamic GHRH activates the differentiation and proliferation of anterior pituitary somatotrophs, as well as their synthesis and release of GH.[3] GHRH is transcribed from a five exon gene located on chromosome 20q11.2 as prepro-GHRH, a 108 amino acid precursor protein that is alternatively spliced to 40 and 44 amino acid isoforms in cell bodies of the hypothalamic arcuate, dorsomedial, and ventromedial nuclei.[4] The amidated 44 amino acid protein circulates in greater concentration, but both isoforms are of equal potency with full biologic activity residing in the first 29 amino acids and its amidated form.[5] Hypothalamic arcuate axons release GHRH into median eminence capillaries of the pituitary portal system for delivery to the somatotrophs in response to alpha-2 adrenergic agonists such as clonidine and gamma-amino butyric acid beta receptor agonists such as baclofen and galanin. GHRH secretion is inhibited by dopamine, serotonin, muscarinic cholinergic agonists (pyridostigmine), β2 adrenergic antagonists (propranolol), L-arginine and somatostatin.[6]

Binding of the GHRH molecule to a seven transmembrane spanning guanosine triphosphate-coupled Gs-receptor activates adenyl cyclase, cyclic AMP, and protein kinase A.

Table 28.1 Factors regulating growth hormone secretion

Stimulatory	Inhibitory
Physiologic	
Sleep	Psychologic stress
Exercise	Increased fatty acids
Physical stress	Increased glucose
Increased amino acids	
Decreased glucose	
Pharmacologic	
Insulin-induced hypoglycemia	Glucocorticoids
Adrenocorticotropic hormone	Progesterone?
Melanocyte-stimulating hormone (MSH)	Melatonin?
Estradiol	
Vasopressin	
Galanin	
Gastrointestinal and hypothalamic	
hormones	
(motilin, vasoactive intestinal peptide,	
peptide histidine, isoleucine amino,	
glucagon, gastrin releasing peptide,	
secretin, gastrin inhibiting peptide,	
bombesin, cholecystokinin)	
Serotonin precursors	Serotonin antagonists
(5-hydroxytryptamine)	(methysergide)
Dopamine agonists (levodopa)	Dopamine antagonists
	(phenothiazines)
β-Adrenergic antagonists	β-Adrenergic agonists
(propranolol)	(isoproterenol)
α-Adrenergic agonists (clonidine)	α-Adrenergic
	antagonists
	(phentolamine)
Cholinergic agonists	Cholinergic antagonists
(methylcholine)	(imipramine)
γ-Aminobutyric acid (GABA) agonists	
Pathologic	
Starvation	Hypothyroidism
Protein deprivation	Obesity

As Na^+ conductance rises, somatotroph depolarization permits influx of ionized calcium through L-type voltage sensitive membrane channels into somatotroph cytosol, releasing stored GH from intracellular granules. Rising concentrations of protein kinase A phosphorylate the cyclic AMP response element binding protein which in concert with Pit l activates transcription of GH1, increasing GH synthesis.[7] The GHRHR is a 401 amino acid, 45 kDa peptide, with an 108 amino terminal extracellular domain and a 43 amino acid intracellular carboxy terminal domain. The extracellular loops and transmembrane helices of GHRH are primarily responsible for binding of GHRH to its receptor.[3] In addition to several transcription factors present at the 5′ terminus of GHRHR, GHRH itself

exerts both stimulatory and inhibitory effects on its receptor. GHRHR numbers decline when somatotrophs are exposed *in vitro* to GHRH, in part reflecting internalization of the ligand–receptor complex. Patients with loss of function mutations of the GHRHR demonstrate somatotroph hypoplasia with pituitary atrophia; basal GH secretion is substantially but not completely reduced. The frequency of GH spontaneous secretory episodes rises but GH is released in a less orderly pattern (increased entropy). GHRH transcription is increased by thyroid hormones and decreased by estrogen.[7] In healthy adults, continuous GHRH infusion increases GH pulse amplitude through inhibition of somatostatin release; however, repeated bolus injections desensitize somatotroph GHRHR and blunt the GH secretory response to subsequent boluses of GHRH.[8] Administration of a GHRH receptor antagonist, (acetyl-Tyr1,D-Arg2)GHRH 1–29 NH$_2$, reduces GH pulse amplitude, nocturnal GH release and the GH response to administration of GHRH.[9] Administration of GHRH to GH deficient children is able to stimulate linear growth.[10]

Quantitative GH release following GHRH does not differ by age or pubertal stage nor into young adulthood.[8] GH secretion is blunted during increasing or peak somatostatin release and maximal when somatostatinergic tone is low, a pattern that explains the variability of inter- and intra-individual GH response following administration of GHRH.[8] In the rat, somatostatin receptors co-localize with GHRH secreting neurons in the arcuate nucleus.[11] Infusion of somatostatin into young male human subjects suppresses both GH pulse amplitude and frequency, consistent with feedback inhibition of pituitary somatotropin and hypothalamic GHRH.[12] Somatostatin is expressed as 14 and 28 amino acid forms, the latter preferentially binding to subtype V receptors.[13] Somatostatin binds to a family of five specific receptor subtypes to inhibit adenylyl cyclase via Gi, and lowers net calcium influx.[14] GH auto-negative feedback acts at both GH and SRIH receptors with somatostatin inhibiting GH release but not biosynthesis.

Treatment of rat GH receptor with anti-sense RNA augments GH secretion by interrupting inhibitory GH receptor mediated auto-feedback and reducing hypothalamic somatostatin gene expression.[15] Central administration of a growth hormone (GH) receptor mRNA antisense increases GH pulsatility and decreases hypothalamic somatostatin expression in rats.[15] Other neuronal pathways which may influence GH auto-negative feedback include neuropeptide Y and galanin; hypothalamic GHRH gene is modulated by glucocorticoid levels and sex steroids.

GHRELIN AND GROWTH HORMONE SECRETAGOGUES

The discovery of the endogenous ligand, ghrelin, followed the identification of the orphan growth hormone secretagogue (GHS) receptor. In fact, the discovery of the receptor itself followed by 20 years the original observation of synthetic

Table 28.2 Chronology development of peptidyl and nonpeptidyl growth hormone secretagogues

Year of report	GH releasing peptide (GHRP)	Nonpeptidyl GHS	Key discoveries
1977	(D-Trp2)-metenkephalin		Opiate action
1984	GHRP-6 (hexapeptide)		Devoid of opiate action
1991	GHRP-1 (heptapeptide)		
1992		L-692,429	Improved oral bioacitvity
1993	GHRP-2 (heptapeptide)		
1994	Hexarelin (heptapeptide)		
1995		MK-0677	Markedly increased oral bioactivity
1996	EP-51389		
1998	Ipamorelin		
1999		NN-703	
2000		CP-424,391	
2001		SM-130686	
2002		EP-01572	

Adapted from van der Lely et al.[17] (See this review for specific references.)

GHS, which binds specifically to the receptor. The sequence of discovery was in reverse order: synthetic GHS → natural receptor → natural ligand.

Ghrelin is a 28 amino acid peptide produced predominately in the stomach and to lesser amounts in the hypothalamus, pituitary, testes, bowel, pancreas, kidneys, immune system, placenta, and lung.[16,17] Ghrelin is a potent releaser of GH secretion. Its activity is mediated through GH secretagogues receptor type 1a (GHS-R1a). This orphan receptor was specific for a family of synthetic GH secretagogues (peptidyl and nonpeptidyl) (Table 28.2).

Bowers and Momamy synthesized the prototypic hexapeptide (GHRP-6 (His-D-Trp-Ala-Trp-D-Phe-Lys-NH$_2$), and demonstrated its potent GH releasing action.[18,19] Walker et al. demonstrated oral bioactivity of GHRP-6 in rats.[20] This novel observation led to numerous studies of this family of compounds and their oral bioactivity in humans, with the nonpeptidyl compound, MK 0677, having the greatest oral bioavailabilty.[21] MK 0677 resulted in the cloning of the GHS-R.[22]

Ghrelin and the family of GHS also have lesser stimulatory effects on prolactin and ACTH secretion. Other endocrine effects include a negative central and peripheral effect on the pituitary–gonadal axis, stimulation of appetite and positive energy balance, actions on gastric motility and acid secretion, and modulation of pancreatic exocrine and endocrine function. Non-endocrine effects influence sleep and behavior, cardiovascular actions, proliferation of neoplastic cells and immune function. GHS-R is expressed by a single gene at human chromosomal location 3q 26.2.[23,24] Two types of GHS-R cDNAs, likely from alternate processing of pre-mRNA, have been designated as receptors 1a and 1b.[24–26] cDNA 1a encodes a 41 kDa GHS-R1a. The 1b cDNA encodes a shorter form of the receptor, GHS-R1b, which consists of 289 amino acids. GHRS-R1a is highly conserved across species. Motilin receptor is a member of GHS-R

family and has 52% homology. Unlike ghrelin, motilin does not require acylation for activation of its receptor.

GHS binds GHS-R1a and activates the phospholipase C signaling pathway. This in turn increases inositol phosphate turnover and protein kinase C activation, followed by release of Ca^{2+} from intracellular stores.[26,27] GHS-R activation also results in inhibition of K$^+$ channels, allowing entry of Ca^{2+} through voltage-gated L-type, but not T-type channels.[28,29] On the other hand, GHS-R1b does not bind nor respond to GHS thus its function remains unknown.

Among the modulators of ghrelin secretion, the most important appear to be insulin,[30,31] glucose,[32–34] and somatostatin.[35–37] Other possible regulators of ghrelin secretion include GH,[38–43] leptin,[44–49] melatonin,[50] thyroid hormones,[51] glucagon,[52] and even the parasympathetic system.[53,54]

Ghrelin and synthetic GHS have more potent effects in man compared to animals.[26,55–61] In man, only acylated ghrelin is bioactive.[62] GHS stimulate GH release from somatotroph cells in vitro[63,64] through depolarization of the somatotroph membrane and increasing the amount of GH secreted per cell.[65] Less certain is whether there is a stimulatory effect of GHS on GH synthesis.[66] Of significance, the in vitro GH-releasing effect of GHS is less than GHRH.[67] An additive or true synergistic effect of GHS on GHRH-stimulated GH has been reported.[68–72] At the pituitary level GHRH-stimulated GH release is abolished by specific GHS antagonists but not GHRH antagonists.[63,65,72] Somatostatin also inhibits GHS stimulated GH release. GHS-stimulated GH release is greater in pituitary preparations mixed with hypothalamic tissue as opposed to pituitary preparations alone.[73] This is consistent with the observation of a greater in vivo versus in vitro stimulation.[73,74] In animals with pituitary stalk lesions, GHS-stimulated GH is markedly reduced. Other studies using GHRH antagonists,[75–77] dwarf mice[78] and rats[75] but not lit/lit mice (absence of pituitary receptors)[75,79]

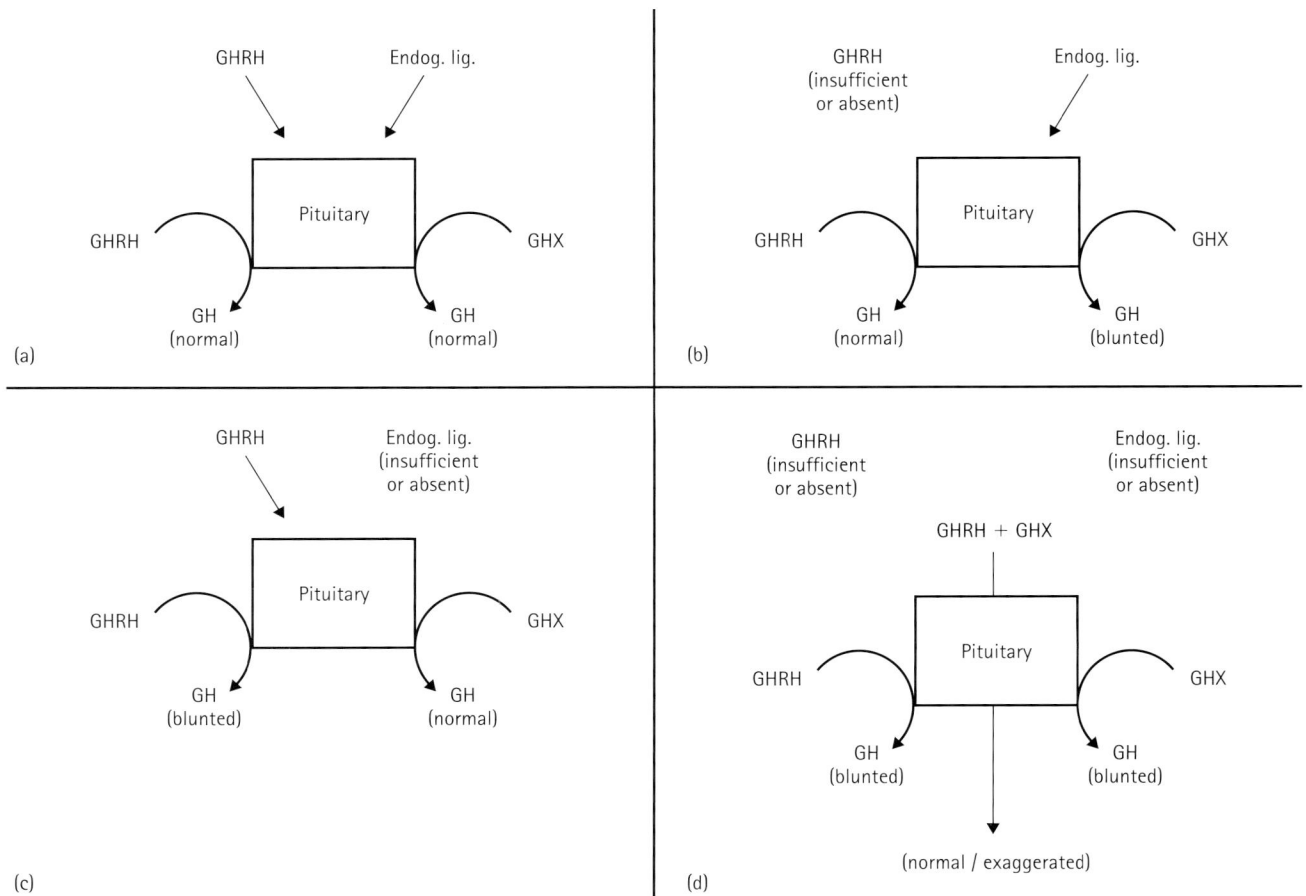

Figure 28.1 Schematic representation of the hypothetical model in support of the complementary relationship of growth hormone releasing hormone (GHRH) and the endogenous ligand for growth hormone releasing peptide (GHRP) or GHRP nonpeptide mimic. See text for discussion of the hypothesis. GHX refers to GHRP or GHRP nonpeptide mimic. From Bercu and Walker.[133]

demonstrate blunted GH release after GHRH stimulation. Prolonged administration of GHS increase IGF-I levels in animals[80–85] and in humans.[86–93] In man, GHS stimulated GH release is inhibited, not eliminated, entirely by GHRH receptor antagonists as well as hypothalamic–pituitary disconnection.[94–97] The most significant action of GHS occurs at the hypothalamic level.[17,98–100] Patients with GHRH receptor deficiency have no increase in GHS stimulated GH release.[101–103] In both animals and humans GHS act as functional somatostatin antagonists.[58,104–107] In humans and animals, desensitization to GHS occur during continuous GHRP infusion,[108–110] but not after intermittent oral or intranasal GHS.[111,112] GHS administrated via parenteral, intranasal or oral routes enhance spontaneous GH pulsatile secretion and IGF-I concentrations in humans.[86–93]

GHS stimulated GH release varies by age. It increases during puberty, plateaus in adulthood and decreases during aging.[58] Enhanced GHS-stimulated GH release at puberty is due to the positive influence of higher estrogen levels, which increase GHS-R expression.[113–118] Hypothalamic GHS-R is reduced during aging in humans. GHS-stimulated GH

release is increased in elderly subjects, but not restored, by supramaximal doses.[115,119] The reduced GHS–GH response during aging is due to age-related alterations in neural control of somatotrophic function including decreased GHRH and increased somatostatinergic activity[120] or perhaps to a decrease in the GHS system (ghrelin release and/or receptor expression).[111–123]

Although ghrelin has a potent GH releasing effect, it is as yet uncertain whether this is the most important physiologic action of ghrelin. GHRH antagonist inhibits 24 h pulsatile GH secretion while not affecting ghrelin levels.[35] In addition, ghrelin does not modulate GH response to provocative stimuli (e.g. insulin-induced hypoglycemia[124,125]) and GH rebound following somatostatin withdrawal.[36] Ghrelin pulsatility is more related to food intake rather than GH pulses.[126]

Combined with GHRH, GHS might be useful as a diagnostic test for testing pituitary reserve and GH deficiency[61,127–131] (see our own hypothesis below). Long-acting orally active GHS have potential application in GH deficiency, as an anabolic treatment in frail elderly subjects, aging adults and osteoporosis.[17]

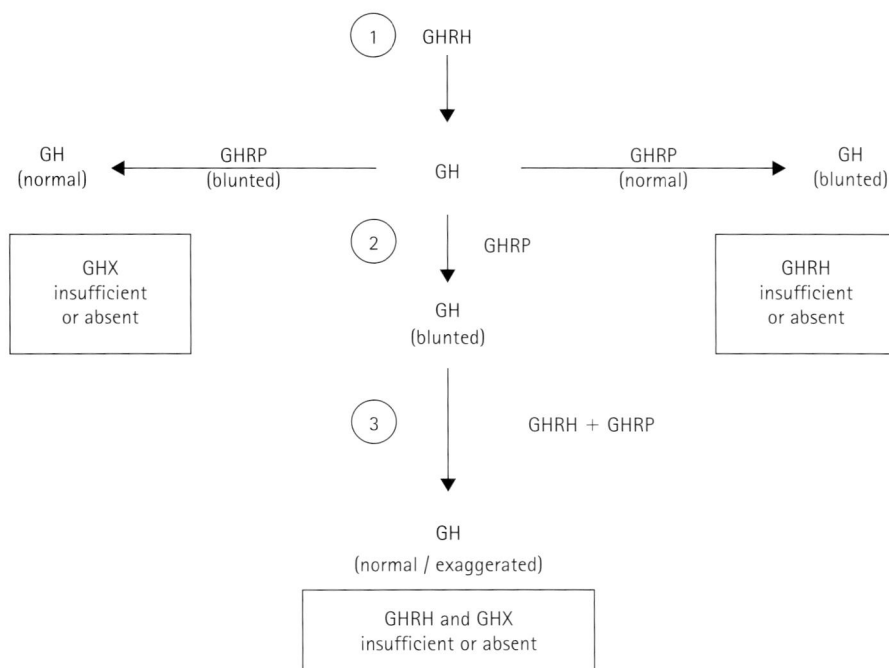

Figure 28.2 A three-step provocative pituitary function test using responses to sequentially administered and co-administered GH secretagogues as diagnostic parameters for determining the neuroendocrine basis of GH secretory dysfunction. From Bercu and Walker.[132]

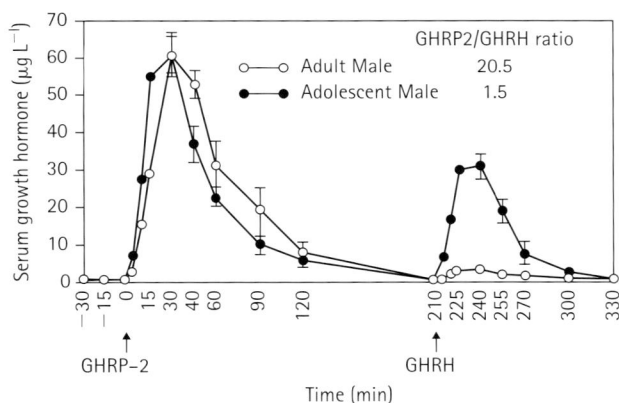

Figure 28.3 Comparison of changes in serum GH concentrations in adult and adolescent males following i.v. sequential administration of GHRP-2 and GHRH ($n = 6$ per group) (mean $\pm$ SEM). From Bercu and Walker.[134a]

USE OF GROWTH HORMONE SECRETAGOGUES AS DIAGNOSTIC TESTS

We hypothesize that GHRH and an endogenous analog to GHRP are complementary GH secretagogues that together provide appropriate stimulation of the pituitary gland to sustain normal GH production and release. Using this logic, GHRH or GHRP could be given alone, or in combination, to diagnose pituitary-based causes of inadequate GH secretion.[132,134] The model (Figs 28.1 and 28.2) assumes that a 'normal' response to GHRP (or GHRP-mimic) stimulation or GHRH requires the presence of its endogenous analog (i.e., GHRH or GHRP, respectively).

A blunted response to either exogenous GH secretagogue is interpreted as indicating a deficiency of its endogenous complement (Fig. 28.1b and c). Blunted responses to both exogenous secretagogues imply deficiencies of both endogenous complements (Fig. 28.1d). This situation can be differentiated from inherent pituitary abnormalities, such as receptor or second-messenger mediated deficits, by a 'normal' response to GHRH and GHRP co-administration. A blunted response following co-administration of both secretagogues would suggest inherent pituitary dysfunction, rather than inadequate endogenous stimuli.

To test our hypothesis, we summarize below the following: (1) use of the diagnostic test in children with altered growth patterns (Table 28.3); (2) use of the diagnostic test in healthy adults and aging subjects (Fig. 28.3); (3) effectiveness of priming with GHRP in aging men to address potential therapy of GH secretagogue(s) in 'normal' aging (Fig. 28.4).

Other clinical investigators have also exploited the ability of GHRPs to release GH by mechanisms separate from GHRH as diagnostic tools[135–139] including in combination with arginine as a somatostatin antagonist.[135]

There is considerable interest in the myriad activities and functioning ghrelin and this family of GHS and receptors that is beyond the scope of this chapter. For further information see van der Lely et al.[17]

Human growth hormone is a 22 kDa, 191 amino acid protein originating from a 217 amino acid prohormone with a 26 amino acid signal peptide. The growth hormone gene, *GH*1, is located on chromosome 17q22–q24, comprising five exons and four introns. Alternative splicing of *GH*1 produces a 20 kDa, 176 amino acid variant of similar biologic activity that contributes 15% of circulating human GH (hGH). The

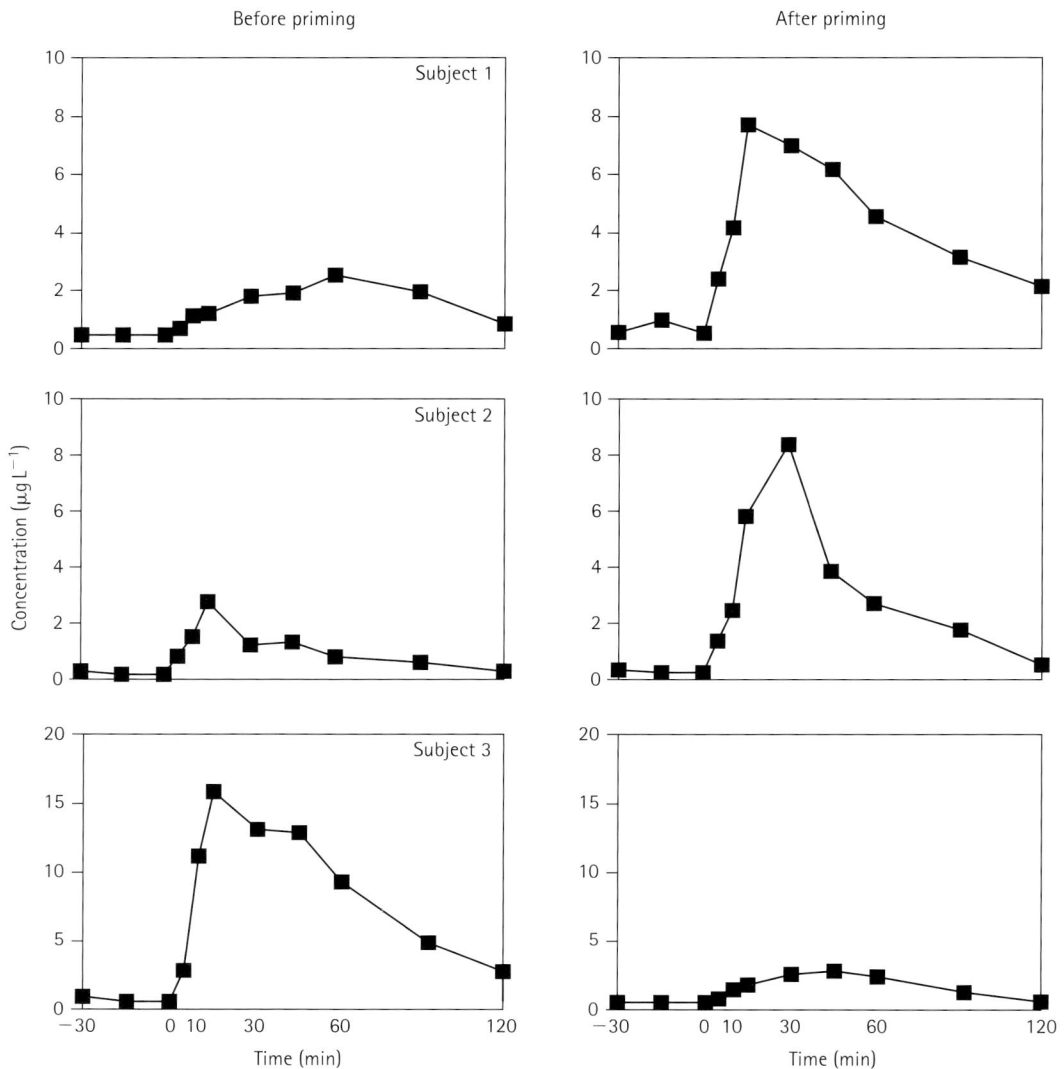

Figure 28.4   Effects of priming (10 consecutive days of subcutaneous administration of GHRP-2) on stimulated GH release in three adult subjects ranging in ages between 37 and 62 years. From Walker and Bercu.[134a]

three-dimensional structure of hGH is comprised of four anti-parallel helices joined by connecting sequences;[140] amino acids Leu45, Arg64, Lys172, Thr175, Phe176 and Arg178 form the functional hGH epitope.[141] The hGH receptor is a single chain polypeptide with extracellular, transmembrane, and intracellular domains; cysteine residues stabilize the amino terminal segment of the extracellular domain. One hGH molecule binds to and links two distinct GH binding sites on the hGHR. Docking first at high affinity hGH receptor site I must precede attachment of the molecule to the lower affinity site II.[140] Differing amino acid sequences at GH binding sites I and II bind essentially the same amino acid array on the hGHR, whose receptor determinants differ by only Asn218 near the carboxyl terminus.[140] Structural realignment intracellularly following hGH binding initiates non-covalent association of Janus kinase 2 (*JAK2*) and phosphorylation of tyrosine residues on moieties of the intracellular domain and adjacent JAK2 molecules. Activated *JAK2* phosphorylates signal transducers and activators of

transcription (*STATs 1,3,5A,5B*) that initiate nuclear gene transcription and excite the Ras mitogen-activated protein kinase (*MAPK*) pathway of gene transcription.[142,143]

NEUROTRANSMITTER REGULATION OF GROWTH HORMONE SECRETION

Cholinergic pathways

In man, muscarinic cholinergic neuroactivation exerts major inhibitory control of hypothalamic somatostatin, playing a key stimulatory role in GH secretion.[144] Cholinergic muscarinic agonists acutely enhance GH release by blunting somatostatinergic tone, perhaps in part by permitting 'rebound release' of GHRH by somatostatinergic synapses on GHRH secreting neurons.[145] Oral administration of the cholinesterase inhibitor, pyridostigmine, for example, doubles daily pulsatile GH mass in men, and partially

Table 28.3 Peak growth hormone (GH) concentrations following GHRP-2 and GHRH in the various groups

Group	Peak GH after GHRP-2 (μg L^{-1})	Peak GH after GHRH (μg L^{-1})	Peak GHRP-2/ GHRH ratio	Area under curve (μg L^{-1}; 90 min) GHRP-2	Area under curve (μg L^{-1}; 90 min) GHRH
GH-deficient children ($n = 15$)	20.1 $\pm$ 5.5 (<0.5->80)	19.6 $\pm$ 5.1 (0.3–70.2)	1.3 $\pm$ 0.4 (0.3–5.6)	995 $\pm$ 371	924 $\pm$ 232
Control children ($n = 8$)	42.2 $\pm$ 4.3 (31.7–62.0)	39.8 $\pm$ 7.8 (19.2–88.9)	1.4 $\pm$ 0.3 (0.4–2.9)	1598 $\pm$ 274	2201 $\pm$ 437
Slowly-growing, non-GH-deficient children ($n = 8$)	63.6 $\pm$ 24.9 (4.9–190.3)	31.4 $\pm$ 8.4 (1.5–78.8)	2.9 $\pm$ 1.3 (0.4–3.3)	2460 $\pm$ 953	1544 $\pm$ 449
Adult volunteers ($n = 7$)	52.0 $\pm$ 15.1 (14.6–123.2)	6.8 $\pm$ 2.4 (2.5–16.3)	15.0 $\pm$ 4.1 (0.9–36.2)	2785 $\pm$ 692	285 $\pm$ 93
Men ($n = 5$)	59.3	3.1	20.5		
Women ($n = 2$)	19.2	16.1	1.2		
Control vs GH-deficient children	$p < 0.02$	$p < 0.05$			$p < 0.01$
Control children vs adult volunteers		$p < 0.01$	$p < 0.01$		$p < 0.02$
GH-deficient children vs adult volunteers	$p < 0.05$		$p < 0.001$	$p < 0.02$	
Slow-growing non-GH-deficient children vs adult volunteers		$p < 0.02$	$p < 0.02$		$p < 0.02$
GH-deficient vs slow-growing, non-GH-deficient children	$p < 0.05$				

From Bercu and Walker[134] and Walker and Bercu.[134a]

re-establishes GH release blunted by repeated GHRH boluses or intravenous treatment with GH. Pyridostigmine also reverses some of the suppressive effect of glucocorticoids on GH release in children, but has little effect in diabetes, where somatostatinergic tone is already low.[146] Pyridostigmine is able to enhance the GH secretory response to GHRH in obese subjects, despite the presence of increased somatostatin tone.[147] Muscarinic receptor antagonists such as methscopolamine, atropine and pirenzepine reduce sleep-associated GH secretion, and extinguish GHRH stimulated GH release, but fail to blunt GH release to insulin induced hypoglycemia.[148,149] In contrast to the GH stimulatory role of muscarinic cholinergic neurotransmitters, nicotinic pathways are inhibitory, as nicotinic receptor blockers such as piperidine augment hypoglycemia or sleep induced GH secretion.[150]

Catecholaminergic pathways

Alpha adrenergic pathways mediate GH stimulatory neurons while beta adrenergic pathways are inhibitory of GH release. Binding of alpha-2 receptors in the median eminence by

agonists clonidine or guanfacine promotes GH release in animals and man by stimulating GHRH and possibly blunting somatostatin tone. In the rat, inactivation of GHRH with passive antibody transfer or arcuate nucleus ablation eliminates the alpha adrenergic GH response.[151] Alpha-2 GH stimulation may also involve somatostatin suppression, as clonidine's stimulatory effects are preserved in human subjects despite GHRH pretreatment abolition of GH response to repeat GHRH boluses. Further, clonidine's GH releasing effects are attenuated in steroid treated adult subjects with augmented somatostatinergic tone.[152]

The neurotransmitter primarily responsible for beta receptor mediated inhibition of GH release is L-epinephrine. Beta adrenergic pathways act by stimulating hypothalamic somatostatin release. For example, somatostatin mediated GH auto-feedback during sleep is blunted by administration of beta adrenergic antagonists.[153]

In short and normal statured children, the beta blocker propranolol augments GH release to hypoglycemia, exercise, glucagon, and GHRH.[154] Salbutamol, a beta-2 adrenergic agonist, is able to override L-arginine and pyridostigmine inhibition of somatostatin to permit GHRH stimulated GH secretion[155] and salbutamol has been shown to diminish the GH response to physical exercise.

GH is acutely released in humans by dopamine and dopaminergic agonists L-dopa, apomorphine, and bromoergocriptine, but is paradoxically inhibited in subjects with acromegaly.[156,157] Gender may affect dopaminergic regulation of GH as significant sex differences are observed in GH responses to the anti-dopaminergic compound metoclopramide;[158] dopaminergic GH stimulation is enhanced by estrogen and likely mediated by GHRH/somatostatin withdrawal. Pretreatment with bromoergocriptine augments GH release to GHRH, but dopaminergic drugs show little effect on GH secretion following insulin-induced hypoglycemia or arginine.[159] Interestingly, the pattern of GH response to dopamine in the rat is often opposite that seen in man.[1]

OTHER GROWTH HORMONE NEUROREGULATORS: PITUITARY ADENYL CYCLASE ACTIVATING PEPTIDE, SUBSTANCE P, BOMBESIN, AND MELATONIN

Serotonin binding to type-1D receptors mediates inhibition of hypothalamic somatostatin and GH release in man. 5-Hydroxytryptophan, a serotonin precursor, augments serum GH concentrations, but also stimulates release of catecholamines.[160] Sumatriptan, a serotonergic agonist that does not act at adrenergic, dopaminergic or GABAergic receptors, is GH stimulatory, while the serotonin antagonist, cyproheptadine, is inhibitory.[161,162] Galanin, a 29 amino acid peptide, is found in high concentration in the median eminence and is present throughout the hypothalamus. Its GTP-coupled receptor is similarly widely distributed in brain. In young male subjects galanin stimulates GH secretion alone and in concert with GHRH. In the arcuate nucleus it co-locates with GHRH.[163] Galanin does not synergistically release GH with hexarelin, however.[164] Women secrete more GH in response to galanin than men, and levels correlate with serum estradiol values;[164] an estrogen response element has also been described on the galanin gene promoter.[165] In the rat, galanin immunoneutralization reduces GH pulse amplitude, extinguishes the normal 3 h periodicity of GH secretion, and augments GH pulse frequency. Paradoxically, galanin appears to inhibit GH secretion in patients with GH secreting adenomas.[166] Calcitonin, synthesized in the thyroid C cells, is also present in the central nervous system with receptors distributed throughout the hypothalamus.[167] The 32-amino acid peptide exerts an inhibitory effect on GH secretion, perhaps through modulations of calcium flux in the pituitary.[168] Opioids inhibit somatostatin release *in vitro* and stimulate GH release in man. They may play a role in stress stimulated GH secretion.[169] Thyrotropin releasing hormone (TRH) is a physiologic GH secretagogue in the rat, but not in healthy man. However, TRH causes paradoxic GH release in various pathologic human conditions including acromegaly, type 1 diabetes mellitus, and renal[170] and hepatic failure.[171–173] TRH suppresses the GH releasing effects of L-dopa, arginine and insulin hypoglycemia probably by augmenting somatostatin release, but fails to inhibit GHRH stimulated GH secretion.[174,175] Neuropeptide Y, an orexigenic hypothalamic peptide that is suppressed by leptin, inhibits GH secretion in the rat and may play a role mediating nutritional effects on the GH and reproductive axes in animals.[176] Its role in human GH secretion remains to be defined. The pineal product melatonin increases basal GH concentrations and the GH response to GHRH when taken orally, suggesting a GH stimulatory effect.

PULSATILE GROWTH HORMONE SECRETION AND GROWTH HORMONE NEUROSECRETORY DYSFUNCTION

Insight into disorders of pulsatile GH secretion comes from studies using cranial radiation. Deleterious effects of cranial radiation on GH secretion are seen in individuals with a variety of neoplastic and hematologic diseases. Early studies assessing the hypothalamic–pituitary effects of cranial radiation were done in male rhesus monkeys. Animals which received central nervous system (CNS) radiation had blunted GH secretion following insulin-induced hypoglycemia (Fig. 28.5). In addition, pulsatile GH secretion was markedly impaired (Fig. 28.6). On the other hand, doubling the dose of insulin from 0.1 to 0.2 unit kg^{-1} normalized GH response, suggesting an intact altered resetting of hypothalamic sensitivity.

In humans, cranial radiation at a lower dose (2400 cGy) has been associated with growth retardation and decreased pulsatile GH secretion in subjects with acute lymphoblastic leukemia (ALL).[177] Twenty-four hour sampling of spontaneous GH secretion is more sensitive for the identification of both quantitative and qualitative abnormalities in GH secretion (reduced GH pulse amplitude and frequency) (Fig. 28.7). Normal GH secretory response to provocative pharmacologic stimuli in patients with a history of cranial radiation in association with abnormal 24 h GH secretion suggests selective defects in neurotransmitter control of GH secretion.[177] GH neurosecretory dysfunction (GHND) was the term used to describe subjects with growth retardation and neural irregularities of GH secretion.

Twenty-four hour studies of spontaneous GH secretion in children who received CNS or total body radiation for ALL, and a variety of other CNS tumors not involving the hypothalamic–pituitary axis demonstrated significant reductions in serum 24 h GH concentrations. Other studies showing blunting of peak GH secretion to a variety of provocative stimuli suggests widespread neuronal damage likely affecting neurotransmitter regulation of GH secretion, e.g. dopaminergic (L-dopa), noradrenergic (clonidine, propranolol), gamma-aminobutyric acid-ergic (GABA-ergic; valproic acid) and cholinergic (pyridostigmine) neurons. On the other hand, GH response to a serotonin-like compound (L-tryptophan) was not significantly affected.[178,179]

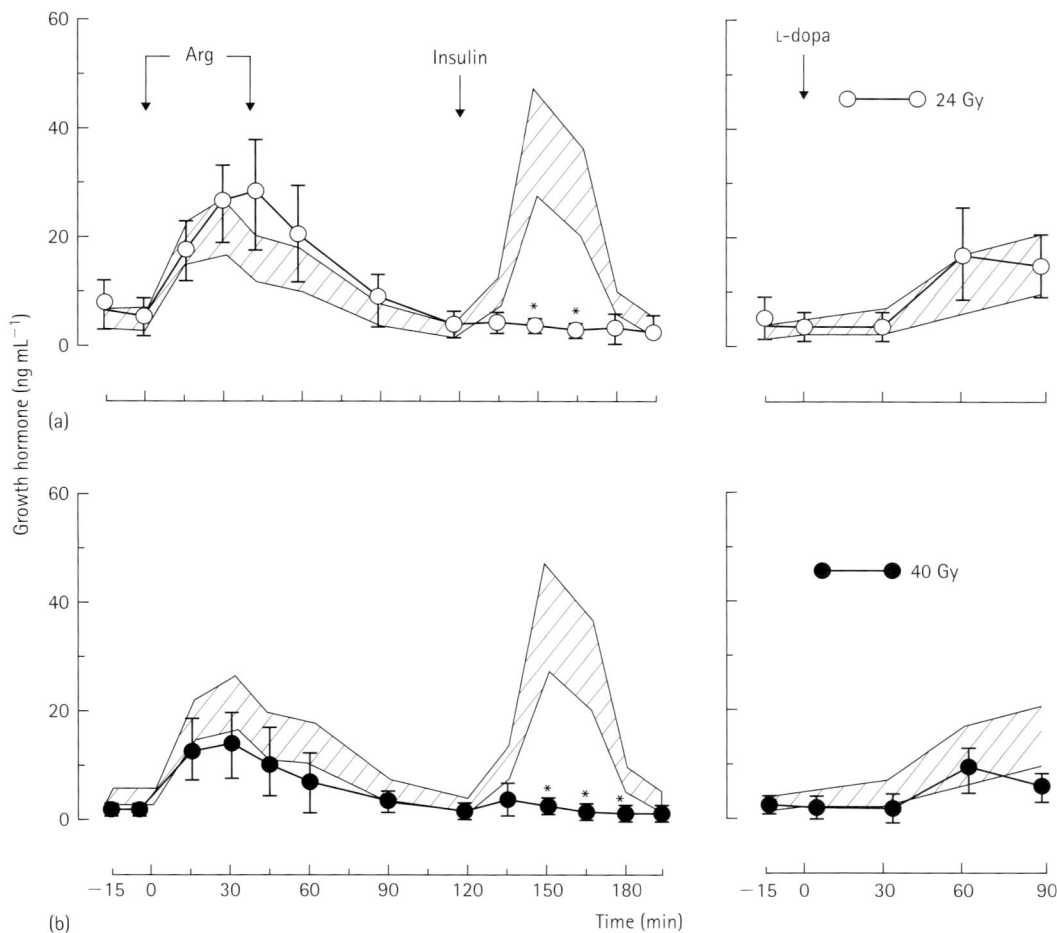

Figure 28.5 Growth hormone responses to arginine (Arg), insulin (Ins) and L-dopa stimulation 50 weeks after cranial irradiation. Primates treated with 24 Gy (open circles, $n = 4$) and 40 Gy (closed circles, $n = 4$) showed a normal response to arginine and L-dopa, but a blunted response to insulin (0.1 U kg^{-1}, i.v.). The shaded area represents the mean $\pm$ SEM from 9 to 13 controls. *$p < 0.001$. From Chrousos et al.[185] (Chrousos GP, Poplack D, Brown T, et al. Effects of cranial radiation on hypothalamic-adenohypophyseal function: Abnormal growth hormone secretory dynamics. *J Clin Endocrinol Metab* 1982; **54**: 1135–9. Copyright 1982, The Endocrine Society.)

In another study of 82 children (0.2–18.9 years; median 4.2 years), following cranial radiation with doses between 2400 and 4500 cGy for primary tumors not involving the hypothalamic–pituitary axis or prophylaxis against CNS leukemia, 74% were thought to be GH deficient based on insulin-induced hypoglycemia. Higher doses in excess of 3000 cGy caused GH deficiency to occur more quickly, with 100% GH deficient within three years (Fig. 28.8).[180] Analysis of GH secretion in 28 children with only ALL, 4.1–10.6 years (median 8.2 years) after prophylactic treatment with 1800 cGy CNS radiation identified 64.3% as GH deficient (using arginine and L-dopa as provocative stimuli); 81.5% has decreased overnight spontaneous GH secretion. Significantly there was a correlation of these biochemical abnormalities with MRI findings (empty sella in one quarter and a reduction in anterior pituitary lobe height). This correlated with peak GH response to arginine and mean overnight GH concentration.[181]

Children, especially those who are younger, are more vulnerable than adults to the effects of ionizing radiation on the central nervous system (CNS).[182] In irradiated children, neurotransmitter control of GH secretion is altered, as evidenced by blunted GH secretion following stimulation with dopaminergic, alpha- and beta-adrenergic, cholinergic, and GABA-ergic agents.[183,184] These studies and others suggest a hierarchy of radiation-induced CNS dysfunction of extrahypothalamic neurotransmitters > hypothalamic neurotransmitters > hypothalamic GHRH, somatostatin and/or ghrelin > pituitary secretion. Spontaneous GH release is also affected by radiation treatment in both primates and man. In monkeys studied prospectively following 1 year of cranial irradiation with 4000 cGy, there was reduction of both frequency and amplitude of GH secretory pulses.[185]

Clinically, slowing of linear growth commonly begins 2 or more years following radiation exposure,[186] and leukoencephalopathy may be present on computed tomography scan of subjects given 2400 cGy of prophylactic CNS irradiation for ALL.[187] Irradiated children may experience precocious sexual development and declines in IGF-I levels due to reduced GH secretion may be masked by increasing

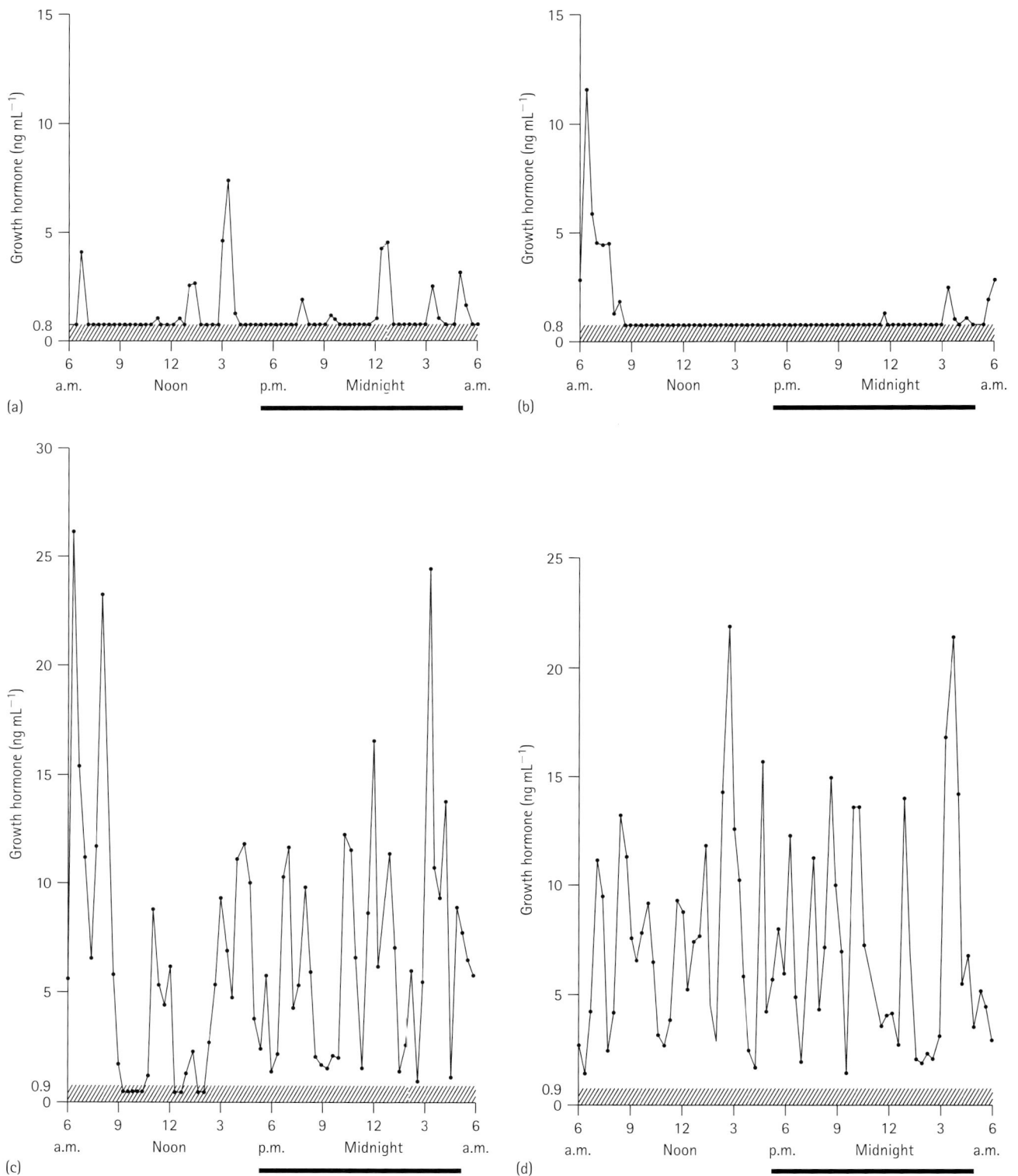

Figure 28.6   Growth hormone secretory pattern over 24 h in two primates treated with cranial irradiation (40 Gy; a,b) and two normal controls (c,d). The study was performed 1 year after treatment. There was a decrease in the number (frequency) and amplitude of secretory spikes in the animals that received radiation. The shaded area represents the detection limit of the assay. The dark period was from 17:00 to 05:00 hours (solid bar). From Chrousos et al.[185] (Chrousos GP, Poplack D, Brown T, et al. Effects of cranial radiation on hypothalamic-adenohypophyseal function: Abnormal growth hormone secretory dynamics. *J Clin Endocrinol Metab* 1982; **54**: 1135–9. Copyright 1982, The Endocrine Society.)

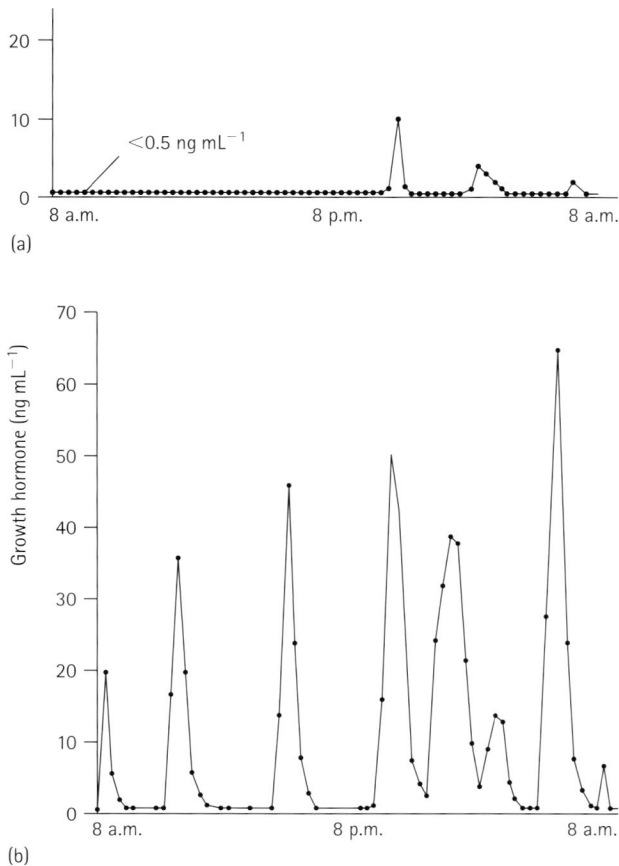

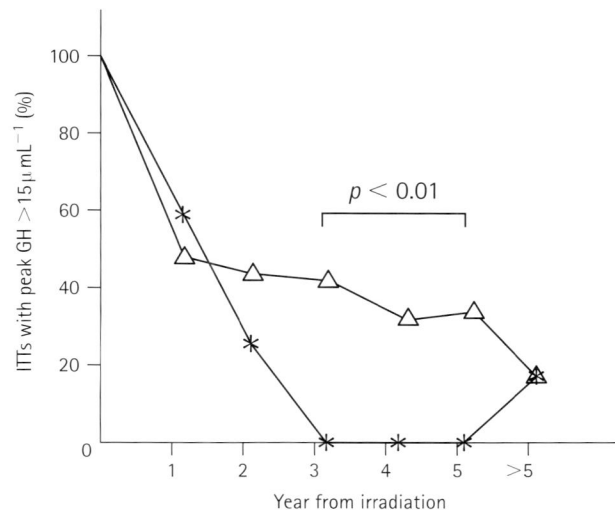

Figure 28.8   Percentage of normal insulin tolerance tests (ITTs) compared with time from irradiation in patients receiving <30 Gy (triangles) or greater than or equal to 30 Gy (asterisks) to the hypothalamic–pituitary axis. From Clayton and Shalet.[180] Copyright, 1984. With permission from Elsevier.

Figure 28.7   Spontaneous pulsatile growth hormone secretion in a representative patient with acute lymphoblastic leukemia who had received central nervous system (CNS) preventive therapy with 24 Gy cranial radiation and intrathecal methotrexate (top panel) and a representative normal child (lower panel). From Blatt et al.[177] Copyright, 1984. With permission from Elsevier.

concentrations of sex steroids. The majority of children who have such early puberty also demonstrate GH insufficiency resulting in attenuated pubertal growth, premature epiphyseal fusion, and eventual adult short stature.[188] Bone marrow transplantation (BMT) effects on neuroendocrine function are multifactorial. GH insufficiency based on pharmacologic testing and spontaneous GH secretion indicate that high radiation therapy doses such as 1000 cGy fractionated over relatively short periods such as 3 days can also result in GH neuroendocrine dysfunction.[189] Studies of these irradiation induced alterations of GH secretory patterns provided the basis for the description of GH neurosecretory dysfunction (GHND) in both CNS irradiated and non-irradiated children.[190]

Biosynthetic GH replacement therapy increased growth velocity in GH deficient children after cranial radiation, but final height was still significantly less than mid-parental height. Such observations demonstrate a lag time before initiation of hGH therapy and the detrimental effects of radiation, especially to the growing spine, in young children.[191]

CIRCULATING METABOLITES AND ABNORMAL GROWTH HORMONE SECRETION

In children and adults, administration of glucose acutely inhibits both basal and stimulated GH release.[192] Oral administration of glucose suppresses serum GH for 1–3 h followed by rebounding GH concentrations at 3–5 h as somatostatin release declines and GHRH levels begin to rise.[1] Modulation of GH through changes in blood glucose concentration do not appear to result from direct pituitary action, but rather are primarily mediated through altered release of hypothalamic somatostatin.[193] Acute hyperglycemia interdicts GHRH stimulated GH release, while GHRH pretreatment eliminates the subsequent GH response to GHRH, but not to hypoglycemia.[194,195] Central cholinergic activation of somatostatin by pyridostigmine blocks the acute inhibitory effect of glucose on GH release.[196] In infancy, however, glucose infusion paradoxically elevates circulating GH concentrations.[197] GH levels change periprandially[198] and acute depression of the blood sugar results in a rapid counter-regulatory release of GH,[199] perhaps through effects on the somatotroph lipid bilayer.[193]

Inherent problems with growth hormone secretory testing

Evaluating infants, children and adolescents with growth disorders may include GH provocative testing and 24 h or 12 h overnight profiles of spontaneous GH release. To date, there is still no 'gold standard' laboratory test to diagnosis GH deficiency. Blunted GH response to known GH secretagogues may help identify subjects with suspected GH deficiency (growth retardation, height less than the third percentile or better less than the first percentile), decreased growth velocity, and delayed bone maturation (bone age)); however, no single stimulation test provides adequate specificity. Thus, a minimum of two provocative tests of GH secretion has been the standard considered necessary to make the diagnosis of GH deficiency.

A subset of children with clinical features of GH deficiency (diminished growth velocity, delayed bone age) was suspected to have abnormalities of GH secretion despite a normal response to provocative GH testing. Children with growth retardation who demonstrate abnormal decreased spontaneous GH secretion but normal provocative tests can have GHND, which is considered a treatable cause of growth retardation (Fig. 28.9).[190,200] Other statistical methods using spontaneous 24h GH secretion and IGF-I levels have improved specificity in identifying children with disorders of GH secretion.[201]

The authors analyzed data collected from three hundred 24h studies of spontaneous GH secretion (sampling every 20 min) in 272 children. Children were further characterized by diagnosis: chronic renal failure, Noonan syndrome, obesity (BMI > 95th percentile for age), precocious puberty, cranial/craniospinal radiation and Turner syndrome (Fig. 28.10). All the above studies done by the authors utilized a standard polyclonal radioimmunoassay for GH.[178,179] Analysis of data using cluster analysis demonstrated preservation of GH pulsatile secretion and uniformity of GH pulse frequency in all subgroups except for obese children. Total spontaneous secretion increased in a linear fashion as BMI increases until the BMI reached 20–25, and has been confirmed by others.[202] Mean 24h GH concentration correlated positively with peak GH response to provocative stimuli (arginine, insulin, L-dopa, clonidine and GHRH;[178,179] Bercu, unpublished data). Significant reductions in mean 24h peak amplitude were seen in CNS radiated and obese subgroups. Serum IGF-I remained normal in obese children, but were decreased in CNS radiated and Turner syndrome children. Another subset of growth-retarded, non-GH deficient children has deceased mean 24h GH concentration, however, without significant changes in mean GH peak amplitude.[178,179]

Spontaneous GH secretory profiles represent a series of complex events with clinical utility. The experience reported here demonstrated decreased GH peak amplitude and frequency in obese children, while cranial irradiated children have decreased GH pulse amplitude. Short, slowly growing, non-GH deficient children also have alterations in their spontaneous GH secretory profiles relative to control children.[178,179]

In children with classical GH deficiency (blunted peak GH response to two or more provocative stimuli and decreased 24h spontaneous secretion), there may be a disturbance in normal dopaminergic inhibitory pathways on prolactin secretion.[185] Pooled 24h prolactin concentrations and 8h daytime pools were higher in children with classical GH deficiency when compared with control and GHND children. There is a bimodal distribution in the GH

deficient group. This suggests variability in anatomic level of disturbance (i.e., hypothalamic versus pituitary) affecting GH secretion[178,179] (Bercu, unpublished data).

Evaluation of growth disorders must include documentation of individual growth velocity, which remains the most useful clinical biologic marker of inadequacy of GH secretion. The authors performed a study on children with growth retardation. Both provocative and 24h spontaneous GH was examined. Three distinct groups based on GH secretory dynamics and pretreatment height velocity were assessed. Regardless of individual GH test results, 88% of those with impaired pretreatment growth velocity (i.e., less than 2 cm year^{-1}), 94% of those with velocities between 2 and 4 cm year^{-1}, and 79% of children with a pretreatment height velocity of greater than 4 cm year^{-1} had increased growth velocities of 2 cm year^{-1} or greater while receiving hGH. There was a significant negative correlation between pre- and post-hGH treatment growth velocities ($r = -0.67$, $p < 0.001$); this observation supports the conclusion that growth velocity remains the most sensitive biological marker of future response to hGH therapy rather than individual GH secretory status.[178,179,203]

Refinements on provocative GH secretory testing

To date GH provocative secretory tests have been used as the gold standard for determining insufficient GH secretion. Spontaneous 24h GH secretory studies and clinical observations have broadened the scope of GH secretory disorders. The timing of the GH secretory pulse affects the peak GH concentration during GH provocative testing[204] (Fig. 28.11). The authors have used somatostatin pretreatment to reduce the variability of GH releasing hormone stimulation testing[204] (Fig. 28.12). This refinement could help by bringing GH secretion to trough level rather than stimulating GH secretion during the up- or down-slope of the GH pulse (Fig. 28.11). It is possible that this model could be applied to all GH provocative tests.

GH secretion is due to a complex series of interactions occurring both in the CNS and in peripheral tissues. Despite an improved understanding of these detailed interactions, clinicians are still hampered by the incomplete understanding of the physiology of growth. Despite improved knowledge of neurotransmitter regulatory control and impact of various pharmacologic agents, clinicians still have no specific way of consistently identifying children who would benefit from exogenous hGH treatment.

Decision-making processes must be viewed in the total clinical setting. The use of overnight and 24h GH secretory profiles, along with GH provocative testing and other accepted biomarkers of GH sufficiency (IGF-I, IGFBPs), supplements physical findings and height velocity. Together all this information aids the clinician in his/her attempt to make the best selection of those children who warrant hGH therapy.

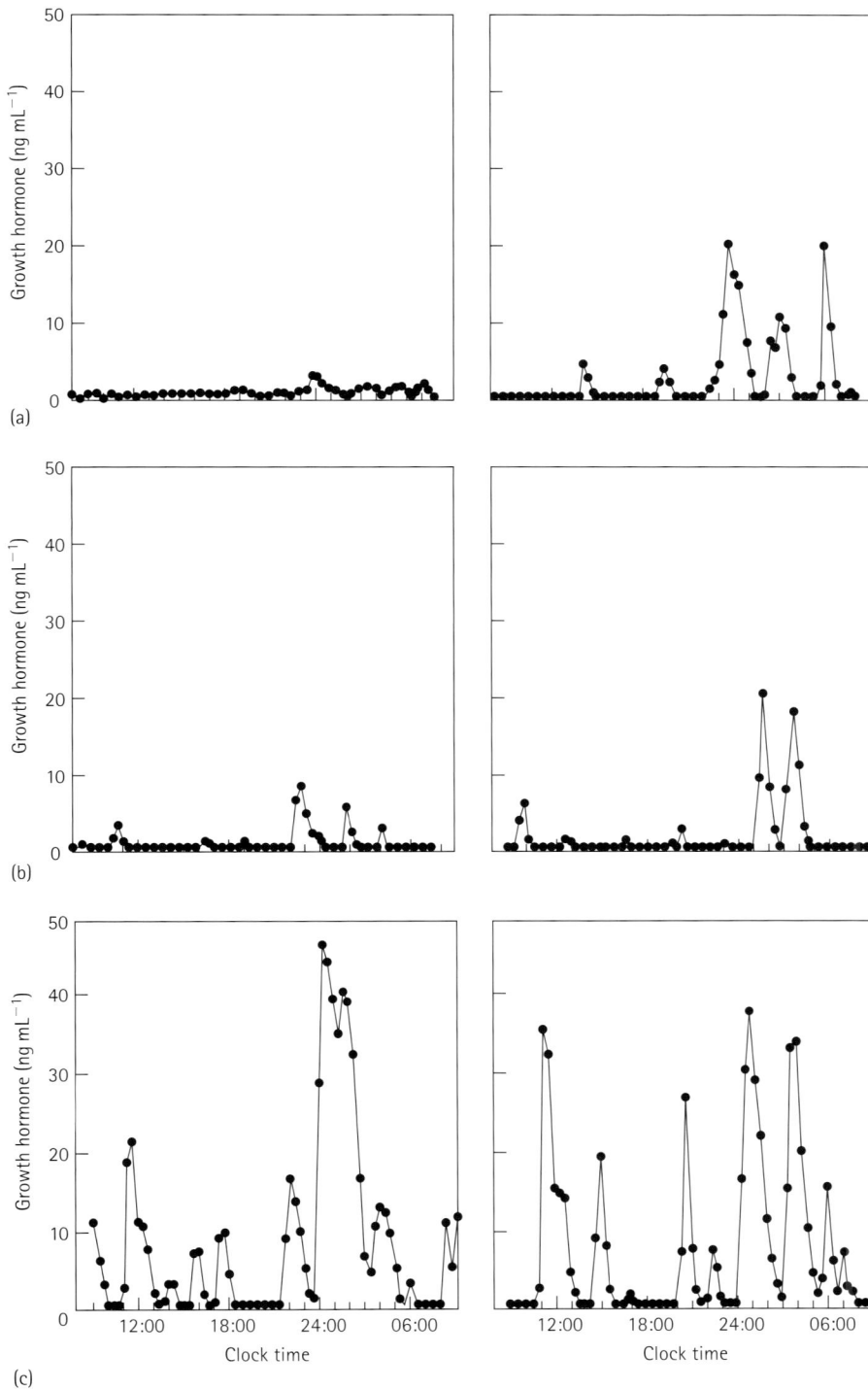

Figure 28.9 Representation 24 h GH secretory patterns in GH-deficient (a, top panel), GH neurosecretory dysfunction (GHND) (b, middle panel) and control subjects (c, lower panel). Control subjects in (c) are Tanner stage I and IV, respectively. Note that a child with classic GH deficiency (right-hand side of (a) had three pulses higher than 10 ng mL^{-1} and two above 20 ng mL^{-1}. This child had a mean endogenous 24 h GH concentration of less than that of two other children with GHND. By definition, the patients with GHND had two or more normal GH provocative tests (peak $\geqslant$ 10 ng mL^{-1}), unlike classic GH-deficient children (two or more GH provocative tests < 10 ng mL^{-1}). The GHND children had a linear growth response to exogenous GH similar to the classic GH-deficient children. From Spiliotis et al.[190]

PHYSIOLOGIC STATES OF ALTERED GROWTH HORMONE RELEASE: AGE, GENDER, SLEEP, AND EXERCISE

Mean spontaneous GH concentrations vary throughout life by three-fold. This is true for spontaneous GH secretion and also to a lesser degree for provocative testing. In full-term newborns GH secretion is high and even higher in premature infants.[205] Immediately after birth, GH levels decrease with lesser peak amplitude and pulse frequency. GH concentrations parallel decreased responsivity of the somatotrope to GHRH stimulation.[206] GH levels remain essentially steady until puberty, when there is a significant increase in GH production, primarily due to burst mass and daytime pulse frequency.[207] During puberty spontaneous GH secretion increases by about 2.5-fold in males and by 2.3-fold in females. Estrogen elevates both basal GH secretion and irregularity of GH pulses, while testosterone

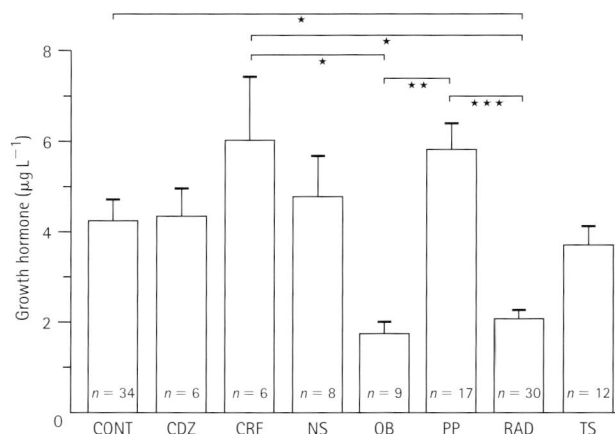

Figure 28.10 Mean 24 h GH concentrations in a variety of conditions associated with growth retardation. CONT, controls; CDZ, chronic disease, including asthma, celiac disease, and thalassemia; CRF, chronic renal failure; NS, Noonan syndrome; OB, obesity; PP, precocious puberty; RAD, CNS irradiation; TS, Turner syndrome. $p < 0.05$; $*p < 0.01$; $***p < 0.001$. From Bercu et al.[178]

Figure 28.11 Timing of growth hormone secretory pulse. Upper panel represents GH responses over time following GHRH administration in children with classical GH deficiency (group I, dashed line/black squares), biochemical GH deficiency and normal growth velocity (group II, solid lines/triangles), biochemical GH sufficiency and subnormal growth velocity (group III, solid line/plus symbols), and GH sufficiency and normal growth velocity (group IV, dotted line/diamonds). Lower panel represents peak GH response (C_{max}, black bar), and area under curve (AUC, stippled bar) after GHRH administration in the four groups. AUC and C_{max} are significantly lower in group I than in group III, respectively ($p < 0.01$). Data are presented as mean $\pm$ SEM. From Cho et al.[204]

causes greater GH pulses.[208] During the third and fourth decades of life, GH declines leading to the ' somatopause', when GH secretion is significantly reduced. GH levels in a 40-year-old are similar to prepubertal levels. The somatopause is due to many factors including decrease GH releasing hormone tone.[209]

Gender is also an important determinant of GH secretion. Females produce more GH than males mostly due to the estrogen effect. Specifically, there is a larger burst mass per peak, with little or no difference in frequency of pulses.[207,210] In females the pulses are both of greater amplitude and longer duration. Prior to puberty females secrete about 30% more GH than males; this difference is continued or accentuated after puberty.[207] Estrogen increases both basal GH production and irregularity (entropy)[208] possibility by alteration of GH-releasing hormone and somatostatin tone.[211] In contrast, testosterone decreases basal GH secretion and pulse frequency whereas testosterone increases pulse amplitude and duration,[212] probably through modulation of GHRH tone.[213] The mechanism of many actions of testosterone may be due to the physiologic conversation to estradiol, since non-aromatizable androgens do not have the same GH augmenting ability as is the case for testosterone.[214]

In adults, a pulse of GH secretion occurs shortly after onset of stage III and IV slow-wave sleep, peaking in 1 h; waking levels are relatively low. In young men, episodic GH release in blood sampled every 30 s correlates closely with onset of stages III and IV slow-wave sleep.[215] In older men, approximately 70% of GH pulses during sleep are coincident with slow-wave sleep. The slow-wave sleep associated increase of GH secretion primarily reflects augmented pulse amplitude as well as higher interpulse (nadir) GH concentrations, consistent with a sleep-associated decline in somatostatin tone.[1] Sleep-associated GH pulse frequency is

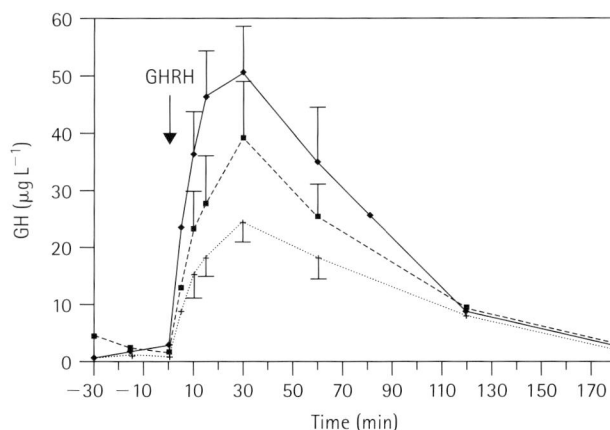

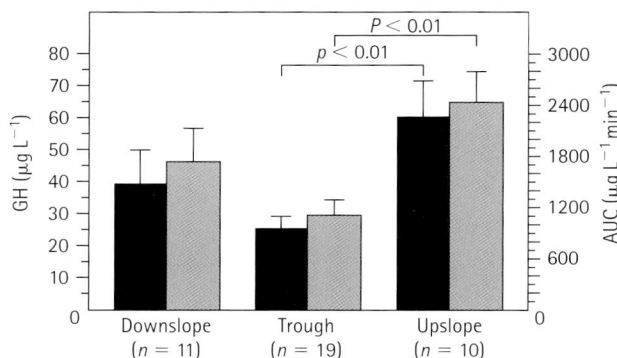

also augmented two-fold compared to waking hours.[216] Enhanced nocturnal GH release to GHRH infusion during slow-wave sleep further supports a withdrawal of somatostatinergic tone during this interval. Injections of GHRH in animals and man decrease wakefulness and augment slow-wave sleep. The GABA agonist, gamma-hydroxybutyrate, also stimulates both GH secretion and slow-wave sleep in young men.[217] With aging, both GH secretion and the quantity of slow-wave sleep decline. Shifts in sleep-onset GH pulses occur with sleep advancement, sleep delay and sleep reversal. Daytime naps, interruptions in sleep, or forced fragmentation of sleep also result in increases in GH secretion after sleep onset.[218]

Exercise induces GH release in response to increased core body temperature[219] with GH levels rising about 15 min after onset of physical activity. Epinephrine, norepinephrine,

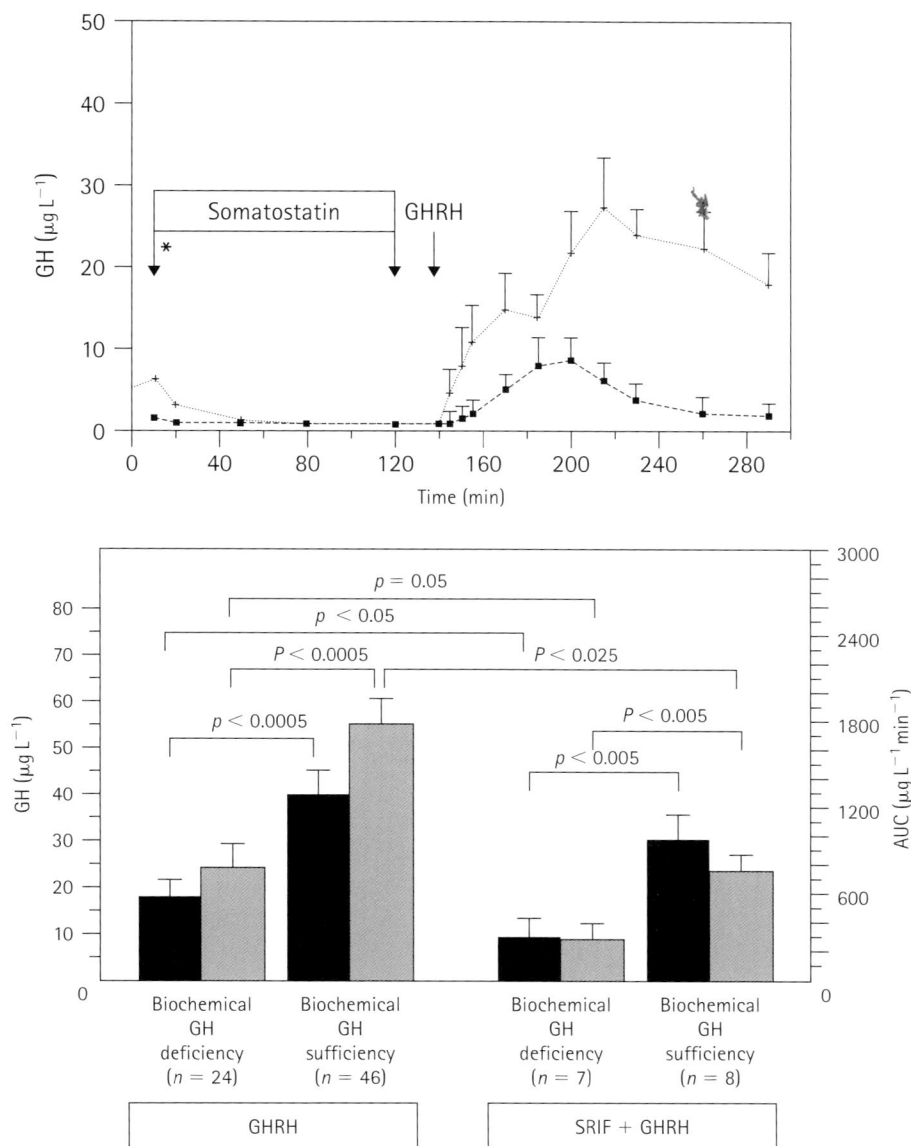

Figure 28.12 Somatostatin infusion. Upper panel represents GH response over time GHRH after GH suppression by somatostatin (SRIF) in the biochemical GH deficient (dotted line) and GH sufficient groups. The asterisk represents the intravenous bolus injection of somatostatin, which was followed by a constant infusion of somatostatin. Lower panel represents area under curve (AUC) (gray) and peak GH response (C_{max}, black) in the biochemical GH sufficiency and deficiency groups after GHRH administration. One group received only GHRH and another group received somatostatin followed by GHRH. In the children with biochemical GH sufficiency there were higher AUC and C_{max} compared to biochemical GH deficiency regardless of somatostatin pretreatment ($p < 0.01$) in both groups. AUC in the biochemical GH sufficient group was significantly lower in the somatostatin/GHRH children when compared to the GHRH alone group ($p < 0.05$). From Cho et al.[204]

acetylcholine and opioids have all been implicated in this process.[220] Integrated 24 h serum GH concentrations in women are also augmented by prolonged exercise training, reflecting an increase in GH pulse amplitude.[221] GH responses vary related to exercise intensity and demonstrate significant inter-subject variability.[222]

GROWTH HORMONE SECRETION DURING ILLNESS AND STRESS

GH concentrations rise quickly during the acute phase of critical illness.[223] There is increased GH pulsatility with augmented inter-pulse secretion.[223] During more protracted severe illness growth hormone concentrations rise quickly during the acute phase of critical illness.[223] During more protracted severe illness, however, a high frequency, low amplitude pattern with lower inter-pulse concentrations

emerges, with low, or normal mildly elevated mean GH concentrations.[224] Acute as well as prolonged critical illness results in reduced circulating concentrations of IGF-I, IGFBP-3 and acid labile subunit (ALS) while IGFBP-3 proteolytic activity is increased.[225] GH neurosecretory abnormalities have been demonstrated in chronic renal failure[226] and high altitudes.[227]

CLINICAL STATES OF ALTERED GROWTH HORMONE SECRETION

Constitutional delay in growth and development (CDGD)

Gender differences in GH secretion in children begin in the peri-pubertal period.[228] As puberty progresses, augmented spontaneous GH secretion related to increased pulse amplitude occurs in both sexes. Spontaneous GH patterns in women reflect more frequent but lower amplitude GH secretory bursts compared to men, whose nadir GH values have been shown to be slightly higher.[228]

CDGD is an altered pattern of growth and pubertal development felt to be a variant of normal. Children present with a gradual slowing of linear growth associated with delay of pubertal development and bone age closer to height age than chronologic age. In untreated children stimulated and spontaneous GH levels have been reported to be normal[229] and reduced.[230] A blunted GH response to provocative testing that normalizes with onset of puberty has also been described.[231] A study of overnight secretion in prepubertal children with CDGD revealed no difference in mean overnight GH levels compared to controls; however, pulse amplitude and frequency were reduced while GH pulses were prolonged. CDGD males had a decreased mass of GH released per burst perhaps reflecting a deficit in GHRH release per secretory event. The pattern results in less GH secretory entropy signifying a more invariant level of GH release.[232] GH levels increase with an increase in GH amplitude at 3 and 12 months in prepubertal boys treated with monthly injections of testosterone enanthate for a year,[233] a pattern that resembles the rise of GH during the pubertal growth spurt,[234] or following androgen priming of peri-pubertal children.[235,236] Prepubertal boys treated with the synthetic androgen oxandrolone, in contrast, demonstrate no change in GH pulse amplitude, but an increase in GH area under the curve (AUC) at 6 months and altered GH pulse frequency, likely reflecting the inability of oxandrolone to aromatize to estrogen.[237]

Obesity

The body mass index of healthy prepubertal children is inversely related to the 24 h daytime and nighttime GH concentrations, as well as to the GH pulse peak amplitude, 24 h AUC, and pulse frequency. These associations are independent of gender differences, and unrelated to chronologic age, bone age, height or weight.[238,239] In girls and female adolescents, the waist/hip ratio, a reflection of visceral fat, is inversely related to nocturnal growth hormone release.[239] In obese children, both spontaneous and stimulated release of GH is reduced.[241–244] This blunting results from augmented somatostatin tone, increased metabolic clearance, and reduced GH secretory burst mass. The ability of pyridostigmine, a somatostatin inhibitor to partially restore GH responsiveness to GHRH in obese subjects supports the presence of an increased somatostatin tone. Fatty acids inhibit GH release directly at the somatotroph.[1] In obese adults, hyposomatotropism reflects alteration of both GH secretion and clearance.[244] For each unit increase in body mass index in adult subjects at a given age, the daily GH secretion rate is decreased by 6%. Reduced GH secretion is partially restored by weight loss.[245] The fat cell hormone leptin is involved in GH regulation. In rodents the leptin receptor is expressed in arcuate and paraventricular nuclear GHRH producing cells[246] and controlling for adiposity, serum leptin concentrations correlate negatively to GH response to GHRH in both lean and obese prepubertal children.

Prader–Willi syndrome

Prader–Willi syndrome, a form of syndromal obesity caused by deletion or uniparental disomy of the 15th chromosome, is associated with infantile hypotonia, hyperphagia with excessive weight gain commencing in the toddler years, hypogonadism and hypomentia. There is mild intrauterine growth retardation, postnatal decline in growth velocity, and blunting of the pubertal growth spurt.[240] Adult height averages 152–162 cm in males and 145–150 cm in females and is reduced to −2.5 SD of reference ranges.[241] Growth hormone responses to provocative testing with insulin, arginine, clonidine and L-dopa are low normal or blunted, as are sleep-induced GH secretion and 24 h integrated GH levels.[242–245] These results are confounded, however, by the suppressive effects of simple obesity on the hypothalamic–pituitary–growth axis. True growth hormone deficiency is postulated given the context of presumed hypothalamic obesity and hypogonadism, the presence of declining growth rate and reduced lean body mass despite progressive obesity, small hands and feet, and relatively low concentrations of insulin-like growth factor compared to values in obese control children.[245,247] Prepubertal children with PWS treated with human growth hormone for periods up to 5 years demonstrate significant catch up growth and adult height predictions increase into the range of parental target height.[248] While improvements in body composition have also been reported, the deaths of several children with PWS receiving GH have led to recommendations against the use of growth hormone in severely obese PWS children and those with respiratory impairment.[249]

Undernutrition and anorexia nervosa

The neuroendocrine regulation of growth hormone secretion is strongly influenced by the state of energy balance. Growth hormone secretion is augmented in fasted human subjects, while concentrations of IGF-I decline.[250] In animal models, undernutrition results in down-regulation of GH binding to hepatic membranes, while postreceptor dysfunction resulting from energy deprivation may also contribute to growth hormone resistance.[251,252] Anorexia nervosa is a severe eating disorder that primarily affects young women and is characterized by substantial weight loss, amenorrhea, and behavioral changes. Basal and GHRH-stimulated growth hormone levels are increased.[253] Thin women with anorexia nervosa manifest decreased levels of growth hormone binding protein (GHBP) and IGFBP-3, and increased concentrations of IGFBP-l and IGFBP-2; these values correct with refeeding.[254] In constitutionally thin women whose BMI is equivalent to anorexia nervosa patients, but whose percent body fat approximates normal weight controls, GH and IGF-I levels are not affected. Ghrelin is a hypothalamic growth hormone secretagogue (GHS) that also acts as a short-term feeding signal when released from the oxyntic cells of the stomach. In both anorexia nervosa and hereditary thinness, morning fasting ghrelin concentrations are increased compared to those in healthy age-matched normal weight women. The 200% increase in ghrelin concentrations observed in subjects with anorexia nervosa return to control values following renutrition. Ghrelin concentrations in anorexia nervosa do not, however, correlate with basal GH secretion.[253]

Intrauterine growth retardation

GH secretion in children born with intrauterine growth retardation (IUGR, SGA) is characterized by a continuum, ranging from GH deficiency, which can be diagnosed at birth, to normal GH secretion. In a Swedish population-based study, 10–15% of children born with low birth weight remained short after 2 years of age.[255] Of 134 children born SGA (97 boys, 37 girls, mean CA = 7.3 ± 0.3 years) 13 had clinical findings consistent with Russell–Silver syndrome (RS); mean birthweight was −2.7 ± 0.1 SDS. At follow-up, all were prepubertal with mean height of −3.0 ± 0.1 SDS; 106 underwent 24 h sampling. The mean estimated secretion rate for GH was lower in the short children born SGA compared with the reference groups born at an appropriate size for gestational age, of either short ($p < 0.05$) or normal stature ($p < 0.001$). In the youngest children born SGA (2–6 years of age) a different pattern of GH secretion was found, with a high basal GH level, low peak amplitude, and high peak frequency. Mean GH secretion rate and AUC were lower in children born SGA compared with children born at the appropriate gestational age (AGA), however, there was overlap. IGF-I and IGFBP-3 concentrations were reduced in SGA children compared with a reference Swedish population. The high baseline levels of GH suggest that short SGA children may have different proportions of the GH isoforms.[256] The proportion of non-22-kDa GH isoforms has been shown to be increased in children born SGA and correlates negatively with height SDS.[257] In a British cohort of 31 SGA children with short stature (17 RS), nine patients (eight with RS) had a single nocturnal GH pulse. Four of 31 had a peak GH $< 20\,\text{mU}\,\text{L}^{-1}$ at night. The results suggest that physiologic GH insufficiency is probably common in children with RS.[258] In Russell–Silver syndrome the adolescent growth spurt occurs early and is reduced in magnitude[259] and many of these children have an inappropriate advance in epiphyseal maturation during middle childhood.[259] In 31 SGA British children six with RS failed to return to the baseline between pulses. Nine had only a single major nocturnal GH peak (a secretory pattern described as 'common' in girls with Turner syndrome)[260] and three showed a fast-frequency pattern with less variation in pulse amplitude than in those with increased frequency. Disordered pulse frequency may be responsible for the low growth velocity in some children who have a normal release of GH following a pharmacologic stimulus.[259]

Hypothalamic lesions

The majority of patients with GH deficiency have a functional hypothalamic disturbance.[261] The presence of a hypothalamic mass lesion with intact pituitary may result in a 'functional stalk section', a disconnection between hypothalamic and pituitary function. In this clinical setting, the release of pituitary hormones following administration of exogenous releasing hormones may be preserved but delayed, or substantially reduced. In hypothalamic hypothyroidism, for example, administration of TRH commonly results in a peak TSH release shifted from 30 to 60 min (and remains elevated at 120 min). In adult subjects with a hypothalamic lesion, GHRH normally provokes GH secretion, but GH secretagogue-induced GH release is blocked and the synergistic action of GHRH and GH secretagogue disappears.[262] In contrast, children with stalk interruption release very little GH following administration of GHRH.[262] Infants with perinatal stress such as breech delivery or birth asphyxia may present with GH deficiency causing hypoglycemic seizures, and microphallus, as the presenting manifestations of panhypopituitarism.[263] MRI changes can include an ectopic posterior pituitary, absent or attenuated pituitary stalk, and atrophic anterior pituitary.[264] In some instances this deformity may result from mechanical transection due to displacement of the brain, while in others a fetal malformational event in the descent and fusion of the neuro- and adenohypophysis may occur.[265,266]

PATHOLOGIC HORMONAL STATES

Glucocorticoids

Physiologic glucocorticoid concentrations are required for maintenance of baseline GH secretory reserve.[267] In Addison's disease due to primary or secondary adrenal insufficiency, the GH secretory response to insulin and arginine is impaired and normal secretion is restored following appropriate steroid replacement.[267] In contrast, hydrocortisone administered to normal men rapidly inhibits the GH release by GHRH, a response that is partially reversed by administration of pyridostigmine, suggesting glucocorticoid stimulation of somatostatinergic tone.[268] Administration of potent synthetic steroids like dexamethasone and prednisone affect GH release in a dose, time and agent dependent manner that may result in early GH release followed by longer term GH suppression. Such biphasic patterns may reflect a varying somatostatinergic state (via enhanced beta-2 adrenergic activity), GHRH rebound, and steroid-induced inhibition of IGF bioactivity.[269,270] Spontaneous and stimulated GH levels are suppressed in prepubertal children receiving long-term glucocorticoid therapy for immunosuppression.[271] In patients with endogenous hypercortisolism (Cushing's syndrome) 24 h mean GH concentrations are reduced and secretory disorder increased; GH peak height and peak area are suppressed, while pulse frequency is not affected.[272] GH secretion following GHRH/GHRP infusion is blunted.[273] Pyridostigmine partially restores GH secretion.[274] Altered GH release may persist for up to 12 months following cure.[272] Hyperglycemia, increased circulating free fatty acids, and obesity that may accompany hypercortisolism contribute to the altered GH secretory dynamics in Cushing's syndrome.

Thyroid hormones

Children with prolonged severe hypothyroidism experience virtual growth arrest; mean nocturnal GH levels may fall by close to half, and IGF-I concentrations decline substantially.[275] 'Catch-up' growth ensues with thyroxine replacement therapy and GH and IGF-I values normalize.[276] Impairment of GH secretory response to provocative stimuli such as insulin hypogycemia, arginine and L-dopa is found in many but not all hypothyroid adults and children and restoration of the euthyroid state results in normalization of GH secretion.[277] The decline in GH concentrations in hypothyroid patients given the anti-somatostatinergic drugs pyridostigmine or arginine points to a primary impairment of GH synthesis in hypothyroidism.[278] In the hypothyroid rat, pituitary GH content, percentage of somatotrophs and somatotroph granulation are all decreased.[279] Deficiency of thyroid hormone is also associated with reductions in hypothalamic GHRH, down-regulation of GHRH receptor numbers, and reduced GHRH binding to pituitary somatotroph receptors.[280] Hyporesponsiveness to GHRH usually corrects within 2 weeks of initiation of L-thyroxine therapy.[281] Reduced GH secretory response to GHRH in hypothyroid rats may in part reflect reduced intra-somatotroph adenyl cyclase activity; levels of pituitary cyclic AMP following GHRH administration to thyroidectomized rats are only 10% those of control animals.[282] Pretreatment of hypothyroid subjects with the beta adrenergic blocking agent propranolol augments the GH response to GHRH and insulin, while pyridostigmine and galanin fail to influence GHRH provoked GH secretion. Significant alterations of GH dynamics also occur in hyperthyroidism. 24 h GH secretory rates are reduced in thyrotoxic adolescents and hyperthyroid men evidence substantially blunted GHRH stimulated GH responses but increased frequency of GH secretory bursts.[283] Return to normal GHRH sensitivity may require up to 3 months of euthyroidism.[268] IGF-I bioactivity is reduced in thyrotoxicosis and increases with achievement of euthyroidism.[234] Hyperglycemic suppression of GH secretion is blunted.[285]

Thyrotropin-releasing hormone (TRH) does not alter GH secretion in healthy individuals, but stimulates GH release in pathologic states such as acromegaly, anorexia and depression.[286]

Insulin and diabetes mellitus

Patients with type l diabetes have an increased secretion of GH compared to healthy controls, especially during the pubertal years.[287–289] This finding has been associated with poor metabolic control, growth retardation, delayed puberty, and diabetic complications such as retinopathy and nephropathy. Increased GH secretion is most evident at Tanner stages 3–4, and is characterized by increases in pulse amplitude, frequency and interpeak concentrations. There is exaggerated GH response to GHRH.[290] These findings may reflect inhibition of somatostatinergic tone as well as catabolism associated reductions in IGF-I feedback.[291,292] Low levels of IGF-I found in type l diabetic patients despite a hyper-somatotrophic state suggest 'GH resistance,' perhaps reflecting down-regulation of hepatic GH receptors by portal hypoinsulinemia and/or altered IGF binding protein milieu influencing IGF-I bioavailability. Reduced concentrations of GH binding protein, the extracellular domain of the GH receptor, further support a GH insensitivity state. Interestingly, diabetics with good metabolic control still manifest diurnal and exercise-stimulated GH hypersecretion.[293] Pretreatment of diabetic subjects with GH fails to limit the GH response to GHRH, suggesting a maximally suppressed endogenous somatostatin pool.[294] Nocturnal GH secretion and the nightly insulin requirements decline in children of different pubertal stages after oral administration of cholinergic antagonists.[295] Mean 24 h GH secretion declines substantially with improved blood glucose control.[296] Four weeks of subcutaneous treatment with IGF-I lowers both serum IGFBP-1 and GH levels in diabetic subjects.[297]

GROWTH HORMONE STIMULATION TESTING

As GH is secreted primarily at night, and its concentrations are frequently low or undetectable between daytime pulses, the diagnosis of GH deficiency has been based historically upon measurements of GH release following stimulation with various pharmacologic secretagogues (insulin, arginine, glucagon, L-dopa, clonidine, etc). More recently, however, experts have questioned relying on stimulation tests as a 'gold standard' for the diagnosis of GH deficiency.[298] In the United States many clinicians use a response of less than $10 \, \text{ng mL}^{-1}$ for the diagnosis of GH deficiency, although this is an arbitrary cut-off that is not adjusted for age, pubertal stage, body composition (obesity), method of GH assay, or provocative agent utilized. Using a cut-off of $10 \, \text{ng mL}^{-1}$ and three different stimulation tests,

Marin demonstrated that 75% of normal-statured prepubertal children with normal heights and growth velocities would be mislabeled as GH deficient (false positives).[299] However, selection of a lower cut-off value, such as $3-5 \, ng \, mL^{-1}$, does appear to increase diagnostic specificity.[300] Furthermore, many small, slowly growing children, who respond to somatotropin therapy with a sustained increase in growth velocity, exceeded $10 \, ng \, mL^{-1}$ on provocative testing (false negatives). GH concentrations are subject to considerable inter-assay variability, are two- to three-fold lower in newer assays,[301,302] and show poor reproducibility in both the short and long term; considerable variability in response may occur based on the timing of stimulation during the pulse cycle.[303] GH stimulation testing using higher cutoffs are poor predictors of growth response to somatotropin therapy, although growth response is substantially better in children with severely blunted GH release ($<3 \, ng \, mL^{-1}$).[304] Our pediatric endocrine division believes that clinicians should continue to perform provocative testing as a means of assessing the entire hypothalamic pituitary axis. We utilize a cocktail that includes arginine, gonadotropin releasing hormone, when age appropriate, TRH when available, and insulin which is also particularly helpful in assessing the hypothalamic–pituitary–adrenal axis. However, the results of provocative testing must be placed in the clinical context of each individual case, and weighed together with significant findings in the child's history and physical examination, growth velocity, bone age X-ray, magnetic resonance imaging of the brain and pituitary, and IGF-l and IGFBP-3 levels.

REFERENCES

1 Giustina A, Veldhuis JD. Pathophysiology of the neuroregulation of growth hormone secretion in experimental animals and the human. *Endocr Rev* 1998; **19**: 717–97.

2 Veldhuis JD, Moorman J, Johnson ML. Deconvolution analysis of neuroendocrine data: waveform-specific and waveform-independent methods and applications. *Methods Neurosci* 1994; **20**: 279–325.

3 Gaylinn BD. Molecular and cell biology of the growth hormone-releasing hormone receptor. *Growth Horm IGF Res* 1999; **9(Suppl A)**: 37–44.

4 Coy DH. In: *Human Growth Hormone Research and Clinical Practice*. Totowa, NJ: Humana Press, 2000: 97–108.

5 Schally AV, Comaru-Schally AM. In: Bercu BB, Walker RF, eds. *Growth Hormone Secretagogues in Clinical Practice*. New York: Marcel Dekker, 1998: 131–43.

6 Root AW, Diamond FB. Regulation and clinical assessment of growth hormone secretion. *Endocrine* 2000; **12**: 137–45.

7 Petersenn S, Shulte HM. Structure and function of the growth-hormone-releasing hormone receptor. *Vitam Horm* 2000; **59**: 35–69.

8 Merriam GR, Cassorla F. *Human Growth Hormone Research and Clinical Practice*. Totowa, NJ: Humana Press, 2000: 297–313.

9 Ocampo-Lim B, Guo W, DeMott-Friberg R, *et al*. Nocturnal growth hormone (GH) secretion is eliminated by infusion of GH-releasing hormone antagonist. *J Clin Endocrinol Metab* 1996; **81**: 4396–9.

10 Borges JL, Blizzard RM, Gelato MC, *et al*. Effects of human pancreatic tumour growth hormone releasing factor on growth hormone and somatomedin C levels in patients with idiopathic growth hormone deficiency. *Lancet* 1983; **ii**: 119–24.

11 Bertherat J, Doumaud P, Berod A, *et al*. Growth hormone-releasing hormone-synthesizing neurons are a subpopulation of somatostatin receptor-labelled cells in the rat arcuate nucleus: a combined in situ hybridization and receptor light-microscopic radioautographic study. *Neuroendocrinology* 1992; **56**: 25–31.

12 Tannenbaum GS, Farhadi-Jou F, Beaudet A. Ultradian oscillation in somatostatin binding in the arcuate nucleus of adult male rats. *Endocrinology* 1993; **133**: 1029–34.

13 Lamberts SWJ, van der Lely AJ, De Herder WW, Hofland LJ. Octreotide. *N Engl J Med* 1996; **25**: 246–9.

14 Holland LJ, Lamberts WE. Somatostatin receptors and disease: role of receptor subtypes. *J Clin Endocrinol Metab* 1996; **10**: 163–76.

15 Pellegrini E, Bluet-Pajot MT, Mounier F, *et al*. Central administration of a growth hormone (GH) receptor mRNA antisense increases GH pulsatility and decreases hypothalamic somatostatin expression in rats. *J Neurosci* 1996; **16**: 8140–8.

16 Kojima M, Hosada H, Date Y, *et al*. Ghrelin is a growth-hormone-releasing acylated peptide from stomach. *Nature* 1999; **402**: 656–60.

17 van der Lely AJ, Tschop M, Herman ML, Ghigo E. Biological, physiological, pathophysiological and pharmacologic aspects of ghrelin. *Endocr Rev* 2004; **25**: 426–57.

18 Momany FA, Bowers CY, Reynolds GA, *et al*. Design, synthesis, and biological activity of peptides which release growth hormone in vitro. *Endocrinology* 1981; **108**: 31–9.

19 Momany FA, Bowers CY, Reynolds GA, *et al*. Coformational energy studies and in vitro and in vivo activity data on growth hormone-releasing peptides. *Endocrinology* 1984; **114**: 1531–6.

20 Walker RF, Codd EE, Barone FC, *et al*. Oral activity of the growth hormone releasing peptide His-D-Trp-Ala-Trp-D-Phe-Lys-NH2 in rats, dogs and monkeys. *Life Sci* 1990; **47**: 29–36.

21 Smith RG, Cheng K, Schoen WR, *et al*. A nonpeptidyl growth hormone secretagogue. *Science* 1993; **260**: 1640–3.

22 Smith RG, Leonard R, Bailey AR, *et al*. Growth hormone secretagogue receptor family members and ligands. *Endocrine* 2001; **14**: 9–14.

23 McKee KK, Tan CP, Palyha OC, *et al*. Cloning and characterization of two human G protein-coupled receptor genes (GPR38 and GPR39) related to the growth hormone secretagogue and neurotensin receptors. *Genomics* 1997; **46**: 426–34.

24 McKee KK, Palyha OC, Feighner SD, *et al*. Molecular analysis of rat pituitary and hypothalamic growth hormone secretagogue receptors. *Mol Endocrinol* 1997; **11**: 415–23.

25 Howard AD, Feighner SD, Cully DF, et al. A receptor in pituitary and hypothalamus that functions in growth hormone release. Science 1996; 273: 974–7.

26 Smith RG, Van der Ploeg LH, Howard AD, et al. Peptidomimetic regulation of growth hormone secretion. Endocr Rev 1997; 18: 621–45.

27 Bednarek MA, Feighner SD, Pong SS, et al. Structure-function studies on the new growth hormone-releasing peptide, ghrelin: minimal sequence of ghrelin necessary for activation of growth hormone secretagogue receptor 1a. J Med Chem 2000; 43: 4370–6.

28 Chen C, Wu D, Clarke IJ. Signal transduction systems employed by synthetic GH-releasing peptides in somatotrophs. J Endocrinol 1996; 148: 381–6.

29 Casanueva FF, Dieguez C. Neuroendocrine regulation and actions of leptin. Front Neuroendocrinol 1999; 20: 317–63.

30 Saad MF, Bernaba B, Hwu CM, et al. Insulin regulates plasma ghrelin concentration. J Clin Metab 2002; 87: 3997–4000.

31 Reimer MK, Pacini G, Ahren B. Dose-dependent inhibition by ghrelin of insulin secretion in the mouse. Endocrinology 2003; 144: 916–21.

32 Tshcop M, Smiley DL, Heiman ML. Ghrelin induces adiposity in rodents. Nature 2000; 407: 908–13.

33 Nakagawa E, Nagaya N, Okumura H, et al. Hyerglycaemia suppresses the secretion of ghrelin, a novel growth-hormone-releasing peptide: responses to the intravenous and oral administration of glucose. Clin Sci (Lond) 2002; 103: 325–8.

34 Shiiya T, Nakazato M, Mizuta M, et al. Plasma ghrelin levels in lean and obese humans and the effect of glucose on ghrelin secretion. J Clin Endocrinol Metab 2002; 87: 240–4.

35 Barkan AL, Dimaraki EV, Jessup SK, et al. Ghrelin secretion in humans is sexually dimorphic, suppresses by somatostatin, and not affected by the ambient growth hormone levels. J Clin Endocrinol Metab 2003; 88: 2180–4.

36 Broglio F, Koetsveld PP, Benso A, et al. Ghrelin secretion is inhibited by either somatostatin or cortistatin in humans. J Clin Endocrinol Metab 2002; 87: 4829–32.

37 Tannenbaum GS, Epelbaum J, Bowers CY. Interreationship between the novel peptide ghrelin and somatostatin/growth hormone-releasing hormone in regultaion of pulsatile growth hormone secretion. Endocrinology 2003; 144: 967–74.

38 Freda PU, Reyes CM, Conwell IM, et al. Serum ghrelin levels in acromegaly: effects of surgical and long-acting octreotide therapy. J Clin Endocrinol 2003; 88: 2037–44.

39 Tschop M, Flora DB, Mayer JP, Heiman ML. Hypophysectomy prevents ghrelin-induced adiposity and increases gastric ghrelin secretion in rats. Obes Res 2002; 10: 991–9.

40 Cappiello V, Ronchi C, Morpurgo PS, et al. Circulating ghrelin levels in basal conditions and during glucose tolerance test in acromegalic patients. Eur J Endocrinol 2002; 147: 189–94.

41 Van der Toorn FM, Janssen JA, De Herder WW, et al. Central ghrelin production does not substantially contribute to systemic ghrelin concentrations; a study in two subjects with active acromegaly. Eur J Endocrinol 2002; 147: 195–9.

42 Muller AF, Lamberts SW, Janssen JA, et al. Ghrelin drives GH secretion during fasting in man. Eur J Endocrinol 2002; 146: 203–7.

43 Murdolo G, Lucidi P, Di Loreto C, et al. Circulating ghrelin levels of visceral obese men are not modified by a short-term treatment with very low doses of GH replacement. J Endocrinol Invest 2003; 26: 244–9.

44 Geloneze B, Tambascia MA, Pilla VF, et al. Ghrelin: a gut-brain hormone: effect of gastric bypass surgery. Obes Surg 2003; 13: 17–22.

45 Kalra SP, Dube MG, Pu S, et al. Interactive appetite-regulating pathways in the hypothalamic regulation of body weight. Endocr Rev 1999; 20: 68–100.

46 Rosicka M, Krsek M, Matoulek M, et al. Serum ghrelin levels in obese patients: the relationship to serum leptin levels and soluble leptin receptor levels. Physiol Res 2003; 52: 61–6.

47 Tolle V, Kadem M, Bluet-Pajot MT, et al. Balance in ghrelin and leptin levels in anorexia nervosa patients and constitutionally thin women. J Clin Endocr Metab 2003; 88: 109–16.

48 Tritos NA, Kokkinos A, Lampadariou E, et al. Cerebral spinal fluid ghrelin is negatively associated with body mass index. J Clin Endocr Metab 2003; 88: 2943–6.

49 Weigle DS, Cummings DE, Newby PD, et al. Roles of leptin and ghrelin in the loss of body weight caused by a low fat, high carbohydrate diet. J Clin Endocrinol Metab 2003; 88: 1577–86.

50 Mustonen AM, Nieminen P, Hyvarinen H. Preliminary evidence that pharmacologic melatonin treatment decreases rat ghrelin levels. Endocrine 2001; 16: 43–6.

51 Riis AL, Hansen TR, Moller N, et al. Hyperthyroidism is associated with suppressed circulating ghrelin levels. J Clin Endocrinol Metab 2003; 88: 853–7.

52 Broglio F, Gottero C, Prodam F, et al. Ghrelin secretion is inhibited by glucose load and insulin-induced hypoglycemia but unaffected by glucagon and arginine in humans. Clin Endocrinol 2004; 61: 503–9.

53 Masuda Y, Tanaka T, Inomata N, et al. Ghrelin stimulates gastric acid secretion and motility in rats. Biochem Biophys Res Commun 2000; 276: 905–8.

54 Sugino T, Yamaura J, Yamagishi M, et al. Involvement of cholinergic neurons in the regulation of the ghrelin secretory response to feeding in sheep. Biochem Biophys Res Commun 2003; 304: 308–12.

55 Arvat E, Di Vito L, Broglio F, et al. Preliminary evidence that ghrelin, the natural GH secretagogue (GHS)-receptor ligand, strongly stimulates GH secretion in humans. J Endocrinol Invest 2000; 23: 493–5.

56 Papotti M, Mucciolo G, Dieguez C, et al. Endocrine activities of ghrelin, a natural growth hormone secretagogue (GHS), in humans: comparison and interactions with hexarelin, a nonnatural peptidyl GHS, and GH-releasing hormone. J Clin Endocrinol Metab 2001; 86: 1169–74.

57 Takaya K, Ariyasu H, Kanamoto N, et al. Ghrelin strongly stimulates growth hormone secretagogues in humans. J Clin Endocrinol Metab 2000; 85: 4908–11.

58 Ghigo E, Arvat E, Giordano R, et al. Biological activities of growth hormone secretagogues in humans. Endocrine 2001; 14: 87–93.

59 Peino R, Baldelli R, Rodriguez-Garcia J, et al. Ghrelin-induced growth hormone secretion in humans. Eur J Endocrinol 2000; 143: R11–4.

60 Seoane LM, Tovar S, Baldelli R, *et al*. Ghrelin elicits a marked stimulatory effect on GH secretion in freely-moving rats. *Eur J Endocrinol* 2000; **1432**: R7–9.

61 Hataya Y, Akamizu T, Takaya K, *et al*. A low dose of ghrelin stimulates growth hormone (GH) release synergistically with GH-releasing hormone in humans. *J Clin Endocrinol Metab* 2001; **86**: 4552–7.

62 Broglio F, Benso A, Gottero C, *et al*. Non-acylated ghrelin does not possess the pituitaric and pancreatic endocrine activity of acylated ghrelin in humans. *J Endocrinol Invest* 2003; **26**: 192–6.

63 Bowers CY, Sartor AO, Reynolds GA, Badger TM. On the actions of the growth hormone-releasing hexapeptide, GHRP. *Endocrinology* 1991; **128**: 2027–35.

64 Sartor O, Bowers CY, Chang D. Parallel studies of His-DTrp-Ala-Trp-D-Phe-Lys-NH2 and human pancreatic growth hormone-releasing factor-44-NH2 in rat primary pituitary cell monolayer culture. *Endocrinology* 1985; **116**: 952–7.

65 Goth MI, Lyons CE, Canny BJ, Thorner MO. Pituitary adenylate cyclase activating polypeptide, growth hormone (GH)-releasing peptide and GH-releasing hormone stimulate GH release through distinct pituitary receptors. *Endocrinology* 1992; **130**: 939–44.

66 Locatelli V, Grilli R, Torsello A, *et al*. Growth hormone-releasing hexapeptide is a potent stimulator of growth hormone gene expression and release in the growth hormone-releasing hormone-deprived infant rat. *Pediatr Res* 1994; **36**: 169–74.

67 Blake AD, Smith RG. Desensitization studies using perifused rat pituitary cells show that growth hormone-releasing hormone and His-D-Trp-Ala-Trp-D-Phe-Lys-NH2 stimulate growth hormone release through distinct receptor sites. *J Endocrinol* 1991; **129**: 11–9.

68 Badger TM, Millard WJ, McCormick GF, *et al*. The effects of growth hormone (GH)-releasing peptides on GH secretion in perifused pituitary cells of adult male rats. *Endocrinology* 1984; **115**: 1432–8.

69 Cheng K, Chan WW, Barreto A Jr, *et al*. The synergistic effects of His-D-Trp-Ala-Trp-D-Phe-Lys-NH2 on growth hormone (GH)-releasing factor-stimulated GH release and intracellular adenosine 3′,5′-monophosphate accumulation in rat primary pituitary cell culture. *Endocrinology* 1989; **124**: 2791–8.

70 Cheng K, Chan WW, Butler B, *et al*. Stimulation of growth hormone release from rat primary pituitary cells by L-692,429, a novel non-peptidyl GH secretagogue. *Endocrinology* 1993; **132**: 2729–31.

71 Wu D, Chen C, Zhang J, *et al*. Effects in vitro of new growth hormone releasing peptide (GHRP-1) on growth hormone secretion from ovine pituitary cells in primary culture. *J Neuroendocrinol* 1994; **6**: 185–90.

72 Wu D, Chen C, Katoh K, *et al*. The effect of GH-releasing peptide-2 (GHRP-2 or KP 102) on GH secretion from primary cultured ovine pituitary cells can be abolished by a specific GH-releasing factor (GRF) receptor antagonist. *J Endocrinol* 1994; **140**: R9–13.

73 Mazza E, Ghigo E, Goffi S, *et al*. Effect of the potentiation of cholinergic activity on the variability in individual GH response to GH-releasing hormone. *J Endocrinol Invest* 1989; **12**: 795–8.

74 Clark RG, Carlsson MS, Trojnar J, Robinson IC. The effects of a growth hormone-releasing peptide and growth hormone-releasing factor in conscious and anaesthetized rats. *J Neuroendocrinol* 1989; **1**: 249–55.

75 Bercu BB, Yang SW, Masuda R, Walker RF. Role of selected endogenous peptides in growth hormone-releasing hexapeptide activity: analysis of growth hormone-releasing hormone, thyroid hormone-releasing hormone, and gonadotropin-releasing hormone. *Endocrinology* 1992; **130**: 2579–86.

76 Conley LK, Teik JA, Deghenghi R, *et al*. Mechanism of action of hexarelin and GHRP-6: analysis of the involvement of GHRH and somatostatin in the rat. *Neuroendocrinology* 1995; **61**: 44–50.

77 Yagi H, Kaji H, Sato M, *et al*. Effect of intravenous or intracerebroventricular injections of His-D-Trp-Ala-Trp-D-Phe-Lys-NH2 on GH release in conscious, freely moving male rats. *Neuroendocrinology* 1996; **63**: 198–206.

78 Korbonits M, Grossman AB. Growth hormone-releasing peptide and its analogues. *Trends Endocrinol Metab* 1995; **6**: 43–9.

79 Dickson SL, Doutrelant-Viltart O, Leng G. GH-deficient dw/dw rats and lit/lit mice show increased Fos expression in the hypothalamic arcuate nucleus following systemic injection of GH-releasing peptide-6. *J Endocrinol* 1995; **146**: 519–26.

80 Sartor O, Bowers CY, Reynolds GA, Momany FA. Variables determining the growth hormone response of His-D-Trp-Ala-Trp-D-Phe-Lys-NH$_2$ in the rat. *Endocrinology* 117: 1441–7.

81 Jacks T, Smith R, Judith F, *et al*. MK-0677, a potent, novel, orally active growth hormone (GH) secretagogue: GH, insulin-like growth factor I, and other hormonal responses in beagles. *Endocrinology* 1996; **137**: 5284–9.

82 Hickey GJ, Jacks TM, Schleim KD, *et al*. Repeat administration of the GH secretagogue MK-0677 increases and maintains elevated IGF-I levels in beagles. *J Endocrinol* 1997; **152**: 183–92.

83 Mazza E, Ghigo E, Goffi S, *et al*. Effect of the potentiation of cholinergic activity on the variability in individual GH response to GH-releasing hormone. *J Endocrinol Invest* 1989; **12**: 795–8.

84 Jacks T, Hickey G, Judith F, *et al*. Effects of acute and repeated intravenous administration of L-692,585, a novel non-peptidyl growth hormone secretagogue, on plasma growth hormone, IGF-I, ACTH, cortisol, prolactin, insulin, and thyroxine levels in beagles. *J Endocrinol* 1994; **143**: 399–406.

85 Walker RF, Yang SW, Masuda R, *et al*. Effects of growth hormone-releasing peptides on stimulated growth hormone secretion in old rats. In: Bercu BB, Walker RF, eds. *Growth Hormone II: Basic and Clinical Aspects*. New York: Springer-Verlag, 1993: 167–192.

86 Chapman IM, Hartman ML, Pezzoli SS, Thorner MO. Enhancement of pulsatile growth hormone secretion by continuous infusion of a growth hormone-releasing peptide

mimetic, L-692,429, in older adults – a clinical research center study. *J Clin Endocrinol Metab* 1996; **81**: 2874–80.

87   Chapman IM, Bach MA, Van Cauter E, *et al.* Stimulation of the growth hormone (GH)-insulin-like growth factor I axis by daily oral administration of a GH secretogogue (MK-677) in healthy elderly subjects. *J Clin Endocrinol Metab* 1996; **81**: 4249–57.

88   Copinschi G, Van Onderbergen A, L'Hermite-Baleriaux M, *et al.* Effects of a 7-day treatment with a novel, orally active, growth hormone (GH) secretogogue, MK-677, on 24-hour GH profiles, insulin-like growth factor I, and adrenocortical function in normal young men. *J Clin Endocrinol Metab* 1996; **81**: 2776–82.

89   Huhn WC, Hartman ML, Pezzoli SS, Thorner MO. Twenty-four-hour growth hormone (GH)-releasing peptide (GHRP) infusion enhances pulsatile GH secretion and specifically attenuates the response to a subsequent GHRP bolus. *J Clin Endocrinol Metab* 1993; **76**: 1202–8.

90   Jaffe CA, Ho, PJ, DeMott-Friberg R, *et al.* Effects of a prolonged growth hormone (GH)-releasing peptide infusion on pulsatile GH secretion in normal men. *J Clin Endocrinol Metab* 1993; **77**: 1641–7.

91   Ghigo E, Arvat E, Gianotti L, *et al.* Short-term administration of intranasal or oral hexarelin, a synthetic hexapeptide, does not desensitize the growth hormone responsiveness in human aging. *Eur J Endocrinol* 1996; **135**: 407–12.

92   Hayashi S, Okimura Y, Yagi H, *et al.* Intranasal administration of His-D-Trp-Ala-Trp-D-Phe-LysNH2 (growth hormone releasing peptide) increased plasma growth hormone and insulin-like growth factor-I levels in normal men. *Endocrinol Jpn* 1991; **38**: 15–21.

93   Laron Z, Frenkel J, Deghenghi R, *et al.* Intranasal administration of the GHRP hexarelin accelerates growth in short children. *Clin Endocrinol (Oxf)* 1995; **43**: 631–5.

94   Hickey GJ, Drisko J, Faidley T, *et al.* Mediation by the central nervous system is critical to the in vivo activity of the GH secretagogue L-692,585. *J Endocrinol* 1996; **148**: 371–80.

95   Popovic V, Damjanovic S, Micic D, *et al.* Blocked growth hormone-releasing peptide (GHRP-6)-induced GH secretion and absence of the synergic action of GHRP-6 plus GH-releasing hormone in patients with hypothalamopituitary disconnection: evidence that GHRP-6 main action is exerted at the hypothalamic level. *J Clin Endocrinol Metab* 1995; **80**: 942–7.

96   Pandya N, DeMott-Friberg R, Bowers CY, *et al.* Growth hormone (GH)-releasing peptide-6 requires endogenous hypothalamic GH-releasing hormone for maximal GH stimulation. *J Clin Endocrinol Metab* 1998; **83**: 1186–9.

97   Popovic V, Miljic D, Micic D, *et al.* Ghrelin main action on the regulation of growth hormone release is exerted at hypothalamic level. *J Clin Endocrinol Metab* 2003; **88**: 3450–3.

98   Deghenghi R, Boutignon F, Luoni M, *et al.* Small peptides as potent releasers of growth hormone. *J Pediatr Endocrinol Metab* 1995; **8**: 311–3.

99   Thorner MO, Vance ML, Rogol AD, *et al.* Growth hormone-releasing hormone and growth hormone-releasing peptide as potential therapeutic modalities. *Acta Paediatr Scand Suppl* 1990; **367**: 29–32.

100   Bluet-Pajot MT, Tolle V, Zizzari P, *et al.* Growth hormone secretagogues and hypothalamaic networks. *Endocrine* 2001; **14**: 1–8.

101   Maheshwari HG, Pezzoli SS, Rahim A, *et al.* Pulsatile growth hormone secretion persists in genetic growth hormone-releasing hormone resistance. *Am J Physiol Endocrinol Metab* 2002; **282**: E943–51.

102   Maheshwari HG, Rahim Asahlet SM, Baumann G. Selective lack of growth hormone (GH) response to the GH-releasing peptide hexarelin in patients with GH-releasing peptide deficiency. *J Clin Endocrinol Metab* 1999; **84**: 956–9.

103   Gondo RG, Aguiar-Oliveira MH, Hayashida CY, *et al.* Growth hormone-releasing peptide-2 stimulates GH secretion in GH-deficient patients with mutated GH-releasing hormone receptor. *J Clin Endocrinol Metab* 2001; **86**: 3279–83.

104   Ghigo E, Arvat E, Giordano R, *et al.* Biologic activities of growth hormone secretagogues in humans. *Endocrine* 2001; **14**: 87–93.

105   Tannenbaum GS, Bowers CY. Interactons of growth hormone secretagogues and growth hormone-releasing hormone/somatostatin. *Endocrine* 2001; **14**: 21–7.

106   Broglio F, Arvat E, Benso A, *et al.* Endocrine activities of cortistatin-14 and its interaction with GHRH and ghrelin in humans. *J Clin Endocrinol Metab* 2002; **87**: 3783–90.

107   Di Vito L, Broglio F, Benso A, *et al.* The GH-releasing effect of ghrelin, a natural GH secretagogue, is only blunted by the infusion of exogenous somatostatin in humans. *Clin Endocrinol (Oxf)* 2002; **56**: 643–8.

108   Bell WK, Pezzoli SS, Thorner MO. Growth hormone (GH) secretion during continuous infusion of GH-releasing peptide: partial response attenuation. *J Clin Endocrinol Metab* 1991; **72**: 1312–6.

109   Huhn WC, Hartman ML, Pezzoli SS, Thorner MO. Twenty-four-hour growth hormone (GH)-releasing peptide (GHRP) infusion enhances pulsatile GH secretion and specifically attenuates the response to a subsequent GHRP bolus. *J Clin Endocrinol Metab* 1993; **76**: 1202–8.

110   Jaffe CA, Ho PJ, DeMott-Friberg R, *et al.* Effects of a prolonged growth hormone (GH)-releasing peptide infusion on pulsatile GH secetion in normal men. *J Clin Endocrinol Metab* 1993; **77**: 1641–7.

111   Sartorio A, Conti A, Ferrero S, *et al.* GH responsiveness to repeated GHRH or hexarelin administration in normal adults. *J Endocrinol Invest* 1995; **18**: 7718–22.

112   Ghigo E, Arvat E, Gianotti L, *et al.* Growth hormone-releasing activity of hexarelin, a new synthetic hexapeptide, after intravenous, subcutaneous, intranasal, and oral administration in man. *J Clin Endocrinol Metab* 1994; **78**: 693–8.

113   Kamegai J, Wakabayashi I, Kineman RD, Frohman LA. Growth hormone-releasing hormone receptor (GHRH-R) and growth hormone secretagogue receptor (GHS-R) mRNA levels during postnatal development in male and female rats. *J Neuroendocrinol* 1999; **11**: 299–306.

114   Arvat E, Gianotti L, Broglio F, *et al.* Oestrogen replacement does not restore the reduced GH-releasing activity of hexarelin, a synthetic hexapeptide, in post-menopausal women. *Eur J Endocrinol* 1997; **136**: 483–7.

115 Arvat E, Camanni F, Ghigo E. Age-related growth hormone-releasing activity of growth hormone secretagogues in humans. *Acta Paediatr Suppl* 1997; **423**: 92–6.

116 Carmignae DF, Bennett PA, Robinson IC. Effects of growth hormone secretagogues on prolactin release in anesthesized dwarf (dw/dw) rats. *Endocrinology* 1998; **139**: 3590–6.

117 Loche S, Colao A, Cappa M, *et al.* The growth hormone response to hexarelin in children: reproducibility and effect of sex steroids. *J Clin Endocrinol Metab* 1997; **82**: 861–4.

118 Bellone J, Aimaretti G, Bartolotta E, *et al.* Growth hormone-releasing activity of hexarelin, a new synthetic hexapeptide before and during puberty. *J Clin Endocrinol Metab* 1995; **80**: 1090–4.

119 Arvat E, Ceda GP, Di Vito L, *et al.* Age-related variations in the neuroendocrine control, more than impaired receptor sensitivity, cause the reduction in GH-releasing activity of GHRPs in human aging. *Pituitary* 1998; **1**: 51–8.

120 Giustina A, Velhuis JD. Pathophysiology of the neuroregulation of growth hormone secretion in experimental animals and the human. *Endocr Rev* 1998; **19**: 717–97.

121 Muccioli G, Ghe C, Ghigo MC, *et al.* Specific receptors for synthetic GH secretagogues in the human brain and pituitary gland. *J Endocrinol* 1998; **157**: 99–106.

122 Bowers CY. Unnatural growth hormone-releasing peptide begets natural ghrelin. *J Clin Endcrinol Metab* 2001; **86**: 1464–9.

123 Thorner MO, Chapman IM, Gaylinn BD, *et al.* Growth hormone-releasing hormone and growth hormone-releasing peptide as therapeutic agents to enhance growth hormone secretion in disease and aging. *Recent Prog Horm Res* 1997; **52**: 215–46.

124 Flanagan DE, Evans ML, Monsod TP, *et al.* The influence of insulin on circulating ghrelin. *Am J Physiol Endocrinol Metab* 2003; **284**: E313–6.

125 Lucidi P, Murdolo G, Di Loreto C, *et al.* Ghrelin is not necessary for adequate hormonal counterregulation of insulin-induced hypoglycemia. *Diabetes* 2000; **51**: 2911–4.

126 Tolle V, Bassant MH, Zizzari P, *et al.* Ultradian rhythmicity of ghrelin secretion in relation with GH, feeding behavior, and sleep-wake patterns in rats. *Endocrinology* 2002; **143**: 1353–61.

127 Broglio F, Benso A, Castiglioni C, *et al.* The endocrine response to ghrelin as a function of gender in humans in young and elderly subjects. *J Clin Endocrinol Metab* 2003; **88**: 1537–42.

128 Leal-Cerro A, Garcia E, Astorga R, *et al.* Growth hormone (GH) responses to the combined administration of GH-releasing hormone plus GH-releasing peptide 6 in adults with GH deficiency. *Eur J Endocrinol* 1995; **132**: 712–5.

129 Ghigo E, Arvat E, Aimaretti G, *et al.* Diagnostic and therapeutic uses of growth hormone-releasing substances in adult and elderly subjects. *Baillieres Clin Endocrinol Metab* 1998; **12**: 341–58

130 Popovic V, Leal A, Micic D, *et al.* GH-releasing hormone and GH-releasing peptide-6 for diagnostic testing in GH-deficient adults. *Lancet* 2000; **356**: 1137–42.

131 Aimaretti G, Baffoni C, Brogiol F, *et al.* Endocrine responses to ghrelin in adult patients with isolated childhood-onset growth hormone deficiency. *Clin Endocrinol (Oxf)* 2002; **56**: 765–71.

132 Bercu BB, Walker RF. Evaluation of pituitary function in children using growth hormone secretagogues. *J Pediatr Endocrinol* 1996; **9**: 325–32.

133 Bercu BB, Walker RF. Novel growth hormone secretagogues: Clinical applications. *Endocrinologist* 1997; **7**: 51–64.

134 Bercu BB, Walker RF. Effectiveness of growth hormone secretagogues in the diagnosis and treatment of GH deficiency. In: Dieguez C, Ghigo E, Boghen M, *et al.* eds. *Growth Hormone Secretagogues: Basic Findings and Clinical Implications.* Amsterdam: Elsevier Science BV, 1999: 157–81.

134a Walker RF, Bercu BB. Effectiveness of growth hormone (GH) secretagogues in diagnosing and treating GH secretory deficiency in aging men. *J Anti Aging Med* 1998; **1**: 219–28.

135 Ghigo E, Aimaretti G, Arvat E, Camanni F. Growth hormone-releasing hormone combined with arginine or growth hormone secretagogues for the diagnosis of growth hormone deficiency in adults. *Endocrine* 2001; **15**: 29–38.

136 Baldelli R, Otero XL, Camina JP, *et al.* Growth hormone secretagogues as diagnostic tools in disease states. *Endocrine* 2001; **14**: 95–9.

137 Shalet SM, Toogood A, Rahim A, Brennan BM. The diagnosis of growth hormone deficiency in children and adults. *Endocr Rev* 1998; **19**: 203–23.

138 Root AW, Diamond FB Jr. Regulation and clinical assessment of growth hormone secretion. *Endocrine* 2000; **12**: 137–45.

139 Bercu BB, Walker RF. Growth hormone secretagogues in children with altered growth. *Acta Paediatr Suppl* 1997; **423**: 102–6.

140 de Vos AM, Ultsch M, Kossiakoff AA. Human growth hormone and extracellular domain of its receptor: cyclic structure of the complex. *Science* 1992; **255**: 306–12.

141 Pearce KH, Wells JA. Activation of the human growth hormone receptor. In: Smith RG, Thorner MO, eds. *Human Growth Hormone Research and Clinical Practice.* Totowa, NJ: Humana Press, 2000: 131–43.

142 Ayling RM, Roos R, Towner P, *et al.* A dominant-negative mutation of the growth hormone receptor causes familial short stature. *Nat Genet* 1997; **16**: 13–4.

143 Guan R, Zhang Y, Jiang J, *et al.* Phorbol ester- and growth factor-induced growth hormone receptor protolysis and GH-binding protein shredding relationship to GH down regulation. *Endocrinology* 2001; **142**: 1137–47.

144 Giustina A, Girelli A, Alberti D, *et al.* Effects of pyridostigmine on spontaneous and growth hormone-releasing hormone stimulated growth hormone secretion in children on daily glucocorticoid therapy after liver transplantation. *Clin Endocinol (Oxf)* 1991; **35**: 391–8.

145 Casanueva FF, Villannueva L, Cabranes JA, *et al.* Cholinergic mediation of growth hormone secretion elicited by arginine, clonidine and physical exercise in man. *J Clin Endocrinol Metab* 1984; **59**: 526–30.

146 Ismail IS, Scanlon MF, Peters JR. Cholinergic control of growth hormone (GH) responses to GH-releasing hormone in insulin dependent diabetics: evidence for attenuated hypothalamic somatostatinergic tone and decreased GH autofeedback. *Clin Endocoirnol (Oxf)* 1993; **38**: 149–57.

147 Wehrenberg WB, Wiviott, SD, Voltz DM, Giustina A. Pyridostigmine-mediated growth hormone release, evidence for somatostatin involvement. *Endocrinology* 1992; **130**: 1445–50.

148 Massara F, Ghigo E, Emislis K, *et al.* Cholinergic involvement in the growth hormone releasing hormone-induced growth hormone release: studies in normal and acromegalic subjects. *Neuroendocrinology* 1986; **43**: 675–9.

149 Evans PJ, Dieguez C, Rees LH, *et al.* The effect of cholinergic blockade on the growth hormone and prolactin response to insulin hypoglycemia. *Clin Endocrinol (Oxf)* 1985; **22**: 733–7.

150 Mendelson WB, Lantigua RA, Wyatt RJ, *et al.* Piperidine enhances sleep-related and insulin-induced growth hormone secretion: further evidence for a cholinergic secretory mechanism. *J Clin Endocinol Metab* 1981; **52**: 409–15.

151 Miki N, Onon M, Shizume K. Evidence that opionergic and alpha-adrenergic mechanisms stimulate rat GH release via growth hormone-releasing factor (GRF). *Endocrinology* 1984; **114**: 1950–2.

152 Giustina A, Buffoli MG, Bussi AR, *et al.* Comparative effects of clonidine and growth hormone (GH)-releasing hormone on GH secretion in adult patients on chronic glucocorticoid therapy. *Horm Metab Res* 1992; **24**: 240–3.

153 Kelijman M, Frohman LA. Beta-adrenergic modulation of growth hormone (GH)-autofeedback on sleep-associated and pharmacologically induced GH secretion. *J Clin Endocrinol Metab* 1989; **69**: 1187–93.

154 Chihara K, Kodama H, Kaji H, *et al.* Augmentation by propranolol of growth hormone releasing hormone (1-44) NH2-induced growth hormone release in normal short and normal children. *J Clin Endocrinol Metab* 1985; **61**: 229–33.

155 Ghigo E, Arvat E, Gianotti L, *et al.* Interaction of salbutamol with pyridostigmine and arginine on both basal and GHRH-stimulated GH secretion in humans. *Clin Endocrinol (Oxf)* 1994; **40**: 799–802.

156 Page MD, Dieguez C, Valcavi R, *et al.* Growth hormone (GH) responses to arginine and L-dopa alone and after GHRH pretreatment. *Clin Endcrinol (Oxf)* 1988; **28**: 551–8.

157 Liuzzi A, Chiodini PG, Botalla L, *et al.* Decreased plasma growth hormone (GH) levels in acromegalics following CB 154 (2-Br-alpha-ergocryptide) administration. *J Clin Endocrinol Metab* 1974; **38**: 910–2.

158 Chiodera P, Coiro V, Zanardi G, *et al.* Effect of metoclopramaide on serum GH levels in normal women. *Horm Metab Res* 1982; **14**: 103–4.

159 Wolf PD, Lantigua R, Lee LA. Dopamine inhibition of stimulated growth hormone secretion: evidence for dopaminergic modulation of insulin and L-dopa induced growth hormone secretion in man. *J Clin Endocrinol Metab* 1979; **49**: 326–30.

160 Imura H, Nakai I, Yoshimi T. Effect of 5-hydroxytryptophan on growth hormone and ACTH release in man. *J Clin Endocrinol Metab* 1973; **39**: 1–5.

161 Delitala G, Devilla L, Bkiolnda S, *et al.* Suppression of human GH secretion by cyproheptadine. *Metabolism* 1973; **26**: 931–5.

162 Biwens CH, Levovitz HE, Feldman JM. Inhibition of hypoglycemia-induced GH secretion by serotonin antagonists cyproheptadine and methysergide. *N Engl J Med* 1973; **289**: 236–8.

163 Nimi M, Takhana J, Sato M, Kawanishik K. Immunohistochemical identification of galanin and growth hormone-releasing factor neurons projecting to the median eminence in the rat. *Neuroendocrinology* 1990; **51**: 571–5.

164 Giustina A, Veldhuis JD. Pathophysiology of the neuroregulation of growth hormone secretion in experimental animals and the human. *Endocr Rev* 1998; **19**: 717–97.

165 Howard G, Peng L, Hyde JF. An estrogen receptor binding site within the human galanin gene. *Endocrinology* 1997; **11**: 4649–56.

166 Giustina A, Bresciana E, Bussi AR, *et al.* Characterization of the paradoxical growth hormone inhibitory effect of galanin in acromegaly. *J Clin Endocrinol Metab* 1995; **80**: 1333–40.

167 Leicht E, Biro G, Weinges KF. Inhibition of releasing-hormone induced secretion of TSH and LH by calcitonin. *Horm Metab Res* 1974; **6**: 410–4.

168 Borle AB. Regulation of cellular calcium metabolism and calcium transport by calcitonin. *J Membr Biol* 1975; **21**: 125–46.

169 Moretti C, Fabbri A, Gnessi L, *et al.* Naloxone inhibits exercise-induced release of PRL and GH in athletes. *Clin Endocrinol (Oxf)* 1983; **18**: 135–8.

170 Ramirez G, Bittle PA, Sanders RD, Bercu BB. Hypothalamo-hypophyseal thyroid and gonadal function before and after erthyropoietin therapy in dialysis patients. *J Clin Endocrinol Metab* 1992; **74**: 517–24.

171 Giustina A, Doga M, Bresciani E, *et al.* Effect of glucocorticoids on the paradoxical growth hormone response to thyrotropin-releasing hormone in patients with acromegaly. *Metabolism* 1995; **44**: 379–83.

172 Valentinir U, Cimino A, Rotondi A, *et al.* Growth hormone response to thyrotropin releasing hormone and placebo in a group of insulin-dependent diabetic patients. *J Endocrinol Invest* 1989; **12**: 643–6.

173 Czernichow P, Dauzet MC, Broyer M, Rappaport R. Abnormal TSH, PRL and GH responses to TSH-releasing factor in chronic renal failure. *J Clin Endocrinol Metab* 1976; **43**: 630–7.

174 Maeda K, Kato Y, Chihara K, *et al.* Suppression by thyrotropin releasing hormone (TRH) of growth hormone release induced by arginine and insulin-induced hypoglycemia in man. *J Clin Endocrinol Metab* 1976; **43**: 453–6.

175 Jordan V, Dieguez C, Valcavi R, et al. Lack of effect of muscarinic cholinergic blockade on the GH response to GRF-1-29 and TRH in acromegalic subjects. Clin Endocrinol (Oxf) 1986; 24: 291–8.

176 Bergendahl M, Veldhuis JD. Altered pulsatile gonadotropin signaling in nutritional deficiency in the male. Trends Endocinol Metab 1995; 6: 145–9.

177 Blatt J, Bercu BB, Gillin JC, et al. Reduced pulsatile growth hormone secretion in children after therapy for acute lymphoblastic leukemia. J Pediatr 1984; 104: 182–6

178 Bercu BB, Heinze HJ, Walker RF. Use of growth hormone in non-growth hormone deficient children: physiologic, pharmacologic and ethical issues. In: Blackman MR, Harman SM, Roth J, Shapiro JR, eds. GHRH, GH, and IGF-I: Basic and Clinical Advances. New York: Springer-Verlag Inc., 1995: 143–68.

179 Jorgensen EV, Shulman DI, Diamond FB, et al. Spontaneous growth hormone secretion in children with normal and abnormal growth. In: Bercu BB, Walker RF, eds. Basic and Clinical Aspects of Growth Hormone II. New York: Springer-Verlag Inc., 1994: 286–98.

180 Clayton PE, Shalet SM. Dose dependency of time of onset of radiation-induced growth hormone deficiency. J Pediatr 1991; 118: 226–8.

181 Cicognani A, Cacciari E, Carla G, et al. Magnetic resonance imaging of the pituitary area in children treated for acute leukemia with low-dose (18-Gy) cranial radiation. Relationships to growth and growth hormone secretion. Am J Dis Child 1992; 146: 1343–8.

182 Sklar CA, Constine LS. Chronic neuroendocrinological sequelae of radiation therapy. Int J Radiat Oncol Biol Phys 1995; 31: 1113–21.

183 Jorgensen EV, Schwartz ID, Hvizdala E, et al. Neurotransmitter control of GH secretion on children after cranial radiation therapy. J Clin Pediatr Endocrol 1993; 6: 131–42.

184 Shulman DI, Hu C-S, Root AW, Bercu BB. Assessment of prolactin secretion in children undergoing evaluation for growth hormone deficiency. J Clin Endocrinol Metab 1989; 69: 1261–7.

185 Chrousos GP, Poplack D, Brown T, et al. Effects of cranial radiation on hypothalamic-adenohypophyseal function: Abnormal growth hormone secretory dynamics. J Clin Endocrinol Metab 1982; 54: 1135–9.

186 Shalet S. Irradiation induced growth failure. Clin Endocrinol Metab 1986; 15: 591–606.

187 Bode U, Oliff A, Bercu BB, et al. Absence of CT brain scan abnormlities with less intensive CNS prophylaxis. Am J Pediatr Hematol Oncol 1980; 2: 21–4.

188 Didcock E, Davies HA, Did M, et al. Pubertal growth in young adult survivors of childood leukemia. J Clin Oncol 1995; 13: 2503–7.

189 Ogilvy-Stuart AI, Clark DJ, Wallace WH, et al. Endocrine deficit after fractionated total body irradiation. Arch Dis Child 1992; 67: 1107–10.

190 Spiliotis B, August G, Hung W, et al. Growth hormone neurosecretory dysfunction: A treatable cause of short stature. JAMA 1984; 251: 2223–30.

191 Ogilvy-Stuart AL, Shalet SM. Effect of chemotherapy on growth. Acta Paediatr Suppl 1995; 411: 52–6.

192 Masuda A, Shibasaki T, Nakahara M, et al. The effect of glucose on growth hormone and (GH)-releasing hormone-mediated GH secretion in man. J Clin Endocrinol Metab 1985; 60: 523–6.

193 Devesa J, Lima L, Tresguerre JAF. Neuroendocrine control of growth hormone secretion in humans. Trends Endocrinol Metab 1992; 71: 1581–3.

194 Delitalia G, Tomasi PA, Palermo M, Fresu P. Interaction of glucose and pyrigostimine on the secretion of growth hormone (GH) induced by GH-releasing hormone (GHRH). Endocrinol Invest 1990; 13: 653–6.

195 Shibasaki T, Hotta M, Masuda A, et al. Plasma response to GHRH and insulin-induced hypoglycemia in man. J Clin Endocrinol Metab 1985; 60: 1265–7.

196 Penalva A, Burgurea B, Casabiel X, et al. Activation of cholinergic neurotransmission by pyridostigmine. Neuroendocrinology 1989; 49: 551–4.

197 Cornblath M, Parker ML, Reisner SH, et al. Secretion and metabolism of growth hormone in premature and full-term infants. J Clin Endocrinol 1965; 25: 209–18.

198 Quabbe H-J. Hypothalamic control of GH secretion: pathophysiology and clinical implications. Acta Neurochir 1985; 75: 60–71.

199 Imaki T, Shibasaki T, Shizume K, et al. The effect of free fatty acids on growth hormone (GH) releasing hormone-mediated GH secretion in man. J Clin Endocrinol Metab 1985; 60: 290–3.

200 Bercu BB. Disorders of growth hormone neurosecretion. In: Lifshitz F, ed. Pediatric Endocrinology. New York: Marcel Dekker, 1990: 43–60.

201 Oerter KE, Sobel AM, Rose SR, et al. Combining insulin-like growth factor-1 and mean spontaneous nighttime growth hormone levels for the diagnosis of growth hormone deficiency. J Clin Endocrinol Metab 1992; 75: 1413–20.

202 Veldhuis JD, Iranmanesh A, Ho KKY, et al. Dual defects in pulsatile growth hormone secretion and clearance subserve the hyposomatotrophism of obesity in man. J Clin Endocrinol Metab 1991; 72: 51–9.

203 Schwartz ID, Hu CS, Shulman DI, et al. Relationship of endogenous GH secretion to linear growth response after exogenous GH treatment in children with short stature. Am J Dis Child 1990; 144: 1092–7.

204 Cho KH, Yang SW, Hu CS, Bercu BB. Growth hormone (GH) response to growth hormone–releasing hormone (GHRH) varies with intrinsic growth hormone secretory rhythm in children; Reduced variability using somatostatin pretreatment. J Pediatr Endocrinol 1992; 5: 155–6.

205 Miller JD, Esparza A, Wright NM, et al. Spontaneous growth hormone release in term infants: changes during the first four days of life. J Clin Endocrinol Metab 1993; 76: 1058–62.

206 Shibasaki T, Shizume K, Nakahara M, et al. Age-related changes in plasma growth hormone response to growth-hormone releasing factor in man. J Clin Endocrinol Metab 1984; 58: 212–4.

207 Roemmich JN, Clark PA, Mai V, et al. Alterations in growth and body composition during puberty. III. Influence of maturation, gender, body composition, fat distribution, aerobic fitness, and energy expenditure on nocturnal growth hormone release. J Clin Endocrinol Metab 1998; 83: 1440-7.

208 Veldhuis JD, Roemmick JN, Rogol AD. Gender and sexual maturation-dependent contrasts in the neuroregulation of growth hormone secretion in prepubertal and late adolescent males and females – A general clinical research center-based study. J Clin Endocrinol Metab 2003; 85: 2385-94.

209 Russell-Aulet M, Jaffe CA, Demott-Friberg R, Barkan AL. In vivo semiquantification of hypothalamic growth hormone releasing (GHRH) output in humans: evidence for relative GHRH deficiency in aging. J Clin Endocrinol Metab 1999; 84: 3490-7.

210 Van den Berg G, Veldhuis JD, Frolich M, Roelfsema F. An amplitude-specific divergence in the pulsatile mode of growth hormone (GH) secretion underlies the gender difference in mean GH concentrations in men and postmenopausal women. J Clin Endocrinol Metab 1996; 81: 2460-7.

211 Veldhuis JD. Neuroendocrine control of pulsatile growth hormone release in the human: relationship with gender. Growth Horm IGF Res 1998, 8(Suppl B): 49-59.

212 Jansson JO, Frohman LA. Differential effects of neonatal and adult androgen exposure on the growth hormone secretory pattern in male rats. Endocrinology 1987; 120: 1551-7.

213 Bonddanelli M, Ambrosio MR, Margutti A, et al. Activation of the somatotropic axis by testosterone in adult men: evidence for a role of hypothalamic growth hormone-releasing hormone. Neuroendocrinology 2003; 77: 380-7.

214 Styne DM. The regulation of pubertal growth. Horm Res 2003; 60(Suppl 1): 22-6.

215 Holl RW, Hartman ML, Veldhuis JD, et al. Thirty second sampling of plasma growth hormone in man: correlation with sleep stages. J Clin Endocrinol Metab 1991; 72: 854-61.

216 Van Cauter E, Kerkhofs M, Caufriez A, et al. A quantitative estimation of growth hormone secretion in normal man: reproducibility and relation to sleep and time of day. J Clin Endocrinol Metab 1992; 74: 1442-50.

217 Van Cauter E, Scharf MB, Leproult R, et al. Simultaneous stimulation of slow-wave sleep and growth hormone secretion by gamma-hydoxybutyrate in normal young men. J Clin Invest 1997; 100: 745-53.

218 Bercu B, Diamond FB Jr. Growth hormone neurosecretory dysfunction. Clin Endocrinol Metab 1986; 15: 537-87.

219 Weeke J, Gundersen HJG. The effect of heating and central cooling on serum TSH, GH and norepinephrine in resting normal man. Acta Physiol Scand 1983; 117: 33-9.

220 Lassarre C, Girard F, Durand J, Raynaud J. Kinetics of human growth hormone during submaximal exercise. J Appl Physiol 1974; 37: 826-30.

221 Weltman A, Weltman JY, Schurrer R, et al. Endurance training amplifies the pulsatile release of growth hormone effects of training intensity. J Appl Physiol 1992; 76: 2188-96.

222 Raynaud J, Capderou A, Martineaud JP, et al. Intersubject variability in growth hormone time course during different types of work. J Appl Physiol 1986; 55: 1682-7.

223 Ross R, Miell J, Freeman E, et al. Critically ill patients have high basal growth hormone levels with attenuated oscillatory activity associated with low levels of insulin-like growth factor-I. Clin Endocrinol (Oxf) 1991; 35: 47-54.

224 Van den Berghe G, de Zegher F, Veldhuis JD, et al. The somatotrophic axis in critical illness: effect of continuous growth hormone (GH) releasing hormone and GH-releasing peptide-2-infusion. J Clin Endocrinol Metab 1997; 82: 590-9.

225 Baxter RC. Changes in the IGF-IGFBP axis in critical illness. Best Pract Res Clin Endocrinol Metab 2001; 15: 421-34.

226 Ramirez G, Bittle PA, Sanders H, et al. The effects of corticotropin and growth hormone releasing hormones in their respective secretory axes in chronic hemodialysis patients before and after correction of anemia with recombinant human erythropoietin. J Clin Endocrinol Metab 1994; 78: 63-9.

227 Ramirez G, Herrera R, Bittle PA, et al. The effects of high altitude on hypothalamic-pituitary secretory dynamics in men. Clin Endocrinol 1995; 43: 11-8.

228 Rose SR, Municchi G, Barnes KM, et al. Spontaneous growth hormone secretion increases during puberty in normal girls and boys. J Clin Endocrinol Metab 1991; 73: 428-35.

229 Lanes R, Bohorquez L, Leal V, et al. Growth hormone secretion in patients with constitutional delay of growth and pubertal development. J Pediatr 1986; 109: 781-3.

230 Bierich JR. Treatment of consitutional delay in growth and adolescence with human growth hormone. Klin Padiatr 1983; 195: 309-16.

231 Gourmelen M, Pham-Huu-Trung MT, Gerard F. Transient partial hGH deficiency in prepubertal children with delay of growth. Pediatr Res 1979; 13: 221-4.

232 Kerrigan JR, Martha PM Jr, Veldhuis JD, et al. Altered growth hormone secretory dynamics in prepubertal males with constitutional delay of growth. Pediatr Res 1993; 33: 278-83.

233 Crowne EC, Wallace WHB, Moore C, et al. Effect of low dose oxandrolone and testosterone treatment on the pituitary-testicular and GH axes in boys with constitutional delay of growth and puberty. Clin Endocrinol 1997; 46: 209-16.

234 Martha PM Jr, Rogol AD, Veldhuis JD, et al. Alterations in the pulsatile properties of circulating growth hormone during puberty in boys. J Clin Endocrin Metab 1989; 69: 563-70.

235 Rose SR, Kibarian M, Gelato M, et al. Sex steroids increase spontaneous growth hormone secretion in short children. J Pediatr Endocrinol 1988; 3: 1-5.

236 Mauras N, Blizzard RM, Link K, et al. Augmentation of growth hormone secretion during puberty: Evidence for a

pulse amplitude-modulated phenomenon. *J Clin Endocrinol Metab* 1987; **64**: 596–601.

237 Ho KY, Evans WS, Blizzard RM, *et al.* Effects of sex and age on the 24-hour profile of growth hormone secretion in man: Importance of endogenous estradiol concentrations. *J Clin Endocrinol Metab* 1987; **64**: 51–8.

238 Martin-Hernandez T, Glavez MD, Cuadro AT, Herrera-Justinia E. Growth hormone secretion in normal prepubertal children: importance of relations between endogenous secretion, pulsatility and body mass. *Clin Endocrinol* 1996; **44**: 327–34.

239 Vahl N, Jorgensen JOL, Skjaerbaek C, *et al.* Abdominal adiposity rather than age and sex predits mass and regularity of GH secretion in healthy adults. *Am J Physiol* 1997; **272**: E 1108–16.

240 Butler M, Meaney F. Standards for selected anthropometric measurements in Prader-Willi syndrome. *Pediatrics* 1991; **88**: 853–60.

241 Wollmann HA, Schultz U, Grauer M, Ranke MB. Reference values for height and weight in Prader-Willi syndrome based on 315 patients. *Eur J Pediatr* 1998; **157**: 634–42.

242 Bray G, Dahms W, Swerdloss R, *et al.* The Prader–Willi syndrome. A study of 40 patients and a review of the literataure. *Medicine* 1983; **62**: 59–80.

243 Costerff H, Horm V, Ruvalcaba R, Shaver J. Growth hormone secretion in Prader-Willi syndrome. *Acta Paediatr Scand* 1990; **79**: 1059–62.

244 Cappa M, Grossi A, Borelli P, *et al.* Growth hormone (GH) response to combined pyridostigime and GH-releasing hormone administration in patients with Prader–Labhart–Willi syndrome. *Horm Res* 1993; **39**: 51–5.

245 Angulo M, Castro-Magana M, Uy J. Pituitary evaluation and growth hormone treatment in Prader-Willi syndrome. *J Pediatr Endocrinol* 1991; **4**: 167–72.

246 Tannenbaum GS, Gurd W, Lapointe M. Leptin is a potent stimulator of spontaneous pulsatile growth hormone (GH) secretion and the GH response to GH-releasing hormone. *Endocrinology* 1998; **139**: 3871–5.

247 Eiholzer U, Bachmann S, l'Allemand D. Is there growth hormone deficiency in Prader-Willi Syndrome. *Horm Res* 2000; **53(Suppl 3)**: 44–52.

248 Eiholzer U, l'Allemand D. Growth hormone normalises height, prediction of final height, and hand length in children with Prader-Willi syndrome. Swedish National Growth Hormone Advisory Group. *Acta Paediatr Suppl* 1999; **88**: 109–11.

249 Eiholzer U, Nordmann Y, l'Allemand D. Fatal outcome of sleep apnea in PWS during the initial phase of growth hormone treatment. A case report. *Horm Res* 2002; **58(Suppl 3)**: 24–6.

250 Stoving RK, Veldhuis JD, Flyvbjerg A, *et al.* Jointly amplified basal and pulsatile growth hormone (GH) secretion and increased process irregularity in women with anorexia nervosa: indirect evidence for disruption of feedback regulation with the GH-insulin-like growth factor I axis. *J Clin Endocrinol Metab* 1999; **84**: 2056–63.

251 Maes M, Underwood LE, Ketelslergers JM. Plasma Somatomedin C in fasted and refed rats: close relationship with changes in lilver somatogenic but not lactogenic binding sites. *J Endocrinol* 1983; **97**: 243–52.

252 Thissen JP, Triest S, Underwood LE, *et al.* Divergent responses of serum insulin-like growth factor-I and liver growth hormone receptors to exogenous GH in protein restricted rats. *Endocrinology* 1990; **126**: 908–13.

253 Counts DR, Gwirtsman H, Carlsson LMS, *et al.* The effect of anorexia nervosa and refeeding on growth hormone-binding protein, the insulin-like growth factors (IGFs), and the IGF-binding proteins. *J Clin Endocrinol Metab* 1992; **75**: 762–7.

254 Tolle V, Kadem M, Bluet-Pajot M-T, *et al.* Balance in ghrelin and leptin plasma levels in anorexia nervosa patients and constitutionally thin women. *J Clin Endocrinol Metab* 2003; **88**: 109–16.

255 Albertsson-Wikland K, Wennergren G, Wennergren M, *et al.* Longitudinal follow-up of growth in children born small for gestational age. *Acta Paediatr* 1993; **82**: 438–43.

256 Albertsson-Wikland K, Boguszerski M, Karlbert J. Children born small-for-gestational age: postnatal growth and hormonal status. *Horm Res* 1998; **49(Suppl 2)**: 7–13.

257 Boguszerski CL, Boguszewski JC, Carlsson LMS. Increased proportion of circulating non-22 kilodalton growth hormone isoforms in short children: A possible mechanism for growth failure. *J Clin Endocrinol Metab* 1997; **82**: 2944–9.

258 Stanhope R, Ackland F, Hamill G, *et al.* Physiologic growth hormone secretion and response to growth hormone treatment in children with short stature and intrauterine growth retardation. *Acta Paediatr Scand Suppl* 1989; **349**: 47–52.

259 Ackland FM, Stanhope R, Eyre C, *et al.* Physiologic growth hormone secretion in children with short stature and intrauterine growth retardation. *Horm Res* 1988; **30**: 241–5.

260 Wit JM, Massarano AA, Kamp GA, *et al.* Growth hormone secretion in Turner's syndrome as determined by time series analysis. *Acta Endocrinol* 1992; **127**: 7–12.

261 Pombo M, Barreiro J, Penalva A, *et al.* Absence of growth hormone (GH) secretion after the administration of either GH-releasing hormone (GHRH), GH-releasing peptide (GHRP-6), or GHRH plus GHRP-6 in children with neonatal pituitary stalk transection. *J Clin Endocrinol Metab* 1995; **80**: 3180–4.

262 Popovic V, Damjanovic S, Micic D, *et al.* Blocked growth hormone-releasing peptide (GHRP-6) induced GH secretion and the absence of the synergic action of GHRP-6 plus GH-releasing hormone in patients with hypothalamo-pituitary disconnection: evidence that GHRP-6 main action is exerted at the hypothalamic level. *J Clin Endocrinol Metab* 1995; **80**: 942–7.

263 Kikuchi K, Fujisawa I, Momoi T, *et al.* Hypothalamic-pituitary function in growth hormone-deficient patients with pituitary stalk transection. *J Clin Endocrinol Metab* 1988; **67**: 817–22.

264   Root AW. Magnetic resonance imaging in hypopituitarism. *J Clin Endocrinol Metab* 1991; **72**: 10–11.

265   Sheehan HL, Whitehead R. The neurohypophysis in post-partum hypopituitarism. *J Path Bacteriol* 1963; **85**: 146–9.

266   Kaufman BA, Kaufman B, Mapstoen TB. Pituitary stalk agenesis: magnetic resonance imaging of 'ectopic posterior lobe' with surgical correlation. *Pediatr Neurosci* 1988; **14**: 140–4.

267   Giustina A, Romanelli G, Candrina R, Giustina G. Growth hormone deficiency in patients with idiopathic adrenocorticotrophin deficiency resolves during glucocorticoid replacement. *J Clin Endocrinol Metab* 1989; **68**: 120–4.

268   Giustina A, Girelli A, Doga M, *et al.* Pyridostigmine blocks the inhibitory effect of glucocorticoids on growth hormone releasing hormone stimulated growth hormone secretion in normal men. *J Clin Endocrinol Metab* 1990; **71**: 580–4.

269   Pralong FP, Miell JP, Corder R, Gaillard RC. Dexamethasone treatment in man induces changes in 24-hour growth hormone (GH) secretion profile without altering total GH released. *J Clin Endocrinol Metab* 1991; **73**: 1191–6.

270   Kauffmann S, Jones KI, Wehrenberg WB, Culler, FL. Inhibition by prednisone of growth hormone (GH) response to GH-releasing hormone in normal men. *J Clin Endocrinol Metab* 1988; **67**: 1258–61.

271   Pennisi AJ, Costin G, Phillips LS. Somatomedin and growth hormone studies in pediatric renal allograft recipients who receive daily prednisone. *Am J Dis Child* 1979; **133**: 950–4.

272   Magiakow M, Mastorakos G, Gomez MT, *et al.* Suppressed spontaneous and stimulated growth hormone secretion in patients with Cushing's disease before and after surgical cure. *J Clin Endocrinol Metab* 1994; **78**: 131–7.

273   Leal-Cero A, Pumar A, Garcia-Garcia E, *et al.* Inhibition of growth hormone release after the combined administration of GHRH and GHRP-6 in patients with Cushing's syndrome. *Clin Endocrinol (Oxf)* 1994; **41**: 649–54.

274   Giustina A, Bossoni S, Bodini C, *et al.* Pyridostigmine enhances even if it does not normalize the growth responses to growth hormone-releasing hormone in patients with Cushing's disease. *Horm Res* 1991; **35**: 99–103.

275   Chernausek SD, Turner R. Attenuation of spontaneous, nocturnal growth hormone secretion in children with hypothyroidism and its correlation with plasma insulin-like growth factor-1 concentration. *J Pediatr* 1989; **114**: 968–72.

276   Iwatsubo H, Omori K, Okado Y, *et al.* Human growth hormone secretion in primary hypothyroidism before and after treatment. *J Clin Endocrinol Metab* 1967; **27**: 1751–4.

277   Chernausek SD, Underwood LE, Utiger RD, Van Wyk JJ. Growth hormone secretion and plasma somatomedin C in primary hypothyroidism. *Clin Endocrinol* 1983; **19**: 337–44.

278   Giustina A, Wehrenberg WB. Influence of thyroid hormones on the regulation of growth hormone secretion. *Eur J Endocrinol* 1995; **133**: 646–53.

279   Diamond FB Jr, Root AW. Interrelated interactions of pituitary growth hormone and the hypothalamic-pituitary-thyroid axis. *J Pediatr Endocrinol Metab* 1992; **5**: 121–7.

280   Devesa J, Lima L, Tresguerres JAF. Neuroendocrine control of growth hormone secretion in humans. *Trends Endocrinol Metab* 1992; **3**: 175–83.

281   Valcavi R, Zini M, Portioli I. Thyroid hormones and growth hormone secretion. *J Endocrinol Invest* 1992; **15**: 313–30.

282   Katakami H, Downs TR, Frohman LA. Decreased hypothalamic growth hormone-releasing hormone content and pituitary responsiveness in hypothyroidism. *J Clin Invest* 1986; **77**: 1704–10.

283   Iranmanesh A, Lizarralde G, Johnson ML, Veldhuis JD. Nature of altered growth hormone secetion in hyperthyroidism. *J Clin Endocrinol Metab* 1991; **72**: 108–15.

284   Miell JP, Taylor AM, Zini M, *et al.* Effects of hypothyroidism and hyperthyroidism on insulin-like growth factors (IGFs) and growth hormone (GH) and IGF binding proteins. *J Clin Endocrinol Metab* 1993; **76**: 950–5.

285   Ortigosa JL, Mendoza F, Argote RM, *et al.* Propranolol effect on plasma glucose, free fatty acid, insulin and growth hormone in Graves' disease. *Metabolism* 1976; **25**: 1201–7.

286   Harvey S. Thyrotropin-releasing hormone: a growth hormone-releasing factor. *J Endocrinol* 1990; **125**: 345–58.

287   Aman J, Kroon M, Karlsson I, *et al.* Reduced growth hormone secretion improved insulin sensitivity in adolescent girls with type 1 diabetes. *Acta Paediatr* 1996; **85**: 31–7.

288   Johansen K, Hansen AP. Diurnal growth hormone levels in poorly and well controlled juvenile diabetics. *Diabetes* 1971; **20**: 239–45.

289   Press M, Tamborlane WV, Sherwin RS. Importance of raised growth hormone levels in mediating the metabolic derangements of diabetes. *N Engl J Med* 1989; **310**: 810–5.

290   Krassowski J, Felber JP, Rogala H, *et al.* Exaggerated growth hormone response to growth hormone-releasing hormone in type 1 diabetes mellitus. *Acta Endocrinol (Copenh)* 1988; **117**: 225–9.

291   Martha PM, Clarke WL. Alterations in growth hormone secretion and clearance in adolescent boys with insulin-dependent diabetes mellitus. *J Clin Endocrinol Metab* 1993; **77**: 638–43.

292   Asplin CM, Faria ACS, Carlsen EC, *et al.* Alterations in the pulsatile mode of growth hormone release in men and women with insulin-dependent diabetes mellitus. *J Clin Endocrinol Metab* 1989; **69**: 239–45.

293   Giustina A, Wehrenberg WB. Growth hormone neuroregulation in diabetes mellitus. *Trends Endocrinol Metab* 1994; **5**: 73–8.

294   Schaper NC, Tamsma JT, Sluiter WJ, *et al.* Growth hormone autoregulation in type 1 diabetes mellitus. *Acta Endocrinol (Copenh)* 1990; **122**: 32–9.

295   Edge JA, Matthews DR, Dunger DB. The dawn phenomenon is related to overnight growth hormone release in adolescent diabetics. *Clin Endocrinol (Oxf)* 1990; **33**: 729–37.

296   Salgado LR, Semer M, Nery M, *et al.* Effect of glycemic control on growth hormone and IGFBP-1 secretion in patients with type 1 diabetes mellitus. *Endocrinol Invest* 1996; **19**: 433–40.

297 Quantrin T, Thraikill K, Baker L, *et al.* Dual hormonal replacement with insulin and recombinant human insulin-like growth factor I in insulin dependent diabetes mellitus effects of glycemic control, IGF-I levels and safety profile. *Diabetes Care* 1997; **20**: 374–80.

298 Gandrud LM, Wilson DM. Is growth hormone stimulation testing in children still appropriate? *Growth Horm IGF-I Res* 2004; **14**: 185–94.

299 Marin G, Domene HM, Barnes KM, *et al.* The effects of estrogen priming and puberty on the growth hormone response to standardized treadmill exercise and arginine-insulin in normal girls and boys. *J Clin Endocrinol Metab* 1994; **79**: 537–41.

300 Ghigo E, Bellone J, Aimaretti G, *et al.* Reliability of provocative tests to assess growth hormone secretory status: .study in 472 normally growing children. *J Clin Endocrinol Metab* 1996; **81**: 3323–7.

301 Guyda HJ. Growth hormone testing and the short child. *Pediatr Res* 2000; **48**: 579–80.

302 Granda ML, Sanmarti A, Lucas A, *et al.* Assay-dependent results of immunoassayable spontaneous 24-h growth hormone secretion in short children. *Acta Paediatr Scand Suppl* 1990; **370**: 63–70.

303 Zadik Z, Chalew SA, Gilula Z, Kowarski AA. Reproducibility of growth hormone testing procedures: a comparison between 24-h integrated concentration and pharmacological stimulation. *J Clin Endocrinol Metab* 1990; **71**: 1127–30.

304 van den Broeck J, Arends N, Hokken-Koelaga A. Growth response to recombinant human growth hormone (GH) in children with idiopathic growth retardation by level of maximum GH peak during GH stimulation tests. *Horm Res* 2000; **53**: 267–73.

29

Abnormalities of growth hormone action

KATIE WOODS, RON ROSENFELD

INTRODUCTION

Over the past 20 years, it has become recognized increasingly that poor growth may be caused not only by defects in growth hormone (GH) secretion, but also by defects in GH action, or GH insensitivity (GHI). The first description of GHI was by Laron and colleagues in 1966, who reported 'three siblings with hypoglycemia and other clinical and laboratory signs of GH deficiency, but with abnormally high concentrations of immunoreactive serum GH'.[1] The underlying cause of this condition, known as GHI syndrome (GHIS) or Laron syndrome, was not determined until 1989, however, when Godowski and co-workers cloned the human GH receptor gene and identified a partial GH gene deletion in three such patients.[2] A wide range of GH receptor gene mutations and deletions have now been identified in GHIS subjects.

Following binding to and activation of the cell-surface bound GH receptor, GH mediates its effects by activating an intracellular signaling cascade which ultimately leads to the synthesis of insulin-like growth factor (IGF)-I, the main effector hormone of growth (Fig. 29.1). Abnormal functioning of molecules involved at any stage in this pathway, either through genetic defects, or acquired disease, may also potentially lead to GHI. A classification of GHI was first developed in 1993, dividing the condition into 'primary' (or genetic) and 'secondary' (or acquired) forms.[3] An updated and expanded version of this classification is presented in Table 29.1. At the time the classification was devised, only defects in the GH receptor gene were known to cause primary GH insensitivity. However, 12 years later, gene defects in several key molecules involved in downstream GH action have been identified. These include IGF-I,[4,5] acid labile subunit (ALS),[6,7] and the STAT 5b gene[8,9] (Fig. 29.1). In addition to broadening the phenotypes associated with GHI, these fascinating 'experiments of nature' have furthered our understanding of the action of GH and the IGFs in man.

At present, many of the patients evaluated for growth failure in the endocrine clinic are labeled as having unexplained, or 'idiopathic' short stature, on the basis of having sufficient GH secretion as judged by the currently available tests, and the absence of an identifiable syndrome. Although such patients have less severe short stature than most of the patients discussed below, it is highly possible that such children have mild abnormalities in the functioning of molecules involved in mediating GH action. As discussed below, several recent avenues of research lend support to this hypothesis, promising in time to lead to a more considered approach to the evaluation and management of short stature in childhood than is currently the standard.

THE GROWTH HORMONE RECEPTOR AND ITS SIGNALING

The human GH receptor (GHR) gene is located on chromosome 5p13.1–p12,[10] contains 10 exons, and encodes a 638 amino acid peptide including an 18 residue leader

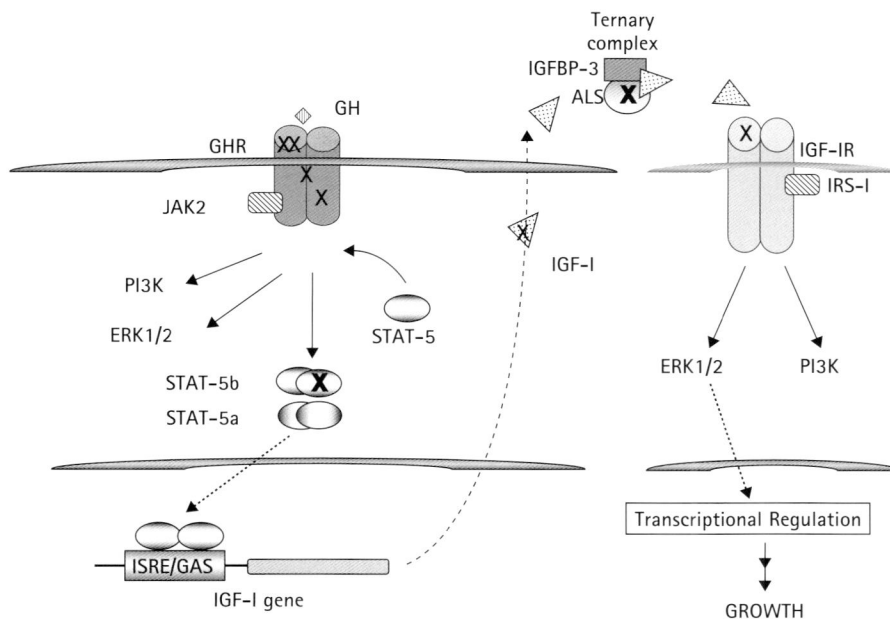

Figure 29.1   Schematic diagram of the GH–IGF-I axis, showing identified defects. Defects leading to GH insensitivity have been identified in the GH receptor gene (affecting GH receptor binding, dimerization, the transmembrane domain and the intracellular domain), the STAT 5b gene, the IGF-I gene, and the ALS gene. Defects in the IGF-I receptor gene associated with intrauterine growth retardation, postnatal growth failure and elevated IGF-I levels have also been reported. Abbreviations: GH = growth hormone, JAK 2 = Janus associated kinase 2, STAT-5 = signal transducer and activator of transcription 5, PI3K = phosphatidylinositol-3 kinase, ERK = extracellular signal regulated kinase, ISRE = interferon-stimulated response element, GAS = interferon–gamma activated sequences, IGFBP-3 = insulin-like growth factor binding protein-3, ALS = acid labile subunit, IGF-I = insulin-like growth factor-I, IGF-IR = IGF-I receptor, IRS = insulin receptor substrate. From *Eur J Endo*, 2004; **151**: S11–S15. Copyright Society of the European Journal of Endocrinology (2004). Reproduced with permission.

Table 29.1   Classification of growth hormone insensitivity (GHI) associated with IGF deficiency ('primary' IGF deficiency)

Primary GH insensitivity (hereditary gene defects)

1. GH receptor deficiency (GHRD) or GH insensitivity syndrome (GHIS)
    i. Defects of the extracellular domain
        a. Associated with decreased GH binding protein (GHBP)
            - Impaired GH receptor binding
            - Impaired receptor trafficking to cell surface
        b. Associated with normal GHBP
            - Impaired receptor dimerisation
    ii. Defects of the transmembrane domain
        a. Associated with elevated GHBP
            - Impaired GHR stabilization in cell membrane
    iii. Defects of the intracellular domain
        a. Associated with normal GHBP
            - Impaired GHR signaling
) Dominant negative mutations (exon 9 splice site)
) Recessive mutations (truncation beyond box 1)
2. Abnormalities in GH signal transduction
    STAT 5b gene defect
3. Primary defects in IGF-I synthesis
    IGF-I gene defect

Secondary GH insensitivity (acquired conditions: may be transitory)

    i. Circulating antibodies to growth hormone that inhibit GH action
    ii. Malnutrition
    iii. Liver disease
    iv. Chronic disease

sequence[11] (Fig. 29.2). The mature 620 amino acid transmembrane receptor molecule is ubiquitously found in the human body. It consists of three domains: (1) a 246 amino acid extracellular, hormone binding domain; (2) a 24 amino acid transmembrane domains; and (3) a 350 amino acid cytoplasmic, or intracellular domain. The GHR is part of a receptor 'superfamily', having significant structural and sequence homology with a variety of other hormone receptors, including those for prolactin, the interleukins 2–7, erythropoietin, granulocyte-macrophage colony stimulating factor (GM-CSF), and interferon.[12]

Interestingly, the extracellular domain of the GHR also circulates in plasma as a GH binding protein (GHBP), which, in humans, is shed from the membrane-bound GHR by proteolytic cleavage.[13,14] The physiologic significance of this circulating GHBP remains unclear, although measurement of GHBP can prove useful in differentiating the causes of GHI, as discussed below.

Mature GHRs exist on the cell surface as loosely associated preformed dimers (Fig. 29.1). The conformational change caused by binding of GH stabilizes the GHR dimer and results in receptor activation. GH signal transduction is mediated through at least three pathways: phosphatidylinositol-3 kinase (PI3K), extracellular signal related kinases (ERK) 1 and 2, and the Janus associated kinase-STAT (JAK-STAT) pathway.[15,16] The JAK-STAT pathway appears to be centrally involved in mediating the growth promoting actions of GH.[17,18] Activated STAT 5b

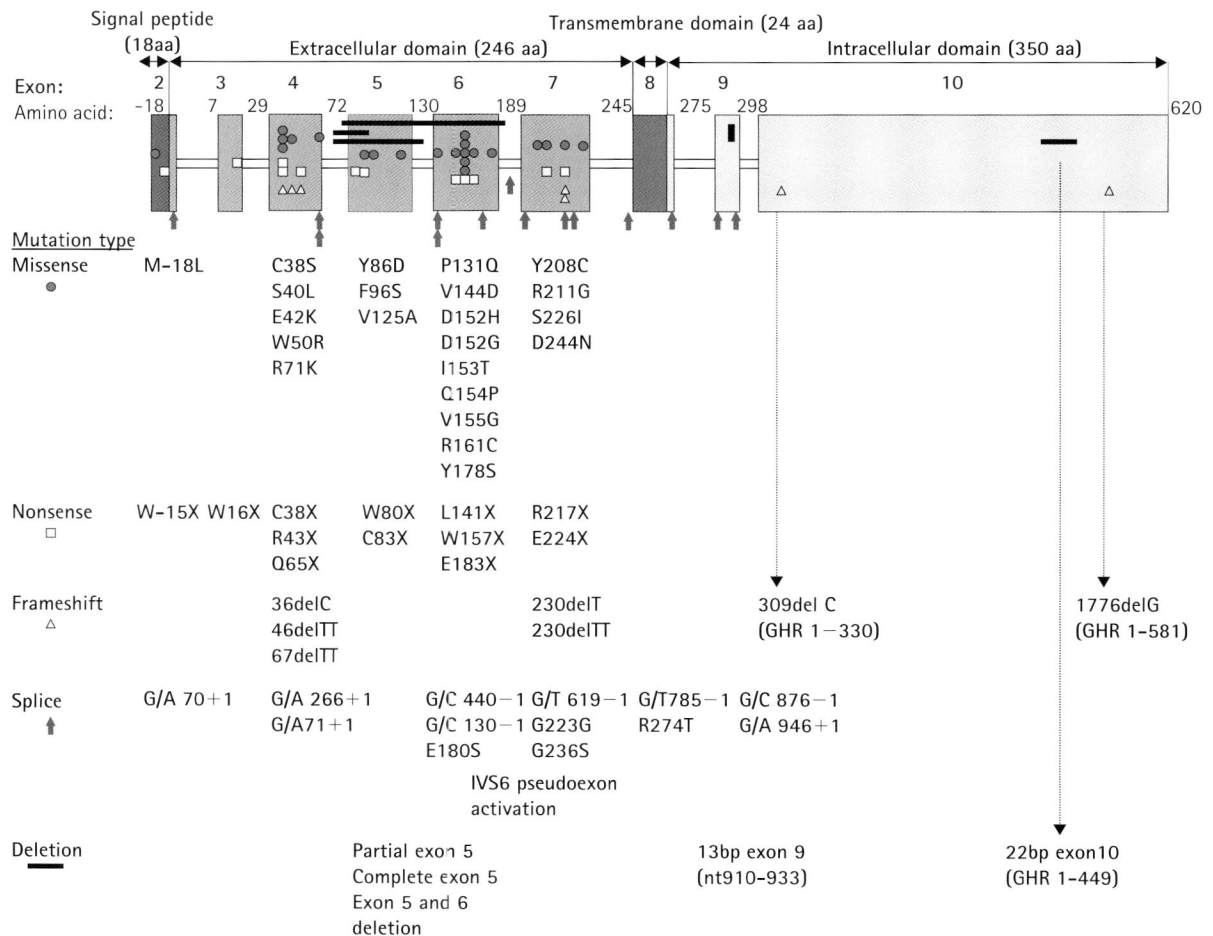

Figure 29.2 Structure of the growth hormone (GH) receptor gene and mutations identified in GH insensitivity syndrome (or Laron syndrome). The GH receptor gene contains nine coding exons, which code for the signal peptide, extracellular (hormone binding) domain, transmembrane domain, and intracellular domain of the GH receptor protein. Sixty distinct GH receptor gene mutations have now been described in GH insensitivity syndrome, the majority of which are clustered in the region of the gene encoding the extracellular domain. Missense and nonsense mutations are numbered by position of amino acid change (using standard amino acid code abbreviations), frameshift mutations by the position of nucleotide change. Data obtained from Laron Z, *JCEM*, 2004, the Human Genome Mapping Database at http://archive.uwcm.ac.uk/uwcm/mg/hgmd0.html (Stenson *et al.*, 2003, The Human Gene Mutation Database (HGMD): 2003 update, *Hum Mut* 2003; 21: 577–581, and Online Mendelian Inheritance in man (OMIM) at http://www.ncbi.nlm.nih.gov. Abbreviations: aa = amino acid, IVS = intervening sequence (or introns), GHR = growth hormone receptor, bp = base pair, del = deletion.

translocates into the nucleus, and has been recently demonstrated to bind to promoter elements in the IGF-I gene and stimulate IGF-I gene transcription.[19] As discussed in more detail below, the recent discoveries of two patients with molecular defects in STAT 5b, and the clinical phenotype of severe GHIS further supports this hypothesis.[8]

The liver has a high concentration of GHRs, and synthesizes most of the IGF-I measurable in the circulation. However, as GHRs are ubiquitiously expressed, IGF-I is also produced locally, producing autocrine/paracrine effects at the tissue level. At present, the relative growth promoting contribution of circulating IGF-I versus local production of IGF-I is a matter of some debate.

EPIDEMIOLOGY OF GROWTH HORMONE INSENSITIVITY SYNDROME

GH insensitivity syndrome (GHIS) is a rare cause of growth retardation, with only around 300 patients described to date wordwide.[20–22] The majority of patients originate from inbred cohorts, or consanguineous unions, reflecting the autosomal recessive nature of the disease in most cases. Three large cohorts of GHIS patients have been reported. Laron, who identified the original cases of GHIS, has followed 60 patients in Israel, in whom 11 different mutations of the GH receptor gene have been identified, including six patients with the first described abnormalities of the

GH receptor gene, deletion of exons 3, 5, and 6 (see above). He has recently reported on his personal experience caring for and studying these patients over the past 45 years.[22] In the mountainous Loja and El Oro regions of southern Ecuador, a large cohort of GHIS patients have been discovered, and thoroughly described by Guevarra-Aguirre and colleagues.[23,24] All but one of these patients have the same mutation of the GH receptor gene (E180S), suggesting a founder effect.[20,25] This geographically isolated group, now thought to number around 80 affected patients in total (Guevarra-Aguirre J, personal communication), is a highly inbred population, believed to be of Spanish descent. Interestingly, one of the patients identified in Israel, an Israeli Jew of Moroccan heritage, is homozygous for E180S, providing some support for the hypothesis that the Ecuadorian cohort may be of Jewish ancestry.[26] A 'European' cohort of GHIS patients has also been described.[21,27] This group, consisting of 82 patients, includes patients residing in a wide range of European countries, and also a few non-European countries, including Australia, Japan, Saudi Arabia, South America, and South Africa. It exhibits the widest range of genetic heterogeneity, with 19 different GHR mutations identified to date. Again, consanguinity is very common, and in many cases, families originate in the Middle East or the Indian subcontinent, possibly reflecting the high rate of consanguinity in these populations.

In addition to these larger cohorts, reports of patients with GHIS secondary to GHR defects continue to appear in the medical literature. These reported cases now total over 100 patients, and in all probability underestimate the total number of sporadic cases, as only those with novel mutations are likely to be reported in the literature.

At present, GHIS secondary to defects in genes other than the GH receptor remains exceptionally rare, with only six cases reported in the literature (discussed in more detail below).

GROWTH HORMONE INSENSITIVITY SYNDROME SECONDARY TO DEFECTS OF ITS RECEPTOR

It was initially postulated that GHIS may be secondary to bioinactive GH.[1] However, the observation that exogenous GH could not stimulate IGF-I production in GHIS,[28,29] and the finding, in 1984, that hepatocytes from two GHI patients were unable to bind GH,[30] suggested that defects in the GH receptor were the cause of GHIS. In 1989, this hypothesis was proved correct, with the discovery of a large deletion of the portion of the gene encoding the extracellular domain of the receptor, involving exons 3, 5, and 6, in three GHIS subjects.[2,31] Originally, this deletion was thought to involve exon 3 in addition to 5 and 6. However, it is now understood that the loss of exon 3 is a normal GH receptor variant, with just over one-third of GH receptor alleles

encoding a sequence that results in the skipping of exon 3 from the GHR messenger RNA.[32] The exon 5, 6 deletion of the GHR gene also results in a frameshift, producing a premature translational stop signal in exon 7, and consequently encodes a receptor effectively lacking all but the early part of the extracellular domain. Not surprisingly, given the severity of the molecular defect, these patients had the classical clinical features of GHIS, including undetectable serum concentrations of GHBP. Shortly after this report, Amselem and co-workers described the first point mutation of the GHR gene in four severely growth retarded children, born to a consanguineous Tunisian family.[33] These patients were found to be homozygous for a nucleotide substitution (thymidine to cytosine) in codon 96 of exon 5, resulting in the replacement of phenylalanine with serine (F96S). Functional studies of this mutation indicate that it abolishes GH binding, thus leading to the severe phenotype observed in the affected children.[34]

Sixty distinct mutations have now been described in patients with GHIS (Fig. 29.2). Interestingly, although the extracellular domain contains only 40 percent of the total amino acids, just under 90 percent of the mutations described (53/60) are located in this region. To date, six mutations have been described solely affecting the intracellular domain. These include two splice site mutations,[35,36] two small deletions,[37,38] and two frameshift mutations,[39,40] all of which result in truncation of the intracellular domain. Functional studies of these mutations are providing useful information about the mechanism of GHR intracellular signalling. The most recently described mutation is a frameshift mutation at the 1776 nucleotide position of exon10, predicted to result in a GHR truncation to 581 amino acids (from the normal 630 amino acids) with a nonsense sequence between residues 560 and 581.[40] Functional studies of this mutation indicated it reduces STAT 5 activation by 50 percent, while retaining the ability of the GHR to activate STAT3. The two splice site mutations identified in exon 9 are the only GHR mutations which act in a dominant negative manner. Both mutations have the same functional effect, producing a greatly truncated GHR protein (GHR 1–277) which lacks most of the intracellular domain, yet retains the transmembrane and extracellular domain. The dominant negative effect is thought to occur secondary to the dimerization of mutant GHR molecules with normal GHR, reducing the available functional receptors.[35,36] Although several polymorphisms in the intracellular domain have been described,[41] no convincing missense mutations have been identified in this region, perhaps suggesting a greater degree of redundancy of amino acid sequence in this region of the GH receptor protein.

Mutations in a number of genes other than the GH receptor have now been identified in patients with GHIS. These patients all present with growth failure and biochemical GH insensitivity, but have a clinical phenotype distinct from patients with GHIS due to GHR defects. These defects are discussed in the relevant sections below.

Table 29.2 Growth and development in primary growth hormone insensitivity

Growth
- Birth weight within 2 SD of normal
- Birth length mildly reduced
- Severe postnatal growth failure (−3.8 to −12 SD)
- Delayed bone age, but advanced for height age
- Segmental ratios and arm span normal for bone age
- Small hands and feet

Craniofacial characteristics
- Sparse hair early in childhood
- Head size normal, but large relative to face and body, giving the impression of a large head
- Hypoplastic nasal bridge; shallow orbits
- Prominent forehead; small, sculpted chin
- Decreased vertical dimension of face
- 'Setting sun sign' in 25 percent of children
- Blue sclerae
- Prolonged retention of primary dentition

Sexual development
- Small phallus in childhood: proportional to body size in adults
- Puberty delayed (3–7 years)
- Normal adult sexual function and fertility

Clinical features of GHIS secondary to GHR deficiency

The major clinical features of classical GHIS are listed in Table 29.2. As originally noted by Laron in his 1966 report,[1] patients with GHI due to mutations of the GH receptor gene are clinically indistinguishable from patients with severe congenital GH deficiency. These observations provide good clinical evidence that GH actions are mediated entirely through the GH receptor.

PRENATAL GROWTH

The most striking feature of GHIS due to GHRD is postnatal growth retardation, demonstrating the primacy of IGF-I in mediating growth during childhood and adolescence. By contrast, in most patients, birth size is only mildly, if at all reduced. In the European cohort of 82 patients, a mild reduction in both birth length standard deviation score (SDS) (average − 1.01) and weight SDS (average − 0.36) was noted, when compared to UK standards.[21] However, birth lengths and weights greater than 2 SDs above the mean were also recorded in some patients, demonstrating that a wide range of sizes at birth is compatible with a diagnosis of GHIS. Amongst the Ecuadorian cohort, birth weight was within normal range for North American infants in 31/34 patients, and below −3 SD in three patients.[20]

Amongst the cohort reported by Laron, however, a reduction in birth length was more common, with 12/20 newborns reported to have birth lengths greater than 2 SDs below the mean.[42]

Overall, as in patients with congenital GH deficiency, it appears that although there may be a minor reduction in prenatal growth in GHIS, severe growth failure does not usually occur until after birth, suggesting that prenatal growth is not largely dependent on GH. As discussed in more detail below, IGF-I, in contrast, is a fetal growth factor.

POSTNATAL GROWTH AND PUBERTY

Laron has published growth curves for GHIS, based on the growth patterns in the Israeli cohort.[3] A fall-off in growth is typically observed within the first 6 months of birth. In the Ecuadorian cohort, height during childhood ranges between −6.8 and −9.6 SDS,[24] and in the Israeli cohort, between −4 and −10 SDS.[22] Based on the growth of the more heterogeneous European group, heights in childhood ranged from −2.2 to −10.4 SD.[21] Although osseous maturation is typically markedly delayed, the profound statural deficit results in advancement in bone age for height age, with bone–age to height–age ratios ranging from 1.6 to 6.4 in the Ecuadorian cohort.[43] Epiphyseal closure in the Israeli group occurred between 20 and 22 years in boys and 16 to 18 years in girls.[22]

Puberty is often delayed, more so in boys than girls, and the pubertal growth spurt is absent or blunted.[25] In the Ecuadorian group, 50 percent of patients went through puberty at the expected time for peers, with the remaining 50 percent having delays of up to 7 years. Amongst the Israeli GHIS boys, testicular enlargement was noted between 13 and 16 years, axillary hair at 16 years, and first conscious ejaculation between 17 and 21 years (average age for this milestone is normally 13.5 years).[44] Timing of menarche in the females of this group was less delayed, at between 13 and 16 years of age.

Adult stature in the Israeli group is reported as between 116 and 142 cm in males and 108 and 136 cm in females.[22] In the Ecuadorian group adult height ranged between −5.3 to −12 SD (95–124 cm in women, and 106–141 cm in men). This considerable variation in stature is particularly interesting in the Ecuadorian group, considering that all (but one) patient share the same GHR mutation, which presumably disrupts GH receptor function to the same extent in each individual. Despite this, stature correlates significantly with serum concentrations of IGF-I. Evidently, some individuals are able to generate IGF-I and grow through GH-independent mechanisms better than others. Unlike other genetic short stature conditions, such as Turner syndrome, although parental height SDS in GHIS does not correlate with patient height SDS,[21] suggesting the mechanisms underlying the variation in growth in GHIS are different, at least in part, from those contributing to the variation in growth in normal individuals.

CRANIOFACIAL CHARACTERISTICS

GHIS is typically characterized by a striking appearance of the facial features, namely a prominent forehead, depressed nasal bridge, shallow orbits, sparse hair, decreased vertical dimension to the face, and a small, sculpted chin.[45] The 'setting sun sign' (the presence of sclera above the iris when looking straight ahead) is seen in many patients (25 percent of the Ecuadorian cohort).[25] Closure of the fontanelles is also delayed. These findings have led to some patients being erroneously misdiagnosed with hydrocephalus. The abnormal craniofacial appearance in GHIS may reflect the fact that growth of the cranium (and brain) is less GH dependent than the facial bones, such that cranial size is disproportionately large relative to facial size. In the Ecuadorian cohort, affected individuals are often identified by knowledgeable family members at birth, suggesting that this disproportionate action of GH on the craniofacial region is already in effect in late gestation.

Other facial features seen in GHIS include blue sclerae, thought to be due to decreased thickness of the scleral connective tissue, and occasional unilateral ptosis or facial asymmetry. These features may represent the consequences of muscular hypoplasia and weakness, as discussed below. Defective dentition is also common, with prolonged retention of the primary teeth, frequent dental decay, and frequent crowding and/or hypodontia of the permanent teeth.[22,46]

SEXUAL DEVELOPMENT

The phallus was noted to be small on clinical examination in 12/29 (41 percent) of males in the European cohort,[21] and below −2 SD for bone age in all 10 pre-pubertal boys examined from the Ecuadorian cohort.[20] As discussed above, onset of puberty is generally later than normal, but full sexual maturation is achieved in both sexes. In males, phallic growth and testicular enlargement occur as normal during puberty. In the Israeli cohort, final length of the penis in males was reported as between 8 and 10 cm, and testicular volume 5–9 mL.[44] Fertility has been documented in both males and females.

INTELLECTUAL FUNCTION AND MAGNETIC RESONANCE IMAGING

Although it is clear that severe GHIS is compatible with normal intelligence, in both the Israeli and European cohorts there is evidence of reduced intellectual function in some patients. Israeli GHIS patients were found to have an overall lower intelligence quotient (IQ) than the general population, with greater deficits in performance IQ than the verbal IQ.[22] MRI imaging of nine adult and three children in the Israeli GHIS cohort revealed mild parenchymal loss in one child and all adults.[47] In the European study, 13.5 percent of patients were reported to have some degree of mental retardation, although formal tests of intellectual function were not performed.[21] One possibility is that reduced mental functioning in some patients may occur as a result of severe untreated hypoglycemia in infancy/early childhood. In the European cohort, however, patients with mental retardation did not report hypoglycemic episodes in

childhood more frequently than those with normal intellectual function (11 percent versus 20 percent). Somewhat in contrast to the above findings, anecdotal reports from Ecuador indicate that many patients with GHIS have exceptional school performance, particularly females.[48] Formal testing of the intellectual function of this group in 1998, using intelligence tests designed to minimize the effects of physical size, motor coordination, and cultural background, demonstrated that the intelligence of patients was no different to that of relatives and community controls.[49] As yet, there is no clear explanation to the apparent protection of the Ecuadorian patients from reduced mental functioning.

MUSCULOSKELETAL DEVELOPMENT AND SKIN

Hypomuscularity has been noted on radiographs of the lower extremities in GHIS, presumably explaining the delayed walking noted in 70 percent of the Ecuadorian patients.[43] Reduced muscle force and endurance has been noticed in adults with GHIS.[50] High pitched voices have been noticed in all affected children and many adults.[20] This may reflect the small size of the larynx in these individuals, as documented in the Israeli cohort.[51] In the Ecuadorian cohort, limited elbow extension was observed in 85 percent of the Ecuadorian cohort over the age of 5 years, and avascular necrosis of the femoral head in 25 percent.[25] These abnormalities have not been noted in the Israeli patients. The skin is frequently thin and prematurely wrinkled in adults, with reduced elastin fibers noted on histopathologic examination.[52]

BODY COMPOSITION AND BONE MINERAL DENSITY

As has been well described in the adult population, GH has a number of metabolic effects, including the promotion of anabolism and lipolysis. Consistent with this GH effect, GHIS patients appear clinically to have an increase in adiposity from infancy,[53] but weight for height is not typically increased until after puberty, when females, in particular, have a very high (>50 percent) increase in body fat.[20]

The bones of patients with GHIS often appear osteopenic on X-ray, and dual-energy X-ray absorptiometry (DEXA) scans on patients in the Israeli cohort initially were reported to confirm low bone mineral density.[54] However, correction for bone size with volumetric bone density measurements,[55] and histomorphometry with bone biopsies, indicated that this initial assumption was incorrect, and, in fact, bone mineral density is normal in GHIS.

GLUCOSE AND LIPID HOMEOSTASIS

As in congenital GH deficiency, hypoglycemia during infancy and early childhood appears common in GHIS, with as many of 50 percent of the Ecuadorian cohort reporting symptoms consistent with hypoglycemia in childhood,[20] and 75 percent of the European cohort.[21] Many patients also have asymptomatic hypoglycemia, as was found when patients were carefully monitored prior to starting recombinant human IGF-I therapy. With increasing age, hypoglycemia reduces in frequency, presumably reflecting a reduced reliance on the counter-regulatory effects of GH to maintain fasting glucose in the normal range. Interestingly, in later life, glucose intolerance, and even diabetes mellitus may develop, possibly reflecting insulin resistance secondary to increasing obesity.[56]

Following a similar pattern, total and LDL-cholesterol levels are generally low in childhood, but increase progressively in adulthood with increasing obesity to above-normal levels.[53]

CARDIOPULMONARY DEFECTS AND LONGEVITY

Cardiomicra, reduced cardiac muscle width, reduced left ventricular output, and reduced maximal exercise capacity have been noted in adult GHIS patients.[57,58] Higher than expected rates of atherosclerotic heart disease have been reported in the Ecuadorian, but not the Israeli, cohort.

Patients surviving into the 70s have been described in both the Ecuadorian and Israeli cohorts. In the Ecuadorian cohort, a high number of deaths in early childhood has been reported,[25] possibly due to unrecognized hypoglycemia in some cases.

Biochemical features of classical GHIS

GROWTH HORMONE

Both basal and stimulated GH levels are elevated in GHIS, consistent with the loss of negative hypothalamic feedback as a consequence of low IGF-I levels. In the Ecuadorian GHIS cohort, random GH levels in all children exceeded 10 ng mL^{-1}, with some as high as 200 ng mL^{-1}, and a mean level of 32 ng mL^{-1}.[20] In adult GHIS subjects in this group, GH levels were also elevated, although less so than in childhood (mean 11 ng mL^{-1}). GH is normally secreted in a pulsatile manner, and GH profiles in GHIS subjects demonstrate that GH pulsatility is preserved, with increases in basal GH levels, peak height and peak number.[59] GH release can be further stimulated by traditional GH secretagogues, including arginine, insulin-induced hypoglycemia and GH releasing hormone.[42,60] Suppression of GH release with somatostatin infusion, or IGF-I administration in GHIS subjects indicates that GH secretion in this condition remains subject to normal regulatory dynamics.[59,61]

GROWTH HORMONE BINDING PROTEIN

As discussed above, GHBP is a cleavage product of the extracellular domain of the human GH receptor, which retains the ability to bind GH.[13,14] The most commonly used assay for GHBP is a ligand-mediated immunofunctional assay (LIFA),[62] which measures the ability of serum GHBP to bind GH, and as such provides a useful circulating proxy of GH receptor binding activity. It was initially reported to be undetectable in GHIS.[63,64] However, as the number of reported cases of GHIS has increased, it became apparent that some patients with this condition have normal, or even elevated GHBP levels, so called 'GHBP positive' GHIS. Amongst the heterogeneous European group of GHIS patients, around 75 percent of patients were GHBP negative (low or undetectable GHBP).[21,27] In such patients, it can be assumed that a GHR mutation is highly probable, and that this mutation either impairs receptor binding, or reduces GHR cell surface expression. For example, the first missense mutation to be described in the GH receptor, F96S, has been demonstrated to both impair GH binding and to inhibit transport to the cell surface.[34,65] A mutation in the GH receptor promoter region or in genes that modulate GH receptor expression is also possible in this group, but has yet to be described.

Patients with GHBP positive GHIS form an interesting subgroup. In the European cohort, such patients had a milder phenotype, in general, with less severe short stature (mean height SDS of −4.9 SD in the GHBP positive patients versus −6.5 SD in those with low levels of GHBP). This condition has a wider potential etiology, encompassing defects in the GH receptor gene which affect GH receptor signaling rather than binding, or defects in genes other than the GH receptor which are involved in modulating GH receptor function, such as STAT 5b or ALS, as discussed in more detail below. One of the first GH receptor mutations to be described in GHBP positive GHIS caused an amino acid substitution which disrupted receptor dimerisation.[66] Two families have been described with classical GHIS yet elevated GHBP levels. In both cases, a splice site mutation was identified which resulted in the deletion of the intracellular and transmembrane domains of the GH receptor, resulting in the production of a severely truncated mutant receptor which highly resembles naturally occurring GHBP.[67,68]

INSULIN–LIKE GROWTH FACTORS

Extremely low levels of IGFs, which do not increase after administration of GH, are characteristic of GHIS. This was first demonstrated in 1969, before the term 'IGF' had been coined, when Daughaday and co-workers reported low serum sulfation factor activity in his GHIS patients, which did not rise with the administration of GH.[69] In the Ecuadorian cohort, serum IGF-I concentrations in prepubertal children were invariably less than 7 ng mL^{-1}, with a mean concentration of only 3 ng mL^{-1}.[20] Interestingly, a significant rise in IGF-I levels during puberty (as seen in normal individuals) also occurred in Ecuadorian patients, with adults having mean IGF levels of 25 ng mL^{-1} (normal 96–270 ng mL^{-1}), despite the lower GH levels in Ecuadorian GHIS adults compared with levels in GHIS children. These observations suggest that some component of the pubertal rise in IGF-I in both GHIS and normal individuals is GH independent.

In the European cohort, patients were characterized as GHIS with the use of a scoring system, taking into account height, basal GH, IGF-I and IGFBP-3 levels pre- and post-GH administration, and GHBP levels.[27] Mean IGF-I levels were less than 20 ng mL^{-1} (the lowest limit of detection in the assay used), with the highest IGF-I level recorded being 82 ng mL^{-1}.[21]

Serum IGF-II concentrations have also been found to be significantly reduced in GHIS, although not as dramatically as those of IGF-I, suggesting they are partially GH dependent.[20] However, it is also possible that IGF-II is reduced secondary to the low levels of IGFBP-3 in GHIS (see below).

INSULIN–LIKE GROWTH FACTOR BINDING PROTEINS

IGF-I and IGF-II circulate in plasma complexed to a family of six structurally related proteins, IGF binding protein (IGFBP) 1 through 6.[70] Insulin-like growth factor 3 (IGFBP-3) is considered to be the principal binding protein for circulating IGF in human serum, binding around 75–80 percent of the IGF content of serum under normal conditions as part of a ternary complex that includes a molecule of IGF peptide, a molecule of IGFBP-3, and a molecule of acid labile subunit (ALS). Thus complexed, the half-life of IGF in serum is increased from 15 min to 12–15 h.

In patients with GHIS secondary to defects of the GHR, both IGFBP-3 and ALS levels are reduced. In the Ecuadorian population, where serum IGFBP-3 concentrations in pooled normal adult serum were 2665 ng mL^{-1} in men and 2347 ng mL^{-1} in women, the mean serum IGFBP-3 levels were only 226 ng mL^{-1} in pre-pubertal patients and 433 ng mL^{-1} in adults.[20] ALS was also profoundly reduced, averaging less than 1 μg mL^{-1}, compared to normal levels of 16–20 μg mL^{-1}.[71] In the European cohort, all of whom were pre- or peripubertal, mean IGFBP-3 levels were 435 ng mL^{-1} (range 95–1762), or −8.5 (−1.4 to −14.9) SD below the mean for age.[21] Interestingly, in both the Ecuadorian and European cohorts, IGFBP-3 levels correlated with height SDS.

Aside from the loss of GH action, one possible mechanism for the reduction of IGFBP-3 and ALS in GHIS may be the extremely low IGF-I levels, reducing ternary complex formation and thus stability of IGFBP-3 and ALS in the serum. However, administration of IGF-I to subjects with GHIS does not increase serum concentrations of IGFBP-3 and ALS, to any great extent, arguing against this hypothesis.[59,72,73] Furthermore, as discussed below, the subject with IGF-I gene deletion had normal IGFBP-3 and ALS levels, despite profoundly low serum IGF-I.[4]

Unlike IGFBP-3, serum concentrations of both IGFBP-1 and IGFBP-2 tend to show modest elevations in GHIS, possibly reflecting the relative insulinopenia of this condition.[20] Consequently, these lower molecular weight IGFBPs

account for most of the IGF-carrying capacity of patients with GHR deficiency.[74]

GROWTH HORMONE INSENSITIVITY SECONDARY TO DEFECTS IN GENES OTHER THAN THE GROWTH HORMONE RECEPTOR

As discussed above, a small number of cases of primary GHIS have now been described associated with defects in genes other than the GH receptor. These include two subjects with IGF-I gene defects, two cases of STAT 5b gene defects, and two cases of ALS deficiency. Although their numbers are small, these human 'experiments of nature' provide significant insights into our understanding of GH–IGF-I physiology.

IGF–I gene deficiency

There are now two reported cases of homozygous mutations of the IGF-I gene. The first, described by Woods and co-workers in 1996, was a 15-year-old boy with a homozygous deletion of exons 4 and 5 of the IGF-I gene, resulting in a mature IGF-I peptide truncated from 70 to 25 amino acids, followed by an additional out-of-frame nonsense sequence of eight residues and a premature stop codon.[4] Recently, a second patient with an IGF-I gene defect has been described, a 55-year-old man with a homozygous missense mutation in IGF-I gene (G274A) which leads to a valine to methionine substitution at residue 44 of the mature IGF-I molecule, resulting in almost complete loss of binding affinity for the IGF-I receptor. Although the clinical features of this second patient have not yet been published, it appears that both patients had a history of severe pre- and postnatal growth failure, biochemical GH insensitivity, deafness, and mental retardation. Despite some common features with classical GHIS caused by GHR deficiency, the phenotype of these two patients differs in a number of important ways from that of GHR deficiency. Comparison of the similarities and differences between these patients and individuals with GHIS provides important insights into the differential effects of GH and IGF-I on growth and development.

GROWTH AND PUBERTY IN *IGF–I* GENE DEFICIENCY

Both cases of IGF-I gene deficiency were associated with a severe reduction in size at birth. The patient described by Woods and co-workers had severe, symmetrical growth retardation at birth (birth length −5.4 SD, birth weight −3.9 SD, head circumference −4.9 SD). The presence of prenatal growth failure in these patients, not usually seen to any great extent in GHR deficiency, is in keeping with the effects observed in the mouse of targeted knockout of the IGF-I gene, where fetal growth was greatly reduced from around midgestation onwards.[75,76] Thus, these cases appear to confirm that IGF-I is a prominent fetal growth factor in man, largely generated by GH-independent means *in utero*.

Postnatal growth of the first described patient with IGF-I gene deficiency was slow, and by the time of diagnosis at 15.75 years, his height SDS was −6.9, and weight SDS −6.5, similar to height deficits seen in classical GHIS. Bone age was delayed 18 months. He was in early puberty at the time of diagnosis (Tanner–Whitehouse classification: genitalia 2, pubic hair stage 1, testes 4 mL bilaterally), indicating a delay in pubertal onset, as seen frequently in classical GHIS. Gonadotrophin levels and testosterone levels were appropriate for pubertal stage.

PHYSICAL APPEARANCE IN *IGF-I* GENE DEFICIENCY

The patient described by Woods and co-workers did not have the typical facial appearance of GHIS. His head size was proportionately reduced when compared to his body, and his facial features did not look small compared to the size of the head. The patient had some mild dysmorphic features, including mild micrognathia, and clinodactyly, not seen in classical GHIS.

NEUROLOGIC FUNCTION IN *IGF-I* GENE DEFICIENCY

Sensorineural deafness and mild mental retardation were noted in both cases of IGF-I gene deficiency. No history of hypoglycemia was present (or would be expected, see below) in these patients, suggesting that the mental retardation is most likely a direct effect of IGF-I on CNS development. As many patients with GHIS or congenital GH deficiency are of normal intelligence, this effect of IGF-I on the brain would appear to be largely GH independent.

METABOLIC FEATURES OF *IGF-I* GENE DEFICIENCY

Unlike GHIS during childhood, where relative insulinopenia is present, the patient described by Woods *et al.* had significant insulin resistance, as documented by marked elevations in fasting insulin, first phase insulin response, and the modified Bergman intravenous glucose tolerance test. Insulin sensitivity improved upon administration of IGF-I, most likely secondary to the lowering of GH secretion induced by this therapy (see below).[77]

BIOCHEMICAL FEATURES OF *IGF-I* GENE DEFICIENCY

The patient described by Woods and co-workers had clear biochemical evidence of GH resistance, with undetectable circulating IGF-I levels, which did not increase after 5 days of GH administration. GH response to insulin-induced hypoglycemia was exaggerated (peak 61 ng mL^{-1}: 122 mU L^{-1}), and an overnight GH profile demonstrated extremely high peaks (maximum 342 mU L^{-1}, 171 ng mL^{-1}) with a failure of GH levels to suppress completely (as is normally seen)

between the troughs. As would be expected, GHBP levels were normal. Interestingly, IGFBP-3 levels were also normal (3.3 mg dL^{-1}, normal for age 2.3–5.2), and ALS levels mildly elevated, suggesting that generation of IGFBP-3 and ALS is a direct effect of GH. It is arguable that IGFBP-3 levels should have been more elevated, given the high GH levels. Possibly, lack of IGF-I, and the consequent lack of ternary complex formation reduced the stability of IGFBP-3 in the circulation to a greater extent than ALS. IGF-II levels were mildly elevated in this patient (1430 ng mL^{-1}, compared with 1010 ng mL^{-1} in a normal serum pool): possibly IGF-II, signaling through the IGF-I receptor (albeit with reduced affinity when compared with IGF-I) may account for some of the growth achieved by this patient despite a profound absence of circulating or locally produced IGF-I.

STAT–5b gene deficiency

The first case of a defect in GHR signaling, a homozygous STAT 5b gene deficiency, has recently been described.[8] As discussed above, STAT 5b is a key signaling molecule in GHR signaling, becoming activated after binding of JAK2 to the GHR. As GH also activates a number of other signaling cascades, it has been unclear how critical the JAK-STAT pathway is for GH function. Knockout of the STAT 5b gene is the mouse produces a 30 percent reduction in size of the male, but not the female, mouse.[78] The affected female patient described by Kofoed and colleagues had a homozygous missense mutation of STAT 5b (A630P) within the critical src homology 2 (SH2) domain of STAT 5b, necessary for docking of STATs to activated receptors. The phenotype of this 16.5-year-old female is remarkable for its similarity with severe GHR deficiency, providing strong evidence that the effects of GH on growth and IGFs in man, at least, are predominantly, if not exclusively, mediated through STAT 5b signaling. She was mildly growth retarded at birth, with a birth weight of 1.4 kg at 33 weeks (−2.0 SD). Birth length was not known. Postnatally, she exhibited profound postnatal growth failure, with a height of 117.8 cm (−7.5 SD) at 16.5 years of age. Clinical examination revealed a prominent forehead, saddle nose, and high-pitched voice. At the time of diagnosis (16.5 years), she was in early puberty, indicating delay in pubertal onset. GH secretion was exaggerated after insulin-induced hypoglycemia (peak 53.8 ng mL^{-1} or 107.2 U L^{-1}), and both IGF-I and IGBP-3 levels were very low (IGF-I: 38 ng mL^{-1}, IGFBP-3 levels: 874 ng mL^{-1}), and failed to increase after exogenous GH administration. GHBP levels were normal.

In addition to the above findings, all typical of classical GHIS, this patient also has evidence of immunodeficiency, not typical of either classical GHIS or IGF-I gene deficiency. After progressive respiratory problems during childhood lymphoid interstitial pneumonia, and *Pneumocystis carinii* lung infection were identified at the age of 10 years, suggesting problems with cell-mediated immunity. This finding points to an important role for STAT 5b in T-cell functioning, not altogether surprising given the fact that STAT 5b is activated in the downstream signaling pathway of many cytokines.[79,80]

A second patient with a molecular defect in the STAT 5b gene has now been identified.[9] This patient, a 16-year-old female of Turkish origin, has a very similar clinical phenotype to the first reported individual, with severe growth retardation (−7.8 SD), very low IGF-I and IGFBP-3 levels unresponsive to GH, and immune dysfunction (hypergammaglobulinemia and pulmonary fibrosis). Sequencing of the STAT 5b gene demonstrated a homozygous insertion of a single nucleotide in exon 10 (which encodes part of the DNA binding domain), causing a frameshift and hence early protein truncation 15 amino acids downstream from the insertion site.

Acid labile subunit deficiency

As discussed above, ALS is a GH-dependent glycoprotein which stabilizes the IGF–IGFBP-3 complex, forming the so-called 'ternary' complex.[81] This 150 kDa complex reduces the passage of IGF-I to the extravascular compartment, and extends its half-life. Inactivation of the ALS gene in the mouse has a profound effect on IGF-I levels (66 percent reduction), IGFBP-3 levels (88 percent reduction), yet only a minor effect on growth (13 percent reduction).[82] In 2004, the first case of human ALS gene deficiency was described by Domené and co-workers.[6] This case demonstrates remarkable similarity to the mouse ALS knockout, with relatively mild growth failure despite profound reductions in IGFs and ALS. The patient, an Argentinian male, was mildly growth retarded when first investigated at 14.6 years of age (height 145.2 cm, height SDS −2.05 by Argentinian standards), weight 35.9 kg (−2.34 SDS). He was noted to have mild micrognathia and truncal obesity, and puberty was delayed (G1, PH1, testes 3 mL bilaterally). By 19 years of age, he had completed puberty spontaneously, and height had increased to 166.4 cm (−0.94 SDS).[83] Size at birth was not known, but at one week of age (when the patient was adopted) weight was 2.5 kg and length 47 cm. Data on the height of biologic parents, unfortunately, were unavailable. Circulating IGF-I (31 ng mL^{-1}, 5.3 SD below the mean for age) and IGFBP-3 (220 ng mL^{-1}; 9.7 SD below the mean for age) were markedly reduced. ALS was undetectable. GH responses to provocative testing were normal (peak 31 ng mL^{-1}), but spontaneous nocturnal GH secretion was elevated. Oral glucose tolerance testing revealed an increase in basal and peak insulin levels, yet normal glucose levels, suggesting insulin resistance. Six months of GH therapy had no effect on IGF-I, IGFBP-3, ALS or insulin levels. Sequencing of the ALS gene demonstrated a homozygous frameshift mutation (1338delG) which predicts a mutant ALS protein retaining only seven amino-terminal residues of mature ALS, and completely lacking the IGFBP-3 binding domain, likely a functional null mutation.

One of the most interesting questions raised by this case is the reason why his growth is apparently so unaffected (final height SDS of −0.94, by Argentinian standards) with a reduction in circulating IGFs compatible with severe GHIS or GH deficiency. With no data on parental heights available, it is difficult to assess whether this patient had any reduction in final height over expected at all. The elevated GH secretion suggests that the pituitary hypothalamic feedback loop was intact and responded to low levels of IGF-I although the GH elevations (in the order of two-fold) are not as high as are typically seen in severe GHRD or IGF gene deficiency. There are two main theories to explain this finding. Firstly, it is possible that free IGFs may be relatively preserved in ALS deficiency, due to the absence of ternary complex formation, and these free IGFs may be more important than bound IGF for growth. Secondly, it may be that locally produced IGFs, theoretically unaffected in ALS deficiency, are able to compensate for the loss of circulating IGF-I, possibly driven by the elevation in GH secretion. In the ALS knockout mice, free IGFs have been reported to be normal, lending support to the first theory.[84] However, preliminary data on the patient described by Domené and co-workers indicate that free IGF-I levels are low, suggesting that locally produced IGF-I may be the explanation for the near-normal height of their patient.[83]

A second case of ALS deficiency has recently been reported.[7] The patient, a 14-year-old male of Turkish origin, demonstrated mild short stature (height 144.6 cm at 14 years, −2.12 SD), an exaggerated GH response to stimulation, and very low levels of IGF-I (25 ng mL^{-1}; normal range, 242–660) and IGFBP-3 (322 ng mL^{-1}; normal range, 2500–4800) which did not increase upon GH administration. ALS was undetectable in serum either by immunoassay or immunoblot. Sequencing of the ALS gene of this patient is currently under way.

'PARTIAL' GROWTH HORMONE INSENSITIVITY

Classical GHIS is typically associated with severe homozygous mutations of the gene involved, leading to almost complete lack to gene effect, and a severe phenotype. However, it became apparent when studying the European GHIS cohort, a heterogeneous group of patients identified using a scoring system, that some individuals had a milder phenotype, with less severe short stature, a more normal facial appearance, and less severe reductions in IGF levels.[21,85] GHR mutations have also been identified in such 'atypical' GHIS patients, in one subject acting in a dominant negative manner,[35] and in another family affecting GHR splicing.[86] These, and other, findings have raised the question of whether 'partial' GH resistance, caused by mild defects in the GHR, could be the cause of the short stature in patients who have apparently normal GH secretion, patients usually labeled as 'idiopathic' short stature (ISS). This hypothesis is supported by the finding that children with ISS have lower IGF-I and GHBP levels than normal statured controls of the same age.[87] Furthermore, those 20 percent of ISS patients with GHBP levels more than 2 SD below the mean have lower IGF-I levels, and higher mean GH levels.[88] Goddard and co-workers analysed the GH receptor gene in 100 patients with ISS, and identified eight patients with GH receptor mutations, all but one of which were heterozygous.[89,90] Subsequent studies of the GHR gene in ISS have found heterozygous GHR mutations in 1/17,[91] 1/26,[92] and 1/14[93] subjects, suggesting an overall prevalence of heterozygous GHR mutations in ISS of around 5 percent. However, in some cases, family members carrying the same heterozygous GHR mutation as the affected patient were not short, suggesting that the mutation identified may not have been sufficient, in and of itself, to cause short stature. Possibly, heterozygous GH receptor mutations may be deleterious to growth only in certain genetic backgrounds, perhaps when GH receptor expression level is low, or GH signaling is suboptimal. Carriers of the E180S mutation, for example, are shorter than non-carriers by an average of 0.75 SD.[94] Interestingly, a recently described common polymorphism in the GHR gene, which determines whether exon 3 of the GHR gene is included in the GHR transcript, has been shown to predict response to GH therapy in patient with ISS.[32,95]

Partial GH resistance in ISS could also be mediated by postreceptor deficits, for example a mild defect in one of the key GH signaling molecules such as STAT 5b. It could be argued that this has already been demonstrated in the one described case of ALS deficiency, although it remains to be seen whether there is a true growth deficiency phenotype in this condition. Interestingly, Salerno and co-workers found reduced GH-induced protein tyrosine phosphorylation in the peripheral blood mononuclear cells in 2/14 patients with ISS.[93] These patients differed from the other 12 ISS patients in that they failed to significantly increase IGF-I levels after GH administration.

GROWTH HORMONE INSENSITIVITY WITH NORMAL LEVELS OF IGF-I: DEFECTS BEYOND THE *IGF-I* GENE

The cases discussed above all focus on individuals with normal to elevated GH secretion, yet low levels of IGF-I, the typical biochemical pattern of GH insensitivity. However, defects in the GH–IGF pathway distal to the IGF-I gene can be thought of as a form of GH insensitivity, despite the fact that they may be associated with normal, or even elevated, IGF-I levels. As illustrated in Fig. 29.1, IGF-I mediates its effects through the IGF-I receptor (also known as the type 1 IGF receptor). The fundamental growth promoting role of this receptor is illustrated by the severe prenatal growth retardation (birth weight 45 percent of normal) seen in mice with homozygous disruption of the IGF-I receptor gene.[75,76] IGF-I receptor nullizygotes also died within the first few days of life, raising the possibility that complete loss of IGF-I receptor function in man may also be incompatible with postnatal survival. To date, no human subject with complete loss of IGF-I receptor function has been described. However, in 2003, two patients with IGF-I receptor gene mutations predicted to partially disrupt IGF-I receptor function were reported by the same group.[96] Both individuals were small for gestational age at birth and demonstrated postnatal growth deficiency. However, biochemical evidence of GH resistance was clearly present only in one of the two cases reported. This patient, a female, was a compound heterozygote for two different missense mutations in exon 2 of the IGF-I receptor gene, which encodes the hormone binding extracellular domain, and functional studies of the patient's fibroblasts demonstrated reduced binding of IGF-I and reduced phosphorylation of the IGF-I receptor by IGF-I, suggesting the mutations reduced the affinity of the receptor for IGF-I without completely abolishing IGF-I signaling. Her birth weight was 1.4 kg (−3.5 SD) and adult height was 134.1 cm (−4.8 SD). GH levels were elevated both on provocative testing and overnight sampling, and at 12 years of age, baseline IGF-I levels were over twice the upper limit of the normal range, IGFBP-3 levels were high normal, and ALS levels were almost twice the upper limit of normal. High dose (0.375 mg kg^{-1} week^{-1}) GH therapy produced only a mild acceleration of the growth rate, despite increasing her IGF-I levels further to over three times the upper limit of normal. The patient also demonstrated some behavioral abnormalities, and had a wide discrepancy between verbal and performance IQ, suggesting a non-verbal learning disorder. Puberty was not delayed, and there was no hearing deficit, as seen in patients with IGF-I defects.

The second patient, a boy, was found to have a heterozygous nonsense mutation in exon 2 of the IGF-I receptor gene, predicting one IGF-I receptor allele to be severely truncated and non-functional receptor. No mutation was identified in the other IGF-I receptor allele. Patient fibroblast studies demonstrated reduced IGF-I receptor number, and the authors suggest that IGF-I receptor haploinsufficiency in this case caused the clinical phenotype. The patient demonstrated growth retardation and microcephaly at birth (weight 2 kg, −3.5 SD; length 40 cm, −5.8 SD; head circumference 31 cm, −4.6 SD). Despite some postnatal catch-up he remained short (−2.6 SD) at 5.3 years. He had mild dysmorphic features, including a receding hairline, bushy eyebrows, a broad nasal bridge, a long philtrum, thin upper lip, short fingers, and clinodactyly, and there was mild delay in motor and verbal milestones. However, biochemical evidence of GH or IGF-I resistance was limited. Peak GH levels in response to insulin (5.7 ng dL^{-1}) and arginine (6.0 ng dL^{-1}) were low, and response to GHRH was within normal limits at 21.1 ng dL^{-1}. Serum IGF-I levels ranged from +1.1 to +2.3 SD above the mean for age, whereas IGFBP-3 levels were within normal limits. Given the lack of biochemical evidence for GH resistance and/or IGF-I resistance in this patient, it is also possible that his growth deficiency may have another, as yet undetermined cause. The subject's mother was also heterozygous for this mutation, and although she was short (adult height, −2.4 SD) with a history of low birth weight (birth weight, -2.4 SD), her birth length was within normal limits (-1.6 SD). Of note, heterozygous IGF-I receptor knockout mice did not exhibit a discernible phenotype.[75,76]

A number of cases of IGF-I receptor gene haploinsufficiency associated with structural defects of chromosome 15 (where the IGF-I receptor gene is located) have been reported in the literature. These patients typically present with pre- and postnatal growth retardation, dysmorphic features, and developmental delay, providing some support to the hypothesis that heterozygous IGF-I receptor defects may be associated with a growth deficiency phenotype in man. However, as these cases all involved losses of genes contiguous to the IGF-I receptor gene it is difficult to ascertain the contribution of the loss of IGF receptor function to the clinical phenotype.[97,98] Elevations in GH, IGF-I, and IGFBP-3 levels have been reported in some, but not all, cases, and fibroblast studies demonstrated a reduction in IGF-I receptor number by around 50 percent in those patients in whom fibroblasts were studied. However, despite the quantitative deficiency of IGF-I receptor number, defects in IGF-I receptor signaling have not been clearly demonstrated.

CONCLUSION

From the original discovery of defects in the GH receptor gene as a cause of GH insensitivity 16 years ago, recent years have seen rapid advances in our understanding of the cellular pathways linking the activation of the GH receptor by GH to the initiation of growth. Defects in an expanding list of genes encoding key molecules in this pathway have been found to be associated with a variety of growth deficiency phenotypes, which share a common biochemical finding of GH resistance. Furthermore, it is becoming increasingly apparent that insensitivity to GH may not only be caused by defects that impair the ability of GH to generate IGF-I, or 'primary IGF-I deficiency',[99] but also by insensitivity to IGF-I. One of the major challenges that now faces the pediatric endocrinologist is to apply these findings in the clinical setting, in order to improve the diagnosis and management of the child presenting in the growth clinic with unexplained, or 'idiopathic' short stature.

KEY LEARNING POINTS

- The GH receptor is found ubiquitously in the human body. Signal transduction is mediated through at least three pathways.
- GH insensitivity syndrome is rare, and the majority of patients originate from inbred cohorts or consanguineous unions.
- Defects in the growth hormone receptor are considered mainly to be the causes of growth hormone insensitivity syndrome.

- A small number of cases of primary growth hormone insensitivity are associated with genes other than the growth hormone receptor.
- Classical growth hormone insensitivity syndrome is associated with severe homozygous mutations in the gene involved, but there is a heterogeneous group of patients who have a milder phenotype and less severe reduction in IGF-I levels.
- Defects in the GH–IGF-I pathway distal to the IGF-I gene can be considered as a form of GH insensitivity.

REFERENCES

● = Seminal primary article

◆ = Key review paper

● 1 Laron Z, Pertzelan A, Mannheimer S. Genetic pituitary dwarfism with high serum concentration of growth hormone – a new inborn error of metabolism? *Isr J Med Sci* 1966; **2**: 152–5.

● 2 Godowski PJ, *et al.* Characterization of the human growth hormone receptor gene and demonstration of a partial gene deletion in two patients with Laron-type dwarfism. *Proc Natl Acad Sci USA* 1989; **86**: 8083–7.

3 Laron Z, Lilos P, Klinger B. Growth curves for Laron syndrome. *Arch Dis Child* 1993; **68**: 768–70.

● 4 Woods KA, Camacho-Hubner C, Savage MO, Clark AJ. Intrauterine growth retardation and postnatal growth failure associated with deletion of the insulin-like growth factor I gene. *N Engl J Med* 1996; **335**: 1363–7.

5 Denley A, *et al.* Structural and functional characteristics of the Val44Met IGF-I missense mutation: correlation with effects on growth and development. *Mol Endocrinol* 2005; **19**: 711–21.

● 6 Domene HM, *et al.* Deficiency of the circulating insulin-like growth factor system associated with inactivation of the acid-labile subunit gene. *N Eng J Med* 2004; **350**: 570–7.

● 7 Hwa V, *et al.* Idiopathic short stature and growth hormone insensitivity (GHI) associated with an absence of acid labile subunit (ALS) [Abstract]. The Endocrine Society Annual Meeting, 2005.

● 8 Kofoed EM, *et al.* Growth hormone insensitivity associated with a STAT5b mutation. *N Engl J Med* 2003; **349**: 1139–47.

9 Hwa V, *et al.* Stat 5b mutations associated with growth hormone insensitivity [Abstract]. The Endocrine Society Annual Meeting, 2005.

10 Barton DE, Foellmer BE, Wood WI, Francke U. Chromosome mapping of the growth hormone receptor gene in man and mouse. *Cytogenet Cell Genet* 1989; **50**: 137–41.

● 11 Leung DW, *et al.* Growth hormone receptor and serum binding protein: purification, cloning and expression. *Nature* 1987; **330**: 537–43.

12 Kelly PA, Djiane J, Postel-Vinay MC, Edery M. The prolactin/growth hormone receptor family. *Endocr Rev* 1991; **12**: 235–51.

13 Trivedi B, Daughaday WH. Release of growth hormone binding protein from IM-9 lymphocytes by endopeptidase is dependent on sulfhydryl group inactivation. *Endocrinology* 1988; **123**: 2201–6.

14 Conte F, *et al.* Identification of a region critical for proteolysis of the human growth hormone receptor. *Biochem Biophys Res Commun* 2002; **290**: 851–7.

15 Herrington J, Carter-Su C. Signaling pathways activated by the growth hormone receptor. *Trends Endocrinol Metab* 2001; **12**: 252–7.

16 Carter-Su C, Rui L, Herrington J. Role of the tyrosine kinase JAK2 in signal transduction by growth hormone. *Pediatr Nephrol* 2000; **14**: 550–7.

17 Herrington J, Smit LS, Schwartz J, Carter-Su C. The role of STAT proteins in growth hormone signaling. *Oncogene* 2000; **19**: 2585–97.

18 Frank SJ. Growth hormone signalling and its regulation: preventing too much of a good thing. *Growth Horm IGF Res* 2001; **11**: 201–12.

19 Woelfle J, Billiard J, Rotwein P. Acute control of insulin-like growth factor-I gene transcription by growth hormone through Stat5b. *J Biol Chem* 2003; **278**: 22696–702.

20 Rosenfeld RG, Rosenbloom AL, Guevara-Aguirre J. Growth hormone (GH) insensitivity due to primary GH receptor deficiency. *Endocr Rev* 1994; **15**: 369–90.

21 Woods KA, *et al.* Phenotype: genotype relationships in growth hormone insensitivity syndrome. *J Clin Endocrinol Metab* 1997; **82**: 3529–35.

22 Laron Z. Laron syndrome (primary growth hormone resistance or insensitivity): the personal experience 1958–2003. *J Clin Endocrinol Metab* 2004; **89**: 1031–44.

23 Rosenbloom AL, Guevara AJ, Rosenfeld RG, Fielder PJ. The little women of Loja–growth hormone-receptor deficiency in an inbred population of southern Ecuador. *N Engl J Med* 1990; **323**: 1367–74.

24 Guevara-Aguirre J, Rosenbloom AL, Fielder PJ, Diamond FB Jr, Rosenfeld RG. Growth hormone receptor deficiency in Ecuador: clinical and biochemical phenotype in two populations. *J Clin Endocrinol Metab* 1993; **76**: 417–23.

25 Rosenbloom AL, Guevara-Aguirre J, Rosenfeld RG, Francke U. Growth hormone receptor deficiency in Ecuador. *J Clin Endocrinol Metab* 1999; **84**: 4436–43.

26 Berg MA, *et al.* Receptor mutations and haplotypes in growth hormone receptor deficiency: a global survey and identification of the Ecuadorean E180splice mutation in an oriental Jewish patient. *Acta Paediatr Suppl* 1994; **399**: 112–4.

27 Savage MO, *et al.* Clinical features and endocrine status in patients with growth hormone insensitivity (Laron syndrome). *J Clin Endocrinol Metab* 1993; **77**: 1465–71.

28 Laron Z, Pertzelan A, Karp M, Kowadlo-Silbergeld A, Daughaday WH. Administration of growth hormone to patients with familial dwarfism with high plasma immunoreactive growth hormone: measurement of sulfation factor, metabolic and linear growth responses. *J Clin Endocrinol Metab* 1971; **33**: 332–42.

29 van den Brande JL, *et al.* Primary somatomedin deficiency. Case report. *Arch Dis Child* 1974; **49**: 297–304.

30 Eshet R, Laron Z, Pertzelan A, Arnon R, Dintzman M. Defect of human growth hormone receptors in the liver of two patients with Laron-type dwarfism. *Isr J Med Sci* 1984; **20**: 8–11.

31 Meacham LR, *et al.* Characterization of a noncontiguous gene deletion of the growth hormone receptor in Laron's syndrome. *J Clin Endocrinol Metab* 1993; **77**: 1379–83.

32 Dos Santos C, *et al.* A common polymorphism of the growth hormone receptor is associated with increased responsiveness to growth hormone. *Nat Genet* 2004; **36**: 720–4.

33 Amselem S, *et al.* Laron dwarfism and mutations of the growth hormone-receptor gene. *N Engl J Med* 1989; **321**: 989–95.

34 Edery M, *et al.* Lack of hormone binding in COS-7 cells expressing a mutated growth hormone receptor found in Laron dwarfism. *J Clin Invest* 1993; **91**: 838–44.

35 Ayling RM, *et al.* A dominant-negative mutation of the growth hormone receptor causes familial short stature. *Nat Genet* 1997; **16**: 13–14.

36 Iida K, *et al.* Growth hormone (GH) insensitivity syndrome with high serum GH-binding protein levels caused by a heterozygous splice site mutation of the GH receptor gene producing a lack of intracellular domain. *J Clin Endocrinol Metab* 1998; **83**: 531–7.

37 Milward A, *et al.* Growth hormone (GH) insensitivity syndrome due to a GH receptor truncated after Box1, resulting in isolated failure of STAT 5 signal transduction. *J Clin Endocrinol Metab* 2004; **89**: 1259–66.

38 Gastier JM, Berg MA, Vesterhus P, Reiter EO, Francke U. Diverse deletions in the growth hormone receptor gene cause growth hormone insensitivity syndrome. *Hum Mutat* 2000; **16**: 323–33.

39 Kaji H, *et al.* Novel compound heterozygous mutations of growth hormone (GH) receptor gene in a patient with GH insensitivity syndrome. *J Clin Endocrinol Metab* 1997; **82**: 3705–9.

40 Tiulpakov A, *et al.* A novel C-terminal growth hormone receptor (GHR) mutation results in impaired GHR-STAT5 but normal STAT-3 signaling. *J Clin Endocrinol Metab* 2005; **90**: 542–7.

41 Kou K, Lajara R, Rotwein P. Amino acid substitutions in the intracellular part of the growth hormone receptor in a patient with the Laron syndrome. *J Clin Endocrinol Metab* 1993; **76**: 54–9.

42 Laron Z. Laron-type dwarfism (hereditary somatomedin deficiency): a review. *Ergeb Inn Med Kinderheilkd* 1984; **51**: 117–50.

43 Rosenbloom AL, Savage MO, Blum WF, Guevara-Aguirre J, Rosenfeld RG. Clinical and biochemical characteristics of growth hormone receptor deficiency (Laron syndrome). *Acta Paediatr Suppl* 1992; **383**: 121–4.

44 Laron Z, Sarel R, Pertzelan A. Puberty in Laron type dwarfism. *Eur J Pediatr* 1980; **134**: 79–83.

45 Schaefer GB, *et al*. Facial morphometry of Ecuadorian patients with growth hormone receptor deficiency/Laron syndrome. *J Med Genet* 1994; **31**: 635–9.

46 Sarnat H, Kaplan I, Pertzelan A, Laron Z. Comparison of dental findings in patients with isolated growth hormone deficiency treated with human growth hormone (hGH) and in untreated patients with Laron-type dwarfism. *Oral Surg Oral Med Oral Pathol* 1988; **66**: 581–6.

47 Kornreich L, Horev G, Schwarz M, Karmazyn B, Laron Z. Craniofacial and brain abnormalities in Laron syndrome (primary growth hormone insensitivity). *Eur J Endocrinol* 2002; **146**: 499–503.

48 Guevara-Aguirre J, Rosenbloom AL. In: *Lessons from Laron Syndrome 1966–1992*. Laron Z, Parks JS, eds. Basel: Karger, 1993: 61–4.

49 Kranzler JH, Rosenbloom AL, Martinez V, Guevara-Aguirre J. Normal intelligence with severe insulin-like growth factor I deficiency due to growth hormone receptor deficiency: a controlled study in a genetically homogeneous population. *J Clin Endocrinol Metab* 1998; **83**: 1953–8.

50 Brat O, Ziv I, Klinger B, Avraham M, Laron Z. Muscle force and endurance in untreated and human growth hormone or insulin-like growth factor-I-treated patients with growth hormone deficiency or Laron syndrome. *Horm Res* 1997; **47**: 45–8.

51 Kornreich L, Horev G, Schwarz M, Karmazyn B, Laron Z. Laron syndrome abnormalities: spinal stenosis, os odontoideum, degenerative changes of the atlanto-odontoid joint, and small oropharynx. *AJNR Am J Neuroradiol* 2002; **23**: 625–31.

52 Abramovici A, Josefsberg Z, Mimouni M, Liban E, Laron Z. Histopathological features of the skin in hypopituitarism and Laron-type dwarfism. *Isr J Med Sci* 1983; **19**: 515–9.

53 Laron Z, Klinger B. Body fat in Laron syndrome patients: effect of insulin-like growth factor I treatment. *Horm Res* 1993; **40**: 16–22.

54 Laron Z, Klinger B. IGF-I treatment of adult patients with Laron syndrome: preliminary results. *Clin Endocrinol (Oxf)* 1994; **41**: 631–8.

55 Benbassat CA, Eshed V, Kamjin M, Laron Z. Are adult patients with Laron syndrome osteopenic? A comparison between dual-energy X-ray absorptiometry and volumetric bone densities. *J Clin Endocrinol Metab* 2003; **88**: 4586–9.

56 Laron Z, Avitzur Y, Klinger B. Carbohydrate metabolism in primary growth hormone resistance (Laron syndrome) before and during insulin-like growth factor-I treatment. *Metabolism* 1995; **44**: 113–8.

57 Feinberg MS, Scheinowitz M, Laron Z. Echocardiographic dimensions and function in adults with primary growth hormone resistance (Laron syndrome). *Am J Cardiol* 2000; **85**: 209–13.

58 Ben Dov I, Gaides M, Scheinowitz M, Wagner R, Laron Z. Reduced exercise capacity in untreated adults with primary growth hormone resistance (Laron syndrome). *Clin Endocrinol (Oxf)* 2003; **59**: 763–7.

59 Vaccarello MA, *et al*. Hormonal and metabolic effects and pharmacokinetics of recombinant insulin-like growth factor-I in growth hormone receptor deficiency/Laron syndrome. *J Clin Endocrinol Metab* 1993; **77**: 273–80.

60 Laron Z, Pertzelan A, Karp M. Pituitary dwarfism with high serum levels of growth hormone. *Isr J Med Sci* 1968; **4**: 883–94.

61 Cotterill AM, Holly JM, Snodgrass GA, Savage MO. Regulation of growth hormone secretion in patients with growth hormone insensitivity. *Acta Paediatr Scand Suppl* 1991; **377**: 92–5.

62 Carlsson LM, Rowland AM, Clark RG, Gesundheit N, Wong WL. Ligand-mediated immunofunctional assay for quantitation of growth hormone-binding protein in human blood. *J Clin Endocrinol Metab* 1991; **73**: 1216–23.

● 63 Baumann G, Shaw MA, Winter RJ. Absence of the plasma growth hormone-binding protein in Laron-type dwarfism. *J Clin Endocrinol Metab* 1987; **65**: 814–6.

● 64 Daughaday WH, Trivedi B. Absence of serum growth hormone binding protein in patients with growth hormone receptor deficiency (Laron dwarfism). *Proc Natl Acad Sci USA* 1987; **84**: 4636–40.

65 Duquesnoy P, Sobrier ML, Amselem S, Goossens M. Defective membrane expression of human growth hormone (GH) receptor causes Laron-type GH insensitivity syndrome. *Proc Natl Acad Sci USA* 1991; **88**: 10272–6.

66 Duquesnoy P, *et al*. A single amino acid substitution in the exoplasmic domain of the human growth hormone (GH) receptor confers familial GH resistance (Laron syndrome) with positive GH-binding activity by abolishing receptor homodimerization. *EMBO J* 1994; **13**: 1386–95.

67 Woods KA, Fraser NC, Postel-Vinay MC, *et al*. A homozygous splice site mutation affecting the intracellular domain of the growth hormone (GH) receptor resulting in Laron syndrome with elevated GH-binding protein. *J Clin Endocrinol Metab* 1996; **81**: 1686–90.

68 Silbergeld A, *et al*. Intronic mutation in the growth hormone (GH) receptor gene from a girl with Laron syndrome and extremely high serum GH binding protein: extended phenotypic study in a very large pedigree. *J Pediatr Endocrinol Metab* 1997; **10**: 265–74.

69 Daughaday WH, Laron Z, Pertzelan A, Heins JN. Defective sulfation factor generation: a possible etiological link in dwarfism. *Trans Assoc Am Physicians* 1969; **82**: 129–40.

70 Lamson G, Giudice LC, Rosenfeld RG. Insulin-like growth factor binding proteins: structural and molecular relationships. *Growth Factors* 1991; **5**: 19–28.

71 Burren CP, *et al*. Serum levels of insulin-like growth factor binding proteins in Ecuadorean children with growth hormone insensitivity. *Acta Paediatr Suppl* 1999; **88**: 185–91.

● 72 Guevara-Aguirre J, *et al*. A randomized, double blind, placebo-controlled trial on safety and efficacy of recombinant human insulin-like growth factor-I in children with growth hormone receptor deficiency. *J Clin Endocrinol Metab* 1995; **80**: 1393–8.

73 Guevara-Aguirre J, *et al*. Two-year treatment of growth hormone (GH) receptor deficiency with recombinant

insulin-like growth factor I in 22 children: comparison of two dosage levels and to GH-treated GH deficiency. *J Clin Endocrinol Metab* 1997; **82**: 629–33.

74   Gargosky SE, *et al*. The composition and distribution of insulin-like growth factors (IGFs) and IGF-binding proteins (IGFBPs) in the serum of growth hormone receptor-deficient patients: effects of IGF-I therapy on IGFBP-3. *J Clin Endocrinol Metab* 1993; **77**: 1683–9.

75   Baker J, Liu JP, Robertson EJ, Efstratiadis A. Role of insulin-like growth factors in embryonic and postnatal growth. *Cell* 1993; **75**: 73–82.

76   Liu JP, Baker J, Perkins AS, *et al*. Mice carrying null mutations of the genes encoding insulin-like growth factor I (Igf-1) and type 1 IGF receptor (Igf1r). *Cell* 1993; **75**: 59–72.

77   Woods KA, *et al*. Effects of insulin-like growth factor I (IGF-I) therapy on body composition and insulin resistance in IGF-I gene deletion. *J Clin Endocrinol Metab* 2000; **85**: 1407–11.

78   Udy GB, *et al*. Requirement of STAT5b for sexual dimorphism of body growth rates and liver gene expression. *Proc Natl Acad Sci USA* 1997; **94**: 7239–44.

79   Moriggl R, Sexl V, Piekorz R, *et al*. Stat5 activation is uniquely associated with cytokine signaling in peripheral T cells. *Immunity* 1999; **11**: 225–30.

80   Welte T, *et al*. STAT5 interaction with the T cell receptor complex and stimulation of T cell proliferation. *Science* 1999; **283**: 222–5.

81   Baxter RC. Circulating levels and molecular distribution of the acid-labile (alpha) subunit of the high molecular weight insulin-like growth factor-binding protein complex. *J Clin Endocrinol Metab* 1990; **70**: 1347–53.

82   Ueki I, *et al*. Inactivation of the acid labile subunit gene in mice results in mild retardation of postnatal growth despite profound disruptions in the circulating insulin-like growth factor system. *Proc Natl Acad Sci USA* 2000; **97**: 6868–73.

83   Domene HM, Martinez AS, Jasper H. Circulating IGF-I deficiency and inactivation of the acid-labile subunit gene [Letter]. *New Engl J Med* 2004; **350**: 18.

84   Yakar S, *et al*. Circulating levels of IGF-I directly regulate bone growth and density. *J Clin Invest* 2002; **110**: 771–81.

85   Burren CP, *et al*. Clinical and endocrine characteristics in atypical and classical growth hormone insensitivity syndrome. *Horm Res* 2001; **55**: 125–30.

86   Metherell LA, *et al*. Pseudoexon activation as a novel mechanism for disease resulting in atypical growth-hormone insensitivity. *Am J Hum Genet* 2001; **69**: 641–6.

87   Carlsson LM, Attie KM, Compton PG, *et al*. Reduced concentration of serum growth hormone-binding protein in children with idiopathic short stature. National Cooperative Growth Study. *J Clin Endocrinol Metab* 1994; **78**: 1325–30.

88   Attie KM, Carlsson LM, Rundle AC, Sherman BM. Evidence for partial growth hormone insensitivity among patients with idiopathic short stature. The National Cooperative Growth Study. *J Pediatr* 1995; **127**: 244–50.

89   Goddard AD, *et al*. Mutations of the growth hormone receptor in children with idiopathic short stature. The Growth Hormone Insensitivity Study Group. *N Engl J Med* 1995; **333**: 1093–8.

90   Goddard AD, *et al*. Partial growth-hormone insensitivity: the role of growth-hormone receptor mutations in idiopathic short stature. *J Pediatr* 1997; **131**: S51–5.

91   Sanchez JE, Perera E, Baumbach L, Cleveland WW. Growth hormone receptor mutations in children with idiopathic short stature. *J Clin Endocrinol Metab* 1998; **83**: 4079–83.

92   Sjoberg M, *et al*. Study of GH sensitivity in chilean patients with idiopathic short stature. *J Clin Endocrinol Metab* 2001; **86**: 4375–81.

93   Salerno M, *et al*. Abnormal GH receptor signaling in children with idiopathic short stature. *J Clin Endocrinol Metab* 2001; **86**: 3882–8.

94   Woods KA, Buckway CK, Pratt KL, *et al*. Growth hormone (GH) receptor gene haploinsufficiency in Ecuador is associated with both impaired growth and reduced GH binding protein levels [Abstract]. The Endocrine Society Annual Meeting, 2004.

95   Pantel J, *et al*. Heterozygous nonsense mutation in exon 3 of the growth hormone receptor (GHR) in severe GH insensitivity (Laron syndrome) and the issue of the origin and function of the GHRd3 isoform. *J Clin Endocrinol Metab* 2003; **88**: 1705–10.

96   Abuzzahab MJ, *et al*. IGF-I receptor mutations resulting in intrauterine and postnatal growth retardation. *N Engl J Med* 2003; **349**: 2211–22.

97   Hammer E, *et al*. Mono-allelic expression of the IGF-I receptor does not affect IGF responses in human fibroblasts. *Eur J Endocrinol* 2004; **151**: 521–9.

98   De Lacerda L, *et al*. In vitro and in vivo responses to short-term recombinant human insulin-like growth factor-1 (IGF-I) in a severely growth-retarded girl with ring chromosome 15 and deletion of a single allele for the type 1 IGF receptor gene. *Clin Endocrinol (Oxf)* 1999; **51**: 541–50.

99   Rosenfeld RG, Hwa V. New molecular mechanisms of GH resistance. *Eur J Endocrinol* 2004; **151(Suppl 1)**: S11–5.

30

Growth and thyroid disorders

ANNETTE GRÜTERS

PATHOPHYSIOLOGY

In the process of endochondral bone formation, which results in longitudinal growth, the chondrocytes of the growth plate differentiate to hypertrophic chondrocytes. Subsequently the newly formed cartilage is invaded by blood vessels and bone cell precursors, which remodel the hypertrophic zone cartilage into bone.[1] The result is that new bone tissue is progressively created at the bottom of the growth plate, resulting in bone elongation. Longitudinal bone growth is dependent on endocrine signals, including growth hormone, insulin-like growth factor I (IGF-I), glucocorticoid, thyroid hormone, estrogen, androgen, vitamin D, and leptin. Some of these hormones regulate the growth plate directly, e.g., by influencing the production and secretion of paracrine peptides like Indian hedgehog (Ihh) and parathyroid hormone-related protein (PTHrP), but at the same time may also influence the secretion of other endocrine signals of the regulatory network.[2] It is well known from animal studies and human thyroid disorders that thyroid hormones are necessary for normal skeletal growth and maturation. Hypothyroidism slows longitudinal bone growth and endochondral ossification, while it is accelerated by hyperthyroidism.

Some of the skeletal effects of thyroid hormones appear to be related to a direct effect on the growth plate. In cell culture, thyroid hormones stimulate hypertrophic differentiation of the chondrocytes.[3] In hypothyroid animals, there is a decrease in the heights of the proliferative and hypertrophic zones, and a decrease in chondrocyte hypertrophy as well as in vascularization. The direct action of thyroid hormones at the growth plate is supported by the fact that the growth plate chondrocytes express thyroid hormone receptor (TR) isoforms TR-α1, α2, and β1.[4] However, the targeted deletion of TR-β isoforms in mice has little effect on growth. In humans, so far, the only published family with a homozygous deletion of TR-β showed epiphyseal stippling and some delayed skeletal maturation, resembling some effects of hypothyroidism, but longitudinal growth was reported to be normal. Most cases of human thyroid hormone resistance caused by dominant-negative mutations of the TR-β gene have been shown to have variable skeletal effects, but not as severe as in untreated congenital or acquired juvenile hypothyroidism.

Thus in humans, TR-β mediates some of the effects of thyroid hormones, but not in mice. In contrast, ablation of TR-α in mice impairs longitudinal bone growth and endochondral ossification, but so far no case of human mutation of the TR-α has been described.

In rats, a sexual dimorphism in the catch-up growth capacity, after restoring long-term thyroid hormone deficiency to normal hormone levels, was observed, with complete catch-up of the growth deficit in the female[5] compared with an incomplete catch-up in the male rat.[6] The decreased ability for catch-up growth in male compared with female rats points to the important role of estrogens in growth velocity dependent on bone maturation. The negative impact of thyroid hormone deficiency on growth results from the lack of stimulatory effects on growth hormone and IGF/IGF binding protein-3 secretion, direct damage to the growth plates and variability of catch-up growth capacities. Evidence for the sexual dimorphism of catch-up growth observed in rats has not been described in humans.

It is well known that, in addition to its local action on the growth plate, thyroid hormones have indirect effects on longitudinal growth by modulating the secretion of growth hormone (GH) and IGF-I. In hypothyroidism in humans and mice, serum GH and IGF-I concentrations are decreased and substitution of GH stimulated longitudinal bone growth occurs in hypothyroid rats. Hypothyroidism leads to a decrease in mRNA levels of pituitary growth hormone and pituitary growth hormone content, which can be restored by thyroid hormone replacement.[7] The increase of pituitary GH by thyroid hormones may be mediated by transcription regulatory elements that are responsive to thyroid hormones, which have been identified in the rat growth hormone gene.[8,9] However, in hypothyroid animal models GH did not restore the defects of endochondral ossification.

Most recently, by studying thyroid-stimulating hormone (TSH) receptor KO mice evidence for an inhibitory direct effect of TSH on osteoclast formation as well as on osteoblast differentiation was provided.[10] However, the relevance for human pathophysiology is so far unclear, but may explain direct effects of primary hypothyroidism at the growth plate level.

GROWTH AND HYPOTHYROIDISM IN HUMANS

Untreated congenital or juvenile hypothyroidism causes growth arrest, delayed bone age, and epiphyseal dysgenesis and some patients with resistance to thyroid hormone (RTH), caused by dominant negative mutant thyroid hormone receptor β (TR-β) proteins, suffer from developmental abnormalities of bone and growth retardation.[11] Studies of the long-term effects of childhood hypothyroidism on linear growth indicate that catch-up growth after thyroxine (T$_4$) replacement is incomplete because bone age advances faster than height.[12] However, when evaluating the effects of thyroid hormone deficiency on growth, it has to be taken into account that hypothyroidism is caused by different disturbances of thyroid function, that these disturbances may present at different ages, and that the effects may be influenced by the duration of hypothyroidism. Therefore, a distinction has to be made between congenital and acquired forms of hypothyroidism. Usually, it is assumed that replacement therapy with thyroxine will compensate completely for the decrease in longitudinal growth by a period of catch-up growth with accelerated growth velocity. This was substantiated by the description of a catch-up growth spurt in infants with congenital hypothyroidism detected on clinical grounds before the introduction of screening programs.[13] However, more recent reports[12,14] indicate that children with long-standing hypothyroidism will fail to achieve normal adult stature despite a remarkable catch-up growth after the initiation of thyroid hormone replacement.[15] Since the effects of thyroid hormones on growth at the cellular or molecular level are still not entirely understood and, especially as studies on cases of acquired juvenile hypothyroidism are scarce, it is difficult

to understand the mechanisms that lead to a persistent impairment of longitudinal growth and growth plate formation in patients with thyroid hormone deficiency.

Growth failure observed in children with hypothyroidism is partly explained by a decrease in GH secretion and a subsequent decrease in insulin-like growth factors (IGFs) and IGF-binding proteins (IGFPBs).[16–18] However, in general, this is reversible by thyroid hormone administration.[19,20]

In addition, hypothyroidism in humans has been described to induce reversible damage to the cartilage growth plates.[21] This is reflected by the radiological finding of a stippled appearance of the epiphyseal centers of ossification (epiphyseal dysgenesis) and disproportionately short limbs in infants with untreated congenital hypothyroidism.

PRE-NATAL GROWTH IN CONGENITAL HYPOTHYROIDISM

Congenital hypothyroidism does not seem to affect pre-natal linear growth, because several studies have reported normal lengths and weights at birth in newborn infants with congenital hypothyroidism irrespective of disease severity or delay of skeletal maturation.[22,23] A normal length at birth is also observed in most newborn infants with congenital GH deficiency. This finding can possibly be explained by the transplacental passage of maternal thyroid hormones, which can maintain fetal growth, and the importance of other factors such as placental nutrition and placental hormones, which are more important for fetal growth than growth hormone or the thyroid hormones.

In 94 patients with congenital hypothyroidism, who were detected using the newborn screening program in Berlin, pre-natal growth was unaffected by hypothyroidism. Mean length at birth in girls ($n = 69$) was 50.9 ± 2.8 cm and in boys ($n = 25$) 51.5 ± 3.0 cm. Comparable data of a Norwegian and Swedish cohort of newborn infants with congenital hypothyroidism have been published recently.[24]

However, a possible role for thyroid hormones in fetal growth was evidenced by a unique patient with fetal and maternal hypothyroidism caused by pit-1 deficiency and untreated maternal hypothyroidism during late gestation.[25] This infant had a length of 46 cm at 38 weeks of gestation (3rd percentile) and the authors concluded, from this case, that transplacental passage of maternal thyroxine is necessary to maintain normal growth in the hypothyroid fetus.

POST-NATAL LONGITUDINAL GROWTH IN CONGENITAL HYPOTHYROIDISM

A normal post-natal growth was observed in most patients with early treated congenital hypothyroidism in most studies.[22,26–28] However, a slight decrease in longitudinal growth compared with normal infants was observed in a few studies during the first year of life.[24,29,30] A French study[23] found a decrease in growth velocity directly after birth with a catch-up growth in the subsequent 6 months. However, final height in correlation to target height is unaffected by congenital hypothyroidism as long as thyroid hormone supplementation and compliance to treatment is adequate.[31,32]

The author's group has analyzed the growth of the 94 patients detected using the newborn screening program. Treatment was initiated at a median age of 9 days (3–42 days) with a median dose of L-thyroxine of $14 \mu g \ kg^{-1} \ day^{-1}$. The age of the patients at the last available growth assessment ranged from 1.5 to 17 years; 10 patients were aged 1–3 years, 52 between 3 and 10 years, and 32 between 11 and 17 years. Their standard deviation scores (SDS) of height are depicted in Fig. 30.1. There was no correlation with height and severity or type of hypothyroidism or with the age at onset of treatment.

To evaluate the attained height in an individual patient, it is necessary to compare the patient's height with his or her target height predicted by the presumably unaffected parents. Therefore, the author's group correlated the actual heights with the target heights (Fig. 30.2).

Attained heights correlated well with target heights ($r = 0.75$, $p < 0.0001$). A decreased height of more than

1 SD compared with target height was observed in only six children (five boys and one girl) with an age of 3–10 years, which was not attributed to poor compliance or other accompanying diseases or problems. The number of boys in this group is remarkable, especially in the face of a female preponderance of 2.75:1 in the whole group. As several patients with congenital hypothyroidism, even after an early onset of treatment, were diagnosed as having GH deficiency,[33,34] it has been speculated that patients with congenital hypothyroidism have to recover from fetal GH deficiency, reflected by significantly lower GH levels at birth compared with normal controls; the authors have suggested that some patients might have a limited GH reserve. In none of the current author's patients with congenital hypothyroidism and early treatment was GH deficiency diagnosed as an additional problem. A decrease of the SDS for height during puberty, which had been described in a recent study,[35] was not observed in these patients.

These data indicate that normal longitudinal growth is maintained throughout childhood and adolescence in patients with congenital hypothyroidism and that they reach their genetic potential if hypothyroidism is treated early and as long as adequate compliance is guaranteed, which is reflected by normal TSH and thyroid hormone concentrations during longitudinal follow-up. Untoward effects of pubertal development were not observed and growth in the vast majority of the patients was in the expected range for the target heights.

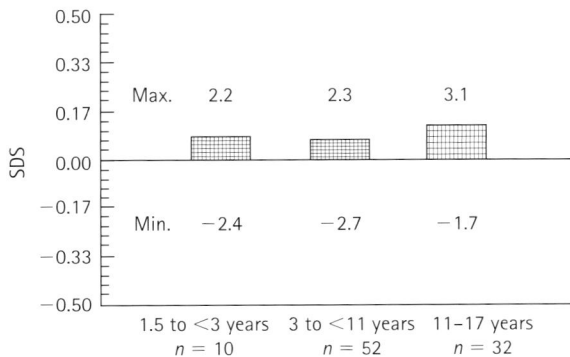

Figure 30.1 Standard deviation score (SDS) of achieved height in patients with early treated congenital hypothyroidism detected by the screening program in Berlin.

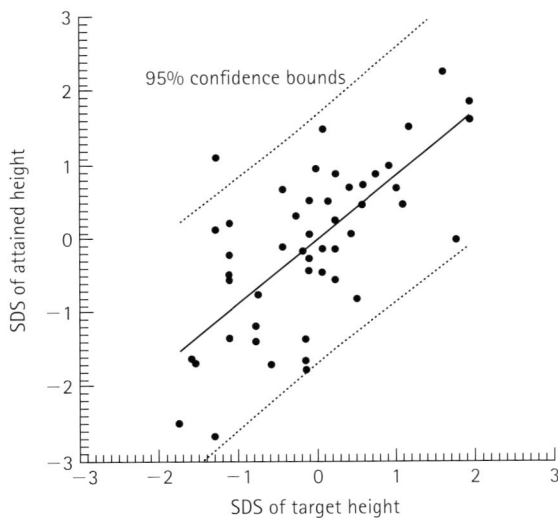

Figure 30.2 Correlation of achieved height (SDS) and target height (SDS) in patients with early treated congenital hypothyroidism detected by the screening program in Berlin.

GROWTH IN ACQUIRED JUVENILE HYPOTHYROIDISM

Juvenile hypothyroidism is a different disease entity. In contrast to congenital hypothyroidism, which results from thyroid dysgenesis in most of the patients, the major cause of juvenile acquired hypothyroidism is autoimmune thyroiditis. Decreasing growth velocity and arrest of statural growth are key symptoms of juvenile hypothyroidism. Studies of long-term growth results in patients with acquired hypothyroidism are rare. It has been assumed that catch-up growth is complete after replacement of thyroid hormones and that normal final heights will be achieved.[13,36] However, recent reports have shown that catch-up growth in some patients with acquired juvenile hypothyroidism is not complete and short stature cannot be prevented.[12,14] The hypotheses on causes for an incomplete catch-up growth after prolonged hypothyroidism in childhood that have been put forward include:[12]

- Prolonged hypothyroidism may directly diminish the reserve for catch-up growth.
- Over-treatment with thyroxine, which leads to a more rapid increase of skeletal maturation than increase in statural height.
- The initiation of replacement at puberty in particular, might accelerate skeletal maturation more than growth velocity.

In one report on four patients with prolonged hypothyroidism, it has been suggested that the third explanation corresponded best, because failure to achieve a normal final height was observed in the three patients who entered puberty shortly after the start of therapy, whereas, in the patient who showed pubertal signs only 4 years after onset of replacement therapy, catch-up growth leading to normal height was observed.[15] Therefore, the authors speculated that the outcome of statural growth would have been better if gonadal suppression had been achieved by administration of gonadotrophin-releasing hormone (GnRH) analogues in order to delay pubertal development in the other three patients; this was because a single case report had described improved height gain in a patient with prolonged hypothyroidism, after simultaneous administration of growth hormone and a GnRH analogue with thyroid hormone replacement.[37] The use of growth hormone and gonadotropin-releasing hormone agonist in addition to L-thyroxine was again recently reported to be successful in attaining normal adult height in two patients with severe Hashimoto's thyroiditis presenting at the ages of 13 and 14 years.[38]

This type of treatment seems to offer a possibility to patients with a substantial growth deficit and iniminent start of puberty; however, long-term results on the improvement in final height are not available.

The age at onset of hypothyroidism may also affect the reserve for catch-up growth. In four patients with an early onset of hypothyroidism caused by autoimmune thyroiditis (age 9 months to 2 years), a normalization of statural growth was achieved.[39] However, in these patients the duration of hypothyroidism was short. The deficit in adult height appears to be related more to the duration of untreated hypothyroidism and to the degree of growth delay at the start of treatment, than to the age at onset of replacement therapy or to the effect of pubertal onset, because failure to achieve predicted adult height was also observed in patients with prolonged hypothyroidism who did not enter puberty during the first 2 years after treatment[12] or in patients with congenital hypothyroidism who were treated late and remained pre-pubertal during therapy.

Two cases of acquired hypothyroidism with substantial permanent growth impairment after long-term hypothyroidism have been observed by the author's group. They remained pre-pubertal during treatment, supporting the hypothesis that factors other than the discrepancy between advancement of pubertal development and skeletal maturation contribute to the growth failure observed in some patients with long-standing hypothyroidism.

Patient 1

This patient was born in the Ukraine and had severe delay in growth and maturation. He was unable to walk until the age of 3 years and speech development only occurred at the age of 5 years. At the age of 4 years hypothyroidism was diagnosed in the Ukraine and he was treated with thyroid extracts. He presented to the author's outpatient clinic after emigration to Germany at the age of 9.5 years. His height was 90.7 cm and his bone age was assessed as 2 years. The appearance was disproportionate with short limbs. His mental and motor development was equivalent to 3 years. His thyroid function tests proved hypothyroidism: TSH of 220 U L^{-1}, T$_4$ of 1.6 pg dL^{-1} and T$_3$ of 0.8 ng mL^{-1} despite treatment with the thyroid extracts. Determination of the content of T$_4$ in the tablet gave a value of 3.8 μg per tablet, which was the daily dose administered.

After replacement with a recommended T$_4$ dose of 75 μg day^{-1}, he underwent a remarkable catch-up growth, with 13.2 cm in the first and 8 cm in the second year (Fig. 30.3). Bone age after 1.5 years of treatment was 6 years, with a progression of 4 years over this period. Interestingly, the radiologist mentioned signs of demineralization of the bone. Levels of IGF-I in the patient were repeatedly low (median 65 ng mL^{-1}) despite treatment and catch-up growth. Growth hormone secretion in the arginine stimulation test resulted in a subnormal peak of 3.2 ng mL^{-1}. The predicted adult height at 11 years was 152 cm, which is 20 cm below his target height of 172 cm, and he was still completely pre-pubertal. Therefore, GH treatment was instituted at the age of 12.5 years, because his IGF-I was low and growth hormone stimulation tests revealed growth hormone deficiency. This treatment resulted in a significant catch-up growth and improvement of final height (161.2 cm), which is still reduced correlated to target height (Fig. 30.3). A diminished GH reserve has been reported in some other patients with prolonged hypothyroidism.[33,34]

Patient 2

This Turkish boy was born and lived in Turkey until he was brought to the author's clinic because of short stature at the age of 11 years by his relatives during a vacation. He had a hoarse voice and dry skin and complained of constipation; his school performance was unremarkable. Hypothyroidism caused by autoimmune thyroiditis, with a TSH of 324 mU L^{-1}, a T$_4$ of 2.5 μg dL^{-1} and a T$_3$ of 0.5 ng mL^{-1}, was diagnosed. Thyroid ultrasonography revealed an enlarged gland with a volume of 12 mL, a hypodense echo pattern and positive anti-thyroid peroxidase antibodies (2000 U L^{-1}) in addition to anti-thyroglobulin antibodies (800 U L^{-1}). His height was 122 cm (11 cm below the 3rd percentile) and his bone age was only 6 years. After initiation of thyroid hormone replacement, he had an insufficient catch-up growth with a growth velocity of 7 cm in the first year and 5 cm in the second year of treatment (Fig. 30.4); there was an advancement of bone age to 9 years at the age of 14 years, when he was still pre-pubertal. His IGF-I level was low (68 ng mL^{-1}) and the stimulation of GH secretion with arginine resulted in a subnormal maximal response of 5.4 ng mL^{-1}, and stimulation with insulin-induced hypoglycemia gave 5.9 ng mL^{-1}. Therefore,

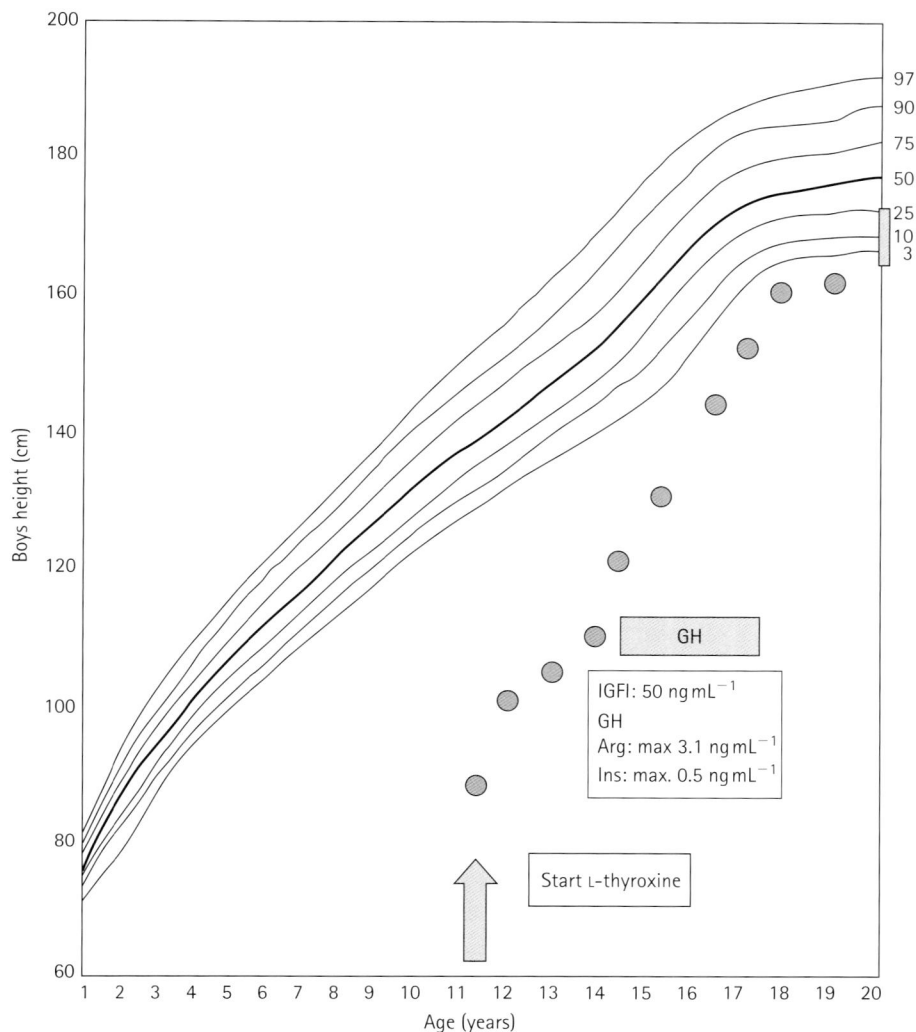

Figure 30.3 Patient with congenital hypothyroidism, delayed thyroid hormone replacement and decreased growth hormone secretion.

it was assumed that the insufficient catch-up growth was caused by a limited GH reserve; therapy with recombinant human growth hormone was initiated at the age of 14 years. In the first 9 months of treatment, growth velocity increased to 15.9 cm year^{-1}, but he failed to achieve his target height of 175 cm and has a final height of 167 cm.

In summary, these cases demonstrate that, in contrast to patients with congenital hypothyroidism who are treated early, an attainment of a final height in the range of the target height might not be possible despite initial catch-up growth in patients who have prolonged hypothyroidism in childhood. The duration of hypothyroidism and the magnitude of decrease in statural growth seem to be the major determinants of growth failure. The molecular and cellular mechanisms, however, remain unclear.

HYPERTHYROIDISM

Childhood thyrotoxicosis causes accelerated growth and advanced bone age, which may lead to craniosynostosis, premature growth plate closure, and eventual short stature.[1,3,4] Besides reports on single cases, studies on growth in patients with juvenile hyperthyroidism, caused by Graves' disease, Hashimoto's thyroiditis, non-autoimmune hyperthyroidism or during treatment with excessive doses of T_4, are very rare. In most studies on the outcome of juvenile hyperthyroidism, statural height has not been reported[40–42] and, when growth has been mentioned, a height within normal limits (1 SD) has been reported.[43] However, acceleration of bone maturation has been observed in children and adolescents with hyperthyroidism[44,45] and after over-treatment with L-thyroxine.[46] In a more recent studies an acceleration of growth and bone age maturation leading to an increased final height was reported.[47] In 25 patients with Graves' disease, who were followed at the author's institution, with a median age of manifestation of 13 years (6–17 years), no significant change in growth velocity, statural height or predicted adult height was observed.

In contrast, in patients with non-autoimmune congenital hyperthyroidism, a remarkable acceleration of fetal bone age has been reported,[48,49] which usually leads to premature craniosynostosis. Also, in patients with neonatal Graves'

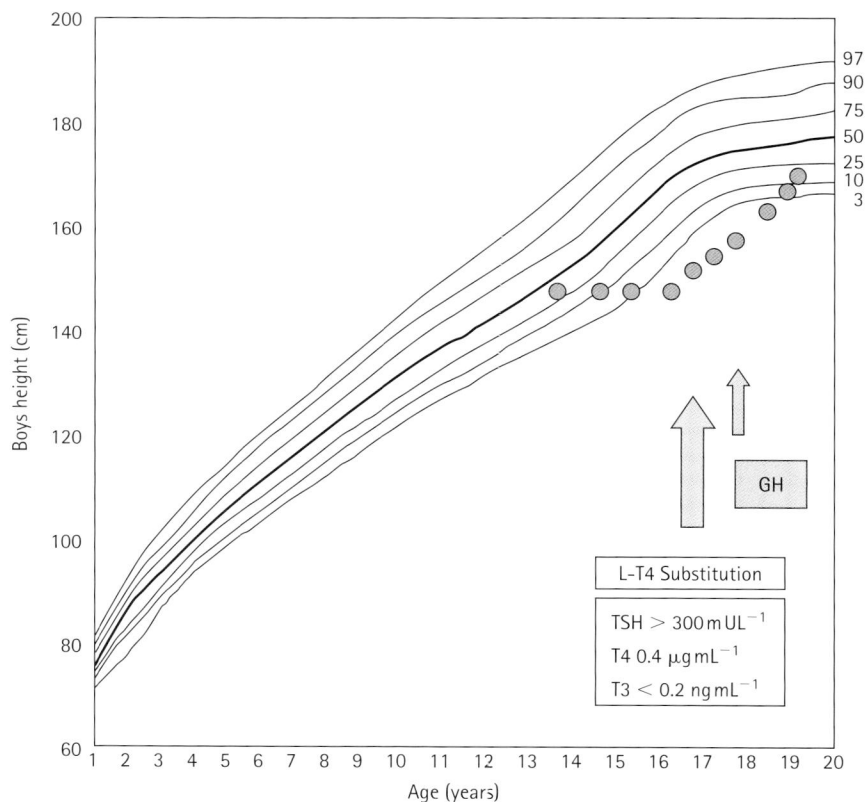

Figure 30.4   Patient with acquired hypothyroidism due to autoimmune thyroiditis and impaired growth hormone secretion.

disease, acceleration of skeletal maturation has been observed,[50] but fetal growth is retarded in most patients with neonatal thyrotoxicosis. Intrauterine growth retardation is a common feature of both autoimmune and non-autoimmune congenital hypothyroidism.[51,52] Therefore, in congenital hyperthyroidism skeletal maturation is advanced, but growth significantly retarded, most probably because of the adverse effects of excessive hormones on energy expenditure and metabolic rate. Maternal Graves' disease also leads to negative effects on placental perfusion and fetal nutrition.

CONCLUSION

A normal growth and final height are achievable in patients with congenital hypothyroidism or with a short duration of hypothyroidism of later onset who are treated early. In contrast, in long-standing hypothyroidism, a limited GH reserve might be responsible for a diminished catch-up growth, which could result from problems in the regulation of the GH gene, a direct effect of hypothyroidism on the growth plate or the effects of gonadal steroids. More studies are necessary to elucidate the pathogenic mechanisms involved in the effects of prolonged hypothyroidism on growth, to establish new treatment strategies for affected patients.

In addition, the molecular mechanisms of thyroid hormone excess, which lead to pre-natal and post-natal acceleration of bone maturation, are unknown, but may be similar to those leading to osteoporosis in adults after prolonged overtreatment with thyroid hormones.

REFERENCES

1   Harper J, Klagsbrun M. Cartilage to bone-angiogenesis leads the way. *Nat Med* 1999; **5**: 617–8.

2   Kindblom JM, Nilsson O, Ohlsson C, Savendahl L. Expression and localization of Indian hedgehog (Ihh) and parathyroid hormone related protein (PTHrP) in the human growth plate during pubertal development *J Endocrinol* 2002; **174**: 1–6.

3   Robson H, Siebler T, Stevens SH, *et al.* Thyroid hormone acts directly on growth plate chondrocytes to promote hypertrophic differentiation and inhibit clonal expansion and cell proliferation. *Endocrinology* 2000; **141**: 3887–97.

4   O'Shea PJ, Bassett JH, Sriskantharajah S, *et al.* Contrasting skeletal phenotypes in mice with an identical mutation targeted to thyroid hormone receptor 1 or β. *Mol Endocrinol* 2005; **19**: 3045–59.

5   Meisami E. Complete recovery of growth deficits after reversal of PTU-induced postnatal hypothyroidism in the female rat: a model for catch-up growth. *Life Sci* 1984; **34**: 1487–96.

6   Mosier HD, Dearden LC, Jansons RA, Hill RR. Growth hormone, somatomedin C and cartilage sulfation in failure of catch-up growth after prolonged PTU-induced hypothyroidism in the rat. *Endocrinology* 1977; **100**: 1644–51.

7   Franldyn JA, Cynam T, Docherty K, *et al.* Effect of hypothyroidism on pituitary cytoplasmic concentrations of mRNA encoding TSH-r3 and alpha subunits, prolactin and growth hormone. *J Endocrinol* 1986; **108**: 43–7.

8 Flug F, Copp RP, Casanova J. Cis acting element of the rat growth hormone gene which mediates basal and regulated expression by thyroid hormone. *J Biol Chem* 1987; **262**: 6373–82.

9 Ye ZS, Samuels HH. Cell and sequence specific binding of nuclear proteins to S-flanking DNA of the rat growth hormone gene. *J Biol Chem* 1987; **262**: 6313–7.

10 Abe E, Marians RC, Yu W, *et al*. TSH is a negative regulator of skeletal remodelling. *Cell* 2003; **115**: 151–62.

11 Weiss RE, Refetoff S. Effect of thyroid hormone on growth: Lessons from the syndrome of resistance to thyroid hormone. *Endocrinol Metab Clin North Am* 1996; **25**: 719–30.

12 Rivkees S, Bode HH, Crawford JD. Longterm growth in juvenile hypothyroidism – The failure to achieve normal adult stature. *New Engl J Med* 1988; **318**: 599–602.

13 Harnack GA, Tanner JM, Whitehouse RH, Rodriguez CA. Catch-up growth in height and skeletal maturation in children on long-term treatment for hypothyroidism. *Z Kinderheilkd* 1972; **112**: 1–17.

14 Pantsiotou S, Stanhope R, Uruena M, *et al*. Growth prognosis and growth after menarche in primary hypothyroidism. *Arch Dis Child* 1991; **66**: 838–40.

15 Boersma B, Otten BJ, Stoelinga GBA, Wit JM. Catch-up growth after prolonged hypothyroidism. *Eur J Pediatr* 1996; **155**: 362–7.

16 Chernausek SD, Underwood LE, Utiger RD. Growth hormone secretion and plasma somatomedin C in primary hypothyroidism. *Clin Endocrinol* 1983; **19**: 337–44.

17 Buchanan CR, Stanhope R, Adlard P, *et al*. Gonadotrophin, growth hormone and prolactin secretion in children with primary hypothyroidism. *Clin Endocrinol* 1988; **29**: 427–36.

18 Arnao *et al*. 1997.

19 Valcavi R, Jordon V, Kieguez C. Growth hormone responses to GRF in patients before and during replacement therapy with thyroxine. *Clin Endocrinol* 1986; **24**: 693–6.

20 Cavaliere H, Knobel M, Medeiros G, Neto G. Effect of thyroid hormone therapy on plasma IGF 1 in normal subjects, hypothyroid patients and endemic cretinism. *Horm Res* 1987; **25**: 132–9.

21 Lewinson D, Harel Z, Shenzer P, *et al*. Effect of thyroid hormone and growth hormone on the recovery from hypothyroidism of epiphyseal growth plate cartilage and adjacent bone. *Endocrinology* 1989; **124**: 937–45.

22 Bucher H, Prader A, Lug R. Head circumference, height, bone age and weight in 103 children with congenital hypothyroidism before and during growth hormone replacement therapy. *Helv Paediatr Acta* 1985; **40**: 305–16.

23 Leger J, Czernichow P. Congenital hypothyroidism: decreased growth velocity in the first weeks of life. *Biol Neonate* 1989; **55**: 218–23.

24 Heyerdahl S, Iilicki A, Karlberg J. Linear growth in early treated children with congenital hypothyroidism. *Acta Paediatr* 1997; **86**: 478–83.

25 de Zegher F, Pernasetti F, Vanhole C, *et al*. The prenatal role of thyroid hormone evidenced by fetomaternal pit-1 deficiency. *J Clin Endocrinol Metab* 1995; **80**: 3127–30.

26 Hulse JA, Grant DB, Jackson D, Clayton B. Growth, development and reassessment of hypothyroid children diagnosed by screening. *BMJ* 1982; **284**: 1435–7.

27 New England Collaborative. Characteristics of infantile hypothyroidism discovered on neonatal screening. *J Pediatr* 1984; **104**: 539–44.

28 Grant DB. Growth in early treated congenital hypothyroidism. *Arch Dis Child* 1994; **70**: 464–8.

29 Aronson R, Ehrlich RM, Bailey JD, Rovet JF. Growth in children with congenital hypothyroidism detected by newborn screening. *J Pediatr* 1990; **116**: 33–7.

30 Chiesa A, Papendieck LG, Keselman A, *et al*. Growth follow-up in 100 children with congenital hypothyroidism before and during treatment. *J Pediatr Endocrinol* 1994; **7**: 211–7.

31 Bain *et al*. 2002.

32 Salerno *et al*. 2001.

33 de Zegher F, Vanderschueren Lodeweyckx M, Suarez P, *et al*. Congenital hypothyroidism and growth hormone deficiency. *Lancet* 1988; **ii**: 1489–90.

34 Lazarus JA. Hughes IA. Congenital abnormalities and congenital hypothyroidism. *Lancet* 1988; **ii**: 52.

35 Gurrado R, Zecchino C, Iannicelli G, *et al*. Transversal and longitudinal growth in early treated congenital hypothyroidism. *Horm Res* 1997; **48**: 163.

36 Tanner JM. Catch-up growth in man. *Br Med Bull* 1981; **37**: 233–8.

37 Minamitani K, Murata A, Ohnishi H, *et al*. Attainment of normal height in severe juvenile hypothyroidism. *Arch Dis Child* 1994; **70**: 429–31.

38 Quintas JB, Sals M. Use of growth hormone and gonadotropin releasing hormone agonist in addition to L-thyroxine to attain normal adult height in two patients with severe Hashimoto's thyroiditis. *Pediatr Endocrinol Metab* 2005; **18**: 515–21.

39 Foley TP, Abassi V, Copeland KC, Draznin MB. Hypothyroidism caused by chronic autoimmune thyroiditis in very young infants. *New Engl J Med* 1994; **330**: 466–8.

40 Hamburger JI. Management of hyperthyroidism in children and adolescents. *J Clin Endocrinol Metab* 1985; **60**: 1019–24.

41 Lippe BM, Landraw EM, Kaplan SA. Hyperthyroidism in children treated with longterm medical therapy: twenty-five percent remission every two years. *J Clin Endocrinol Metab* 1987; **64**: 1241–5.

42 Perrild H, Grüters A, Feldt-Rasmussen U, *et al*. Diagnosis and treatment of thyrotoxicosis in children: A European questionnaire study. *Eur J Endocrinol* 1994; **131**: 467–73.

43 Karidi I, Maniati M, Chiotis D, *et al*. Hyperthyroidism in childhood: Longterm resuits. *Horm Res* 1997.

44 Johnsonbaugh RE, Bryan RN, Hieriwimmer UR, Georges LP. Premature craniosynostosis: a common complication of juvenile thyrotoxicosis. *J Pediatr* 1978; **93**: 188–91.

45 Lazar L, Kalter-Leibovici O, Pertzelan A, *et al*. Thyrotoxicosis in prepubertal children compared with pubertal and postpubertal patients. *J Clin Endocrinol Metab* 2000; **85**: 3678–82.

46   Penfold JL, Simpson DA. Premature craniosynostosis – complication of thyroid replacement therapy. *J Pediatr* 1975; **86**: 360–3.

47   Wong GW, Lai J, Cheng PS. Growth in childhood thyrotoxicosis. *Eur J Pediatr* 1999; **158**: 776–9.

48   Kopp P, van Sande J, Parma J. *et al.* Congenital hyperthyroidism caused by a mutation in the TSH receptor gene. *New Engl J Med* 1995; **332**: 150–4.

49   Schwab KO, Söhlemann P, Geruch M, *et al.* Mutations of the TSH receptor as a cause of congenital hypothyrcidism. *Exp Clin Endocrinol Diabetes* 1996; **104**: 124–8.

50   Daneman D, Howard NJ. Neonatal thyrotoxicosis, intellectual impairment and craniosynostosis in later years. *J Pediatr* 1980; **97**: 257–9.

51   Hollingsworth D, Mabry CC. Congenital Graves' disease. *Am J Disease Child* 1976; **130**: 148–55.

52   de Roux N, Polak M, Couet J, *et al.* Neomutation of the TSH receptor in severe neonatal hypothyroidism. *J Clin Endocrinol Metab* 1996; **81**: 2023–6.

31

Adrenal disorders

HELEN L STORR, MARTIN O SAVAGE

INTRODUCTION

Abnormalities of adrenal function in childhood may be associated with significant disturbance of linear growth. There are several potential mechanisms responsible for this. First, the adrenal disorder may be a component of a dysmorphic syndrome, of which tall or short stature is a feature. This is the case with some ACTH resistance syndromes and the IMAGe association. Secondly, the underlying defect may cause excess secretion of androgens or estrogens, which stimulate linear growth but also advance skeletal maturation leading potentially to adult short stature. This is the case with virilizing congenital adrenal hyperplasia and some adrenal tumors. Thirdly, excess secretion of glucocorticoids, as in Cushing's syndrome, may retard skeletal maturation and suppress linear growth. The management of each condition needs to be assessed independently in order to normalize growth where possible and achieve optimal adult height.

AUTOIMMUNE ADDISON'S DISEASE

Childhood Addison's disease is not usually associated with marked disturbance of growth. As many patients present with salt-depletion, growth prior to the diagnosis may be compromised and in the series reported by Grant from Great Ormond Street Hospital in London, height at presentation was usually below average.[1] Growth rates on steroid replacement were generally normal, but only one of 14 patients achieved an adult height above the 50th centile.[1] Pubertal growth was on the whole normal, except in patients with multiple autoimmune endocrinopathy who had sex steroid secreting cell autoantibodies which caused impairment of pubertal development.

ACTH RESISTANCE SYNDROMES

Familial glucocorticoid deficiency (FGD) is a rare autosomal recessive disorder characterized by resistance to ACTH leading to glucocorticoid but not mineralocorticoid deficiency.[2] Many cases described in the literature report that the patients were unusually tall at the time of clinical presentation.[3,4]

The primary defect in FGD consists of mutations of the *MC-2R* gene in approximately 25% patients[5] with functional studies demonstrating defective ACTH binding and/or signalling.[2] Many patients, however, have a similar clinical phenotype, but have a normal *MC2-R* gene coding sequence. Clark *et al.* have used the term FGD type 1 to describe patients with *MC-2R* mutations and FGD type 2 to describe those without mutations of this gene. The majority of patients with this syndrome who are tall have *MC-2R* gene mutations (FGD type 1) and those without mutations generally have normal stature.[2]

In a report from Clark's group,[6] five unrelated patients are described, three with novel mutations and one with a previously described mutation of the *MC2-R*. All these patients had tall stature (Fig. 31.1). Most patients with this association are inappropriately tall for their mid-parental height at the time of diagnosis. They also have large occipito-frontal head circumferences. There was a suggestion that growth rate declined with glucocorticoid replacement (Fig. 31.1) and that the greatly elevated circulating ACTH may have a role in the generation of this abnormality. No

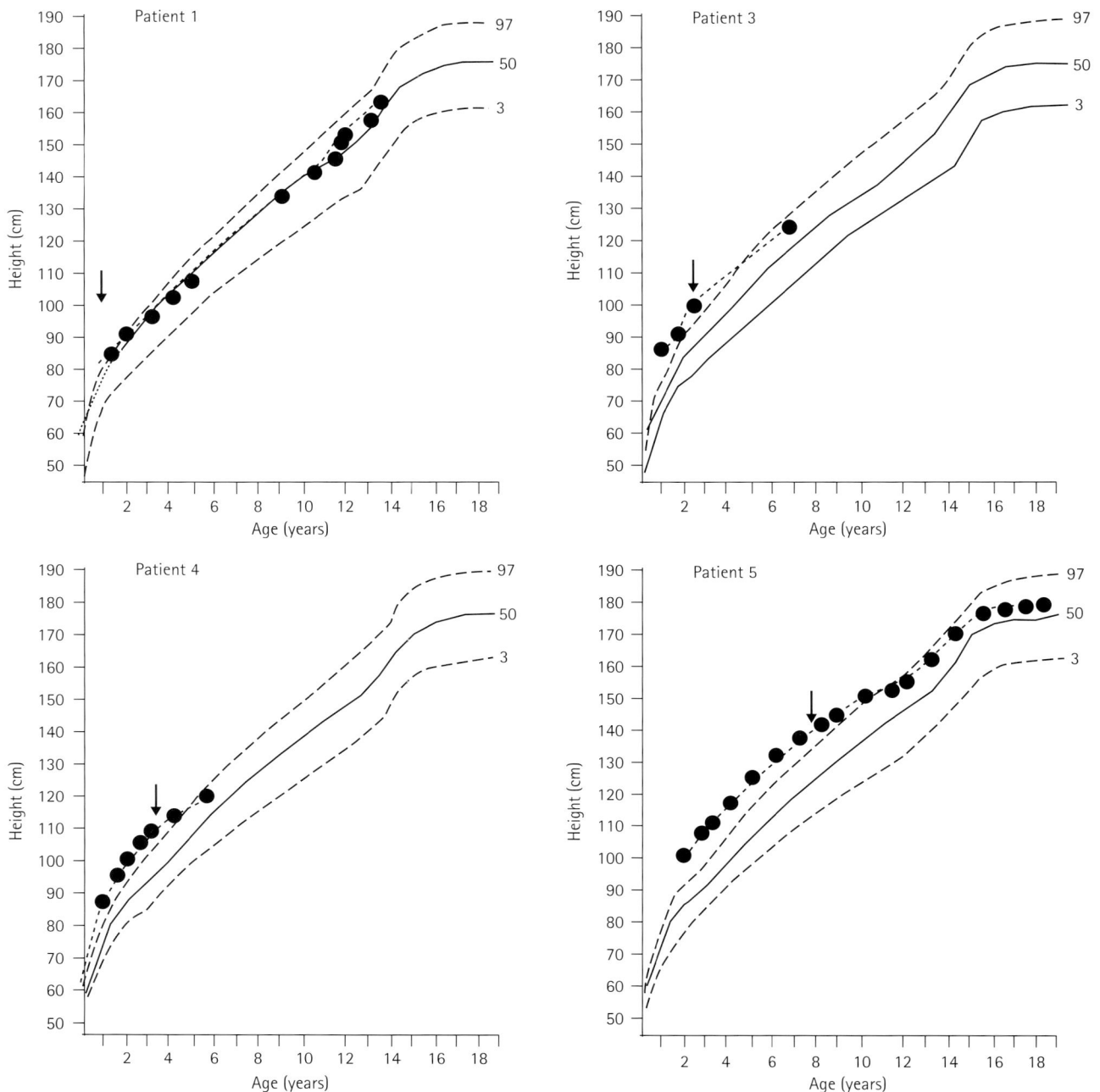

Figure 31.1 Growth charts of four patients with ACTH resistance, demonstrating tall stature and the point at which glucocorticoid replacement was started (vertical arrow).

abnormalities in the GH-IGF axis have been reported in such patients to date.

The combined features of advance in growth and bone age and increased head circumference are also compatible with Sotos syndrome, as is neonatal hypoglycemia and jaundice.[7] Some patients also have an unusual facies with frontal prominence, hypertelorism, and an anti-mongoloid slant to the eyes.[6] However, ACTH resistance is not part of Sotos syndrome. The phenomenon of excessive growth in patients with ACTH resistance is therefore of great interest and remains unexplained. It seems probable that the action of ACTH and the role of the *MC2-R* is more complex than it first appears, and that understanding of this

phenomenon may provide unexpected insights into aspects of growth control.

IMAGe ASSOCIATION

The IMAGe association consists of a series of abnormal features, two of which are adrenal insufficiency and short stature. The syndrome was first described by Vilain *et al.* in 1999[8] and the full features are: intrauterine growth retardation (I), metaphyseal dysplasia (M), congenital adrenal hypoplasia (A), and micropenis or hypospadias (Ge). There are therefore two reasons for short stature to be present, namely the metaphyseal dysplasia and the intrauterine growth retardation. The adrenal failure usually becomes manifest in the neonatal period when hyponatremia presents associated with increased serum ACTH. The basic pathogenesis of the adrenal failure is not explained and no genetic explanation exists for the link between short stature and adrenal failure.

CONGENITAL ADRENAL HYPERPLASIA

It has long been recognized that adult height may be compromised in congenital adrenal hyperplasia related to 21-hydroxylase deficiency.[9] There are several reasons why growth can be disturbed. Firstly, if adrenal androgen secretion is not adequately suppressed with glucocorticoid replacement therapy, high levels of androgens will stimulate linear growth and advance skeletal maturation. Secondly, central precocious puberty may develop as a result of androgen-mediated activation of the hypothalamic–pituitary–gonadal axis. Both factors result in premature epiphyseal fusion and ultimately adult short stature.

Finally, CAH treatment with glucocorticoids may result in growth suppression. This is often due to excessive steroid treatment particularly in the first years of life. In this situation, some catch-up growth may occur with reduction in steroid dose, but full catch-up to normal height is rarely achieved and long-term short stature usually results. Steroid administration even at replacement doses has also been associated with poor growth and many CAH patients with adequate hormonal control do not reach their target height.[10] Several long-term studies of growth in congenital adrenal hyperplasia have been performed. A detailed analysis by Jääskeläinen and Voutilainen[11] of 92 Finnish patients showed some interesting findings. First, the birth length of patients diagnosed at birth was greater than the national mean ($p < 0.001$). Mean relative length diminished from +0.8 SDS at birth to −1.0 SDS at 1 year of age, indicating a suppression of growth in infancy. Adult height was −1.0 SDS in men and −0.8 SDS in women. Another series reports impaired early growth (0–3 years) followed by normal childhood growth in salt-wasting patients. In contrast, patients with simple virilizing forms of CAH had normal growth in early childhood but above standard growth subsequently.[12]

Pubertal growth has been analyzed in several series and has been shown to be suppressed. An analysis of a large database of over 500 patients from central Europe[12] has shown that pubertal growth is more impaired in patients with simple virilizing congenital adrenal hyperplasia, who may present in later childhood compared to salt-wasting patients who will present earlier. This is presumably related to the damaging effect of advanced bone age on the pubertal growth spurt.

Early diagnosis of CAH (<1 year) and early initiation treatment with more physiological doses of steroid, particularly in the first year of life has been shown to improve height outcome.[13] As has adequate mineralocorticoid therapy in all patients with classical forms of CAH.[13,14] Growth hormone therapy in combination with GnRH analogues is a treatment

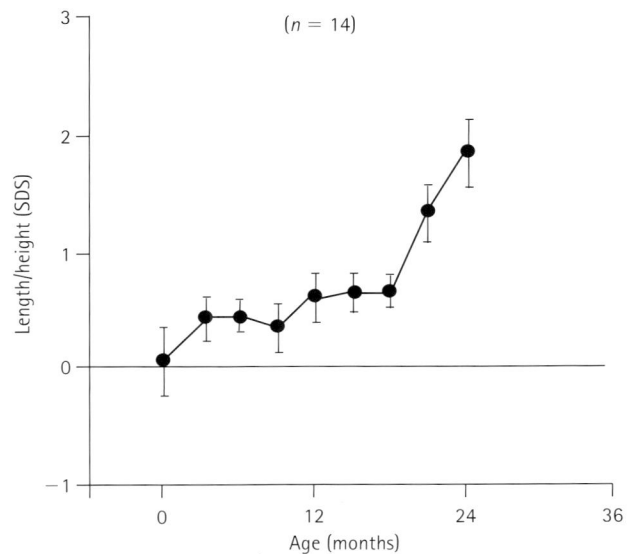

Figure 31.2 Height SDS for 14 children with 21-hydroxylase deficiency diagnosed after 2 years of age. During the first 28 months of age all patients were untreated. Advanced growth compared to a reference normal population was not seen until 2 years of age. From Thilén et al.[15]

strategy which may improve final height in some patients with CAH.[10,14]

Growth in untreated congenital adrenal hyperplasia

We had the opportunity to follow a child with non-salt-losing 21-hydroxylase deficiency, whose parents refused to accept treatment. Despite very high levels of 17-hydroxy progesterone, androstenedione and testosterone linear growth and bone age were not advanced until 18 months of age. This case was published together with a retrospective analysis of growth in untreated patients, diagnosed with late-onset disease from Sweden,[15] who showed a similar pattern of normal infantile growth (Fig. 31.2).

These data suggest that there is a certain degree of androgen resistance, similar to that seen with the neonatal testosterone surge, in early childhood. This would strengthen the argument that only small doses of glucocorticoids are required in infancy and that larger doses, as described earlier, have the potential to cause suppression of growth with long-term consequences for childhood and adult height.

VIRILIZING ADRENAL TUMORS

Virilizing adrenal tumors are known to present with advanced growth and skeletal maturation. After successful removal of the tumor, growth tends to normalize. In a report of nine girls with virilizing tumors,[16] mean height at presentation was 1.23 ± 0.42 SDS, whereas height at a mean follow-up interval of 9.5 years was 1.67 ± 0.37 SDS and mean final height in three patients was 1.30 ± 0.45 SDS.

In a child with advanced growth due to a virilizing adrenal tumor, we have seen the phenomenon of true precocious puberty occurring after successful removal of the tumor.

CUSHING'S SYNDROME

Cushing's syndrome is known to be associated with suppression of linear growth.[17] There are several potential causes for this. Exposure to supraphysiological free circulating glucocorticoids delays skeletal maturation and suppresses growth hormone secretion. Growth hormone action may also be impaired with a decrease in circulating levels of free IGF-I and a target tissue resistance to IGF-I and other growth factors.[18]

Primary nodular adrenal hyperplasia

As potentially in all causes of pediatric Cushing's syndrome, growth was impaired in most patients with primary nodular adrenal hyperplasia (PNAH). In the series of six pediatric patients we recently reported,[19] five had height SDS values below the mean and in four height velocity was subnormal varying from 2.5 to 3.9 cm year^{-1}. Catch-up growth was also seen in three of the patients after successful bilateral adrenalectomy.

Cushing's disease

In a series of 17 patients with pediatric Cushing's disease,[20] mean height SDS at presentation was −1.81 (range −0.28 to

−4.17). Fifty-three percent of patients had a height SDS < −1.8. Height velocity was subnormal in six subjects (0.9–3.8 cm year^{-1}). An important auxological diagnostic feature of Cushing's disease was the discrepancy between height SDS and BMI SDS, which in contrast to height, was always above 0, with a mean value of 2.29 (range, 1.72–5.06) (Fig. 31.3).

Linear growth following successful treatment of Cushing's disease has been studied in detail in our unit.[21] Retrospective analysis of 10 patients demonstrated that in the short-term post-operative period, catch-up growth did not occur. This has been previously reported from the NIH where growth and final height in these patients has been disappointing.[22] In our pediatric CD series there is a high prevalence of growth hormone deficiency after successful treatment, either by transsphenoidal surgery or pituitary radiotherapy and may persist for many years.[23] Fourteen pediatric and adolescent CD patients were treated with growth hormone, four in combination with a GnRH analogue.[24] This resulted in good catch-up growth with a significant improvement ($p < 0.01$) in the difference between final or latest height SDS and target height SDS of −1.2 (−3.3 to 0.5) compared with this parameter at presentation of −2.4 (−3.9 to −0.5) (Figs 31.4 and 31.5). Several of these patients were still growing, but it seems that final height within the target range can be achieved with early diagnosis and treatment of GH deficiency.

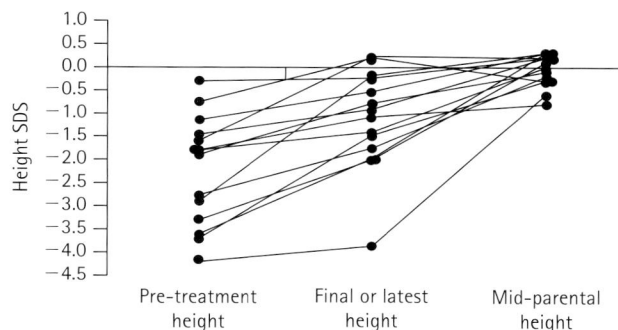

Figure 31.4 Pre-treatment height, final height and mid-parental height SDS values in 14 patients with Cushing's disease. Eleven of the patients were treated with growth hormone, four of which had GnRH analogue therapy in addition.

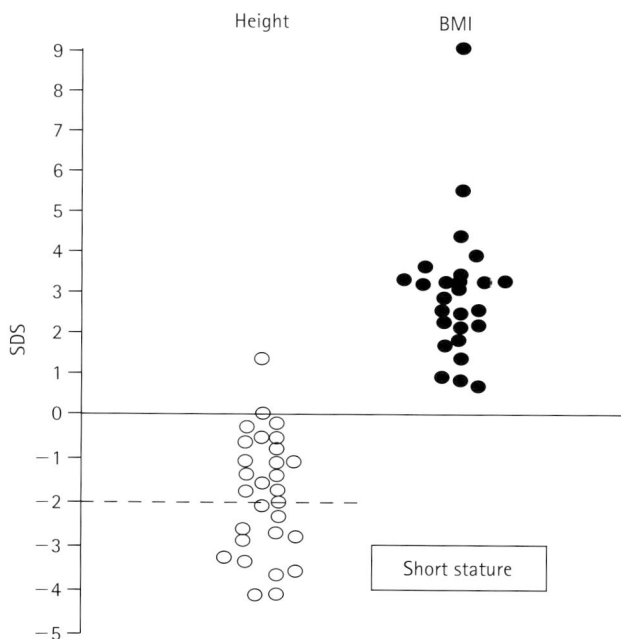

Figure 31.3 Height and body mass index (BMI) standard deviation scores (SDS) at diagnosis in 30 children and adolescents with Cushing's disease.

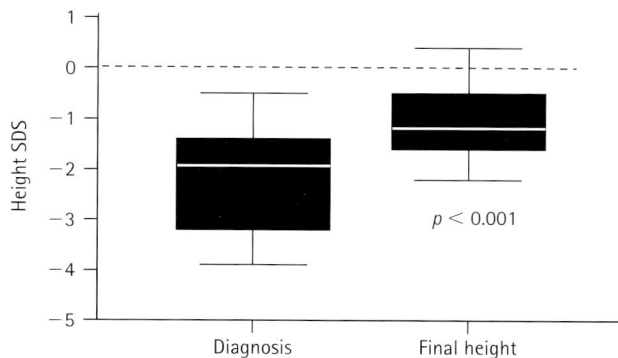

Figure 31.5 Height SDS at diagnosis and at final height compared to mid-parental height SDS in 14 patients with Cushing's disease.

CONCLUSIONS

Linear growth may thus be disturbed in childhood adrenal disease associated with either endocrine hypo- or hyperfunction. Abnormal growth may be a useful diagnostic feature in some disorders, such as ACTH resistance syndromes or the IMAGe association. Abnormal secretion of steroids from the adrenal cortex may significantly stimulate or suppress linear growth so that normal final adult height is potentially compromised. In a wide range of adrenal disorders, management of abnormal growth is an important component of the overall treatment of the primary condition.

REFERENCES

♦ = Key review paper

1 Grant DB, Barnes ND, Moncrieff MN, Savage MO. Clinical presentation, growth and pubertal development in Addison's disease. *Arch Dis Child* 1985; **60**: 405–6.
♦ 2 Clark AJL, Weber A. Adrenocorticotropin insensitivity syndromes. *Endocri Rev* 1998; **19**: 828–43.
3 Migeon CJ, Kenny FM, Kowarski A, *et al.* The syndrome of congenital adrenocortical unresponsiveness to ACTH. Report of six cases. *Pediatr Res* 1968; **2**: 501–13.
4 Thistlethwaite D, Darling JAB, Fraser R, *et al.* Familial glucocorticoid deficiency: studies of diagnosis and pathogenesis. *Arch Dis Child* 1975; **50**: 291–7.
5 Clark AJL, McLoughlin L, Grossman AB. Familial glucocorticoid deficiency caused by a point mutation in the ACTH receptor. *Lancet* 1993; **341**: 461–2.
6 Elias LLK, Huebner A, Metherell LA, *et al.* Tall stature in familial glucocorticoid deficiency. *Clin Endocrinol* 2000; **53**: 423–30.
♦ 7 Opitz JM, Weaver DW, Reynolds JF Jr. The syndromes of Sotos and Weaver: report and review. *Am J Med Genet* 1998; **79**: 294–304.
♦ 8 Vilain E, Le Merrer M, Lecointre C, *et al.* IMAGe, a new clinical association of intrauterine growth retardation, metaphyseal dysplasia, adrenal hypoplasia congenita, and genital anomalies. *J Clin Endocrinol Metab* 1999; **84**: 4335–40.
9 Urban MD, Lee PA, Migeon CJ. Adult height and fertility in men with congenital virilizing adrenal hyperplasia. *New Engl J Med* 1978; **299**: 1392–6.
♦ 10 New MI. An update of congenital adrenal hyperplasia. *Ann NY Acad Sci* 2004; **1038**: 14–43.
11 Jääskeläinen J, Voutilainen R. Growth of patients with 21-hydoxylase deficiency: An analysis of the factors influencing adult height. *Pediatr Res* 1997; **41**: 30–3.
12 Frisch H, Waldhauser F, Lebl J, *et al.* and the MEWPE-CAH Study Group Congenital Adrenal Hyperplasia: Lessons from a multinational study. *Horm Res* 2002; **57(Suppl 2)**: 95–101.
13 Balsamo A, Cicognani A, Baldazzi L, *et al.* CYP21 genotype, adult height, and pubertal development in 55 patients treated for 21-hydroxylase deficiency. *J Clin Endocrinol Metab* 2003; **88**: 5680–8.
14 Hughes IA. Congenital adrenal hyperplasia: transitional care. *Growth Horm IGF Res* 2004; **14(Suppl A)**: S60–6.
15 Thilén A, Woods KA, Perry LA, *et al.* Early growth is not increased in untreated moderately severe 21-hydroxylase deficiency. *Acta Paediatr* 1995; **84**: 894–8.
16 Salt AT, Savage MO, Grant DB. Growth patterns after surgery for virilising adrenocortical adenoma. *Arch Dis Child* 1992; **67**: 234–6.
17 Weber A, Trainer PJ, Grossman AB, *et al.* Investigation, management and therapeutic outcome in 12 cases of childhood and adolescent Cushing's syndrome. *Clin Endocrinol* 1995; **43**: 19–28.
18 Unterman TG, Phillips LS. Glucocorticoid effects on somatomedins and somatomedin inhibitors. *J Clin Endocrinol Metab* 1985; **61**: 618–26.
19 Storr HL, Mitchell H, Swords FM, *et al.* Clinical features, diagnosis, treatment and molecular studies in paediatric Cushing's syndrome due to primary nodular adrenocortical hyperplasia. *Clin Endocrinol* 2005; **61**: 553–9.
20 Savage MO, Storr HL, Grossman AB, Krassas GE. Growth and growth hormone secretion in paediatric Cushing's syndrome. *Hormones* 2003; **2**: 93–7.
21 Lebrethon M-C, Grossman AB, Afshar F, *et al.* Linear growth and final height after treatment for Cushing's disease in childhood. *J Clin Endocrinol Metab* 2000; **85**: 3262–5.
22 Magiakou MA, Mastorakos G, Gomez MT, *et al.* Suppressed spontaneous and stimulated growth hormone secretion in patients with Cushing's disease before and after surgical care. *J Clin Endocrinol Metab* 1994; **78**: 131–7.
23 Carroll P, Monson JP, Grossman AB, *et al.* Successful treatment of childhood-onset Cushing's disease is associated with persistent reduction in growth hormone secretion. *Clin Endocrinol* 2004; **60**: 169–74.
24 Davies JH, Storr HL, Davies K, *et al.* Final adult height and body mass index after cure of paediatric Cushing's disease. *Clin Endocrinol* 2005; **62**: 466–72.

32

Gonadal disorders

S FAISAL AHMED

INTRODUCTION

Longitudinal growth is controlled by the activity of chondrocytes in the epiphyseal growth plates of long bones and many hormones; growth factors as well as nutritional status are involved in the regulation of this process. Among these, sex steroids are of crucial importance and the most obvious demonstration of their effect on human growth is the initiation, maintenance, and decline of the pubertal growth spurt. Adequate levels of thyroid hormone and cortisol continue to be prerequisites, but the gonadal steroid hormones play a pre-eminent role in controlling pubertal growth. However, it is possible that low-level estrogen production of the infantile ovary may play a part in influencing pre-pubertal growth and skeletal maturation as suggested by the relatively faster maturation of bones of female infants.[1]

Although the growth hormone/insulin-like growth factor-I (GH/IGF-I) axis and gonadal steroids continue to exert independent effects, it is the interaction between these two that underlines the dramatic alterations in growth and skeletal development. The observation that puberty, itself, is delayed in boys and girls with GH deficiency or insensitivity, and that, rhGH treatment reduces this delay shows that the relationship between the gonadal and the GH/IGF-I axes is truly bi-directional.[2,3]

The gonadal disorders that are associated with abnormal growth are primarily those that present with abnormal puberty but it is increasingly recognized that abnormal growth is also a feature of a number of disorders of gonadal development. A thorough understanding of the abnormal growth that accompanies many gonadal disorders requires the interpretation of the effects of steroid hormones on growth as well as other factors that influence chondrogenesis and skeletal development (see Chapter 3). The effect of sex steroids on growth can be examined in detail at two levels, the systemic level and at the local level of the growth plate. Current knowledge about the mechanisms by which these hormones influence growth is, therefore, summarized, before dealing, specifically, with the growth problems associated with gonadal disorders.

It has to be borne in mind, however, that abnormal statural growth is only one of the many problems that are encountered by children with disorders of gonads and sex steroid production. Whilst growth, per se, may not lead to any functional problems, it is quite likely that its recognition may allow the identification of the gonadal disorder and the associated problems that may exist long-term, in bone, cardiovascular, psychosocial or reproductive health. Some of these conditions, such as Turner syndrome and congenital adrenal hyperplasia are covered in other chapters.

SYNTHESIS AND ACTION OF SEX STEROIDS

Although the gonads are the major source of circulating levels of sex steroids in the body, several mammalian peripheral tissues, including growth plate chondrocytes, contain enzymes that are present in the gonads and which are also capable of formation of active androgens and estrogens in the peripheral tissues.[4-6] Dihydroepiandrosterone (DHEA), its sulfate, DHEAS, and androstenedione (A4) are the most abundant 19-carbon steroids, circulating products of the adrenal glands. The androgenic activity of DHEA (and DHEAS) and A4 is 20 times and 10 times less than that of testosterone (T), respectively. Although, the production of

T by the adrenal is minimal and the androgenic activity of the circulating adrenal-derived 19-carbon steroids is very low, the latter can, nevertheless, act as substrate for the formation of T in peripheral tissues, a clear example of intracrinology where the major enzymes involved include type I and II 17β-hydroxysteroid dehydrogenase (HSD), steroid sulfatase (STS) and 3β-HSD. Finally, 5α-reductase irreversibly convedrts T into dihydrotestosterone (DHT) which has a 3 times higher androgenic activity than T. Peripheral synthesis of estrogens can also occur from adrenal derived androgens using the same enzymes that are involved in estrogen synthesis in the ovary. The aromatase p450 mediates the conversion of the androgens, A4 and T, into the estrogens, estrone (E1) and estradiol (E2). Type I 17β-HSD converts E$_1$ to E$_2$, whereas type II 17β-HSD catalyzes the conversion in the opposite direction.

SEX STEROIDS AND THE GROWTH PLATE

A number of studies have unequivocally demonstrated the presence of the androgen receptor (AR) and both estrogen receptors, ERα and ERβ, in growth plate tissue at the mRNA and protein level in several species, including rat, rabbit, and human,[7] suggesting that androgens and estrogens can directly regulate processes in the growth plate. Although, androgens may have direct effects on growth plate cartilage and, thus, on longitudinal bone growth, this has been difficult to prove. Non-aromatizable androgens, such as DHT have been shown to regulate both proliferation and differentiation of cultured human epiphyseal chondrocytes, probably by promoting local IGF-I synthesis and increasing IGF-I receptor expression.[8,9]

Estrogen has a number of effects on the growth plate. First, estrogen has separate and independent effects on chondroblast proliferation and on active epiphyseal fusion. Second, it has a biphasic effect on proliferation, which is stimulated by low levels and inhibited by high levels.[10] The latter predominate in late adolescence in both sexes, leading initially to growth cessation and subsequently to active fusion.[11] This dual effect of estrogen has only recently become clear and has often been overlooked because the second effect is much easier to demonstrate radiographically than the first, and it is also contrary to popular thinking that growth cessation occurs following epiphyseal fusion.[12]

SEX STEROIDS AND THE SYSTEMIC GH/IGF–I AXIS

At the level of the hypothalamic–pituitary axis, sex steroids have both organizational and activational effects on the GH axis. These effects range from modulating the number of hypothalamic neurons controlling GH secretion, their responsiveness to later exposure to sex steroids, and the synaptic connectivity and neuropeptide production, to modulation of somatotroph numbers in the anterior pituitary

and their responsiveness to inputs controlling GH synthesis and secretion.[13] During puberty, a 1.5- to three-fold increase in the pulsatile secretion of GH occurs, together with over a three-fold increase in serum IGF-I concentration, which peaks at 14.5 years in girls and 1 year later in boys.[14] The rise in mean 24 h GH levels during puberty results from an increase in the maximal GH secretory rate (pulse amplitude) and in the mass of GH per secretory burst.[15,16] The differential increase in GH secretion between boys and girls at puberty mirrors the pattern of change in growth velocity. Girls show a significant rise in circulating GH levels beginning at Tanner breast stage 2, with the highest levels found at Tanner breast stage 3–4. In boys, the increase in GH levels occurs later and the peak coincides with Tanner genital stage 4.[17] By the time adolescent development is complete, the levels of GH and IGF-I decrease to prepubertal values in both genders.

Androgens

Androgens are known to stimulate growth during childhood and adolescence, but large doses will also restrict future growth, evidenced by an acceleration of bone age in excess of chronological age. The latter is very much a matter of the amount and type of androgen administered and the potential for conversion to estradiol. When considering the effects on growth, androgens can be divided into two major functional classes: those that can be aromatized to estrogens (e.g., testosterone) and those that cannot (e.g., dihydrotestosterone and several synthetic androgens). The former may have a dual action – as androgens and (after aromatization) as estrogens. Oxandrolone, a non-aromatizable androgen may also stimulate growth (e.g., boys with delayed puberty), but it seems to do this without the typical increase in GH and IGF-I levels seen after testosterone administration.[18–20] DHT, another non-aromatizable androgen may even lower GH and IGF-I levels.[21,22] For these reasons, it could be hypothesized that the increase in GH and IGF-I blood levels, and also the advancement of bone age, which are seen after testosterone administration are to a large extent an effect of estrogens, and that 'pure', non-aromatizable androgens stimulate growth through other mechanisms – possibly directly on the growth cartilage. The impaired long bone growth in mice with androgen receptor deficiency has been reported to relate to low circulating concentrations of IGF-I.[23] Although testosterone plays an important role in augmenting spontaneous GH secretion and production,[24] the ability of testosterone to stimulate pituitary GH secretion is primarily via its aromatization to estrogen;[22] in addition, this GH promoting effect is transient and only evident during puberty despite high testosterone concentrations in adulthood.

Estrogens

In contrast, the effect of estrogen on GH secretion is variable; low doses of estrogen stimulate GH secretion and

IGF-I production whereas higher doses inhibit IGF-I production at the hepatic level.[25] This response also depends on the form of estrogen itself.[26] In addition, some forms of estrogens such as those produced endogenously may also increase GH sensitivity in peripubertal children.[27] The condition, androgen insensitivity syndrome (AIS) has proved that, even in the complete absence of androgen action, there is a pronounced pubertal growth spurt at the time of surging estrogens, with a timing and magnitude between that of males and females.[28] Estrogens can also enhance the GH response to acute provocation tests.[29] The stimulatory effect of estrogen on GH secretion in both sexes has been confirmed by studies using non-aromatizable androgens or estrogen-receptor antagonists in pubertal boys showing decreased GH and IGF-I levels.[30,31] Conversely, use of the androgen-receptor antagonist flutamide is associated with increasing circulating GH concentrations.[32] The stimulatory effect of estrogen on GH secretion is mediated via the ERα and ERβ receptors which are expressed in the anterior pituitary as well as the hypothalamus. Female mice with a knock-out of ERα (ERKO) have decreased femur length and this decrease is associated with lower serum IGF-I.[33] Conversely, knock-out of ERβ (BERKO) in mice results in an increased length of femur with an increase of serum IGF-I.[34] It is possible that these inhibitory effects on appendicular growth may be sex and age specific and require further investigation in primates.[35] Interestingly, the length of femur and serum levels of IGF-I were, in female double ER knock-out (DERKO) mice, intermediate between ERKO and BERKO mice.[34] These experiments suggest that the opposing effects of estrogen via the two receptors are related to differential effects on circulating IGF-I levels. Clinically, raloxifene, the selective estrogen receptor modulator that selectively acts as an ERβ agonist acts peripherally at the hepatic level to reduce IGF-I production and recently has been described as an adjunct to treatment in acromegaly.[36] However, the rapid decline in the growth of girls with tall stature who have been treated with large doses of estrogens is only associated with a moderate decrease in circulating IGF-I[37] highlighting the importance of estrogen at the level of the growth plate.

Two rare syndromes have amply demonstrated that, even in the male, estrogens are needed for completing epiphyseal closure and full bone mineralization. Smith[38] described a man with a homozygous null mutation in the ERα gene, which rendered him insensitive to estrogenic hormones. He was of mean height at age 15, but in spite of normal male sexual maturation and puberty, he never stopped growing and was 206 cm at 28 years of age. Radiological examination revealed non-ossified physeal growth plates and osteoporosis. Second, a recently described man with a genetic deficiency of aromatase activity (therefore unable to synthesize estrogens) showed a similar clinical picture: tall stature, non-ossified growth plates (bone age of 14 years at a chronological age of 24 years) and osteoporosis. He was treated with estrogens in an attempt to improve bone mineral status and stop his growth.[39] These two clinical syndromes, as well as AIS, suggest that, in humans, not only does estrogen increases growth rate, but also that it may cause physeal ossification, and thus terminates the growth period.

DISORDERS OF PUBERTY

Premature sexual maturation

Early maturation is defined as the development of sexual characteristics before the age of 8 years in girls and 9 years in boys. The prominent clinical feature of premature sexual maturation is breast development in girls and testicular development in boys. Also, the occurrence of menarche in girls before age 10 years indicates sexual precocity. In the US, these criteria were reconsidered following a community-based study of more than 17 000 girls showing a trend towards earlier breast development in otherwise healthy girls.[40,41] Interestingly, the 50th percentile for menarcheal age was unchanged from previous standards at 12.7 years, indicating that earlier onset of breast development might be associated with slower progression of puberty. In countries other than the US, there is no evidence of recent reduction in age at onset of female or male puberty although it is recognized that detecting early signs of breast development in girls, especially those who are overweight can be difficult.[42]

PREMATURE THELARCHE AND THELARCHE VARIANT

Isolated premature thelarche is a common disorder, characterized by breast development in girls, usually under the age of 2 years and with no other signs of puberty. Growth and bone age are normal unless accompanied by excess adiposity. The extent of the breast development may be asymmetrical and commonly fluctuates up and down. This condition is self-limiting over a few years and it is likely that most girls are following a familial predisposition towards early puberty and age at menarche may be at the lower end of the normal range;[43] final height is, however, unaffected and within the parental target range.[44] In girls, there are other forms of premature sexual development that exist as a continuum between isolated premature thelarche and central precocious puberty, with a gradation of endocrinology and ovarian ultrasound appearance which have been variably termed as slowly progressive precocious puberty or thelarche variant[45,46] and approximately 15 percent of girls with isolated premature thelarche may progress via this continuum to central precocious puberty.[47] Thelarche variant may be associated with the presence of pubic hair and detectable serum estradiol but the LH-predominant response to LHRH-stimulation, that is typically seen in central precocious puberty, is absent. These girls do, however have an advanced bone age and an increased height velocity[46] but current studies suggest that final height is unaffected.[48]

ISOLATED PREMATURE MENARCHE

Repeated vaginal bleeding in girls without any other signs of sexual development is described as premature menarche. Ovarian follicular cysts have been reported in these girls. However, it is important to exclude the presence of a local lesion of the genital tract, McCune–Albright syndrome (premature menarche may rapidly be followed by vulvovaginal and breast changes), exogenous administration of estrogens and child abuse. Premature menarche seems to be a benign and self-limiting condition and final height does not seem to be affected.[49]

PREMATURE ADRENARCHE

Premature adrenarche is defined as premature development of sexual hair (pubic hair, axillary hair or both) before 8 years of age in girls or 9 years of age in boys, with no other signs of sexual maturation, with a peak of frequency between the ages of 5 and 8 years. The etiology is unknown, but there is premature activation of adrenal androgen secretion from the zona reticularis of the adrenal cortex with plasma levels of dehydroepiandrosterone (DHEA-S), androstenedione and urinary 17-ketosteroids in the range normally seen in older pubertal children. The term 'premature pubarche' is reserved for the scenario where the premature development of sexual hair is not associated with any other signs of sexual maturation or biochemical evidence of excess androgen secretion. The condition is more commonly reported in girls than in boys and in children of South Asian or Afro-Caribbean origin. Familial transmission is rare. At presentation, children may be taller and have an advanced bone age. Pre-pubertal growth in affected girls is enhanced with respect to normal controls, and this enhancement may be compensated for by a reduction of the pubertal growth component leading to a final height in accordance with the target height.[50,51]

CENTRAL PRECOCIOUS PUBERTY

In central precocious puberty (CPP) or gonadotrophin dependent precocious puberty, premature cascade activation of the hypothalamic pituitary gonadal system results in virilization in boys and feminization in girls, with acceleration of linear growth and bone maturation in both sexes. CPP is by far much more frequent in girls than in boys. In boys, typically, CPP is associated with a clearly identifiable underlying pathological entity and in this situation it does not present a therapeutic or a diagnostic dilemma; this is in contrast to CPP in girls where an underlying pathology is much rarer and the benefits of therapy may not be as clear. CPP will cause an acceleration of growth rate but these children will also show premature ossification and fusion of the growth cartilage and early cessation of growth. Although it has been reported that girls with very early puberty presenting before 6 years of age will, on average, lose 12–15 cm in final height, whereas girls with puberty between 6 and 9 years lose 7–10 cm,[52] the risk of short stature may have been overestimated and more recently, there is some concern about over-treatment of the condition.[41,53] The risk of short stature is greater in children who may have accompanying GH insufficiency or limited potential to grow due to cranial or craniospinal irradiation. Early puberty may result in a higher sitting height to leg length ratio as a final sign of the premature bone maturation. The interpretation of height gain data in CPP patients must take into account the inaccuracy of adult height predictions which are based on bone age estimation, a technique based on reference data from normal healthy children. Furthermore, considering that CPP is at one extreme of a continuum of a group of conditions of premature sexual maturation, it is not surprising that the tempo of pubertal advance and bone age advance may be variable and the response to treatment will be influenced by these features.[54–56] In some cases, the case for intervention may be more influenced by the need to ameliorate any behavioral or pyschosocial upset in the child.[56]

GONADOTROPHIN-INDEPENDENT PRECOCIOUS PUBERTY

Gonadotrophin-independent precocious puberty (GIPP) is characterized by pubertal sex steroid concentrations with pre-pubertal or suppressed gonadotrophins. The possibility of disorders of the gonad or adrenal gland or an autonomous secretion of gonadotrophins by a tumor should be excluded. GIPP has been described in girls with McCune–Albright syndrome characterized by irregular areas of skin pigmentation and polyostotic fibrous dysplasia. In this condition, the accelerated growth may also be due to coexisting hyperthyroidism or GH excess. GIPP may also occur in children with primary hypothyroidism; in affected girls, there is usually isolated breast development and cystic ovarian enlargement without a growth spurt. Boys with primary hypothyroidism may have a larger testicular volume than would be expected for their stage of sexual maturation or rate of growth. Thyroxine treatment may be associated with catch-up growth and normalization of the lack of consonance of normal puberty but final height may be shorter owing to a rapid advance in epiphyseal maturation.[57] In males, another cause of GIPP which is associated with increased linear growth is testotoxicosis or familial male precocious puberty (FMPP).[58] The timing of the onset of central, gonadotrophin puberty can be predicted by the degree of skeletal maturation as there is a remarkable degree of synchrony between timing of central puberty and skeletal maturation across the various disorders of puberty.[59] In all these cases, the clinical picture is dominated by the signs of excess sex steroid production for age, including accelerated growth rate. The final height may be compromised depending on the time of diagnosis and the success of the treatment. However, in a recently reported case that was untreated, a prolonged period of a marked growth spurt of 12.5 cm year^{-1} from the age of 3.8 years to 9.0 years ensured that the boy's final height, which was reached at the age of 13, was within the target height.[60]

PRE-PUBERTAL GYNECOMASTIA

Gynecomastia in pre-pubertal children may occur due to a number of reasons.[61] Most boys with idiopathic gynecomastia are tall and relatively obese and it is possible that they have a higher peripheral aromatase activity that explains their tall stature.[62] Aromatase excess that is detectable by routine endocrine assays may be responsible for this condition in about 10 percent of cases.[63] These cases of aromatase excess, which may be associated with gain of function mutations in the aromatase gene[64] are reported to have an increase in height velocity in contrast to those who have gynecomastia without apparent increased aromatase activity.[63,65]

Delayed sexual maturation

Sexual maturation may be delayed due to a delay in activation of the hypothalamic–pituitary trigger of gonadal function or due to a primary defect of the gonad, itself. The former is the commonest and is typically diagnosed in generally healthy adolescents. This primary, physiological state of transient hypogonadotrophic hypogonadism in otherwise well children needs to be differentiated from the secondary delayed growth and puberty that is often seen in children with chronic disease, as well as defects of GH synthesis and action.

PRIMARY DELAY OF GROWTH AND PUBERTY

Often referred to as constitutional delayed growth and puberty, this diagnosis should be reserved for, otherwise, healthy adolescents when stature is reduced for chronological age but is generally appropriate for stage of pubertal development and bone maturation, both of which are usually delayed. There is, usually, a relatively short upper body segment, both at presentation and at final height.[66] Although the final height in patients with primary delayed growth and puberty is predicted to be normal based on bone age estimation, it is possible that some do not reach the third percentile or remain in the lowest part of their family's target range.[66–68] This condition is often associated with a family history of delayed puberty and it is much more common in boys than in girls; the condition also seems to be commoner in children with a past history of atopy.[69] Sex steroid treatment will induce a growth spurt which, after the onset of spontaneous puberty, will be sustained in the post-treatment period and become indistinguishable from the spontaneous growth spurt of puberty. Low-dose sex steroid therapy does not decrease or increase the height potential.[70,71] However, it is possible that aromatase inhibitors may increase the adult height of boys with delayed puberty.[72]

SECONDARY DELAY OF GROWTH AND PUBERTY

Virtually every child with any chronic disease could present with delayed puberty (due to recurrent infections, immunodeficiency, gastrointestinal disease, renal disturbances, respiratory illnesses, chronic anemia, endocrine disease, eating disorders, exercise and a number of miscellaneous abnormalities).[73] The degree to which growth and pubertal development are affected in chronic illness depends upon the type of disease as well as other factors such as the age, duration of illness and its severity, nutritional status and concurrent medications. The earlier its onset and the longer and more severe the illness, the greater the effect on growth and pubertal development. This form of delayed puberty has often been mistaken for primary or constitutional delayed growth and puberty which is a temporary phenomenon and not as profound or protracted. However, its clinical importance is relevant due to the larger number of children with chronic disorders who are now surviving past the age of puberty and expect a better quality of life. Considering that adults with a history of primary delay in growth and puberty may be relatively short, it is not surprising that there are reports of continuing short stature in the third decade in some adults with childhood onset chronic disease, and especially those who have had treatment with glucocorticoids.[74,75]

HYPOGONADAL ENDOCRINOPATHY

These can be divided into three broad categories, hypogonadotrophic hypogonadism, hypergonadotrophic hypogonadism and finally, the hypogonadism that is described in association with other endocrine disorders.

Hypogonadotrophic hypogonadism

In hypogonadotrophic hypogonadism, such as Kallman's syndrome, there may be a complete absence of puberty, including absence of the pubertal growth spurt. If human growth is illustrated by the so-called infancy–childhood–puberty (ICP) model,[76] the pubertal component will be missing while the childhood component will be normal. The growth rate will decline in an asymptotic fashion, so that by age 15 or 16 years it may be down to 3 cm year^{-1} or less. However, growth will not cease completely until late in the third decade, and the final height may be taller than average in untreated cases. The price of this is abnormal ('eunuchoid') body proportions, illustrating the observation that sex hormones tend to mature the skeleton in a centripetal fashion – from the periphery towards the central parts. Although initially stature tends to be low for chronological age but normal for bone age, sex steroid replacement results in normal final height.[77]

Primary hypogonadism

Inability of the gonads to respond to gonadotrophins to produce sufficient amounts of sex steroids will cause the same disordered growth as described under hypogonadotrophic hypogonadism. The most common cause of primary hypogonadism in boys, Klinefelter syndrome (47,XXY) is, however, associated with tallness in itself and does not therefore manifest itself as short stature – rather the opposite! Growth of pre-pubertal Klinefelter syndrome boys is increased all through childhood, even before androgen deficiency is manifest. Actually, pre-pubertal boys with Klinefelter syndrome are not androgen deficient; on the contrary, testosterone levels in saliva from Klinefelter syndrome boys have been found to be higher than in those of controls until early puberty. Thereafter, testicular involution and androgen deficiency become obvious.[78]

In pre-natal testicular atrophy, such as in the case of 'the vanishing testes' (sometimes incorrectly named testicular aplasia), the childhood component of growth seems to be normal, illustrating that the normal low baseline secretion of testicular androgens in childhood is of little importance for linear growth.

In the most common form of ovarian dysgenesis, Turner syndrome, the growth pattern is influenced by both the skeletal problems inherent to the absence of one X chromosome (including mildly disproportionate short stature) and the absence or deficiency of estrogens during adolescence. If the ovaries completely lack follicles, the previous deterioration of growth rate will be further accentuated in puberty, as a result of the lack of a growth spurt. In those cases of Turner mosaicism, when one cell line includes a Y chromosome (e.g., 45,X/46,XY or girls with mixed gonadal dysgenesis), final height is significantly higher than in pure 45,X individuals.

Hypogonadism with other endocrinopathy

Patients with GH deficiency or a GH receptor defect are often reported to have delayed puberty. The common feature in these conditions is a low IGF-I level or lack of IGF-I function. Therefore, one of the factors that switch on puberty is believed to be the amount of IGF-I secretion.[2,3] Delayed puberty was also reported previously in children with type 1 diabetes mellitus (T1DM) but more recent studies do not confirm this finding and do not show any evidence of restricted final height. However, there is some evidence to suggest that the pubertal growth spurt may be attenuated in T1DM.[79] Primary hypothyroidism is associated with subnormal responses of LH to GnRH administration and normal response to hCG.[80] Thyroid hormone is known to affect sex hormone-binding hormonal globulin (SHBG) concentrations and free testosterone concentrations which may be low seem to normalize after thyroid hormone replacement. Hypothyroidism may delay the onset of puberty or menarche and treatment with levothyroxine reverses this pattern. Even though growth may continue for a longer period after start of therapy, final height may be permanently restricted.[81] Cushing's syndrome can cause delayed onset or arrest of puberty which can be corrected by removal of the source.[82,83]

DISORDERS OF GONADAL AND SEXUAL DEVELOPMENT

Some of these conditions have already been covered under the section on 'primary hypogonadism'. In boys with mixed gonadal dysgenesis (45,X/46,XY), short stature during the childhood growth phase is generally not the result of androgen deficiency, but rather the result of their 45,X cell line which causes short stature, which is dependent on the degree of mosaicism, similar to the situation for girls with Turner syndrome.

Other sex chromosome abnormalities in girls include 46,XY pure gonadal dysgenesis, 47,XXX (triple X syndrome) and androgen insensitivity syndrome (AIS). In addition to the influence of abnormal sex hormone production or sensitivity in puberty, their growth may also be influenced by other growth-enhancing genes (of unknown nature) of the Y and the X chromosomes. The Y chromosome as well as the supernumerary X chromosomes in males will be associated with tall stature. The final height of 47,XXX girls has been reported to be similar to that of controls,[78] although 46,XY girls with complete AIS end up with a height in between that of normal women and men.[28,84] Girls with complete AIS with intact gonads have a normal, female pubertal growth spurt despite lack of androgen action.[28] Ogata and Matsuo[85] compared the adult height of published cases of patients with XX gonadal dysgenesis (XXGD) and those with XY gonadal dysgenesis (XYGD) and found that the mean adult height of XYGD patients was significantly greater than that of XXGD patients. This finding supports the existence of Y specific growth genes that promote statural growth independently of the effects of gonadal sex steroids.[86] Early gonadectomy does not alter the childhood component of growth emphasizing the relative lack of importance of sex steroids in the pre-pubertal phase of normal growth.[87]

> ## KEY LEARNING POINTS
>
> - Sex steroids are crucial for growth primarily through their effect on the initiation, maintenance and decline of the pubertal growth spurt.
> - The bi-directional interaction between sex steroids, primarily estrogen, and GH/IGF-I axis at the systemic level and at the local level of the growth plate underlines the dramatic alterations in growth and skeletal development.
> - Cessation of longitudinal bone growth may precede epiphyseal fusion.
> - The sex chromosomes may have a sex-steroid independent influence on linear growth.
> - The likelihood of short stature in children with premature sexual maturation, particularly older girls with isolated gonadotrophin-dependent precocious puberty may have been overestimated in the past.
> - Delayed puberty occurs commonly in children with chronic disease and these children may have a shorter final height than expected for their target height.

REFERENCES

● = Seminal primary article

◆ = Key review paper

● 1   Hochberg Z. *Endocrine Control of Skeletal Maturation: Annotation to Bone Age Readings.* Basel: Karger AG, 2002.

● 2   Laron Z, Sarel R, Pertzelan A. Puberty in Laron type dwarfism. *Eur J Pediatr* 1980; **134**: 79–83.

3   Tanaka T, Cohen P, Clayton PE, *et al.* Diagnosis and management of growth hormone deficiency in childhood and adolescence – part 2: growth hormone treatment in growth hormone deficient children. *Growth Horm IGF Res* 2002; **12**: 323–41.

4   Labrie F, Luu-The V, Lin SX, *et al.* Intracrinology: role of the family of 17β-hydroxysteroid dehydrogenases in human physiology and disease. *J Mol Endocrinol* 2000; **25**: 1–16.

5   Simpson E, Rubin G, Clyne C, *et al.* The role of local estrogen biosynthesis in males and females. *Trends Endocrinol Metab* 2000; **11**: 184–8.

● 6   Van Der Eerden BC, Van De Ven J, Lowik CW, *et al.* Sex steroid metabolism in the tibial growth plate of the rat. *Endocrinology* 2002; **143**: 4048–55.

◆ 7   Vanderschueren D, Vandenput L, Boonen S, *et al.* Androgens and bone. *Endocr Rev* 2004; **25**: 389–425.

8   Blanchard O, Tsagris L, Rappaport R, *et al.* Age-dependent responsiveness of rabbit and human cartilage cells to sex steroids in vitro. *J Steroid Biochem Mol Biol* 1991; **40**: 711–6.

9   Krohn K, Haffner D, Hugel U, *et al.* 1,25(OH)2D3 and dihydrotestosterone interact to regulate proliferation and differentiation of epiphyseal chondrocytes. *Calcif Tissue Int* 2003; **73**: 400–10.

◆ 10   Frank GR. Role of estrogen and androgen in pubertal skeletal physiology. *Med Pediatr Oncol* 2003; **41**: 217–21.

● 11   Weise MS, De-Levi KM, Barnes RI, *et al.* Effects of estrogen on growth plate senescence and epiphyseal fusion. *Proc Natl Acad Sci USA* 2001; **98**: 6871–6.

◆ 12   Parfitt MM. Misconceptions (1): Epiphyseal fusion causes cessation of growth. *Bone* 2002; **30**: 337–9.

13   Chowen JA, Frago LM, Argente J. The regulation of GH secretion by sex steroids. *Eur J Endocrinol* 2004; **151(Suppl 3)**: U95–100.

14   Juul A, Bang P, Hertel NT, *et al.* Serum insulin-like growth factor-I in 1030 healthy children, adolescents, and adults: relation to age, sex, stage of puberty, testicular size, and body mass index. *J Clin Endocrinol Metab* 1994; **78**: 744–52.

● 15   Martha PM Jr, Gorman KM, Blizzard RM, *et al.* Endogenous growth hormone secretion and clearance rates in normal boys, as determined by deconvolution analysis: relationship to age, pubertal status, and body mass. *J Clin Endocrinol Metab* 1992; **74**: 336–44.

16   Rose SR, Municchi G, Barnes KM, *et al.* Spontaneous growth hormone secretion increases during puberty in normal girls and boys. *J Clin Endocrinol Metab* 1991; **73**: 428–35.

● 17   Albertsson-Wikland K, Rosberg S, Karlberg J, Groth T. Analysis of 24-hour growth hormone profiles in healthy boys and girls of normal stature: relation to puberty. *J Clin Endocrinol Metab* 1994; **78**: 1195–201.

18   Ulloa-Aguirre A, Blizzard RM, Garcia-Rubi E, *et al.* Testosterone and oxandrolone, a nonaromatizable androgen, specifically amplify the mass and rate of growth hormone (GH) secreted per burst without altering GH secretory burst duration or frequency or the GH half-life. *J Clin Endocrinol Metab* 1990; **71**: 846–54.

19   Malhotra A, Poon E, Tse WY, *et al.* The effects of oxandrolone on the growth hormone and gonadal axes in boys with constitutional delay of growth and puberty. *Clin Endocrinol (Oxf)* 1993; **38**: 393–8.

20   Crowne EC, Wallace WH, Moore C, *et al.* Effect of low dose oxandrolone and testosterone treatment on the pituitary-testicular and GH axes in boys with constitutional delay of growth and puberty. *Clin Endocrinol (Oxf)* 1997; **46**: 209–16.

21   Eakman GD, Dallas JS, Ponder SW, Keenan BS. The effects of testosterone and dihydrotestosterone on hypothalamic regulation of growth hormone secretion. *J Clin Endocrinol Metab* 1996; **81**: 1217–23.

● 22   Keenan BS, Richards GE, Ponder SW, *et al.* Androgen-stimulated pubertal growth: The effect of testosterone and dihydrotestosterone on GH and IGF-I in the treatment of short stature and delayed puberty. *J Clin Endocrinol Metab* 1993; **76**: 996–1001.

23   Vanderschueren D, Van Herck E, Suiker AM, *et al.* Bone and mineral metabolism in the androgen-resistant (testicular feminized) male rat. *J Bone Miner Res* 1993; **8**: 801–9.

24   Martha PM Jr, Rogol AD, Veldhuis JD, *et al.* Alterations in the pulsatile properties of circulating growth hormone concentrations during puberty in boys. *J Clin Endocrinol Metab* 1989; **69**: 563–70.

25   Ho KY, Evans WS, Blizzard RM, *et al.* Effects of sex and age on the 24-hour profile of growth hormone secretion in man: importance of endogenous estradiol concentrations. *J Clin Endocrinol Metab* 1987; **64**: 51–8.

◆ 26   Leung KC, Johannsson G, Leong GM, Ho KK. Estrogen regulation of growth hormone action. *Endocr Rev* 2004; **25**: 693–721.

27   Coutant R, de Casson FB, Rouleau S, *et al.* Divergent effect of endogenous and exogenous sex steroids on the insulin-like growth factor I response to growth hormone in short normal adolescents *J Clin Endocrinol Metab* 2004; **89**: 6185–92.

28   Zachmann M, Prader A, Sobel EH, *et al.* Pubertal growth in patients with androgen insensitivity: Indirect evidence for the importance of estrogens in pubertal growth of girls. *J Pediatr* 1986; **108**: 694–7.

29   Marin G, Domené HM, Barnes KM, *et al.* The effects of estrogen priming and puberty on the growth hormone response to standardized tread-mill exercise and arginine-insulin in normal girls and boys. *J Clin Endocrinol Metab* 1994; **79**: 537–41.

30 Metzger DL, Kerrigan JR. Estrogen receptor blockade with tamoxifen diminishes growth hormone secretion in boys: evidence for a stimulatory role of endogenous estrogens during male adolescence. *J Clin Endocrinol Metab* 1994; **79**: 513–8.

31 Veldhuis JD, Metzger DL, Martha PM Jr, *et al.* Estrogen and testosterone, but not a nonaromatizable androgen, direct network integration of the hypothalamo-somatotrope (growth hormone)-insulin-like growth factor I axis in the human: evidence from pubertal pathophysiology and sex-steroid hormone replacement. *J Clin Endocrinol Metab* 1997; **82**: 3414–20.

32 Metzger DL, Kerrigan JR. Androgen receptor blockade with flutamide enhances growth hormone secretion in late pubertal males: evidence for independent actions of estrogen and androgen. *J Clin Endocrinol Metab* 1993; **76**: 1147–52.

33 Vidal O, Lindberg M, Savendahl L, *et al.* Disproportional body growth in female estrogen receptor-alpha-inactivated mice. *Biochem Biophys Res Commun* 1999; **265**: 569–71.

34 Lindberg MK, Alatalo SL, Halleen JM, *et al.* Estrogen receptor specificity in the regulation of the skeleton in female mice. *J Endocrinol* 2001; **171**: 229–36.

35 Chagin AS, Lindberg MK, Andersson N, *et al.* Estrogen receptor-beta inhibits skeletal growth and has the capacity to mediate growth plate fusion in female mice. *J Bone Miner Res* 2004; **19**: 72–7.

36 Dimaraki EV, Symons KV, Barkan AL. Raloxifene decreases serum IGF-I in male patients with active acromegaly. *Eur J Endocrinol* 2004; **150**: 481–7.

37 Svan H, Ritzén EM, Hall K, *et al.* Estrogens treatment of tall girls: Dose dependency of effects on subsequent growth and IGF-I levels in blood. *Acta Paediatr Scand* 1991; **80**: 328–32.

● 38 Smith E. Estrogen resistance caused by a mutation in the estrogen receptor gene in a man. *New Engl J Med* 1994; **331**: 1056–61.

● 39 Morishima A, Grumbach MM, Simpson ER, *et al.* Aromatase deficiency in male and female siblings caused by a novel mutation and the physiological role of estrogens. *J Clin Endocrinol Metab* 1995; **80**: 3689–98.

40 Herman-Giddens ME, Slora EJ, Wasserman RC, *et al.* Secondary sexual characteristics and menses in young girls seen in office practice: a study from the Pediatric Research in Office Settings Network. *Pediatrics* 1997, **99**: 505–12.

◆ 41 Kaplowitz PB, Oberfield SE, and the Drug and Therapeutics and Executive Committees of the Lawson Wilkins Pediatric Endocrine Society: Reexamination of the age limit for defining when puberty is precocious in girls in the United States: implications for evaluation and treatment. *Pediatrics* 1999, **104**: 936–41.

◆ 42 Parent AS, Teilmann G, Juul A, *et al.* The timing of normal puberty and the age limits of sexual precocity: variations around the world, secular trends, and changes after migration. *Endocr Rev* 2003; **24**: 668–93.

● 43 van Winter JT, Noller KL, Zimmerman D, Melton LJ. Natural history of premature thelarche in Olmsted County, Minnesota, 1940 to 1984. *J Pediatr* 1990; **116**: 278–80.

● 44 Salardi, Cacciari E, Mainetti B, *et al.* Outcome of premature thelarche: relation to puberty and final height. *Arch Dis Child* 1998; **79**: 173–4.

45 Fontoura M, Brauner R, Prevot C, Rappaport R. Precocious puberty in girls: early diagnosis of a slowly progressing variant. *Arch Dis Child* 1989; **64**: 1170–6.

46 Stanhope R, Brook CGD. Thelarche variant: a new syndrome of precocious sexual maturation? *Acta Endocrinol (Copenh)* 1990; **123**: 481–6.

47 Volta C, Bernasconi S, Cisternino M, *et al.* Isolated premature thelarche and thelarche variant: clinical and auxological follow-up of 119 girls. *J Endocrinol Invest* 1998; **21**: 180–3.

48 Palmert MR, Malin HV, Boepple PA. Unsustained or slowly progressive puberty in young girls: initial presentation and long-term follow-up of 20 untreated patients. *J Clin Endocrinol Metab* 1999, **84**: 415–23.

49 Saggese G, Ghirri P, Del Vecchio A, *et al.* Gonadotropin pulsatile secretion in girls with premature menarche. *Horm Res* 1990; **33**: 5–10.

50 Ghizzoni L, Milani S. The natural history of premature adrenarche. *J Pediatr Endocrinol Metab* 2000; **13(Suppl 5)**: 1247–51.

51 Pere A, Perheentupa J, Peter M, Voutilainen R. Follow up of growth and steroids in premature adrenarche. *Eur J Pediatr* 1995; **154**: 346–52.

52 Kletter GB, Kelch RP. Effects of gonadotropin-releasing hormone analogue therapy on adult stature in precocious puberty. *J Clin Endocrinol Metab* 1994; **79**: 331–4.

◆ 53 Oerter Klein K. Precocious puberty: Who has it? Who should be treated? [Editorial]. *J Clin Endocrinol Metab* 1999; **84**: 411–4.

54 Lazar L, Pertzelan A, Weintrob N, *et al.* Sexual precocity in boys: Accelerated versus slowly progressive puberty gonadotropin-suppressive therapy and final height. *J Clin Endocrinol Metab* 2001; **86**: 4127–32.

55 Kreiter M, Burstein S, Rosenfield RL, *et al.* Preserving adult height potential in girls with idiopathic true precocious puberty. *J Pediatr* 1990; **117**: 364–70.

◆ 56 Partsch CJ, Heger S, Sippell WG. Management and outcome of central precocious puberty. *Clin Endocrinol* 2002; **56**: 129–48.

57 Pringle PJ, Stanhope R, Hindmarsh P, Brook CGD. Abnormal pubertal development in primary hypothyroidism. *Clin Endocrinol* 1988; **28**: 479–86.

58 Rosenthal SM, Grumbach MM, Kaplan SL. Gonadotropin-independent familial sexual precocity with premature Leydig and germinal cell maturation (familial testotoxicosis): effects of a potent luteinizing hormone-releasing factor agonist and medroxyprogesterone acetate therapy in four cases. *J Clin Endocrinol Metab* 1983; **57**: 571–9.

59. Weise M, Flor A, Barnes KM, *et al.* Determinants of growth during gonadotropin-releasing hormone analog therapy

for precocious puberty. *J Clin Endocrinol Metab* 2004; **89**: 103–7.

60 Partsch CJ, Krone N, Riepe FG, *et al.* Long-term follow-up of spontaneous development in a boy with familial male precocious puberty. *Horm Res* 2004; **62**: 177–81.

61 Stratakis CA, Batista D, Sabnis G, Brodie A. Prepubertal gynaecomastia caused by medication or the aromatase excess syndrome. *Clin Endocrinol* 2004; **61**: 779–80.

62 Sher ES, Migeon CJ, Berkovitz GD. Evaluation of boys with marked breast development at puberty. *Clin Pediatr* 1998; **37**: 367–71.

63 Einav-Bachar R, Phillip M, Aurbach-Klipper Y, Lazar L. Prepubertal gynaecomastia: aetiology, course and outcome. *Clin Endocrinol* 2004; **61**: 55–60.

64 Shozu M, Sebastian S, Takayama K, *et al.* Estrogen excess associated with novel gain-of-function mutations affecting the aromatase gene. *N Engl J Med* 2003; **348**: 1855–65.

65 Hemsell DL, Edman CD, Marks JF, *et al.* Massive extranglandular aromatization of plasma androstenedione resulting in feminization of a prepubertal boy. *J Clin Invest* 1977; **60**: 455–64.

66 Albanese A, Stanhope R. Predictive factors in the determination of final height in boys with constitutional delay of growth and puberty. *J Pediatr* 1995; **126**: 545–50.

67 Crowne EC, Shalet SM, Wallace WH, *et al.* Final height in girls with untreated constitutional delay in growth and puberty. *Eur J Pediatr* 1991; **150**: 708–12.

68 Sperlich M, Butenandt O, Schwarz HP. Final height and predicted height in boys with untreated constitutional growth delay. *Eur J Pediatr* 1995; **154**: 627–32.

69 Baum WF, Schneyer U, Lantzsch AM, Kloditz E. Delay of growth and development in children with bronchial asthma, atopic dermatitis and allergic rhinitis. *Exp Clin Endocrinol Diabetes* 2002; **110**: 53–9.

● 70 Kelly BP, Paterson WF, Donaldson MD. Final height outcome and value of height prediction in boys with constitutional delay in growth and adolescence treated with intramuscular testosterone 125 mg per month for 3 months. *Clin Endocrinol* 2003; **58**: 267–72.

71 Pozo J, Argente J. Ascertainment and treatment of delayed puberty. *Horm Res* 2003; **60(Suppl 3)**: 35–48.

● 72 Wickman S, Sipila I, Ankarberg-Lindgren C, *et al.* A specific aromatase inhibitor and potential increase in adult height in boys with delayed puberty: a randomised controlled trial. *Lancet* 2001; **357**: 1743–8.

◆ 73 Pozo J, Argente J. Delayed puberty in chronic illness. *Best Pract Res Clin Endocrinol Metab* 2002; **16**: 73–90.

74 Alemzadeh N, Rekers-Mombarg LT, Mearin ML, *et al.* Adult height in patients with early onset of Crohn's disease. *Gut* 2002; **51**: 26–9.

75 Sawczenko A, Ballinger AB, Croft NM, *et al.* Adult height in patients with early onset of Crohn's disease. *Gut* 2003; **52**: 454–5.

76 Karlberg J. On the construction of the infancy–childhood–puberty growth standard. *Acta Paediatr Scand Suppl* 1989; **356**: 26–37.

77 van der Werff ten Bosch JJ, Bot A. Some skeletal dimensions of males with isolated gonadotrophin deficiency. *Neth J Med* 1992; **41**: 259–63.

78 Ratcliffe SG, Butler GE, Jones M. Edinburgh study of growth and development of children with sex chromosome abnormalities. IV. *Birth Defects* 1990; **26**: 1–44.

79 Chiarelli F, Giannini C, Mohn A. Growth, growth factors and diabetes. *Eur J Endocrinol* 2004; **151**: 109–17.

80 Meikle AW. The interrelationships between thyroid dysfunction and hypogonadism in men and boys. *Thyroid* 2004; **14(Suppl 1)**: S17–25.

81 Pantsiouou S, Stanhope R, Uruena M, *et al.* Growth prognosis and growth after menarche in primary hypothyroidism. *Arch Dis Child* 1991; **66**: 838–40.

82 Styne DM, Grumbach MM, Kaplan SL, *et al.* Treatment of Cushing's disease in childhood and adolescence by transsphenoidal microadenomectomy. *N Engl J Med* 1984; **310**: 889–93.

83 Zadik Z, Cooper M, Chen M, Stern N. Cushing's disease presenting as pubertal arrest. *J Pediatr Endocrinol* 1993; **6**: 201–4.

84 Wisniewski AB, Migeon CJ, Meyer-Bahlburg HF, *et al.* Complete androgen insensitivity syndrome: long-term medical, surgical, and psychosexual outcome. *J Clin Endocrinol Metab* 2000; **85**: 2664–9.

85 Ogata T, Matsuo N. Comparison of adult height between patients with XX and XY gonadal dysgenesis: support for a Y specific growth gene(s). *J Med Genet* 1992; **29**: 539–41.

86 Ogata T, Tomita K, Hida A, *et al.* Chromosomal localisation of a Y specific growth gene(s). *J Med Genet* 1995; **32**: 572–5.

87 Hibi I, Tanaka T. Hormonal regulation of growth and maturation II. The effect of hormones and postnatal and pubertal growth. *Clin Pediatr Endocrinol* 1998; **7**: 1–11.

PART 5

TREATMENT OF GROWTH DISORDERS

33

Treatment of growth disorders: Growth hormone deficiency

RAYMOND L HINTZ

INTRODUCTION

Any review of the treatment of growth hormone deficiency is to a large extent the history of the therapeutic use of growth hormone.[1-4] However, it must also include the use of insulin-type growth factor-I (IGF-I), GH releasing substances such as GHRH, and the GHRP analogues and mimetic compounds. This chapter will cover the use of these substances, and the modulation of sex steroid levels to treat growth hormone deficiency (GHD) (Table 33.1). Even though at least a third of the patients with GHD have other defects in the hypothalamic–pituitary axis, including ADH, TSH, ACTH, and the gonadotropins, the treatment of these additional deficiencies will not be covered here but in other chapters. From evidence in literature and paintings it is likely that growth hormone deficiency, both isolated and as part of pan-hypopituitarism, has existed for as long as human history. Both the Pharaohs of ancient Egypt and the monarchs of seventeenth century Spain delighted in having dwarfed people, including some with proportional dwarfism and therefore likely to have GHD, among their courtiers. Deficiency in the pituitary secretion of GH was long hypothesized to be the cause of some cases of extreme short stature. However, the proof that GHD existed did not come until advances in technology led to two separate and

Table 33.1 Methods of treatment of growth hormone deficiency

- Modulation of sex steroids levels
- IGF-I as a substitute for growth hormone
- Growth hormone releasing hormone
- Growth hormone releasing peptides and related substances

IGF-I: insulin-type growth factor-I.

compelling lines of evidence. The purification of human growth hormone and the successful use of it to treat cases of severe short stature who were felt to have GHD on clinical grounds[5] provided one convincing line of evidence that GHD was responsible for their poor growth. Soon thereafter methods for measuring circulating GH levels in serum were developed[6] and allowed a direct confirmation of the diagnosis of GHD in these patients. The best available data[7] suggest that profound GHD has a prevalence in childhood of approximately 1/2000, about 1/3 of which are due to CNS tumors or their treatment. It is important to emphasize that although GH is a very important factor in the control of growth in childhood, it is by no means the only one.

Control of growth

The control of growth is a complex process, involving many hormonal and nonhormonal components. Many of the hormonal components of growth are controlled via the hypothalamic–pituitary axis,[8] including GH, IGF, thyroid hormones, and the sex steroids. In addition, the secretion of insulin, which is not directly under pituitary control, also plays an important role in the control of cellular growth. Of course, many other factors play major roles in the control of growth, including nutrition and genetic factors. In addition there are many tissue growth factors, such as fibroblast growth factor (FGF), epidermal growth factor (EGF) and nerve growth factor (NGF), whose roles in the overall control of growth are still poorly understood.[3] The interactions of these hormonal and nonhormonal factors result in either normal growth and development, or abnormally slow growth leading to short stature. When other factors are normal, it is the secretion of GH which plays a controlling role in the achievement of normal adult stature.

Growth hormone

Growth hormone is a 191-amino-acid-long polypeptide secreted by special cells in the anterior pituitary gland called somatotropes. Neurohormones control these cells by way of the hypophysial portal system, and both positive effectors of growth hormone secretion and an inhibitor of growth hormone secretion exist.[9] Present data indicate that growth hormone-releasing factor (GRF) is responsible for the rapid pulses of growth hormone secretion seen mainly during the night-time hours and in response to meals and exercise, while the inhibitor of growth hormone secretion, somatostatin (SRIF), appears to be responsible for the underlying tone of growth hormone secretion. In addition, there is a GH releasing peptide hormone (GRP) produced in the lining of the stomach and in the hypothalamus homologous to the synthetic GH releasing peptides (GHRPs) and the non-peptide homologues which bind to the GHRP receptor.[10]

Growth hormone secretion, like that of many other polypeptide hormones, is pulsatile.[11] In addition, growth hormone secretion is strongly associated with sleep. A large number of brain centers and neurotransmitters have been implicated in the control of growth hormone. In addition, there is evidence that at least one of the growth hormone-stimulated peptides, IGF-I, plays a feedback role at the level of both the hypothalamus and the somatotropes on the secretion of growth hormone.[12] The control of GH synthesis and secretion is reviewed in more detail in Chapter 6.

There are two major forms of growth hormone synthesized, stored, and secreted by the somatotropes.[13] The most abundant form (approximately 90 percent) is the 22 kDa molecular weight form. In addition, there is an alternative splicing of the growth hormone messenger RNA, which leads to a minor 20 kDa form of growth hormone whose physiological role is unknown. In addition, there are other minor molecular variants of GH in the circulation, such as 17 kDa and 5 kDa.

After growth hormone is released into the blood stream, a large proportion of it binds to a specific growth hormone-binding protein (GHBP).[14,15] It is now clear that in humans GHBP is the circulating extracellular portion of the growth hormone receptor. Like many receptors for polypeptide hormones, the receptor site for growth hormone consists of three polypeptide domains: an extracellular domain which contains all of the three-dimensional structure necessary for the recognition of the hormone; a transmembrane domain which is highly hydrophobic; and finally, an intracellular domain which contains the three-dimensional structure necessary to lead to the biological action within the cell. In humans it appears that there is a proteolytic cleavage of the extracellular domain of the growth hormone receptor which leads to a circulating polypeptide which plays a major role in protein-binding of growth hormone in the serum. The exact biological role of this binding protein is unclear. However, the circulating levels of GHBP do serve as a useful index to the level of growth hormone receptors in the body.[15] Growth hormone receptors are widely distributed throughout tissues in the body, and it is the binding of the growth hormone ligand to these growth hormone receptors which leads to the biological events within the cells themselves. The chain of GH intracellular action is covered in detail in Chapter 6. There are many direct biological events which are ascribed to growth hormone action, but the modulation of linear growth is mainly through the production of a pair of other polypeptide hormones known as insulin-like growth factors (IGFs).

Insulin–like growth factors

IGF messenger RNA is widely distributed throughout the body, and is under GH control not only in the liver, but in other tissues as well.[16] There are two distinctly different types of insulin-like growth factors known as IGF-I and IGF-II. These insulin-like growth factors bear a strong homology to each other and to insulin. Of the two polypeptides, IGF-I is the most closely related to growth hormone secretion and action. There are two predicted forms of IGF-I prohormone and thus far only one predicted prohormone for IGF-II. All of these prohormone forms contain long carboxyterminal extensions beyond the known structure of the active hormone which are known as E-regions. It appears that in normal circumstances these E-regions are cleaved off very efficiently before insulin-like growth factor is secreted. However, in certain circumstances such as renal failure and tumor-associated hypoglycemia, both circulating prohormone forms and E-peptide segments have been demonstrated.[17] Insulin-like growth factors circulate tightly bound to proteins known as insulin-like growth factor binding proteins (IGFBPs).[18] In most normal circumstances there is little or no free IGF-I or IGF-II polypeptide circulating. There are now known to be a total of at least six distinct but homologous IGFBPs. By far the most abundant form of IGFBP in normal serum is IGFBP-3. This is a glycosylated protein of approximately 40 kDa molecular weight. The combined IGF-peptide/IGFBP-3 complex binds to yet another protein known as the acid labile subunit (ALS) to form a 150 kDa, three-subunit protein complex which is the major circulating form of the IGFs.[19] This 150 kDa complex contains more than 85 percent of the total IGF in the serum in most circumstances. The levels of IGFBP-3, IGFBP-5[20] and the ALS[21] are also under GH control, and thus is the major factor in determining the level of circulating IGF peptides. In addition, GH stimulates the production of IGF-I in a wide variety of tissues and thus can act via a paracrine mechanism as well as an endocrine mechanism.[22] The balance between the endocrine and paracrine actions of IGF at different stages of life and in different clinical circumstances is unclear.

Difficulties in the diagnosis of GH deficiency

The methods of diagnosis of GHD are covered in detail in Chapter 12. The many methods that have been utilized in the diagnosis of GHD are a compelling illustration of the sometimes difficult nature of this apparently straightforward task.[23] However, although people may disagree about the borders of the diagnosis of GH deficiency, there is no doubt that there are patients in whom the endogenous secretion of GH is inadequate, and rate limiting for their growth. Thus, it is not surprising that to a large extent, the history of the treatment of GH deficiency is the also the history of the discovery and therapeutic use of GH.

Methods of treatment of growth hormone deficiency: The use of growth hormone

The spectacular success early in the twentieth century of using non-human insulin in the treatment of patients with diabetes mellitus made it logical to test the use of purified bovine GH to treat patients with severe short stature.[24,25] Unfortunately, it soon became apparent that GH from bovine sources was ineffective in the treatment of patients with the clinical syndrome of GHD. The successful treatment of clinically diagnosed GHD patients with human pituitary GH was first reported by Raben in 1958.[5] At that time, the only source of human GH was the pituitaries of humans that were donated postmortem. After the demonstration of the therapeutic usefulness of human GH, there was initially a chaotic situation with a variety of individual scientists collecting human pituitary glands and purifying the GH for the use of a very few patients. It was soon recognized that the collection of postmortem pituitary glands and the purification and distribution of GH needed to become a coordinated effort. Nationwide cooperative efforts to collect pituitaries, and to purify and distribute GH were developed in the 1960s in several countries including the

UK, France, and the USA.[26–29] These efforts allowed a rapid increase in the number of GHD patients treated with GH. In 1962, four years after the first report of the successful treatment of GHD, there were only approximately 100 GHD patients being treated with human GH in the USA. After the organization of the US National Pituitary Agency in 1963 there was a dramatic increase in the number of pituitary glands collected and the amount of growth hormone available in the United States, and the increase in the number of GHD patients treated was almost logarithmic for the next two decades (Fig. 33.1). In addition to the individual national efforts to collect human pituitary glands and purify GH, several pharmaceutical firms also produced and marketed purified human GH products.[30] By 1985 over 3000 patients in the United States were under treatment with human pituitary growth hormone from both the National Hormone and Pituitary Program (NHPP) and the commercial sources, and a similar number elsewhere in the world. However, even this increase in the supply of GH was insufficient to treat all of the patients with severe GHD. It was estimated in the early 1980s by Dr S. Raiti, the director of the NHPP, that there were at least twice as many growth hormone deficient patients who deserved treatment than were being treated in the United States at that time.[31] The difficult and inadequate supply of hGH was the primary reason why the production of human GH became one of the first developmental goals for the fledgling biotechnology

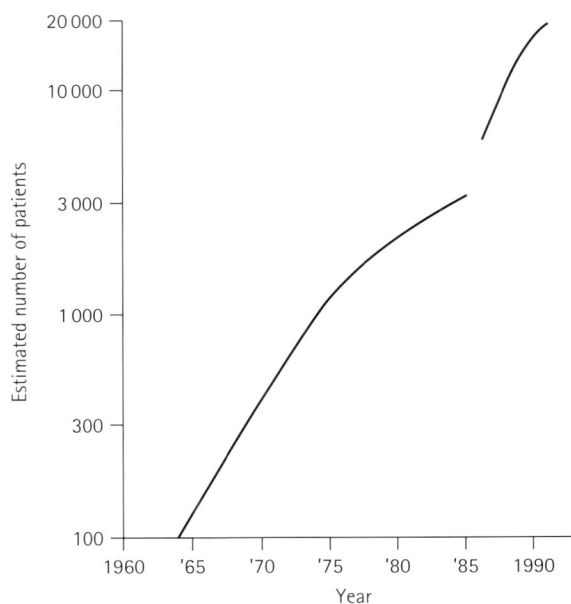

Figure 33.1 The estimated use of growth hormone (GH) in the United States. The data represent the number of patients estimated to be on active treatment with GH in the United States from 1964 until 1992, and derived from the National Hormone and Pituitary Program and commercial sources. The estimated number of patients on active treatment is plotted on a logarithmic scale. (From: Reference 94: Hintz RL. Untoward events in patients treated with GH in the USA. *Hormone Research* 1992; **38(Suppl 1)**: 44–49.)

industry in the later half of the 1970s. Indeed, GH became one of first human genes to be successfully cloned and expressed.[32] Human experiments with biosynthetic GH were begun in 1980,[33] and collaborative studies on the use of synthetic GH in pediatric patients with GHD were conducted in the following years.[34,35] Because of the discovery of cases of Creutzfeldt–Jakob disease associated with use of purified human pituitary GH, the use of pituitary GH was stopped in early 1985 by the NHPP in the United States.[36] At the same time, the UK, and many other countries and commercial sources also stopped the distribution of pituitary GH. For several months, GH was essentially unavailable for the treatment of GHD other than through research protocols. Then in November 1985 the use of synthetic growth hormone was approved by the FDA in the United States. By the end of 1986 the number of patients on growth hormone in the United States had doubled to more than 6000 and a steady increase in the use of growth hormone has continued. At present, it is estimated that at least 50 000 patients are actively on treatment with growth hormone in the USA and more than double that number worldwide, and that since 1960 more than 300 000 children worldwide have been treated with growth hormone of either pituitary or synthetic origin. The use of GH in adults with GHD is younger in its history, so it is more difficult to estimate the numbers of patients being treated. However, the use for this indication is increasing, and may eventually equal or exceed the use of GH for growth promotion.

Therapeutic effects of growth hormone treatment

The GH/IGF hormonal system clearly has a major role in body anabolism. Growth hormone has long been known to have a major controlling influence on linear growth[5,6] and in addition it has well-defined effects on protein, carbohydrate, lipid, bone and mineral metabolism.[33–40] This extensive general list is probably not complete because GH is also reported to have effects on the brain and neurotransmitters,[41] which may explain some of the clinical changes in mood and sense of well-being that has been reported with GH treatment.[42] GH has now been approved for the treatment of severe growth failure in children not only due to inadequate GH secretion, but also Turner syndrome, children with Prader–Willi syndrome, and short stature associated with IUGR.[43–45] In addition, idiopathic short stature (ISS) has recently been approved as an indication for GH treatment in the US.[46] These topics are covered in detail in following chapters. The therapeutic use of GH is not limited to its growth promoting properties. The administration of GH to adults as well as children results in prompt and reproducible effects on metabolism, including protein synthesis, an increase in insulin resistance, and changes in lipid, calcium and mineral metabolism.[47] In addition, it is now clear that GH has major effects on the heart,[48,49] the response of the gonads to gonadotropins,[50] cognition,[51] and quality

of life.[52] Thus, GH continues to play an important role in metabolism long after linear growth has ceased, and adults with GHD have major changes in body composition, morbidity and mortality.[53] It is becoming clear that use of GH therapy for growth promotion in young patients with GHD and the use of GH therapy to normalize the body composition and metabolism of adult patients with GHD are quite different, and therefore these uses of GH will be considered separately.

THERAPEUTIC USE OF GH IN GHD FOR GROWTH PROMOTION

Route

GH has been administered intravenously, intramuscularly, subcutaneously, transdermally and even nasally. The intravenous administration of GH is not practical for routine clinical care, although it has been an effective tool in studying GH pharmacology.[54,55] The most common route of administration for GH was initially intramuscular. However, it is now clear[56–58] that the subcutaneous route of administration is preferable in most instances. It causes less pain upon administration, and it has been demonstrated convincingly that the GH is just as bioavailable as when administered intramuscularly. There is also less risk of a complication of the injection, such as nerve damage, that occasionally happened with intramuscular injection, and it is easier to teach to the parents and/or patient. Thus, the subcutaneous route of administration is the recommended one in the overwhelming percentage of the cases. As is true of insulin, there is some variation between subcutaneous sites of administration with GH[59] but since the onset and duration of the biological action of GH is prolonged, this is not of clinical importance. The search for a practical non-parenteral route of GH administration has so far been unsuccessful. There is some adsorption of GH when it is administered nasally, but the bioavailability of GH administered by the nasal route is very low.[60] Other non-parenteral approaches to the administration of peptides are on the horizon, such as pulmonary, transdermally or orally bound to a matrix that releases the peptide beyond the majority of gastrointestinal peptidase, but as of yet none of these methods of delivery have been proven practical.

Treatment schedule

A wide variety of GH treatment schedules have been explored, from weekly administration to multiple times per day. The original work on frequency of administration in patients found that intramuscular injections three times per week in patients with GHD resulted in a higher growth rate than weekly injections, but they were unable to show a clear advantage of daily injections compared to three times per week.[61,62] Thus, the standard treatment schedule was initially set at three times per week. However, work over the last 15 years has shown that there is a small but definite advantage to treating with GH daily,[63,64] and therefore the most common treatment schedules being used now are either daily or 6 days out of 7. There has been some question from animal experiments[65] of whether GH might be even more effective if it was administered multiple times per day or continuously. However, in humans, the administration of daily subcutaneous injections of GH has been shown to be essentially as effective as continuous infusion[66] or pulsatile overnight infusion[67] of GH, and of course it has the advantage of being much more practical for home use. Work is under way testing chemically modified GHs with long durations of action that could be injected weekly or perhaps even less frequently. It is unclear at this point whether these approaches will be proven practical or not. The one long-acting GH approved by the FDA so far has been withdrawn from the market.[68] During the era of treatment of GHD with pituitary GH the shortage of the supply led to experiments with using GH therapy intermittently. GHD patients grew nearly as well when treated eight months out of the year as they did when treated continuously throughout the year.[69] This observation has been confirmed using synthetic hGH.[70] However, in the absence of any shortage of GH, most endocrinologists prefer a continuous daily regime. There is an effect of the timing of administration of the GH injection. It has been shown that there is an increase in IGF-I and growth rate in patients treated with daily subcutaneous GH injections in the evening as compared to the administration in the morning.[71] This difference may be due to a closer imitation of the natural secretion of GH in association with sleep and during the time of relatively low circulating levels of glucocorticoids. However GH is administered, it is clear that young patients have a better growth response to GH treatment than older patients.[72–74] Thus, early diagnosis and initiation of therapy are important goals for the physicians dealing with young GHD patients.

Dosage

The dose–response curve for the response of GHD patients to GH is relatively flat,[75] so that a doubling of GH dosage does not lead to a doubling in response. In addition, there are individual differences in the response to GH treatment. Thus, the clinician is faced with finding a dose of GH between the minimally effective dose for the individual patient and an upper limit dose defined by the increasing potential for adverse events as the dosage increases, and the increasing expense and decreasing effectiveness/cost ratio. This task is made all the more difficult by the difference in how GH is measured (international units or milligrams) and how dosages are calculated (by weight, by surface area, or flat dosage). In the USA doses of GH are most commonly administered on the basis of milligrams GH per body weight in kilograms ($mg\,kg^{-1}$). Using these systems of measure, the most common starting dose of GH is between $0.025\,mg\,kg^{-1}$ day^{-1} and $0.05\,mg\,kg^{-1}\,day^{-1}$,[43] while in Europe the most common initial dose is $0.05–0.10\,IU\,kg^{-1}$ day^{-1} or $1.5–3\,IU\,m^{-2}$ BSA day^{-1}.[76] There is a difference in the initial mean growth rates achieved by GHD patients treated with these starting dosages, with the higher dose giving higher mean growth rates. However, this difference is less in subsequent years than in the first year of treatment. Studies have also shown that there are better mean growth responses with higher doses of GH during the first year.[76] However, it is unclear whether the higher starting doses of GH are of long-term advantage to the GHD patients. It is clear, however, that the dosages of GH used for children with GHD are too high for use in the treatment of adults with GHD. The use of the doses of GH commonly used in young patients with GHD in adults is associated with a high incidence of side effects,[77,78] and considerably lower doses of GH appear to be biologically effective.[79]

THERAPEUTIC USE OF GH IN GHD AFTER THE CESSATION OF GROWTH

Many endocrinologists long had the clinical impression that adult patients with GHD are weak, have poor energy levels, and have a diminished overall feeling of good health. These patients often complain of lethargy and fatigue despite adequate thyroid, adrenal and gonadal hormone replacement therapy.[80] A retrospective study of 333 patients with childhood onset panhypopituitarism and GH deficiency who had routine standard hormone replacement therapy without GH treatment as adults showed that this group of patients had a cardiovascular death rate nearly twice that of the general population.[81] The authors hypothesized that this increased mortality was a result of GH deficiency and the accompanying hypercholesterolemia. Several controlled studies of GH therapy in GH deficient adults have been published. The majority of these studies have shown significant changes in body composition, exercise capacity, and an enhanced sense of well-being.[82–84] There are major shifts in extracellular fluid compartments,[60,85] and an improvement in the lipid markers of cardiovascular risk.[86,87] There have also been studies demonstrating positive changes in markers of bone and mineral metabolism, and increases in bone density.[40,88,89] In addition, several studies have shown improvement in tests measuring the quality of life.[42,52] These studies are very promising, and controlled long-term intervention trials on the GH treatment of adult GH deficiency have been reported.[90] The use of GH therapy for adults with GH deficiency has been approved in several countries, including the USA. The criteria for the diagnosis of GHD in the adult, and the extent to which GH therapy should be used in adults with GHD is a matter of debate.[53,91] There is a significant difference in the response to GH treatment between those adults who were diagnosed as GHD in childhood, and those GHD patients who were diagnosed as adults.[92] It seems clear that not every patient diagnosed as

GHD during childhood should be routinely treated with GH as adults, particularly when they have isolated GHD.[93]

ADVERSE EVENTS

Human growth hormone has now been used therapeutically for several hundred thousand patient-years over the last four decades. While the overall safety of the synthetic preparations of GH has been very good, a number of adverse events either directly or potentially related to GH therapy have been seen. This topic has been reviewed in detail,[94–98] but safety is an important part of the physician's decision to treat a patient with GHD.

Creutzfeldt–Jakob disease

A total of at least 26 definite cases of Creutzfeldt–Jakob disease (CJD) have been associated with the use of GH purified from pituitaries in the United States, and a total of at least 80 cases have occurred worldwide.[36,99] It is likely that other cases of Creutzfeldt–Jakob disease will continue to appear sporadically for some time to come until there are no more patients who were exposed to pituitary growth hormone. This devastating disease is undoubtedly associated with the use of pituitary growth hormone. In addition to the unique cluster of young patients with Creutzfeldt–Jakob disease among pituitary GH treated patients, one of the monkeys who was injected with suspected lots of pituitary growth hormone has developed Creutzfeldt–Jakob disease after a long incubation period.[100] So far, all of the cases identified in the United States had treatment with pituitary growth hormone initiated before 1970, presumably due to a change in the purification procedures for pituitary GH used by the NHPP in the early 1970s. A recent study found that allelic homozygosity at codon 129 of the chromosome 20 amyloid gene is an additional risk factor in susceptibility to the Creutzfeldt–Jakob disease infectious agent.[101] A survey conducted by the NIH in the late 1980s of the vast majority of pituitary GH treated patients in the United States[102] failed to reveal any cases of Creutzfeldt–Jakob disease not already identified, but cases have continued to appear since that report, and continued careful follow-up of these patients is necessary.[99] There should be no risk of CJD developing associated with the use of synthetic GH.

Antibodies

Antibodies against growth hormone have appeared in patients treated with both pituitary and synthetic growth hormones, and occasionally have caused growth failure.[30] Antibodies have been seen in a variable percentage of patients treated with synthetic growth hormone.[34,103,104] Although a small percentage of patients develop antibodies against synthetic GH, only a few patients have been reported to have growth hormone attenuation as a result of anti-GH antibodies.

Insulin resistance

It has been known since the early years of growth hormone research[105] that growth hormone has marked affects on carbohydrate metabolism by changing the level of insulin resistance. Approximately 10 percent of patients with growth hormone hypersecretion due to acromegaly have clinical evidence of diabetes. The short-term studies with synthetic growth hormone[106] confirmed there is a decrease in insulin sensitivity. Longer-term studies of hypopituitary children treated with growth hormone seem to indicate that the short-term change in insulin resistance is not clinically significant[107] with the doses of GH presently used. Although changes in insulin resistance with GH treatment could clearly be shown in these patients, this again did not appear to be of any clinical significance at the dosages of GH used. Although the picture is reassuring for the use of growth hormone in children at the present dosage levels, the use of GH in adults may have more potential problems.[108]

Sodium and water retention

GH therapy leads to sodium and water retention due to changes in renal handling.[33] Clinically apparent water retention and edema have been relatively uncommon in children being treated with GH with the exception of patients with Turner syndrome who sometimes experience a reappearance of lymphedema. In addition, some children with severe cardiac disease as well as GHD have had an increase in cardiac failure when GH was begun.[94] A number of patients have developed intracranial hypertension when on treatment with GH.[109] In general, the development of symptomatic fluid retention seems to be a more common phenomenon in adults treated with GH, but the use of low doses of GH or short-term treatment with diuretics usually handles this problem.

Growth-related events

Other unfavorable clinical events associated with GH treatment appear to be related to the growth-promoting actions of growth hormone. The occurrence of slipped capital femoral epiphysis (SCFE) in young GHD patients treated with GH has been reviewed.[110,111] The occurrence of SCFE in children receiving GH treatment is similar to the incidence of SCFE in rapidly growing youngsters, and may be related to the rapid growth induced by GH. A few young patients with GHD being treated long-term with GH have been reported to grow excessively and develop features suggestive of acromegaly.[112] These patients had high IGF-I levels, and IGF-I levels may be useful for monitoring the treatment of patients treated with growth hormone.[113] Patients with hypersecretion of growth hormone due to acromegaly frequently develop carpal-tunnel syndrome, apparently because of soft tissue growth induced by growth hormone. This complication appears to be limited to the use of GH treatment in adults,[114,115] and is clearly dose-related.

Leukemia

A source of major concern has been the association of leukemia with growth hormone treatment.[116–118] In the USA and European experience, the incidence of patients developing leukemia other than patients who have already had one oncologic disorder appears to be no different from what would be expected in an untreated population. The present data indicate that treatment with growth hormone is not an added leukemogenic risk to patients with severe growth deficiency who do not have coexisting risk factors.[119,120]

Tumor re-growth

The use of growth hormone in patients treated for brain tumors also has another associated concern, the re-growth of the original tumor. This subject has been extensively reviewed.[121] There are no data in either the United States or the worldwide experience to suggest that patients who have had brain tumors treated and are subsequently treated with growth hormone have any higher incidence of the redevelopment of brain tumors than those brain tumor patients who are not treated with growth hormone.[122]

MODULATION OF SEX STEROIDS LEVELS IN THE TREATMENT OF GHD

Before the demonstration of the effectiveness of human GH in the treatment of GHD, androgen treatment was used to stimulate the growth rate of GHD patients.[25] Growth rates did increase in these patients, but at the cost of early closure of the epiphyses and the loss of final height potential. Even after the introduction of pituitary GH treatment for GHD there were studies on the use of the non-aromatotizable androgen oxandrolone as an adjunct to GH therapy and as a way of extending the short supply of pituitary GH to more patients with severe GHD.[123,124] These experiments were never very successful, and were ultimately abandoned as the supply of GH increased. It is not considered useful as part of the growth management of patients with GHD, although obviously androgen therapy is an important part of the treatment of older male GHD patients who also have gonadotropin deficiency. More recently, there have been investigations of the use of gonadotropin-releasing hormone analogues to decrease the production of gonadotropin and therefore sex steroids in pubertal patients with GHD.[125–127] In theory, this should lengthen the time available for GHD

patients who are going through spontaneous puberty to respond to GH treatment and achieve an adequate final height. Short term results are promising in GHD patients with early pubertal development, There is now published long-term data to support the efficacy and safety of this therapeutic approach in other patients with GHD.[128,129]

IGF–I AS A POTENTIAL SUBSTITUTE FOR GH IN THE TREATMENT OF GHD

Since IGF-I mediates most of the growth promoting actions of GH, it might be thought the IGF-I itself could be useful in the treatment of patients with GHD. The growth response to IGF-I treatment of patients with genetic defects in the GH receptor (Laron syndrome) and therefore unresponsive to GH treatment demonstrates that IGF-I is indeed a potential therapy for GHD.[130] So far, the only experience in treating GHD with IGF-I is in isolated GHD type IA patients who have a deletion of the GH-I gene. These GHD patients frequently become unresponsive to GH treatment because of the development of anti-GH antibodies, and IGF-I treatment of these relatively rare GHD patients has increased their growth rates.[131–133] IGF-I treatment has also been investigated in a short term study in adult GHD.[134] It seems likely that the therapeutic use of IGF-I in the setting of GHD will be limited to the patients with GHD type IA who become unresponsive to GH. There is no clear advantage to using IGF-I in other GHD patients, and IGF-I therapy has been associated with significant side effects.[135,136] In addition, IGF-I is at present only available for experiment use.

THERAPEUTIC EFFECTS OF TREATMENT WITH GROWTH HORMONE RELEASING HORMONE

Many of the children who are diagnosed as GHD do not have absolute GHD on the basis of a tumor or anatomical defect of the CNS. In this group of GHD patients the defect in the production of adequate GH appears to be in the hypothalamic control of GH secretion, and therefore might be responsive to treatment with a GH secretagogue. In the last two decades there have been many studies on the therapeutic use of GHRH 1–44 and GHRH 1–29 in this group of children with GHD not due to organic disease.[137,138] It has been shown in double-blind studies that GHRH can increase the growth rate of patients with GHD, and therefore might be a useful alternative to GH in the treatment of GHD, and it has been approved for this use in the USA. So far the widespread therapeutic use of GHRH in GHD has been limited by several factors. First of all, it is not useful in the one-third of GHD patients in childhood who have organic GHD.[139] Although it is absorbed nasally[140,141] this non-parenteral route of administration has not been proven to be clinically useful. Therefore, it must be administered subcutaneously like GH itself. Direct comparisons of the effectiveness of GH and GHRH in the treatment of GHD have not shown any clear advantage for GHRH.[142] The initial studies suggested that GHRH needed to be administered multiple times per day to be maximally effective,[143] making it less attractive as an alternative to GH. In the absence of any clear indication of any therapeutic or practical advantage in using GHRH, most clinicians stayed with GH as the prime therapeutic agent for the treatment of GHD. Because of poor sales, the company marketing GHRH has taken it off the market and it is now unavailable for clinical use.

PRELIMINARY DATA CONCERNING GROWTH HORMONE RELEASING PEPTIDE AND RELATED SUBSTANCES

Another potential approach to treating GHD in those patients without organic pituitary disease is the use of GHRPs and their non-peptide homologues. The GHRPs are synthetic GH secretagogues that bind to a different receptor from the GHRH receptor. Studies in humans have shown that the GHRPs are active by the intravenous, intramuscular, subcutaneous, nasal and oral routes in increasing the secretion rate of endogenous GH.[144,145] Human trials are under way to test the therapeutic usefulness of these compounds in the treatment of GHD. It has been hypothesized for some time that there must be an endogenous receptor for GHRP, and this has recently been defined using a non-peptide homologue of GHRP as the ligand. The non-peptide homologues are well absorbed and active orally in releasing GH,[146,147] and studies are under way on their usefulness in treating GH deficiency. The data on the GHRPs and non-peptide homologues are too preliminary to allow firm predictions of their therapeutic usefulness in treating GHD. However, they have the potential of having some practical advantages, such as ease of administration and cost, over GH in those young patients who have non-organic GHD.

PERSPECTIVE

The treatment of GHD has advanced tremendously over the last several decades. No longer do physicians have to agonize over treatment decisions because of the scarcity of the supply of pituitary GH, or unwittingly introduce a slow but lethal infectious agent into their patients while attempting to help them achieve a more normal life. Although the therapeutic decisions are still not easy because the diagnosis of GHD is not always crystal clear, at least we have an array of treatments available. First and foremost, of course, is biosynthetic GH itself. This is the best studied and proven agent for the treatment of GHD, and in most cases still the best choice. However, although GH is highly effective as a treatment for GHD, it is an expensive treatment and involves daily injections at least throughout the growing years of a GHD patient until an adequate adult height is achieved. Perhaps lifelong treatment will be needed to maintain normal body composition and quality of life and

to prevent a premature cardiovascular death. Experiments are under way on new methods of delivery of GH, and new therapeutic regimes that may make long-term treatment with GH easier. In addition, as the number of patients treated with GH for adult indications increases, the price of GH treatment may drop. Other treatments for GHD are becoming available. Treatment of GHD with IGF-I seems to be indicated only in those rare patients with Type 1a GHD and resistance to GH because of antibody formation. The modulation of androgen levels also have a rather narrow range of indications in the treatment of GHD, and only in combination with GH treatment. GHRH and the GHRPs and their non-peptide homologues may eventually have wide application in that subset of patients with GHD who have the ability to make and release GH from their pituitaries when stimulated. This wider application will become a reality only if oral forms of GHRPs or their non-peptide homologues are proven as effective as GH in the treatment of these GHD patients, and are shown to be less expensive for the long-term management of GHD. In any case, the developments of the next few years should have just as many improvements in the effective management of patients with GHD as the great advances of the last several decades.

REFERENCES

1   Butenandt O. Therapy of growth hormone deficiency. *Baillieres Clin Endocrinol Metab* 1992; **6**: 547–55.

2   Chipman JJ. Recent advances in hGH clinical research. *J Pediatr Endocrinol* 1993; **6**: 325–8.

3   Hintz RL. Growth factors. *Curr Opin Pediatr* 1990; **2**: 786–93.

4   Tanaka T, Cohen P, Clayton PE, *et al.* Diagnosis and management of growth hormone deficiency in childhood and adolescence – Part 2: Growth hormone treatment in growth hormone deficient children. *Growth Horm IGF Res* 2002; **12**: 323–41.

5   Raben MS. Treatment of a pituitary dwarf with human growth hormone. *J Clin Endocrinol Metab* 1958; **18**: 901–3.

6   Glick SM, Roth J, Yalow RS, Berson SA. Immunoassay of human growth hormone in plasma. *Nature* 1963; **199**: 784–6.

7   Rona RJ, Tanner JM. Aetiology of idiopathic growth hormone deficiency in England and Wales. *Arch Dis Child* 1977; **52**: 197–208.

8   Hintz RL. Disorders of growth. In: Lee P, Sanfilipo J, eds. *Pediatric and Adolescent Gynecology.* Philadelphia: WB Saunders, 1993: 34–43.

9   Reichlin S. Neuroendocrinology. In: Wilson JD, Foster DW, eds. *Williams Textbook of Endocrinology*, 8th edn. Philadelphia: WB Saunders, 1992: 135–219.

10 Kojima M, Hosoda H, Kangawa K. Purification and distribution of ghrelin: the natural endogenous ligand for the growth hormone secretagogue. *Hormone Research* 2001; **56 (Suppl 1)**: 93–7.

11 Muller EE, Locatelli V, Cocchi D. Neuroendocrine control of growth hormone secretion. *Physiol Rev* 1999; **79**: 511–607.

12 Berelowitz M, Szabo M, Frohman LA, *et al.* Somatomedin-C mediates growth hormone negative feed-back by effects on both the hypothalamus and the pituitary. *Science* 1981; **212**: 1279–81.

13 Baumann G. Growth hormone heterogeneity: genes, isohormones, variants, and binding proteins. *Endocr Rev* 1991; **12**: 424–49.

14 Leung DW, Spencer SA, Cachianes G, *et al.* Growth hormone receptor and serum binding protein: purification, cloning and expression. *Nature* 1987; **330**: 537–43.

15 Baumann G. Growth hormone-binding proteins: state of the art. *J Endocrinol* 1994; **141**: 1–6.

16 Holly JMP, Wass JAH. Insulin-like growth factors, autocrine, paracrine or endocrine? New perspectives of the somatomedin hypotheses in the light of recent developments. *J Endocrinol* 1989; **122**: 611–18.

17 Powell DR, Lee PDK, Chang D, *et al.* Antiserum developed for the E peptide region of human IGF-IA prohormone recognizes a 13-19 kilodalton serum protein. *J Clin Endocrinol* 1987; **65**: 868–75.

18 Hintz RL. The role of growth hormone and insulin-like growth factor binding proteins. *Horm Res* 1990; **33**: 105–10.

19 Baxter RC. Insulin-like growth factor binding proteins in the human circulation: a review. *Horm Res* 1994; **42**: 140–4.

20 Ono T, Kanzaki S, Seino Y, *et al.* Growth hormone GH; treatment of GH-deficient children increases serum levels of insulin-like growth factors IGFs, IGF-binding protein-3 and -5, and bone alkaline phosphatase isoenzyme. *J Clin Endocrinol Metab* 1996; **81**: 2111–16.

21 Liu F, Hintz RL, Khare A, *et al.* Immunoblot studies of the IGF-related acid-labile subunit. *J Clin Endocrinol Metab* 1994; **79**: 1883–6.

22 Jones JI, Clemmons DR. Insulin-like growth factors and their binding proteins: biological actions. *Endocr Rev* 1995; **16**: 3–34.

23 Rosenfeld RG, Albertsson-Wikland K, Cassorla F, *et al.* Diagnostic controversy: The diagnosis of childhood growth hormone deficiency revisited. *J Clin Endocrinol Metab* 1995; **80**: 1532–40.

24 Bennett LL, Weinberger H, Escamilla R, *et al.* Failure of hypophyseal growth hormone to produce nitrogen storage in a girl with hypophyseal dwarfism. *J Clin Endocrinol* 1950; **10**: 492–5.

25 Escamilla R, Bennett LL. Pituitary infantilism treated with purified growth hormone, thyroid and sublingual methyltestosterone (case report). *J Clin Endocrinol* 1951; **11**: 221–8.

26 Blizzard RM. The past, present, and future of pituitary growth hormone. *Am J Dis Child* 1963; **106**: 439–40.

27 Frasier SD. The not-so-good old days: working with pituitary growth hormone in North America, 1956 to 1985. *J Pediatr* 1997; **1311(Pt 2)**: S1–4.

28 Milner RCG, Russell-Fraser T, Brook CGD, *et al.* Experience with human growth hormone in Great Britain: the report of the MRC Working Party. *Clin Endocrinol* 1979; **11**: 15–8.

29 Job JC, Joab N, Toublanc JE, Canlorbe P. Resultats a terme des traitements par l'hormone de croissance humanine. *Arch Fr Pediatr* 1984; **41**: 477–82.

30 Underwood LE, Voina SJ, Van Wyk JJ. Restoration of growth by human growth hormone in hypopituitary dwarfs immunized by other growth hormone preparations: clinical and immunological studies. *J Clin Endocrinol Metab* 1974; **38**: 288–97.

31 Raiti S. The national hormone and pituitary program: Achievements and current goals. In: Raiti S, Tolman R, eds. *Human Growth Hormone.* New York: Plenum, 1986: 1–12.

32 Goeddel DV, Heynecker HL, Hozumi T, *et al.* Direct expression in *Escherichia coli* of a DNA sequence coding for human growth hormone. *Nature* 1979; **281**: 544–8.

33 Hintz RL, Rosenfeld RG, Wilson DM, *et al.* Biosynthetic methionyl-human growth hormone is biologically active in adult man. *Lancet* 1982; **1**: 1276–9.

34 Kaplan SL, Underwood LE, August GP, *et al.* Clinical studies with recombinant-DNA derived methionyl-hGH in GH deficient children. *Lancet* 1986; **1**: 697–700.

35 Gunnarsson R, Wilton P. Clinical experience with Genotropin worldwide: an update. *Acta Paediatr Scand Suppl* 1987; **337**: 147–52.

36 Hintz RL. The prismatic case of Creutzfeldt–Jakob disease associated with pituitary growth hormone treatment. *J Clin Endocrinol Metab* 1995; **80**: 2298–301.

37 Wit JM, Kamp GA, Rikken B. Spontaneous growth and response to growth hormone treatment in children with growth hormone deficiency and idiopathic short stature. *Pediatr Res* 1996; **39**: 295–302.

38 Holmes SJ, Shalet SM. Role of growth hormone and sex steroids in achieving and maintaining normal bone mass. *Horm Res* 1996; **45**: 86–93.

39 Kubo T, Tanaka H, Inoue M, *et al.* Serum levels of carboxyterminal propeptide of type I procollagen and pyridinoline crosslinked telopeptide of type I collagen in normal children and children with growth hormone deficiency during GH therapy. *Bone* 1995; **17**: 397–401.

40 Amato G, Izzo G, La Montagna G, Bellastella A. Low dose recombinant human growth hormone normalizes bone metabolism and cortical bone density and improves trabecular bone density in growth hormone deficient adults without causing adverse effects. *Clin Endocrinol* 1996; **45**: 27–32.

41 Burman P, Hetta J, Wide L, *et al.* Growth hormone treatment affects brain neurotransmitters and thyroxine. *Clin Endocrinol* 1996; **44**: 319–24.

42 Stabler B, Clopper RR, Siegel PT, *et al.* Links between growth hormone deficiency, adaptation and social phobia. *Horm Res* 1996; **45**: 30–3.

43 Hintz RL. Current and potential therapeutic uses of growth hormone and insulin-like growth factor I. *Endocrinol Metab Clin North Am* 1996; **25**: 759–73.

44 Allen DB, Carrel AL. Growth hormone therapy for Prader–Willi syndrome: a critical appraisal. *J Pediatr Endocrinol Metab* 2004; **17(Suppl 4)**: 1297–306.

45 Czernichow P. Treatment with growth hormone in short children born with intrauterine growth retardation. *Endocrine* 2001; **15**: 39–42.

46 Wit JM, Rekers-Mombarg LT, Cutler GB, *et al*. Growth hormone treatment to final height in children with idiopathic short stature: evidence for a dose effect. *J Pediatr* 2005; **146**: 45–53.

47 Hoffman AR, Marcus R, Hintz RL, *et al*. The effects of recombinant human insulin-like growth factor-I in human aging. In: Lackman, Harman, Roth, Shapiro, eds. *GHRH, GH and IGF-I: Basic and Clinical Advances*. Berlin: Springer-Verlag, 1995: 266–76.

48 Crepaz R, Pitscheider W, Radetti G, *et al*. Cardiovascular effects of high-dose growth hormone treatment in growth hormone-deficient children. *Pediatr Cardiol* 1995; **16**: 223–7.

49 Kohno H, Ueyama N, Yanai S, *et al*. Beneficial effect of growth hormone on atherogenic risk in children with growth hormone deficiency. *J Pediatr* 1995; **126**: 953–5.

50 Tato L, Zamboni G, Antoniazzi F, Piubello G. Gonadal function and response to growth hormone in boys with isolated GH deficiency and to GH and gonadotropins in boys with multiple pituitary hormone deficiencies. *Fertil Steril* 1996; **65**: 830–4.

51 Sartorio A, Conti A, Molinari E, *et al*. Growth, growth hormone and cognitive functions. *Horm Res* 1996; **45**: 23–9.

52 McGauley G, Cuneo R, Salomon F, Sonksen PH. Growth hormone deficiency and quality of life. *Horm Res* 1996; **45**: 34–7.

53 Juul A, Jorgensen JO, Christiansen JS, *et al*. Metabolic effects of GH: a rationale for continued GH treatment of GH-deficient adults after cessation of linear growth. *Horm Res* 1995; **44(Suppl 3)**: 64–72.

54 Jorgensen JO, Moller N, Lauritzen T, Christiansen JS. Pulsatile versus continuous intravenous administration of growth hormone in GH-deficient patients: effects on circulating insulin-like growth factor-I and metabolic indices. *J Clin Endocrinol Metab* 1990; **70**: 1616–23.

55 Laursen T, Moller J, Jorgensen JO, *et al*. Bioavailability and bioactivity of intravenous vs subcutaneous infusion of growth hormone in GH-deficient patients. *Clin Endocrinol* 1996; **45**: 333–9.

56 Russo L, Moore WW A comparison of subcutaneous and intramuscular administration of human growth hormone in the therapy of growth hormone deficiency. *J Clin Endocrinol Metab* 1982; **55**: 1003–6.

57 Kastrup KW, Christiansen JS, Andersen JK, Orskov H. Increased growth rate following transfer to daily SC administration from three weekly IM injections of hGH in growth hormone deficient children. *Acta Endocrinol* 1983; **104**: 148–52.

58 Wilson DM, Baker B, Hintz RL, Rosenfeld RG. Subcutaneous versus intramuscular growth hormone therapy: Growth and acute somatomedin response. *Pediatrics* 1985; **76**: 361–4.

59 Laursen T, Jorgensen JO, Christiansen JS. Pharmacokinetics and metabolic effects of growth hormone injected subcutaneously in growth hormone deficient patients: thigh versus abdomen. *Clin Endocrinol* 1994; **40**: 373–8.

60 Moller J, Frandsen E, Fisker S, *et al*. Decreased plasma and extracellular volume in growth hormone deficient adults and the acute and prolonged effects of GH administration: a controlled experimental study. *Clin Endocrinol* 1996; **44**: 533–9.

61 Tanner JM, *et al*. Effect of human growth hormone treatment for 1 to 7 years on growth of 100 children with growth hormone deficiency, inherited smallness, Turner's syndrome, and other complaints. *Arch Dis Child* 1971; **46**: 745–82.

62 Frasier SD, Aceto JT, Hayles AB. Collaborative study of the effects of human growth hormone in growth hormone deficiency. V. Treatment with growth hormone administered once a week. *J Clin Endocrinol Metab* 1978; **47**: 686–8.

63 Hindmarsh PC, Stannhope R, Preece MA, Brook CGD. Frequency of administration of GH – an important factor in determining growth response to exogenous GH. *Horm Res* 1990; **33(Suppl 4)**: 83–9.

64 MacGillivray MH, Baptista J, Johanson A. Outcome of a four-year randomized study of daily versus three times weekly somatropin treatment in prepubertal naive growth hormone-deficient children. Genentech Study Group. *J Clin Endocrinol Metab* 1996; **81**: 1806–9.

65 Jansson JO, Albertsson-Wikland K, Eden S, *et al*. Effect of frequency of growth hormone administration on longitudinal bone growth and body weight in hypophysectomized rats. *Acta Physiol Scand* 1982; **114**: 261–5.

66 Laursen T, Jorgensen JO, Jakobsen G, *et al*. Continuous infusion versus daily injections of growth hormone for 4 weeks in GH-deficient patients. *J Clin Endocrinol Metab* 1995; **80**: 2410–8.

67 Cavallo L, De Luca F, Bernasconi S, *et al*. Subcutaneous growth hormone administration in growth-hormone-deficient children. Continuous plus pulsatile overnight versus single daily injection: effects on growth rate velocity. *Horm Res* 1994; **42**: 86–9.

68 Kemp SF, Fielder PJ, Attie KM, *et al*. Pharmacokinetic and pharmacodynamic characteristics of a long-acting growth hormone preparation nutropin depot in GH-deficient children. *J Clin Endocrinol Metab* 2004; **87**: 3234–40.

69 Preece MA, Tanner JM. Results of intermittent treatment of growth hormone deficiency with human growth hormone. *J Clin Endocrinol Metab* 1977; **45**: 169–70.

70 Bougneres P. Efficacy of intermittent therapy in growth hormone-deficient children. *Eur J Endocrinol* 1994; **1305**: 459–62.

71 Zadik Z, Lieberman E, Altman Y, *et al*. Effect of timing of growth hormone administration on plasma growth-hormone-binding activity, insulin-like growth factor-I and growth in children with a subnormal spontaneous secretion of growth hormone. *Horm Res* 1993; **39**: 188–91.

72 Blethen SL, Baptista J, Kuntze J, *et al*. Adult height in growth hormone-deficient children treated with biosynthetic GH. The Genentech Growth Study Group. *J Clin Endocrinol Metab* 1997; **82**: 418–20.

73 Boersma B, Rikken B, Wit JM. Catch-up growth in early treated patients with growth hormone deficiency. Dutch Growth Hormone Working Group. *Arch Dis Child* 1995; **72**: 427–31.

74 Rappaport R, Mugnier E, Limoni C, *et al.* A 5-year prospective study of growth hormone-deficient children treated with GH before the age of 3 years. French Serono Study Group. *J Clin Endocrinol Metab* 1997; **82**: 452–6.

75 Frasier SD, Costin G, Lippe BM, *et al.* A dose–response curve for human growth hormone. *J Clin Endocrinol Metab* 1981; **53**: 1213–7.

76 de Muinck Keizer-Schrama SM, Rikken B, Hokken-Koelega A, *et al.* Comparative effect of two doses of growth hormone for growth hormone deficiency. The Dutch Growth Hormone Working Group. *Arch Dis Child* 1994; **71**: 12–8.

77 Hintz RL, Hoffman AR, Butterfield G, Marcus R. Effects and side effects of growth hormone treatment in the adult. In: Laron Z, Butenandt O, eds. *Growth Hormone Replacement Therapy in the Adult: Pros and Cons.* Tel Aviv, London: Freund Publishing, 1993: 157–70.

78 Cohn L, Feller AG, Draper MW, *et al.* Carpal tunnel syndrome and gynaecomastia during growth hormone treatment of elderly men with low circulating IGF-I concentrations. *Clin Endocrinol* 1993; **39**: 417–25.

79 de Boer H, Blok GJ, Voerman B, *et al.* The optimal growth hormone replacement dose in adults, derived from bioimpedance analysis. *J Clin Endocrinol Metab* 1995; **80**: 2069–76.

80 Powrie J, Weissberger A, Sonksen P. Growth hormone replacement therapy for growth hormone-deficient adults. *Drugs* 1995; **49**: 656–63.

81 Rosen T, Bengtsson B-A. Premature mortality due to cardiovascular disease in hypopituitarism. *Lancet* 1990; **336**: 285–8.

82 Jorgensen JO, Thuesen L, Muller J, *et al.* Three years of growth hormone treatment in growth hormone-deficient adults: near normalization of body composition and physical performance. *Eur J Endocrinol* 1994; **130**: 224–8.

83 Hansen TB, Vahl N, Jorgensen JO, *et al.* Whole body and regional soft tissue changes in growth hormone deficient adults after one year of growth hormone treatment: a double-blind, randomized, placebo-controlled study. *Clin Endocrinol* 1995; **43**: 689–96.

84 Lonn L, Johansson G, Sjostrom L, *et al.* Body composition and tissue distributions in growth hormone deficient adults before and after growth hormone treatment. *Obes Res* 1996; **4**: 45–54.

85 Hoffman DM, Crampton L, Sernia C, *et al.* Short-term growth hormone treatment of GH-deficient adults increases body sodium and extracellular water, but not blood pressure. *J Clin Endocrinol Metab* 1996; **81**: 1123–8.

86 Leonsson M, Oscarsson J, Bosaeus I, *et al.* Growth hormone therapy in GH-deficient adults influences the response to a dietary load of cholesterol and saturated fat in terms of cholesterol synthesis, but not serum low density lipoprotein cholesterol levels. *J Clin Endocrinol Metab* 1999; **84**: 1296–303.

87 O'Halloran DJ, Wieringa G, Tsatsoulis A, Shalet SM. Increased serum lipoprotein concentrations after growth hormone treatment in patients with isolated GH deficiency. *Ann Clin Biochem* 1996; **33(Pt 4)**: 330–4.

88 Johannsson G, Rosen T, Bosaeus I, *et al.* Two years of growth hormone treatment increases bone mineral content and density in hypopituitary patients with adult-onset GH deficiency. *J Clin Endocrinol Metab* 1996; **81**: 2865–73.

89 Hansen TB, Brixen K, Vahl N, *et al.* Effects of 12 months of growth hormone treatment on calciotropic hormones, calcium homeostasis, and bone metabolism in adults with acquired GH deficiency: a double blind, randomized, placebo-controlled study. *J Clin Endocrinol Metab* 1996; **81**: 3352–9.

90 Gotherstrom G, Svensson J, Koranyi J, *et al.* A prospective study of 5 years of GH replacement therapy in GH-deficient adults: sustained effects on body composition, bone mass, and metabolic indices. *J Clin Endocrinol Metab* 2001; **86**: 4657–65.

91 Brook CGD. Growth hormone replacement treatment in adult patients. *Clin Endocrinol* 1996; **44**: 317.

92 Attanasio AF, Lamberts SW, Matranga AM, *et al.* Adult growth hormone-deficient patients demonstrate heterogeneity between childhood onset and adult onset before and during human GH treatment. Adult growth hormone deficiency study group. *J Clin Endocrinol Metab* 1997; **82**: 82–8.

93 Tauber M, Moulin P, Pienkowski C, *et al.* Growth hormone retesting and auxological data in 131 GH-deficient patients after completion of treatment. *J Clin Endocrinol Metab* 1997; **82**: 352–6.

94 Hintz RL. Untoward events in patients treated with GH in the USA. *Horm Res* 1992; **38(Suppl 1)**: 44–9.

95 Blethen SL. Complications of growth hormone therapy in children. *Curr Opin Pediatr* 1995; **7**: 466–71.

96 Blethen SL, Allen DB, Graves D, *et al.* Safety of recombinant deoxyribonucleic acid-derived growth hormone: The National Cooperative Growth Study experience. *J Clin Endocrinol Metab* 1996; **81**: 1704–10.

97 Cowell CT, Dietsch S. Adverse events during growth hormone therapy. *J Pediatr Endocrinol Metab* 1995; **8**: 243–52.

98 Czernichow P. Complications of treatment with growth hormone. *Arch Pediatr* 1996; **3(Suppl 1)**: 156s–57.

99 Mills JL, Schonberger LB, Wysowski DK, *et al.* Long-term mortality in the United States cohort of pituitary-derived growth hormone recipients. *J Pediatr* 2004; **144**: 430–6.

100 Gibbs CJ Jr, Asher DM, Brown PW, *et al.* Creutzfeldt–Jakob disease infectivity of growth hormone derived from human pituitary glands. *New Engl J Med* 1993; **328**: 358–9.

101 Brown P, Cervenakova L, Goldfarb LG, *et al.* Iatrogenic Creutzfeldt–Jakob disease: an example of the interplay between ancient genes and modern medicine. *Neurology* 1994; **44**: 291–3.

102 Fradkin JE, Schonberger LB, Mills JL, *et al.* Creutzfeldt–Jakob disease in pituitary growth hormone recipients in the United States. *JAMA* 1991; **265**: 880–4.

103 Pirazzoli P, Cacciari E, Mandini M, *et al.* Follow-up of antibodies to growth hormone in 210 growth hormone-deficient children treated with different commercial preparations. *Acta Paediatr* 1995; **84**: 1233–6.

104 Massa G, Vanderschueren-Lodeweyckx M, Bouillon R. Five-year follow-up of growth hormone antibodies in growth hormone deficient children treated with recombinant human growth hormone. *Clin Endocrinol* 1993; **38**: 137–42.

105 Young FG. The pituitary gland and carbohydrate metabolism. *Endocrinology* 1940; **26**: 345–51.

106 Rosenfeld RG, Wilson DM, Dollar LA, *et al.* Both human pituitary growth hormone and recombinant DNA derived human growth hormone cause insulin resistance at a post-receptor level. *J Clin Endocrinol Metab* 1989; **54**: 1033–8.

107 Walker J, Chaussiam JL, Bougneses PF. Growth hormone treatment of children with short stature increases insulin secretion but does not impair glucose disposal. *J Clin Endocrinol Metab* 1989; **69**: 253–8.

108 Abdul Shakoor SK, Shalet SM. Effects of GH replacement on metabolism and physical performance in GH deficient adults. *J Endocrinol Invest* 2003; **26**: 911–8.

109 Malozowski S, Tanner LA, Wysowski DK, *et al.* Benign intracranial hypertension in children with growth hormone deficiency treated with growth hormone. *J Pediatr* 1995; **126**: 996–9.

110 Rappaport EB, Fife D. Slipped capital femoral epiphysis in growth hormone-deficient patients. *Am J Dis Child* 1985; **136**: 396–9.

111 Loder RT, Wittenberg B, DeSilva G. Slipped capital femoral epiphysis associated with endocrine disorders. *J Pediatr Orthop* 1995; **15**: 349–56.

112 Baens-Bailon R, Foley TP, Hintz RL, Lee PA. Excessive growth hormone dosing in GH deficiency. *Pediatr Res* 1992; **31**: 73A.

113 Lee KW, Cohen P. Individualized growth hormone therapy in children: advances beyond weight-based dosing. *J Pediatr Endocrinol Metab* 2003; **16(Suppl 3)**: 625–30.

114 Johanson AJ, Blizzard RM. Low somatomedin-C levels in older men rise in response to growth hormone administration. *Johns Hopkins Med J* 1981; **149**: 115–7.

115 Salomon F, Cuneo RC, Hesp R, Sönksen PH. The effects of treatment with recombinant human growth hormone on body composition and metabolism in adults with growth hormone deficiency. *N Engl J Med* 1989; **321**: 1797–803.

116 Rogers PC, Komp D, Rogol A, Sabio H. Possible effects of growth hormone on development of acute lymphoblastic leukaemia. *Lancet* 1977; **2**: 434–5.

117 Watanabe S, Yamaguchi N, Tsunematsu Y, Komiyama A. Risk factors for leukemia occurrence among growth hormone users. *Japan J Cancer Res* 1989; **80**: 822–5.

118 Stahnke N, Zeisel HJ. Growth hormone therapy and leukaemia. *Eur J Pediatr* 1989; **148**: 591–6.

119 Ogilvy-Stuart AL. Safety of growth hormone after treatment of a childhood malignancy. *Horm Res* 1995; **44(Suppl 3)**: 73–9.

120 Nishi Y, Tanaka T, Takano K, *et al.* Recent status in the occurrence of leukemia in growth hormone-treated patients in Japan. GH Treatment Study Committee of the Foundation for Growth Science. *Japan J Clin Endocrinol Metab* 1999; **84**: 1961–5.

121 Rappaport R, Brauner R. Growth and endocrine disorders secondary to cranial irradiation. *Pediatr Res* 1989; **25**: 561–7.

122 Ogilvy-Stuart AL, Ryder WD, Gattamaneni HR, *et al.* Growth hormone and tumour recurrence. *BMJ* 1992; **304**: 1601–5.

123 Raiti S, Trias E, Levitsky L, Grossman MS. Oxandrolone and human growth hormone. *Am J Dis Child* 1973; **126**: 597–600.

124 Romshe CA, Sotos JF. Combined effect of growth hormone and oxandrolone in patients with GH-deficiency. *J Pediatr* 1980; **96**: 127–31.

125 Saggese G, Cesaretti G, Andreani G, Carlotti C. Combined treatment with growth hormone and gonadotropin-releasing hormone analogues in children with isolated growth hormone deficiency. *Acta Endocrinol* 1992; **127**: 307–12.

126 Cara JF, Kreiter ML, Rosenfield RL. Height prognosis of children with true precocious puberty and growth hormone deficiency: effect of combination therapy with gonadotropin releasing hormone agonist and growth hormone. *J Pediatr* 1992; **120**: 709–15.

127 Adan L, Souberbielle JC, Zucker JM, *et al.* Adult height in 24 patients treated for growth hormone deficiency and early puberty. *J Clin Endocrinol Metab* 1997; **82**: 229–33.

128 Tanaka T, Satoh M, Yasunaga T, *et al.* When and how to combine growth hormone with a luteinizing hormone-releasing hormone analogue. *Acta Paediatr Suppl* 1999; **88**: 85–8.

129 Mericq MV, Eggers M, Avila A, *et al.* Near final height in pubertal growth hormone GH-deficient patients treated with GH alone or in combination with luteinizing hormone-releasing hormone analog: results of a prospective, randomized trial. *J Clin Endocrinol Metab* 2000; **85**: 569–73.

130 Carel JC, Chaussain JL, Chatelain P, Savage MO. Growth hormone insensitivity syndrome Laron syndrome: main characteristics and effects of IGF1 treatment. *Diabetes Metab* 1996; **22**: 251–6.

131 Nishi Y, Hamamoto K, Kajiyama M, *et al.* Treatment of isolated growth hormone deficiency type IA due to GH-I gene deletion with recombinant human insulin-like growth factor I. *Acta Paediatr* 1993; **82**: 983–6.

132 Youlton R. Growth hormone gene deletion: results of treatment with recombinant human insulin-like growth factor I. *Acta Paediatr Suppl* 1994; **399**: 150–1.

133 Backeljauw PF, Underwood LE. Prolonged treatment with recombinant insulin-like growth factor-I in children with growth hormone insensitivity syndrome – a clinical research center study. GHIS Collaborative Group. *J Clin Endocrinol Metab* 1996; **81**: 3312–7.

134 Thoren MC, Wivall-Helleryd IL, Blum WF, Hall KE. Effects of repeated subcutaneous administration of recombinant human insulin-like growth factor I in adults with growth hormone deficiency. *Eur J Endocrinol* 1994; **131**: 33–40.

135 Ranke MB, Wilton P. Adverse events during treatment with recombinant insulin-like growth factor I in patients with growth hormone insensitivity. *Acta Paediatr Suppl* 1994; **399**: 143–5.

136 Thompson JL, Butterfield GE, Marcus R, *et al*. The effects of recombinant human insulin-like growth factor-I and growth hormone on body composition in elderly women. *J Clin Endocrinol Metab* 1995; **80**: 1845–52.

137 Chen RG, Shen YN, Yei J, *et al*. A comparative study of growth hormone and GH-releasing hormone(1-29)-NH2 for stimulation of growth in children with GH deficiency. *Acta Paediatr Suppl* 1993; **388**: 32–5.

138 Lievre M, Chatelain P, Van Vliet G, *et al*. Treatment with growth hormone-releasing hormone (GHRH) 1-44 in children with idiopathic growth hormone deficiency: a randomized double-blind dose-effect study. The GHRH European Multicenter Study (GEMS) Group. *Fundam Clin Pharmacol* 1992; **6**: 359–66.

139 Pombo M, Barreiro J, Penalva A, *et al*. Absence of growth hormone secretion after the administration of either GH-releasing hormone (GHRH), GH-releasing peptide (GHRP-6), or GHRH plus GHRP-6 in children with neonatal pituitary stalk transection. *J Clin Endocrinol Metab* 1995; **80**: 3180–4.

140 Hummelink R, Sippell WG, Benoit KG, *et al*. Intranasal administration of growth hormone-releasing hormone(1-29)-NH2 in children with growth hormone deficiency: effects on growth hormone secretion and growth. *Acta Paediatr Suppl* 1993; **388**: 23–6.

141 Laron Z, Frenkel J, Gil-Ad I, *et al*. Growth hormone releasing activity by intranasal administration of a synthetic hexapeptide (hexarelin). *Clin Endocrinol* 1994; **41**: 539–41.

142 Neyzi O, Yordam N, Ocal G, *et al*. Growth response to growth hormone-releasing hormone(1-29)-NH2 compared with growth hormone. *Acta Paediatr Suppl* 1993; **388**: 16–21.

143 Thorner MO, Rogol AD, Blizzard RM, *et al*. Acceleration of growth rate in growth hormone-deficient children treated with human growth hormone-releasing hormone. *Pediatr Res* 1988; **24**: 145–51.

144 Bowers CY, Alster DK, Frentz JM. The growth hormone releasing activity of a synthetic hexapeptide in normal men and short statured children after oral administration. *J Clin Endocrinol Metab* 1992; **74**: 292–8.

145 Saenger P. Oral growth hormone secretagogues – better than Alice in Wonderland's growth elixir? *J Clin Endocrinol Metab* 1996; **81**: 2773–5.

146 Camanni F, Ghigo E, Arvat E. Growth hormone-releasing peptides and their analogs. *Front Neuroendocrinol* 1998; **19**: 47–72.

147 Ghigo E, Arvat E, Giordano R, *et al*. Biologic activities of growth hormone secretagogues in humans. *Endocrine* 2001; **14**: 87–93.

34

Idiopathic short stature

J M WIT

EVIDENCE SCORING OF THERAPY

     *   Non-randomized controlled trials, cohort study, etc.
   **   One or more well-designed randomized controlled trials
***   Systematic review or meta-analysis

INTRODUCTION

Idiopathic short stature (ISS) is a purely descriptive term that refers to a child, adolescent or adult with a height below the age reference for population and sex, in whom with current diagnostic tools no etiological diagnosis is made.

In this chapter six aspects of ISS will be discussed. First, the definition will be dealt with. Special attention will be given to the notion that the key issue of ISS is that other causes of short stature are excluded, but that there appears little consensus about which investigations should be performed to reach this goal.

Second, the natural history of ISS is described, both in terms of stature and possible psychological effects of shortness. Third, the effects of growth hormone (GH) therapy, either alone or in combination with GnRH analogues (GnRHa) are discussed, both on growth and on psychosocial adjustment. Fourth, a short summary is given of effects of alternative forms of therapy. Fifth, potential risks of GH treatment are reviewed, followed by a sixth section with some considerations about economic and ethical aspects.

DEFINITION AND DIAGNOSIS

Definition

It is generally assumed that growth is regulated by a multitude of genes and epigenetic mechanisms in interaction with influences from the internal and external milieu. ISS can then be considered as a condition in which the net effect of growth-inhibiting and growth-promoting factors is a height below the lower limit of the population's normal range. Depending on the mixture of genes determining the tempo of growth, final height can be either low or normal.

According to this assumption, height in the population should have an approximately Gaussian distribution, similar to many other polygenetic traits. In fact, height distribution for age is almost perfectly Gaussian in large-scale growth studies, although the numbers of individuals measured are insufficient to accurately determine the extreme centiles. Theoretically, one would expect that the left tail of the distribution might be a bit more stretched than the right-hand tail, as height can more easily be severely inhibited than strongly increased. Individuals with a height shorter than the -2.0 SD cut-off limit of the population distribution can either be considered as the necessary 2 percent shortest part of the 'normal' distribution, or as individuals with a disorder that restricts growth. In essence, both notices do not necessarily contradict each other if we accept the multifactorial nature of growth.

In short individuals the prevalence of known growth disorders is obviously much higher than in the total population, but these still constitute the minority. In most short children no diagnosis can be made, and the label 'idiopathic short stature' is used. According to an expert workshop,[1] ISS is defined as a condition in which the height of the individual is more than 2 SD below the corresponding mean height for a given age, sex, and population group, and in which no identifiable disorder is present. ISS is subclassified into familial short stature (the child is short compared with the relevant population, but remains within the expected target range for his or her family) or non-familial short stature (NFFS) (the child is short for the population as well as for the familial target range).

In the expert meeting it was discussed how to deal with the issue of maturational (developmental) delay. There are two parameters for developmental delay: before the onset of puberty only bone age is available, and after pubertal onset both the age at pubertal onset and bone age. The traditionally used terms 'constitutional delay in growth and development (CDGD), puberty (CDGP) or adolescence (CDGA)' illustrate that this can easily lead to confusion. It is a clinical observation that some children who present with bone age delay pre-pubertally enter into puberty at a normal age, and vice versa.[2] Furthermore, for a clear subclassification one can not use more than one criterion. It was thus decided at the expert meeting that only the onset of puberty should be used for further subclassification of FSS and NFSS (normal or delayed onset of puberty).

It was also discussed whether a subdivision in short children with or without decreased growth velocity as proposed by Darendeliler et al.[3] would make sense. It was decided that the variability of growth velocity is so great[4] that such distinction would be arbitrary.

ISS is a condition that remains after exclusion of other conditions. However, two conditions are difficult to exclude, and their demarcations from ISS are and probably always will remain hazy. Most well-known are the problems in distinguishing ISS from growth hormone deficiency (GHD).[5,6] Extreme forms of GHD, usually presenting in infancy or early childhood with severe growth retardation, and in many cases with additional pituitary deficiencies, are easy to diagnose, but the distinction between isolated partial GHD and ISS is, to a great extent, arbitrary. There is no 'gold standard' for GHD, as all parameters have arbitrary cut-off levels and a low accuracy. In particular, a GH provocation test is an unreliable tool for the diagnosis of GHD, for several reasons: high inter-test variation, high inter-assay variation, divergent standards, the effect of age and body mass index on maximal serum GH levels, the arbitrary age-limits beyond which sex steroid priming is advocated,[7] etc. Also, serum insulin growth factor-I (IGF-I) and IGF binding protein-3 (IGFBP-3) measurements may not be as predictive as initially thought.[8]

This situation probably implies that a number of children who are labelled 'partially GH deficient' may in fact not really have a diminished GH secretion. Studies on retesting cases diagnosed as GHD in childhood when they are adults have shown that a substantial portion of them have a normal GH peak after provocation.[9] This probably reflects false-positive results of the initial GH provocation tests rather than a 'transient' GHD. There is little reason to think that there are no false-negative results, which are now labelled ISS but in reality may have restricted growth because of a diminished GH secretion (for a given GH sensitivity).

Many clinicians have become accustomed to think not in terms of yes or no statements about GHD, but rather in terms of a range of probabilities (likelihoods) from 0 to 100 percent, that the growth retardation may be caused by a decreased GH secretion. The likelihood is estimated on the basis of auxology, the medical history, bone age delay, additional pituitary deficiencies, magnetic resonance imaging (MRI), genetic investigations, plasma IGF-I and IGFBP-3, and maximum GH levels after provocation tests. Above a certain likelihood of GHD the condition is treated with GH and theoretically the growth response can serve as a final test to confirm or not that GH insufficiency was the rate-limiting factor for growth in this individual.[10] In practice, however, on the regular GH dosage as used in the United States (approx twice the estimated spontaneous secretion) virtually every short child, classically GH deficient or not, shows an increased growth rate, including children with Turner syndrome, chronic renal failure, persistent short stature after being born small for gestational age (SGA) and ISS.

On this basis, it follows that in some children considered as GHD, GH secretion may in fact not be the rate-limiting step, while in others considered as non-GHD (and thus ISS), a limited GH secretion may well be involved. An example is the recent discovery of a range of haplotypes of the GH promoter, with a functionality of three times lower to three times higher than the most frequent (wild-type) promoter.[11,12] Many of these children have a normal GH peak after provocation, so they may be examples of the hypothetical neurosecretory dysfunction that has been postulated on the basis of 24 h profiles.[13]

Another condition which cannot be delineated sharply from ISS is persistent short stature after being born SGA. The usual definition of SGA includes that weight and/or length is < -2 SD for gestational age. Usually the etiology of low birth size is unknown. The 'and/or' part of this definition implies that the chance availability of information about birth length can decide whether a child with a birth weight slightly higher than the lower cut-off limit of the normal range may fall under the definition of SGA or ISS: a low birth length would make him SGA, an unknown birth length ISS. Thus, some children labelled ISS may well have a birth weight > -2.0 SDS but a short birth length about which no information is available. Another reason to assume that the distinction between idiopathic SGA and ISS is arbitrary is that the Gaussian distribution of birth weight and birth length in ISS is shifted to the left by 1 SD.[14]

Although it is becoming clear that many genes are involved in growth regulation, one can assume that in proportionate short stature disturbances in the GH–IGF-I axis may play a major role. Often these disturbances are divided into two gross categories: subnormal GH secretion and subnormal GH sensitivity (responsiveness). By definition, in ISS patients the GH peak after provocation is normal, so that a classical GHD is ruled out. Still, most children with ISS have a relatively low IGF-I and IGFBP-3. Some of them may have subtle abnormalities of GH secretion, detected by a 12 h or 24 h GH profile (and possibly caused by a subfunctional promoter region of the GH gene), which can be termed 'neuro-secretory dysfunction'. Others may have a heterozygous mutation in the translated part of the GH receptor (GHR) gene or a defect in GH signalling.[15–21] However, so far there is little evidence that heterozygous GHR mutations have a clinical phenotype. In recent years abnormalities downstream from the GHR have been found, such as a mutation of STAT5B[22] and of IKappaB.[23] In both conditions there are immunological disturbances, but these may be very mild.

Disturbances in the IGF-I gene, resulting in a deletion (leading to undetectable IGF-I) or a missense mutation (high radioimmunoassayable IGF-I),[24,25] or heterozygous mutations in the IGFIR gene (IGF-I high or in the upper normal range)[26] are associated with low birth size, so such abnormalities may be found in genetic testing of SGA patients. However, heterozygous carriers of the IGF-I mutation are significantly shorter at birth (but still within the normal range) and postnatally than non-carrier family members.[25] So, some apparently ISS cases may in fact be heterozygous IGF-I deletions or mutations.

A final point is how children adopted from non-industrialized countries into families living in the industrialised part of the world should be classified. They may be normal for their ethnic background, but usually no up-to-date and reliable growth references are available. If there are reference data, and height falls within the expected range, one could consider their height indeed normal for ethnicity, but they are still short for the population where they live. In contrast, a child of short parents of the same ethic origin who immigrated some time ago, is usually labeled 'familial short stature'. In a multicultural society the distinction between 'normal for ethnic origin' and 'familial short stature' is arbitrary.

Diagnosis

In textbooks the issue of which disorders should be excluded before the label idiopathic may be given is usually not dealt with in detail. However, if one questions pediatric endocrinologists which tests they use for the work-up of a short child without further abnormalities in its medical history and at physical examination, there is a wide variation. Even in some countries where consensus guidelines were prepared, the compliance of physicians to such guidelines is rather poor.[26a] An additional problem is that the guidelines are mostly consensus-based, with surprisingly little scientific evidence.

Table 34.1 Laboratory investigations proposed for screening purposes in children with short stature without diagnostic clues from the medical history and physical examination (adapted from the Dutch Consensus Guidelines on Short Stature.[27])

Laboratory investigation	Diseases diagnosed
Blood	
Hemoglobin, hematocrit, cell indices, leukocyte differentiation, erythrocyte sedimentation rate (ferritin)	Anemia, infections, celiac disease, cystic fibrosis
Alanine aminotransferase, aspartate transaminase, gamma-glutamyl transferase	Liver diseases
Albumin, creatinine, sodium, potassium, calcium, phosphate, alkaline phosphatase, acid–base equilibrium	Renal diseases
IgA-anti-endomysium, IgA-anti-gliadin, IgA-anti-tissue glutaminase,† total IgA	Celiac disease
Thyroid stimulating hormone, thyroxine	Hypothyroidism
IGF-I, IGFBP-3	Growth hormone deficiency
Follicle stimulating hormone‡	Turner syndrome
Urine	
pH, glucose, protein, blood and sedimentation	Renal diseases

†IgA-anti-endomysial and anti-tissue transglutaminase antibodies have replaced the previously used anti-gliadin antibodies.
‡FSH is only used as a screening parameter in girls younger than 1 year or older than 8 years. In all short girls in whom no diagnosis is made, a chromosomal analysis is advised.

In Table 34.1 the laboratory investigations are shown that were proposed in the Dutch consensus guidelines,[27] in combination with guidelines about auxological screening. We recently reported that the auxological screening guidelines, particularly in terms of growth velocity, would lead to far too many referrals[28] and that the distance between height SDS and target height SDS is a better screening parameter for Turner syndrome than height SDS as such or the change in height SDS over time.[29**]

Unfortunately, the list of laboratory investigations in Table 34.1 is still far from evidence-based, with probably just one exception (celiac disease). A literature review of studies on the percentage of celiac disease patients detected by measuring anti-endomysial and anti-gliadin antibodies in asymptomatic short children[30**] showed that this investigation is essential before the diagnosis ISS is considered.

An important additional dimension is how far genetic testing should go before one is sufficiently sure that the condition is idiopathic. For example, a heterozygous deletion or mutation of *SHOX* has been described in about 2.5 percent of ISS children without abnormalities in body proportions,[31,32] but in many cases this was not tested in children considered ISS. There is no unanimity about the cost-effectiveness of ordering a fluorescence *in situ* hybridization assay (FISH), if necessary followed by mutation analysis. For further information about genetic testing in short stature we refer to a recent review.[33] However, one should be aware that scientific knowledge in this area is rapidly expanding.

The same applies to the additional investigation of a 12 h or 24 h GH profile, or an IGF-I generation test. If in all children with a low IGF-I and IGFBP-3 (below an arbitrary cut-off limit) and a normal GH peak in a provocation test the clinician decides to perform a GH profile, there will certainly be children who show a low spontaneous secretion (again, below an arbitrary cut-off).[34,35] These children will be labeled GH deficient, while a similar child who is not tested will be labeled ISS. Similarly, children with the combination of a high GH peak in a provocation test and a low IGF-I and IGFBP-3 can be tested or not with an IGF-I generation test. This should theoretically distinguish between mutations in the translated part of the *GH* gene on the one hand and GHR or post-receptor defects on the other. However, there is uncertainty about the cut-off limits of the test and the predictive power. So far, the prevalence of such disorders appears very low[36–40] and these investigations are only carried out in a few potential candidates.

Thus some children labeled ISS may have an organic disorder that has not been excluded (for example celiac disease), a genetic disorder that has not been studied (for example *SHOX* haploinsufficiency), a low spontaneous GH secretion that has not been detected, a dysfunctional GH promoter or an abnormal GH molecule that has not been tested, or some form of decreased responsiveness to GH by a genetic defect in GH signaling. Of these, theoretically children with GH secretion disorders or an abnormal GH molecule should respond to a substitution dose of GH as favorably as children with classical GHD. Children with *SHOX* haploinsufficiency and partial GH unresponsiveness respond less, but still significantly, to a higher GH dose. It is foreseeable that in the coming years more identifiable clinical conditions will be discovered that nowadays are still residing under the cover of the term 'idiopathic'.

NATURAL HISTORY

Somatic development

Over the last 20 years more data have become available about the spontaneous growth pattern of ISS. Reports written before 1996 on final height have been described in several papers and reviews.[2,41–44] In one of these studies, the classification as proposed by the expert panel[1] was used, subdividing children into FSS and NFSS, and both into two further

subdivisions according to puberty onset. Male and female subjects with FSS had a mean final height of 2.1 and 0.6 cm less than target height, respectively. Final height SDS was very similar to pre-pubertal height SDS. For male and female subjects with NFSS, the mean final height was 8.3 and 6.8 cm less than target height, respectively, but substantially higher than initial height SDS.[2] Mean final height was a few centimeters less than the predicted adult height (based on bone age readings) in most studies.[43] In a later study, we observed that while mean final height is quite similar to mean predicted height in ISS, there is a large interindividual variation that is primarily correlated with bone age delay: a large delay gives a large overprediction, and a small delay an underprediction.[45**]

Psychosocial adjustment

About the question to what extent short children, adolescents, and adults suffer from their shortness, and how they cope, many studies have been performed, which are summarized in various reviews and editorials.[46–53] In essence, one can say that in some studies social immaturity, infantilization, low self-esteem, and behavioral problems appear associated with short stature, while in other studies it is concluded that short children are functioning quite well.

These varying results are probably mainly due to a number of methodological factors.[54] The most important one may be the choice of the study population (medically referred or not).[55,56] A second important aspect is which outcome parameter is assessed: psychosocial stressors, psychosocial adaptation, or psychopathology,[57] and which investigational tools (generic or complaint-specific) are used.[58] Thirdly, it is of relevance who are targeted as respondents (the children or adolescents themselves, parents, or teachers).[59] Finally, age and gender appear to play a role.

With regard to the population studied, most children and adolescents with ISS who have been studied had been medically referred. When such children were compared with non-referred short children and normal size controls, only the referred short children showed some behavioral problems.[56*] Similarly, in a longitudinal population-based study short healthy children did not show psychosocial problems, although they were bullied more often than their taller peers.[53,55] Also, adults with ISS, who in their childhood were referred to a pediatrician, reported a negative impact of short stature on their social functioning, their personality, and on finding a partner or a proper job, whereas non-referred short adults showed no impairments in quality of life.[60*,61,62] Thus, people who consult a pediatrician for their short stature, tend to have more psychosocial problems than those who do not: they are a select sample from the short population.

With respect to the level at which the impact of short stature can be measured three levels have been distinguished:[57] (1) stress exposure due to short stature, such as being teased or juvenilized because of being short; (2) quality of coping responses (adaptational process); such as impact on body image and self-esteem; and (3) occurrence of psychopathology (adjustment outcome).

Height-related psychosocial stressors, such as being teased and being juvenilized, have been reported in 14–28 percent of cases in two Dutch studies[63,63a] and up to 50–70 percent in the US.[64] A growth disorder-specific questionnaire for parents may be more sensitive to pick up growth related stressors than generic questionnaires.[58] With regard to psychosocial adaptation, contrasting reports have appeared on body image and self-esteem. Satisfaction with physical appearance was found to be decreased in some studies, and normal in others.[65–68] Perceived height appeared a stronger predictor of psychosocial functioning than measured height.[69]

With respect to potential psychopathology, usually parental reports on the Child Behavior Check List (CBCL) have been used. A common finding has been a lower social competence or social problems, compared to children with normal stature.[47,66,68,70–74] However, in studies using reports from teachers and peers[65,67] no deviations were found in social competence in children with ISS. In terms of potential behavior problems, some studies found indications for aggressive, hostile and defiant behavior or externalizing problems in general,[66,70–72,75] but many other studies could not confirm this. With respect to internalizing behavior problems, withdrawn behavior among children with ISS, as well as somatic complaints and anxious and depressive behavior, were reported,[66,70–72] but not confirmed by others. Intelligence and scholastic competence generally appear normal, but in some studies a decrease was observed.[73] Some indications were found for attention problems (based on CBCL-scores).[72,74]

As mentioned above, the impact of short stature in adulthood appears strongly dependent on whether they were referred as a child to the clinic or not. In two referred groups of individuals, a relatively low percentage of marriages, a relatively high percentage of unemployment, and self-reported problems in social functioning were found,[60,76] but this was not found in two other studies.[77,78] In the study on quality of life of short young adults due to different conditions using utility measures like the standard gamble and time trade off, the loss of quality of life (QOL) was about 4 percent in all patient categories,[60] including ISS (referred cases), GHD, Turner syndrome and chronic renal failure (CRF). In non-referred cases with ISS there were no signs that their short stature had any impact on quality of life. Treated and untreated young adults had a similar and normal quality of life.[79*]

In conclusion, the subgroup of children with ISS who visit a pediatrician typically reports being teased and juvenilized, and tends to show a lower social competence and slightly more than normal behavioral problems. The large inter-individual differences in adaptation to short stature and in the impact of being short may be a function of several risk and protective factors, including parental attitudes and prevailing cultural opinions.[63a]

EFFECT OF GROWTH HORMONE THERAPY

The effect of growth hormone alone on growth

Pediatricians and pediatric endocrinologists are confronted with short children and their parents who ask: 'Can something be done?' Clinicians usually consider this as a signal that short stature is felt as a problem to some extent, and may tend to respond positively. The aim of such treatment would then be to increase height velocity to such an extent that height becomes normal for age in childhood and adolescence, and that final height reaches the normal range for young adults. The assumption, both of child, parents and clinician, is that this would have a positive impact on the individual, both in youth and in adulthood.

Since 1985 many clinical trials have been performed to study the efficacy of GH treatment in ISS. Many of these studies cannot be rated highly on the hierarchy of evidence, and do not comply with the strict rules that can be applied to clinical trials.[80,81] In most instances, the design was to administer a fixed dose per kilogram body weight or square meter body surface from childhood up to near final height. Other designs include a regimen of a dose increment after the first year of treatment, a high dose GH restricted to the pre-pubertal period and a combination of GH with a gonadotropin releasing hormone analogue (GnRHa) in adolescence. Outcome measures are height velocity (as change in height SDS or as velocity per se (centimeters per year or SDS), bone age advance, final height and measures of psychosocial adjustment.

GH treatment in ISS in almost all children leads to an increase of height velocity in the first year, which then gradually tapers off in subsequent years. The acceleration of growth velocity is already substantial at a dosage close to a substitution dosage (0.66 mg m^{-2} body surface day^{-1}, approximately equivalent to 0.17 mg kg^{-1} week^{-1}),[82,83**] and slightly, but statistically significantly, more on higher dosages.[84*] These results indicate that in the wide majority of children either the endogenous GH secretion is suboptimal for normal growth, or that the GH sensitivity is only slightly decreased and can be overcome by administration of GH substitution doses on top of the spontaneous GH secretion. In fact, the response to GH in ISS is quite similar to the growth response to GH in Turner syndrome and SGA. GH does not only have an effect on body stature, but also on body composition. In general, lean body mass is increased more than fat mass, and bone mineral density may also be increased.[85]

Differing results have been obtained with regard to the influence of GH on the rate of bone age advancement and the onset and pace of puberty. In the randomized placebo-controlled study[86**] with a dosage of 0.22 mg kg^{-1} week^{-1} and a British randomized controlled study[87**] using approx 0.33 mg kg^{-1} week^{-1} no effect was observed, while in the randomized controlled study with a dosage of 0.50 mg kg^{-1} week^{-1} a significant advancement of bone age and onset of puberty was seen.[88**] Besides the dosage, also the age at onset of GH therapy may have an impact on the effect of GH on these two markers of maturation.

In the last years several cohorts have reached final height, so that now a global picture has emerged of the long-term efficacy. However, the analysis of final height results is quite complex. Final height, as such, usually expressed as SDS for the population and sex, would appear to be the logical outcome parameter, but final height is correlated with a number of clinical and auxological variables, which have to be entered into the analysis of variance. The individual prediction of final height is rather inaccurate. At a group level, besides final height SDS as such, the difference between final height and predicted final height (on the basis of height and bone age at the start of GH treatment), the difference between final height and height SDS at start of therapy, the difference between final height and target height, and the change in height SDS (for ISS) can be used as surrogate parameters to evaluate the 'success' of treatment. However, each of these outcome measures is again strongly correlated with one or more baseline auxological features. The parameter used most is the difference between final height and predicted adult height, but there is a marked intra- and inter-observer error in bone age readings, different bone age methods yield different results,[89] and the accuracy of the prediction is strongly dependent on the severity of bone age advance.[45]

This methodological issue is particularly important if studies are not designed as randomized clinical trials. We found that when final height SDS as such is used, initial height SDS and bone age delay at start should be assessed as covariates.[45] Children with NFSS tend to end up with a somewhat lower adult height SDS than children with FSS.[45,90*] The difference between final height SDS and initial height SDS (height SDS gain) is quite different between FSS and NFSS subgroups and dependent on bone age delay. Final height SDS minus the predicted adult height (PAH) at baseline in controls has little precision, being strongly dependent on bone age delay, and can only be used if bone age is >6 years. Finally, final height minus target height of untreated children with ISS is much lower in non-FSS and IUGR than in FSS. From these observations it is clear that for a proper analysis of the result of pharmacological therapy a suitable control group (preferably randomized) is needed. A multiple regression analysis should then be performed to tease out the effect of GH from the effects of various covariates.[45]

While the dose–effect with respect to short-term growth response is of modest size, there appears to be a stronger dose–response relationship if final height is taken as outcome measure. On an initial dosage range between 0.17 and 0.25 mg kg^{-1} week^{-1}, even if the dosage is increased in later years,[45] the average effect on final height is approximately 3–4 cm. This was found in the only placebo-controlled trial, in which GH was administered three times per week in a weekly dosage[86] of 0.22 mg kg^{-1} week^{-1} as well as in studies using historical controls or in controlled trials.[43,45,91–95]

In one study it was even suggested that final height might be lower than would have been attained naturally.[96]

All studies using a dosage of approx 0.35 mg kg^{-1} week^{-1} from start until near final height have shown an average final height gain of about 7 cm.[45,87,93,97–101*] In one of these studies[45**,101**] the effect of dosage (0.35 versus 0.25 mg kg^{-1} week^{-1}) was studied in a randomized trial, in the other studies it was the only dosage given. This dosage is about twice the theoretically calculated substitution dosage, which is used for GHD in many countries, but equal to the dosage for GHD in the US. It is also equal to the dosage generally used in Turner syndrome and chronic renal failure. The effect on final height in ISS is of similar size as the effect on final height in Turner syndrome, if treatment is started in mid or late childhood.[102**]

It is remarkable that a regimen in which the dose in the first year was 0.25 mg kg^{-1} week^{-1} and then increased to 0.35 mg kg^{-1} did not result in a better final height result than the dosage of 0.25 mg kg^{-1} week^{-1} over the whole treatment period.[45,101] Similarly, doubling the dosage from 0.17 to 0.35 mg kg^{-1} week^{-1} after 1 year in children responding relatively poorly, did not lead to a good final height gain.[45] Thus, the initial dosage appears the key to a good final height gain.

In my view all available data on this issue are reasonably unequivocal in this respect, so that little doubt remains about the efficacy of GH in ISS in this dosage. Still, one should be aware that there is no placebo-controlled trial, or even a trial with untreated controls, that has studied the long-term effect of this dosage regimen. Furthermore, in virtually all studies there is a considerable loss to follow-up, which may theoretically give rise to selection bias. On the other hand, we found in the intention-to-treat analysis similar results as in the per protocol analysis.[84] Also, with other statistical methods we have demonstrated that selection bias appears minimal, in spite of considerable loss to follow-up.[101]

Recently, the US Food and Drug Administration (FDA) has registered ISS as an indication for two GH preparations, the first one based on the combination of two studies: the placebo-controlled study with the relatively low-dose, administered at low frequency[86] having an effect of approximately 3 cm, and the long-term dose–response study showing that the high dosage was significantly more efficacious than the lower dosage regimens.[45,101]

An alternative therapeutical regimen is a high-dose GH treatment (approx 0.50 mg kg^{-1} week^{-1}) limited to the prepubertal period.[88**,103] However, its efficacy is doubtful, because the interim analysis after 5 years showed that height SDS for bone age and predicted adult height had not changed in comparison to untreated controls. On this regimen we also observed an earlier onset of puberty,[88] which was not observed on dosages of 0.25 or 0.35 mg kg^{-1} week^{-1}.[87,103a] It may thus well be that the dosage of 0.35 mg kg^{-1} week^{-1} is close to the optimum dosage for this condition.

In all studies it has been observed that there is considerable interindividual variation in the long-term growth response.

Probably this is also the case for the effect on final height, but this is difficult to prove due to the uncertainty about the best outcome measure. Various predictive variables at onset of therapy have been reported, including age, initial height SDS, pre-treatment growth velocity, target height minus initial height SDS, the integrated concentration of GH, maximum GH response to provocative tests, serum IGF-I and IGFBP-3 and bone age delay.[83,104–107] Gender does not appear to have a significant effect on growth response.[14] In the first year of treatment height velocity response correlates with bone alkaline phosphatase and/or procollagen type III N-terminal propeptide[108,109] and the result of an IGF-I generation test.[103,110,111] It is likely that a multitude of genetic factors may be involved in GH responsiveness. An example may be the polymorphism in the GHR, which leads to a GHR molecule of which exon 3 is skipped (d3). In GHD the d3 variant shows a better response to GH than the full-length variant.[112] Possibly, in the future the use of prediction models may facilitate the decisions about whether the growth response of an individual child is appropriate or not.[113] With respect to final height, we found that a longer initial bone age delay appeared to increase the final height gain.[45,101]

The effect of GnRHa in combination with growth hormone on growth

In children with ISS and in patients born SGA growth hormone may stimulate a rapid progression through puberty, which is expected to reduce final height gain.[114] Therefore, the effect of GH might be improved by adding a GnRHa or another inhibitor of sex steroid effect on the growth plate.

In a randomized controlled trial the effect of 3 years therapy of GH and GnRHa was assessed versus no treatment in 36 children with ISS or IUGR.[115**] At discontinuation of treatment the estimated effect on PAH was 8.0 cm for girls and 10.4 cm in boys, and the ratio between sitting height/height decreased significantly. Final height gain was 5 cm greater than in controls.

A prospective study to compare the effect of GH alone or GH plus GnRHa in girls with ISS and a relatively early puberty indicated that both regimens increased predicted adult height, but the combination therapy appeared more effective.[116*] Other (uncontrolled) studies on the effect of the combination therapy reported a gain in final height prediction between −0.5 and 10 cm.[117–121] A similar effect was seen in two randomized studies in short adopted girls with early puberty, in which GnRHa plus GH was compared with GnRHa alone.[122**,123**] After 2 and 3 years the mean PAH in the combination groups was 2.7 and 4.5 cm taller, respectively.

From the accumulated evidence it is apparent that the duration of the treatment period is important with regard to the effect on final height. The study by Balducci et al.[124**] showed a gain in PAH after 2 years of 4.4 cm, whereas the mean completed height was only 1.4 cm higher than the

PAH. In contrast, the study by Pasquino et al.[116] used a mean treatment period of 4.6 years, and reported a PAH gain of 10.5 cm, of which only 0.5 cm was lost when the girls were followed to completion of growth.

The aim of this form of treatment is not to increase height in the first year of therapy, as height SDS remains the same in comparison to untreated controls. This regimen only aims at extending the available time to grow by several years, which should enable the body to reach a taller final height. This obviously has an effect on the balance of pros and cons: one advantage of GH treatment (short-term growth acceleration) is taken away, and a disadvantage is added (postponement of pubertal development).[125] As an alternative to the combination of GH + GnRHa, aromatase inhibitors have been administered, and preliminary results indicate that this may increase final height.[126**] Previously, the combination of GH and cyproterone acetate was studied, which did not have a positive effect on final height.[127]

Effect of growth hormone therapy on psychosocial functioning

As shown in a previous paragraph, the effect of short stature on psychological adjustment is generally mild. This implies that there is little room for improvement of psychosocial functioning by any form of treatment. In fact, most studies on the effect of GH therapy have shown little effect on psychological variables. For example, GH therapy (without GnRHa) does not seem to affect social competence, behavior problems, self-esteem, perceived physical appearance, personality and cognitive functioning/scholastic competence.[79,128–132] Only in one study did social and behavioral functioning appear to improve.[131] One study showed a decrease in some aspects of quality of life, as reported by the children themselves.[132**] Still, most parents and children reported that they experienced the treatment as positive,[79,129,132] in spite of the daily injections and regular visits to the clinic.

The effect of GH treatment on quality of life parameters in young adulthood has been described in only a few studies. In a follow-up study of GH-treated ISS individuals, compared with untreated (historical) controls, both groups were found to have a normal quality of life.[79] Most treated individuals said that they were satisfied with the treatment, and they would do it again and would ask for it for their children. This may be an expression of a general tendency in people, i.e., to explain away their decisions.

Few data are available yet with respect to the psychosocial consequences of a combined growth hormone and GnRHa treatment in children with short stature. In a study in which the psychosocial effects of this combined treatment is studied in adopted children with early puberty,[133**] it was concluded that the treatment had no negative effects on psychosocial well being. In our randomized controlled study on the effect of GH + GnRHa we also investigated psychosocial adjustment. Essentially the results in both groups were normal, but the improvement in various parameters observed in the control group (that went through puberty) was not noticed in the treated group.[133a] Long term effects of combined GH/GnRHa treatment on psychosocial functioning will become available soon.[133b]

OTHER MEDICATION

An opposite approach is the administration of androgens to boys with short stature, with or without a delayed puberty. In pre-pubertal boys there is considerable experience with oxandrolone, an anabolic with little virilizing effects.[134–136] Although the absence of controlled studies makes a definite conclusion impossible, it is likely that this treatment does increase height velocity in the first years of treatment, but that bone age accelerates correspondingly, which probably results in no effect on final height. Thus, if one considers improving growth in adolescence as most important, oxandrolone can be given; if one assumes that improving final height is more relevant, oxandrolone is not indicated.

A more logical approach appears to be the administration of testosterone esters to boys with delayed puberty. The primary aim of this treatment is to initiate or increase physical signs of maturation, at the same time as increasing height velocity. This treatment can have a great psychological benefit[77] and is probably too often withheld. If the dosage is kept low, there is no effect on final height.[137]

In children with idiopathic short stature without precocious puberty the effect of GnRHa alone appears limited to 0–4 cm.[138–140**] There is a statistically significant, though clinically modest, effect of GnRHa alone on final height SDS of girls adopted from nonindustrialized countries.[141]

In the 1980s and early 1990s several drugs with a GH stimulatory effect were investigated, such as oral arginine, clonidine, ornithine 2-oxoglutarate and cyproheptadine. In spite of several short-term positive results, clinical trials of longer duration have shown that these agents are ineffective. More recently, short-term clinical trials with GHRH or GH-releasing peptides (GHRPs) have been performed, which appear to have led to some increase of height velocity.[142–145] However, no long-term results have been reported.

POTENTIAL RISKS OF GROWTH HORMONE TREATMENT

So far, GH treatment seems remarkably safe, at least during treatment. In controlled studies, as well as in pharmaceutical surveillance programmes (KIGS, National Cooperative Growth Study) no serious adverse effects have been discovered as yet.[146–155] Still, the potential influence of GH on carbohydrate metabolism and possible associations between GH, IGF-I, and various neoplastic diseases underscore the need for continued surveillance of the safety of GH. The speculations about an effect on tumor formation are based on laboratory findings that IGF-I can stimulate tumor cell

growth *in vitro*, and on the increased prevalence of certain tumors, particularly of the intestines, in acromegaly.[156] For further reading on this topic there is a large number of recent reviews available.[155,157–162,163**]

A possible adverse effect of the combination of GH and GnRHa is a decreased bone mineral density. This was observed in a study in a heterogeneous group of GHD and non-GHD patients.[140] Whether this will be confirmed in randomized controlled trials in ISS is still unknown. In GHD patients the effect of the combination of GH and a GnRHa has only a transient effect on bone mineral density.[164**]

ECONOMIC AND ETHICAL CONSIDERATIONS

GH treatment for children with ISS has been heavily debated over the last decades, particularly the economic and ethical issues.[165–170] It has often been called an example of cosmetic medicine, partially because it was often emphasized that these children were 'normal' (hence the terms 'normal variant short stature' and 'constitutional short stature'). It has been noted that 'a focus on final height attainment ignores the important psychological components of being short, the concerns about possible harm that may arise from such invasive intervention, and the important role that parents must assume in their child's development.' 'The motivation for GH therapy may say much more about parental hopes than any aspirations expressed by the child'.[171,172] It was also emphasized that 'we must not impose our goals on them, either in thought or in action, ... our suggestion that he should be taller can also do harm'.[165] These important notes of warning, urge the clinician to carefully balance the possible benefits of enhancing growth in adolescence and adulthood against possible psychosocial consequences of GH treatment and (in the case of a combined treatment) delay of pubertal development.

Essentially, the argument is: 'Why treat normal children for a somatic characteristic that can not be called a disease or disorder, and that does not lead to substantial loss of quality of life? Particularly if the financial consequences are considerable!'. In this discussion often the term 'heightism' is used, denominating a tendency in society to label a tall height positively. It is also emphasized that GH treatment for ISS 'is sought by parents who believe that two things are true: first, that GH will make children taller and, second, that being taller will benefit the child',[165,173] while the last assumption is not proven.

With regard to the economics of GH treatment in ISS, there is no doubt that biosynthetic GH is expensive. The annual cost for one child weighing 30 kg is about US$ 19 000,[174] so that the treatment from mid-childhood to final height for the average ISS child will cost about US$ 100 000–150 000. The high costs arise partly because, in the US and many other countries, the GH dosage is calculated per kilogram body weight. If the dosage is calculated per square meter body surface, which is theoretically a more rational approach, this saves much money in adolescence. These figures make it clear that a nationwide decision to reimburse GH treatment for ISS has a considerable impact on healthcare resources.

In my opinion, the primary task of pediatric endocrinologists, as a group, on this issue has been and still is to collect evidence about the efficacy (in all domains, thus both biomedical and psychosocial) and adverse effects of GH treatment. When these data are assembled and properly reviewed at expert meetings, decision-making is the next step, at various levels. First, in the clinic the individual child and his/her parents, who ask medical advice about short stature, are counseled about possible GH treatment. Second, at a regional or national level decisions can be made within the pediatric endocrine professional bodies, about a common guideline. Third, at the level of governmental bodies and insurance companies decisions can be made whether the expected gains of reimbursing GH medication to ISS are worth the financial investment, in the light of other social constraints and necessities in healthcare. At the first and second level, the pediatric endocrinologist is directly involved. At the third level, at best (s)he is consulted for advice, and his or her advice may have a greater or lesser impact on decision-making.

Let us first look at the available evidence. In previous paragraphs the presently available data on efficacy and possible adverse effects are reviewed. In summary, a dosage of $0.35 \, \mathrm{mg \, kg^{-1} \, week^{-1}}$ leads to an average 7 cm final height gain; no adverse effects have been detected yet; most short children cope rather well with their shortness, but some psychosocial stress can be detected; during therapy psychosocial adjustment remains basically the same; and short adults (that is to say, those who were referred to a doctor in childhood) would have liked to be taller. These data are quite similar to the available evidence on GH treatment in Turner syndrome (TS), CRF and SGA, although remarkably few studies have been performed in these medical conditions, for which GH therapy has been registered for some time (TS, CRF) or recently (SGA). Even in GHD patients, certainly children with partial GHD, the facts and figures may be quite similar.

Then how to deal with this evidence in the clinic? It is my experience that, after proper diagnostic steps (including an estimate of the likelihood that an insufficient GH secretion may be the rate-limiting factor), a thorough inventory of the degree of apparent suffering and predictive variables for response in the individual case,[51] as well as a full explanation of the available clinical evidence on effects and side effects (including the financial issue) (see Table 34.2), will usually lead to a consensus among child, parents and clinician about the strategy to be followed. If the child, parents and clinician agree that this particular child might benefit substantially from GH treatment, enough to accept the known downsides of treatment and the unknown possible long-term side effects, it will then depend on the local and national situation (and on the financial resources of the parents) whether the child can be treated. In many instances, however,

Table 34.2 Arguments in favor of and against growth hormone (GH) therapy in children with idiopathic short stature (ISS). (Adapted from Wit.[180])

Points arguing in favor

1. GH in a supraphysiological dosage generally increases height velocity in childhood, leads to less height deficit in childhood and adolescence, and to an adult height which is on average 7 cm higher
2. GH administration can be felt to be rewarding for the child, parents and clinician because they have the feeling that something is being done
3. GH injections are generally well tolerated
4. Significant adverse events have not been observed
5. GH may increase bone mass density
6. Some children labeled ISS may have a form of GH insufficiency (e.g., neurosecretory dysfunction, abnormal GH molecule, inactive GH promoter, etc)

Points arguing against

1. Even with a supraphysiological dosage the average effect on final height is modest (final height still below or in the lower half of the normal distribution of the population and lower than target height)
2. The growth response is variable, and cannot be predicted with acceptable accuracy
3. Most studies on psychosocial adjustment in short children and adults have failed to demonstrate a significant negative effect of shortness, and have failed to show significant changes during therapy
4. GH treatment leads to medicalization (daily injections, regular clinic visits)
5. Theoretical risk of unwanted long-term sequelae of elevated serum GH and IGF-I
6. Large-scale use at the present price would consume an important part of the health budget
7. Ethical considerations that GH treatment in allegedly short 'normal' children is an unacceptable form of cosmetic medicine

the result of the consultation will be a joint decision that the ultimate effect in terms of final height gain may not be sufficient to take the trouble of daily injections for many years, with many doctor's visits and unknown long-term side effects.

How to deal with the issue at the second and third levels? The still limited evidence and uncertainties on this issue, as well as divergent opinions about the ethical aspects, make it likely that among pediatricians and pediatric endocrinologists varying opinions exist. The wealth of a country and the organization of the health system also are expected to have an impact on the decision whether all children with ISS, or only extreme cases, or none at all, are considered suitable candidates for GH treatment. Inquiries among pediatric endocrinologists have indeed shown varying opinions, as well as a great variation in practice.[175,176] Large international databases show a similar picture.[177–179] Since 2002, in the

USA, GH treatment for ISS has been approved by the FDA, but it is not universally reimbursed by insurance companies and health maintenance organizations. In other countries the registration is still under review.

For the future it is expected that better diagnostic procedures will become available, which can better distinguish whether short stature is primarily due to an impaired GH secretion, or to partial GH insensitivity or other causes. In the meantime, a pragmatic approach could be to restrict GH treatment to cases of severe short stature in whom there is sufficient indication that an insufficient GH secretion or an abnormal GH molecule may be the cause. A therapeutic trial for 6–12 months with GH, with measurements of IGF-I, IGFBP-3 and various metabolic markers may serve as a practical tool to help to make the decision to maintain therapy up to final height. However, for a proper assessment of GH sensitivity a substitution dosage (approx 0.17–$0.23\,\mathrm{mg\,kg^{-1}\,week^{-1}}$) may be most rational, while it is now clear that for long-term treatment a higher GH dosage of about $0.35\,\mathrm{mg\,kg^{-1}\,week^{-1}}$ from the onset of therapy should be given in order to reach a substantially taller final height.

As clinicians we have the duty to serve the best interests of the patients, and to act as their advocates. As advisors to regional or national health organizations, we can outline the pros and cons of GH treatment for ISS and leave it to others to decide whether this treatment with some impact on the full lifetime can stand up against all kinds of other medical treatment at all ages. What we might ask at least is that other medical treatments are scrutinized in the same explicit way as has been done for ISS.

usually coping mechanisms are sufficient to prevent low self-esteem, psychopathology and behaviour problems. Short children referred to the clinic have more problems than non-referred short children.

- In general, short young adults have adapted quite well, but some of them attribute their problems to being short.
- The effect of GH on growth velocity and on final height gain is dose-dependent. On dosages of 0.17–$0.25\,\mathrm{mg\,kg^{-1}}$ body weight $\mathrm{week^{-1}}$ average final height gain is approximately 3–4 cm, on $0.35\,\mathrm{mg\,kg^{-1}\,week^{-1}}$ approximately 7 cm. On a higher dosage ($0.50\,\mathrm{mg\,kg^{-1}\,week^{-1}}$) bone age advance and earlier pubertal onset was observed, leading to unchanged predicted adult height.
- In children entering puberty when their present and predicted height SDS is low, the combination of GH and a GnRH analogue appears to increase final height by approx 5 cm.
- GH is tolerated well in general and psychosocial functioning shows little change.
- No serious adverse effects have been observed of GH therapy in ISS, but continued surveillance remains indicated, particularly with regard to neoplastic diseases and carbohydrate metabolism.
- A carefully balanced approach to GH therapy in ISS is necessary, and should involve all pros and cons that are currently available. This applies to individual clinical care as well as national health policy.

KEY LEARNING POINTS

- Idiopathic short stature is a diagnosis of exclusion, but there exists no consensus about which other diagnoses should be excluded in the absence of clinical symptoms and signs.
- The delineation of ISS from GH deficiency is hazy. For the individual child, the combination of clinical, auxological and biochemical data can only provide an estimate of the likelihood that the diminished growth is causally associated with a decreased GH secretion.
- Untreated children with familial short stature usually reach an adult height SDS close to height SDS in childhood and to target height. Children with non-familial idiopathic short stature reach a final height SDS substantially higher than height SDS in childhood, but 7–8 cm below target height.
- Short stature in children and adolescents exposes them to some stress (teasing, juvenilization), but

REFERENCES

● = Seminal primary article
◆ = Key review paper
✳ = First formal publication of a management guideline

✳ 1 Ranke MB. Towards a consensus on the definition of idiopathic short stature. Summary. *Horm Res* 1996; **45(Suppl 2)**: 64–6.

2 Rekers-Mombarg LTM, Wit JM, Massa GG, *et al.* Spontaneous growth in idiopathic short stature. *Arch Dis Child* 1996; **75**: 175–80.

3 Darendeliler F, Hindmarsh PC, Brook CGD. Non-conventional use of growth hormone: European experience. *Horm Res* 1990; **33**: 128–36.

● 4 Voss LD, Wilkin TJ, Bailey BJR, Betts PR. The reliability of height and height velocity in the assessment of growth (the Wessex Growth Study). *Arch Dis Child* 1991; **66**: 833–7.

◆ 5   Rosenfeld RG, Albertsson-Wikland K, Cassorla F, *et al.* Diagnostic controversy: The diagnosis of childhood growth hormone deficiency revisited. *J Clin Endocrinol Metab* 1995; **80**: 1532–40.

◆ 6   Consensus guidelines for the diagnosis and treatment of growth hormone (GH) deficiency in childhood and adolescence: summary statement of the GH Research Society. GH Research Society. *J Clin Endocrinol Metab* 2000; **85**: 3990–3.

   7   Marin G, Domene HM, Barnes KM, *et al.* The effects of estrogen priming and puberty on the growth hormone response to standardized treadmill exercise and arginine-insulin in normal girls and boys. *J Clin Endocrinol Metab* 1994; **79**: 537–41.

   8   Mitchell H, Dattani MT, Nanduri V, *et al.* Failure of IGF-I and IGFBP-3 to diagnose growth hormone insufficiency. *Arch Dis Child* 1999; **80**: 443–7.

   9   Tauber M, Moulin P, Pienkowski C, *et al.* Growth hormone (GH) retesting and auxological data in 131 GH-deficient patients after completion of treatment. *J Clin Endocrinol Metab* 1997; **82**: 352–6.

  10   Wit JM. Growth hormone therapy for the growth hormone deficient child. In: Wass JAH, Shalet SM, eds. *Oxford Textbook of Endocrinology and Diabetes.* Oxford: Oxford University Press, 2002: 1008–18.

● 11   Millar DS, Lewis MD, Horan M, *et al.* Novel mutations of the growth hormone 1 (GH1) gene disclosed by modulation of the clinical selection criteria for individuals with short stature. *Hum Mutat* 2003; **21**: 424–40.

● 12   Horan M, Millar DS, Hedderich J, *et al.* Human growth hormone 1 (GH1) gene expression: complex haplotype-dependent influence of polymorphic variation in the proximal promoter and locus control region. *Hum Mutat* 2003; **21**: 408–23.

● 13   Spiliotis BE, August GP, Hung W, *et al.* Growth hormone neurosecretory dysfunction. A treatable cause of short stature. *JAMA* 1984; **251**: 2223–30.

  14   Wit JM. Growth hormone treatment of idiopathic short stature in KIGS. In: Ranke MB, Wilton P, eds. *Growth Hormone Therapy-10 Years' Experience.* Heidelberg: Johann Ambrosius Barth Verlag, 1999: 225–43.

  15   Clayton PE, Freeth JS, Norman MR. Congenital growth hormone insensitivity syndromes and their relevance to idiopathic short stature. *Clin Endocrinol (Oxf)* 1999; **50**: 275–83.

  16   Monson JP, Rosenfeld RG. Sensitivity to growth hormone – the perspective. Round table discussion. *Horm Res* 2001; **55(Suppl 2)**: 65–7.

  17   Salerno M, Balestrieri B, Matrecano E, *et al.* Abnormal GH receptor signaling in children with idiopathic short stature. *J Clin Endocrinol Metab* 2001; **86**: 3882–8.

  18   Rosenfeld RG, Buckway CK. Growth hormone insensitivity syndromes: lessons learned and opportunities missed. *Horm Res* 2001; **55(Suppl 2)**: 36–9.

  19   Savage MO, Burren CP, Blair JC, *et al.* Growth hormone insensitivity: pathophysiology, diagnosis, clinical variation and future perspectives. *Horm Res* 2001; **55(Suppl 2)**: 32–5.

  20   Rosenfeld RG, Hwa V. New molecular mechanisms of GH resistance. *Eur J Endocrinol* 2004; **151(Suppl 1)**: S11–5.

  21   Rosenfeld RG, Hwa V. Toward a molecular basis for idiopathic short stature. *J Clin Endocrinol Metab* 2004; **89**: 1066–7.

● 22   Kofoed EM, Hwa V, Little B, *et al.* Growth hormone insensitivity associated with a STAT5b mutation. *N Engl J Med* 2003; **349**: 1139–47.

● 23   Janssen R, van Wengen A, Hoeve MA, *et al.* The same IkappaBalpha mutation in two related individuals leads to completely different clinical syndromes. *J Exp Med* 2004; **200**: 559–68.

● 24   Woods KA, Camacho-Hubner C, Savage MO, Clark AJ. Intrauterine growth retardation and postnatal growth failure associated with deletion of the insulin-like growth factor I gene. *N Engl J Med* 1996; **335**: 1363–7.

● 25   Walenkamp MJE, Karperien M, Pereira AM, *et al.* Homozygous and heterozygous expression of a novel IGF-I mutation. *J Clin Endocrinol Metab* 2005; **90**: 2855–64.

● 26   Abuzzahab MJ, Schneider A, Goddard A, *et al.* IGF-I receptor mutations resulting in intrauterine and postnatal growth retardation. *N Engl J Med* 2003; **349**: 2211–22.

 26a   Grote FK, Oostdijk W, de Muinck Keizer-Schrama SMPF, *et al.* Growth monitoring and diagnostic work-up of short stature: an international inventarisation. *J Ped Endocrinol Metab* 2005; **18**: 1031–8.

  27   Muinck Keizer-Schrama SM. Consensus 'diagnosis of short stature in children'. National Organization for Quality Assurance in Hospitals. *Ned Tijdschr Geneeskd* 1998; **142**: 2519–25.

  28   Van Buuren S, Bonnemaijer-Kerckhoffs DJ, Grote FK, *et al.* Many referrals under Dutch short stature guidelines. *Arch Dis Child* 2004; **89**: 351–2.

  29   Van Buuren S, Van Dommelen P, Zandwijken GR, *et al.* Towards evidence based referral criteria for growth monitoring. *Arch Dis Child* 2004; **89**: 336–41.

  30   van Rijn JC, Grote FK, Oostdijk W, Wit JM. Short stature and the probability of coeliac disease, in the absence of gastrointestinal symptoms. *Arch Dis Child* 2004; **89**: 882–3.

  31   Rappold GA, Fukami M, Niesler B, *et al.* Deletions of the homeobox gene SHOX (short stature homeobox) are an important cause of growth failure in children with short stature. *J Clin Endocrinol Metab* 2002; **87**: 1402–6.

◆ 32   Munns CF, Glass IA, Flanagan S, *et al.* Familial growth and skeletal features associated with SHOX haploin sufficiency. *J Pediatr Endocrinol Metab* 2003; **16**: 987–96.

  33   Kant SG, Wit JM, Breuning MH. Genetic analysis of short stature. *Horm Res* 2003; **60**: 157–65.

  34   Dammacco F, Boghen MF, Camanni F, *et al.* Somatotropic function in short stature: evaluation by integrated auxological and hormonal indices in 214 children. *J Clin Endocrinol Metab* 1993; **77**: 68–72.

  35   Rogol AD, Blethen SL, Sy JP, Veldhuis JD. Do growth hormone (GH) serial sampling, insulin-like growth factor-I (IGF-I) or auxological measurements have an advantage

over GH stimulation testing in predicting the linear growth response to GH therapy? *Clin Endocrinol (Oxf)* 2003; **58**: 229–37.

36 Cotterill AM, Camacho-Hubner C, Duquesnoy P, Savage MO. Changes in serum IGF-I and IGFBP-3 concentrations during the IGF-I generation test performed prospectively in children with short stature. *Clin Endocrinol (Oxf)* 1998; **48**: 719–24.

◆ 37 Lopez-Bermejo A, Buckway CK, Rosenfeld RG. Genetic defects of the growth hormone-insulin-like growth factor axis. *Trends Endocrinol Metab* 2000; **11**: 39–49.

38 Buckway CK, Guevara-Aguirre J, Pratt KL, *et al.* The IGF-I generation test revisited: a marker of GH sensitivity. *J Clin Endocrinol Metab* 2001; **86**: 5176–83.

39 Buckway CK, Selva KA, Pratt KL, *et al.* Insulin-like growth factor binding protein-3 generation as a measure of GH sensitivity. *J Clin Endocrinol Metab* 2002; **87**: 4754–65.

40 Selva KA, Buckway CK, Sexton G, *et al.* Reproducibility in patterns of IGF generation with special reference to idiopathic short stature. *Horm Res* 2003; **60**: 237–46.

41 Heitmann BL, Sorensen TIA, Keiding N, Skakkebaek NE. Predicting the adult height of short children. *BMJ* 1994; **308**: 360.

42 Ranke MB, Grauer ML, Kistner K, *et al.* Spontaneous adult height in idiopathic short stature. *Horm Res* 1995; **44**: 152–7.

◆ 43 Wit JM, Kamp GA, Rikken B. Spontaneous growth and response to growth hormone treatment in children with growth hormone deficiency and idiopathic short stature. *Pediatr Res* 1996; **39**: 295–302.

44 Price DA. Spontaneous adult height in patients with idiopathic short stature. *Horm Res* 1996; **45(Suppl 2)**: 59–63.

45 Wit JM, Rekers-Mombarg LT. Final height gain by GH therapy in children with idiopathic short stature is dose dependent. *J Clin Endocrinol Metab* 2002; **87**: 604–11.

46 Sandberg DE. Caring for the short, endocrinologically normal child. *Curr Probl Pediatr* 1995; **25**: 163–70.

47 Sandberg DE, Kranzler J, Bukowski WM, Rosenbloom AL. Psychosocial aspects of short stature and growth hormone therapy. *J Pediatr* 1999; **135**: 133–4.

48 Sandberg DE, MacGillivray MH. Growth hormone therapy in childhood-onset growth hormone deficiency: adult anthropometric and psychological outcomes. *Endocrine* 2000; **12**: 173–82.

49 Sandberg DE, Voss LD. The psychosocial consequences of short stature: a review of the evidence. *Best Pract Res Clin Endocrinol Metab* 2002; **16**: 449–63.

50 Haverkamp F, Ranke MB. The ethical dilemma of growth hormone treatment of short stature: a scientific theoretical approach. *Horm Res* 1999; **51**: 301–4.

51 Haverkamp F, Eiholzer U, Ranke MB, Noeker M. Symptomatic versus substitution growth hormone therapy in short children: from auxology towards a comprehensive multidimensional assessment of short stature and related interventions. *J Pediatr Endocrinol Metab* 2000; **13**: 403–8.

52 Voss LD. Growth hormone therapy for the short normal child: who needs it and who wants it? The case against growth hormone therapy. *J Pediatr* 2000; **136**: 103–6.

◆ 53 Voss LD, Sandberg DE. The psychological burden of short stature: evidence against. *Eur J Endocrinol* 2004; **151(Suppl 1)**: S29–33.

◆ 54 Wiklund I, Erling A, Albertsson-Wikland K. Critical review of measurement issues in quality of life assessment for children with growth problems. In: Drotar D, ed. *Measuring Health-related Quality of Life in Children and Adolescents. Implications for Research and Practice.* Mahwah, New Jersey: Lawrence Erlbaum Associates, 1998: 255–71.

55 Downie AB, Mulligan J, Stratford RJ, *et al.* Are short normal children at a disadvantage? The Wessex growth study. *BMJ* 1997; **314**: 97–100.

56 Kranzler JH, Rosenbloom AL, Proctor B, *et al.* Is short stature a handicap? A comparison of the psychosocial functioning of referred and nonreferred children with normal short stature and children with normal stature. *J Pediatr* 2000; **136**: 96–102.

57 Noeker M, Haverkamp F. Adjustment in conditions with short stature: a conceptual framework. *J Pediatr Endocrinol Metab* 2000; **13**: 1585–94.

58 Haverkamp F, Noeker M. 'Short stature in children' – a questionnaire for parents: a new instrument for growth disorder-specific psychosocial adaptation in children. *Qual Life Res* 1998; **7**: 447–55.

59 Theunissen NC, Vogels TG, Koopman HM, *et al.* The proxy problem: child report versus parent report in health-related quality of life research. *Qual Life Res* 1998; **7**: 387–97.

60 Busschbach JJ, Rikken B, Grobbee DE, *et al.* Quality of life in short adults. *Horm Res* 1998; **49**: 32–8.

61 Rikken B, van Busschbach J, le Cessie S, *et al.* Impaired social status of growth hormone deficient adults as compared to controls with short or normal stature. Dutch Growth Hormone Working Group [see comments]. *Clin Endocrinol (Oxf)* 1995; **43**: 205–11.

62 Ulph F, Betts P, Mulligan J, Stratford RJ. Personality functioning: the influence of stature. *Arch Dis Child* 2004; **89**: 17–21.

63 Huisman J, Slijper FM, Sinnema G, *et al.* (Good things come in small packages? Psychosocial aspects of small stature). Klein maar fijn? De psychosociale aspecten van een kleine gestalte. Nederlandse werkgroep 'Psycholen en Groeihormoon'. *Tijdschr Kindergeneeskd* 1992; **60**: 139–46.

63a Visser-van Balen H, Geenen R, Kamp GA, *et al.* Motives for growth enhancing hormone treatment in young adolescents with idiopathic short stature or intra-uterine growth retardation: a questionnaire and structured interview study. *BMC Pediatrics* 2005; **5**: 15.

64 Sandberg DE MP. Psychosocial stress related to short stature: does their presence imply psychological dysfunction? In: Drotar D, ed. *Measuring Health-related Quality of Life in Children and Adolescents; Implications for Research and Practice.* Mahwah, New Jersey: Lawrence Erlbaum Associates, 1998: 287–312.

65   Gilmour J, Skuse D. Short stature – the role of intelligence in psychosocial adjustment. *Arch Dis Child* 1996; **75**: 25–31.

66   Gordon M, Crouthamel C, Post EM, Richman RA. Psychosocial aspects of constitutional short stature: social competence, behavior problems, self-esteem, and family functioning. *J Pediatr* 1982; **101**: 477–80.

67   Richman RA, Gordon M, Tegtmeyer P, Crouthamel C, Post EM. Academic and emotional difficulties associated with constitutional short stature. In: Stabler B, Underwood LE, eds. *Slow Grows the Child: Psychosocial Aspects of Growth Delay*. Hillsdale, New Jersey: Lawrence Erlbaum Associates, 1986: 13–26.

68   Young-Hyman D. Effects of short stature on social competence. In: Stabler B, Underwood LE, eds. *Slow Grows the Child: Psychosocial Aspects of Growth Delay*. Hillsdale, New Jersey: Lawrence Erlbaum Associates, 1986: 27–45.

69   Hunt L, Hazen RA, Sandberg DE. Perceived versus measured height. Which is the stronger predictor of psychosocial functioning? *Horm Res* 2000; **53**: 129–38.

70   Frankel SA. Psychological complications of short stature in childhood. Some implications of the role of visual comparisons in normal and pathological development. *Psychoanal Study Child* 1996; **51**: 455–74.

71   Holmes CS, Karlsson JA, Thompson RG. Longitudinal evaluation of behavior patterns in children with short stature. In: Stabler B, Underwood LE, eds. *Slow Grows the Child: Psychosocial Aspects of Growth Delay*. Hillsdale, New Jersey: Lawrence Erlbaum Associates, 1986: 1–12.

72   Sandberg DE, Brook AE, Campos SP. Short stature: a psychosocial burden requiring growth hormone therapy? *Pediatrics* 1994; **94**: 832–40.

73   Stabler B, Clopper RR, Siegel PT, *et al*. Academic achievement and psychological adjustment in short children. The National Cooperative Growth Study. *J Dev Behav Pediatr* 1994; **15**: 1–6.

74   Skuse D, Gilmour J, Tian CS, Hindmarsh P. Psychosocial assessment of children with short stature: a preliminary report. *Acta Paediatr Suppl* 1994; **406**: 11–6.

75   Siegel P. The psychological adjustment of short children and normal controls. In: Stabler B, Underwood LE, eds. *Growth, Stature, and Adaptation*. Chapel Hill, North Carolina: University of North Carolina, 1994: 123–34.

76   Sartorio A, Morabito F, Peri G, *et al*. The social outcome of adults with constitutional growth delay. *J Endocrinol Invest* 1990; **13**: 593–5.

77   Crowne EC, Shalet SM, Wallace WHB, *et al*. Final height in boys with untreated constitutional delay in growth and puberty. *Arch Dis Child* 1990; **65**: 1109–12.

78   Zimet GD, Owens R, Dahms W, *et al*. The psychosocial functioning of adults who were short as children. In: Eiholzer U, Haverkamp F, Voss L, eds. *Growth, Stature and Psychosocial Wellbeing*. Seattle: Hogrefe & Huber Publishers, 1999: 47–55.

79   Rekers-Mombarg LT, Busschbach JJ, Massa GG, *et al*. Quality of life of young adults with idiopathic short stature: effect of growth hormone treatment. Dutch Growth Hormone Working Group. *Acta Paediatr* 1998; **87**: 865–70.

80   Hindmarsh PC. Evidence-based decisions in growth hormone therapy. In: Hindmarsh PC, ed. *Current Indications for Growth Hormone Therapy*. Basel: Karger, 1999: 1–12.

81   Farewell VT, Cook RJ. Methodological issues for clinical trials in growth hormone therapy. In: Hindmarsh PC, ed. *Current Indications for Growth Hormone Therapy*. Basel: Karger, 1999: 13–32.

82   Wit JM, Rietveld DH, Drop SL, *et al*. A controlled trial of methionyl growth hormone therapy in prepubertal children with short stature, subnormal growth rate and normal growth hormone response to secretagogues. *Acta Paediatr Scand* 1989; **78**: 426–35.

83   Wit JM, Fokker MH, de Muinck Keizer-Schrama SMPF, *et al*. Effects of two years of methionyl growth hormone therapy in two dosage regimens in prepubertal children with short stature, subnormal growth rate and normal growth hormone response to secretagogues. *J Pediatr* 1989; **115**: 720–5.

84   Rekers-Mombarg LT, Massa GG, Wit JM, *et al*. Growth hormone therapy with three dosage regimens in children with idiopathic short stature. European Study Group Participating Investigators. *J Pediatr* 1998; **132**: 455–60.

85   Lanes R, Gunczler P, Weisinger JR. Decreased trabecular bone mineral density in children with idiopathic short stature: normalization of bone density and increased bone turnover after 1 year of growth hormone treatment. *J Pediatr* 1999; **135**: 177–81.

86   Leschek EW, Rose SR, Yanovski JA, *et al*. Effect of growth hormone treatment on adult height in peripubertal children with idiopathic short stature: a randomized, double-blind, placebo-controlled trial. *J Clin Endocrinol Metab* 2004; **89**: 3140–8.

87   McCaughey ES, Mulligan J, Voss LD, Betts PR. Randomised trial of growth hormone in short normal girls. *Lancet* 1998; **351**: 940–4.

88   Kamp GA, Waelkens JJ, De Muinck Keizer-Schrama SM, *et al*. High dose growth hormone treatment induces acceleration of skeletal maturation and an earlier onset of puberty in children with idiopathic short stature. *Arch Dis Child* 2002; **87**: 215–20.

89   Brämswig JH, Fasse M, Holthoff ML, *et al*. Adult height in boys and girls with untreated short stature and constitutional delay of growth and puberty: Accuracy of five different methods of height prediction. *J Pediatr* 1990; **117**: 886–91.

90   Rekers Mombarg LT, Wit JM, Massa GG, *et al*. Spontaneous growth in idiopathic short stature. European Study Group. *Arch Dis Child* 1996; **75**: 175–80.

91   Guyda HJ. Growth hormone treatment of non-growth hormone deficient subjects: the International Task Force report. *Clin Pediatr Endocrinol* 1996; **5(Suppl 7)**: 11–8.

92   Hintz RL. Growth hormone treatment of idiopathic short stature. *Horm Res* 1996; **46**: 208–14.

93   Kamp GA, Wit JM. High-dose growth hormone therapy in idiopathic short stature. *Horm Res* 1998; **49(Suppl 2)**: 67–72.

94 Hindmarsh PC, Brook CGD. Final height of short normal children treated with growth hormone. *Lancet* 1996; **348**: 13–6.

95 Cowell CT, Craig ME, Ambler GR. Use of growth hormone in idiopathic short stature. In: Hindmarsh PC, ed. *Current Indications for Growth Hormone Therapy*. Basel: Karger, 1999: 68–86.

96 Kawai M, Momoi T, Yorifuji T, *et al*. Unfavorable effects of growth hormone therapy on the final height of boys with short stature not caused by growth hormone deficiency [see comments]. *J Pediatr* 1997; **130**: 205–9.

97 Hintz RL, Attie KM, Baptista J, Roche A. Effect of growth hormone treatment on adult height of children with idiopathic short stature. Genentech Collaborative Group. *N Engl J Med* 1999; **340**: 502–7.

98 Buchlis JG, Irizarry L, Crotzer BC, *et al*. Comparison of final heights of growth hormone-treated vs. untreated children with idiopathic growth failure. *J Clin Endocrinol Metab* 1998; **83**: 1075–9.

99 Lopez-Siguero JP, Garcia-Garcia E, Carralero I, Martinez-Aedo MJ. Adult height in children with idiopathic short stature treated with growth hormone. *J Pediatr Endocrinol Metab* 2000; **13**: 1595–602.

100 Finkelstein BS, Imperiale TF, Speroff T, *et al*. Effect of growth hormone therapy on height in children with idiopathic short stature: a meta-analysis. *Arch Pediatr Adolesc Med* 2002; **156**: 230–40.

101 Wit JM, Rekers-Mombarg LTM, Cutler GB Jr, *et al*. on behalf of the European Idiopathic Short Stature Study Group. Growth hormone treatment to final height in children with idiopathic short stature: evidence for a dose effect. *J Pediatr* 2005; **146**: 45–53.

102 Rosenfeld RG, Frane J, Attie KM, *et al*. 6-Year results of a randomized, prospective trial of human growth hormone and oxandrolone in Turner syndrome. *J Ped* 1992; **121**: 49–55.

103 Kamp GA, Zwinderman AH, van Doorn J, *et al*. Biochemical markers of growth hormone (GH) sensitivity in children with idiopathic short stature: individual capacity of IGF-I generation after high-dose GH treatment determines the growth response to GH. *Clin Endocrinol (Oxf)* 2002; **57**: 315–25.

103a Crowe BJ, Rekers-Mombarg LTM, Roberts K, *et al*. for the European Idiopathic Short Stature Group. Effect of growth hormone dose on bone maturation and puberty in children with idiopathic short stature. *J Clin Endocrinol Metab* 2006; **91**: 169–75.

104 Zadik Z, Landau H, Limoni Y, Lieberman E. Predictors of growth response to growth hormone in otherwise normal short children. *J Ped* 1992; **121**: 44–8.

105 Kristrom B, Jansson C, Rosberg S, Albertsson-Wikland K. Growth response to growth hormone (GH) treatment relates to serum insulin-like growth factor I (IGF-I) and IGF-binding protein-3 in short children with various GH secretion capacities. Swedish Study Group for Growth Hormone Treatment. *J Clin Endocrinol Metab* 1997; **82**: 2889–98.

106 Rikken B, van Doorn J, Ringeling A, *et al*. Plasma levels of insulin-like growth factor (IGF)-I, IGF-II and IGF-binding protein-3 in the evaluation of childhood growth hormone deficiency. *Horm Res* 1998; **50**: 166–76.

107 Ranke MB, Guilbaud O, Lindberg A, Cole T. Prediction of the growth response in children with various growth disorders treated with growth hormone: analyses of data from the Kabi Pharmacia International Growth Study. International Board of the Kabi Pharmacia International Growth Study. *Acta Paediatr Suppl* 1993; **82(Suppl 391)**: 82–8.

108 Tapanainen P, Risteli L, Knip M, *et al*. Serum aminoterminal propeptide of type III procollagen: a potential predictor of the response to growth hormone therapy. *J Clin Endocrinol Metab* 1988; **67**: 1244–9.

109 Crofton PM, Stirling HF, Kelnar CJ. Bone alkaline phosphatase and height velocity in short normal children undergoing growth-promoting treatments: longitudinal study. *Clin Chem* 1995; **41**: 672–8.

110 Thalange NK, Price DA, Gill MS, *et al*. Insulin-like growth factor binding protein-3 generation: an index of growth hormone insensitivity. *Pediatr Res* 1996; **39**: 849–55.

● 111 Attie KM, Carlsson LM, Rundle AC, Sherman BM. Evidence for partial growth hormone insensitivity among patients with idiopathic short stature. The National Cooperative Growth Study. *J Pediatr* 1995; **127**: 244–50.

● 112 Dos SC, Essioux L, Teinturier C, *et al*. A common polymorphism of the growth hormone receptor is associated with increased responsiveness to growth hormone. *Nat Genet* 2004; **36**: 720–4.

113 Ranke MB, Lindberg A, Chatelain P, *et al*. The potential of prediction models based on data from KIGS as tools to measure responsiveness to growth hormone. *Horm Res* 2001; **55(Suppl 2)**: 44–8.

114 Leger J, Reynaud R, Czernichow P. Do all girls with apparent idiopathic precocious puberty require gonadotropin-releasing hormone agonist treatment? *J Pediatr* 2000; **137**: 819–25.

115 Kamp GA, Mul D, Waelkens JJ, *et al*. A randomized controlled trial of three years growth hormone and gonadotropin-releasing hormone agonist treatment in children with idiopathic short stature and intrauterine growth retardation. *J Clin Endocrinol Metab* 2001; **86**: 2969–75.

116 Pasquino AM, Pucarelli I, Roggini M, Segni M. Adult height in short normal girls treated with gonadotropin-releasing hormone analogs and growth hormone. *J Clin Endocrinol Metab* 2000; **85**: 619–22.

117 Job JC, Toublanc JE, Landier F. Growth of short normal children in puberty treated for 3 years with growth hormone alone or in association with gonadotropin-releasing hormone agonist. *Horm Res* 1994; **41**: 177–84.

118 Satoh M, Tanaka T, Horikawa R, *et al*. The effect of combined gonadal suppression and growth hormone (GH) treatment on bone maturation in boys with non-endocrine short stature (NESS). *Clin Pediatr Endocrinol* 1994; **3**: 79–83.

119 Tanaka T, Satoh M, Yasunaga T, *et al.* GH and GnRH analog treatment in children who enter puberty at short stature. *J Pediatr Endocrinol Metab* 1997; **10**: 623–8.

120 Lanes R, Gunczler P. Final height after combined growth hormone and gonadotrophin-releasing hormone analogue therapy in short healthy children entering into normally timed puberty. *Clin Endocrinol (Oxf)* 1998; **49**: 197–202.

121 Saggese G, Cesaretti G, Barsanti S, Rossi A. Combination treatment with growth hormone and gonadotropin-releasing hormone analogs in short normal girls. *J Pediatr* 1995; **126**: 468–73.

122 Tuvemo T, Gustafsson J, Proos LA. Growth hormone treatment during suppression of early puberty in adopted girls. Swedish Growth Hormone Advisory Group. *Acta Pediatr* 1999; **88**: 928–32.

123 Mul D, Wit JM, Oostdijk W, Van den BJ. The effect of pubertal delay by GnRH agonist in GH-deficient children on final height. *J Clin Endocrinol Metab* 2001; **86**: 4655–6.

124 Balducci R, Toscano V, Mangiantini A, *et al.* Adult height in short normal adolescent girls treated with gonadotropin-releasing hormone analog and growth hormone. *J Clin Endocrinol Metab* 1995; **80**: 3596–600.

125 Kaplowitz PB. If gonadotropin-releasing hormone plus growth hormone (GH) really improves growth outcomes in short non-GH-deficient children, then what? *J Clin Endocrinol Metab* 2001; **86**: 2965–8.

126 Wickman S, Sipila I, Ankarberg-Lindgren C, *et al.* A specific aromatase inhibitor and potential increase in adult height in boys with delayed puberty: a randomised controlled trial. *Lancet* 2001; **357**: 1743–8.

127 Kawai M, Momoi T, Yorifuji T, *et al.* Combination therapy with GH and cyproterone acetate does not improve final height in boys with non-GH-deficient short stature. *Clin Endocrinol (Oxf)* 1998; **48**: 53–7.

128 Boulton TJ, Dunn SM, Quigley CA, *et al.* Perceptions of self and short stature: effects of two years of growth hormone treatment. *Acta Paediatr Scand Suppl* 1991; **377**: 20–7.

129 Pilpel D, Leiberman E, Zadik Z, Carel CA. Effect of growth hormone treatment on quality of life of short-stature children. *Horm Res* 1995; **44**: 1–5.

130 Downie AB, Mulligan J, McCaughey ES, *et al.* Psychological response to growth hormone treatment in short normal children. *Arch Dis Child* 1996; **75**: 32–5.

131 Stabler B, Siegel PT, Clopper RR, *et al.* Behavior change after growth hormone treatment of children with short stature. *J Pediatr* 1998; **133**: 366–73.

132 Theunissen NC, Kamp GA, Koopman HM, *et al.* Quality of life and self-esteem in children treated for idiopathic short stature. *J Pediatr* 2002; **140**: 507–15.

133 Mul D, Versluis-den Bieman HJ, Slijper FM, *et al.* Psychological assessments before and after treatment of early puberty in adopted children. *Acta Paediatr* 2001; **90**: 965–71.

133a Visser-van Balen H, Geenen R, Moerbeek M, *et al.* Psychosocial functioning of adolescents with idiopathic short stature or intrauterine growth retardation during

three years of combined growth hormone and gonadotropin-releasing hormone against treatment. *Horm Res* 2005; **64**: 77–87.

133b Visser-van Balen H, Geenen R, Kamp GA, *et al.* Young adults after hormone treatment for idiopathic short stature or persistent short stature born small for gestational age: a long-term follow-up evaluation of psychosocial functioning. *Acta Paediatr* (in press).

134 Joss EE, Schmidt HA, Zuppinger KA. Oxandrolone in constitutionally delayed growth, a longitudinal study up to final height. *J Clin Endocrinol Metab* 1989; **69**: 1109–15.

135 Tse WY, Buyukgebiz A, Hindmarsh PC, *et al.* Long term outcome of oxandrolone treatment in boys with constitutional delay of growth and puberty. *J Pediatr* 1990; **117**: 588–91.

136 Blizzard RM, Hindmarsh PC, Stanhope R. Oxandrolone therapy: 25 years experience. *Growth Genet Horm* 1991; **7**: 1–6.

137 Martin MM, Martin ALA, Mossman KL. Testosterone treatment of constitutional delay in growth and development: effect of dose on predicted versus definitive height. *Acta Endocrinol* 1986; **113(Suppl 279)**: 147–52.

138 Lindner D, Job JC, Chaussain JL. Failure to improve height prediction in short-stature pubertal adolescents by inhibiting puberty with luteinizing hormone-releasing hormone analogue. *Eur J Pediatr* 1993; **152**: 393–6.

139 Carel JC, Hay F, Coutant R, *et al.* Gonadotropin-releasing hormone agonist treatment of girls with constitutional short stature and normal pubertal development. *J Clin Endocrinol Metab* 1996; **81**: 3318–22.

140 Yanovski JA, Rose SR, Municchi G, *et al.* Treatment with a luteinizing hormone-releasing hormone agonist in adolescents with short stature. *N Engl J Med* 2003; **348**: 908–17.

141 Mul D, Oostdijk W, Waelkens JJ, *et al.* Gonadotrophin releasing hormone agonist treatment with or without recombinant human GH in adopted children with early puberty. *Clin Endocrinol (Oxf)* 2001; **55**: 121–9.

142 Hernandez M, Fragoso J, Barrio R, *et al.* Subcutaneous treatment with growth hormone-releasing hormone for short stature. *Horm Res* 1988; **30**: 252–7.

143 Kirk JM, Trainer PJ, Majrowski WH, *et al.* Treatment with GHRH(1-29)NH2 in children with idiopathic short stature induces a sustained increase in growth velocity. *Clin Endocrinol (Oxf)* 1994; **41**: 487–93.

144 Laron Z. Growth hormone secretagogues. Clinical experience and therapeutic potential. *Drugs* 1995; **50**: 595–601.

145 Grunt JA, Schwartz ID, Buchanan C, Howard CP. Effects of long-term growth hormone releasing hormone 1-29 in significantly short children. *Acta Paediatr* 1995; **84**: 631–3.

◆ 146 Ritzen EM, Czernichow P, Preece M, *et al.* Safety of human growth hormone therapy. *Horm Res* 1993; **39**: 92–3.

147 Tuffli GA, Johanson A, Rundle AC, Allen DB. Lack of increased risk for extracranial, nonleukemic neoplasms in recipients of recombinant deoxyribonucleic acid growth hormone. *J Clin Endocrinol Metab* 1995; **80**: 1416–22.

148 Blethen SL, Allen DB, Graves D, *et al.* Safety of recombinant deoxyribonucleic acid-derived growth hormone: The National Cooperative Growth Study experience. *J Clin Endocrinol Metab* 1996; **81**: 1704–10.

149 Allen DB, Rundle AC, Graves DA, Blethen SL. Risk of leukemia in children treated with human growth hormone: review and reanalysis. *J Pediatr* 1997; **131**: S32–6.

150 Van Loon K. Safety of high doses of recombinant human growth hormone. *Horm Res* 1998; **49(Suppl 2)**: 78–81.

151 Price DA, Wilton P, Jonsson P, *et al.* Efficacy and safety of growth hormone treatment in children with prior craniopharyngioma: an analysis of the Pharmacia and Upjohn International Growth Database (KIGS) from 1988 to 1996. *Horm Res* 1998; **49**: 91–7.

152 Saenger P, Attie KM, DiMartino-Nardi J, *et al.* Metabolic consequences of 5-year growth hormone (GH) therapy in children treated with GH for idiopathic short stature. Genentech Collaborative Study Group. *J Clin Endocrinol Metab* 1998; **83**: 3115–20.

153 Wilton P. Adverse events during GH treatment: 10 years' experience in KIGS, a pharmacoepidemiological survey. In: Ranke MB, Wilton P, eds. *Growth Hormone Therapy in KIGS-10 Years' Experience.* Heidelberg: Johann Ambrosius Barth Verlag, 1999: 349–64.

154 Maneatis T, Baptista J, Connelly K, Blethen S. Growth hormone safety update from the National Cooperative Growth Study. *J Pediatr Endocrinol Metab* 2000; **13(Suppl 2)**: 1035–44.

155 Critical evaluation of the safety of recombinant human growth hormone administration: statement from the Growth Hormone Research Society. *J Clin Endocrinol Metab* 2001; **86**: 1868–70.

156 Cohen P, Clemmons DR, Rosenfeld RG. Does the GH–IGF axis play a role in cancer pathogenesis? *Growth Horm IGF Res* 2000; **10**: 297–305.

157 Clayton PE, Cowell CT. Safety issues in children and adolescents during growth hormone therapy – a review. *Growth Horm IGF Res* 2000; **10**: 306–17.

◆ 158 Khandwala HM, McCutcheon IE, Flyvbjerg A, Friend KE. The effects of insulin-like growth factors on tumorigenesis and neoplastic growth. *Endocr Rev* 2000; **21**: 215–44.

159 Furstenberger G, Senn HJ. Insulin-like growth factors and cancer. *Lancet Oncol* 2002; **3**: 298–302.

160 Shulman DI. Metabolic effects of growth hormone in the child and adolescent. *Curr Opin Pediatr* 2002; **14**: 432–6.

161 Ali O, Cohen P, Lee KW. Epidemiology and biology of insulin-like growth factor binding protein-3 (IGFBP-3) as an anti-cancer molecule. *Horm Metab Res* 2003; **35**: 726–33.

162 Ogilvy-Stuart AL, Gleeson H. Cancer risk following growth hormone use in childhood: implications for current practice. *Drug Saf* 2004; **27**: 369–82.

163 Renehan AG, Zwahlen M, Minder C, *et al.* Insulin-like growth factor (IGF)-I, IGF binding protein-3, and cancer risk: systematic review and meta-regression analysis. *Lancet* 2004; **363**: 1346–53.

164 Mericq V, Gajardo H, Eggers M, *et al.* Effects of treatment with GH alone or in combination with LHRH analog on bone mineral density in pubertal GH-deficient patients. *J Clin Endocrinol Metab* 2002; **87**: 84–9.

165 Diekema DS. Is taller really better? Growth hormone therapy in short children. *Perspect Biol Med* 1990; **34 I**: 109–23.

166 Allen DB, Brook CGD, Bridges NA, *et al.* Therapeutic controversies: growth hormone (GH) treatment of non-GH deficient subjects. *J Clin Endocrinol Metab* 1994; **79**: 1239–48.

167 Considerations related to the use of recombinant human growth hormone in children. American Academy of Pediatrics Committee on Drugs and Committee on Bioethics. *Pediatrics* 1997; **99**: 122–9.

168 Kelnar CJ, Albertsson-Wikland K, Hintz RL, *et al.* Should we treat children with idiopathic short stature? *Horm Res* 1999; **52**: 150–7.

169 Bolt LL, Mul D. Growth hormone in short children: beyond medicine? *Acta Paediatr* 2001; **90**: 69–73.

◆ 170 Allen DB, Fost NC. Ethical issues in growth hormone therapy: where are we now? *Endocrinologist* 2001; **11(Suppl 1)**: 1S–89.

171 Underwood LE, Rieser PA. Is it ethical to treat healthy short children with growth hormone? *Acta Paediatr Scand Suppl* 1989; **362**: 18–23.

172 Guyda HJ. Growth hormone therapy for non-growth hormone-deficient children with short stature. *Curr Opin Pediatr* 1998; **10**: 416–21.

173 Guyda HJ. Idiopathic short stature. In: Kelnar CJH. Savage MO, Stirling HF, Saenger P, eds. *Growth Disorders. Pathophysiology and Treatment.* London: Chapman & Hall, 1998: 609–21.

174 Burch KJ, Alvarado-Hughes M. Selection of a human growth hormone product. *Clin Pharm* 1988; **7**: 239–40.

175 Wyatt DT, Mark D, Slyper A. Survey of growth hormone treatment practices by 251 pediatric endocrinologists [see comments]. *J Clin Endocrinol Metab* 1995; **80**: 3292–7.

176 Cuttler L, Silvers JB, Singh J, *et al.* Short stature and growth hormone therapy. A national study of physician recommendation patterns [see comments]. *JAMA* 1996; **276**: 531–7.

177 Guyda HJ. Use of growth hormone in children with short stature and normal growth hormone secretion, a growing problem. *Trends Endocrinol Metab* 1994; **5**: 334–40.

178 Tachibana K, on behalf of of ICGS Japan. Demographic data of the International Cooperative Growth Study (ICGS) in Japan. *Clin Pediatr Endocrinol* 1994; **3(Suppl 5)**: 11–18.

179 Cowell CT, Dietsch S, Greenacre P. Growth hormone therapy for 3 years: the OZGROW experience. *J Paediatr Child Health* 1996; **32**: 86–93.

◆ 180 Wit JM. Growth hormone therapy. *Best Pract Res Clin Endocrinol Metab* 2002; **16**: 483–503.

35

Turner and Noonan syndromes: Disease-specific growth and growth-promoting therapies

MICHAEL B RANKE

EVIDENCE SCORING OF THERAPY

* Non-randomized controlled trials, cohort study, etc.
** One or more well-designed randomized controlled trials

TURNER SYNDROME

Introduction

In 1938, Henry H. Turner described a disorder found in seven girls, which was characterized by sexual infantilism, pterygium colli, cubitus valgus, and short stature. As early as 1930, however, Otto Ullrich had recognized the same disorder as being a specific entity. The disorder, which is currently known to be caused by the complete or partial absence of one of the X chromosomes, is commonly termed Turner syndrome. Turner syndrome is rather frequent (about one in 2500 live born girls). It is characterized by three main clinical features: (1) abnormal external appearance and abnormalities of certain internal organs; (2) malformation of the ovaries; and (3) short stature (Fig. 35.1). In about 50 percent of cases, karyotype analysis of peripheral lymphocytes reveals the complete loss of one X chromosome (karyotype 45,X) whereas the remaining patients display a multitude of chromosomal abnormalities, including part absence of one X chromosome or mosaicism. In 60 percent of cases it is the paternal X that is lost during meiosis.[1]

Short stature is the most familiar feature in Turner syndrome. It is invariably present, irrespective of karyotype, and is occasionally the only obvious symptom. Short stature

in Turner syndrome has been associated with haplo-insufficiency of a critical chromosomal region (distal of Xp22.2), which escapes inactivation (pseudoautosomal region of X and Y), and in which the short stature homeobox (SHOX) gene resides (Xp22.33). The latter encodes for two isoforms of a protein (SHOXa and SHOXb), whose function is as yet unclear (putative transcription factor).[2] During human embryogenesis, the SHOX gene is predominantly expressed in the limbs. SHOX defects are known to cause mesomelic short stature associated with varied phenotypical features. The heterozygous state causes Léri–Weill dyschondrosteosis, which is characterized by mesomelic short stature and Madelung deformity, whereas the homozygous type causes Langer's osteodysplasia.[3] Ogata and Matsuo have suggested that a higher frequency of Madelung deformations in women with Léri–Weill dyschondrosteosis is caused by the effects of estrogens, which are either absent or low in Turner syndrome.[4] Zinn and colleagues[5] have also suggested that there is a locus in the interval Xp11.1–p22 encoding for the gene (or genes) pertinent to stature, and have proposed that the transcription factor ZFX is the likely candidate gene. From a schematic perspective, growth in Turner syndrome can formally be divided into four phases:[6,7]

1. The occurrence of intrauterine growth retardation: Turner syndrome girls born close to term are about 3 cm shorter than normal newborns.
2. Growth during infancy and early childhood is lower than normal.[8,9]
3. Between the ages of about 3 and 12 years, children with Turner syndrome lose about 15 cm in height compared with normal girls.

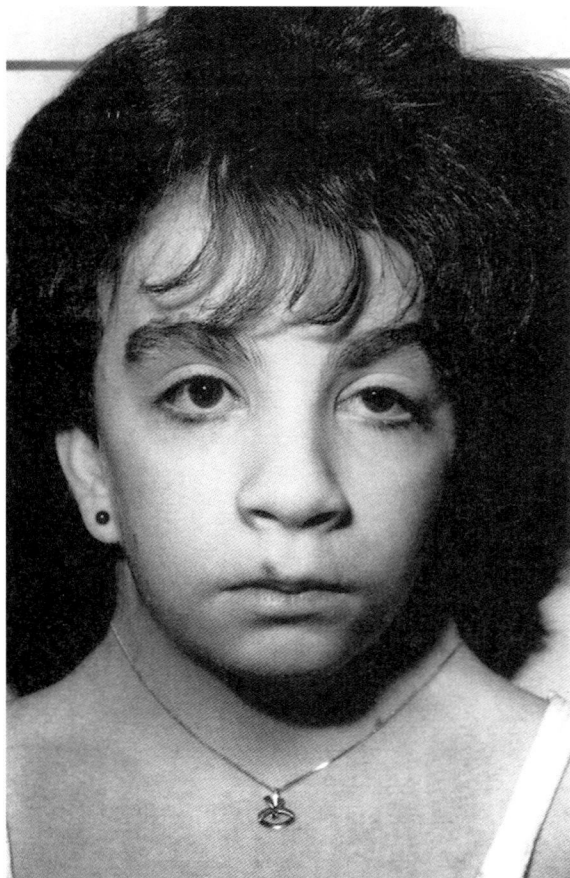

Figure 35.1   Typical appearance of a girl with Turner syndrome.

4. In most cases, the pubertal growth spurt does not occur; instead, the total growth phase is prolonged. The combined effect of these circumstances is that only a minor loss in height is observable during this phase. This leads to the assumption that the significance of sex steroids in growth regulation in Turner syndrome is rather limited during this period.[10]

Pre-natal growth

The fact that the birth length of a newborn child already represents about 20–30 percent of its final height, implies that investigations on pre-natal growth are of considerable relevance in understanding the eventual outcome. Accurate data exemplifying the entire pre-natal growth process in Turner syndrome are not available. There is evidence that a substantial number of fetuses bearing the Turner syndrome karyotype are spontaneously aborted.[11,12] Amniocentesis provides the opportunity to diagnose pre-natal disorders and it is likely that, in the future, this method of testing, combined with sonography, will enable physicians to follow pre-natal growth more closely. A number of reports are available on size at birth in children born after the 30th week of gestation. These data show that full-term Turner syndrome babies (i.e., after 38 or more weeks of pregnancy) are about 3 cm shorter and weigh 500 g less than normal

female newborns. As lymphoedema is a characteristic feature of Turner syndrome, weight at birth (which can be measured more accurately than length) may appear to be rather high. It is a known fact that approximately one-third of liveborn neonates are small for gestational age (SGA). There is no evidence indicating that size at birth is associated with a particular karyotype.

Post-natal growth

Post-natal growth in Turner syndrome has been studied by a number of groups (for a review see Ranke and Grauer[13] and Ranke[14]). The data reported are mostly based on retrospective analyses in which longitudinal and cross-sectional data are combined. The presenting symptoms of Turner syndrome may be karyotype, dysmorphology, short stature, delayed puberty or even infertility. The diagnosis can, therefore, be made pre-natally in some cases, but, in other cases, the syndrome may remain unnoticed until adolescence or even adulthood. In addition, the numbers investigated are limited in comparison to studies aimed at defining normal growth of a given population. Thus, although it can be claimed that post-natal growth in Turner syndrome is probably the best described of all known syndromes, a few uncertainties concerning the spontaneous growth process still need to be clarified.

A steady decrease in growth velocity leads to a progressive loss in height, and about 75 percent of height loss occurs during childhood. As the estrogen-related pubertal growth phase is absent in about 90 percent of patients,[15*,16] growth continues to be characteristic of the childhood component,[17] and the total duration of growth extends into the late teens. The greatest difference in height between Turner syndrome girls and healthy children, therefore, is evident at about the age of 14 (Fig. 35.2). The pattern of height development that emerged in several large series is surprisingly analogous. Similarities have also been observed between the variability in height for Turner syndrome girls for a given age (one standard deviation [SD] amounts to approximately 4.7 percent of a given age mean) and the range for normal children.[6,18]

Few published studies providing height velocity reference values are available, mainly owing to the fact that such data are more difficult to collect. Based on our earlier data, the author's group assumes that a continuous decline in height velocity prevails towards the end of growth.[6] In a later study, involving 738 cases, conclusive evidence was found that two minor growth spurts take place: the first occurs during the pre-pubertal (adrenarche?) stage, and the second during the pubertal phase (Fig. 35.3).[19] The latter was also observed by Haeusler et al.[20] even in the absence of recognizable breast development. These findings, coupled with cautious consideration of the above reasoning, lead to the assumption that the factors regulating growth in normal children are also relevant to the growth process in Turner syndrome.

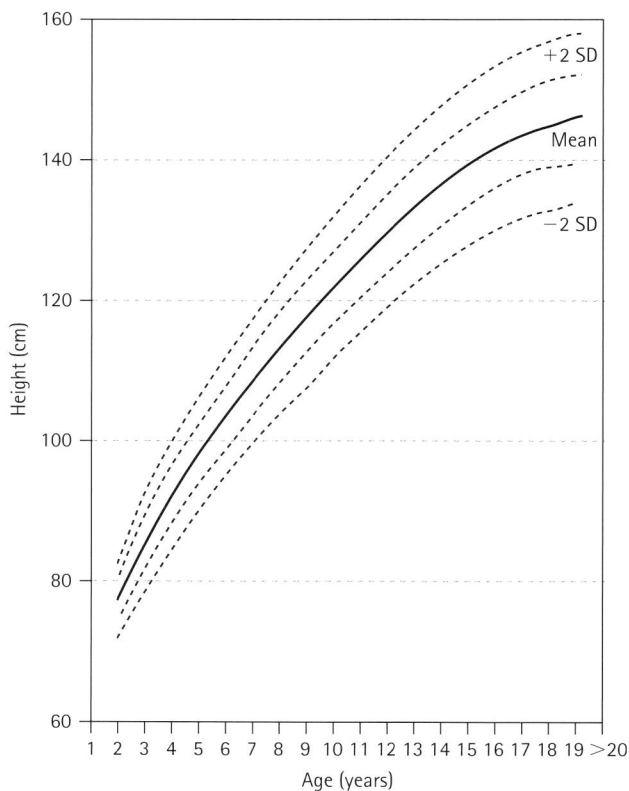

Figure 35.2 Reference values for height in Turner syndrome (From: Ranke *et al.*[6]).

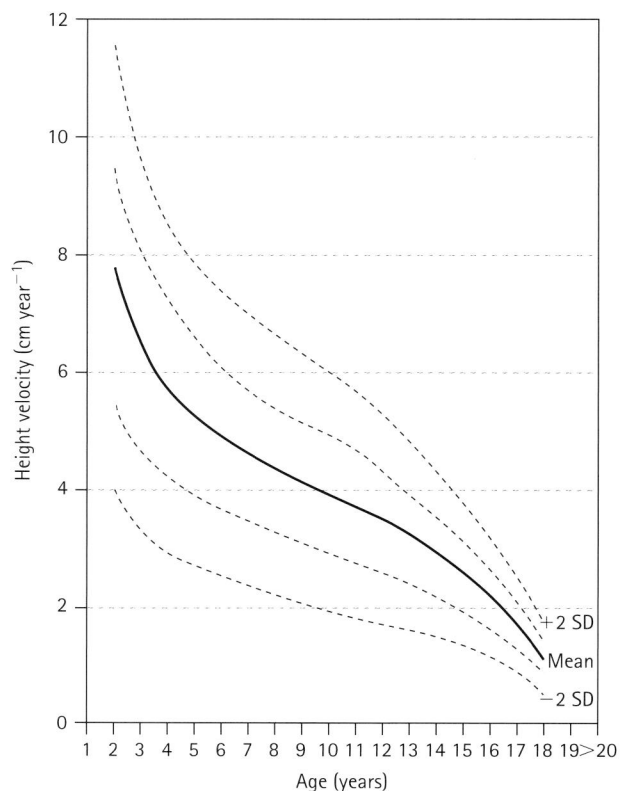

Figure 35.3 Reference values for height velocity in Turner syndrome (From: Ranke *et al.*[6]).

Adult height

The collection of data on adult height in patients who at no time received substances influencing growth (e.g., growth hormone, anabolic steroids such as oxandrolone, or estrogen) is difficult, because their unavailability is a direct consequence of the fact that therapy is now the standard approach taken. Values for adult height vary from one published report to another (Table 35.1). The mean adult stature of Turner syndrome patients of white European origin ranges from about 142 cm to 147 cm. A comparison of reports on adult height in Turner syndrome shows a difference of 20 cm between average normal female adult height and adult height in Turner syndrome within the same population (for references see Ranke and Grauer[13]). The degree of variability of adult height is similar to that of the normal population. There is a positive correlation between final adult height and parental height.[10,13,21]

A survey on adult height, involving 661 patients from several European countries, showed an association between differences in adult height and geographical origin:[13] patients from the northern regions are generally taller than those in the southern regions. It can be argued that these differences are most probably related to the height differences characteristic of the underlying populations, owing to a high overall correlation between target height and adult height. In patients with the 45,X karyotype, there appears to be a higher

correlation to maternal height,[22] a finding which is compatible with the suggestion that, in 45,X Turner syndrome, the paternal X chromosome is predominantly lost.[23] This study also did not reveal any essential differences between karyotypes. Whether there is a secular growth trend in Turner syndrome, as is well described in normal children, is uncertain.[24]

Other auxological parameters

On radiographs, differences in bone structure and spontaneous bone age development are evident in Turner syndrome compared with the normal population.[6,19,25–28] Cautious evaluation of radiographs in Turner syndrome is particularly called for, because errors of judgement are not uncommon in rating bone age, and, in Turner syndrome, structural abnormalities of the bones pose difficulties. During childhood, up to an age of about 12 years, bone age is retarded by about 1 year but progresses about 1 year per year (Fig. 35.4, Table 35.2). Thereafter, bone age slows down progressively, probably partly as a result of the absence or very low levels of ovarian steroids. Weight tends to be increased for a given height, particularly after the age of 10 years.[27*, 29,30] To date, only a few reports on other body proportions are available[31–34] which validate the observations that the lower body segment is comparatively shorter than the upper, that head circumference is not significantly

Table 35.1   Auxological reference values for Turner syndrome

Age (years)	Height (cm)[a] mean	(SD)	Height (cm)[b] mean	(SD)	Height velocity (cm year^{-1})[b] mean	(SD)	Sitting height (cm)[c] mean	SD	Bone age[d] TW2-RUS (CASAS) mean ± SD
2	74.9	(4.3)	77.3	(2.6)	7.8	(1.9)			
3	83.1	(4.4)	85.1	(3.5)	6.5	(1.6)	53.0	(2.1)	2.3 ± 0.7
4	88.3	(4.7)	91.6	(3.8)	5.7	(1.4)	55.4	(2.2)	3.4 ± 0.9
5	92.7	(5.4)	97.3	(4.0)	5.3	(1.3)	57.5	(2.3)	4.5 ± 1.0
6	97.8	(4.0)	102.5	(4.2)	4.9	(1.2)	59.5	(2.4)	5.6 ± 1.9
7	102.3	(5.1)	107.4	(4.4)	4.6	(1.1)	62.5	(2.5)	6.8 ± 1.2
8	105.2	(4.6)	111.9	(4.6)	4.3	(1.1)	64.5	(2.6)	7.9 ± 1.2
9	112.5	(4.9)	116.2	(4.8)	4.1	(1.0)	66.5	(2.7)	8.9 ± 1.2
10	116.7	(4.6)	120.3	(5.0)	3.9	(1.0)	68.5	(2.7)	9.8 ± 1.2
11	119.8	(4.6)	124.2	(5.1)	3.8	(0.9)	70.0	(2.8)	10.8 ± 1.1
12	123.0	(6.6)	128.0	(5.3)	3.5	(0.9)	71.6	(2.9)	11.6 ± 1.3
13	128.1	(6.0)	131.5	(5.4)	3.2	(0.8)	73.0	(2.9)	12.4 ± 1.0
14	131.3	(6.3)	134.7	(5.5)	2.9	(0.7)	74.5	(3.0)	13.0 ± 0.9
15	134.2	(5.9)	137.6	(5.7)	2.6	(0.6)	75.9	(3.0)	13.6 ± 0.8
16	138.3	(5.8)	140.1	(5.8)	2.1	(0.5)			14.0 ± 0.7
17	139.1	(5.2)	142.2	(5.9)	1.7	(0.4)			14.3 ± 0.6
18	139.2	(3.8)	143.9	(5.9)	1.1	(0.3)			14.4 ± 0.6
19	142.8	(3.7)	145.0	(6.0)					
>20	143.2	(4.5)	146.3	(6.1)					

[a]From Lyon et al.[18]; [b]From Ranke et al.[91]; [c]From Herdach[34]; [d]From Schwarze et al.[28]

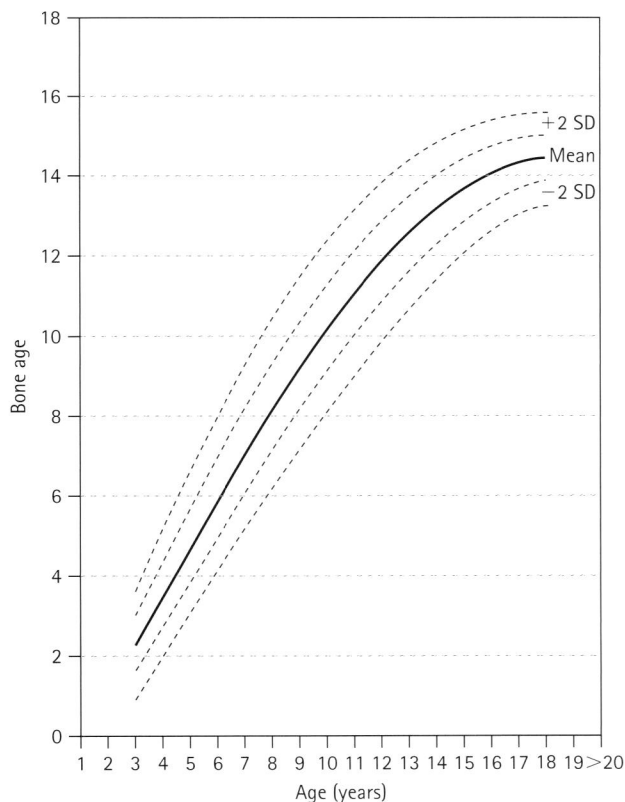

Figure 35.4   Reference values for bone age in Turner syndrome (From: Ranke et al.[19]).

Table 35.2   Comparison of bone age

Study and groups	n	CA at start	PAH (cm)	Final height (cm)	Gain over PAH (cm)
Rosenfeld et al.[43]					
GH	17	9.1	142.1	150.4	
GH + Ox	43	9.1	141.8	152.1	
Control	25	9.1	144.2	144.2	0.0
van Pareren et al.[56]					
A	19	6.5	145.7	157.6	11.9
B	20	6.9	147.2	162.9	15.7
C	21	6.5	146.6	163.9	16.9

GH, growth hormone; PAH, predicted adult height; CA, chronological age; Ox, oxandrolone.

reduced[6] and that arm span corresponds to height (Figs 35.5 and 35.6).

Prediction of adult height

In normal children, mean parental height can be used in making a rough estimate of adult height[35]. This approach assumes that both parents' genetic influences on adult height are of equal magnitude, which may not, however,

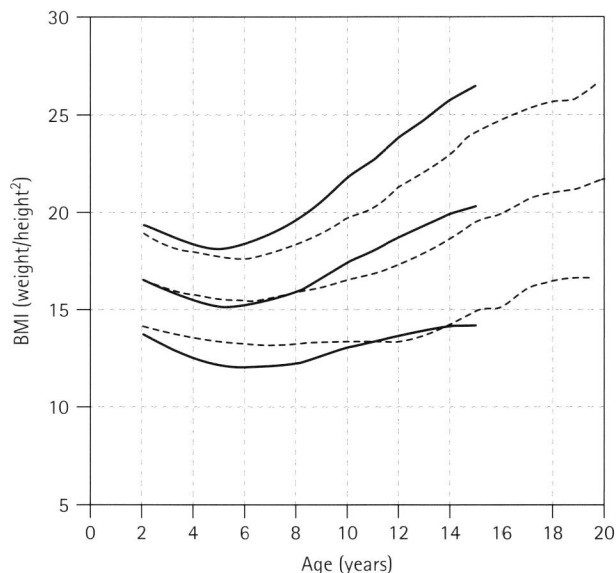

Figure 35.5 Reference values for body mass index in Turner syndrome (From: Herdach[34]).

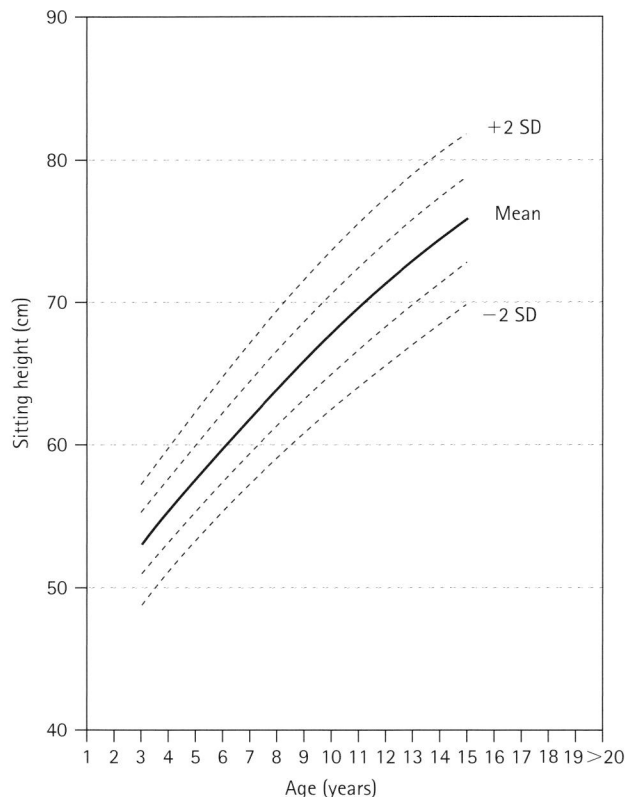

Figure 35.6 Reference values for sitting height in Turner syndrome (From: Herdach[34]).

necessarily apply to Turner syndrome. Nevertheless, as a high correlation exists between parental stature and height in Turner syndrome, this approach may be useful during counselling.[13,36]

Several methods have been devised to predict the adult height of individuals more accurately.[17,37,38] The most popular model involves plotting the growth of an individual girl with Turner syndrome on a growth chart specific for Turner syndrome and to extend this line following the individual percentile to a 'projected final height'. This assumes that childhood growth in Turner syndrome follows the channel of targeted height,[37] and that individual influences on a child's growth (e.g., parental height) are already expressed in the deviation of height from the disease-specific mean for a given age. The validity of this approach for predicting adult height is supported by empirical evidence.[17,37] In the author's view, this appears to be quite a sound approach, and has become the basis for evaluating the efficacy of treatment modalities. Methods based on bone age, which are commonly used in predicting height in several types of growth disorders, have not yet proved to be a better alternative for height prediction in Turner syndrome,[38,39] perhaps owing to the fact that the basis of disease-specific bone age is still too small.

Evaluation of the growth response to treatment

The main objective in treating short stature is to improve a patient's height by narrowing the gap between their height and that of the normal population. It is therefore essential, during treatment, to evaluate whether the mode of treatment applied concurs with this goal. Obviously, an

increase in height velocity is not very applicable in judging whether this goal is being achieved – not even if appropriate data specific for Turner syndrome on spontaneous height velocity are used. The extent of growth is not only expressed by height velocity but also by the tempo of growth (e.g., slow growth over a longer period of time may result in higher stature than fast growth during a shorter time). The effect of treatment must, therefore, be evaluated by selecting a parameter that clearly indicates changes in the tempo of growth. During normal growth, bone age development is a suitable indicator, because the relationship between height and bone age reflects the tempo and the potential of growth. Spontaneous bone age development in Turner syndrome is dissimilar to that of the normal population,[6,19,25,28] which is why it remains unclear whether bone age values employed in height predictions in Turner syndrome provide valid information relating to the actual growth potential. In attempting to fulfil the expectations of patients, which rest on height values relating to the normal population, treatment should be aimed at achieving growth within the normal limits during childhood and adolescence as well as adult height attainment within the normal range. Thus, in order to evaluate any mode of treatment, the crucial issue is whether the approach chosen demonstrably improves height only in terms of disease-specific standards or whether it, in fact, undoubtedly normalizes height.

Treatment with growth hormone

The pathogenesis of the growth disorder in Turner syndrome is still unknown. Changes in GH secretion and in the age-related levels of IGF-I have been associated with it, but it can be assumed that such alterations result from either gonadal dysgenesis or obesity. When pituitary human growth hormone became available, an attempt to treat a few Turner syndrome patients was undertaken.[40,41] The results of these trials were largely disappointing. The advances in the recombinant technique made growth hormone available in abundant amounts, and it has been possible to conduct carefully-designed studies aiming at a re-evaluation of this approach. The prototype of all recent studies is the one designed by the Genentech Study Group, of which successive reports have been published.[42,43] In this study, a representative cohort of Turner syndrome girls was treated with recombinant human growth hormone. A total of 70 patients entered the study at a mean age of 9.1 years. They either received exclusive treatment with 0.375 mg growth hormone per kg body weight per week ($n = 17$) or growth hormone combined with oxandrolone at a dosage of 0.125–0.065 mg kg^{-1} body weight per day. The group which received only growth hormone reached a mean height of 150.4 (5.5) cm, the average gain being 8.4 cm over projected height; while the group with combined treatment reached 152.1 (5.9) cm, averaging a gain of 10.3 cm over projected height. A historical control group comprising 25 patients reached 144.2 (6.0) cm which was almost identical to projected height. Similar, but in general, comparatively inferior results were reported from a number of studies and surveys designed in the 1980s,[44*–52,48*,50*,51*] mainly due to the fact that, in most of these studies, the patients were older when growth hormone therapy started and, in addition, the dosage was relatively low. In a recently published controlled trial with untreated patients, the growth-promoting effect of this regimen was confirmed.[53] It is now a widely accepted fact that both the dose of growth hormone and age at therapy start are the most important factors.[54*,55,56**]

In a recent Dutch study,[56**] 68 patients were randomized into three groups at a mean age of 6.6 years, after they had received growth hormone during the first year at a dose of 45 μg kg^{-1} day^{-1}. This dose was maintained in group A, whereas it was increased to 68 μg kg^{-1} day^{-1} in groups B and C. In the third year, the dose was further increased to 90 μg kg^{-1} day^{-1} only in group C. The final height achieved in groups A, B and C, are (in means and SD scores) 157.6 (6.5), 162.9 (6.1) and 163.6 (6.0) cm, respectively (Table 35.2). The influential factors in this study were the growth hormone dose, age at start of growth hormone therapy (the younger, the better) and height velocity during the first year. The responsiveness to growth hormone treatment during the first year[55] is clearly one of the main determinants of the final outcome. On the other hand, disproportion is an unfavorable condition in terms of the outcome.[50*]

Without intending to discuss the details of the various study designs, the methods used in evaluating the growth response or the results of each individual study, a brief outline of the knowledge acquired through the studies is given:[1,57*]

- Growth hormone given in higher-than-substitutive doses (0.7–1.5 IU kg^{-1} week^{-1}; prescribed as equal daily subcutaneous injections) leads to an increase in adult height in Turner syndrome patients. Many patients who received such treatment attained a final height exceeding 150 cm, which is a socially acceptable height for adult women.
- The gain in height correlates positively with the dose given.
- The highest increment in height is observable during the first 3 years of treatment.
- The individual response is highly variable and, so far, not predictable.
- The statural outcome correlates negatively with age at start of growth hormone treatment. The limited experience available concerning the treatment of children younger than 7 years of age makes it difficult to pinpoint the optimal age for starting with growth hormone treatment in this age group.
- Adjuvant use of the anabolic steroid, oxandrolone, enhances GH treatment (0.0625–0.05 mg kg^{-1} day^{-1}) in that it increases the tempo of growth, thus shortening the total duration of GH treatment to final height. Oxandrolone also probably improves the total gain in height. The mechanism of its action is, however, still unclear. The non- or limited availability of oxandrolone in many countries has impeded further studies of this substance.
- Estrogens are required in order to induce feminisation at an appropriate age. There is, however, no evidence available of the growth-promoting effect of estrogens in Turner syndrome.[58*,59*] The optimization of growth in Turner syndrome is still an on-going process; and it is, therefore, essential that the treatment of patients is documented systematically.

Risks of growth-promoting therapy

The potential risks of growth-promoting therapies are posed by the following: (1) specific factors related to Turner syndrome; (2) specific side-effects of the drugs used; (3) the dosage and duration of the drugs used; and (4) a combination of these factors.

In spite of the risk potential of GH therapy with supraphysiological doses, the incidence of adverse events observed in Turner syndrome is not essentially different from that of idiopathic GH deficiency.[54*,60] Growth hormone therapy during childhood and adolescence, however, must be seen within the wider, life-span perspective that is now emerging, in which consideration is given to the development of a Turner syndrome girl into an adult woman.[61,62–64*] Impaired glucose tolerance and a disposition towards high blood pressure (even in the absence of cardiac failure) are well-documented abnormalities in Turner syndrome (for a review see references 65–69). High doses of growth hormone may increase the risk of developing diabetes mellitus. Although recent studies have shown that the negative effects of growth hormone on glucose tolerance are transient,[65,70,71] the long-term risks cannot be predicted. Oxandrolone has been in use for decades and appears to be rather safe when given in low doses. The hazards posed by long periods of application with oxandrolone have, however, by no means been ruled out. As the dose–risk potential may be age-dependent, caution is recommended during the treatment of younger patients.

NOONAN SYNDROME

Long before Ullrich and Turner described the syndrome that became associated with their names, descriptions of male patients with a phenotype similar to Turner syndrome had been published.[72] The term 'male Turner syndrome' was frequently used when a phenotype resembling Ullrich–Turner syndrome was observed in males.[73] In 1963, during a review of children with congenital heart defects, Noonan and Ehmke described nine patients – six boys and three girls – having supravalvular pulmonary stenosis and a distinct clinical appearance.[74] These children were characterized by short stature, mild mental handicap, and, in some instances, by ptosis, undescended testes, and skeletal malformations.[73,75] The term Noonan syndrome is now generally accepted for children fitting this description, and the nosological incoherence in the literature has meanwhile been clarified.[76–78]

In recent years, several excellent reviews on the Noonan syndrome have been published.[75,76–80] Although this syndrome shares a multitude of findings with the Ullrich–Turner syndrome, it is now well established that both syndromes have a different cause[76,79*,81] After the gene for Noonan syndrome was mapped to chromosome 12,[82] Tartaglia et al.[83] identified a missense mutation in protein-tyrosine phosphatase, non-receptor-type 11 (PTPN11). The specific gene protein product, SHP-2, has a role in the signalling cascade of growth factors and a role in the migration, differentiation and proliferation of cells.[83,84] The observed mutations, which are found in about 50 percent of the individuals identified with Noonan syndrome are gain-of-function mutations. Cardiological abnormalities are a typical observation among patients with a documented mutation.[85–87*,88*] The role of excessive SHP-2 in the pathophysiology of Noonan syndrome is, however, not yet understood. In only about 20 percent of the cases could familiarity be documented. The phenotype of the Noonan syndrome is, however, related to developmental changes and its expression is highly variable. The incidence of Noonan syndrome is estimated to be in the range of about 1 in 1000–5000 live births.[76] In most clinical studies, the frequency of male and female patients was similar. As sufficient data are not available, it

cannot yet be proved whether or not a sex difference in the expression of the disorders exists. In boys there seems to be a higher prevalence of gonadal anomalies. However, these findings may be fictitious, because disorders such as maldescended testes are easy to diagnose. Likewise, the higher incidence of microcephaly in boys observed in the author's study requires substantiation with higher numbers.

Nature of symptoms and frequency of occurrence

The most characteristic symptoms and frequency of occurrence in patients with Noonan syndrome, compared with those found in patients with Turner syndrome, are listed in Table 35.3. A clear overlap of the symptoms is evident in both syndromes, although, in Noonan syndrome, the cardiac defect is characteristically located on the right side and mental handicap is more frequent. More recently, it was discovered that feeding difficulties during infancy, similar to those found in Turner syndrome, are also common to Noonan syndrome. Further, there are indications of an abnormality in bleeding, possibly related to a deviation from normal of the intrinsic pathway.[89] A typical example of the outward appearance of Noonan syndrome in boys is shown in Fig. 35.7.

Growth parameters in Noonan syndrome

Statural development has been reported from two large cohorts of patients.[90,91] Weight and length (mean $\pm$ SD) of children born between weeks 38 and 42 of gestation were ($n = 55$) 3482 ± 1052 g and ($n = 44$) 51.0 ± 1.9 cm, respectively, for boys and ($n = 37$) 3219 ± 745 g and ($n = 39$) 51.1 ± 2.4 cm, respectively, for girls. These data do not differ significantly from those of the normal population. Size at birth thus differs markedly from that in Turner syndrome, where both weight and length are diminished by about 1 SD in children born near term.[6]

As has been shown by Witt et al.[90] and by the author's group,[92] reduced height (length) is a regular feature of patients with Noonan syndrome. The American collaborative study[93] was based on cross-sectional measurements of 112 patients (64 boys, 48 girls) and a total of 173 measurements. The German collaborative study was based on 392 cross-sectional measurements in boys and 355 measurements in girls. As shown in Table 35.4, the data obtained from both studies are remarkably similar. Compared with the normative growth standards of Tanner et al.,[94,95] the mean height in both sexes is about equivalent to the 3rd centile until the start of puberty in normal children. A further decline follows, which results from delayed pubertal development. With the onset of puberty, mean height again begins to draw near the 3rd centile. Adult height is evidently reached at the end of the second decade of life. Adult height in men ($n = 20$)

Table 35.3 A comparison of frequency of symptoms (percent) between Noonan (*n* = 410) and Turner syndrome (*n* = 387), using data collected from various sources

Abnormal symptoms: area	Noonan syndrome (percent)	Turner syndrome (percent)
Eyes	87	29
Ears	63	58
High arched palate	51	61
Neck/pterygium colli	41	67
Low-set hairline	61	80
Thorax	64	76
Cubitus valgus	67	50
Skin	32	72
Cardiac defect (all)	56	20
Pulmonary stenosis	42	Rare
Coarctation	3	14
Renal	25	57
Gonads		
Male	72	–
Female	Rare	95
Mental handicap	44	11

and women (*n* = 18) was (mean ± SD) 162.5 ± 5.4 cm and 152.7 ± 5.7 cm, respectively. There is no statistical evidence to support the view that women reach a relatively greater adult height than men. The variation of height around the mean values is of the same order of magnitude as in normal children and in patients with Turner syndrome. Reference curves for patients with Noonan syndrome have been published.[90,92] Height in patients with Noonan syndrome, compared with the normal range, is illustrated in Fig. 35.8.

To the author's knowledge, sufficient data are at present not available in the literature about height velocity in Noonan syndrome. Such data require longitudinal observations. If height velocity is deduced from mean height data (see Fig. 35.2), it is evidently always below the 50th centile of the normal population. During most of childhood, the velocity remains constant, at about the 10th to 25th centile of normal children. In girls, height velocity during childhood tends to be slightly higher than in Turner syndrome. The pubertal growth spurt is of minor magnitude, even if compared with that of normal children with delayed puberty. The maximum pubertal velocity is reached with a delay of about 2 years.

The ratio of weight to height was found to be normal in Noonan syndrome. This finding differs from observations in Turner syndrome, in which weight tends to exceed ideal weight with progressing age. The information on bone age development in Noonan syndrome is rather limited. In the author's study[92] 119 measurements in male and 78 measurements in female patients were analysed using the method devised by Greulich and Pyle. These data are not sufficient for developing solid references for bone age in this disorder. Bone age was, however, generally found to be lower

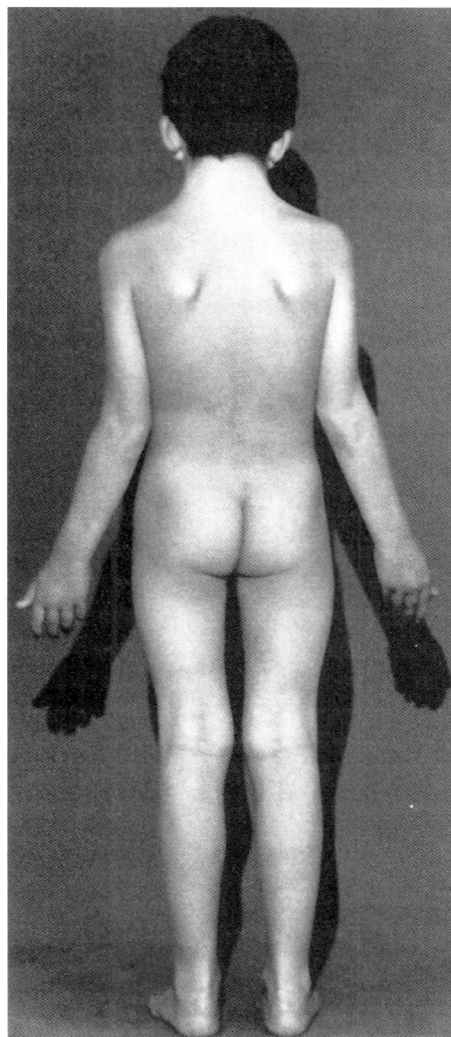

Figure 35.7 Typical appearance of a child with Noonan syndrome.

than chronological age in both sexes, regardless of age. After 5 years of age, bone age tended to be delayed by about 2 years. Head circumference was found to be normal in all (*n* = 10) females but was below the 3rd centile in 13 of 23 (57 percent) males.[92]

Growth promotion in Noonan syndrome

The pathogenesis of the growth disorder in Noonan syndrome is at present not known. It is very likely, however, that the disorder does not primarily involve the GH–IGF axis. Attempts to treat Noonan syndrome with growth hormone – in analogy to Turner syndrome – have been made, but results are still very limited and no definite conclusions can be drawn from the results available.

Ahmed *et al.*[96] treated six children with a dose of 0.6 IU kg^{-1} day^{-1} and observed a height increase of 1 SDS in 1 year, plus a doubling of the basal height velocity. Cotterill

Table 35.4   Height (mean ± SD) in patients with Noonan syndrome

Age (years)	Ranke et al.[91] Males	Females	Witt et al.[90] Males	Females
1	70.8 ± 3.2	68.4 ± 3.1	± 3.3	66.0 ± 4.2
2	80.1 ± 3.6	78.1 ± 3.5	± 3.3	79.0 ± 4.3
3	94.3 ± 4.2	86.0 ± 3.9		
4	100.0 ± 4.5	92.7 ± 4.2	86.5 ± 5.6	90.0 ± 8.6
5	105.4 ± 4.7	98.6 ± 4.4		
6	110.1 ± 5.0	104.1 ± 4.7	109.0 ± 7.5	107.0 ± 9.2
7	115.0 ± 5.2	109.3 ± 4.9		
8	120.7 ± 5.4	114.3 ± 5.1	113.0 ± 6.0	121.0 ± 5.4
9	125.3 ± 5.6	119.1 ± 5.4		
10	125.3 ± 5.6	123.8 ± 5.6	124.0 ± 4.7	120.0 ± 6.0
11	130.8 ± 5.9	128.4 ± 5.8		
12	135.1 ± 6.1	133.0 ± 6.0	132.5 ± 9.1	122.0 ± 4.7
13	139.2 ± 6.3	137.9 ± 6.2		
14	143.1 ± 6.4	142.9 ± 6.4	142.0 ± 7.5	136.0 ± 9.4
15	148.1 ± 6.7	146.9 ± 6.6		
16	153.5 ± 6.9	149.3 ± 6.7	151.5 ± 7.1	144.0 ± 9.1
17	157.5 ± 7.1	150.3 ± 6.8		
18	159.7 ± 7.2	150.7 ± 6.9	161.0 ± 8.5	150.5 ± 6.2
19	161.4 ± 7.3	151.0 ± 6.8		

et al.[97] treated 14 children (growth hormone dose: 28 IU m^{-2} week^{-1}) and observed a mean increase in height velocity from 3.8 to 10.5 cm year^{-1}. Otten[98] analyzed children treated within the Kabi International Growth Study (KIGS), and observed that, in the 55 children treated for 1 year (GH dose: 0.6 IU kg^{-1} day^{-1}), an increase in height velocity from 4.3 to 7 cm year^{-1} occurred. The predicted height in the 24 cases followed longitudinally rose by 0.6 SDS. Analysis in the first year showed that the response followed the prediction model developed for Turner syndrome girls rather than that for children with GH deficiency. Thomas et al.[99]* treated five patients, starting at a mean age of 3.9 years, over 3 years with a dose of recombinant human growth hormone (rhGH) of 0.15 IU kg^{-1} day^{-1}, and observed an increase from −3.3 SDS to 2.4 SDS. Romano et al.[93] analysed the Noonan syndrome patients enrolled in the National Collaborative Growth Study (NCGS). On a mean dose of growth hormone of 0.31 mg kg^{-1} week^{-1} they observed a sustained increase in height velocity over baseline even after 4 years. Otten and Noordam[100]* observed an increment from −3.0 to 2.7 SDS on a dose of 0.21 mg kg^{-1} week^{-1} when analysing the first year growth of 101 children in the KIGS database. Kirk et al.[101]* observed a gain in height SDS from 2.9 to 2.6 SDS during the first year on 26 mg kg^{-1} week^{-1} in 66 patients. Noordam et al.[102]** reported a gain of 0.5 SDS in 17 patients

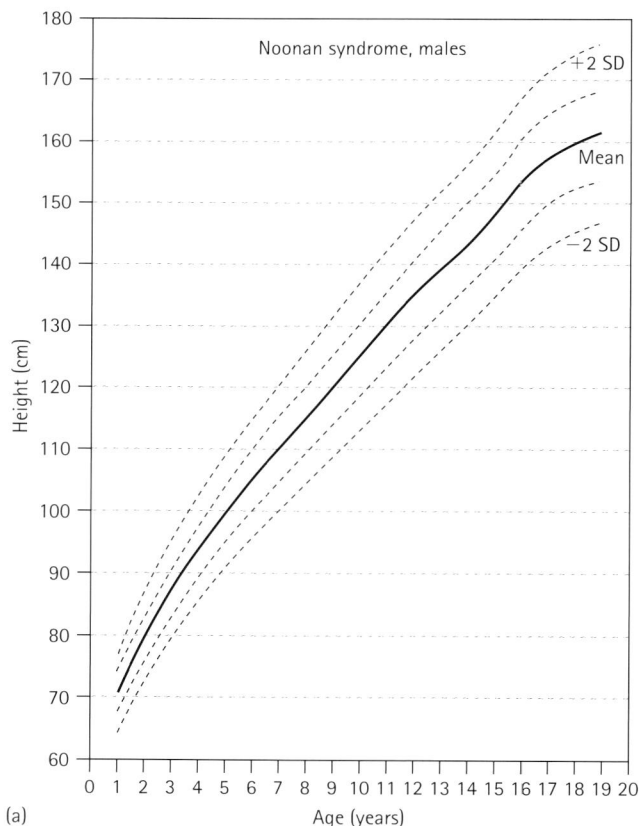

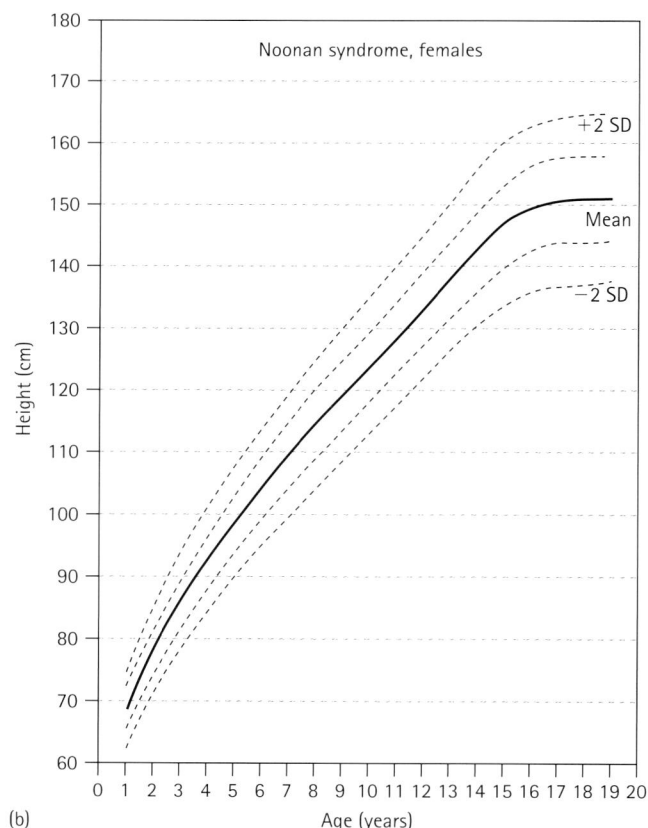

Figure 35.8   (a) Reference values for height in boys with Noonan syndrome, (b) Reference values for height in girls with Noonan syndrome.

who received a growth hormone dose of 33 mg kg^{-1} week^{-1}. These results mirror the data of MacFarlane *et al.*[103**]

To date, few data have been reported about the final height outcome in Noonan syndrome. In a series reported by Romano *et al.*,[104*] 40 individuals who were treated with a dose of 33 mg kg^{-1} week^{-1} showed a gain in height from −3.6 to −2.3 SDS. The 18 patients in the KIGS series[100*] had achieved a gain from −3.7 to −2.1 SDS. So far no systematic increase in side-effects attributable to growth hormone treatment have been observed, particularly with reference to cardiac events. The effect of growth hormone in hypertrophic cardiomyopathy is of specific concern in this group of patients.

The overall effect of growth hormone treatment on growth in children with Noonan syndrome is rather variable, but appears to be less pronounced than in, for instance, girls with Turner syndrome.[105] This may partly be explained by the fact that the dosages used have been relatively low. It may, however, also be attributed to an intrinsically lower sensitivity to growth hormone.[106,107] Methods need to be developed to identify Noonan syndrome patients who are sensitive to growth hormone in order to avoid unnecessary treatment in those who are less responsive.

KEY LEARNING POINTS

TURNER SYNDROME

- Turner syndrome (TS) is caused by the presence of only one X chromosome (or parts of it) and is characterized by short stature, gonadal dysgenesis and variable dysmorphic features.
- TS must be suspected in any short girl. Almost all girls with TS are short. Adult height is 20 cm below the mean female population.
- About 3/4 of shortness are caused by the absence of the SHOX gene.
- Height can be normalized in most patients by means of growth hormone therapy given in supra-physiological doses (approx. >50 μg kg^{-1} day^{-1}). Individualization is essential.
- Treatment in childhood is aimed at assuring normal physical and psychosocial well-being.
- Long-term care in TS needs to be focussed on medical issues (hypertension, diabetes type 2, thyroiditis), gynecological issues (estrogen replacement, fertility) and issues of cognitive functioning (hearing).

NOONAN SYNDROME

- Noonan syndrome is characterized by clinical features only superficially resembling those of Turner syndrome.

- The disorder is frequent (incidence 1:1000) and affects both sexes. Familial occurrence is occasional.
- Typical features for the Noonan syndrome are a Turner-like phenotype, abnormalities of the heart (right-sided), short stature (50% of the individuals), and mild mental retardation.
- In about 50% of cases there is a missense mutation of the protein-tyrosine phosphatase, non-receptor-type 11 (PTPN11), whose complex function in the disorder is still enigmatic.
- The effect of growth promotion with GH in short individuals has so far not been fully investigated.

REFERENCES

● = Seminal primary article

◆ = Key review paper

◆ 1 Ranke MB, Saenger P. Turner's syndrome. *Lancet* 2001; **28**: 309–14.

● 2 Rao E, Weiss B, Fukami M, *et al.* Pseudoautosomal deletions encompassing a novel homeobox gene cause growth failure in idiopathic short stature and Turner syndrome. *Nature Genet* 1997; **16**: 54–63.

3 Belin V, Cusin V, Viot G, *et al.* SHOX mutations in dyschondrosteosis (Léri–Weill syndrome). *Nature Genet* 1998, **19**: 67–9.

◆ 4 Ogata T, Matsuo N. Sex chromosome aberrations and stature: deduction of the principal factors involved in the determination of adult height. *Hum Genet* 1993; **91**: 551–62.

5 Zinn AR, Ross JL. Critical regions for Turner syndrome phenotypes on the X chromosome. In: Saenger P, Pasquino AM, eds. *Optimizing Health Care for Turner Patients in the 21st Century*. Amsterdam: Elsevier, 2000: 19–28.

● 6 Ranke MB, Pflueger H, Rosendahl W, *et al.* Turner syndrome: spontaneous growth in 150 cases and review of the literature. *Eur J Paediatr* 1983; **141**: 81–8.

7 Ranke MB, Blum WF, Frisch H. The acid-stable subunit of insulin-like growth factor binding protein (IGFBP-3) in disorders of growth. In: Drop SLS, Hintz RL, eds. *Insulin-like Growth Factor Binding Proteins*. Amsterdam: Excerpta Medica, 1989: 103–12.

8 Karlberg J, Albertsson-Wikland K, Naeraa RW, *et al.*, in collaboration with the Swedish and the Dutch Study Group for GH Treatment. Reference values for spontaneous growth in Turner girls and its use in estimating treatment effects. In: Hibi I, Takano K, eds. *Basic and Clinical Approach to Turner Syndrome*. International Congress Series 1014, Amsterdam: Excerpta Medica, 1993: 83–92.

9 Davenport ML, Punyasavatsut N, Stewart PW, *et al.* Growth failure in early life: an important manifestation of Turner syndrome. *Horm Res* 2002; **57**: 157–64.

10 Massa G, Vanderschueren-Lodeweyckx M, Malvaux P. Linear growth in patients with Turner syndrome: influence of spontaneous puberty and parental height. *Eur J Pediatr* 1990; **149**: 246–50.

11 Golbus MS. Prenatal diagnosis and fetal loss. In: Rosenfeld RG, Grumbach MM, eds. *Turner Syndrome.* New York: Marcel Dekker, 1990: 101–7.

12 Hall J. The relationship between karyotype and growth in Turner syndrome. In: Rosenfeld RG, Grumbach MM, eds. *Turner Syndrome.* New York: Marcel Dekker, 1991: 9–13.

13 Ranke MB, Grauer ML. Adult height in Turner syndrome: results of a multinational survey 1993. *Horm Res* 1994; **42**: 90–4.

◆ 14 Ranke MB. Disease-specific standards in congenital syndrome. *Horm Res* 1996; **45**: 35–41.

15 Hibi I, Tanae A, Tanaka T, *et al.* Spontaneous puberty in Turner syndrome: its incidence, influence on final height and endocrinological features. In: Ranke MB, Rosenfeld RG, eds. *Turner Syndrome: Growth Promoting Therapies.* Amsterdam: Excerpta Medica, 1991: 75–81.

16 Pasquino AM, Passeri F, Pucarelli I, *et al.* Spontaneous pubertal development in Turner's syndrome. Italian Study Group for Turner's Syndrome. *J Clin Endocrinol Metab* 1997; **82**: 1810–13.

17 Karlberg J, Albertsson-Wikland K, Naeraa RW, on behalf of the Swedish Pediatric Study Group for GH treatment. In: Ranke MB, Rosenfeld RG, eds. *Turner Syndrome: Growth Promoting Therapies.* Amsterdam: Excerpta Medica, 1991: 89–94.

● 18 Lyon AJ, Preece MA, Grant DB. Growth curve for girls with Turner syndrome. *Arch Dis Child* 1985; **60**: 932–5.

19 Ranke MB, Chavez-Meyer H, Blank B, *et al.* Spontaneous growth and bone age development in Turner syndrome: results of a multicentric study 1990. In: Ranke MB, Rosenfeld RG, eds. *Turner Syndrome: Growth Promoting Therapies.* Amsterdam: Excerpta Medica, 1991: 101–6.

20 Haeusler G, Schemper M, Frisch H, *et al.* Spontaneous growth in Turner syndrome: evidence for a minor pubertal growth spurt. *Eur J Pediatr* 1992; **151**: 283–7.

21 Brook CG, Gasser T, Werder EA, *et al.* Height correlations between parents and mature offspring in normal subjects and in subjects with Turner's and Klinefelter's and other syndromes. *Ann Hum Biol* 1977; **4**: 17–22.

◆ 22 Ranke MB. Growth disorders in Ullrich–Turner syndrome. *Bailliere's Clin Endocrinol Metab* 1992; **6**: 603–19.

23 Connor JM, Loughlin SAR. Molecular genetic analysis in Turner syndrome. In: Ranke MB, Rosenfeld RG, eds. *Turner Syndrome: Growth Promoting Therapies.* Amsterdam: Excerpta Medica, 1991: 3–8.

24 Hauspie RC, Vercauteren M, Susanne C. Secular changes in growth. *Horm Res* 1996; **45**: 8–17.

● 25 Brook CG, Murset G, Zachmann M, Prader A. Growth in children with 45,XO Turner's syndrome. *Arch Dis Child* 1974; **49**: 789–95.

26 Rochiccioli P, Pienkowski C, Tauber MT. Spontaneous growth in Turner syndrome: a study of 61 cases. In: Ranke MB, Rosenfeld RG, eds. *Turner Syndrome: Growth Promoting Therapies.* Amsterdam: Excerpta Medica, 1991: 107–12.

27 Price DA, Albertsson-Wikland K. Demography, auxology and response to recombinant human growth hormone treatment in girls with Turner's syndrome in the Kabi Pharmacia International Growth Study. *Acta Paediatr Scand Suppl* 1993; **391**: 69–74.

28 Schwarze CP, Arens D, Haber HP, *et al.* Bone age in 116 untreated patients with Turner's syndrome rated by a computer-assisted method (CASAS). *Acta Paediatr* 1998; **87**: 1146–50.

29 Ranke MB, Haug F, Blum WF, *et al.* Effect on growth of patients with Turner's syndrome treated with low estrogen doses. *Acta Endocrinol (Copenh) Suppl* 1986; **279**: 153–6.

◆ 30 Gravholt CH. Medical problems of adult Turner's syndrome. *Horm Res* 2001; **56(Suppl 1)**: 44–50.

31 Neufeld ND, Lippe BM, Kaplan SA. Disproportionate growth of the lower extremities. A major determinant of short stature in Turner's syndrome. *Am J Dis Child* 1978; **132**: 296–8.

32 Hughes PC, Ribeiro J, Hughes IA. Body proportions in Turner's syndrome. *Arch Dis Child* 1986; **61**: 506–7.

33 Rongen-Westerlaken C, Rikken B, Vastrick P, *et al.* Body proportions in individuals with Turner syndrome. The Dutch Growth Hormone Working Group. *Eur J Pediatr* 1993; **152**: 813–17.

34 Herdach F. Proportionen im Verlauf bei Ullrich–Turner-Syndrom. Inaugural dissertation, Medizinische Fakultät, Universität Tübingen, 1997.

35 Preece MA. Genetic contribution to stature. *Horm Res* 1996; **45**: 56–8.

36 Salerno MC, Job JC. La taille dans le syndrome de Turner: correlation avec la taille des parents. *Archives Francaises de Pédiatrie (Paris)* 1987; **44**: 863–5.

◆ 37 Frane JW, Sherman BM and the Genentech Collaborative Group. Predicted adult height in Turner syndrome. In: Rosenfeld RG, Grumbach MM, eds. *Turner Syndrome.* New York: Marcel Dekker, 1990: 405–16.

38 Naeraa RW, Nielsen J. Standards for growth and final height in Turner's syndrome. *Acta Paediatr Scand* 1990; **79**: 182–90.

39 Joss E. Evaluation of hormonal treatment on linear growth and skeletal maturation: methods of predicting final height in Turner syndrome. In: Ranke MB, Rosenfeld RG, eds. *Turner Syndrome: Growth Promoting Therapies.* Amsterdam: Excerpta Medica, 1991: 83–8.

40 Hutchings J, Escamilla R, Li C, Forsham P. Human growth hormone administration in gonadal dysgenesis. *Am J Dis Child* 1965; **109**: 318–21.

41 Tzagournis M. Response to long-term administration of human growth hormone in Turner's syndrome. *JAMA* 1969; **210**: 2373–76.

42 Rosenfeld RG, Frane J, Attie KM, *et al.* Six year results of a randomized, prospective trial of human growth hormone

and oxandrolone in Turner syndrome. *J Pediatr* 1992; **121**: 49–55.

◆ 43 Rosenfeld RG, Attie KM, Frane J, *et al.* Growth hormone therapy of Turner's syndrome: beneficial effect on adult height. *J Pediatr* 1998; **132**: 319–24.

44 Heinrichs C, De Schepper J, Thomas M, *et al.* and members of the Belgian Study Group for Pediatric Endocrinology. Final height in 46 girls with Turner syndrome treated with growth hormone in Belgium: evaluation of height recovery and predictive factors. In: Albertsson-Wikland K, Ranke MB, eds. *Turner Syndrome in a Life-span Perspective: Research and Clinical Aspects*. Amsterdam: Excerpta Medica, 1995: 137–47.

45 Massa G, Van den Broeck J, Attanasio A, Wit JM, on behalf of the Lilly European Turner Study Group. Final height results of the Lilly European Turner studies. In: Albertsson-Wikland K, Ranke MB, eds. *Turner Syndrome in a Life-span Perspective: Research and Clinical Aspects*. Amsterdam: Excerpta Medica, 1995: 155–9.

46 Ranke MB, Price DA, Maes M, *et al.* Factors influencing final height in Turner syndrome following GH treatment: results of the Kabi International Growth Study (KIGS). In: Albertsson-Wikland K, Ranke MB, eds. *Turner Syndrome in a Life-span Perspective: Research and Clinical Aspects*. Amsterdam: Excerpta Medica, 1995: 161–5.

47 Rochiccioli P, Chaussain JL. Final height in patients with Turner syndrome treated with growth hormone ($n = 117$). In: Albertsson-Wikland A, Ranke MB, eds. *Turner Syndrome in a Life-span Perspective: Research and Clinical Aspects*. Amsterdam: Excerpta Medica, 1995: 123–8.

48 Tillmann V, Price DA, Bucknall JL, Clayton PE. Experience within the Manchester Growth Clinic of growth treatment of girls with Turner syndrome: the influence of duration of treatment on final height. In: Albertsson-Wikland K, Ranke MB, eds. *Turner Syndrome in a Life-span Perspective: Research and Clinical Aspects*. Amsterdam: Excerpta Medica, 1995: 149–54.

49 Nilsson KO, Albertsson-Wikland K, Alm J, *et al.* Growth promoting treatment in girls with Turner syndrome: final height results according to three different Turner syndrome growth standards. In: Albertsson-Wikland K, Ranke MB, eds. *Turner Syndrome in a Life-span Perspective: Research and Clinical Aspects*. Amsterdam: Excerpta Medica, 1995: 89–94.

50 Schweizer R, Ranke MB, Binder G, *et al.* Experience with growth hormone therapy in Turner syndrome in a single centre: low total height gain, no further gains after puberty onset and unchanged body proportions. *Horm Res* 2002; **53**: 228–38.

51 Ranke MB, Partsch CJ, Lindberg A, *et al.* Adult height after GH therapy in 188 Ullrich–Turner syndrome patients: results of the German IGLU Follow-up Study 2001. *Eur J Endocrinol* 2002; **147**: 625–33.

52 Cave CB, Bryant J, Milne R. Recombinant growth hormone in children and adolescents with Turner syndrome. *Cochrane Database System Rev* 2003; CD003887.

53 Stephure DK. Impact of growth hormone supplementation on adult height in Turner syndrome: results of the Canadian randomized controlled trial. *J Clin Endocrinol Metab* 2005; **90**: 3360–6.

54 Wilton P. Adverse events during GH treatment: 10 years' experience in KIGS, a pharmacoepidemiological survey. In: Ranke MB, Wilton P, eds. *Growth Hormone Therapy in KIGS: 10 years' Experience*. Heidelberg: Johann Ambrosius Barth Verlag, 1999: 349–64.

● 55 Ranke MB, Lindberg A, Chatelain P, *et al.* Prediction of long-term response to recombinant human growth hormone in Turner syndrome: development and validation of mathematical models. KIGS International Board. Kabi International Growth Study. *J Clin Endocrinol Metab* 2000; **85**: 4212–8.

56 van Pareren YK, de Muinck Keizer-Schrama SMPF, Stijnen T, *et al.* Final height in girls with Turner syndrome after long-term growth hormone treatment in three dosages and low dose estrogens. *J Clin Endocrinol Metab* 2003; **88**: 1119–25.

57 Saenger P, Albertsson-Wikland K, Conway GS, *et al.* Recommendations for the diagnosis and management of Turner syndrome. *J Clin Endocrinol Metab* 2001; **86**: 3061–69.

58 Kastrup KW. Oestrogen therapy in Turner's syndrome. *Acta Paediatr Scand Suppl* 1988; **343**: 43–6.

59 Quigley CA, Crowe BJ, Anglin DG, Chipman JJ. Growth hormone and low dose estrogen in Turner syndrome: results of a United States multi-center trial to near-final height. *J Clin Endocrinol Metab* 2002; **87**: 2033–41.

60 Wilton P. Adverse events during growth hormone treatment: 5 years' experience in the Kabi International Growth Study. In: Ranke MB, Gunnarsson R, eds. *Progress in Growth Hormone Therapy – 5 Years of KIGS*. Mannheim: J & J Verlag, 1994: 291–307.

61 Landin-Wilhelmsen K, Bryman I, Windh M, Wilhelmsen L. Osteoporosis and fractures in Turner syndrome – importance of growth promoting and oestrogen therapy. *Clin Endocrinol (Oxf)* 1999; **51**: 497–502.

◆ 62 Elsheikh M, Dunger DB, Conway GS, Wass JA. Turner's syndrome in adulthood. *Endocr Rev* 2002; **23**. 120–40.

63 Gravholt CH. Turner syndrome and the heart: cardiovascular complications and treatment strategies. *Am J Cardiovasc Drugs* 2002; **2**: 401–13.

64 Ostberg JE, Conway GS. Adulthood in women with Turner syndrome. *Horm Res* 2003; **59**: 211–21.

65 Wilson DM, Frane JW, Sherman B, *et al.* Carbohydrate and lipid metabolism in Turner syndrome: effect of therapy with growth hormone, oxandrolone, and a combination of both. *J Pediatr* 1988; **112**: 210–17.

66 Chiumello G, Bognetti E, Bonfanti R, *et al.* Glucose metabolism in Turner syndrome. In: Ranke MB, Rosenfeld RG, eds. *Turner Syndrome: Growth Promoting Therapies*. Amsterdam: Excerpta Medica, 1991: 47–9.

67 Monti LD, Brambilla P, Caumo A, *et al.* Glucose turnover and insulin clearance after growth hormone treatment in girls with Turner's syndrome. *Metabolism* 1997; **46**: 1482–8.

68 Burgert TS, Vuguin PM, DiMartino-Nardi J, *et al.* Assessing insulin resistance: application of a fasting glucose to insulin ratio in growth hormone-treated children. *Horm Res* 2002; **57**: 37–42.

69 Gravholt CH, Naeraa RW, Brixen K, *et al.* Short-term growth hormone treatment in girls with Turner syndrome decreases fat mass and insulin sensitivity: a randomized, double-blind, placebo-controlled, crossover study. *Pediatrics* 2002; **110**: 889–96.

70 Sippell WG, Partsch CJ, Steinkamp H, on behalf of the German Pfrimmer-Kabi UTS Study Group. Biosynthetic growth hormone (Genotropin) therapy in girls with the Ullrich–Turner-syndrome (UTS). In: Ranke MB, Rosenfeld RG, eds. *Turner Syndrome: Growth Promoting Therapies.* Amsterdam: Excerpta Medica, 1991: 237–40.

71 Stahnke N, Stubbe P, Keller E, Zeisel HJ and Serono Study Group Hamburg. Effects and side-effects of GH plus oxandrolone in Turner syndrome. In: Ranke MB, Rosenfeld RG, eds. *Turner Syndrome: Growth Promoting Therapies.* Amsterdam: Excerpta Medica, 1991: 241–7.

72 Opitz JM, Pallister PD. Brief historical note: the concept of 'gonadal dysgenesis'. *Am J Med Genet* 1979; **4**: 333–43.

73 Flavell G. Webbing of neck with Turner's syndrome in the male. *Br J Surg* 1943; **31**: 150–3.

● 74 Noonan JA, Ehmke DA. Associated noncardiac malformations in children with congenital heart disease. *J Pediatr* 1963; **63**: 468–70.

◆ 75 Mendez HM, Opitz JM. Noonan syndrome: a review. *Am J Med Genet* 1985; **21**: 493–506.

● 76 Nora JJ, Sinha AK. Direct familial transmission of the Turner phenotype. *Am J Dis Child* 1968; **116**: 343–50.

77 Nora JJ, Nora AH, Sinha AK, *et al.* The Ullrich–Noonan syndrome (Turner phenotype). *Am J Dis Child* 1974; **127**: 48–55.

78 Elders MJ, Char F. Possible etiologic mechanisms of the short stature in the Noonan syndrome. *Birth Defects* 1976; **12**: 127–33.

79 Char FC, Rodriguez-Fernandez HL, Scott C, *et al.* The Noonan syndrome – a clinical study of forty-five cases. *Birth Def* 1972; **8**: 110–8.

80 Allanson JE. Noonan syndrome. *J Med Genet* 1987; **24**: 9–13.

81 Summitt RL. Turner syndrome and Noonan's syndrome. *J Pediatr* 1969; **74**: 155–6.

● 82 Jamieson CR, van der Burgt L, Brady AF, *et al.* Mapping a gene for Noonan syndrome to the long arm of chromosome 12. *Nature Genet* 1994; **8**: 357–60.

● 83 Tartaglia M, Mehler EL, Goldberg R, *et al.* Mutations in PTPN11, encoding the protein tyrosine phosphatase SHP-2, cause Noonan syndrome. *Nature Genet* 2001; **29**: 465–8.

84 Tartaglia M, Kalidas K, Shaw A, *et al.* PTPN11 mutations in Noonan syndrome: molecular spectrum, genotype–phenotype correlation, and phenotypic heterogeneity. *Am J Hum Genet* 2002; **70**: 1555–63.

85 Kosaki K, Suzuki T, Muroya K, *et al.* PTPN11 (protein-tyrosine phosphatase, nonreceptor-type 11) mutations in seven Japanese patients with Noonan syndrome. *J Clin Endocrinol Metab* 2002; **87**: 3529–33.

86 Maheshwari M, Belmont J, Fernbach S, *et al.* PTPN11 mutations in Noonan syndrome type I: detection of recurrent mutations in exons 3 and 13. *Hum Mutat* 2002; **20**: 298–304.

87 Musante L, Kehl HG, Majewski F, *et al.* Spectrum of mutations in PTPN11 and genotype–phenotype correlation in 96 patients with Noonan syndrome and five patients with cardio-facio-cutaneous syndrome. *Eur J Hum Genet* 2003; **11**: 201–6.

88 Zenker M, Buheitel G, Rauch R, *et al.* Genotype–phenotype correlations in Noonan syndrome. *J Pediatr* 2004; **144**: 368–74.

● 89 Sharland M, Patton MA, Talbot S, *et al.* Coagulation-factor deficiencies and abnormal bleeding in Noonan's syndrome. *Lancet* 1992; **339**: 19–21.

● 90 Witt DR, Keena BA, Hall JG, Allanson JE. Growth curves for height in Noonan syndrome. *Clin Genet* 1986; **30**: 150–3.

● 91 Ranke MB, Heidemann P, Knupfer C, *et al.* Noonan syndrome: growth and clinical manifestations in 144 cases. *Eur J Paediatr* 1988; **148**: 220–7.

92 Ranke MB, Stubbe P, Majewski F, Bierich JR. Spontaneous growth in Turner's syndrome. *Acta Paediatr Scand Suppl* 1988; **343**: 22–30.

93 Romano AA, Blethen SI, Dana K, Noto RA. Growth hormone treatment in Noonan syndrome: the National Cooperative Growth Study experience. *J Pediatr* 1996; **128**: 518–21.

94 Tanner JM, Whitehouse RH, Takaishi M. Standards from birth to maturity for height, weight, height velocity and weight velocity. British children, 1965, I. *Arch Dis Child* 1966; **41**: 454–71.

95 Tanner JM, Whitehouse RH, Takaishi M. Standards from birth to maturity for height, weight, height velocity and weight velocity. British children, 1965, II. *Arch Dis Child* 1966; **41**: 613–35.

96 Ahmed ML, Foot AB, Edge JA, *et al.* Noonan's syndrome: abnormalities of the growth hormone-IGF-I axis and the response to treatment with human biosynthetic growth hormone. *Acta Paediatr Scand* 1991; **80**: 446–50.

97 Cotterill AM, McKenna WJ, Elsawi M, *et al.* The effect of GH (Saizen) therapy (28 IU/sqm/wk) on linear growth and cardiac morphology in short children with Noonan syndrome. *Pediatr Res* 1993; **(Suppl 5)**: Abstract 240.

98 Otten BJ. Short stature in Noonan syndrome: Demography and response to growth hormone therapy in the Kabi International Growth Study. In: Ranke MB, Gunnarsson R, eds. *Progress in Growth Hormone Therapy – 5 Years of KIGS.* Mannheim: J & J Verlag, 1994: 206–15.

99 Thomas BC, Stanhope R. Long-term treatment with growth hormone in Noonan's syndrome. *Acta Paediatr Scand* 1993; **82**: 853–5.

100 Otten BJ, Noordam K. Short stature in Noonan syndrome: demography and response to growth hormone treatment in KIGS. In: Ranke MB, Wilton P, eds. *Growth Hormone*

Therapy in KIGS: 10 Years' Experience. Heidelberg: Johann Ambrosius Barth Verlag, 1999: 269–80.

101 Kirk JM, Betts PR, Butler GE, *et al*. Short stature in Noonan syndrome: response to growth hormone therapy. *Arch Dis Child* 2001; **84**: 440–3.

102 Noordam C, van der Burgt I, Sengers RC, *et al*. Growth hormone treatment in children with Noonan's syndrome: four year results of a partly controlled trial. *Acta Paediatr* 2001; **90**: 889–94.

103 MacFarlane CE, Brown DC, Johnston LB, *et al*. Growth hormone therapy and growth in children with Noonan's syndrome: results of 3 years' follow-up. *J Clin Endocrinol Metab* 2001; **86**: 1953–6.

104 Romano AA, Blethen SI, Dana K. Adult height after growth hormone in patients with Noonan syndrome: the National Cooperative Growth Study experience [Abstract]. *Pediatr Res* 2001; **(Suppl)**: P1–421.

105 Kelnar C. Growth hormone therapy in Noonan syndrome. *Horm Res* 2000; **53(Suppl 1)**: 77–81.

106 Noordam K, van der Burgt I, Brunner HG, Otten BJ. The relationship between clinical severity of Noonan's syndrome and growth, growth hormone (GH) secretion and response to GH treatment. *J Pediatr Endocrinol Metab* 2002; **15**: 175–80.

107 Binder G, Neuer K, Ranke MB, Wittekindt NE. PTPN11 mutations are associated with mild growth hormone resistance in individuals with Noonan syndrome. *J Pediatr Endocrinol Metab* 2005; **90**: 5377–81 (E-pub).

36

Prader–Willi syndrome: Disease-specific auxology and therapy

ANN CHRISTIN LINDGREN

EVIDENCE SCORING OF THERAPY

*   Non-randomized controlled trials, cohort study, etc.
**   One or more well-designed randomized controlled trials
*** Systematic review or meta-analysis

INTRODUCTION

In 1956, Prader, Labhart and Willi made the first description of the Prader–Willi syndrome by reporting nine children with muscular hypotonia, hypomentia, hypogonadism, obesity, and diabetes.[1,2]

GENETICS

Prader–Willi syndrome (PWS) is a genetic disorder characterized by both mental and physical abnormalities. Occurring in 70–75 percent of affected individuals, the principal genetic mutation associated with the condition is deletion of a segment of the paternally derived chromosome 15 (15q11–q13). Several other abnormalities have also been linked with the syndrome, 20–25 percent of patients with PWS exhibit maternal disomy of the same region of chromosome 15q, 2–5 percent have imprinting center mutations and approximately 1 percent of affected individuals have a balanced translocation.[3–5] All these abnormalities result in an absence of paternally expressed genes localized in the 15q11–q13 region. The individual gene or genes from within 15q11–q13 that cause the condition have yet to be identified but two genes involved in the development of central nervous system functioning have been demonstrated to be absent in PWS, namely the small nuclear ribonucleoprotein polypeptide N (*SNRPN*) gene and *Necdin* gene.[5–7]

CLINICAL MANIFESTATIONS OF PRADER–WILLI SYNDROME

Clinically, PWS is characterized by a range of mental and physical symptoms. These include short stature, muscular hypotonia, excessive appetite with progressive obesity, hypogonadism, mental retardation, behavioral abnormalities, sleep disturbances (including sleep apnea), and dysmorphic features.[8] The photograph of a boy with PWS illustrates the typical physical features of the condition (Fig. 36.1).

Diagnosis of PWS is made according to a set of consensus clinical criteria published in 1993[9] (Table 36.1). On this basis, it is estimated that one child in every 10 000 to 25 000 live births suffers from the syndrome.[10–12] However, as it relies on subjective identification of characteristic symptoms and signs, it is likely that this figure is not completely accurate. Recently, a paper revising the clinical criteria to help to identify the appropriate patients for DNA testing for PWS has been published[13] (Table 36.2).

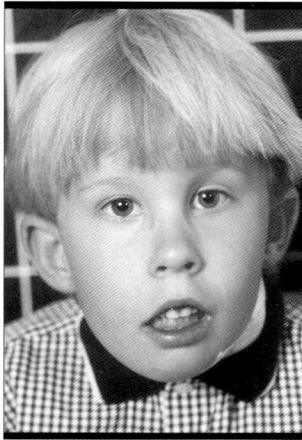

Figure 36.1   A boy with Prader–Willi syndrome. Please see Plate 21.

In the newborn child, PWS first manifests as muscular hypotonia. It is often so pronounced that babies are described as 'floppy'. They frequently have feeding difficulties due to a poor suck and thus require tube feeding for several weeks or months.[4,8,9]

As a consequence of their insatiable appetite and compulsive eating, children with PWS usually become overweight by the age of 4 years.[14] Unfortunately, obesity progresses with age[15–17] and historically we have observed that about one-third of individuals with PWS are more than twice their ideal body weight.[18,19] Obesity is a risk factor for many other serious conditions including cardiovascular disease and diabetes, hence it is a major cause of increased morbidity and mortality among patients with PWS.[20,21]

During their first 6 years of life, children with PWS often do not achieve normal levels of cognitive, motor, and language development. Indeed, according to most studies, these individuals have a below average IQ of about 70.[22] A review of cognitive ability among 575 affected individuals confirms this, showing that just 5 percent of patients had a normal IQ (i.e., >85).[23] Borderline mental retardation was observed in 28 percent of patients, while 34 percent, 27 percent, and 5 percent, respectively, were mildly, moderately or severely mentally retarded. In addition to impaired mental development, many subjects with PWS display a range of behavioral problems,[4] including excessive appetite and lack of food selectivity, and also a high incidence of stubbornness, verbal perseverance, skin picking, and temper tantrums. Furthermore, affected individuals have a tendency toward depression, and a diminished ability to initiate and maintain social contacts. A high pain threshold is also characteristic of the condition and sleep apnea and excessive daytime sleepiness are particularly common among older children. Given these problems it is understandable that many children with PWS experience learning disabilities often requiring special education services.[9]

The handicaps associated with PWS have significant implications in later life as many of those affected are incapable of independent living. According to a large survey of

Table 36.1   Clinical diagnostic criteria for Prader–Willi syndrome (adapted from Holm et al.[9]): 5 points (⩾ 4 points from major criteria) strongly suggests Prader–Willi syndrome in children ⩽3 years of age, whereas 8 points (⩾5 points from major criteria) are indicative in older individuals

Major criteria (1 point each)
- Neonatal and infantile hypotonia
- Infantile feeding problems or failure to thrive
- Excessive or rapid weight gain between the ages of 1 and 6 years
- Characteristic facial features, including narrow face, almond-shaped eyes, small-appearing mouth with thin upper lip, down-turned corners of the mouth (three or more required)
- Hypogonadism (impaired function of the gonads) with under-developed genitalia and/or impaired pubertal development
- Developmental delay, mental retardation or learning problems
- Hyperphagia, food foraging or obsession with food
- Deletion 15q11–q13 on high resolution cytogenetic analysis or other abnormality of the Prader–Willi chromosome region

Minor criteria (0.5 point each)
- Decreased fetal movement or infantile lethargy
- Typical behavioral problems: temper tantrums, violent outbursts; obsessive/compulsive behavior, argumentative, rigid, possessive, stubborn, manipulative, stealing, lying (five or more required)
- Sleep disturbances or sleep apnea
- Short stature for family by the age of 15 years
- Fairer eyes, skin and hair than expected
- Smaller hands and feet than expected for height and age
- Narrow hands with straight ulnar border
- Esotropia or myopia
- Viscous saliva
- Speech articulation defects
- Skin picking

Supportive criteria (0 points, but help to confirm diagnosis)
- High pain threshold
- Reduced incidence of vomiting
- Temperature control problems
- Scoliosis or kyphosis
- Early adrenarche
- Osteoporosis
- Unusual skill with jigsaw puzzles
- Normal neuromuscular findings

adults with the condition,[20] the majority lived in group homes or with their family. Over a third (35 percent) did not work; of those who did work, the vast majority were employed in a sheltered environment.

AUXOLOGY IN PRADER–WILLI SYNDROME

Restriction of growth is also a frequently observed sequel of PWS; approximately 90 percent of affected individuals have a short final stature.[10] Specific growth charts for PWS

Table 36.2 Suggested new criteria to prompt DNA testing for Prader–Willi syndrome (adapted from Gunay-Aygun et al.[13])

Age at assessment	Features sufficient to prompt DNA testing
Birth to 2 years	1. Hypotonia with poor suck
2–6 years	1. Hypotonia with history of poor suck 2. Global developmental delay
6–12 years	1. History of hypotonia with poor suck (hypotonia often persists) 2. Global developmental delay 3. Excessive eating (hyperphagia; obsession with food) with central obesity if uncontrolled
13 years through adulthood	1. Cognitive impairment; usually mild mental retardation 2. Excessive eating (hyperphagia; obsession with food) with central obesity if uncontrolled 3. Hypothalamic hypogonadism and/or typical behavior problems (including temper tantrums and obsessive-compulsive features)

are available. In the American chart based on a study of the weight and height of 71 Caucasian Americans, aged 4–24 years, with PWS compared with healthy subjects, the 50th centile for height in the patient group fell below the normal 5th centile by the age of 12–14 years, whereas the 50th centile for weight in the affected individuals approximated the 95th centile in the healthy population.[24] As a result of their feeding difficulties, affected infants often fail to thrive and, during the first year, this may result in growth below the 3rd percentile. Thereafter, linear growth is only slightly compromised, remaining at the 10th percentile or below until the age of 10 years for females and 12 years for males, after which height velocity often declines relative to the norm at these ages, due to a lack of growth spurt.[10,24] This growth pattern may vary in the individual child, partly as a consequence of evolving obesity or dietary interventions. Thus, it is not uncommon to see temporary growth arrest when caloric restrictions take effect after late diagnosis, or, conversely, an improvement in growth rate may be seen when obesity develops. Cassidy reports that the mean adult heights achieved by men and women with PWS are 155 and 148 cm respectively.[4] However, in the study by Wollmann et al. the mean height was slightly higher – 162 and 150 cm for men and women, respectively[16] – while Hauffa and colleagues noticed a near final mean height of 159 cm in boys and 149 cm in girls[25] (Fig. 36.2).

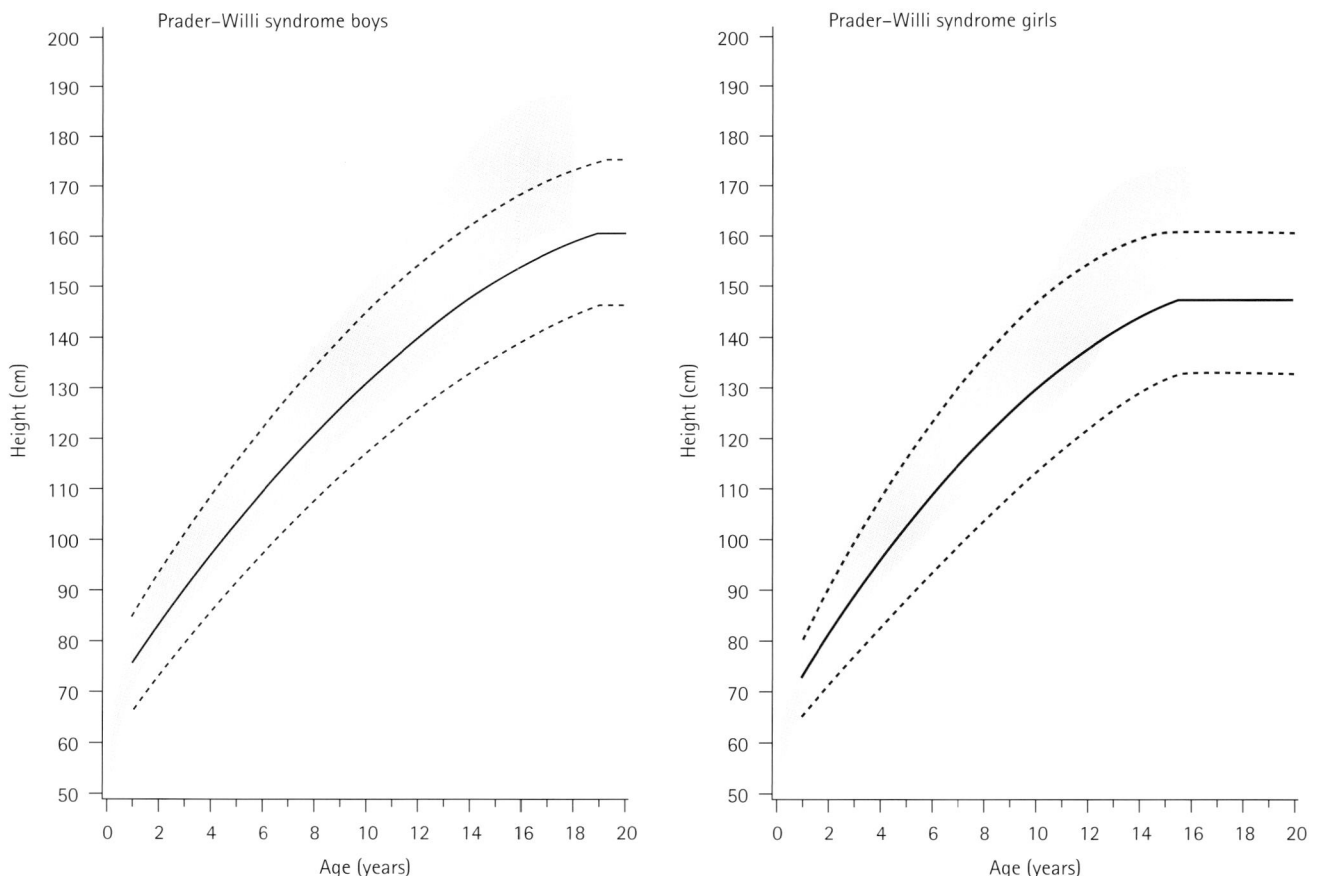

Figure 36.2 Growth charts for children with Prader–Willi syndrome. Adapted from Hauffa et al.[25] With permission from Blackwell Publishing.

Evaluation of body composition in PWS has shown that PWS is associated with high body fat mass and low muscle mass when compared with healthy controls. Studies have shown that the mean percent body fat in PWS was 42 percent to 51 percent.[15,26,27] In contrast to healthy children and young adults, mean percent body fat was only 11 percent in males, 15.5 percent in girls less than 15 years old, and 24 percent in females older than 15 years.[28,29]

Brambilla and co-workers[15] have show that patients with PWS had a low lean body mass (LBM) as well as a higher ratio of fat mass to lean body mass compared with both healthy individuals of normal weight and, importantly, those with simple obesity (Fig. 36.3). The study also shows that LBM declines further with age. Young children with PWS (less than 12 years old) had an LBM that was 81–93 percent of that found in the children of normal weight, whereas in older patients, LBM was only 63–83 percent of the normative values. Limb areas appeared to be most compromised. In addition, bone mineral content was found to be lower than in the healthy obese and normal weight populations. Notably, Eiholzer and co-workers have shown that even in the first years of life children with PWS have an abnormally low LBM.[30]

The low LBM associated with PWS is likely to reflect a reduced muscle mass and thus it may contribute to the observed moderate clinical hypotonia and poor physical performance of these individuals.[15,31] Muscle is a metabolically active tissue and a small mass of this tissue, in conjunction with reduced physical activity,[26] may explain the low energy expenditure found in patients with PWS.[31–35] In one study, patients with the condition expended approximately 50 percent less energy than healthy obese controls.[18]

NATURAL HISTORY OF PRADER–WILLI SYNDROME

PWS is associated with increased morbidity and premature mortality, the main cause of which is thought to be obesity.[20,21] Many of the medical complications of obesity

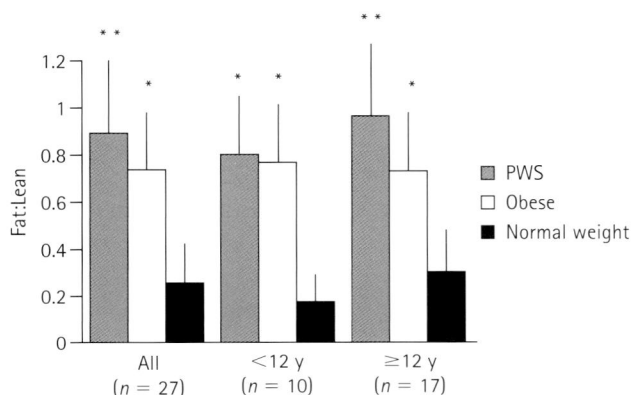

Figure 36.3   The ratio of fat mass to lean mass in children and adolescents (10 who were younger than 12 years) with Prader-Willi syndrome. (From Brambilla *et al.*[15] Reproduced with permission by the American Journal of Clinical Nutrition. Copyright *Am J Clin Nutr*. American Society for Clinical Nutrition.)

including type II diabetes mellitus, hypertension, atherosclerosis, hyperlipidemia, compromised cardiopulmonary function, sleep disturbance, and psychological problems such as depression and lack of self-esteem[36–40] have also been described in PWS.[41,42] Affected individuals are also at risk of developing scoliosis, and this may be a concern when considering GH therapy to improve growth rate. Up to 80 percent of patients are reported to have a scoliosis exceeding 10° and 15–20 percent have clinically significant scoliosis.[43] Similarly, the incidence of osteoporosis is higher among patients with PWS, to which reduced GH secretion and hypogonadism could contribute.[44] Lastly, given their high risk of co-morbidity, mental retardation, lack of employment and limited social and personal relationships, poor quality of life is a major concern for patients with PWS.[4,22]

Glucose intolerance is a significant co-morbid condition found in PWS and several reports suggest that glucose tolerance is abnormal in individuals with PWS. Fasting plasma insulin concentration and the insulin response to glucose are often increased in affected individuals, suggesting insulin resistance.[45] A reduction in the number of insulin receptors on monocytes has also been described in the syndrome, echoing a similar abnormality seen in patients with simple obesity.[46]

The reported prevalence of diabetes mellitus among patients with PWS varies. For example, in children with PWS the prevalence of diabetic glucose tolerance varies from 35 to 41 percent and diabetes from 7 to 21 percent.[17,41,47] However, diabetes is more common in older patients and the prevalence in the literature varies from 17 percent to 41 percent, the majority of whom required insulin therapy.[20,21,41,48] Clinically, the diabetes presented is type II, which responded to weight reduction and oral hypoglycemic agents.

The differing rates of diabetes reported could result from differences in age and body weight between the study groups. In most of the above studies, however, a large proportion of patients were grossly obese.

In contrast to these reports, some recent studies involving children with PWS who are of normal weight or only moderately obese, have demonstrated low insulin levels combined with normal serum glucose concentrations.[49–52] As subjects with 'simple' obesity generally have elevated insulin levels these results suggest that patients with PWS have increased insulin sensitivity, which is different from that of the grossly obese. One interpretation of these findings would be that some degree of GH insufficiency in PWS increases insulin sensitivity. Additionally, the high prevalence of diabetes cited in earlier reports may be secondary to gross obesity, rather than a feature of the syndrome itself, but this is an area where more data are needed.[41]

The high risk of vascular disease in adults with PWS is another significant co-morbid condition. The prevalence of hypertension in the literature varies from 17 percent to 32 percent[20,48] and these studies showed that co-morbidity was related to weight gain, as hypertension, heart problems and respiratory difficulties were all correlated with obesity but also secondary to the present growth hormone deficiency.[42,53–56] Furthermore, it also remains to be established whether hyperlipidemia is a feature of PWS, as both normal and elevated lipid levels have been reported.[42,57–60]

Impaired respiratory function is frequently observed in patients with PWS.[61] In the literature restrictive lung disease commonly affects individuals over the age of 30 years[48] and cor pulmonale has been shown to be the most common cause of death among patients with the condition.[21] A further complication seen in affected patients with reduced lung function is hypercapnia.[61] Until recently this was thought to be a secondary effect of respiratory muscle weakness or the result of Pickwickian syndrome brought about by increased abdominal and thoracic fat. However, it has been found that affected individuals with PWS have an impaired response to short periods of hypercapnia and a reduced ventilatory volume, indicating that the sensitivity of peripheral chemoreceptors to changes in blood oxygen and carbon dioxide is decreased.[62–64] In addition, the pharyngeal narrowness found in children with PWS may together with the respiratory abnormalities play an important role in the high mortality rate reported in children with PWS, regardless of whether they are on growth hormone therapy.[65] Thus, it seems that impaired respiratory function in PWS is not caused solely by obesity or muscle weakness but due to a hypothalamic abnormality and anatomical abnormalities.[65,66]

GH/IGF–I STATUS IN PRADER–WILLI SYNDROME

There are many data indicating reduced GH secretion in patients with PWS. Low peak GH response to stimulation tests, decreased spontaneous GH secretion and low serum insulin-like growth factor I (IGF-I) levels have been documented in at least 14 studies involving about 300 affected children.[49,60,67–78***] Depending on the stimulation test used, 40–100 percent of children with this condition fulfill the criteria for GH deficiency (GHD), which is generally defined as 'peak-GH levels of less than $10 \mu g \ L^{-1}$ in response to one or two stimulation tests'. The majority of affected children also have low GH secretion when measured by frequent blood sampling over 24 h. However, healthy, obese individuals also show reduced GH secretion during provocation tests, when compared with healthy, 'lean' controls.[79] The cause of reduced GH secretion in obesity is not fully understood, and both free fatty acids[80] and insulin have been proposed as mediators of this effect.[81] At least one study has shown elevated levels of free IGF-I in individuals with 'simple' obesity, suggesting a negative feed-back at the pituitary/hypothalamic level.[82] However, normal levels of free IGF-I have been found in other studies of subjects with the same condition.[83] As a result of these findings, it has been argued that the apparent GH insufficiency in patients with PWS simply reflects their obesity. In order to determine whether this is in fact the case, a detailed comparison of the two conditions with respect to GH-related parameters and clinical features is required.

Firstly, the GH response to GH-releasing hormone (GHRH) in obese individuals is enhanced by simultaneous administration of a cholinesterase inhibitor, such as pyridostigmine.[84] This effect is probably the result of reducing somatostatinergic tone. In contrast, when these agents are co-administered to patients with PWS, 13 out of 18 still showed a blunted GH response, suggestive of genuine GHD.[85] In children with GHD and most, but not all, children with PWS, serum IGF-I levels are reduced, whereas healthy children with simple obesity have normal or slightly elevated IGF-I levels. Furthermore, the level of IGF-I has been shown to correlate with body mass index (BMI) in obese children.[83,86] This is not the case in children with PWS, where low IGF-I and GH levels are not limited to those who are severely obese but have also been found in patients who are of normal weight. Lastly, in contrast to healthy obese children,[80,83,87] affected individuals[49] have depressed levels of IGF-binding protein 3.

Clinical features of the condition also support the presence of GHD in PWS. Both PWS and GHD are characterized by short stature, obesity with extra fat deposits over the abdomen, abnormal body composition with reduced muscle mass, decreased bone density and, in some patients, retarded bone age.[9,15,88] Conversely, children with simple obesity are often tall for their age, have an increased absolute fat free mass and an advanced bone age.[89,90] In summary then, available data suggest that, as a group, patients with PWS are GH deficient, though the degree of GHD may vary from mild to severe insufficiency.

The occurrence of reduced GH secretion and hypogonadotropic hypogonadism in the majority of children with PWS, together with abnormal appetite control and high pain threshold, suggest hypothalamic–pituitary dysfunction. Autopsies of five patients with PWS performed by Swaab and co-workers, indicated that the hypothalamic paraventricular nucleus was reduced in size and there were fewer oxytocin-expressing neurons[91] than in healthy subjects. In a later publication, Swaab identified further hypothalamic irregularities associated with PWS, these included a 30 percent reduction in GHRH-releasing neurons in the nucleus arcuatus, a down regulation of neuropeptide Y, and a deficiency in vasopressin.[92] Magnetic resonance imaging has also revealed an abnormal bright spot in the posterior pituitary lobe of some affected individuals, this is considered to be a sign of hypothalamic dysfunction.[93]

SEX HORMONES IN PRADER–WILLI SYNDROME

In addition to insufficient GH secretion, the majority of individuals with PWS have a dysfunctional hypothalamic–pituitary–gonadal axis, which manifests as retarded or incomplete sexual development. Neonatal hypogonadism is difficult to assess in girls, but boys affected by the syndrome often have a small penis and/or undescended testicles, both of which are indications of prenatal hypogonadotropic hypogonadism.[10] Detailed studies of gonadal structure and function in neonatal and prepubertal patients with PWS are lacking.

Puberty is generally delayed in children with PWS and in some individuals it may never occur at all,[44,48] although there have been at least two reported cases of precocious puberty.[94,95] In fact, many children experience premature adrenarche characterized by growth of axillary and pubic hair, this being particularly common in obese individuals.[96] Premature adrenarche has also been reported in children with hyperinsulinism, suggesting that they are predisposed to metabolic 'syndrome X'.[97] However, these observations do not reflect the situation in PWS, which is generally associated with low serum insulin levels. In many affected individuals puberty fails to progress beyond this stage. One study has shown that just 39 percent of these patients experienced menarche.[20] It seems that very obese girls with PWS may be more likely to experience puberty. A possible explanation for this is that aromatization of androgens in the fat tissue of these subjects, produces sufficient amounts of estrogen to prompt maturation.[10] However, even if menses do occur, bleeding is usually irregular and it is unlikely to be associated with a normal menstrual cycle. Furthermore, spontaneous breast development is difficult to assess in PWS because normal glandular development may be confused with increasing fat tissue, particularly in obese girls. Pubertal growth spurt and bone maturation are also compromised in the syndrome. Reduced levels of circulating sex hormones fail to provide the trigger for GH secretion, which may itself be depressed.

Hypogonadism associated with PWS is generally due to insufficient gonadotropin secretion, i.e., it is hypogonadotropic hypogonadism. In confirmation of this diagnosis, investigators have found that most affected individuals demonstrate a poor response to GnRH.[98–100,101***] that improves after prolonged clomiphene administration. These findings point to a hypothalamic dysfunction in the regulation of gonadotropin secretion. However, it should be noted that some individuals showed a normal gonadotropin response to GnRH and that some males may reached testosterone levels within the normal range. Testicular biopsies in males with PWS have shown atrophy of seminiferous tubules, few germ cells to no spermatogonia, some thickening of the tubular basement membranes and seemingly normal Leydig cells.[101,102]

These scattered observations in male patients with PWS may be the result of hypogonadotropic hypogonadism combined with primary testicular dysgenesis manifesting as very poor spermatogenesis.[98] Gonadotropin secretion may improve in early adulthood, leading to atrophy and hyalinization of seminiferous tubules. Furthermore, some male patients have poor Leydig cell function. Hypothetically, in the early years of life, this could be explained by a lack of LH stimulation, but in later years it may be secondary to seminiferous tubular damage caused by present or previous cryptorchidism.

Until recently it was thought that all individuals with PWS were sterile. However, we are now aware of two women with the syndrome who have become pregnant.[103,104] In one case a woman with maternal disomy gave birth to a healthy girl, whereas the other woman, who had a deletion of 15q11–q13, gave birth to a child with Angelman syndrome.

It is possible that the tempo of gonadal maturation varies between individuals, thereby increasing the heterogeneity of patient groups in the various studies. There is some evidence for delayed gonadal maturation, as the normalization of testosterone levels in blood in affected men over the age of 20 years has been observed (personal observations). Furthermore, one affected woman, reported to have given birth at the age of 33 years, had primary amenorrhea until the age of 29 years.[103]

OTHER HORMONAL AXES

Thyroid hormones and baseline TSH levels are normal or slightly elevated[8,99] in affected patients. Spontaneous cortisol and ACTH levels are usually normal, as is the response to i.v. ACTH.[8,44,99] Basal and TRH-stimulated prolactin levels are also within the normal range.[96] It has been reported that levels of both dehydroepiandrosterone (DHEA) and its sulfate (DHEAS) are elevated in PWS.[105]

TREATMENT OF PATIENTS WITH PRADER–WILLI SYNDROME

Currently, there is no cure for PWS, but several of the problems associated with the condition can be managed effectively if treatment begins early. This is now possible by using molecular genetic methods to identify affected children in the neonatal period. If the quality of life of patients with PWS is to be improved, a holistic approach to their treatment is needed. Before discussing the potential for endocrine hormone replacement, some of the other therapies which may be required for successful management of the condition are described.

Enteral gastric tube feeding is indicated in many neonates with PWS. Feeding difficulties commonly occur and may lead to malnutrition if not addressed. Training of balance and motor abilities is also important from an early age, as is physical training to increase muscle strength and energy consumption later in life. Other conditions such as scoliosis, hyperopia/myopia and cryptorchidism should be treated if present. The behavior of affected children may be improved by imposition of regular routines and the strict reinforcement of behavioral limits. Affected children may also benefit from special education. However, the most important aspect of treating PWS is control of excessive weight gain, specifically with respect to fat. As indicated previously, individuals afflicted by this condition seem to have similar complications to those experienced by healthy obese people. Thus, weight reduction could be expected to have beneficial effects on morbidity and mortality. A strictly controlled diet, in conjunction with eating-habit training and regular exercise, is important from an early age and remains the basis for all therapeutic interventions. To date, appetite suppressants have been mostly unsuccessful in controlling weight gain, as have surgical procedures, such as gastric banding, small-intestine by-pass and jaw wiring.[10,41] A comprehensive team to manage the various components of medical, psychological and sociological care is required for individuals with PWS.

Effects of treatment with growth hormone on stature

The GH-deficient state commonly associated with PWS, as evidenced by reduced GH secretion, low serum IGF-I levels and clinical features typical of GHD, has provided a rationale for trials assessing the efficacy of GH treatment. Recently, treatment with growth hormone has become an approved indication in Europe, US, and Japan based on the experience of three controlled randomized studies.[60,106,107**] However, up to now the duration of treatment is limited. Longitudinal growth has been shown to increase by GH treatment.[60,72,75,106–114] The initial positive effects on height velocity appear to be sustained throughout treatment. Furthermore, a report involving children treated with GH over a period of 7.5 years and other reports of shorter duration of GH treatment show that growth continues to improve with the result that target height SDS can be reached.[110–113*] The currently approved dosage of GH is $0.033\,\mathrm{mg\,kg^{-1}\,day^{-1}}$.

Effects of treatment with growth hormone on body composition and muscle function

The effect of GH treatment on body composition in PWS has been assessed in several studies,[26,75,107–109*] including two controlled studies.[106,113**] In these studies, a controlled diet was initiated before commencement of GH therapy and maintained throughout the trial. The results show that GH treatment leads to an overall improvement in body composition by reducing fat mass and increasing muscle mass (Figs 36.4 and 36.5). Follow-up of long-term treatment of GH treatment has shown a reduction in fat mass and a sustained increase in LBM. However, LBM did not reach values observed in healthy children.[111,112–114*] Improved motor performance and agility have also been documented in children with PWS who received GH.[106,108,109,113*] Furthermore, some reports suggest that such treatment has beneficial effects on physical appearance, energy, and

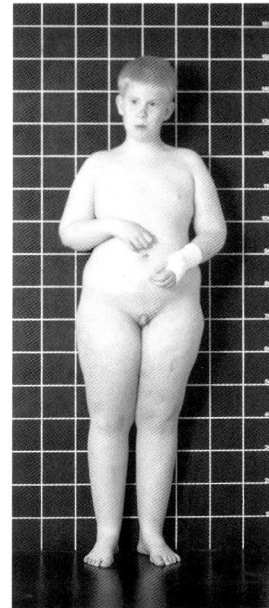

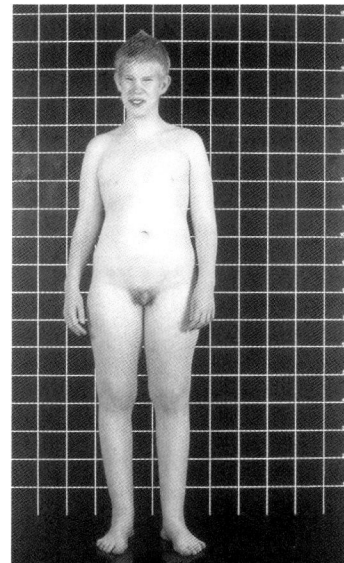

Figure 36.4   A boy before the start of growth hormone treatment and 1 year after commencing treatment. Please see Plate 22.

endurance, thus improving the psycho-social functioning of affected children.[60,106,111,112,115*] In a note of caution, it is recognized that many of these observations are based on spontaneous reports by parents and attending physicians, therefore further studies are required to confirm these particular benefits.

Other effects of treatment with growth hormone

There are studies that have shown that GH treatment can improve respiratory function in children with PWS[116] by

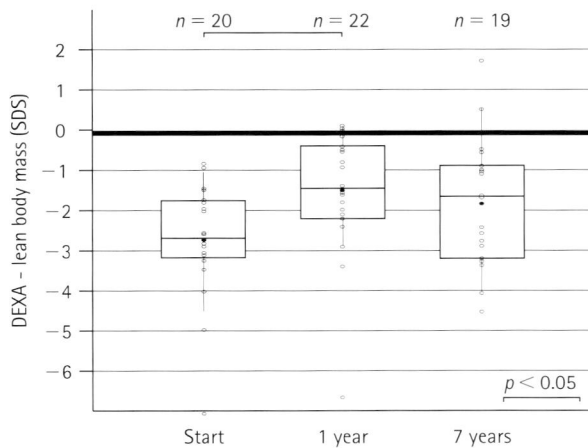

Figure 36.5 Sustained body composition (lean body mass) after 7 years of growth hormone treatment in Prader–Willi syndrome. (From Lindgren.[112])

improving respiratory muscle strength.[60,113] Treatment with GH has also been shown to have a direct or indirect effect on the central respiratory regulatory system resulting in increased ventilation and sensitivity of peripheral chemoreceptors to carbon dioxide.[64]

Side effects of treatment with growth hormone

The reported adverse events during GH treatment of patients with PWS are generally similar to those observed during treatment of children with classic GHD, Turner syndrome or chronic renal insufficiency. Recent studies have shown that insulin levels in children with PWS are lower than in obese controls at baseline, but increase during GH treatment. Glucose levels tend to remain unchanged or increase within the normal reference range.[49–51,117] However, considering the limited experience of prolonged GH treatment in these patients and the increased incidence of diabetes mellitus associated with the condition, carbohydrate metabolism (glucose, HbA_{1c}) should be closely monitored in patients receiving GH.

Attributed to a combination of obesity and muscular hypotonia, scoliosis is common in both children and adolescents with PWS. The rapid growth associated with GH may aggravate this spinal deformity, therefore the occurrence and development of scoliosis should be monitored during therapy. If quantification of scoliosis is difficult, in advanced obesity for example, X-ray monitoring should be used. In the controlled randomized studies performed the majority of the patients had a mild scoliosis ($<20°$) occurring equally between the control and treatment groups.[60,106] Furthermore, there was no significant worsening of the condition in either group during the studies and not during the

follow-ups.[110,112–114] Recently, several publications have reported an increased mortality rate in children with PWS, irrespective of GH treatment.[65,118] The disturbed body composition with obesity, the insufficient ventilation due to muscle weakness and central nervous respiratory abnormalities together with anatomical pharyngeal narrowness seem to play an important role.[65] Thus, before start of GH treatment a vigorous weight control of the patients with PWS must be introduced and followed, as well as polysomnography and an otorhinolaryngologic examination which will be repeated during GH treatment and have the patients to undergo tonsillectomy if necessary.[65]

Sex hormone replacement therapy

Treatment of hypothalamic–pituitary–gonadal failure in PWS remains a controversial issue. However, most clinicians agree that cryptorchidism should be corrected in order to enable detection of testicular malignancies (fertility may not be a goal in PWS). The true incidence of hypogonadism in adults with PWS is unknown but in the literature, less than 50 percent of males and one-third of females received sex hormone replacement therapy.[10,17] Sex hormone replacement therapy may be beneficial to hypogonadic patients in a number of ways. Obviously the development of secondary sexual characteristics would be encouraged but there is also potential for improvements in bone mineral content and bone mineral density. Possibly as a result of decreased estrogen and androgen production these parameters are abnormally low in patients with PWS from a relatively early age.[15,119]

Systematic studies of sex hormone replacement therapy in adolescents or adults with PWS are lacking and until such studies are published, these patients should be treated as other hypogonadal individuals. Thus, the current suggestion is that if hypogonadism prevails to the age of 17–18 years in a man with PWS, a low dose of testosterone substitution should be offered. Its subsequent effect on activity, strength, endurance, and quality of life should then be followed. If aggressiveness increases, the substitution could be stopped. In female patients, bone mineral density should be monitored during and after adolescence. Estrogen therapy should be considered if it becomes low normal. In very obese patients, peripheral conversion of adrenal androgens to estrogen might be sufficient for the basic needs. However, in the increasing number of lean adolescent and adult patients with this syndrome, the estrogen status should be monitored yearly. The need for substitution therapy should be judged individually against the background of the development of bone mineral density, general activity and quality of life.[41] Given the recent reports of pregnancy in two women with PWS, carers should be aware of the possible need for contraceptives.

KEY LEARNING POINTS

- Prader–Willi syndrome (PWS) is a neurogenetic disorder caused by the lack of paternally expressed gene or genes on chromosome 15q11–q13.
- Many of the symptoms present in PWS are a result of hypothalamic–pituitary dysfunction.
- Muscular hypotonia, delayed psychomotor development, insatiable appetite resulting in obesity, compromised growth and puberty, resulting in short final height and incomplete sexual development, and dysmorphic features are characteristic symptoms in PWS.
- Subjects with PWS have compromised growth and abnormal body composition with increased fat mass, decreased lean body mass, and low bone density resembling a growth hormone deficient status.
- Growth hormone treatment with a dose of $0.033 \, \text{mg} \, \text{kg}^{-1} \, \text{day}^{-1}$ has a beneficial effect on growth with increased final height and an improvement and maintenance of body composition.
- Vigorous weight control is important before and during GH therapy.
- Before starting GH therapy polysomnography and an otorhinolaryngologic examination are recommended.
- Substitution with sex hormones should be considered in young adults with PWS.
- A comprehensive team to manage the various components of medical, psychological, and sociological care is required for individuals with PWS.

REFERENCES

- • = Seminal primary article
- ◆ = Key review paper
- ✳ = First formal publication of a management guideline

- 1 Prader A, Labhart A, Willi H. Ein syndrome von adipositas, kleinwuchs, kryptorchismus und oligophrenie nach myotonieartigem zustand im neugeborenenalter. *Schweiz Med Wochenschr* 1956; **86**: 1260–1.
- 2 Prader A, Labhart A, Willi H. Das syndrome von Imbezilliat, Adipositas Muskelhypotonie, Hypogenitalismus und Diabetes mellitus mit 'myatonic'-Anamnese. In: *Proceedings of Second International Congress on Mental Retardation*. Vienna: S Karger, 1961.
- 3 Wharton RH, Loechner KJ. Genetic and clinical advances in Prader–Willi Syndrome. *Curr Opin Pediatr* 1996; **8**: 618–24.
- 4 Cassidy SB. Prader–Willi Syndrome. *J Med Genet* 1997; **34**: 917–23.
- ◆ 5 Nicholls RD, Ohta T, Gray TA. Genetic abnormalities in Prader–Willi syndrome and lessons from mouse models. *Acta Paediatr Suppl* 1999; **88**: 99–104.
- 6 MacDonald HR, Wevrick R. The Necdin gene is deleted in Prader–Willi syndrome and is imprinted in human and mouse. *Hum Mol Genet* 1997; **6**: 1873–8.
- 7 Muscatelli F, Abrous DN, Massacrier A, *et al.* Disruption of the mouse Necdin gene results in hypothalamic and behavioral alterations reminiscent of the human Prader–Willi syndrome. *Hum Mol Genet* 2000; **9**: 3101–10.
- • 8 Cassidy SB. Prader–Willi Syndrome. *Curr Probl Pediatr* 1984; **14**: 1–55.
- • 9 Holm VA, Cassidy SB, Butler MG, *et al.* Prader–Willi syndrome. Consensus diagnostic criteria. *Pediatrics* 1993; **91**: 398–402.
- • 10 Bray GA, Dahms WT, Swerdloff RS, *et al.* The Prader–Willi syndrome. A study of 40 patients and a review of the literature. *Medicine* 1983; **62**: 59–80.
- 11 Burd L, Vesely B, Martsolf J, Kerbeshian J. Prevalence study of Prader–Willi syndrome in North Dakota. *Am J Med Genet* 1990; **37**: 97–9.
- 12 Ehara H, Ohno K, Takeshita K. Frequency of the Prader–Willi syndrome in the San-in district, Japan. *Brain Dev* 1995; **17**: 324–6.
- 13 Gunay-Aygun M, Schawartz S, Heeger S, *et al.* The changing purpose of Prader–Willi syndrome clinical diagnostic criteria and proposed revised criteria. *Pediatrics* 2001; **108**: e92.
- 14 Laurance BM. Prader–Willi Syndrome. *Pediatric Res Commun* 1993; **7**: 77–91.
- 15 Brambilla P, Bosio L, Manzoni P, *et al.* Peculiar body composition in patients with Prader–Labhart–Willi syndrome. *Am J Clin Nutr* 1997; **65**: 1369–74.
- 16 Wollmann HA, Schultz U, Grauer ML, Ranke MB. Reference values for height and weight in Prader–Willi syndrome based on 315 patients. *Eur J Pediatr* 1998; **157**: 634–42.
- 17 Hall DM, Smith DW. Prader–Willi Syndrome. *J Pediatr* 1972; **81**: 286–93.
- 18 Schoeller DA, Levitsky LL, Bandibi LG, *et al.* Energy expenditure and body composition in Prader–Willi syndrome. *Metabolism* 1988; **37**: 115–20.
- 19 Meaney FJ, Butler MG. Assessment of body composition in Prader–Lubhart–Willi syndrome [Abstract]. *Clin Genet* 1989; **35**: 300.
- 20 Greenswag L. Adults with Prader–Willi syndrome. A survey of 232 cases. *Dev Med Child Neurol* 1987; **29**: 145–52.
- • 21 Laurance BM, Brito A, Wilkinson J. Prader–Willi syndrome after the age of 15 years. *Arch Dis Child* 1981; **56**: 181–6.
- 22 Dykens EM, Cassidy SB. Prader–Willi syndrome. Genetic, behavioral, and treatment issues. *Child Adolesc Psychiatr Clin N Am* 1996; **5**: 913–27.
- 23 Curfs LMG, Fryns J-P. Prader–Willi syndrome: a review with special attention to cognitive and behavioral profile. *Birth Def (Original Article Series)* 1992; **28**: 99–104.
- • 24 Butler MG, Meaney FJ. Standards for selected anthropometric measurements in Prader–Willi syndrome. *Pediatrics* 1991; **88**: 853–60.
- 25 Hauffa BP, Schlippe G, Roos M, *et al.* Spontaneous growth in German children and adolescents with genetically

confirmed Prader–Willi syndrome. *Acta Paediatr* 2000; **89**: 1302–11.

26 Davies PSW, Joughlin C. Using stable isotopes to assess reduced physical activity of individuals with Prader–Willi syndrome. *Am J Ment Retard* 1993; **3**: 349–53.

27 Lee PD, Hwu K, Henson H, *et al*. 3 Body composition studies in Prader–Willi syndrome: effects of growth hormone therapy. *Basic Life Sci* 199; **60**: 201–5.

28 Boot AM, Bouquet J, de Ridder MAJ, *et al*. Determinants of body composition measured by dual-energy x-ray absorptiometry in Dutch children and adolescents. *Am J Clin Nutr* 1997; **66**: 232–8.

29 Ogle GD, Allen JR, Humphries IR, *et al*. Body composition assessment by dual-energy x-ray absorptiometry in subjects aged 4-26. *Am J Clin Nutr* 1995; **61**: 746–53.

30 Eiholzer U, Blum WF, Molinari L. Body fat determined by skinfold measurements is elevated despite underweight in infants with Prader–Lubhart–Willi syndrome. *J Pediatr* 1999; **134**: 222–5.

31 Davies PSW, Joughin C, Cole TJ, *et al*. Total energy expenditure in the Prader–Willi syndrome. *Am J Clin Genet* 1992; **44**: 75–8.

✻ 32 Coplin SS, Hine J, Gormican A. Outpatient dietary management in the Prader–Willi syndrome. *J Am Diet Assoc* 1976; **68**: 330–4.

33 Nelson RA, Anderson LF, Gastineau CF, *et al*. Physiology and natural history of obesity. *JAMA* 1973; **223**: 627–30.

34 van Mil EG, Westerterp KR, Kester AD, *et al*. Activity related energy expenditure in children and adolescents with Prader–Willi syndrome. *Int J Obes Relat Metab Disord* 2000; **24**: 429–34.

35 van Mil EG, Westerterp KR, Gerver WJ, *et al*. Energy expenditure at rest and during sleep in children with Prader–Willi syndrome is explained by body composition. *Am J Clin Nutr* 2000; **71**: 752–6.

36 Klish WJ. Childhood obesity: Pathophysiology and treatment. *Acta Paediatr Jpn* 1995; **37**: 1–5.

37 Rosengren A, Wedel H, Wilhelmsen L. Body weight and weight gain during adult life in men in relation to coronary heart disease and mortality. A prospective population study. *Eur Heart J* 1999; **20**: 269–77.

38 Csabi G, Torok K, Jeges S, Molnar D. Presence of metabolic cardiovascular syndrome in obese children. *Eur J Pediatr* 2000; **159**: 91–4.

39 Karason K, Lindroos AK, Stenlof K, Sjostrom L. Relief of cardiorespiratory symptoms and increased physical activity after surgically induced weight loss: results from the Swedish Obese Subjects study. *Arch Intern Med* 2000; **160**: 1797–802.

40 Anonymous. Overweight, obesity and health risk. National task force on the prevention and treatment of obesity. *Arch Intern Med* 2000; **160**: 898–904.

◆ 41 Burman P, Ritzén EM, Lindgren AC. Endocrine dysfunction in Prader–Willi syndrome: A review with special reference to GH. *Endocr Rev* 2001; **22**: 787–99.

42 Höybye C, Hilding A, Jacobsson H, Thorén M. Metabolic profile and body composition in adults with Prader–Willi

syndrome and severe obesity. *J Clin Endocrinol Metals* 2002; **87**: 3590–7.

43 Holm VA, Laurnen EL. Prader–Willi syndrome and scoliosis. *Dev Med Child Neurol* 1981; **23**: 192–201.

44 Lee PDK. Endocrine and metabolic aspects of Prader–Willi syndrome. In: Greenswag LR, Alexander RC, eds. *Management of Prader–Willi Syndrome*. New York: Springer-Verlag, 1995: 32–57.

45 Tze WJ, Dunn HG, Rothstein R. The endocrine profiles and metabolic aspects of Prader–Willi syndrome. In: Holm VA, Sulzbacher S, Pipes PL, eds. *Prader–Willi Syndrome*. Baltimore: University Park Press, 1981: 281–91.

46 Kousholt AM, Beck-Nielsen H, Lund HT. A reduced number of insulin receptors in patients with Prader–Willi syndrome. *Acta Endocrinol* 1983; **104**: 345–51.

47 Illig R, Tschumi A, Vischer D. Glucose intolerance and diabetes mellitus in patients with the Prader–Labhart–Willi syndrome. *Mod Probl Pediatr* 1975; **12**: 203–10.

48 Cassidy SB, Devi A, Mukaida C. Aging in Prader–Willi syndrome: 22 patients over age 30 years. *Proc Greenwood Genet Center* 1994; **13**: 102–3.

49 Eiholzer U, Stutz K, Weinmann C, *et al*. Low insulin, IGF-I and IGFBP-3 levels in children with Prader–Labhart–Willi syndrome. *Eur J Pediatr* 1998; **157**: 890–3.

● 50 Lindgren AC, Hagenas L, Ritzen EM. Growth hormone treatment of children with Prader–Willi syndrome: effects on glucose and insulin hemostasis. Swedish National Growth Hormone Advisory Group. *Horm Res* 1999; **51**: 157–61.

51 Zipf WB. Glucose homeostasis in Prader–Willi syndrome and potential implications of growth hormone therapy. *Acta Paediatr Suppl* 1999; **433**: 115–7.

52 Schuster DP, Osei K, Zipf WB. Characterization of alterations in glucose and insulin metabolism in Prader–Willi subjects. *Metabolism* 1996; **12**: 1514–20.

53 Reed WB, Ragsdale W, Curtis AC, Rickards HJ. Acantosis nigricans in association with various genodermatosis. *Acta Dem Venereol (Stockh)* 1968; **149**: 963–4.

54 Lamb AS, Johnson WM. Premature coronary artery atherosclerosis in a patient with Prader–Willi syndrome. *Am J Med Genet* 1987; **28**: 873–80.

55 Juul J, Dupont A. Prader–Willi syndrome. *J Ment Deficiency Res* 1967; **11**: 12–22.

56 Bassali R, Hoffman WH, Chen H, Tuck-Muller CM. Hyperlipidemia, insulin-dependent diabetes mellitus, and rapidly progressive diabetic retinopathy and neuropathy in Prader–Willi syndrome with del. (15) (q11.2q13). *Am J Med Genetics* 1997; **71**: 267–70.

57 Laurance BM. Hypotonia, mental retardation, obesity, and cryptorchidism associated with dwarfism, and diabetes in children. *Arch Dis Child* 1967; **42**: 126–39.

58 Bier DM, Kaplan SL, Havel RJ. The Prader–Willi syndrome, regulation of fat transport. *Diabetes* 1977; **26**: 874–80.

59 Butler MG, Swift LL, Hill JO. Fasting plasma lipid, glucose, and insulin levels in Prader–Willi syndrome and obese individuals. *Dysmorphol Clin Genet* 1990; **4**: 23–6.

60 Carrel AL, Myers SE, Whitman BY, Allen DB. Growth hormone improves body composition, fat utilization, physical strength and agility, and growth in Prader–Willi syndrome: a controlled study. *J Pediatr* 1999; **134**: 215–21.

61 Hakonarson H, Moskovitz J, Daigle KL, *et al.* Pulmonary function abnormalities in Prader–Willi syndrome. *J Pediatr* 1995; **126**: 565–70.

62 Arens R, Gozal D, Burrell BC, *et al.* Arousal and cardiorespiratory responses to hypoxia in Prader–Willi syndrome. *Am J Respir Crit Care Med* 1996; **153**: 283–7.

63 Schluter B, Buscbatz D, Trowitzsch E, *et al.* Respiratory control in children with Prader–Willi syndrome. *Eur J Pediatr* 1997; **156**: 65–8.

● 64 Lindgren AC, Hellström LG, Ritzén EM, Milerad J. Growth hormone treatment increases CO(2)-response, ventilation and central respiratory drive in children with Prader–Willi syndrome. *Eur J Pediatr* 1999; **158**: 936–40.

65 Eiholzer U. Deaths in children with Prader–Willi syndrome. *Horm Res* 2005; **63**: 33–9.

◆ 66 Nixon GM, Brouillette RT. Sleep and breathing in Prader–Willi syndrome. *Pediatr Pulmonol* 2002; **34**: 209–17.

67 Fesseler WH, Bierich JR. Untersuchungen beim Prader–Labhart–Willi-syndrome. *Monatsschr Kinderheilkd* 1983; **131**: 844–7.

68 Costeff H, Holm VA, Ruvalcaba R, Shaver J. Growth hormone secretion in Prader–Willi syndrome. *Acta Paediatr Scand* 1990; **79**: 1059–62.

69 Calisti L, Giannessi N, Cesaretti G, Saggese G. Studio endocrino nella sindrome di Prader–Willi. A proposito di 5 casi. *Minerva Pediatr* 1991; **43**: 587–93.

70 Huw K, Klish WJ, Henson H, *et al.* Endocrine status, growth hormone therapy and body composition in Prader–Willi syndrome. Abstracts of the 74th Annual Meeting of the Endocrine Society (abstract 710). 1992: 229.

71 Cappa M, Grossi A, Borrelli P, *et al.* Growth hormone (GH) response to combined pyridostigmine and GH-releasing hormone administration in patients with Prader–Labhardt–Willi syndrome. *Horm Res* 1993; **39**: 51–5.

72 Angulo M, Castro-Magana M, Mazur B, *et al.* Growth hormone secretion and effects of growth hormone therapy on growth velocity and weight gain in children with Prader–Willi syndrome. *J Pediatr Endocrinol Metab* 1996; **3**: 393–9.

73 Grosso S, Cioni M, Buoni S, *et al.* Growth hormone secretion in Prader–Willi syndrome. *J Endocrinol Invest* 1998; **21**: 418–22.

74 Grugni G, Guzzaloni G, Moro D, *et al.* Reduced growth hormone (GH) responsiveness to combined GH-releasing hormone and pyridostigmine and administration in the Prader–Willi syndrome. *Clin Endocrinol (Oxf)* 1998; **48**: 769–75.

● 75 Lindgren AC, Hagenäs L, Müller J, *et al.* Growth hormone treatment of children with Prader–Willi syndrome affects

linear growth and body composition favourably. *Acta Paediatr* 1998; **87**: 28–31.

76 Sipilä I, Alanne S, Apajasalo M, Hietanen H. Growth hormone therapy in children with Prader–Willi syndrome. A preliminary report of one year treatment in 19 children (abstract). *Horm Res* 1998; **50(Suppl 3)**: 1–150.

77 Thacker MJ, Hainline B, St Dennis-Feezle L, *et al.* Growth failure in Prader–Willi syndrome is secondary to growth hormone deficiency. *Horm Res* 1998; **49**: 216–20.

78 Corrias A, Bellone J, Beccaria L, *et al.* 2000 GH/IGF-I axis in Prader–Willi syndrome: evaluation of IGF-I levels and of the somatotroph responsiveness to various provocative stimuli. Genetic Obesity Study Group of Italian Society of Pediatric Endocrinology and Diabetology. *J Endocrinol Invest* 2000; **23**: 84–9.

79 Williams T, Berelowitz M, Joffe SN, *et al.* Impaired growth hormone responses to growth hormone-releasing factor in obesity: a pituitary defect reversed by weight reduction. *N Engl J Med* 1984; **311**: 1403–7.

80 Scacchi M, Pincelli AI, Cavagnini F. Growth hormone in obesity. *Int J Obes Relat Metab Disord* 1999; **23**: 260–71.

81 Lanzi R, Luzi L, Caumo A, *et al.* Elevated insulin levels contribute to the reduced growth hormone (GH) response to GH-releasing hormone in obese subjects. *Metabolism* 1999; **48**: 1152–6.

82 Nam SY, Lee EJ, Kim KR, *et al.* Effect of obesity on total and free insulin-like growth factor (IGF)-I, and their relationship to IGF-binding protein (BP)-1, IGFBP-2, IGFBP-3, insulin, and growth hormone. *Int J Obes Relat Metab Disord* 1997; **21**: 355–9.

83 Park MJ, Kim HS, Kang JH, *et al.* Serum levels of insulin-like growth factor (IGF)-I, free IGF-I, IGF binding protein (IGFBP)-I, IGFBP-3 and insulin in obese children. *J Pediatr Endocrinol Metab* 1999; **12**: 139–44.

84 Ghigo E, Mazza E, Corrias A, *et al.* Effect of cholinergic enhancement by pyridostigmine on growth hormone secretion in obese adults and children. *Metabolism* 1989; **38**: 631–3.

85 Beccaria L, Benzi F, Sanzari A, *et al.* Impairment of GH responsiveness to GH releasing hormone and pyridostigmine in patients affected with Prader–Labhardt–Willi syndrome. *J Endocrinol Invest* 1996; **19**: 687–92.

86 Bideci A, Cinaz P, Hasanoglu A, Elbeg S. Serum levels of insulin-like growth factor-I and insulin-like growth factor binding protein-3 in obese children. *J Pediatr Endocrinol Metab* 1997; **10**: 295–9.

87 Radetti G, Bozzola M, Pasquino B, *et al.* Growth hormone bioactivity, insulin-like growth factors (IGFs) and IGF binding proteins in obese children. *Metabolism* 1998; **47**: 1490–3.

88 Rosenbaum M, Gerner J, Leibel R. Effects of systemic (GH) administration on regional adipose tissue distribution in GH deficient children. *J Clin Endocrinol Metab* 1989; **69**: 1274–81.

89 Vignolo M, Naselli A, Di Battista E, *et al.* Growth and development in simple obesity. *Eur J Pediatr* 1988; **147**: 242–4.

90 Vanderschueren-Lodeweyckx M. The effect of simple obesity on growth and growth hormone. *Horm Res* 1993; **40**: 23–30.

91 Swaab DF, Purba JS, Hofman MA. Alterations in the hypothalamic paraventricular nucleus and its oxytocin neurones (putative satiety cells) in Prader–Willi syndrome. A study of five cases. *J Clin Endocrinol Metab* 1995; **80**: 573–9.

92 Swaab DF. Prader–Willi syndrome and the hypothalamus. *Acta Pediatr Suppl* 1997; **423**: 50–4.

93 Miller L, Angulo M, Price D, Taneja S. MR of the pituitary in patients with Prader–Willi syndrome: Size determinations and imaging findings. *Pediatr Radiol* 1996; **26**: 43–7.

94 Kauli R, Prager-Lewin R, Laron Z. Pubertal development in the Prader–Labhart–Willi syndrome. *Acta Paediatr Scand* 1978; **67**: 763–7.

95 Vanelli MD, Bernasconi S, Caronna N V, *et al.* Precocious puberty in a male with Prader–Labhart–Willi syndrome. *Helv Paediat Acta* 1984; **39**: 373–7.

96 Garty B, Shuper A, Mimouni M, *et al.* Primary gonadal failure and precocious adrenarche in a boy with Prader–Labhart–Willi syndrome. *Eur J Pediatr* 1982; **139**: 201–3.

97 Ibanez L, Potau N, Marcos MV, deZegher F. Exaggerated adrenarche and hyperinsulinism in adolescent girls born small for gestational age. *J Clin Endocrinol Metab* 1999; **84**: 4739–41.

98 Jeffcoate WJ, Laurance BM, Edwards CRW, Besser GM. Endocrine function in the Prader–Willi syndrome. *Clin Endocrinol* 1980; **12**: 81–9.

99 Ritzén EM, Bolme P, Hall K. Endocrine physiology and therapy in Prader–Willi syndrome. NATO ASI Series H61, 1992; 153–69.

100 Tolis G, Lewis W, Verdy M, *et al.* Anterior pituitary function in the Prader–Labhart–Willi syndrome. *J Clin Endocrinol Metab* 1974; **39**: 1061–66.

101 Wannarachue N, Ruvalcaba HA. Hypogonadism in Prader–Willi syndrome. *Am J Ment Defic* 1975; **79**: 592–603.

102 Katcher ML, Bargman GJ, Gilert EF, Opitz JM. Absence of spermatogonia in the Prader–Willi syndrome. *Eur J Pediatr* 1977; **124**: 257–60.

103 Akefeldt A, Tornhage CJ, Gillberg C. A woman with Prader–Willi syndrome gives birth to a healthy baby girl. *Dev Med Child Neurol* 1999; **41**: 789–90.

104 Schulze A, Mogensen H, Hamborg-Petersen B, *et al.* Fertility in Prader–Willi syndrome: a case report with Angelman syndrome in the offspring. *Acta Paediatr* 2001; **90**: 455–9.

105 L'Allemand D, Eiholzer U, Rousson V, *et al.* Increased adrenal androgen levels in patients with Prader–Willi syndrome are associated with insulin, IGF-I and leptin, but not with measures of obesity. *Horm Res* 2002; **58**: 215–22.

106 Lindgren AC, Hagenäs L, Müller J, *et al.* Effects of growth hormone treatment on growth and body composition in Prader–Willi syndrome: a preliminary report. *Acta Paediatr Suppl* 1997; **423**: 60–2.

107 Hauffa BP. One-year results of growth hormone treatment of short stature in Prader–Willi syndrome. *Acta Paediatr Suppl* 1997; **423**: 63–5.

108 Davies PSW, Evens S, Broomhead S, *et al.* Effect of growth hormone on height, weight, and body composition in Prader–Willi syndrome. *Arch Dis Child* 1998; **78**: 474–6.

109 Eiholzer U, Gisin R, Weinmann C, *et al.* Treatment with human growth hormone in patients with Prader–Labhart–Willi syndrome reduces body fat and increases muscle mass and physical performance. *Eur J Pediatr* 1997; **157**: 368–77.

110 Lindgren AC, Ritzén EM. Five years of growth hormone treatment in children with Prader–Willi syndrome. *Acta Paediatr Suppl* 1999; **433**: 109–111.

111 Eiholzer U, l'Allemand D. Growth hormone normalizes height, prediction of final height and hand length in children with Prader–Willi syndrome after 4 years of therapy. *Horm Res* 2000; **53**: 185–92.

112 Lindgren AC. Long-term growth hormone therapy in children with Prader–Willi syndrome. Proceedings from 36th International Symposium: GH and Growth Factors in Endocrinology and Metabolism, 14–15 May 2004, Geneva.

113 Myers SE, Carrel AL, Whitman BY, Allen DB. Sustained benefit after 2 years of growth hormone on body composition, fat utilization, physical strength and agility, and growth in Prader–Willi syndrome. *J Pediatr* 2000; **137**: 42–9.

114 Carrel AL, Myers SE, Whitman BY, Allen DB. Benefits of long-term GH therapy in Prader–Willi syndrome: A 4-year study. *J Clin Endocrinol Metals* 2002; **87**: 1581–5.

115 Whitman BY, Myers S, Carrel A, Allen D. The behavioral impact of growth hormone treatment for children and adolescents with Prader–Willi syndrome: A 2-year controlled study. *Pediatrics* 2002; **109**: E35.

116 Haqq AM, Stadler DD, Jackson RH, *et al.* Effects of growth hormone on pulmonary function, sleep quality, behavior, cognition, growth velocity, body composition and resting energy expenditure in Prader–Willi syndrome *J Clin Endocrinol Metals* 2003; **88**: 2206–12.

117 L'Allemand D, Eiholzer U, Schlumpf M, *et al.* Carbohydrate metabolism is not impaired after 3 years of growth hormone therapy in children with Prader–Willi syndrome. *Horm Res* 2003; **59**: 239–48.

118 Schrander-Stumpel CTRM, Curfs LMG, Sastrowijoto P, *et al.* Causes of death in an international series of 27 cases. *Am J Med Genet* 2004; **124A**: 333–8.

119 Rubin K, Cassidy SB. Hypogonadism and osteoporosis. In: Greenswag LR, Alexander RC, eds. *Management of Prader–Willi Syndrome*. New York: Springer-Verlag, 1988: 23–3.

37

Obesity in children and adolescents

LOUISE A BAUR, ELIZABETH DENNEY-WILSON

EVIDENCE SCORING OF CLINICAL INTERVENTIONS

* Non-randomized controlled trial, cohort study
** One or more well-designed randomized controlled trials
*** Systematic review or meta-analysis

THE DEFINITION OF OVERWEIGHT AND OBESITY IN CHILDHOOD AND ADOLESCENCE

Body mass index: A measure of total body fatness

Body mass index (BMI; weight/height^2), is a simple, cost-effective measure of body fatness in both adulthood and childhood.[1] Among adults, a person with a BMI of 25.00–29.99 kg m^{-2} is considered overweight, while those with a BMI >30.00 kg m^{-2} are classified as obese, cut-points that relate to the point at which health risks rise steeply, at least in adult European populations.[2] Among children there is insufficient evidence to provide an absolute definition of health-related overweight. BMI also varies dramatically with age and sex during childhood and adolescence, rising in the first year, falling during pre-school years before then rising once more into adolescence, the point at which BMI starts to increase again, between 4 and 7 years of age, being termed the point of 'adiposity rebound' (see Fig. 37.1a and b).

Until recently, no standard definitions of overweight and obesity existed for children and adolescents. In the late 1990s, the International Obesity TaskForce (IOTF) recommended that BMI, based on centile curves that at age 18 pass through the adult cut-points of 25 kg m^{-2} and 30 kg m^{-2}, be used to define overweight and obesity among children and adolescents.[3] Subsequently, in 2000, Cole and his colleagues developed a table of age- and sex-specific cut-points based upon a compilation of nationally representative cross-sectional growth studies from a number of countries[4] (see Table 37.1). These cut-points are used in epidemiological research to classify overweight and obesity and allow international comparison of trends in overweight and obesity. The IOTF definition is not designed for clinical use.

Another definition in widespread use is based on the revised United States growth charts from the Centers for Disease Control and Prevention (CDC) (see Fig. 37.1a and b).[5] In this, the 85th and 95th centiles on the BMI-for-age charts are used as the cut-points for defining 'at risk of overweight' and 'overweight', respectively.[6] Advantages of such a definition are that it can be readily adapted to clinical use, it accords with conventions used in other growth charts and the reference population is well documented. Disadvantages include the relatively arbitrary nature of the cut-points, the use of a United States reference population which is potentially bigger than many other populations, and the fact that 'obesity', as such, is not defined!

Several countries have developed their own BMI-for-age growth charts and these can be used clinically in order to chart an individual's BMI and monitor changes over time.[7–9]

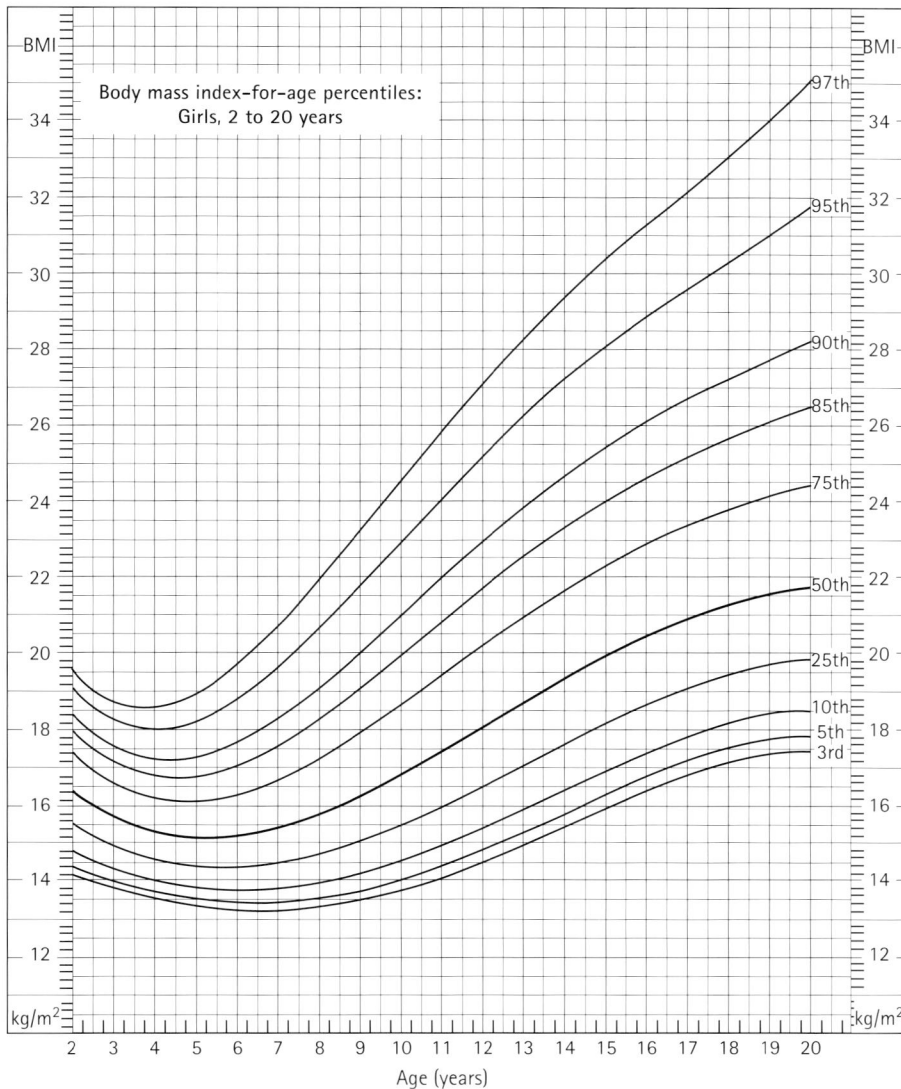

Figure 37.1 (a) Body mass index for age chart for girls aged 2–20 years. From: Kuczmarski et al.[5]

At present the decision as to which specific centile lines denote overweight and obesity remains arbitrary.

Waist circumference: A measure of fat distribution

In adults, abdominal fatness is strongly linked to a range of metabolic and cardiovascular risk complications[10] and both waist circumference and waist–hip ratio are approximate anthropometric measures of abdominal fatness.[11] No globally applicable cut-points for waist circumference are available. Table 37.2 shows sex-specific waist circumference cut-points and risk of metabolic complications for obesity in an adult Caucasian population.[12]

In children and young people, waist circumference is also correlated with abdominal fat, as well as with cardiovascular risk factors.[13] Waist circumference charts have been published for some individual countries, including Italy,[14] Spain,[15] and the United Kingdom.[16] As yet there are no internationally accepted criteria for high- or low-risk waist circumference in this age group. Nationally developed waist circumference-for-age charts can be used to monitor clinical progress of an individual patient.

Racial and ethnic variations in definition

A further consideration is that racial and ethnic variations exist in the biological response to excess adiposity. Among adults, Asians generally have a higher percentage body fat for a given BMI, and an associated increased health risk at lower BMI values, compared with Europeans, whereas Pacific populations generally have a lower percentage body fat and a decreased health risk at the same BMI levels.[17,18] In the United States, Mohawk Indian, Mexican–American and African–American children have increased abdominal fat compared with white children at the same BMI.[19] Such differences may ultimately require the development of ethnic- or race-specific definitions or criteria for obesity.

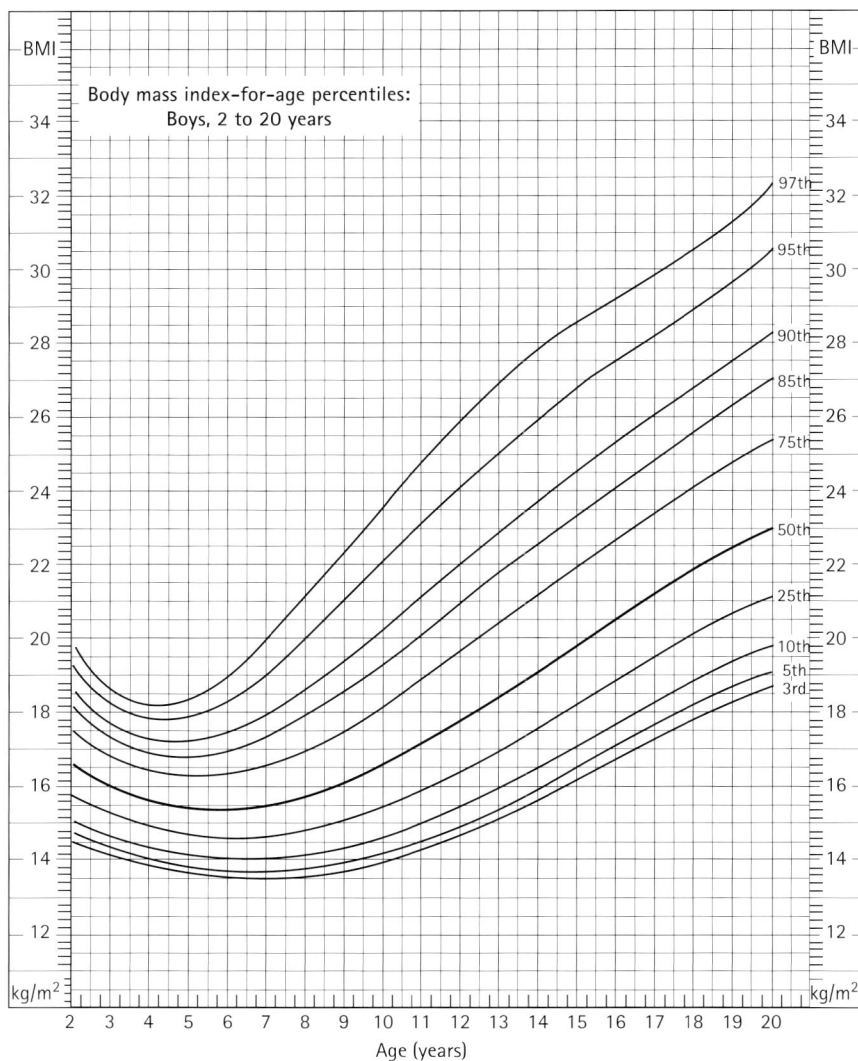

Figure 37.1 (b) Body mass index for age chart for boys aged 2–20 years. From: Kuczmarski *et al.*[5]

Table 37.1   Cut-points for defining overweight and obesity in children and adolescents aged 2–18 years (International Obesity TaskForce)*

Age (years)	Body mass index 25 kg m^{-2}		Body mass index 30 kg m^{-2}	
	Males	Females	Males	Females
2	18.41	18.02	20.09	19.81
2.5	18.13	17.76	19.80	19.55
3	17.89	17.56	19.57	19.36
3.5	17.69	17.40	19.39	19.23
4	17.55	17.28	19.29	19.15
4.5	17.47	18.19	19.26	19.12
5	17.42	17.15	19.30	19.17
5.5	17.45	17.20	19.47	19.34
6	17.55	17.34	19.78	19.65
6.5	17.71	17.53	20.23	20.08
7	17.92	17.75	20.63	20.51
7.5	18.16	18.03	21.09	21.01
8	18.44	18.35	21.60	21.57

(continued)

Table 37.1 (Continued)

Age (years)	Body mass index 25 kg m^{-2}		Body mass index 30 kg m^{-2}	
	Males	Females	Males	Females
8.5	18.76	18.69	22.17	22.18
9	19.10	19.07	22.77	22.81
9.5	19.46	19.45	23.39	23.46
10	19.84	19.86	24.00	24.11
10.5	20.20	20.29	24.57	24.77
11	20.55	20.74	25.10	25.42
11.5	20.89	21.20	25.58	26.05
12	21.22	21.68	26.02	26.67
12.5	21.56	22.14	26.43	27.24
13	21.91	22.58	26.84	27.76
13.5	22.27	22.98	27.25	28.20
14	22.62	23.34	27.63	28.57
14.5	22.96	23.66	27.98	28.87
15	23.29	23.94	28.30	29.11
15.5	23.60	24.17	28.60	29.29
16	23.90	24.37	28.88	29.43
16.5	24.19	24.54	29.14	29.56
17	24.46	24.70	29.41	29.69
17.5	24.73	24.85	29.70	29.84
18	25	25	300	30

*From Cole et al.[4] (Cole TJ, Bellizzi MC, Flegal KM, Dietz WH. Establishing a standard definition for child overweight and obesity worldwide: international survey. BMJ 2000; 320: 1240–3. With permission of the BMJ Publishing Group.)

Table 37.2 Sex-specific waist circumference and risk of metabolic complications associated with obesity in Caucasian adults*

Risk of metabolic complications	Waist circumference (cm)	
	Men	Women
Increased	≥94	≥80
Substantially increased	≥102	≥88

* Presented in the WHO Report[1] and based upon a study of 4881 adults in the Netherlands.[12] Note that the identification of risk using waist circumference cut-points is population-specific and applies only to adults.

THE PREVALENCE OF OVERWEIGHT AND OBESITY AMONG CHILDREN AND ADOLESCENTS

International prevalence rates and secular trends

A recent report from the International Obesity Task Force (IOTF) demonstrates that the pediatric obesity epidemic has spread throughout the world, with some countries in economic transition having prevalence rates higher than those in the United States.[2] Using the IOTF definition, the worldwide prevalence of overweight (including obesity) in children and young people aged 5–17 years is approximately 10 percent, with that of obesity alone being 2–3 percent.[2] Certain regions and countries have particularly high rates of pediatric obesity. More than 30 percent of children and adolescents in the Americas, and approximately 20 percent of those in Europe, are overweight or obese, with much lower prevalence rates being seen in sub-Saharan Africa and Asia (Fig. 37.2a and b).

The IOTF report shows that the prevalence of overweight and obesity in childhood and adolescence has risen rapidly in many countries in several continents over the past three decades (Fig. 37.3). This is the case even for China, with its relatively low overall obesity prevalence (although note the caveats about the definition of obesity mentioned above). A related finding is that not only is the prevalence of obesity increasing in several countries, but overweight children are heavier than in the past.[20,21]

Data from the United Kingdom show that mean waist circumference increased by 6.9 cm among boys and 6.2 cm among girls aged 11–16 over the 20 years between 1977 and 1997.[22] This implies that total body fat and central adiposity have both increased in this pediatric population – a finding that is also likely to apply to other countries.

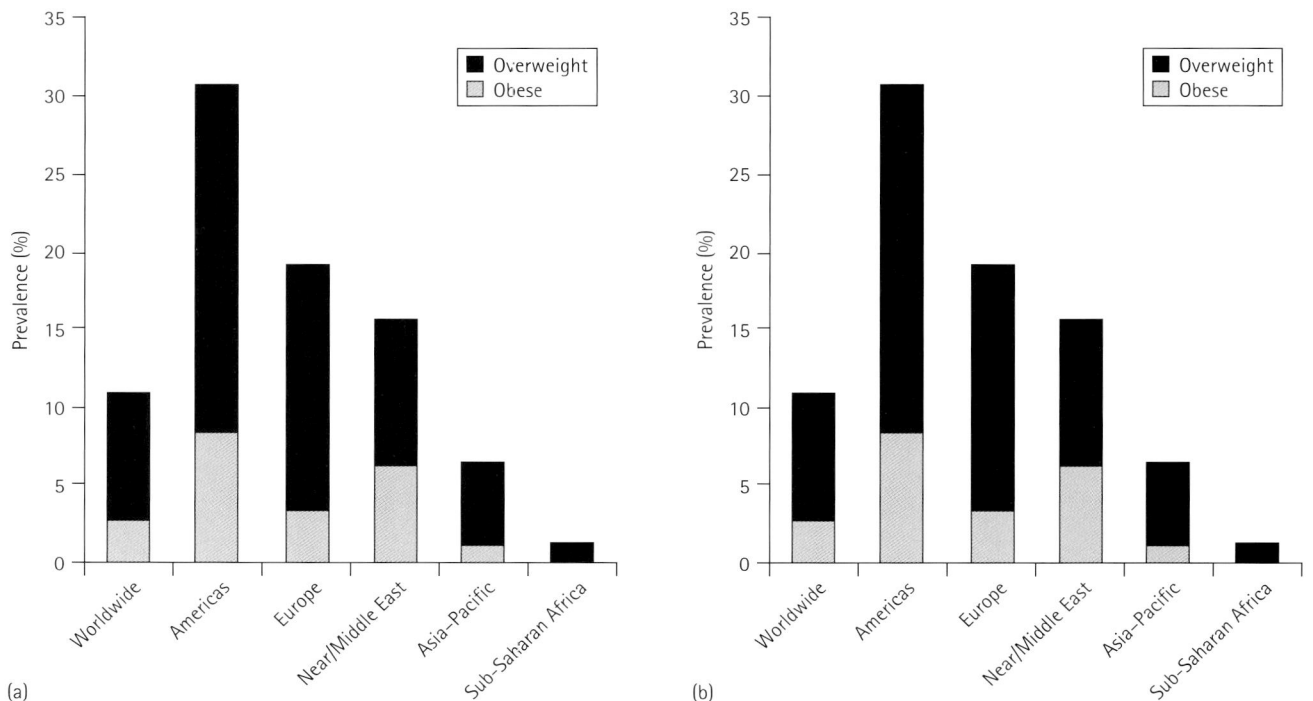

(a)

(b)

Figure 37.2 (a) Prevalence of overweight and obesity among boys aged 5–17 years by global region. Overweight and obesity defined by International Obesity Task Force (IOTF) criteria. (b) Prevalence of overweight and obesity among girls aged 5–17 years by global region. Overweight and obesity defined by IOTF criteria. From: Lobstein *et al.*[2] (Lobstein T, Baur L, Uauy R. Obesity in children and young people: A crisis in public health. Report of the International Obesity Task Force Childhood Obesity Working Group. *Obes Rev* 2004; **5(Suppl. 1)** 4–85. With permission of Blackwell Publishing.)

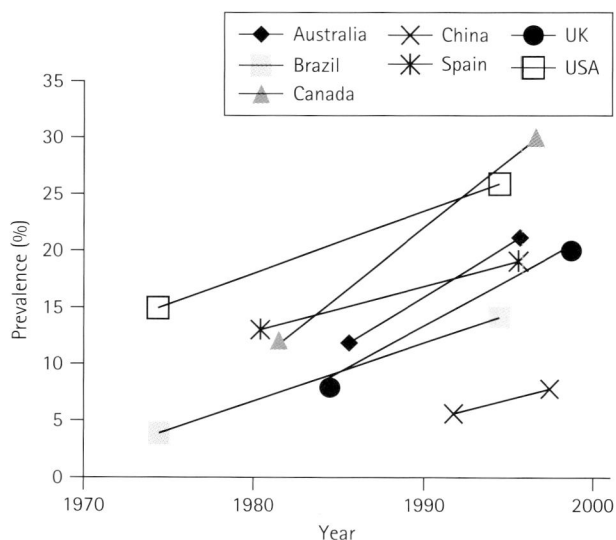

Figure 37.3 Trends in the prevalence of overweight, 1970–2000. Overweight defined by International Obesity Task Force criteria. Children's ages (in years): Australia: 2–18; Canada: 7–13; China: 6–18; Spain: 6–14; UK: 7–11; USA 6–18. From: Lobstein *et al.*[2] (Lobstein T, Baur L, Uauy R. Obesity in children and young people: A crisis in public health. Report of the International Obesity Task Force Childhood Obesity Working Group. *Obes Rev* 2004; **5(Suppl. 1)** 4–85. With permission of Blackwell Publishing.)

Sociodemographic differences in the prevalence of obesity

Overweight is high among the poorer children in developed countries and the richer children in developing countries.[2,23] For example, data from the United States indicate that socio-demographic differences in prevalence of obesity exist among Hispanic (21.8 percent), African–American (21.5 percent) and white children (12.3 percent), with the sharpest increases occurring among African–American and Hispanic children.[24] An inverse social gradient between overweight and socio-economic group in both boys and girls has also been shown in other westernized countries such as Germany,[25] the United Kingdom,[26] and France.[27] However, among countries in economic transition, the association between overweight prevalence and socio-economic group is reversed: obesity is more prevalent among higher income groups and in urban, compared with rural, communities.[23] Potential contributors to obesity in urbanized developing countries include increased availability of cheap energy-dense foods and widespread access to television which would favor a more sedentary, indoor lifestyle.[28]

OBESITY-ASSOCIATED COMPLICATIONS

The potential complications of obesity among children and adolescents have been extensively reviewed[29,30] and are summarized in Table 37.3. They affect many organ systems and may be immediate (i.e., affecting the obese child or young person), or may not manifest until the medium- to long-term.

Complications associated with the endocrine system

Endocrine complications are among the most serious and long-term problems confronting even the young obese person. Morbidity in other organ systems is strongly associated with endocrine complications and as such is covered in this section.

SHORT-TERM COMPLICATIONS

Elevated fasting insulin may be the first indication of endocrine complications in the obese child. Data from the Bogalusa Heart Study indicate that overweight children are

Table 37.3 Potential obesity-associated complications among children and adolescents

System	Health problems
Psychosocial	Social isolation and discrimination, decreased self esteem, learning difficulties, body image disorder, bulimia *Medium- and long-term*: Poorer social and economic 'success', bulimia
Respiratory	Obstructive sleep apnea, asthma, poor exercise tolerance
Orthopedic	Back pain, slipped femoral capital epiphyses, tibia vara, ankle sprains, flat feet
Hepatobiliary	Non-alcoholic fatty liver disease, gallstones
Reproductive	Polycystic ovary syndrome, menstrual abnormalities
Cardiovascular	Hypertension, adverse lipid profile (low HDL cholesterol, high triglycerides, high LDL cholesterol) *Medium- and long-term*: Increased risk of hypertension and adverse lipid profile in adulthood, increased risk of coronary artery disease in adulthood, left ventricular hypertrophy
Endocrine	Hyperinsulinemia, insulin resistance, impaired glucose tolerance, impaired fasting glucose, type 2 diabetes mellitus *Medium- and long-term*: Increased risk of type 2 diabetes mellitus and metabolic syndrome in adulthood
Neurological	Benign intracranial hypertension
Skin	Acanthosis nigricans, striae, intertrigo

12.6 times more likely to have elevated fasting insulin concentrations than their lean peers.[31] In apparently healthy white children, obesity accounts for 55 percent of the variance in insulin sensitivity[32] and in a hyperinsulinemic euglycemic clamp study of pre-adolescent children, obese children had decreased insulin sensitivity and hyperinsulinemia when compared to non-obese children of the same age.[33]

Impaired glucose tolerance and impaired fasting glucose have been documented in obese children and adolescents in a range of heterogeneous studies. For example, in a Unites States study involving 439 obese children and young people, 17 percent had impaired glucose tolerance at baseline, with eight developing type 2 diabetes mellitus when followed longitudinally over a mean of 21.5 months.[34]

Originally extremely rare among children and adolescents, the incidence of type 2 diabetes mellitus is increasing and is linked to the prevalence of obesity among young people. In the late 1970s and early 1980s, the first reports of type 2 diabetes in Native American and Canadian First Nation young people were published, with subsequent reports in the 1990s noting an increased prevalence, especially among Hispanics and black Americans.[35] There are now affected children and young people with type 2 diabetes in most countries where there has been an increase in obesity. Youth with type 2 diabetes are generally in the adolescent age-group, are obese, have acanthosis nigricans, have a family history of type 2 diabetes and are female.[36]

The metabolic syndrome, a term describing a cluster of highly prevalent disorders in western countries which appear linked to insulin resistance and central obesity, was initially identified among adults,[37] and a definition has recently been developed by the International Diabetes Federation.[38,39] Although slightly different definitions have been used among young people, abdominal obesity in childhood is also highly correlated with risk factors such as elevated fasting insulin and lipid concentrations[40] and, among adolescents in the United States, the overall prevalence is approximately 10 percent. However, among overweight adolescents in the United States, the metabolic syndrome affects almost one-third of individuals.[41]

Reproductive system complications are also associated with insulin resistance in young obese individuals, in particular the early onset of puberty and menarche, menstrual irregularities and polycystic ovary disease. There is a strong association between abdominal fat, increased levels of the androgenic hormones, hirsutism, insulin resistance and polycystic ovaries which, grouped together, is termed polycystic ovary syndrome.[42] Polycystic ovary syndrome is associated with infertility among adult women, with weight loss improving fertility outcomes.[43]

Acanthosis nigricans is characterized by thickened areas of hyper-pigmentation, with later development of hypertrophy and sometimes papillomatosis. The skin lesions typically occur in intertriginous regions such as the base of the neck, axillae, groin, antecubital and popliteal fossae, and umbilicus.[44] The condition is more frequently seen in darker-skinned ethnic groups and may cause embarrassment to the affected young person.

LONG-TERM ENDOCRINE AND METABOLIC COMPLICATIONS

Individuals who are overweight as children have an increased risk of endocrine and metabolic complications as adults. A 33 year follow-up of a birth cohort from Singapore showed that BMI at age 11 years predicted diabetes in adulthood.[45] Results from the Bogalusa Heart Study show that childhood obesity is the strongest predictor of the development, in adulthood, of the metabolic syndrome: those children who were in the top quartile of BMI were 11 times more likely to develop the metabolic syndrome as adults than their lean peers.[46]

Complications of the cardiovascular system

SHORT-TERM COMPLICATIONS

Risk factors for cardiovascular disease are one of the most common problems facing the obese young person. In the Bogalusa Heart Study, 60 percent of overweight 5- to 10-year-olds had one cardiovascular risk factor, such as hypertension, high LDL cholesterol or high triglycerides; while over 20 percent had two or more risk factors.[31] Overall, when compared with their lean peers, overweight children were 2.4 times as likely to have elevated total cholesterol and diastolic blood pressure; and 4.5 times as likely to have elevated systolic blood pressure. Similar findings have been reported from the Taipei Children's Heart study, which showed a significant association between obesity and higher blood pressure, blood glucose and blood lipids.[47] A central fat distribution is particularly associated with the clustering of cardiovascular risk factors.[19] Additional evidence of the association between overweight and cardiovascular risk, is shown in a study of asymptomatic overweight and normal weight children aged 9–12 years who underwent non-invasive assessment of vascular structure and function: the overweight children had significantly lower flow-mediated endothelial dilatation and increased carotid intima-media thickness when compared with the non-obese children.[48]

LONG-TERM CARDIOVASCULAR COMPLICATIONS

Obesity in childhood and adolescence is associated with increased risk of heart disease in adulthood. For example, non-invasive assessments of vascular structure in three long-term cohort studies have shown that adult carotid intima-media thickness is associated with a variety of child or adolescent cardiovascular risk factors, especially obesity.[49–51] In a cohort in the United Kingdom followed up over a 57 year period, both all-cause and cardiovascular mortality was associated with higher childhood BMI.[52] Study participants who, as children, were heavier than the 75th centile

for BMI were twice as likely to die from ischemic heart disease than those who as children had a BMI between the 25th and 75th centiles. In a similar long-term (55 year) follow-up of a US cohort of adolescents, overweight in adolescence was a significant predictor of morbidity and mortality from cardiovascular disease, independent of adult weight status.[53]

Hepatobiliary complications

Obese children and adolescents may experience a range of gastrointestinal and hepatobiliary disorders, the most significant being non-alcoholic fatty liver disease (NAFLD). NAFLD is an umbrella term that includes steatosis as well as steatohepatitis. In adults, NAFLD is a leading cause of chronic liver disease, with such serious potential outcomes as cirrhosis and end stage liver disease.[54]

NAFLD is increasingly recognized as a complication of pediatric obesity, with liver steatosis (on ultrasound) being noted in up to 47 percent of obese patients in an Italian pediatric obesity clinic, and 77 percent of patients in a Hong Kong clinic.[55] NAFLD typically presents as an asymptomatic elevation of transaminases. The degree of steatosis is associated with the severity of obesity, a central fat distribution, hypertriglyceridemia, insulin resistance and the presence of raised transaminases, with a raised alanine aminotransaminase being most specific for steatosis.[55–57] A retrospective review of patients with NAFLD in a pediatric hepatology clinic in the United States showed that such patients were mostly male, Hispanic, obese and had insulin resistance.[58] Liver fibrosis and even evolving cirrhosis have been identified in liver biopsy findings of patients with NAFLD in an Australian pediatric hepatology service.[59]

There is a well-recognized association between cholelithiasis and obesity in adults, with the prevalence being especially high in those with the highest BMI.[60] The increased prevalence of cholesterol gallstones is most likely due to supersaturation of bile with cholesterol, as a result of increased synthesis by the liver and secretion into the bile. Several clinical audits from pediatric surgical units have now also demonstrated an association between cholesterol cholelithiasis and pediatric obesity.[61]

Psychosocial complications

SHORT-TERM COMPLICATIONS

The most common consequences of obesity in childhood and adolescence are those related to psychosocial dysfunction and social isolation.[29,30,63] Pre-adolescent children associate overweight body shape (on silhouette) with poor social functioning, impaired academic success and reduced fitness and health.[64] In pre-adolescent children, physical appearance and athletic competence self-esteem are lower than in their normal weight peers, but global self-esteem appears to be preserved.[65]

In adolescent girls, increased BMI is significantly related to body dissatisfaction, drive for thinness and bulimia as measured by the Eating Disorders Inventory.[66] Cross-sectional studies of teenagers consistently show an inverse relationship between weight and both global self-esteem and body-esteem.[63]

Obesity is related to bullying behaviors. In a large Canadian population study in which bullying and BMI were self-reported by boys and girls aged 11–16 years, overweight and obese youths generally had greater relative odds of being victims of aggression (both relational and overt victimization) than normal weight youths.[67] Obese youths aged 15 and 16 years were also more likely to perpetrate bullying than their normal weight peers.

Recent studies of health-related quality of life in children and adolescents show differences between obese and non-obese children. Severely obese children and adolescents aged 5 to 18 years in a clinical setting report significantly reduced health-related quality of life compared with healthy children, and similar quality of life scores to children diagnosed with cancer.[68] In a randomly sampled population of Australian primary school children, the physical and social domains of health-related quality of life for obese children were lower than for children who were not overweight, although less significantly reduced than seen in a clinical sample using the same measure.[69]

LONG-TERM PSYCHOSOCIAL COMPLICATIONS

Overweight in adolescence may also be associated with later social and economic problems. A large prospective study from the United States showed that obese adolescent females and young women are more likely, as adults, to have lower family incomes, higher rates of poverty and lower rates of marriage than women with other forms of chronic physical disability but who were not overweight, a finding suggesting that discrimination plays a role in adverse outcomes.[70] However, in a long-term follow-up of a British cohort, obesity limited to childhood was not associated with adverse socioeconomic, educational, social, and psychological outcomes in adulthood.[71] Persistent obesity in women, but not men, was associated with a higher risk of never having been employed and not having a current partner.

Orthopedic complications

Orthopedic complications are well recognized in obese children. For example, in a large international multi-center study, 63 percent of children with slipped capital femoral epiphyses had a body weight which was greater than or equal to the 90th centile for age.[72] In that study, obese patients had an earlier onset of slippage than in non-obese patients. Obesity may also be associated with the development of Blount disease (tibia vara) in which there is a deformity of the medial portion of the proximal tibial metaphysis.[73] This deformity arises as a result of increased, and possibly unconventional, weight bearing on cartilaginous bone with subsequent compensatory overgrowth and bowing of the tibia.[74] Young people who are overweight or obese have low bone area and bone mass relative to their body weight, making them more prone to fractures than lean individuals.[75]

More minor orthopedic abnormalities are also seen, including knock knee (genu valgum) and a decreased recovery from soft tissue ankle injuries.[76] Obese children have flat, wide feet with increased static and dynamic plantar pressures;[77] this may put them at risk of a range of minor orthopedic problems.

Neurological complications

Idiopathic raised intracranial pressure (pseudotumor cerebri) is a rare but potentially very serious complication of obesity. In adult case series, obesity is very strongly associated with idiopathic intracranial hypertension,[78] but it is less commonly seen in pediatric patients with the same problem (about one-third of cases in a pediatric Miami clinic).[79] The role obesity plays in the pathogenesis of the disorder is unknown.

Asthma and sleep-disordered breathing

Respiratory outcomes can be poor in obese children. For example, 30 percent of obese children have asthma, and when compared with lean children with asthma, overweight and obese children use more anti-asthma medications, have more wheezing episodes and experience more unscheduled visits to hospital.[80] Among school-aged boys but not girls, obesity is significantly associated with newly diagnosed asthma (relative risk, 2.87; 95 percent CI, 1.35–3.88).[81] Obese children also have a lower exercise tolerance than their lean peers, possibly compounding their obesity.[82]

Potentially more serious is the complication of obstructive sleep apnea. This is characterized by snoring, adenotonsillar hypertrophy and periods of partial or complete airway obstruction while asleep, leading to recurrent hypoxia and sleep deprivation. The prevalence of obstructive sleep apnea in cohort studies of obese children varies, depending upon the definition of obstructive sleep apnea and of obesity, with rates of 13–26 percent being reported.[83] Obstructive sleep apnea is associated with severity of obesity, insulin resistance and dyslipidemia among children and adolescents and increases in severity in association with increased fasting insulin.[84,85] Profound hypoventilation and even sudden death have been reported in severe cases of sleep apnea associated with obesity.[86]

Skin complications

Obese children suffer from over-heating as their fat tissue acts as insulation, resulting in profuse sweating with any physical activity. Thrush occurs more commonly in obese subjects, especially in such moist, over-heated areas as skin folds or the groin. Striae can also occur, particularly on the abdomen and thighs.

Obesity in adulthood

The most significant health risk faced by obese young people is that they are at risk of becoming obese adults, and therefore at increased risk of cardiovascular disease, diabetes, and some cancers. Tracking of obesity from childhood and adolescence through to adulthood is more likely with a family history of parental obesity, the presence of obesity in late childhood or adolescence or with increased severity of obesity.[87] However, as the epidemic of obesity among children is a relatively recent phenomenon, studies to date examining the prevalence of tracking of weight status into adulthood were necessarily done in a population with a relatively lower prevalence of overweight during their childhood, and who were living in a less obesogenic environment than provided in current twenty-first century westernized communities. As BMI in childhood is highly correlated with BMI in adulthood,[88] and both obesity-related behaviors and BMI track into adulthood,[89] it is possible that an even greater proportion of the adult population will be overweight or obese in the future.

ETIOLOGY OF OBESITY

Obesity is a multi-faceted condition with interactions between genetic, metabolic, behavioral, and environmental factors all contributing to its development.

Physiological basis of obesity

Obesity is a chronic disorder affecting energy imbalance, i.e., there is a perturbation in the balance between energy intake and energy expenditure (see Fig. 37.4). This balance

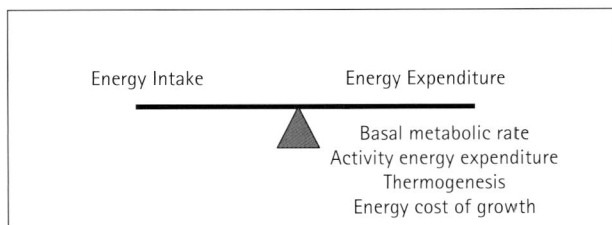

Figure 37.4 Key elements of the energy balance system. Obesity develops if energy intake chronically exceeds that of energy expenditure. Energy expenditure consists of basal metabolic rate, activity energy expenditure, thermogenesis and the energy cost of growth. The latter two are relatively minor contributors to daily energy expenditure.

is influenced by a complex set of physiological pathways, of which the hypothalamus acts as the central regulator of energy homeostasis and energy intake. The arcuate nucleus, which has a key role in this system, has two sets of neurones. The first set is orexigenic, producing neuropeptide Y and agouti-related protein, which promote food intake and reduce energy expenditure. The other set is anorexigenic, producing pro-opiomelanocortin (POMC) and cocaine- and amphetamine-related transcript, which have the opposite effect.[90]

Circulating peripherally derived factors modulate this system. These include long-term signals of energy stores (leptin, insulin) and short-term hunger (ghrelin), as well as satiety signals derived from the gastrointestinal system (cholecystokinin, glucagon-like peptide, peptide YY_{3-36}).[91] The central arcuate nucleus then processes these hormonal signals through signaling to second-order down-stream effector neurones (ultimately influencing dietary intake and energy expenditure), which also receive modifying inputs from dopamine, serotonin and endocannabinoid signals. These effector neurones express receptors including melanocortin 4 receptor (MC4R).[92]

The resultant energy regulation system is very protective against weight loss, which has been the dominant physiological threat to the individual until the past couple of decades in most westernized societies. However, the system is not protective against weight gain. With increasing body fatness, the resultant increase in circulating leptin (the principal fat store size signal) has only a limited effect on reducing food intake, presumably due to cellular resistance to leptin signaling.[92]

Genetic associations of obesity

THE HERITABILITY OF OBESITY

There is a strong familial association with obesity, with numerous studies indicating that a major part of this association is via a shared genetic predisposition. In multiple twin studies, correlations in body composition for monozygotic twins are in the range 0.6 to 0.9, with values for dizygotic twins being of the level seen in other first-degree relatives.[93] Adoption studies have shown that adoptees resemble their biological relatives in body composition, rather than members of their adoptive family. Studies of twins reared apart confirm these findings.[94,95] In Stunkard's classic paper, intra-pair correlation coefficients of the values for BMI of identical twins reared apart were 0.70 for men and 0.66 for women, and were only slightly lower than those for identical twins reared together.[94] In that study, only the environmental influences unique to the individual, and not those shared by family members, was important, accounting for about 30 percent of the variance in BMI. However, family studies show an overall lower heritability of BMI and body composition than that seen in twin studies, with values of 25–50 percent being suggested.[93]

GENES ASSOCIATED WITH COMMON (POLYGENIC) OBESITY

The Human Obesity Gene Map summarizes the literature on this and is updated on an annual basis.[96] As of October 2004, 135 different candidate genes were associated with obesity-related phenotypes, of which 18 had been replicated in five or more studies, and eight in 10 or more studies (see Table 37.4). The range of actions, or presumed actions, of the many gene products of candidate genes is extremely varied, reflecting the many physiological pathways influencing total body energy balance and fat distribution. Genes influencing appetite and satiety signals, fat cell signaling, adrenal action, resting metabolic rate, diet-induced thermogenesis, nutrient partitioning, peripheral insulin action, deposition of visceral fat, and obesity-related co-morbidities are all the subject of intense investigation.[92,96,97]

MONOGENIC FORMS OF OBESITY

Mutations in several genes that encode proteins with probable roles in central appetite regulation have been described. In the 2004 update of the Human Obesity Gene Map single-gene mutations in 10 different genes had been reported, involving 173 individuals with obesity.[96,97] Most of the mutations, with the exception of mutations in the MC4R gene, are associated with severe early onset obesity and have a recessive form of inheritance.

1997 saw the first report of a single gene mutation causing severe early-onset obesity, congenital leptin deficiency.[98] To date, two United Kingdom families of Pakistani origin, one Turkish family and one unrelated Canadian child of Pakistani origin have been described with leptin gene mutations.[99] Affected individuals are homozygous for the leptin gene mutation and have severe early onset obesity (e.g., BMI of 53–72 kg m^{-2} at age 13–19 years), marked hyperphagia,

Table 37.4 Selected candidate genes associated with the obesity phenotype*

Gene	Gene name	Location	Phenotype
ADRB2	Beta-2 adrenergic receptor	5q31–q32	Waist:hip ratio, BMI, body weight increase, BMI change, fat mass change, percent body fat change, sum of eight skin folds, body weight, waist circumference, leptin
ADRB3	Beta-3 adrenergic receptor	8p12–p11.2	Body weight, body weight increase, BMI, abdominal (visceral or subcutaneous) fat, fat mass, waist circumference, waist:hip ratio
GNB3	Beta polypeptide 3 guanine nucleotide binding protein (G protein)	12p13.31	Obesity, pregnancy weight gain, BMI, weight loss with sibutramine, waist circumference, skin folds, birth weight, fat mass change, body weight
LEPR	Leptin receptor	1p31	BMI, fat mass, fat-free mass, sagittal abdominal diameter, extreme obesity, 24 h energy expenditure, adipocyte size (subcutaneous abdominal), percent body fat, abdominal fat (total, subcutaneous)
NR3C1	Nuclear receptor subfamily 3, group C, member 1 (glucocorticoid receptor)	5q31	Abdominal visceral fat, BMI waist-to-hip ratio, leptin, BMI, waist circumference, sum of skin folds, body weight gain, lean mass
PPARG	Peroxisome proliferative activated receptor gamma	3p25	BMI, leptin, waist circumference, BMI change, fat mass, waist-to-hip ratio, morbid obesity, weight increase, 24 h lipid oxidation, ponderal index at birth, abdominal fat (visceral, subcutaneous)
UCP2	Uncoupling protein-2	11q13.3	24 h energy expenditure, spontaneous physical activity, respiratory quotient, BMI, resting energy expenditure, glucose oxidation rate, lipid oxidation rate, body weight increase, percent body fat, body weight, sum of skin folds
UCP3	Uncoupling protein-3	11q13	BMI, respiratory quotient, lean body mass, waist-to-hip ratio, fat mass, lean mass, percent body fat, resting energy expenditure, leptin, sum of skin folds, body weight

*Adapted from Perusse et al.[96]
Candidate genes for which markers have been shown to be associated with obesity-related phenotypes in >10 studies.

hyperinsulinemia, hyperlipidemia, hypothalamic hypothyroidism, and hypogonadism. Daily subcutaneous injections of recombinant leptin have led to complete reversal of clinical and biochemical abnormalities in four affected individuals.[99]

Other genes for which specific mutations associated with early onset obesity, hyperphagia, and recessive inheritance have been identified include leptin receptor, melanocortin 3 receptor, POMC, proprotein convertase subsilin/kexin 1, corticotrophin-releasing hormone receptors 1 and 2, single-minded homolog 1, and G protein-coupled receptor 24.[96,97]

By far the most common monogenic form of obesity is due to a mutation in the gene that encodes MC4R.[100–102] MC4R deficiency usually has an autosomal dominant mode of inheritance and may be present in 1–6 percent of individuals with severe early onset obesity in a range of different ethnic groups.[103] Carriers have severe obesity, increased linear growth, hyperphagia, and hyperinsulinemia, with retained reproductive function. In children with the MC4R gene mutation, the severity of obesity and hyperphagia are associated with the degree of impairment in MC4R cell signaling.[103] However, during adolescence, the significant sense of hunger and degree of hyperinsulinemia become less marked, with adult carriers of the gene mutation not being phenotypically different from obese adults who are non-carriers.[103] MC4R knockout mice that are fed low-fat diets are not hyperphagic, but become hyperphagic after the introduction of diets with increased fat content,[104] suggesting that gene–environment interactions may be important in the manifestation of the phenotype.

SYNDROMIC FORMS OF OBESITY

Many rare syndromes have obesity as one of a constellation of physical and development abnormalities. To date, causal genes, or likely candidate genes, have been identified for most of the 36 such obesity-associated Mendelian syndromes.[96,97] Selected Mendelian syndromes are summarized in Table 37.5. The most frequent of these syndromes is Prader–Willi

Table 37.5   Selected obesity-related Mendelian disorders*

Syndrome	Locus	Candidate gene	Additional clinical features
Autosomal dominant			
Albright hereditary osteodystrophy	20q13.1–13.3	GNAS	Short stature, brachydactyly, subcutaneous calcifications, other skeletal abnormalities, impaired olfaction
Multiple endocrine neoplasia, type 1 (MEN1) with Cushing's disease	11q13	MEN1(Menin)	Pituitary and adrenal tumors, elevated cortisol level
Prader–Willi syndrome	15q11–q12	GABRG3, IPW, MAGEL2, NDN, PWCR1, SNRPN, ZNF127	Fetal hypotonia, mental retardation, short stature, hypothalamic hypogonadism, characteristic facial and skeletal phenotype (almond-shaped palpebral fissures, narrow bifrontal diameter, small hands and feet, tapering fingers), hyperphagia
Ulnar-mammary (Schinzel) syndrome	12q24.1	TBX2	Ulnar defects, delayed puberty, hypoplastic nipples
Autosomal recessive			
Alstrom syndrome	2p13–p12	ALMS1	Retinal dystrophy, neurosensory deafness, diabetes
Bardet–Biedl syndrome	11q13	BBS1	Mental retardation, retinal degeneration, polydactyly, structural abnormalities of the kidneys, renal impairment, hypogonadism
	16q21	BBS2	
	3p13–p12	BBS3 (ARL6)	
	15q22.3–q23	BBS4	
	2q31	BBS5	
	20p12	MKKS	
	4q26–q27	BS7 or BBS2L1	
	14q32.1	BBS8	
Cohen syndrome	8q22	COH1	Prominent central incisors, ophthalmopathy, microcephaly
X-linked			
Borjeson–Forssman–Lehmann syndrome	Xq26–q27	PHF6	Mental retardation, hypogonadism, large ears
Fragile X syndrome with Prader–Willi-like phenotype	Xq27.3	FMR-1	Mental retardation, short stature, stubby hands and feet, regional hyperpigmentation, full face
Mental retardation, X-linked, syndromic 16	Xq28	MECP2	Mental retardation, resting tremors
Simpson–Golabi–Behmel 1	Xq26.1	GPC3	Mental retardation, pre- and post-natal overgrowth, macroglossia, renal and skeletal abnormalities

*Adapted from Perusse et al.,[96] the Obesity Gene Map Database,[97] and Online Mendelian Inheritance in Man.[105]

syndrome, characterized by diminished fetal activity, obesity, muscular hypotonia, mental retardation, short stature, hypogonadotropic hypogonadism, and small hands and feet, as well as a number of other features.[105]

Environmental and behavioral associations of obesity

Genetic factors make a major contribution to an individual's susceptibility to the development of obesity. However, unless the 'correct' environmental conditions exist, an individual's genetic predisposition for obesity may not be fully expressed – a situation that presumably was the norm in most countries prior to the last decades of the twentieth century. The increased prevalence of obesity in recent decades in genetically stable populations highlights the central role of recent important environmental trends in the development of the obesity epidemic.[92] Table 37.6 summarizes the strength of the evidence for factors associated with promotion of, or protection against, the development of obesity in both adult and pediatric populations, as outlined in a WHO report.[106]

TELEVISION VIEWING

The association between television viewing and obesity in childhood and adolescence has been demonstrated in both cross-sectional and longitudinal studies.[107–109] Of particular interest is the finding in some prospective studies that television viewing is associated with an increased incidence of new cases of obesity, as well as a decrease in remission rates of established obesity.[108,109] Further evidence for an association between television viewing and obesity comes from a school-based intervention aimed at decreasing

television, videotape, and videogame use in 3rd and 4th graders in the Unites States, which led to a statistically significant decrease in measures of body fatness in the intervention children compared with non-intervention control children.[110] There are, however, no clear data linking viewing of interactive videogames, computers, or other 'small-screen' time with the development of obesity. Possible mechanisms for the association between television viewing and obesity include the following:

- Increased exposure of children to food marketing[111]
- Increased snacking of energy-dense foods and drinks while watching television[111]
- Displacement of time spent in more physical activities
- Reinforcement of sedentary behavior
- Reduction in basal metabolic rate while watching television[112]
- Television viewing may be a proxy measure of a generally obesogenic lifestyle

DIETARY INTAKE AND EATING PATTERNS

The increased prevalence of obesity in recent decades has resulted, in part, from changes in dietary intake, such as an increase in the consumption of energy-dense, micronutrient-poor foods or in sugar-sweetened drinks.[113] Consumption of soft (soda) drinks at baseline is associated with increased weight gain over the next 19 months in young adolescents.[114] In a cross-sectional study of 4746 adolescents in the United States, eating at fast-food restaurants was positively associated with total energy intake and daily soft drink consumption, and negatively associated with consumption of fruit, vegetables, and milk, but there was no association with weight status.[115] In longitudinal studies of adolescent girls and women, eating fast food meals once or more per

Table 37.6 Summary of strength of evidence on factors that might promote or protect against weight gain and obesity*

Evidence	Decreased risk	No relationship	Increased risk
Convincing	Regular physical activity High dietary intake of NSP# (dietary fiber)		Sedentary lifestyles High intake of energy-dense micronutrient-poor foods
Probable	Home and school environments that support healthy food choices for children Breast feeding		Heavy marketing of energy-dense foods and fast-food outlets High intake of sugars – sweetened soft drinks and fruit juices Adverse socioeconomic conditions
Possible	Low glycemic index foods	Protein content of diet	Large portion sizes High proportion of food prepared outside the home (developed countries) 'Rigid restraint/periodic disinhibition' eating patterns
Insufficient	Increasing eating frequency		Alcohol

*Adapted from a WHO report.[106]

#NSP: non-starch polysaccharides

week has been associated with BMI and weight gain.[116,117] The relative contributions of dietary fat (versus energy) intake, glycemic index, portion sizes, and specific eating patterns to the development of obesity remains unclear, although all may play an important role.

A systematic review has highlighted the small but protective effect of breastfeeding against obesity, with some evidence of a dose-dependent effect of breast-feeding duration the prevalence of obesity.[118] A comprehensive review of on parental feeding styles has shown that parental feeding restriction, but no other feeding domain, is associated with increased child eating and weight status.[119] It is possible that parental (especially maternal) feeding restriction may promote over-eating in the young child.

PHYSICAL ACTIVITY AND SEDENTARY BEHAVIOR

Ecological studies, largely in adult populations, suggest that low levels of physical activity are associated with increasing obesity.[120] A review of physical activity and obesity in childhood has shown that lower physical activity levels and sedentary behaviors are associated with a higher prevalence of obesity in children.[121] Prospective studies in childhood suggest that physical activity may have a protective effect on the development of excess weight gain in childhood. For example, in a 3 year study of young children, higher levels of baseline aerobic activity were associated with a subsequent lower weight gain.[122] In a prospective study of children from the Framingham Children's Study, followed from pre-school to first grade and assessed using accelerometers and skin-fold measurements, those with low levels of physical activity at baseline had substantially more subcutaneous fat at follow-up than did more active children.[123]

Other factors associated with obesity

GROWTH PATTERNS DURING INFANCY AND CHILDHOOD

Several growth patterns, perhaps reflecting a combination of dietary intake at critical periods, genetic programming and intra-uterine growth, are associated with an increased risk of subsequent obesity. Thus, an earlier adiposity rebound is associated with increased BMI or body fatness in mid-childhood and adolescence.[124] In a large-scale prospective study of English children, rapid catch-up growth between birth and age 2 years, weight Z-score at 8 months or 18 months, and weight gain in the first year, were all associated with an increased risk of obesity at age 7 years.[109]

ADDITIONAL PARENTAL FACTORS

The association between parental and child obesity is well known, a consequence of a range of genetic and environmental factors. Whitaker et al.[87] showed that parental obesity more than doubles the risk of adult obesity among both obese and non-obese children aged less than 10 years, and

Reilly et al.[109] showed that having two obese parents increases the risk of mid-childhood obesity by more than 10 when compared with children where neither parent is obese.

Parental eating behavior also influences the development of excess weight gain in the child. In a study of pre-schoolers, maternal dietary disinhibition was associated with the daughter's subsequent excess weight gain.[125] A 6 year outcome study of children aged 3–5 years at baseline showed that parental dietary disinhibition was associated with greater increases in body fatness.[126]

Obesity secondary to medical conditions or drug therapy

Obesity may occur secondary to a range of medical conditions including several endocrine disorders (e.g., hypothyroidism, hypercortisolism, growth hormone deficiency or resistance), central nervous system damage (i.e., hypothalamic–pituitary damage due to surgery, trauma or cranial irradiation) and post-malignancy (acute lymphoblastic leukemia).[127] A range of pharmacological agents has obesity as a recognized complication and includes glucocorticoids, some anti-epileptics (e.g., sodium valproate),[128] antipsychotics (e.g., risperidone, olanzapine),[129] and insulin.

THE MANAGEMENT OF CHILD AND ADOLESCENT OBESITY

The clinical assessment and management of the obese child or adolescent is outlined below. Readers are also referred to several national guidelines[130,131] or reviews[2,29,132] for additional information.

Clinical assessment

CLINICAL HISTORY

The features that should be covered in a clinical history are outlined in Table 37.7. They include a sensitive exploration of the implications of obesity for the young person and family and of their motivation for behavioral change. A family history of obesity and disorders associated with insulin resistance (e.g., type 2 diabetes, hypertension, dyslipidemia, premature heart disease, and obstructive sleep apnea) should be obtained. There should also be a detailed exploration of the factors influencing physical activity, sedentary behavior, and dietary intake.

ANTHROPOMETRY

Height and weight should be precisely and accurately measured; BMI is calculated as weight/height^2 and then plotted on a BMI-for-age chart. Although recommended as a form of assessment in only one national guideline to date,[131] waist

Table 37.7 History to be sought as part of clinical assessment of the obese patient

General history	• Pregnancy details, including maternal gestational diabetes • Early medical history • Ethnicity
Weight history	• History of obesity including onset and duration of obesity • Pubertal history (including menstrual history if relevant) • Impact of obesity on the life of the patient and his/her family • Reasons for seeking clinical help
Complications history	• Psychological effects of obesity, including teasing and bullying • Presence of sleep apnea/disturbed sleep • Asthma • Specific symptoms such as knee/hip pain • Menstrual history (girls) • Exercise tolerance
Family history of obesity and disorders associated with insulin resistance	• BMI or BMI percentile for first degree relatives; relative weights of other family members • Family history of obesity, type 2 diabetes, cardiovascular and cerebrovascular disease, fatty liver disease and obstructive sleep apnea
Lifestyle history	• Physical activity, including transport to/from school, participation in organized sports or other activities, access to recreation space or equipment for games, availability of friends or family for games or play • Sedentary activities including TV, video games, computer use, other passive entertainment time, mobile phone use • Dietary history including meal patterns, fast food intake and snacks, soft drink intake

Table 37.8 Features to be sought on physical examination of the obese patient

Element of physical examination	Comments
Anthropometry	Height, weight, BMI (charted), waist circumference (charted if possible)
Pubertal stage	
Blood pressure	Use appropriately sized cuff and age-appropriate reference values
Skin	Acanthosis nigricans; striae; intertrigo; skin chafing; hirsutism
Abdominal examination	Hepatomegaly; right upper quadrant tenderness (gallstones)
Respiratory and ear, nose, and throat examination	Clinical signs of asthma; tonsillar enlargement
Musculoskeletal examination	Gait; mobility; clinical signs of hip, knee or ankle problems; bowing of tibia
Neurological	Papilloedema
Warning signs for presence of rare causes of obesity	Short stature; dysmorphic features; intellectual disability, visual disturbances or other neurological signs

circumference should be measured. Ideally, waist circumference should be plotted on a waist circumference for age chart.[15,16] BMI and waist circumference are most useful in the clinical assessment of the individual patient when measured serially and used to monitor change over time.

PHYSICAL EXAMINATION

Features to be sought on physical examination are outlined in Table 37.8 and include hypertension (ensure that cuff width is adequate),[134] acanthosis nigricans, striae, intertrigo, adenotonsillar hypertrophy, hepatomegaly (fatty liver), and an abnormal gait due to joint problems. Findings on physical examination which may indicate other causes for obesity and which call for further assessment include short stature, dysmorphic features, violaceous striae, intellectual disability, and visual or neurological defects indicative of a central nervous system lesion.

LABORATORY INVESTIGATIONS

For overweight and mildly obese children, laboratory investigations are generally not necessary. However, if a child or adolescent is very obese (especially if centrally obese), has a family history of disorders associated with insulin resistance, or history and examination suggesting the presence of complications of obesity or other risk factors, then the following biochemical screening for dyslipidemia, insulin resistance, glucose intolerance, and liver abnormalities has been recommended in one national guideline:[131]

- Fasting lipid profile (total cholesterol, LDL cholesterol, HDL cholesterol, triglycerides)
- Fasting glucose
- Liver function tests (specifically alanine aminotransaminase)
- Consider fasting insulin
- Consider oral glucose tolerance test

Further assessment of liver function (e.g., liver ultrasound, exclusion of other causes of liver dysfunction) may be required. More detailed endocrinological assessment is usually not needed, unless there is other evidence of endocrine disease, such as short stature, hirsutism or menstrual

Table 37.9   Defining weight management outcomes

Improvement in complications or behavior	Improvement in adiposity
Resolution of medical complications, e.g., sleep apnea, hypertension, insulin resistance, glucose intolerance, dyslipidemia, non-alcoholic fatty liver disease	Weight: slowing in rate of weight gain, weight maintenance, weight loss
Improvement in self-esteem and psychosocial functioning Increase in healthy lifestyle behaviors (related to eating, physical activity, sedentary behavior)	Waist circumference: decrease
Increase in level of fitness or aerobic capacity Improvement in family functioning	

Table 37.10   Basic elements of behavioural management of obesity in childhood and adolescence

Clarification of treatment outcomes

Family involvement

Developmentally appropriate approach
- Pre-adolescent children: focus on parents
- Adolescents: consider separate sessions for the young person and parent(s)

Long-term dietary change
- Energy reduction
- Food choices that are lower in fat and have a lower glycemic index
- Reduction in high-sugar foods and drinks
- Water as the main beverage
- Avoidance of severe dietary restriction
- Appropriate portion sizes
- Modified eating patterns (regular meals, eat together as a family, avoid eating while watching the television)

Increase in physical activity
- Incidental activity
- Active transport options (e.g., walking, cycling, using public transport)
- Lifestyle activities
- Organized activities
- Improved access to recreation spaces and play equipment

Decrease in sedentary behavior
- Television, computer, playstation and other small-screen use
- Alternatives to motorized transport

irregularities. Where there is clinical suspicion of obstructive sleep apnea then referral for polysomnography is warranted.

Defining treatment outcomes

When treating a child or adolescent with obesity the goals of therapy should be initially clarified (Table 37.9) with the parents or young person, as appropriate. Markers of a successful outcome of therapy may include an improvement in morbidity (e.g., sleep apnea, hypertension, insulin resistance, dyslipidemia), psychosocial functioning, healthy lifestyle behaviors, aerobic capacity, or family functioning. While weight loss may be an appropriate goal in obese older children and adolescents, in younger children weight maintenance or a reduced rate of weight gain during a growth spurt may be the most achievable approach; in effect, pre-pubertal or peripubertal children may be able to 'grow in' to an appropriate weight adjusted for height. A decrease in waist circumference ('waist loss') is a useful indicator of reduction in abdominal obesity.

Education of the family and, where appropriate, the young person, about the nature of obesity, including the realization that it is a chronic disorder of energy balance, is also important, as the need for long-term changes in behavior will then be more readily apparent. In helping the family or young person, small, achievable goals are important: examples may include aiming initially for one extra walk per week, or reducing television viewing by 1 h per day every few weeks.

Broad principles of management

Systematic reviews of the treatment of obesity in children have shown that there are only a limited number of randomized controlled trials to guide clinical decision-making.[135,136]

Published studies have usually had small samples sizes with varying attrition rates, have measured outcomes almost exclusively in terms of degree of overweight, rather than including broader medical, psychosocial, and behavioral outcomes, and have usually involved fairly homogeneous patient samples managed in a tertiary care setting. Thus, the evidence to support effective intervention is limited and may not be generalizable to other clinical settings. Nevertheless, the broad principles of management are well-recognized[2,135] (Table 37.10):

- Family involvement
- A developmentally appropriate approach
- Long-term behavior modification
- Dietary change
- Increased physical activity
- Decreased sedentary behavior

Conventional treatment approaches

FAMILY FOCUS (***)

A systematic review of the involvement of family members in weight control interventions has highlighted the importance of parental involvement when managing obese children, although the data for management of obese adolescents are limited.[137] Several studies have now shown that long-term maintenance of weight loss (i.e., from 2 to 10 years) can be achieved when the intervention is family-based (**).[135,138,139] Long-term weight control 'success' in childhood obesity is associated with such factors as the amount of weight the parent loses in the initial phase, the use of reinforcement techniques such as parental praise, and a change in eating habits, such as eating meals at home or a moderate reduction in fat intake.[138] Such findings imply that altered food and physical activity patterns within the whole family, as well as support of the child and parental reinforcement of a healthy lifestyle, are important factors in successful outcomes.

A DEVELOPMENTALLY APPROPRIATE APPROACH: PRE-ADOLESCENT CHILDREN (**)

Treatment of pre-adolescent obesity with the parents as the exclusive agents of lifestyle change appears superior to a child-centered approach (**).[140–142] An Israeli study randomized obese children aged 6–11 years and their parents to either an experimental intervention where only the parents attended group sessions (with an emphasis on general parenting skills), or a control intervention where only the children attended group sessions.[140,141] At 12 months, there was a greater reduction in overweight in the children in the experimental group, with children in the control group having higher rates of reported anxiety and of withdrawal from the program.[140] At the 7 year follow-up from this study, when children were aged 14–19 years, the mean reduction in children's overweight was 29 percent in the parent-only group, versus 20 percent in the child-only group ($p < 0.05$).[142] At that point, 60 percent of the children in the parent-only group, versus 31 percent of those in the child-only group, were classified as non-obese. These data suggest that when dealing with the obese pre-adolescent child, sessions involving the parent or parents alone, without the child being present, are likely to be the most effective.

ADOLESCENT-FOCUSSED INTERVENTIONS (**)

To date, eight randomized controlled trials of obesity management among adolescents have been published (**).[143–150] All except one were performed in North America, and all involved intense behavioral management support, with most follow-up periods being for 6 months or less. Four used conventional dietary modification, increased physical activity and support for behavioral change and three showed modest success in the short term.[143–145,148] One of these showed at least short-term success in management of adolescent obesity with a novel phone- and mail-based behavioral intervention initiated in a primary care setting.[148] In two of the other studies, significant weight loss at 6 months was seen in patients receiving sibutramine versus placebo[146,149] or at 12 months in patients receiving orlistat

versus placebo.[150] The final study resulted in greater weight loss at 6 months in patients on a low glycemic load diet compared with those receiving a conventional reduced fat diet.[147] Such studies provide some guidance as to the efficacy of treatment interventions for adolescents in resource-intensive settings, but there is only limited evidence to guide effective weight management interventions at an intensity that would be sustainable in most health care settings.

BEHAVIOR MODIFICATION (** AND ***)

Psychological interventions, and particularly behavioral and cognitive behavioral interventions, are well-recognized components of effective weight management in adults and are primarily useful when combined with diet and exercise strategies, resulting in additional weight loss.[151] Several studies have incorporated a range of behavioral modification strategies in the management of childhood obesity, including the following: monitoring behavior, setting goals, rewarding successful changes in behavior and controlling the environment (**).[132,152,153] The nature of each of these strategies will vary depending upon the age and developmental status of the patient. Thus, an adolescent will take responsibility for setting at least some of the goals around weight management and will likewise monitor his or her behavior. However, the parent would be responsible for these strategies when the patient is a young child.[132]

DIETARY MANAGEMENT

There have been several systematic reviews of the macronutrient composition of weight reduction diets in adults. Low-fat diets appear as efficacious as other weight-reducing diets for achieving sustained weight loss in adults (***).[154] There is insufficient evidence to make recommendations concerning low carbohydrate diets in weight management; however, of the published studies, weight loss while using low-carbohydrate diets is principally associated with a decrease in energy intake and increased diet duration, but not with reduced carbohydrate content.[155] Likewise, the evidence of the effectiveness of a low glycemic-index diet in adults is also limited, with medium-term studies suggesting that there is no specific advantage of low glycemic-index over high glycemic-index diets, although this area remains controversial (**).[156,157] These data are not surprising. Ultimately, energy reduction is the key modification required for a change in the 'input' arm of the energy balance equation and many factors will affect which dietary strategy is most suitable for a particular patient.

In the past, more prescriptive dietary approaches were used in the treatment of child and adolescent obesity, but the current approach generally involves education about healthy nutrition and healthy food choices.[2,132] There is no direct evidence for which dietary modification is most effective for weight management in children and adolescents. In the management of childhood obesity, a moderate restriction in fat intake in the initial phase of therapy is associated with sustained treatment effects (*).[139] There is one randomized controlled trial of a low glycemic index diet versus a calorie-reduced low fat diet in adolescents aged 13–21 years which showed a greater reduction in BMI and fat mass at 12 months (**).[147]

What recommendations should currently be given? Dietary interventions should follow national nutrition guidelines and have an emphasis on regular meals, eating together as a family, food choices which are lower in fat and have a lower glycemic-index, increased vegetable and fruit intake, healthier snack food options and, very probably, decreased portion sizes.[2,132] A reduction in soft drink or fruit juice intake, with a move to water as the main beverage, may also be important in decreasing total energy intake.[114,158] Involvement of the entire family in making the change to a sustainable and healthy food intake is vital. This is because changes in shopping and cooking practices, and altered attitudes to snacking and mealtimes, are required.[132] The focus should be on behavior change, healthier food choices, and a reduction in the consumption of energy-dense, micronutrient-poor foods and high-sugar drinks. Avoidance of severe dietary restriction may be an important strategy in both helping the development of the child's capacity to self-regulate dietary intake[119] and in avoiding the subsequent development of disordered eating.[159] Nevertheless, a flexible and individualized menu plan may be useful in helping a family or young person to make the transition to sustained healthy eating habits.

PHYSICAL ACTIVITY AND SEDENTARY BEHAVIOR

A meta-analysis of weight loss studies in adults has shown that an aerobic exercise program produces relatively modest weight loss compared with caloric restriction, although when added to a dietary intervention it improves weight loss outcomes when compared with diet alone (***).[160] Physical activity also appears to be crucial for maintaining weight loss in previously obese adults.[161] A meta-analysis of several small studies of lifestyle interventions in childhood obesity has shown that a combined exercise–diet intervention improved weight outcomes when compared with diet intervention alone (***).[162]

Epstein and colleagues have shown that participation of obese children in a lifestyle program (e.g., walking, running, cycling or swimming, based on the family's preference) led to greater reductions in percentage overweight at 6 months and 17 months when compared with a program of isocaloric programmed aerobic exercise (**).[163] A study of similar design, but including a third control group involved in calisthenics, and with follow-up for 10 years, showed that the lifestyle and aerobic exercise programs were superior in terms of percentage overweight reduction to the calisthenics control group (**).[164]

Epstein's group have also addressed the issue of targeting sedentary behavior. For example, in one study, 90 families of obese children aged 8–12 years, were assigned to different arms of a behavioral weight control program which differed in whether sedentary or physically active behaviors were targeted and the degree of behavior change required (**).[165] Results at the 2 year follow-up showed that targeting either decreased sedentary behavior or increased physical activity was associated with significant and similar decreases in percentage overweight and body fat and improved aerobic fitness.

What recommendations can be given in terms of physical activity and sedentary behavior reduction? Families and young people need to be reminded that increased physical activity may best result from a change in incidental activity (e.g., walking or cycling for transport, playing with friends or family) and not necessarily from organized activities such as school sport or gym programs. Importantly, children and adolescents should be encouraged to choose activities that they enjoy and which are therefore likely to be more sustainable. Limiting television viewing to fewer than 2 h per day may be very strategic.[158] Parental involvement is vital if an increase in physical activity or a decrease in sedentary behavior is to occur. This may include monitoring television use, role-modeling of healthy behaviors, encouragement and providing access to recreation areas or recreational equipment.[132]

Non-conventional approaches to therapy

As yet, there is little information to guide the use of more aggressive treatment approaches such as very-low-calorie diets, drug therapy or bariatric surgery in the treatment of severe pediatric obesity. Such therapies should occur in the context of a behavioral weight management program and be restricted to specialist centers with expertise in managing severe obesity.

VERY-LOW-CALORIE DIETS

A systematic review of commercial weight loss therapies in adults found one randomized trial and several case series of medically supervised very-low-calorie diet programs (***).[166] Patients who completed treatment lost approximately 15–25 percent of initial weight. The limitations of such programs include high costs, high attrition rates, and a high probability of regaining 50 percent or more of lost weight in 1–2 years. There are case series, although no randomized controlled trials, of the use of very-low-calorie-diets in adolescents and older children showing that rapid weight loss can be produced, at least at 12 months follow-up (*).[167]

PHARMACOLOGICAL THERAPY

Both the pancreatic lipase inhibitor, orlistat, and the serotonin- and noradrenaline-reuptake inhibitor, sibutramine, have been shown to aid weight loss and limit weight regain in large placebo-controlled randomized controlled trials in adults (**).[168,169] No pharmacological agents are currently approved for the treatment of pediatric obesity, although therapeutic trials are under way. Berkowitz *et al.*[146] performed a randomized controlled trial of sibutramine in 82 adolescents with BMI 32–44 kg m^{-2}. The addition of sibutramine to a comprehensive behavioral program resulted in a significantly greater mean weight loss at 6 months (7.8 kg, SD 6.3 kg) than in the group treated with the behavioral program and placebo (3.2 kg, SD 6.1 kg); however, 23 of 82 patients required a lower dose and ten ceased treatment because of hypertension (**). Similar weight loss findings were reported by Godoy-Matos *et al.*[149] in another study of sibutramine in adolescents, although in that study no participant withdrew because of adverse events (**).

A trial of orlistat, given to adolescents in the context of a diet and exercise behavioral therapy program, showed a significant improvement in BMI at 12 months in those on orlistat compared with those on placebo (0.55 kg m^{-2} decrease versus 0.31 kg m^{-2} increase, $p = 0.001$) (**).[150] Generally, mild-to-moderate gastrointestinal tract adverse events occurred in 9–50 percent of the orlistat group and in 1–13 percent of the placebo group. There is little information on factors that may improve adherence to orlistat therapy in adolescent patients.

Recent studies have considered the use of metformin versus placebo in non-diabetic hyperinsulinemic obese adolescents and have shown at least short-term (2–6 months) improvement in body composition and metabolic parameters (* and **).[170,171] Metformin therapy should be considered in the obese adolescent with significant hyperinsulinemia who has a family history of diabetes.

Existing national guidelines on management of overweight and obesity in children provide little guidance on the use of pharmacological therapy, reflecting the paucity of clinical studies.[130,131] Sibutramine and orlistat can be used in obese young people with complications who have failed conventional management; such therapy should be given in the context of a behavioral management program, with specialist supervision, and only when there is a reasonable expectation of benefit over risk.

OBESITY (BARIATRIC) SURGERY

Bariatric surgery is increasingly seen as an important form of therapy for adults with severe obesity, especially if medical therapy has failed.[1] Several forms of bariatric surgery are available: gastric banding (including the laparoscopic adjustable gastric band), gastric bypass, gastroplasty and biliopancreatic diversion or duodenal switch. A systematic review of the outcomes of bariatric surgery in adults has shown that the surgery leads to a mean percentage weight loss of 61.2 percent, with higher weight losses, and higher operative mortalities, reported for those procedures associated with malabsorption (***).[172] In the majority of reported patients, bariatric surgery leads to either resolution or significant improvements in diabetes, hyperlipidemia, hypertension and obstructive sleep apnea.[172]

There are several case reports or case series of bariatric surgery in adolescents, with as yet no randomized controlled trials to guide management decisions (*).[173,174] A United States expert consensus report has recommended that bariatric surgery should be considered in adolescent patients who are very obese (BMI $\geqslant$40 kg m^{-2}), have attained skeletal maturity (girls $\geqslant$13 years; boys $\geqslant$15 years), have obesity-associated co-morbidities and who have experienced failure of 6 months of organized weight loss therapy attempts.[175] The panel also recommends that patients should be referred to centers with multidisciplinary weight management teams and that surgery should be performed in tertiary institutions experienced in bariatric surgery. The varied response to these recommendations, which are reasonably conservative, highlights the different views on surgical management of severely obese adolescents existing in the bariatric surgery, pediatric surgery and pediatric medicine professional communities.[176–178]

Settings for treatment intervention

There have been few studies looking at the effectiveness, in adult obesity, of different types of interventions (e.g., group programs, individual counselling sessions, sessions delivered by different types of health care professional) or interventions delivered in different settings (e.g., primary care, community health centers, tertiary institutions).[179] When dealing with obese children and adolescents, there is some evidence that time-efficient interventions such as group sessions, holiday camps or mail- and phone-based behavioral interventions do at least as well as individual sessions (*).[148,180]

PRIMARY PREVENTION OF CHILD AND ADOLESCENT OBESITY

Effective primary prevention strategies are ultimately required in order to curb the obesity epidemic. The Cochrane review on the prevention of obesity in children included a number of school-based interventions and noted that the majority of studies were short-term (***).[181] Some studies that focused on dietary or physical activity approaches showed a small but positive impact on BMI status, and nearly all studies included resulted in some improvement in diet or physical activity.[181] These findings are supported by a series of systematic reviews looking at interventions around physical activity and nutritional intake in children and young people (***).[182–186] The reviews identified the following:

- Multifaceted school-based interventions (e.g., school curricula, mass media, cafeteria changes, parent mailing) can alter food intake of children and young people in the short-term.
- Children's nutritional intake can be altered when their food source in modified.
- Educational interventions designed to decrease sedentary behavior appear more effective at changing behavior than those increasing physical activity.

- Shifting the balance from skill development to aerobic activity increases physical activity among students.
- Multi-component interventions including an environmental as well as an educational component directed at improving nutrition and increasing physical activity levels in children were the most effective at changing these behaviors.

Interventions simply focussing on educating individuals and communities about behavior change have had limited or no success in modifying obesity prevalence.[1,2] This is because the broader environment in many communities does not readily support healthy food choices for physically active lifestyles. Up-stream factors (physical, economic, and socio-cultural) contributing to obesity in individuals can operate at both a micro-environmental level (i.e., the settings where individuals live, eat, play or go to school) as well as at a macro-environmental level (i.e., the broader sectors that ultimately influence dietary intake and physical activity and which are beyond the ability of an individual to influence).[187] Table 37.11 lists examples of the settings that may be important in influencing the development of obesity. It is apparent that opportunities exist for a range of prevention strategies in a given community or country. These might include:

- Development of town planning policies which promote active transport or public transport over motorized transport
- Regulation of the nature and amount of food marketing directed at children
- Provision of high-quality recreation areas
- Regulation of the types of food and drink provided in school canteens
- Provision of innovative and inclusive physical education programs in schools
- Improvement in public transport
- Subsidies on vegetables and fruits
- Provision of safe cycle paths and safe street lighting in local neighborhoods
- Provision of economic incentives for the production and distribution of vegetables and fruit
- Support of walk-to-school programs

Such interventions will require inter-sectoral and inter-governmental cooperation, supported by adequate resourcing and significant community ownership.

Table 37.11   Examples of microenvironment settings and macroenvironment sectors for the prevention of obesity*

Microenvironment settings	Macroenvironment sectors
Homes	Technology and design (e.g., labor-saving devices, architecture)
Schools	Food production and importing
Community groups (e.g., clubs, churches)	Food manufacturing and distribution
Community places (e.g., parks, shopping malls)	Food marketing (e.g., fast-food advertising)
Institutions (e.g., boarding schools)	Food catering services
Food retailers (e.g., supermarkets)	Sports and leisure industry (e.g., instructor training programs)
Food service outlets (e.g., canteens, lunch bars, restaurants)	Urban and rural development (e.g., town planning, local government)
Recreation facilities (e.g., pools, gyms)	Transport system (e.g., public transportation systems)
Neighborhoods (e.g., cycle paths, street safety)	Health system
Local health care	

*From Swinburn et al.[187] (Reprinted from *Preventative Medicine*, vol. **29**, Swinburn G, Effer G, Fezeela R. Dissecting obesogenic environments: the development and application of a framework for identifying and prioritising environmental interventions for obesity. pp. 563–570, copyright 1999, with permission from Elsevier.)

KEY LEARNING POINTS

- Body mass index (weight/height^2) and waist circumference are reasonable measures of body fatness, and fat distribution, respectively, in children and adolescents. They should be adjusted for age and sex.
- Obesity-associated complications may be either immediate or long-term, psychosocial or medical. Insulin resistance and related disorders (e.g., dyslipidemia, obstructive sleep apnea, non-alcoholic fatty liver disease, the metabolic syndrome) are prevalent in obese children and adolescents.
- The heritability of body mass index and body composition in the general population is approximately 25–50%.
- The most common, although still rare, monogenic form of obesity is melanocortin 4 receptor deficiency.
- The increased prevalence of obesity in recent decades is a result of major environmental change, particularly affecting genetically predisposed individuals.
- There is convincing or probable evidence of an increased risk of obesity with sedentary lifestyles, a high-intake of energy-dense, micronutrient-poor diets, a high intake of sugar-sweetened drinks and heavy marketing of energy-dense foods and fast-food outlets. Regular physical activity, breastfeeding and home and school environments that

support healthy food choices for children appear protective against obesity.

- The basic principles of weight management are family involvement, a developmentally appropriate approach, long-term behavior modification, dietary change, increased physical activity and decreased sedentary behavior.
- Non-conventional treatments (pharmacological therapy, very-low-calorie diets, bariatric surgery) should occur in the context of a behavioral weight management program and be restricted to specialist centers with expertise in managing severe obesity.
- Primary prevention of obesity requires modification of both micro-environmental and macro-environmental factors influencing dietary intake and physical activity.

REFERENCES

● = Seminal primary article
◆ = Key review paper
❋ = First formal publication of a management guideline

◆ 1   WHO. *Obesity: Preventing and Managing the Global Epidemic.* Report of a WHO consultation on obesity. Geneva: WHO, 1998.
◆ 2   Lobstein T, Baur L, Uauy R. Obesity in children and young people: A crisis in public health. Report of the International Obesity TaskForce Childhood Obesity Working Group. *Obes Rev* 2004; **5(Suppl 1)**: 4–85.
3   Bellizzi MC, Dietz WH. Workshop on childhood obesity: summary of the discussion. *Am J Clin Nutr* 1999; **70**: 173S–5S.
● 4   Cole TJ, Bellizzi MC, Flegal KM, Dietz WH. Establishing a standard definition for child overweight and obesity worldwide: international survey. *BMJ* 2000; **320**: 1240–3.
● 5   Kuczmarski RJ, Ogden CL, Grummer-Strawn LM, *et al.* CDC growth charts: United States. *Advance Data* 2000; **341**: 1–27. Web-site: *http://www.cdc.gov/growthcharts*
❋ 6   Himes JH, Dietz WH. Guidelines for overweight in adolescent preventive services: recommendations from an expert committee. The Expert Committee on Clinical Guidelines for Overweight in Adolescent Preventive Services. *Am J Clin Nutr* 1994; **59**: 307–16.
7   Cole TJ, Roede MJ. Centiles of body mass index for Dutch children aged 0-20 years in 1980 – a baseline to assess recent trends in obesity. *Ann Hum Biol* 1999; **26**: 303–8.
8   Cole TJ, Freeman JV, Preece MA. British 1990 growth reference centiles for weight, height, body mass index and head circumference fitted by maximum penalized likelihood. *Stat Med* 1998; **17**: 407–29.

9   Leung SS, Cole TJ, Tse LY, Lau JT. Body mass index reference curves for Chinese children. *Ann Hum Biol* 1998; **25**: 169–74.
10   Pi-Sunyer FX. The epidemiology of central fat distribution in relation to disease. *Nutr Rev* 2004; **62(7 Pt 2)**: S120–6.
11   Ross R, Leger L, Morris D, *et al.* Quantification of adipose tissue by MRI: relationship with anthropometric variables. *J Appl Physiol* 1992; **72**: 787–95.
12   Han TS, Seidell JC, Currall JE, *et al.* The influences of height and age on waist circumference as an index of adiposity in adults. *Int J Obes* 1997; **21**: 83–9.
13   Maffeis C, Pietrobelli A, Grezzani A, *et al.* Waist circumference and cardiovascular risk factors in prepubertal children. *Obes Res* 2001; **9**: 179–87.
14   Zannolli R, Morgese G. Waist percentiles: a simple test for atherogenic disease? *Acta Paediatr* 1996; **85**: 1368–9.
15   Morenoa LA, Fleta J, Mur L, *et al.* Waist circumference values in Spanish children – gender-related differences. *Eur J Clin* 1999; **53**: 429–33.
16   McCarthy HD, Jarrett KV, Crawley HF. The development of waist circumference percentiles in British children aged 5.0-16.9y. *Eur J Clin Nutr* 2001; **55**: 902–7.
17   Wang J, Thornton JC, Russell M, *et al.* Asians have lower body mass index (BMI) but higher percent body fat than do whites: comparison of anthropometric measurements. *Am J Clin Nutr* 1994; **60**: 23–8.
◆ 18   WHO Expert Consultation. Appropriate body-mass index for Asian populations and its implications for policy and intervention strategies. *Lancet* 2004; **363**: 157–63.
19   Goran MI, Gower BA. Relation between visceral fat and disease risk in children and adolescents. *Am J Clin Nutr* 1999; **70**: 149S–56S.
20   Troiano RP, Flegal KM. Overweight children and adolescents: description, epidemiology and demographics. *Pediatrics* 1998; **(Suppl 2)**: 497–504.
21   Lazarus R, Wake M, Hesketh K, Waters E. Change in body mass index in Australian primary school children, 1985-1997. *Int J Obes* 2000; **24**: 679–84.
22   McCarthy HD, Ellis SM, Cole TJ. Central overweight and obesity in British youth aged 11-16 years: cross sectional surveys of waist circumference. *BMJ* 2003; **326**: 624.
● 23   Wang Y, Monteiro C, Popkin BM. Trends of obesity and underweight in older children and adolescents in the United States, Brazil, China, and Russia. *Am J Clin Nutr* 2002; **75**: 971–7.
24   Strauss RS, Pollack HA. Epidemic increase in childhood overweight, 1986-1998. *JAMA* 2001; **286**: 2845–8.
25   Danielzik S, Czerwinski-Mast M, Langnase K, *et al.* Parental overweight, socioeconomic status and high birth weight are the major determinants of overweight and obesity in 5-7 year-old children: baseline data of the Kiel Obesity Prevention Study (KOPS). *Int J Obes* 2004; **28**: 1494–502.
26   Jebb SA, Rennie KL, Cole TJ. Prevalence of overweight and obesity among young people in Great Britain. *Pub Health Nutr* 2004; **7**: 461–5.

27 Klein-Platat C, Wagner A, Haan MC, et al. Prevalence and sociodemographic determinants of overweight in young French adolescents. Diabetes Metab Res Rev 2003; 19: 153–8.

28 Caballero B. A nutrition paradox – underweight and obesity in developing countries. N Engl J Med 2005; 352: 1514–6.

◆ 29 Ebbeling CB, Pawlak DB, Ludwig DS, Childhood obesity: Public health crisis, common sense cure. Lancet 2002; 360: 473–82.

◆ 30 Must A, Strauss RS. Risks and consequences of childhood and adolescent obesity. Int J Obesity 1999; 23(Suppl 2): S2–S11.

● 31 Freedman DS, Dietz WH, Srinivasan SR, Berenson GS. The relation of overweight to cardiovascular risk factors among children and adolescents: The Bogalusa Heart Study. Pediatrics 1999; 103: 1175–82.

32 Anonymous. Type 2 diabetes in children and adolescents. American Diabetes Association. Diabetes Care 2000; 23: 381–9.

● 33 Caprio S, Bronson M, Sherwin RS, Rife F. Co-existence of severe insulin resistance and hyperinsulinaemia in pre-adolescent obese children. Diabetologia 1996; 39: 1489–99.

● 34 Weiss R, Dziura J, Burgert TS, et al. Obesity and the metabolic syndrome in children and adolescents. N Engl J Med 2004; 350: 2362–74.

35 Pinhas-Hamiel O, Dolan LM, Daniels SR, et al. Increased incidence of non-insulin-dependent diabetes mellitus among adolescents. J Pediatr 1996; 128: 608–15.

● 36 Fagot-Campagna A, Pettitt DJ, Engelgau MM, et al. Type 2 diabetes among North American children and adolescents: an epidemiologic review and a public health perspective. J Pediatr 2000; 136: 664–72.

37 Reaven GM. Banting lecture 1988. Role of insu in resistance in human disease. Diabetes 1988; 37: 1595–607.

38 Zimmet PZ, Alberti KGMM, Shaw JE. Mainstreaming the metabolic syndrome: a definitive definition. Med J Aust 2005; 183: 175–6

39 International Diabetes Federation. The IDF consensus worldwide definition of the metabolic syndrome. Brussels: IDF, 2005. Available at: http://www.idf.org/webdata/docs/ IDF_ Metasyndrome_definition.pdf (accessed May 2005).

40 Gustat J, Elkasaany A, Srinivasan S, Berenson GS. Relation of abdominal height to cardiovascular risk factors in young adults: the Bogalusa heart study. Am J Epidemiol 2000; 151: 885–91.

● 41 De Ferranti SD, Gauvreau K, Ludwig DS, et al. Prevalence of the metabolic syndrome in American adolescents: findings from the Third National Health and Nutrition Examination Survey. Circulation 2004; 110: 2494–7.

42 Driscoll DA. Polycystic ovary syndrome in adolescence. Semin Reprod Med 2003; 21: 301–7.

43 Norman RJ, Davies MJ, Lord J, Moran LJ. The role of lifestyle modification in polycystic ovary syndrome. Trends Endocrinol Metab 2002; 13: 251–7.

44 Hermanns-Le T, Scheen A, Pierard GE. Acanthosis nigricans associated with insulin resistance: pathophysiology and management. Am J Dermatol 2004; 5: 199–203.

45 Cheung YB, Machin D, Karlberg J, Khoo KS. A longitudinal study of pediatric body mass index values predicted health in middle age. J Clin Epidmiol 2004; 57: 1316–22.

● 46 Srinivasan SR, Myers L, Berenson GS. Predictability of childhood adiposity and insulin for developing insulin resistance syndrome (syndrome X) in young adulthood: The Bogalusa Heart Study. Diabetes 2002; 51: 204–9.

47 Chu NF. Prevalence and trends of obesity among school children in Taiwan – the Taipei Children Heart Study. Int J Obesity 2001; 25: 170–6.

48 Woo KS, Chook P, Yu CW, et al. Overweight in children is associated with arterial endothelial dysfunction and intima-media thickening. Int J Obesity 2004; 28: 852–7.

49 Mahoney LT, Lauer RM, Lee J, Clarke WR. Factors affecting tracking of coronary heart disease risk factors in children. The Muscatine Study. Ann NY Acad Sci 1991; 623: 120–32.

50 Bao W, Srinivasan SR, Wattigney WA, Berenson GS. Persistence of multiple cardiovascular risk clustering related to syndrome X from childhood to young adulthood. The Bogalusa Heart Study. Arch Intern Med 1994; 154: 1842–7.

51 Davis PH, Dawson JD, Riley WA, Lauer RM. Carotid intimal-medial thickness is related to cardiovascular risk factors measured from childhood through middle age: The Muscatine Study. Circulation 2001; 104: 2815–9.

52 Gunnell DJ, Frankel SJ, Nanchahal K, et al. Childhood obesity and adult cardiovascular mortality: A 57-y follow-up study based on the Boyd Orr cohort. Am J Clin Nutr 1998; 67: 1111–8.

● 53 Must A, Jacques PF, Dallal GE, et al. Long-term morbidity and mortality of overweight adolescents. A follow-up of the Harvard Growth Study of 1922 to 1935. New Engl J Med 1992; 327: 1350–5.

54 Hui JM, Kench JG, Chitturi S, et al. Long-term outcomes of cirrhosis in nonalcoholic steatohepatitis compared with hepatitis C. Hepatology 2003; 38: 420–7.

55 Guzzaloni G, Grugni G, Minocci A, et al. Liver steatosis in juvenile obesity: correlations with lipid profile, hepatic biochemical parameters and glycemic and insulinemic responses to an oral glucose tolerance test. Int J Obes 2000; 24: 772–6.

56 Chan DF, Li AM, Chu WC, et al. Hepatic steatosis in obese Chinese children. Int J Obes 2004; 28: 1257–63.

57 Fishbein MH, Miner M, Mogren C, Chalekson J. The spectrum of fatty liver in obese children and the relationship of serum aminotransferases to severity of steatosis. J Pediatr Gastroenterol Nutr 2003; 36: 54–61.

58 Schwimmer JB, Deutsch R, Rauch JB, et al. Obesity, insulin resistance, and other clinicopathological correlates of pediatric nonalcoholic fatty liver disease. J Pediatr 2003; 143: 500–5.

59 Manton ND, Lipsett J, Moore DJ, et al. Non-alcoholic steatohepatitis in children and adolescents. Med J Aust 2000; 173: 476–9.

60 Erlinger S. Gallstones in obesity and weight loss. *Eur J Gastroenterol Hepatol* 2000; **12**: 1347–52.

61 Honore LH. Cholesterol cholelithiasis in adolescent females: its connection with obesity, parity, and oral contraceptive use – a retrospective study of 31 cases. *Arch Surg* 1980; **115**: 62–4.

62 Schweizer P, Lenz MP, Kirschner HJ. Pathogenesis and symptomatology of cholelithiasis in childhood. A prospective study. *Digest Surgery* 2000; **17**: 459–67.

◆ 63 French SA, Story M, Perry CL. Self-esteem and obesity in children and adolescents: a literature review. *Obes Res* 1995; **3**: 479–90.

64 Hill AJ, Silver EK. Fat, friendless and unhealthy: 9 year old children's perception of body shape stereotypes. *Int J Obes* 1995; **19**: 423–30.

65 Phillips RG, Hill AJ. Fat, plain, but not friendless: self-esteem and peer acceptance of obese pre-adolescent girls. *Int J Obesity* 1998; **22**: 287–93.

66 Freidman MA, Wilfley DE, Pike KM, *et al.* The relationship between weight and psychological functioning among adolescent girls. *Obes Res* 1995; **57**: 57–62.

67 Janssen I, Craig WM, Boyce WF, Pickett W. Associations between overweight and obesity with bullying behaviors in school-aged children. *Pediatrics* 2004; **113**: 1187–94.

68 Schwimmer JB, Burwinkle TM, Varni JW. Health-related quality of life of severely obese children and adolescents. *JAMA* 2003; **289**: 1813–9.

69 Williams J, Wake M, Hesketh K, *et al.* Health-related quality of life of overweight and obese children. *JAMA* 2005; **293**: 70–6.

● 70 Gortmaker SL, Must A, Perrin JM, *et al.* Social and economic consequences of overweight in adolescence and young adulthood. *N Engl J Med* 1993; **329**: 1008–12.

71 Viner RM, Cole TJ. Adult socioeconomic, educational, social, and psychological outcomes of childhood obesity: a national birth cohort study. *BMJ* 2005: **330**; 1354.

72 Loder RT. The demographics of slipped capital femoral epiphysis. An international multicenter study. *Clin Orthop* 1996; **322**: 8–27.

73 Dietz WH Jr, Gross WL, Kirkpatrick JA Jr. Blount disease (tibia vara): another skeletal disorder associated with childhood obesity. *J Pediatr* 1982; **101**: 735–7.

74 Henderson RC, Greene WB. Etiology of late-onset tibia vara: is varus alignment a prerequisite? *J Pediatr Orthoped* 1994; **14**: 143–6.

75 Goulding A, Taylor RW, Jones IE, *et al.* Overweight and obese children have low bone mass and area for their weight. *Int J Obes* 2000; **24**: 627–32.

76 Timm NL, Grupp-Phelan J, Ho ML. Chronic ankle morbidity in obese children following an acute ankle injury. *Arch Pediatr Adol Med* 2005; **159**: 33–6.

77 Dowling AM, Steel JR, Baur LA. Does obesity influence foot structure and plantar pressure patterns in prepubescent children? *Int J Obes* 2001; **25**: 845–52.

78 Galvin JA, Van Stavern GP. Clinical characterization of idiopathic intracranial hypertension at the Detroit Medical Center. *J Neurol Sci* 2004; **223**: 157–60.

79 Scott IU, Siatkowski RM, Brodsky MC, Lam BL. Idiopathic intracranial hypertension in children and adolescents. *Am J Ophthalmol* 1997; **124**: 253–5.

80 Belmarich PF, Luder E, Kattan M, *et al.* Do obese inner-city children with asthma have more symptoms than nonobese children with asthma? *Pediatrics* 2000; **106**: 1436–41.

81 Gilliland FD, Berhane K, Islam T, *et al.* Obesity and the risk of newly diagnosed asthma in school-age children. *Am J Epidemiol* 2003; **158**: 406–15.

82 Reybrouck T, Mertens L, Schepers D, *et al.* Assessment of cardiorespiratory exercise function in obese children and adolescents by body mass-independent parameters. *Eur J Appl Physiol Occup Physiol* 1997; **75**: 478–83.

83 Ng DK, Lam YY, Kwok KL, Chow PY. Obstructive sleep apnoea syndrome and obesity in children. *Hong Kong Med J* 2004; **10**: 44–8.

84 Redline S, Tishler PV, Schluchter M, *et al.* Risk factors for sleep-disordered breathing in children. Associations with obesity, race, and respiratory problems. *Am J Resp Crit Care Med* 1999; **159**: 1527–32.

85 de la Eva RC, Baur LA, Donaghue K, Waters KA. Metabolic correlates with obstructive sleep apnea. *J Pediatr* 2002; **140**: 654–9.

86 Riley DJ, Santiago TV, Edelman NH. Complications of obesity-hypoventilation syndrome in childhood. *Am J Dis Child* 1976; **130**: 671–4.

● 87 Whitaker RC, Wright JA, Pepe MS, *et al.* Predicting obesity in young adulthood from childhood and parental obesity. *New Engl J Med* 1997; **337**: 869–73.

88 Wattigney WA, Webber LS, Srinivasan SR, Berenson GS. The emergence of clinically abnormal levels of cardiovascular disease risk factor variables among young adults: The Bogalusa Heart Study. *Prev Med* 1995; **24**: 617–26.

89 Kvaavik E, Tell GS, Klepp KI. Predictors and tracking of body mass index from adolescence into adulthood: follow-up of 18 to 20 years in the Oslo Youth Study. *Arch Pediatr Adol Med* 2003; **157**: 1212–8.

90 Barsh GS, Schwartz MW. Genetic approaches to studying energy balance: perception and integration. *Nat Rev Genet* 2002; **3**: 589–600.

91 Spiegelman BM, Flier JS. Obesity and the regulation of energy balance. *Cell* 2001; **104**: 531–43.

◆ 92 Bell CG, Walley AJ, Froguel P. The genetics of human obesity. *Nat Rev Genet* 2005; **6**: 221–34.

93 Bouchard C, Perusse L. Genetic aspects of obesity. *Ann NY Acad Sci* 1993; **699**: 26–35.

● 94 Stunkard AJ, Harris JR, Pederson NL, McClearn GE. The body-mass index of twins who have been reared apart. *N Engl J Med* 1990; **322**: 1483–7.

95 Price RA, Gottesman II. Body fat in identical twins reared apart: roles for genes and environments. *Behav Genetics* 1991; **21**: 1–7.

◆ 96 Perusse L, Rankinen T, Zuberu A, *et al.* The human obesity gene map: 2004 update. *Obesity Res* 2005; **13**: 381–490.

◆ 97 Obesity Gene Map Database. http://obesitygene.pbrc.edu/

● 98 Montague CT, Farooqi IS, Whitehead JP, *et al.* Congenital leptin deficiency is associated with severe early-onset obesity. *Nature* 1997; **387**: 903–8.

99 Gibson WT, Farooqi IS, Moreau M, *et al.* Congenital leptin deficiency due to homozygosity for the Delta133G mutation: report of another case and evaluation of response to four years of leptin therapy. *J Clin Endocrinol Metab* 2004; **89**: 4821–6.

100 Hinney A, Schmidt A, Nottebom K, *et al.* Several mutations in the melanocortin-4 receptor gene including a nonsense and a frameshift mutation associated with dominantly inherited obesity in humans. *J Clin Endocrinol Metab* 1999; **84**: 1483–6.

101 Vaisse C, Clement K, Durand E, *et al.* Melanocortin-4 receptor mutations are a frequent and heterogeneous cause of morbid obesity. *J Clin Invest* 2000; **106**: 253–62.

102 Farooqi IS, Yeo GS, Keogh JM, *et al.* Dominant and recessive inheritance of morbid obesity associated with melanocortin 4 receptor deficiency. *J Clin Invest* 2000; **106**: 271–9.

● 103 Farooqi IS, Keogh JM, Yeo GS, *et al.* Clinical spectrum of obesity and mutations in the melanocortin 4 receptor gene. *N Engl J Med* 2003; **48**: 1085–95.

104 Butler AA, Cone RD. Knockout studies defining different roles for melanocortin receptors in energy homeostasis. *Ann NY Acad Sci* 2003; **994**: 240–5.

105 OMIM – Online Mendelian Inheritance in Man. http://www.ncbi.nlm.nih.gov/entrez/query.fcgi?db=OMIM

◆ 106 World Health Organization. *Diet, Nutrition and the Prevention of Chronic Diseases: report of a joint WHO/FAO expert consultation.* WHO technical report series: 916. Geneva: WHO; 2003.

● 107 Dietz WH, Gortmaker SL. Do we fatten our children at the television set? Obesity and television viewing in children and adolescents. *Pediatr* 1985; **75**: 807–12.

◆ 108 Robinson TN. Television viewing and childhood obesity. *Pediatr Clin North Am* 2001; **48**: 1017–25.

● 109 Reilly JJ, Armstrong J, Dorosty AR, *et al.* Avon Longitudinal Study of Parents and Children Study Team. Early life risk factors for obesity in childhood: cohort study. *BMJ* 2005; **330**: 1357.

● 110 Robinson TN. Reducing children's television viewing to prevent obesity: a randomized controlled trial. *JAMA* 1999; **282**: 1561–7.

◆ 111 Cook KA, Tucker KL. Television and children's consumption patterns. A review of the literature. *Minerva Paediatr* 2002; **54**: 423–36.

112 Klesges RC, Shelton ML, Klesges LM. Effects of television viewing on metabolic rate: potential implications for childhood obesity. *Pediatr* 1993; **91**: 281–6.

◆ 113 Astrup A, Grunwald GK, Melanson EL, *et al.* The role of low-fat diets in body weight control: a meta-analysis of *ad libitum* dietary intervention. *Int J Obes* 2000; **24**: 1545–52.

● 114 Ludwig DS, Peterson KE, Gortmaker SL. Relation between consumption of sugar-sweetened drinks and childhood obesity: a prospective, observational analysis. *Lancet* 2001; **357**: 505–8.

115 French SA, Story M, Neumark-Sztainer D, *et al.* Fast food restaurant use among adolescents: associations with nutrient intake, food choices and behavioral and psychosocial variables. *Int J Obes* 2001; **25**: 1823–33.

116 Thompson OM, Ballew C, Resnicow K, *et al.* Food purchased away from home as a predictor of change in BMI z-score among girls. *Int J Obes* 2004; **28**: 282–9.

117 Ball K, Brown W, Crawford D. Who does not gain weight? Prevalence and predictors of weight maintenance in young women. *Int J Obes* 2002; **26**: 1570–8.

◆ 118 Arenz S, Ruckerl R, Koletzko B, von Kries R. Breast-feeding and childhood obesity – a systematic review. *Int J Obes* 2004; **28**: 1247–56.

◆ 119 Faith MS, Scanlon KS, Birch LL, *et al.* Parent-child feeding strategies and their relationships to child eating and weight status. *Obes Res* 2004; **12**: 1711–22.

◆ 120 Jebb SA, Moore MS. Contribution of a sedentary lifestyle and inactivity to the etiology of overweight and obesity: current evidence and research issues. *Med Sci Sports Exerc* 1999; **31(Suppl 11)**: S534–41.

121 Steinbeck KS. The importance of physical activity in the prevention of overweight and obesity in childhood: a review and an opinion. *Obes Rev* 2001; **2**: 117–30.

122 Klesges RC, Klesges LM, Eck LH, Shelton ML. A longitudinal analysis of accelerated weight-gain in preschool-children. *Pediatrics* 1995; **95**: 126–30.

123 Moore LL, Nguyen USDT, Rothman KJ, *et al.* Preschool physical-activity level and change in body fatness in young-children – the Framingham Childrens Study. *Am J Epidemiol* 1995; **142**: 982–8.

● 124 Rolland-Cachera MF, Deheeger M, Bellisle F, *et al.* Adiposity rebound in children: a simple indicator for predicting obesity. *Am J Clin Nutr* 1984; **39**: 129–35.

125 Cutting TM, Fisher JO, Grimm-Thomas K, Birch LL. Like mother, like daughter: familial patterns of overweight are mediated by mother's dietary disinhibition. *Am J Clin Nutr* 1999; **69**: 608–13.

126 Hood MY, Moore LL, Sundarajan-Ramamurti A, *et al.* Parental attitudes and the development of obesity in children: the Framingham Children's Study. *Int J Obes* 2000; **24**: 1319–25.

127 Reilly JJ, Kelly A, Ness P, *et al.* Premature adiposity rebound in children treated for acute lymphoblastic leukaemia. *J Clin Endocrinol Metab* 2001; **86**: 2775–8.

128 Jallon P, Picard F. Bodyweight gain and anticonvulsants: a comparative review. *Drug Saf* 2001; **24**: 969–78.

129 Virk S, Schwartz TL, Jindal S, *et al.* Psychiatric medication induced obesity: an aetiologic review. *Obes Rev* 2004; **5**: 167–70.

❋ 130 National Guideline Clearinghouse Guideline Synthesis. Overweight and obesity in children and adolescents: assessment, prevention, and management. http://www.guideline.gov/Compare/comparison.aspx?file=OBESITY2_Child.inc

＊ 131 National Health and Medical Research Council. Clinical Practice Guidelines for the Management of Overweight and Obesity. Canberra: Commonwealth of Australia, 2003. Web address: www.obesityguidelines.gov.au

◆ 132 Dietz WH, Robinson TN. Overweight children and adolescents. *N Engl J Med* 2005; **352**: 2100–9.

133 Norton K, Olds T, eds. *Anthropometrica*. Sydney: University of NSW Press; 1996.

134 Ingelfinger JR. Pediatric antecedents of adult cardiovascular disease – awareness and intervention. *N Engl J Med* 2004; **350**: 2123–6.

◆ 135 Summerbell CD, Ashton V, Campbell KJ, *et al*. Interventions for treating obesity in children (Cochrane Review). *Cochrane Database Systematic Reviews* 2003, Issue 3. Art No: CD001872. DOI: 10.1002/14651858.CD001872

◆ 136 Glenny A-M, O'Meara S, Melville A, *et al*. The treatment and prevention of obesity: a systematic review of the literature. *Int J Obes* 1997; **21**: 715–37.

◆ 137 McLean N, Griffin S, Toney K, Hardeman W. Family involvement in weight control, weight maintenance and weight-loss interventions: a systematic review of randomised trials. *Int J Obes* 2003; **27**: 987–1005.

● 138 Epstein LH, Valoski A, Wing RR, McCurley J. Ten-year follow-up of behavioural, family-based treatment for obese children. *JAMA* 1990; **264**: 2519–23.

139 Nuutinen O, Knip M. Predictors of weight reduction in obese children. *Eur J Clin Nutr* 1992; **46**: 785–94.

● 140 Golan M, Weizman A, Apter A, Fainaru M. Parents as the exclusive agents of change in the treatment of childhood obesity. *Am J Clin Nutr* 1998; **67**: 1130–5.

● 141 Golan M, Fainaru M, Weizman A. Role of behaviour modification in the treatment of childhood obesity with the parents as the exclusive agents of change. *Int J Obes* 1998; **22**: 1217–24.

● 142 Golan M, Crow S. Targeting parents exclusively in the treatment of childhood obesity: long-term results. *Obes Res* 2004; **12**: 357–61.

143 Brownell KD, Kelman JH, Stunkard AJ. Treatment of obese children with and without their mothers. *Pediatrics* 1983; **71**: 515–23.

144 Mellin LM, Slinkard LA, Irwin CE. Adolescent obesity intervention: validation of the SHAPEDOWN program. *J Am Diet Assoc* 1987; **87**: 333–8.

145 Coates TJ, Jeffery RW, Slinkard LA, *et al*. Frequency of contact and monetary reward in weight loss, lipid change and blood pressure reduction in adolescents. *Behav Ther* 1982; **13**: 175–85.

146 Berkowitz RI, Wadden TA, Tershakovec AM, Cronquist JL. Behaviour therapy and sibutramine for the treatment of adolescent obesity: a randomized controlled trial. *JAMA* 2003; **289**: 1805–12.

147 Ebbeling CB, Leidig MM, Sinclair KB, *et al*. A reduced-glycemic load diet in the treatment of adolescent obesity. *Arch Pediatr Adolesc Med* 2003; **157**: 773–9.

148 Saelens BE, Sallis JF, Wilfley DE, *et al*. Behavioral weight control for overweight adolescents initiated in primary care. *Obes Res* 2002; **10**: 22–32.

149 Godoy-Matos A, Carraro L, Vieira A, *et al*. Treatment of obese adolescents with sibutramine: a randomized, double-blind, controlled study. *J Clin Endocrinol Metab* 2005; **90**: 1460–5.

150 Chanoine JP, Hampl S, Jensen C, *et al*. Effect of orlistat on weight and body composition in obese adolescents: a randomized controlled trial. *JAMA* 2005; **293**: 2873–83.

◆ 151 Shaw K, O'Rourke P, Del Mar C, Kenardy J. Psychological interventions for overweight or obesity. *The Cochrane Database of Systematic Reviews* 2005, Issue 2. Art. No.: CD003818. DOI: 10.1002/14651858.CD003818.pub2.

152 Epstein LH, Paluch RA, Kilanowski CK, Raynor HA. The effect of reinforcement or stimulus control to reduce sedentary behavior in the treatment of pediatric obesity. *Health Psychol* 2004; **23**: 371–80.

153 Epstein LH, Wing RR, Woodall K, *et al*. Effects of family-based behavioural treatment on obese 5-to-8-year-old children. *Behav Ther* 1985; **16**: 205–12.

◆ 154 Pirozzo S, Summerbell C, Cameron C, Glasziou P. Should we recommend low-fat diets for obesity? *Obes Rev* 2003; **4**: 83–90.

◆ 155 Bravata DM, Sanders L, Huang J, *et al*. Efficacy and safety of low-carbohydrate diets: a systematic review. *JAMA* 2003; **289**: 1837–50.

156 Raben A. Should obese patients be counselled to follow a low-glycaemic index diet? No. *Obes Rev* 2002; **3**: 245–56.

157 Pawlak DB, Ebbeling CB, Ludwig DS. Should obese patients be counselled to follow a low-glycaemic index diet? Yes. *Obes Rev* 2002; **3**: 235–43.

158 Whitaker RC. Obesity prevention in pediatric primary care: four behaviors to target. *Arch Pediatr Adolesc Med* 2003; **157**: 725–7.

159 Polivy J. Psychological consequences of food restriction. *J Am Diet Assoc* 1996; **96**: 593–4.

◆ 160 Miller WC, Koceja DM, Hamilton EJ. A meta-analysis of the past 25 years of weight loss research using diet, exercise or diet plus exercise intervention. *Int J Obes* 1997; **21**: 941–7.

● 161 McGuire MT, Wing RR, Klem ML, Hill JO. Behavioral strategies of individuals who have maintained long-term weight losses. *Obes Res* 1999; **7**: 334–41.

◆ 162 Epstein LH, Goldfield GS. Physical activity in the treatment of overweight and childhood obesity. *Med Sci Sports Exerc* 1999; **31**: S553–9.

● 163 Epstein LH, Wing RR, Koeske R, *et al*. A comparison of lifestyle change and programmed exercise on weight and fitness changes in obese children. *Behav Ther* 1982; **13**: 651–65.

● 164 Epstein LH, Valoski A, Wing RR, *et al*. Ten year outcomes of behavioural family-based treatment for childhood obesity. *Health Psychol* 1994; **13**: 373–83.

165 Epstein LH, Paluch RA, Gordy CC, Dorn J. Decreasing sedentary behaviors in treating pediatric obesity. *Arch Pediatr Adolesc Med* 2000; **154**: 220–6.

◆ 166 Tsai AG, Wadden TA. Systematic review: an evaluation of major commercial weight loss programs in the United States. *Ann Int Med* 2005; **142**: 56–66.

167   Sothern M, Udall JN Jr, Suskind RM, *et al.* Weight loss and growth velocity in obese children after very low calorie diet, exercise, and behavior modification. *Acta Paediatr* 2002; **89**: 1036–43.

168   Torgerson JS, Hauptman J, Boldrin MN, Sjostrom L. XENical in the prevention of diabetes in obese subjects (XENDOS) study: a randomized study of orlistat as an adjunct to lifestyle change for the prevention of type 2 diabetes in obese patients. *Diabetes Care* 2004; **27**: 155–61.

169   James WP, Astrup A, Finer N, *et al.* Effect of sibutramine on weight maintenance after weight loss: a randomised controlled trial. STORM Study Group. Sibutramine Trial of Obesity Reduction and Maintenance. *Lancet* 2000; **356**: 2119–25.

170   Freemark M, Bursey D. The effects of metformin on body mass index and glucose tolerance in obese adolescents with fasting hyperinsulinaemia and family history of type 2 diabetes. *Pediatrics* 2001; **107**: e55.

171   Kay JP, Alemzxadeh R, Langley G, *et al.* Beneficial effect of metformin in normoglycaemic morbidly obese adolescents. *Metabolism* 2001; **50**: 1457–61.

◆ 172   Buchwald H, Avidor Y, Braunwald E, *et al.* Bariatric surgery: a systematic review and meta-analysis. *JAMA* 2004; **292**: 1724–37.

173   Inge TH, Garcia V, Daniels S, *et al.* A multidisciplinary approach to the adolescent bariatric surgical patient. *J Pediatr Surg* 2004; **39**: 442–7.

174   Capella JF, Capella RF. Bariatric surgery in adolescence. Is this the best age to operate? *Obesity Surg* 2003; **13**: 826–32.

175   Inge TH, Krebs NF, Garcia VF, *et al.* Bariatric surgery for severely overweight adolescents: concerns and recommendations. *Pediatrics* 2004; **114**: 217–23.

176   Barlow SE. Bariatric surgery in adolescents: For treatment failures or health care system failures? *Pediatrics* 2004; **114**: 252–3.

177   Wiittigrove AC. Surgery for severely obese adolescents: Further insight from the American Society for Bariatric Surgery. *Pediatrics* 2004; **114**: 253–4.

178   Rodgers B. Bariatric surgery for adolescents: A view from the the American Pediatric Surgical Association. *Pediatrics* 2004; **114**: 255–6.

◆ 179   Harvey EL, Glenny A-M, Kirk SFL, Summerbell CD. Improving health professionals' management and the organisation of care for overweight and obese people

(Cochrane review). In: *The Cochrane Library*, Issue 2, 1999. Oxford: Update Software.

180   Braet C, van Winckel M, van Leeuwen K. Follow-up results of different treatment programs for obese children. *Acta Paediatr* 1997; **86**: 397–402.

◆ 181   Summerbell CD, Waters E, Edmunds LD, *et al.* Interventions for preventing obesity in children. *Cochrane Database Systematic Reviews.* 2005, Issue 3. Art No: CD001871. DOI: 10.1002/14651858.CD001871. pub2

◆ 182   Cliska D. Interventions to improve nutritional intake in children and youth. In: Thomas H, Ciliska D, Micucci S, *et al.*, eds. *Effectiveness of Physical Activity Enhancement and Obesity Prevention Programs in Children and Youth.* Hamilton, Ontario: Effective Public Health Practice Project, 2004.

◆ 183   Cliska D. Interventions to reduce physical inactivity in children and youth. In: Thomas H, Ciliska D, Micucci S, *et al.*, eds. *Effectiveness of Physical Activity Enhancement and Obesity Prevention Programs in Children and Youth.* Hamilton, Ontario: Effective Public Health Practice Project, 2004.

◆ 184   Thomas H. Interventions to increase physical activity in children and youth. In: Thomas H, Ciliska D, Micucci S, *et al.*, eds. *Effectiveness of Physical Activity Enhancement and Obesity Prevention Programs in Children and Youth.* Hamilton, Ontario: Effective Public Health Practice Project, 2004.

◆ 185   Thomas H. Interventions to increase physical activity and improve nutritional intake in children and youth. In: Thomas H, Ciliska D, Micucci S, *et al.*, eds. *Effectiveness of Physical Activity Enhancement and Obesity Prevention Programs in Children and Youth.* Hamilton, Ontario: Effective Public Health Practice Project, 2004.

◆ 186   Micucci S. Environmental interventions to improve nutrition and increase physical activity in children and youth. In: Thomas H, Ciliska D, Micucci S, *et al.*, eds. *Effectiveness of Physical Activity Enhancement and Obesity Prevention Programs in Children and Youth.* Hamilton, Ontario: Effective Public Health Practice Project, 2004.

● 187   Swinburn B, Egger G, Fezeela R. Dissecting obesogenic environments: the development and application of a framework for identifying and prioritising environmental interventions for obesity. *Prev Med* 1999; **29**: 563–70.

38

Disorders of growth in the child treated for cancer

MARK F H BROUGHAM, W HAMISH B WALLACE, CHRISTOPHER J H KELNAR

EVIDENCE SCORING OF THERAPY

* Non-randomized controlled trials, cohort study, etc.
** One or more well-designed randomized controlled trials

INTRODUCTION

Childhood cancer is relatively rare, with an incidence of between 70 and 160 cases per million children per year.[1] In contrast to the malignancies commonly observed in the adult population, which are predominantly carcinomas involving lung, breast, prostate or colon, cancers diagnosed in the pediatric age group represent a more heterogeneous group. As demonstrated in Fig. 38.1, acute leukaemia represents approximately one third of all childhood cancers, and around one quarter are tumors involving the central nervous system (CNS). Although survival from these malignancies was very poor in the 1960s, major advances, both in treatment, including multi-agent chemotherapy in combination with radiotherapy and surgery, and in supportive care, have resulted in markedly improved rates of cure over recent decades (Fig. 38.2). Indeed, current data suggest that around 75–80 percent of children with cancer will be alive 5 years from diagnosis.[2] As a result, the number of long-term survivors is increasing, and it has been estimated that by the year 2010, about one in 715 of the adult population will have been treated for cancer in childhood.[3]

Because of this, the emphasis in the management of childhood cancer has changed, from 'cure at any cost' to one in which quality of life after treatment has become

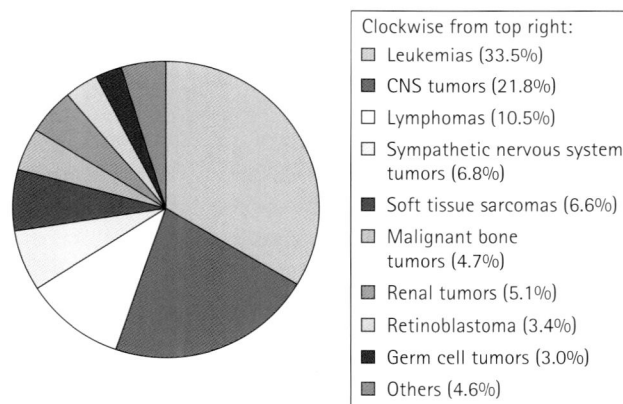

Clockwise from top right:
- Leukemias (33.5%)
- CNS tumors (21.8%)
- Lymphomas (10.5%)
- Sympathetic nervous system tumors (6.8%)
- Soft tissue sarcomas (6.6%)
- Malignant bone tumors (4.7%)
- Renal tumors (5.1%)
- Retinoblastoma (3.4%)
- Germ cell tumors (3.0%)
- Others (4.6%)

Figure 38.1 Relative frequencies of childhood cancers (diagnosed age 14 or below) in Scotland 1975–1999 (Source: Campbell J *et al.* (2004) Childhood cancer in Scotland: trends in incidence, mortality and survival 1975–1999. Edinburgh: Information and Statistics Division.)

increasingly important. Thus whilst continuing to strive for improved survival, attention must be directed towards minimizing the late effects of treatment.

Adverse late effects of childhood cancer treatment are diverse and include growth impairment, disorders of the endocrine system, infertility, abnormalities of cardiac and pulmonary function, renal and hepatic impairment, second malignancies, and cognitive and psychosocial difficulties.

Childhood represents a critical period of growth, particularly within the first year of life and around puberty. Disruption of normal growth during this time may therefore result in permanent impairment, and this has certainly been

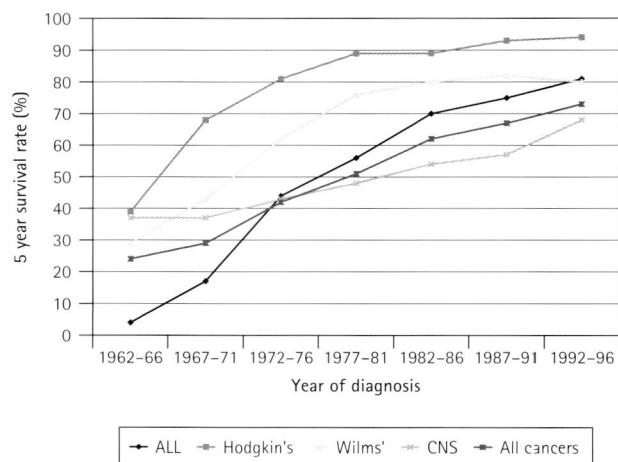

Figure 38.2 Trends in 5-year survival rates (percent) in selected pediatric malignancies from 1962–1996. ALL, acute lymphoblastic leukemia. (Source: National Registry of Childhood Tumours.)

described following treatment for childhood cancer.[4] Normal growth requires a complex interaction between the skeleton, the endocrine system and the overall health of the child, and thus the etiology of poor growth following childhood cancer is usually multi-factorial. However, treatment-related morbidity, secondary to both radiotherapy and chemotherapy, represents the most significant risk factor in this patient group, rather than the underlying pathological diagnosis.

This chapter will focus on the consequences of childhood cancer treatment on growth. Long-term follow-up of these patients is essential, in order that adverse effects are diagnosed early and appropriate counselling and therapeutic intervention is instituted. Awareness of the etiology and prevalence of such late complications will allow modifications of treatment that will improve the quality of life for long-term survivors of childhood cancer.

THE EFFECTS OF RADIOTHERAPY

Radiotherapy can significantly impair growth, either indirectly via disruption of the endocrine system, or via a direct effect on the spine and long bones. Indeed, it is these deleterious effects that limit the use of this therapeutic modality within pediatric oncology, particularly during the first few years of life. However, it does remain an important component of treatment for a number of children, such as those with tumors of the central nervous system (CNS) who may require cranial irradiation, and in the context of conditioning before bone marrow transplantation (BMT) with total body irradiation (TBI).

Hypothalamic–pituitary dysfunction

The hypothalamic–pituitary axis is central to the control of the endocrine system, and therefore disruption of this axis

will have far-reaching consequences, not only on growth but also on other aspects of endocrine function. Cranial irradiation is known to cause hypothalamic–pituitary dysfunction,[5] and the resultant hormone deficiency is dependent on the total dose of radiation received and the fractionation schedule.[6]

Growth hormone (GH) secretion is the most radiosensitive of the pituitary hormones, with doses as low as 18 Gy resulting in GH deficiency.[7] Subsequently, with increasing radiation dose, deficiencies are seen in gonadotrophin, corticotrophin, and thyrotrophin secretion, commonly in that order.[8]

In addition to the dose-dependent effects, hypothalamic–pituitary dysfunction has been demonstrated to become progressively more severe with time since radiation treatment.[8,9] This may, in part, be due to the delayed effects of radiotherapy on the axis as a whole. However, it may also reflect subsequent pituitary dysfunction secondary to earlier hypothalamic damage, as there is increasing evidence that the hypothalamus is more radiosensitive than the pituitary gland.[10]

This latter point has implications with regard to follow-up and investigation of pituitary function. Pituitary function tests currently used rely on pharmacological provocation tests to detect deficiencies. However, there is evidence to suggest that following radiation damage physiological secretion of pituitary hormones is impaired, yet peak responses to provocation tests remain normal.[11,12] This impairment, known as neurosecretory dysfunction, can have clinical significance, particularly during the pubertal growth spurt, when an increased growth hormone secretion is required.

The prevalence of hypopituitarism may therefore be underestimated by standard provocation tests. However, assessment of physiological secretion by overnight profile is difficult in practical terms, and currently remains a research tool. This emphasizes the importance of continued long-term follow-up and clinical vigilance for these patients.

An additional risk factor important in neuroendocrine dysfunction is the age of the child at the time of radiotherapy. There is evidence to suggest that younger children are more sensitive to radiation-induced damage of the hypothalamic–pituitary axis as compared to older children and adults.[13]

Therefore, in summary, pituitary deficiencies are likely to be multiple, and manifest rapidly and completely in younger children, those receiving higher radiation doses or where tumors are centrally positioned. By comparison, deficits may be single, evolve more slowly or be qualitative rather than quantitative in nature following irradiation to more distant tumors or after lower cranial doses. This will result in a cohort of survivors who may require hormone replacement therapy as adults, despite not requiring treatment as children.

Growth hormone deficiency

GH deficiency is the commonest endocrine abnormality following cranial irradiation, and this may contribute to the short stature observed following such treatment. A reduction in final adult height has been documented following cranial and cranio-spinal irradiation,[4] and this is more pronounced with treatment received at a younger age.[14] Although additional factors will certainly contribute to the height loss observed, GH deficiency has an important role.

In addition to effects on height, GH has numerous other physiological roles. Indeed, deficiency of this hormone has also been implicated in causing a reduced lean body mass and increased fat mass,[15] metabolic abnormalities including an adverse lipid profile and impaired glucose tolerance,[16] a reduction in bone mineral density[17] and impaired quality of life.[18]

Whilst many other aspects of both treatment and the disease itself play a role in the deleterious effects listed above, GH deficiency is important, and because of this, replacement with recombinant growth hormone has been advocated. This treatment has resulted in an improved growth response in children with GH deficiency after cranial irradiation.[19**] In addition to the benefits observed in growth, replacement therapy has been demonstrated to reduce fat mass and increase muscle mass, reduce the cardiovascular risk factor profile, increase bone mineral density and improve quality of life.[20-23]

It is therefore now well accepted to treat documented GH deficiency in childhood with replacement doses of recombinant human GH. Unfortunately, the diagnosis of GH deficiency can be problematic, particularly in the early post-irradiation period.[12] Measurements of mean or peak GH secretion will miss deficits confined to qualitative, subtle disturbances in pulsatility and also those in which there is an inability to adequately augment pubertal GH secretion.[24,25] In addition, measurements of insulin-like growth factors and their binding proteins are unreliable indicators of GH secretion in this situation.[26] These difficulties make it imperative that all children are fully assessed following cranial irradiation and GH insufficiency considered.

Due to the evolving nature of GH insufficiency in these children, it is important that treatment with recombinant GH is commenced as early as possible in at risk groups. Indeed, even if the cause of growth impairment is unclear, a trial of GH treatment may be appropriate.

Recombinant GH is usually given as a daily subcutaneous injection. Replacement therapy is normally discontinued once attainment of final height has been achieved. However, given the additional benefits of treatment discussed above, there is some evidence to suggest that replacement therapy, at a reduced dose, should be continued into adulthood.[27**]

Growth hormone, however, is potentially mitogenic, and there have been concerns raised regarding its use in cancer survivors. There was concern that GH therapy could be associated with an increased risk of relapse of leukemia and brain tumors.[28] In addition, a recent report has suggested an increased risk of colorectal cancer in adults treated with human pituitary GH prior to 1985.[29]

Lymphocyte natural killer activity is reduced in some patients with GH deficiency.[30] In addition, lymphocytes possess GH receptors, and therefore if leukemic transformation has occurred GH therapy could potentially accelerate this process. However, much higher concentrations than those used therapeutically are required for this to occur.[31] Indeed, long-term studies of patients treated with physiological replacement doses of recombinant GH have failed to demonstrate any such increased risk,[32-34] although continued surveillance is essential. As discussed above, GH therapy should be commenced early to achieve a maximal response. However, in view of the concerns raised, most centers do not advocate introducing therapy within the first 2 years after cancer treatment, as this is the time of highest relapse rate.

Hypothalamic–pituitary–gonadal axis

Disturbance of the hypothalamic–pituitary–gonadal axis will not only affect gonadal function, but may also disrupt the normal progression of puberty. As pubertal growth is an important determinant of final adult height, this disruption may cause significant long-term consequences.

GONADOTROPHIN DEFICIENCY

With doses of cranial irradiation higher than those associated with GH deficiency, damage to the hypothalamic–pituitary axis can disrupt gonadotrophin secretion. Indeed, patients receiving radiation doses of 35–45 Gy have demonstrated subsequent deficiencies in both follicle stimulating hormone (FSH) and luteinizing hormone (LH) secretion.[6] In addition, as with growth hormone, the prevalence of gonadotrophin deficiency increases with time following irradiation.

The clinical sequelae of gonadotrophin deficiency exhibit a broad spectrum of severity, from subclinical abnormalities detectable only by gonadotrophin releasing hormone (GnRH) testing, to a significant reduction in circulating sex hormone levels and delayed puberty. As discussed earlier, the hypothalamus is more radiosensitive than the pituitary gland and therefore the etiology of hypogonadism in these patients following cranial irradiation is hypothalamic GnRH deficiency.[35*] In view of this, exogenous GnRH can be used as replacement therapy in order to restore gonadal function and fertility.

EARLY AND PRECOCIOUS PUBERTY

In contrast to the situation described above it appears that, paradoxically, lower doses of cranial irradiation can result in premature activation of the hypothalamic–pituitary–gonadal axis, leading to early or precocious puberty. Precocious puberty is defined as the onset of puberty prior to age 8 years in girls and 9 years in boys, whereas early puberty is categorized as onset between 8 and 10 years in girls and 9 and 11 years in boys. The precise etiology of radiation-induced early puberty is thought to be via disinhibition of cortical influences on the hypothalamus.

Before 1992 in the United Kingdom all children with acute lymphoblastic leukemia (ALL) received cranial irradiation as CNS-directed treatment, in order to prevent recurrent CNS disease. The dose used was 18–24 Gy, which is generally lower than that required to treat solid tumors of the CNS. Subsequently, it has been noted that this treatment is associated with a higher incidence of early and precocious puberty, predominantly affecting girls.[36] Indeed, the incidence of early puberty in boys receiving cranial irradiation for ALL is no higher than in the normal population.[37] This is likely to reflect sex differences in the control of the onset of puberty. However, higher doses of cranial irradiation, such as that required for brain tumors can lead to the early onset of puberty in both sexes.[38]

Therefore early puberty as a consequence of cranial irradiation is dose-dependent, and the dose threshold of this effect is gender specific. In addition, with higher doses of irradiation, a patient may enter puberty early but subsequently develop gonadotrophin deficiency as discussed earlier, thus suggesting differential effects of radiotherapy with time. Therefore treatments to delay puberty in this situation should be used with caution.

The timing of pubertal onset is also related to the age of the child at the time of irradiation,[38] with treatment at a younger age resulting in more profound disturbances in the timing of puberty (Fig. 38.3).

The consequence of entering puberty early is a premature pubertal growth spurt followed by early epiphysial fusion and a consequent reduction in final adult height.

As discussed earlier, GH deficiency is common in patients who have received cranial irradiation. Although the duration of puberty is usually normal[14,39] the combination of undiagnosed GH deficiency with early puberty further reduces final height potential by reducing peak height velocity.[39]

In addition to an overall reduction in height, growth in children after treatment is often disproportionate in that much of their height loss is due to a reduction in sitting

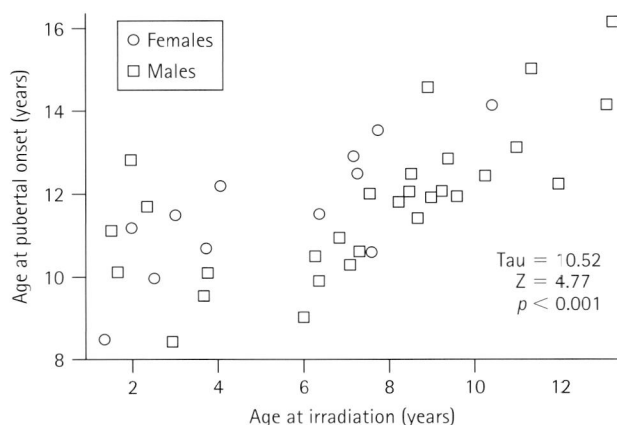

Figure 38.3 Relationship between age at irradiation and age at pubertal onset in 41 children who received cranial/craniospinal irradiation for a brain tumor or irradiation for acute lymphoblastic leukemia.

height.[40] Spinal growth plays an important role during the latter part of the pubertal growth spurt, and early puberty co-incident with undiagnosed GH deficiency clearly has a deleterious effect. In addition, irradiation involving the spine will further disrupt spinal growth, which will only partially respond to GH therapy. It has also been noted that the younger the child is at the time of irradiation the greater the subsequent skeletal disproportion.[41]

As discussed earlier, GH replacement therapy is effective in improving final height. In view of the effects discussed above, if pubertal onset is early it is also advantageous to suppress pubertal progression and delay skeletal fusion with GnRH analogues, in order to ensure height potential can be maximized. Indeed, combined treatment with growth hormone and a GnRH analogue in this situation improves the height prognosis[42*] and final adult height, although the height obtained remains lower than the target height.[43]

It is therefore essential that these patients are followed up indefinitely after treatment with regards to their growth and puberty. This involves 6-monthly clinical assessment of pubertal status and auxology measurements and, when indicated, biochemical assessment of growth hormone and gonadotrophin secretion, and radiological assessment of their bone age.

Thyroid disorders

Thyroid disorders can occur following treatment for childhood cancer, either via disruption of the hypothalamic–pituitary–thyroid axis or following direct damage to the thyroid gland itself. Thyroid function can subsequently be affected, usually with hypothyroidism, which may adversely affect growth. In addition to abnormalities of thyroid function, cancer therapy may also cause thyroid nodules and occasionally secondary thyroid cancer.[44]

Cranial irradiation can disrupt the hypothalamic–pituitary–thyroid axis, resulting in central hypothyroidism.[8] The incidence of radiation induced thyroid stimulating hormone (TSH) deficiency is dose-dependent[6] and, as discussed earlier, this part of the axis appears to be the least vulnerable to radiation damage.[8] In children, disturbances of the hypothalamic–pituitary–thyroid axis are uncommon with doses lower than 40 Gy.[45]

The biochemical diagnosis of central hypothyroidism relies on levels of TSH and thyroid hormone (free T_4). However, there is some evidence to suggest that subtle abnormalities of thyrotrophin secretion, not detected in this manner, can be significant enough to have clinical implications. Thus TSH and free T_4 may fall within the normal range, yet more detailed investigation of TSH dynamics suggests clinically significant central hypothyroidism.[46] This damage may occur at lower doses of irradiation than that suggested above.

The implications of this may be important in deciding thresholds for intervention with thyroxine supplements, and this may be particularly important in the pediatric population as reduced thyroid function may affect growth[47] and physical and intellectual performance. Further investigation is required in order to demonstrate the functional significance of these findings before the criteria for clinical intervention are modified. However, this again demonstrates the importance of follow-up and clinical vigilance in these children after treatment.

Thyroid abnormalities may also occur following direct damage to the thyroid gland itself. This is usually secondary to radiotherapy where the neck falls within the radiation field, including craniospinal irradiation, although chemotherapy can potentiate this radiation-induced damage.[48] Chemotherapy alone rarely affects thyroid function, although damage has been reported following intensive treatment with busulfan and cyclophosphamide,[49] as used for conditioning prior to bone marrow transplantation.

Hypothyroidism is the commonest abnormality following direct thyroid damage,[50] and this is usually initially in the form of compensated hypothyroidism with an elevated TSH and normal thyroxine. Despite this, thyroxine replacement may be justified in order to reduce the theoretical risk of thyroid cancer,[51] thought to be secondary to prolonged stimulation of the thyroid gland. Risk factors for developing hypothyroidism in this manner include higher doses of neck irradiation, female sex and older age at diagnosis. The greatest risk is during the first 5 years following treatment.[50]

Hyperthyroidism is less common but can occur following neck irradiation, with those patients receiving higher doses being at greater risk.[50]

In addition to abnormalities in thyroid function, neoplasms of the thyroid gland, both benign and malignant, are more frequent following irradiation involving the neck.[44,52,53] The risk of developing thyroid neoplasia increases with higher doses of radiotherapy[54] and with younger age at the time of treatment.[55] In addition, females are at higher risk of developing thyroid cancer.[56]

Benign thyroid nodules include adenomas, focal hyperplasia and colloid nodules. Papillary carcinoma is the commonest thyroid cancer that develops secondary to irradiation,[56] which, if detected early, is associated with a high cure rate. Thus long term follow-up of these children must include regular examination of the thyroid gland, and some advocate the use of ultrasound as a screening tool.[57]

Hypothalamic–pituitary–adrenal axis

The hypothalamic–pituitary–adrenal axis appears to be relatively radioresistant.[8] Abnormalities in adrenocorticotrophin hormone (ACTH) or cortisol secretion are uncommon after low dose cranial irradiation.[58] However, ACTH deficiency is potentially life threatening, its symptoms often subtle and it should be considered in patients receiving higher doses of irradiation and in those patients treated for pituitary or closely related tumors.[8] Life-long

replacement is necessary and is particularly problematic if posterior pituitary dysfunction is also present, such as after craniopharyngiomas.

As with the assessment of thyroid function, the incidence of abnormalities may be underestimated due to the diagnostic difficulty in evaluating the hypothalamic–pituitary–adrenal axis. In addition, clinical signs of cortisol deficiency can be non-specific and thus the diagnosis may be missed. The insulin tolerance test is regarded as the gold standard but can be problematic, particularly in the pediatric population due to the consequences of severe hypoglycemia. Excessive tiredness in a patient who has received cranial irradiation should warrant testing of the hypothalamic–pituitary–adrenal axis. Hydrocortisone replacement is essential, and increased doses are required for intercurrent illness and surgery.

Direct radiotherapy-induced effects

Whilst radiotherapy can result in endocrine disorders, which can in turn impair growth, it can also result in direct damage to the skeletal system. Radiotherapy that includes either the spine or the long bones within its field may therefore also compromise growth.

Spinal growth plays an important role in determining final height. Radiotherapy involving the spine, including cranio-spinal irradiation, total body irradiation, and thoracic or abdominal irradiation, may affect this growth, thereby reducing final adult height.[41,59,60]

Radiotherapy causes permanent disruption of the epiphyses, and the consequence of this on spinal growth results in skeletal disproportion, with a greater reduction in sitting height as compared to leg length. This effect is more pronounced the younger the child is at the time of treatment.[41] Cranial irradiation alone can also result in skeletal disproportion[40] due to the endocrine effects discussed earlier, although the consequences are less pronounced (Fig. 38.4).

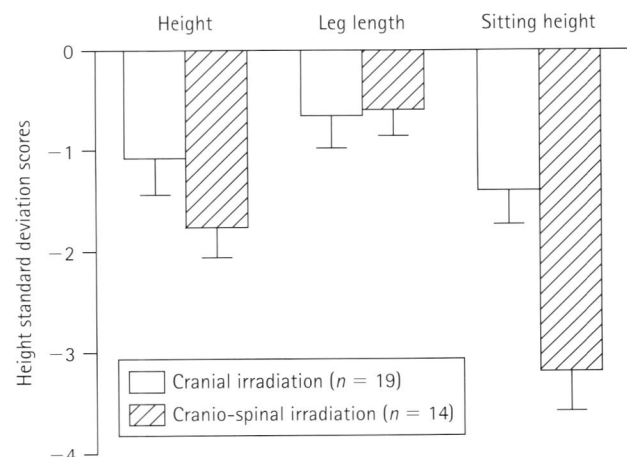

Figure 38.4 Adult height without endocrine therapy of 33 patients irradiated in childhood for brain tumors.

Scoliosis and kyphosis have long been recognized as complications of radiotherapy involving the spine.[61] However, with more modern techniques, in particular the use of megavoltage radiotherapy and symmetrical irradiation of the vertebral bodies, these complications are less frequent[62] although may still occur as radiotherapy can cause asymmetry of the paraspinal muscles.

Thus radiotherapy can have a detrimental effect on spinal growth, and therefore sitting height and spinal curvature should be routinely examined as part of the follow-up for these patients.

In a similar manner, localized radiotherapy can disrupt the growth of a particular area of the body that falls within the radiation field.[63] This may result in skeletal hypoplasia and atrophy of overlying soft tissue, and this can involve areas of the head and neck[63] or the extremities.[64] Whilst this may not affect overall growth, the problems encountered as a result can have a devastating impact upon the child.

Total radiotherapy dose and growth failure

As discussed above, the effects of radiotherapy are dependent upon the age of the patient at the time of treatment, the field of treatment and the dose received. The effects of varying doses on the endocrine system, and subsequently growth, are summarized in Table 38.1.

THE EFFECTS OF CHEMOTHERAPY

As can be seen from the preceding discussion, radiotherapy received during childhood can result in significant, and often permanent, growth impairment. However, although

Table 38.1 Effects of varying doses of radiation on the endocrine system

Dose (Gy)	Effect
Cranial/craniospinal irradiation	
<24	Early puberty GH insufficiency in context of pubertal growth spurt
>24	Early or delayed puberty GH deficiency within 5 years
≈54	GH deficiency within 2 years TSH deficiency
Total body irradiation	
7.5–15.75	GH insufficiency (particularly at puberty) – thyroid dysfunction (direct thyroid damage) Radiation-induced skeletal dysplasia

GH, growth hormone; TSH, thyroid stimulating hormone.

this therapeutic modality is used widely within a number of patient groups, the majority of children with cancer can achieve cure with multi-agent chemotherapy, without the need for additional cytotoxic treatments. Chemotherapeutic agents are, however, also associated with significant toxicity. Indeed because, in general, they target rapidly dividing cells, normal growth and bone activity may also be affected.[65,66]

The impact of chemotherapy on growth

Growth has been extensively studied during and after treatment for acute lymphoblastic leukemia (ALL). ALL is the commonest childhood malignancy and, unlike many other cancers, is treated with ongoing chemotherapy of varying intensity over a prolonged period of time. With current protocols in the United Kingdom, treatment lasts for at least 2 years, extending up to 3 years in boys. Prior to 1992 cranial radiotherapy, to prevent CNS disease, was part of the management for all children with ALL. This is no longer used routinely and therefore the majority of patients will now receive chemotherapy alone in the treatment of their malignancy.

Growth deceleration has been demonstrated during treatment for ALL, and this effect is most marked during the first year of treatment[67] and in younger children.[68] Different studies have reported growth decelerations of varying severity. Kirk et al.[69] reported significant growth retardation following treatment for ALL, with a mean standing height standard deviation score (SDS) of −1.37 six years after diagnosis, compared with −0.44 observed by Clayton et al.[67] after the same time period. Varying intensities of chemotherapy protocols are likely to explain these differences, with patients from the former study having received treatment with the more intensive LSA2L2 protocol.

Obviously many of the longer term studies, such as those discussed above, include children who received radiotherapy in addition to chemotherapy, and as previously noted this will have a detrimental effect on growth. However, studies investigating the role of chemotherapy alone have also demonstrated an impact on growth, although the magnitude of this effect is less marked.[70,71]

The impact of chemotherapy on the growth of long bones has been demonstrated by measurement of lower leg length during different phases of treatment for ALL.[72] In this study growth of the lower leg was effectively stopped during periods of intensive chemotherapy. With less intensive 'maintenance' chemotherapy the growth returned to a rate comparable to that of healthy children, and this was followed by a compensatory 'catch-up' period of accelerated growth velocity following cessation of treatment.

Thus catch-up growth does occur but only after chemotherapy is stopped which, as discussed above, may be up to 3 years after diagnosis. However, there is evidence to suggest that this catch-up growth tends to be complete in patients that receive chemotherapy alone, whereas those who have received radiotherapy still have a sub-optimal final height in adulthood.[73,74]

Bone metabolism

Bone development is maximal during puberty, and peak bone mass is reached at around 20 years of age.[75] This can be disrupted by childhood cancer and its treatment. Indeed, a reduced bone mineral density (BMD), as measured by surrogate two-dimensional measures on dual X-ray absorptiometry (DEXA) scans, has been demonstrated after treatment for childhood ALL[76*] and other malignancies.[77*] These surrogate measures need interpreting with care but any reduction in BMD is important. The etiology of this is likely to be multi-factorial and secondary to both the disease itself as well as its treatment. This can involve alterations in calcium absorption, vitamin D metabolism, insulin-like growth factors and their binding proteins, hypogonadism, and growth hormone deficiency.[78–82]

Various bone markers can be measured in order to assess the impact of chemotherapy on the dynamics of bone turnover and growth. In a prospective study of 22 children with ALL, markers of bone formation, bone resorption, soft tissue turnover, and the growth hormone axis were measured.[78] At diagnosis bone turnover was low, probably secondary to growth hormone resistance associated with the disease itself. During intensive phases of chemotherapy there was further suppression of the markers of bone and soft tissue turnover. However, these markers increased dramatically during periods of less intensive treatment.

Of the chemotherapeutic agents used, steroids and methotrexate have been particularly implicated in playing a pathological role in bone homeostasis.[78] Steroids cause retardation of bone growth, both directly by decreasing osteoblast activity and turnover, and indirectly by altering calcium homeostasis.[83,84] Decreased intestinal absorption and increased urinary excretion of calcium causes secondary hyperparathyroidism and consequently, bone resorption. Methotrexate also inhibits bone growth, probably via inhibition of osteoblast proliferation and differentiation, secondary to folate deficiency.[85,86] In addition to chemotherapy, radiotherapy can also result in reduced bone mineral density. This is most commonly observed in the context of growth hormone deficiency following cranial irradiation.[82]

Because altered bone homeostasis can result in osteopenia, these patients may develop premature osteoporosis, and possibly pathological fractures in later life.[77*,87] Assessment of calcium status and BMD at the end of treatment should enable early identification of those patients with impaired skeletal development, and thus allow the institution of potential therapeutic interventions. Nutritional support, including ensuring an adequate calcium intake, exercise to optimize body weight and physical fitness, and medical intervention with calcitonin, vitamin D,

and bisphosphonate treatment may all improve the BMD in these patients.[76*,77*]

ADDITIONAL FACTORS AFFECTING GROWTH

As discussed, both radiotherapy and chemotherapy received during childhood can result in impaired growth. However, although treatment related morbidity has the most significant impact in this regard, a number of additional factors may also play a role, either directly or indirectly disrupting normal growth and bone metabolism.

Firstly, the disease process itself may lead to growth impairment. This may be demonstrated at diagnosis, although patients with overt cachexia are unusual in the context of pediatric oncology. In addition, tumor recurrence may present as poor growth. Bone metabolism may also be affected by malignancy, particularly in patients with leukemia, as infiltration and expansion of the bone marrow spaces with leukemic cells can destroy the spongiosa. In addition, the leukemic cells themselves may secrete factors such as osteoblast inhibiting factor and parathyroid hormone related peptide, further contributing to the bone loss.[88]

In addition to the direct effects of the disease, other factors in these children are important. Poor nutrition, anorexia and vomiting, reduced physical activity and immobilization, prolonged hospitalization and psychosocial factors may all play a role in certain children, although the relative impact of each of these factors is difficult to ascertain.

Furthermore, adverse effects of treatment can affect growth indirectly. For example, serious infective episodes as a result of myelosuppression may impact on the child's height and weight progression. In addition, both cardiovascular and respiratory disease can occur secondary to childhood cancer treatment, and this may contribute significantly to the late morbidity of disease-free survivors.[89] Cardiovascular damage in this patient group is most commonly due to direct damage from radiotherapy, primarily following mediastinal irradiation or total body irradiation (TBI), and from chemotherapeutic agents, particularly the anthracyclines such as doxorubicin and daunorubicin. Subsequent myocardial dysfunction is related to the cumulative dose received,[90] although even relatively low doses can cause adverse cardiac effects, and the likelihood of these occurring increases over time.[91] In addition to dose, younger age at the time of treatment and female gender are further independent risk factors.[92]

Pulmonary function can also be affected by cancer treatment. Radiotherapy can result in restrictive pulmonary disease and reduced compliance, and these problems are most commonly seen following thoracic radiation, which may be used in the treatment of lymphoma. TBI will also include the lungs within the treatment field, and this may also cause restrictive defects, although at the doses used pulmonary dysfunction is usually subclinical.[93] The lungs are, in general, less sensitive to the effects of chemotherapy, although both carmustine and bleomycin can cause subsequent pulmonary dysfunction,[94] and this may be potentiated by additional use of radiotherapy.

Although there is no evidence at present that cardiopulmonary dysfunction secondary to cancer treatment affects long term growth,[95] long-term follow-up of patients with such complications must include growth assessment. This is of particular importance during puberty, due to the increased demands on cardiac and respiratory function during this period.

OBESITY

Excessive weight gain is a recognized complication of certain childhood malignancies, in particular suprasellar tumors and acute lymphoblastic leukemia. Obesity is an increasing problem within the pediatric community and, in survivors of childhood cancer, as with other patients who become obese, can be associated with significant morbidity.[96] In addition, it is important to note that inappropriate weight gain can result in a 'normal' height velocity at the expense of inappropriately rapid skeletal maturation, resulting in a reduced height prognosis.

Obesity is seen frequently in patients with craniopharyngioma, with one recent study demonstrating severe obesity (defined as a body mass index (BMI) greater than 3 standard deviations above the mean) in 44 percent of patients at follow-up.[97] The etiology of this is likely to be multifactorial, although appears to be associated with hypothalamic damage.[98] This results in hyperinsulinemia secondary to disinhibition of vagal tone at the pancreatic beta cell, and may also result in insensitivity to endogenous leptin,[99] which normally inhibits appetite via hypothalamic receptors. In addition, increased bioavailability of insulin-like growth factor has been implicated.[100]

Obesity is also well documented following treatment for ALL, and a number of risk factors have been postulated. Those children with ALL who received cranial irradiation as part of their treatment have an increased BMI as compared to their peers, and remain at significant risk of becoming overweight in adulthood.[101] GH deficiency, as discussed earlier, is likely to play a role, but other important factors may include damage to areas of the brain that normally control appetite and body composition. Indeed, as with craniopharyngioma, higher leptin levels have been noted in these patients and this may reflect a degree of leptin insensitivity.[102]

Obesity after treatment for ALL has also been described in patients who have not received cranial irradiation,[103] although this has not been demonstrated in all studies.[101] The etiology of excess weight gain in this patient group is likely to be multifactorial, and a number of risk factors have been suggested. Children with ALL are less active than their peers, both during[104] and after[105] treatment, and this appears to be one of the most important factors contributing to the excess weight gain observed.

Obesity in this patient group is also more pronounced in girls[106] and is more likely in those who are younger and thinner at diagnosis.[107] There may also be a familial contribution, with a significant number of obese patients having an obese mother.[108] In addition, pulsed steroids are used throughout ALL treatment regimens, causing a significant increase in energy intake and this further contributes to the prevalence of obesity in these children.[109]

Dietetic input is essential in these patient groups, in order to optimize nutrition and body composition. In addition, the importance of physical activity and a healthy lifestyle must be emphasized.

MONITORING FOR GROWTH PROBLEMS FOLLOWING CANCER TREATMENT

It is clear from the preceding discussion that the degree and nature of long-term growth impairment following treatment for childhood cancer will depend on the underlying malignancy, the type and intensity of the treatment given and the age of the child at the time of treatment. Appropriate investigation and follow-up strategies will therefore vary between patients and between treatment groups. At one extreme, there are survivors who are unlikely to develop significant problems, and therefore minimal follow-up would be required. Such patients would include those treated with surgery alone or low risk chemotherapy (Table 38.2). However, at the other extreme would be patients who have received radiotherapy, bone marrow transplantation or megatherapy. Patients in this group should be seen in a medically supervised late effects clinic at least three times per annum until final height is achieved, and at least annually thereafter (Table 38.2). It is vital that such follow-up is multi-disciplinary, and as such must include a variety of personnel including a pediatric oncologist, endocrinologist, radiation oncologist, specialist nurse, and the general practitioner.

Current recommendations for the monitoring of growth impairment in children who have survived cancer include regular measurements of height in all patients until final adult height is attained.[3] In addition, evaluation of growth in a number of children may also require assessments of bone age and pubertal staging. Patients who have received craniospinal irradiation must also have their sitting height measured, along with an assessment of spinal curvature as part of the clinical examination.

Children with impaired growth velocity noted at follow up require determination of the cause of their impaired growth, and appropriate treatment must be instituted. As discussed previously, patients who have received cranial irradiation are at significant risk of growth hormone deficiency, and therefore may benefit from growth hormone replacement. However, debate persists regarding testing of the hypothalamic–pituitary axis in these patients. Whilst some practitioners favor regular monitoring of growth velocity, with intervention only when the velocity slows,

Table 38.2 Possible levels of follow-up more than 5 years from completion of treatment

Level	Treatment	Method of follow-up	Frequency	Examples
1	Surgery alone Low risk chemotherapy	Post or telephone	1–2 years	Wilms' stage I/II LCH (single system) Germ cell tumors (surgery only)
2	Chemotherapy Low dose cranial irradiation (<24 Gy)	Nurse or primary care led	1–2 years	Majority of patients (e.g., ALL in first remission)
3	Radiotherapy (except above) Megatherapy	Medically supervised late effects clinic	Annual	Brain tumors Post BMT Stage 4 patients (any tumor)

ALL, acute lymphoblastic leukemia; BMT, bone narrow transplantation; LCH, Langerhans cell histiocytosis.

others advocate regular testing of hypothalamic–pituitary function so that any deficiency is detected before significant growth impairment occurs. However, pituitary function tests are both invasive and unpleasant, and therefore their use within this patient group should be considered on an individual basis. In many patients it is appropriate to await clinical evidence of reduced growth before investigation and treatment. Indeed, once growth has slowed it can be argued whether it is appropriate to subject the child to further investigations in order to prove what is clinically apparent in a child at known risk of evolving GH deficiency. In addition, as mentioned previously, poor growth secondary to neurosecretory dysfunction will not be detected using conventional pituitary function tests, emphasizing the importance of clinical vigilance in this patient group.

However, as discussed previously, poor growth in these patients may not solely be due to GH deficiency and therefore other causes must be considered and treated as necessary. Deficiencies of other pituitary hormones may exist, particularly in patients who have received higher doses of cranial irradiation, or those treated at a younger age. In addition, it is essential to assess pubertal progression in these patients due to the consequences related to either early or delayed puberty. With regards to puberty, it is also important to be aware whilst assessing these patients that apparent catch-up growth can actually be due to the pubertal growth spurt.

Patients who have a craniopharyngioma, whether this is treated with surgery alone or additional radiotherapy, are at particular risk of pituitary dysfunction,[110] and as such should have pituitary function testing both at diagnosis and at regular intervals thereafter.[3] In addition, as discussed above, these patients are prone to obesity.

Thus follow-up, with appropriate investigation and subsequent management must be tailored to the requirements of each patient. This will primarily be based on their original diagnosis and treatment received, although additional factors with regard to their overall health must also be considered.

CONCLUSIONS

The successful treatment of childhood cancer is associated with significant morbidity in later life. The major challenge faced by pediatric oncologists today is to sustain the excellent survival rates whilst striving to achieve optimal quality of life. Growth impairment, endocrine dysfunction and disorders of bone metabolism form a significant part of this morbidity, and thus awareness of such complications, with appropriate long-term follow-up and early intervention is essential in the management of these children. Involvement of all members of the multi-disciplinary team, including oncologists, radiotherapists, endocrinologists, specialist nurses, dieticians and many others, is vital in the ongoing care of patients after childhood cancer treatment.

In the United Kingdom strategies are being developed in order to define a comprehensive programme of follow-up,[3] together with the centralization of data to fully evaluate the late effects of childhood cancer therapy.[111] It is hoped that in the future treatment protocols may be further modified in order to reduce the impact of these late effects and subsequently improve the quality of life for these children as they progress into adulthood.

KEY LEARNING POINTS

- As more children survive cancer, long-term side effects of treatment are becoming increasingly important within pediatric oncology.
- Cranial irradiation may result in hypothalamic–pituitary dysfunction; such dysfunction is dependent upon the age of the patient and the total dose received.
- Growth hormone (GH) secretion is particularly radiosensitive, and as such GH replacement therapy may be indicated in this patient group. Studies to date suggest GH therapy is safe within this population, although long-term surveillance is essential.

- Cranial irradiation can affect normal pubertal progression, resulting in either early or delayed puberty. This may further compromise growth and final adult height.
- Thyroid dysfunction, particularly hypothyroidism, may be observed following both cranial irradiation and radiation directly involving the thyroid gland.
- Radiotherapy may directly affect skeletal growth.
- Chemotherapy can also affect growth in childhood, although generally to a lesser extent than radiotherapy.
- Cytotoxic therapy may affect bone metabolism, which can result in premature osteoporosis.
- Malignant disease itself, along with several other associated factors, may also contribute to the growth impairment and reduced bone density observed in these patients.
- Obesity is a recognized complication following cancer treatment, particularly for patients with craniopharyngioma and acute lymphoblastic leukemia.
- Long term multi-disciplinary follow-up, clinical vigilance and awareness of potential problems are essential in the management of this patient group, in order to reduce the impact of growth impairment as these children enter adolescence and adult life.

REFERENCES

● = Seminal primary article
◆ = Key review paper
✳ = First formal publication of a management guideline

1 Stiller CA. Epidemiology and genetics of childhood cancer. *Oncogene* 2004; **23**: 6429–44.
2 Mertens AC, Yasui Y, Neglia JP, *et al.* Late mortality experience in five-year survivors of childhood and adolescent cancer: the Childhood Cancer Survivor Study. *J Clin Oncol* 2001; **19**: 3163–72.
✳ 3 Scottish Intercollegiate Guidelines Network. Guideline 76: *Long Term Follow Up Care of Survivors of Childhood Cancer.* Edinburgh: 2004.
4 Muller HL, Klinkhammer-Schalke M, Kuhl J. Final height and weight of long-term survivors of childhood malignancies. *Exp Clin Endocrinol Diabetes* 1998; **106**: 135–9.
5 Constine LS, Woolf PD, Cann D, *et al.* Hypothalamic–pituitary dysfunction after radiation for brain tumors. *N Engl J Med* 1993; **328**: 87–94.
● 6 Littley MD, Shalet SM, Beardwell CG, *et al.* Radiation-induced hypopituitarism is dose-dependent. *Clin Endocrinol (Oxf)* 1989; **31**: 363–73.
7 Brennan BM, Rahim A, Mackie EM, *et al.* Growth hormone status in adults treated for acute lymphoblastic leukaemia in childhood. *Clin Endocrinol (Oxf)* 1998; **48**: 777–83.
● 8 Littley MD, Shalet SM, Beardwell CG, *et al.* Hypopituitarism following external radiotherapy for pituitary tumours in adults. *Q J Med* 1989; **70**: 145–60.
9 Clayton PE, Shalet SM. Dose dependency of time of onset of radiation-induced growth hormone deficiency. *J Pediatr* 1991; **118**: 226–8.
10 Schmiegelow M, Lassen S, Poulsen HS, *et al.* Growth hormone response to a growth hormone-releasing hormone stimulation test in a population-based study following cranial irradiation of childhood brain tumors. *Horm Res* 2000; **54**: 53–9.
11 Bercu BB, Diamond FB Jr. Growth hormone neurosecretory dysfunction. *Clin Endocrinol Metab* 1986; **15**: 537–90.
12 Spoudeas HA, Hindmarsh PC, Matthews DR, Brook CG. Evolution of growth hormone neurosecretory disturbance after cranial irradiation for childhood brain tumours: a prospective study. *J Endocrinol* 1996; **150**: 329–42.
13 Shalet SM, Beardwell CG, Pearson D, Jones PH. The effect of varying doses of cerebral irradiation on growth hormone production in childhood. *Clin Endocrinol (Oxf)* 1976; **5**: 287–90.
14 Ogilvy-Stuart AL, Shalet SM. Growth and puberty after growth hormone treatment after irradiation for brain tumours. *Arch Dis Child* 1995; **73**: 141–6.
15 de Boer H, Blok GJ, Van der Veen EA. Clinical aspects of growth hormone deficiency in adults. *Endocr Rev* 1995; **16**: 63–86.
16 Talvensaari K, Knip M. Childhood cancer and later development of the metabolic syndrome. *Ann Med* 1997; **29**: 353–5.
17 Kaufman JM, Taelman P, Vermeulen A, Vandeweghe M. Bone mineral status in growth hormone-deficient males with isolated and multiple pituitary deficiencies of childhood onset. *J Clin Endocrinol Metab* 1992; **74**: 118–23.
18 Stabler B. Impact of growth hormone (GH) therapy on quality of life along the lifespan of GH-treated patients. *Horm Res* 2001; **56(Suppl 1)**: 55–8.
19 Vassilopoulou-Sellin R, Klein MJ, Moore BD III, *et al.* Efficacy of growth hormone replacement therapy in children with organic growth hormone deficiency after cranial irradiation. *Horm Res* 1995; **43**: 188–93.
20 Murray RD, Darzy KH, Gleeson HK, Shalet SM. GH-Deficient survivors of childhood cancer: GH replacement during adult life. *J Clin Endocrinol Metab* 2002; **87**: 129–35.
21 Pfeifer M, Verhovec R, Zizek B. Growth hormone (GH) and atherosclerosis: changes in morphology and function of major arteries during GH treatment. *Growth Horm IGF Res* 1999; **9(Suppl A)**: 25–30.
22 Longobardi S, Di Rella F, Pivonello R, *et al.* Effects of two years of growth hormone (GH) replacement therapy on bone metabolism and mineral density in childhood and adulthood onset GH deficient patients. *J Endocrinol Invest* 1999; **22**: 333–9.
23 Lagrou K, Xhrouet-Heinrichs D, Massa G, *et al.* Quality of life and retrospective perception of the effect of growth hormone treatment in adult patients with

childhood growth hormone deficiency. *J Pediatr Endocrinol Metab* 2001; **14(Suppl 5)**: 1249–62.

24 Moell C, Garwicz S, Westgren U, *et al*. Suppressed spontaneous secretion of growth hormone in girls after treatment for acute lymphoblastic leukaemia. *Arch Dis Child* 1989; **64**: 252–8.

25 Crowne EC, Moore C, Wallace WH, *et al*. A novel variant of growth hormone (GH) insufficiency following low dose cranial irradiation. *Clin Endocrinol (Oxf)* 1992; **36**: 59–68.

26 Achermann JC, Hindmarsh PC, Brook CG. The relationship between the growth hormone and insulin-like growth factor axis in long-term survivors of childhood brain tumours. *Clin Endocrinol (Oxf)* 1998; **49**: 639–45.

27 Vahl N, Juul A, Jorgensen JO, *et al*. Continuation of growth hormone (GH) replacement in GH-deficient patients during transition from childhood to adulthood: a two-year placebo-controlled study. *J Clin Endocrinol Metab* 2000; **85**: 1874–81.

28 Watanabe S, Tsunematsu Y, Fujimoto J, Komiyama A. Leukaemia in patients treated with growth hormone (letter). *Lancet* 1988; **1**: 1159–60.

29 Swerdlow AJ, Higgins CD, Adlard P, Preece MA. Risk of cancer in patients treated with human pituitary growth hormone in the UK, 1959-1985: a cohort study. *Lancet* 2002; **360**: 273–7.

30 Kiess W, Doerr H, Eisl E, Butenandt O, Belohradsky BH. Lymphocyte subsets and natural-killer activity in growth hormone deficiency (Letter). *N Engl J Med* 1986; **314**: 321.

31 Zadik Z, Estrov Z, Karov Y, *et al*. The effect of growth hormone and IGF-I on clonogenic growth of hematopoietic cells in leukaemic patients during active disease and during remission – a preliminary report. *J Pediatr Endocrinol* 1993; **6**: 79–83.

32 Ogilvy-Stuart AL, Ryder WD, Gattamaneni HR, *et al*. Growth hormone and tumour recurrence. *BMJ* 1992; **304**: 1601–5.

33 Swerdlow AJ, Reddingius RE, Higgins CD, *et al*. Growth hormone treatment of children with brain tumors and risk of tumor recurrence. *J Clin Endocrinol Metab* 2000; **85**: 4444–9.

34 Sklar CA, Mertens AC, Mitby P, *et al*. Risk of disease recurrence and second neoplasms in survivors of childhood cancer treated with growth hormone: a report from the Childhood Cancer Survivor Study. *J Clin Endocrinol Metab* 2002; **87**: 3136–41.

35 Hall JE, Martin KA, Whitney HA, *et al*. Potential for fertility with replacement of hypothalamic gonadotrophin-releasing hormone in long term female survivors of cranial tumors. *J Clin Endocrinol Metab* 1994; **79**: 1166–72.

36 Leiper AD, Stanhope R, Preece MA, *et al*. Precocious or early puberty and growth failure in girls treated for acute lymphoblastic leukaemia. *Horm Res* 1988; **30**: 72–6.

37 Quigley C, Cowell C, Jimenez M, *et al*. Normal or early development of puberty despite gonadal damage in children treated for acute lymphoblastic leukaemia. *N Engl J Med* 1989; **321**: 143–51.

38 Ogilvy-Stuart AL, Clayton PE, Shalet SM. Cranial irradiation and early puberty. *J Clin Endocrinol Metab* 1994; **78**: 1282–6.

39 Didcock E, Davies HA, Didi M, *et al*. Pubertal growth in young adult survivors of childhood leukaemia. *J Clin Oncol* 1995; **13**: 2503–7.

40 Davies HA, Didcock E, Didi M, *et al*. Disproportionate short stature after cranial irradiation and combination chemotherapy for leukaemia. *Arch Dis Child* 1994; **70**: 472–5.

41 Shalet SM, Gibson B, Swindell R, Pearson D. Effect of spinal irradiation on growth. *Arch Dis Child* 1987; **62**: 461–4.

42 Cara JF, Kreiter ML, Rosenfield RL. Height prognosis of children with true precocious puberty and growth hormone deficiency: effect of combination therapy with gonadotrophin releasing hormone agonist and growth hormone. *J Pediatr* 1992; **120**: 709–15.

43 Adan L, Souberbielle JC, Zucker JM, *et al*. Adult height in 24 patients treated for growth hormone deficiency and early puberty. *J Clin Endocrinol Metab* 1997; **82**: 229–33.

44 Black P, Straaten A, Gutjahr P. Secondary thyroid carcinoma after treatment for childhood cancer. *Med Pediatr Oncol* 1998; **31**: 91–5.

45 Sklar CA, Constine LS. Chronic neuroendocrinological sequelae of radiation therapy. *Int J Radiat Oncol Biol Phys* 1995; **31**: 1113–21.

46 Rose SR, Lustig RH, Pitukcheewanont P, *et al*. Diagnosis of hidden central hypothyroidism in survivors of childhood cancer. *J Clin Endocrinol Metab* 1999; **84**: 4472–9.

47 Rose SR. Isolated central hypothyroidism in short stature. *Pediatr Res* 1995; **38**: 967–73.

48 Livesey EA, Brook CG. Thyroid dysfunction after radiotherapy and chemotherapy of brain tumours. *Arch Dis Child* 1989; **64**: 593–5.

49 Michel G, Socie G, Gebhard F, *et al*. Late effects of allogeneic bone marrow transplantation for children with acute myeloblastic leukaemia in first complete remission: the impact of conditioning regimen without total body irradiation - a report from the Societe Francaise de Greffe de Moelle. *J Clin Oncol* 1997; **15**: 2238–46.

50 Sklar C, Whitton J, Mertens A, *et al*. Abnormalities of the thyroid in survivors of Hodgkin's disease: data from the Childhood Cancer Survivor Study. *J Clin Endocrinol Metab* 2000; **85**: 3227–32.

51 Doniach I, Kingston JE, Plowman PN, Malpas JS. The association of post-radiation thyroid nodular disease with compensated hypothyroidism. *Br J Radiol* 1987; **60**: 1223–6.

52 Kaplan MM, Garnick MB, Gelber R, *et al*. Risk factors for thyroid abnormalities after neck irradiation for childhood cancer. *Am J Med* 1983; **74**: 272–80.

53 Fleming ID, Black TL, Thompson EI, *et al*. Thyroid dysfunction and neoplasia in children receiving neck irradiation for cancer. *Cancer* 1985; **55**: 1190–4.

54 de Vathaire F, Hardiman C, Shamsaldin A, *et al*. Thyroid carcinomas after irradiation for a first cancer during childhood. *Arch Intern Med* 1999; **159**: 2713–9.

55 Ron E, Modan B, Preston D, *et al*. Thyroid neoplasia following low-dose radiation in childhood. *Radiat Res* 1989; **120**: 516–31.

56   Inskip PD. Thyroid cancer after radiotherapy for childhood cancer. *Med Pediatr Oncol* 2001; **36**: 568–73.

57   Crom DB, Kaste SC, Tubergen DG, *et al.* Ultrasonography for thyroid screening after head and neck irradiation in childhood cancer survivors. *Med Pediatr Oncol* 1997; **28**: 15–21.

58   Crowne EC, Wallace WH, Gibson S, *et al.* Adrenocorticotrophin and cortisol secretion after low dose cranial irradiation. *Clin Endocrinol (Oxf)* 1993; **39**: 297–305.

59   Thomas BC, Stanhope R, Plowman PN, Leiper AD. Growth following single fraction and fractionated total body irradiation for bone marrow transplantation. *Eur J Pediatr* 1993; **152**: 888–92.

60   Wallace WH, Shalet SM, Morris-Jones PH, *et al.* Effect of abdominal irradiation on growth in boys treated for a Wilms' tumor. *Med Pediatr Oncol* 1990; **18**: 441–6.

61   Riseborough EJ, Grabias SL, Burton RI, Jaffe N. Skeletal alterations following irradiation for Wilms' tumor: with particular reference to scoliosis and kyphosis. *J Bone Joint Surg Am* 1976; **58**: 526–36.

62   Rate WR, Butler MS, Robertson WW Jr, D'Angio GJ. Late orthopedic effects in children with Wilms' tumor treated with abdominal irradiation. *Med Pediatr Oncol* 1991; **19**: 265–8.

63   Larson DL, Kroll S, Jaffe N, *et al.* Long-term effects of radiotherapy in childhood and adolescence. *Am J Surg* 1990; **160**: 348–51.

64   Gonzalez DG, Breur K. Clinical data from irradiated growing long bones in children. *Int J Radiat Oncol Biol Phys* 1983; **9**: 841–6.

65   Ogilvy-Stuart AL, Shalet SM. Effect of chemotherapy on growth. *Acta Paediatr Suppl* 1995; **411**: 52–6.

66   van Leeuwen BL, Kamps WA, Jansen HW, Hoekstra HJ. The effect of chemotherapy on the growing skeleton. *Cancer Treat Rev* 2000; **26**: 363–76.

67   Clayton PE, Shalet SM, Morris-Jones PH, Price DA. Growth in children treated for acute lymphoblastic leukaemia. *Lancet* 1988; **1**: 460–2.

68   Schriock EA, Schell MJ, Carter M, *et al.* Abnormal growth patterns and adult short stature in 115 long-term survivors of childhood leukaemia. *J Clin Oncol* 1991; **9**: 400–5.

69   Kirk JA, Raghupathy P, Stevens MM, *et al.* Growth failure and growth-hormone deficiency after treatment for acute lymphoblastic leukaemia. *Lancet* 1987; **1**: 190–3.

70   Sklar C, Mertens A, Walter A, *et al.* Final height after treatment for childhood acute lymphoblastic leukaemia: comparison of no cranial irradiation with 1800 and 2400 centigrays of cranial irradiation. *J Pediatr* 1993; **123**: 59–64.

71   Ahmed SF, Wallace WH, Kelnar CJ. An anthropometric study of children during intensive chemotherapy for acute lymphoblastic leukaemia. *Horm Res* 1997; **48**: 178–33.

72   Ahmed SF, Wallace WH, Crofton PM, *et al.* Short-term changes in lower leg length in children treated for acute lymphoblastic leukaemia. *J Pediatr Endocrinol Metab* 1999; **12**: 75–80.

73   Hokken-Koelega AC, van Doorn JW, Hahlen K, *et al.* Long-term effects of treatment for acute lymphoblastic leukaemia with and without cranial irradiation on growth and puberty: a comparative study. *Pediatr Res* 1993; **33**: 577–82.

74   Birkebaek NH, Clausen N. Height and weight patterns up to 20 years after treatment for acute lymphoblastic leukaemia. *Arch Dis Child* 1998; **79**: 161–4.

75   Kroger H, Kotaniemi A, Kroger L, Alhava E. Development of bone mass and bone density of the spine and femoral neck – a prospective study of 65 children and adolescents. *Bone Miner* 1993; **23**: 171–82.

76   Arikoski P, Komulainen J, Voutilainen R, *et al.* Reduced bone mineral density in long-term survivors of childhood acute lymphoblastic leukaemia. *J Pediatr Hematol Oncol* 1998; **20**: 234–40.

77   Arikoski P, Komulainen J, Riikonen P, *et al.* Reduced bone density at completion of chemotherapy for a malignancy. *Arch Dis Child* 1999; **80**: 143–8.

78   Crofton PM, Ahmed SF, Wade JC, *et al.* Effects of intensive chemotherapy on bone and collagen turnover and the growth hormone axis in children with acute lymphoblastic leukaemia. *J Clin Endocrinol Metab* 1998; **83**: 3121–9.

79   Arikoski P, Komulainen J, Riikonen P, *et al.* Alterations in bone turnover and impaired development of bone mineral density in newly diagnosed children with cancer: a 1-year prospective study. *J Clin Endocrinol Metab* 1999; **84**: 3174–81.

80   Halton JM, Atkinson SA, Fraher L, *et al.* Altered mineral metabolism and bone mass in children during treatment for acute lymphoblastic leukaemia. *J Bone Miner Res* 1996; **11**: 1774–83.

81   Henderson RC, Madsen CD, Davis C, Gold SH. Bone density in survivors of childhood malignancies. *J Pediatr Hematol Oncol* 1996; **18**: 367–71.

82   Hoorweg-Nijman JJ, Kardos G, Roos JC, *et al.* Bone mineral density and markers of bone turnover in young adult survivors of childhood lymphoblastic leukaemia. *Clin Endocrinol (Oxf)* 1999; **50**: 237–44.

83   Gaynon PS, Lustig RH. The use of glucocorticoids in acute lymphoblastic leukaemia of childhood. Molecular, cellular, and clinical considerations. *J Pediatr Hematol Oncol* 1995; **17**: 1–12.

84   Atkinson SA, Halton JM, Bradley C, *et al.* Bone and mineral abnormalities in childhood acute lymphoblastic leukaemia: influence of disease, drugs and nutrition. *Int J Cancer Suppl* 1998; **11**: 35–9.

85   Scheven BA, van der Veen MJ, Damen CA, *et al.* Effects of methotrexate on human osteoblasts in vitro: modulation by 1,25-dihydroxyvitamin D3. *J Bone Miner Res* 1995; **10**: 874–80.

86   Uehara R, Suzuki Y, Ichikawa Y. Methotrexate (MTX) inhibits osteoblastic differentiation in vitro: possible mechanism of MTX osteopathy. *J Rheumatol* 2001; **28**: 251–6.

87   Haddy TB, Mosher RB, Reaman GH. Osteoporosis in survivors of acute lymphoblastic leukaemia. *Oncologist* 2001; **6**: 278–85.

88   Halton JM, Atkinson SA, Fraher L, *et al.* Mineral homeostasis and bone mass at diagnosis in children with acute lymphoblastic leukaemia. *J Pediatr* 1995; **126**: 557–64.

89 Truesdell S, Schwartz CL, Clark E, Constine LS. Cardiovascular effects of cancer. In: Schwartz CL, Hobbie WL, Constine LS, Ruccione KS, eds. *Survivors of Childhood Cancer*. St Louis: CV Mosby; 1994:

90 Pihkala J, Saarinen UM, Lundstrom U, *et al*. Myocardial function in children and adolescents after therapy with anthracyclines and chest irradiation. *Eur J Cancer* 1996; **32A**: 97–103.

91 Sorensen K, Levitt G, Bull C, *et al*. Anthracycline dose in childhood acute lymphoblastic leukemia: issues of early survival versus late cardiotoxicity. *J Clin Oncol* 1997; **15**: 61–8.

92 Lipshultz SE, Lipsitz SR, Mone SM, *et al*. Female sex and drug dose as risk factors for late cardiotoxic effects of doxorubicin therapy for childhood cancer. *N Engl J Med* 1995; **332**: 1738–43.

93 Nysom K, Holm K, Hesse B, *et al*. Lung function after allogeneic bone marrow transplantation for leukaemia or lymphoma. *Arch Dis Child* 1996; **74**: 432–6.

94 O'Driscoll BR, Hasleton PS, Taylor PM, *et al*. Active lung fibrosis up to 17 years after chemotherapy with carmustine (BCNU) in childhood. *N Engl J Med* 1990; **323**: 378–82.

95 Sorensen K, Levitt GA, Bull C, *et al*. Late anthracycline cardiotoxicity after childhood cancer: a prospective longitudinal study. *Cancer* 2003; **97**: 1991–8.

✳ 96 Scottish Intercollegiate Guidelines Network. Guideline 69: *Management of Obesity in Children and Young People*. Edinburgh: 2003.

97 Muller HL, Bueb K, Bartels U, *et al*. Obesity after childhood craniopharyngioma – German multi-center study on pre-operative risk factors and quality of life. *Klin Padiatr* 2001; **213**: 244–9.

98 de Vile CJ, Grant DB, Hayward RD, *et al*. Obesity in childhood craniopharyngioma: relation to post-operative hypothalamic damage shown by magnetic resonance imaging. *J Clin Endocrinol Metab* 1996; **81**: 2734–7.

99 Roth C, Wilken B, Hanefeld F, *et al*. Hyperphagia in children with craniopharyngioma is associated with hyperleptinaemia and a failure in the down-regulation of appetite. *Eur J Endocrinol* 1998; **138**: 89–91.

100 Tiulpakov AN, Mazerkina NA, Brook CG, *et al*. Growth in children with craniopharyngioma following surgery. *Clin Endocrinol (Oxf)* 1998; **49**: 733–8.

101 Sklar CA, Mertens AC, Walter A, *et al*. Changes in body mass index and prevalence of overweight in survivors of childhood acute lymphoblastic leukaemia: role of cranial irradiation. *Med Pediatr Oncol* 2000; **35**: 91–5.

102 Brennan BM, Rahim A, Blum WF, *et al*. Hyperleptinaemia in young adults following cranial irradiation in childhood: growth hormone deficiency or leptin insensitivity? *Clin Endocrinol (Oxf)* 1999; **50**: 163–9.

103 Reilly JJ, Blacklock CJ, Dale E, *et al*. Resting metabolic rate and obesity in childhood acute lymphoblastic leukaemia. *Int J Obes Relat Metab Disord* 1996; **20**: 1130–2.

104 Reilly JJ, Ventham JC, Ralston JM, *et al*. Reduced energy expenditure in preobese children treated for acute lymphoblastic leukaemia. *Pediatr Res* 1998; **44**: 557–62.

105 Warner JT, Bell W, Webb DK, Gregory JW. Daily energy expenditure and physical activity in survivors of childhood malignancy. *Pediatr Res* 1998; **43**: 607–13.

106 Odame I, Reilly JJ, Gibson BE, Donaldson MD. Patterns of obesity in boys and girls after treatment for acute lymphoblastic leukaemia. *Arch Dis Child* 1994; **71**: 147–9.

107 Reilly JJ, Ventham JC, Newell J, *et al*. Risk factors for excess weight gain in children treated for acute lymphoblastic leukaemia. *Int J Obes Relat Metab Disord* 2000; **24**: 1537–41.

108 Shaw MP, Bath LE, Duff J, *et al*. Obesity in leukaemia survivors: the familial contribution. *Pediatr Hematol Oncol* 2000; **17**: 231–7.

109 Reilly JJ, Brougham M, Montgomery C, *et al*. Effect of glucocorticoid therapy on energy intake in children treated for acute lymphoblastic leukaemia. *J Clin Endocrinol Metab* 2001; **86**: 3742–5.

110 de Vile CJ, Grant DB, Hayward RD, Stanhope R. Growth and endocrine sequelae of craniopharyngioma. *Arch Dis Child* 1996; **75**: 108–14.

◆ 111 Wallace WHB, Blacklay A, Eiser C, *et al*. Developing strategies for long term follow up of survivors of childhood cancer. *BMJ* 2001; **323**: 271–4.

39

Growth hormone therapy in the short, small-for-gestational age child

LINDA B JOHNSTON

EVIDENCE SCORING OF THERAPY

   * Non-randomized controlled trials, cohort study, etc.
   ** One or more well-designed randomized controlled trials
   *** Systematic review or meta-analysis

DEFINITION OF SMALL FOR GESTATIONAL AGE

It is important to understand the terms used in describing babies who are born small. Small for gestational age (SGA) (or small for dates) and intrauterine growth retardation (IUGR) are both commonly used but are not synonymous terms. IUGR infants may or may not be SGA and vice versa. Sequential antenatal auxology using fetal ultrasonography is essential to make the diagnosis of IUGR as the documentation of a subnormal fetal growth rate is required. However, this is not carried out routinely in the third trimester and therefore fetal growth rates cannot be calculated in the majority of pregnancies. SGA describes an infant's size at birth compared to appropriate population standards for gestational age. This assessment of size at birth is not adequate to determine whether the individual also had IUGR.

Birth size forms a continuum and the definition of SGA is arbitrary. Most growth clinics will define SGA as birth size (weight or length) two or more standard deviations ($\leqslant -2$ SDS) below the mean for gender and gestational age. In the UK birth length is not always available and is often not as reliably measured as birth weight, so the definition of SGA relies on the assessment of birth weight for gender and gestation.

ETIOLOGY OF SMALL FOR GESTATIONAL AGE

The control of normal fetal growth is complex involving the interplay between maternal, fetal, and placental genetic and environmental factors and there is the potential for any abnormality in these systems to adversely influence normal fetal growth.[1] Thus SGA infants are a heterogeneous group.

The SGA infant should always be investigated, preferably shortly after birth, to find an underlying cause because a positive finding will allow counselling of the family regarding the likely prognosis and allow any appropriate specific therapies to be instigated. The etiology of SGA birth size may be apparent from the pregnancy history, e.g., maternal smoking, alcohol abuse or pre-eclampsia, from examination of the newborn or cytogenetic studies, e.g., dysmorphic syndromes, from serological investigation of the newborn, e.g., congenital infection or there may be a family history of SGA babies in siblings or the parents. However, the etiology remains elusive in a large number of cases despite a careful review of the medical history and organization of specific investigations.

CLINICAL PROBLEMS IN THE SMALL-FOR-GESTATIONAL AGE CHILD

The range of clinical needs of short children born SGA is broad and many of these requirements have perhaps been overlooked.[2] Frequently, these patients have good general health and they may be discharged early from medical care. If they are under medical supervision, it is usually because of specific difficulties. There are three predominant areas of need in childhood relating to being born SGA. These are, first, neurological and developmental difficulties; secondly, possible association with dysmorphic features and/or genetic conditions; and thirdly, short stature requiring long-term surveillance, potential treatment, and endocrine safety monitoring. In addition to this there may be complications of prematurity that require additional clinical consideration and attention. The medical supervision of the SGA child might therefore be spread through different pediatric subspecialties but may best be served by seeing a multidisciplinary team within one clinic.

Neurodevelopmental problems

A number of studies have shown that many SGA children, particularly those with symmetrical IUGR, have suboptimal neurological development and intellectual attainment, both in childhood and adult life. A study of intellectual development of children with IUGR at age 7 years showed a highly significant difference in IQ (Wechsler) values between IUGR and normal birth weight subjects.[3] Similarly, an analysis of functional outcomes of SGA subjects at the age of 26 years, showed a significant reduction in scores of professional and managerial skills, a higher rate of manual and un-skilled or semi-skilled occupations and a reduced weekly income compared with subjects with normal birth weight.[4*]

Association with dysmorphic features and genetic disease

Genetic factors have a significant influence on birth weight and length.[1] It is recognized that SGA is a component of many dysmorphic and genetic syndromes and also that many SGA patients have dysmorphic features. This aspect of assessment and investigation of the SGA child may be omitted or not appreciated, particularly if the dysmorphic features are subtle and do not obviously concord with a named syndrome. Careful assessment of these features, linked with appropriate cyto-genetic or molecular investigations may clarify the pathogenesis of SGA in the individual child and help with long-term prognosis and management.

Incidence of short stature in SGA

Studies of the natural growth patterns in children born SGA have demonstrated that the majority will experience

Table 39.1   Percentage of Dutch small-for-gestational age (SGA) children with catch-up growth at 6 months, 1 and 2 years of age[6*]

Age	Premature SGA (n = 423)	Term SGA (n = 301)
At 6 months	40	71
At 1 year	65	81
At 2 years	82.5	87.5

post-natal growth acceleration to 'catch-up' to the normal population standards and their target growth centiles. In a study of 3650 Swedish term singleton SGA infants approximately 87 percent of SGA children experienced catch-up growth to reach heights within the normal population height standards (± 2 SDS) by 2 years of age.[5*] These SGA children with catch-up growth reached a mean final height of -0.7 SDS compared with -1.7 SDS in those SGA children who had not caught up by 2 years. At final height (at 18 years of age) 7.9 percent of the subjects born SGA remained short, thus only a small minority (5 percent) continued to catch up spontaneously during childhood. The best predictors of catch-up growth were longer birth length and taller midparental height.

A significant proportion of SGA infants are born prematurely either spontaneously or are actively delivered early due to obstetric concerns over fetal growth and placental function. These premature SGA infants have a different pattern of post-natal growth where they experience catch-up growth at a later age than term SGA infants.[6*] A Dutch study (see Table 39.1) of 724 SGA children, 423 born prematurely and 301 born at term, showed that although there was no significant difference in the proportion of term and preterm SGA children who had caught up at 2 years, fewer premature SGA had had catch-up growth by 6 months and 1 year. This demonstrates the importance of taking gestational age into account when assessing the early post-natal growth of an SGA child, in order to avoid labeling a premature SGA child as non-catch-up when they may experience delayed catch-up growth.

Although lack of catch-up to normal height in SGA subjects as a whole is relatively infrequent, in the context of children being referred for short stature, patients born SGA account for 21 percent of short pre-pubertal children.[5*]

Etiology of short stature in SGA

The etiology of short stature in an SGA child should always be investigated, in the same way as in any other child presenting with short stature, in order to identify any cause that would be amenable to specific treatment. The specific pathophysiological mechanisms underlying the poor post-natal growth seen in SGA children who do not catch up are not fully understood and, given that these children form a rather heterogeneous group, the mechanisms involved are likely to vary between individuals.

As in other growth disorders the growth hormone (GH)–insulin-like growth factor I (IGF-I) axis has been studied in some detail in short SGA children. In the newborn period GH levels are higher in SGA infants compared to controls but by mid childhood the situation has changed.[7] Studies of spontaneous GH secretion and GH provocation tests have demonstrated that up to half of short SGA children have subnormal peak GH (<20 mU L^{-1}) and/or low mean GH secretion rates compared to normal controls.[8,9]

Cord IGF-I, IGF-II, and insulin levels are lower in the newborn SGA infant than levels in appropriate for gestational age infants.[7,10] This may relate to preceding placental insufficiency in the SGA babies but, in the majority, this reverses within the first few days of life. Serum IGF-I levels in childhood may lie within the normal reference range, but the majority of short SGA children (80 percent in a Swedish study) have IGF-I levels below the 50th centile, supporting the diagnosis of GH and/or IGF-I insufficiency.[11] Defects in the GH–IGF-I axis may thus be obvious on investigation or more subtle and can contribute to poor post-natal catch-up growth.

Further endocrine axes have been investigated in a group of Italian children born SGA comparing those with and without catch-up. These studies found that the non-catch-up SGA children tended to have higher TSH levels and higher cortisol levels.[12,13] Thus subtle defects of the thyroid axis or adrenal axis may also influence post-natal growth in SGA children.

TREATMENT OPTIONS FOR SHORT STATURE IN SMALL–FOR–GESTATIONAL AGE CHILDREN

Short stature in SGA children should be assessed to exclude any treatable cause of growth failure. This assessment should include a detailed history and complete physical examination followed by investigations including full blood count, urea, creatinine and electrolytes, bone and liver profile, celiac screen, chromosomes (in girls to exclude co-existing Turner syndrome) as well as baseline endocrine tests (thyroid function, cortisol, prolactin, IGF-I). Random GH measurements are not useful due to the pulsatile nature of GH secretion. Any specific abnormalities identified in this way can then receive the appropriate specific therapeutic interventions.

The observation of abnormalities in the GH–IGF-I axis led to the first trials of GH therapy, with subsequent observation of growth acceleration, in short SGA children.[14] In 2003 the European Union's Committee on Proprietary Medicinal Products approved recombinant human growth hormone (rGH) for the treatment of short stature in SGA children. This offers a new licensed therapeutic option where no other specific cause for growth failure is identified. A consensus statement on the management of short

SGA children was published by a panel of international experts in 2003 following the licensing of GH for treatment in these children in both Europe and USA.[15] A significant body of evidence was established for approval and research continues in this area. This chapter will give an overview of the evidence base with specific reference to the effectiveness, safety, potential metabolic implications and the selection of patients.

Effectiveness of growth hormone in short, SGA children: Initial growth response

A large number of published trials report on the impact of GH therapy on linear growth in short SGA children. Table 39.2 summarizes the findings of the principal studies where an untreated or placebo treated control group have been included. The doses are shown in comparable units.

Randomized control trials have shown treated subjects have significant growth acceleration in childhood, maximal in the first year but continuing into the second and third years when compared to untreated or placebo treated short SGA controls.[16**–18**] While there is some growth deceleration on discontinuing therapy, the majority of the height gain is retained.[19**,20,21]

The initial growth response is dose dependent with those on higher doses showing more rapid catch-up growth.[16**,18**,22] Advocates of using a higher dose (0.067 mg kg^{-1} day^{-1}) claim the importance of rapid normalization of height and the importance of dose in the growth prediction models justifies the higher IGF-I levels (30 percent of cases have IGF-I SDS >2) seen in these subjects.[23] The commonly used lower dose (0.033 mg kg^{-1} day^{-1}) results in significant gains in linear growth, lower IGF-I levels and a similar gain in final height to the higher dose at lower cost.[16**] The European license thus recommends a dose of 0.035 mg kg^{-1} day^{-1}.

Individual genetic variation may also influence initial growth response to GH in short SGA children. Studies of the GH receptor have identified differing responsiveness to GH therapy dependent on the presence or absence of exon 3.[24,25] The presence of the d3 allele results in greater growth acceleration clinically and greater GH receptor signaling *in vitro*.

A deceleration of growth on stopping GH therapy, less than the preceding growth acceleration, is reported.[20,26] One small study giving intermittent treatment with high doses of GH has shown treatment (alternating 2 years on and 2 years off) resulted in a height gain of 1.7 SDS after 6 years, i.e., four treated and two untreated years.[22] A French study discontinued therapy after 2 years for 2 years and recommended therapy only if the height SDS had dropped by more than 0.5. The European license recommends continuous therapy but schedules for intermittent therapy may be more convenient for patients and more cost-effective. However, further research is required before such protocols can be recommended.

Table 39.2 Growth hormone therapy trials in short small-for-gestational age (SGA) patients with untreated or placebo control groups

Definition, SGA/short	GH dose/protocol (mg kg⁻¹ day⁻¹)	n	At start			Delta height SDS					Final height		Delta bone age	Reference
			Age	Ht SDS	HV SDS	1 y	2 y	3 y	4 y	5 y	n	Ht SDS		
<−2 SDS	Untreated	12	5.18	−2.91		0.07	−0.03	0.18						16**
	0.033	16	4.4	−3.29		1.09	0.45						1	
	0.067	20	4.63	−3.22		1.43	0.7	0.41					1	
<−1.88 SDS	Untreated	29	7.8	−2.6							15	−2.3		18
	0.033	41	7.3	−3						2.2	28	−1.1	1.4	29
	0.067	38	7.2	−3.1						2.6	26	−0.9	1.3	
<−2 SDS	Placebo 6 months then 0.02 for 2.5 y	18	8.24	−3.16	−1.63									54**
	Placebo 6 months then 0.06 for 2.5 y	20	8.16	−3.36	−0.64									
	0.02 for 3 y, 1 y off	15	8.4	−3.1	0.1		0.66	0.77	−0.3				1.15	19
	0.06 for 3 y, 1 y off	40	8.1	−3.2	−1		1.25	1.61	−0.22				1.27	
	0.02 for 2 y, 0.06 for 3rd y, 1 y off	23	7.9	−3.1	−0.7		0.66	0.93	−0.25				1.13	
<−2 SDS/ <−2.5 SDS	Untreated	13	4.9	−3.4	−0.6		0.2							55**
	0.067	20	5.4	−3.5	−0.9		2.1						1.35	
	0.1	19	5.1	−3.7	−0.7		2.5						1.33	
<−SDS/ <−2.5 SDS	Untreated	47	12.8	−3.2							33	−2.7		31**
	0.067	102	12.7	−3.2				−2.1			91	−2.1		
<10th centile, not GHD	Untreated	20	10.7	−1.97							20	−1.9		28**
<10th centile, GHD	0.038	29*	10.9	−2.28							29	−1.8		

Ht, height; HV, height velocity; SGA, small for gestational age.

Two studies compared growth in GH insufficient short SGA children treated with lower doses of GH, with growth in untreated non-GH deficient short SGA children and found no significant gain in final height.[27,28] However, there is no significant difference reported in response between treated short SGA children with and without GH insufficiency.[18**] Thus GH provocation or GH profile testing is not required before treatment with GH as the acquired information on GH secretion status will not change the decision to treat or the recommended GH dose. However, IGF-I and IGF binding protein 3 (IGFBP-3) should always be measured before the start of treatment.

Effectiveness of growth hormone in short SGA children: Final height

The Dutch controlled SGA study followed 54 treated and untreated pre-pubertal SGA children to final height.[29**] This study used GH doses of 0.033 or 0.066 mg kg^{-1} day^{-1} and demonstrated that after 6 years of treatment the final height gain was 2.2 SDS (approx. 12 cm) compared with 0.3 SDS in the untreated control subjects.[18**] In a meta-analysis performed by Novo Nordisk and Pfizer of their joint data, 82 percent of 56 treated patients reached their target height (target height SDS ±1.3 SD). The Swedish SGA study of GH therapy (0.033 μg kg^{-1} day^{-1}) in 77 pre-pubertal children showed a final height gain (adult height minus predicted height pre-treatment) of 1.3 SDS (equivalent to 9 cm) in the whole group.[30**] However, in those children who started GH therapy at least 2 years prior to the onset of puberty the gain was 1.7 SDS. This group concludes that the younger, shorter, and lighter short SGA children have the greatest gains from GH therapy.

Comparison of the Dutch SGA study and a French high dose study where subjects were first treated in adolescence supports the observation in the Swedish study that the gain in final height is greater if the treatment is started at an earlier age.[29**,31**] The Dutch SGA study started treatment at a mean age of seven years with a final height gain of 2.2 SDS (controls 0.3 SDS gain) while the French adolescent subjects were treated for a mean 2.7 years from a mean age of 12.7 and height gain was 1.1 SDS (controls 0.4 SDS gain).[29**,31**] Commencing treatment around the time of puberty results in more modest height gain and higher GH doses may be required. This may be a group that can be identified as requiring a higher initial dose of GH therapy.

Continuous GH therapy is recommended from 4 years of age in order to achieve maximum growth benefit. The published response prediction model, generated from 618 GH treated short SGA subjects and validated in 68 independent patients, supports this.[32] In the first year 52 percent of the variability in growth response can be attributed to the dose of GH given, the mid-parental height, the weight and age at the start of treatment. The first three variables are positively correlated but age is negatively correlated. Individualisation of therapy could be facilitated in

the future through use of such a prediction model in addition to genetic testing of variants known to affect growth response.

The goals of treatment, which are induction of catch-up growth with normalization of childhood height and growth, and increased final adult height can be achieved. Few adverse drug events have been reported which are related to the GH therapy itself. GH thus offers an effective therapeutic option for short SGA children which does not negatively influence body proportions or unduly accelerate skeletal maturation or alter the onset or tempo of puberty or growth during puberty.[18**,21,33***−35**]

Other effects of GH therapy: Body composition

In the Dutch SGA study where body mass index (BMI) in short SGA children was significantly reduced compared to controls (−1.3 SDS) at start, BMI normalized over 5 years.[36**]

A magnetic resonance imaging study in 14 short SGA children during 3 years of GH therapy and 1 year off therapy found that during GH therapy short SGA subjects increased muscle and decreased adipose tissue cross-sectional area.[37] Adipose tissue was similar at the end of three years but the muscle surface area became greater in the SGA children than controls. These changes in muscle and adipose tissue were maintained one year after stopping therapy, suggesting changes in body composition may be long-lasting.

Other effects of growth hormone therapy: Head growth and learning

There is a positive correlation between head circumference at birth and subsequent neurodevelopmental progress.[38] Children born SGA may have a small head circumference and learning difficulties. These features are predicted by the severity of SGA as opposed to just the presence of SGA.[38] Mean HC SDS was significantly lower in the Dutch short SGA subjects born with both low birth length and weight compared to those with only low birth length. Three years of GH therapy resulted in normalization of head circumference as well as height.[39**] Further studies of the intellectual and psychosocial functioning before and after GH therapy showed subnormal measures of IQ at start with normalization during therapy and maintenance after therapy.[40**] Behavior and self-perception scores also improved significantly over this time to become similar levels to those seen in Dutch peers. Furthermore, GH treatment in short SGA children is reported to improve attention capacity and self-esteem measures such that, after 2 years of therapy, there was no difference between cases and controls in scholastic competence, social acceptance, athletic competence, physical appearance, behavioral conduct, and general self-worth.[41,42]

However, a different group have reported adverse effects in perceived scholastic performance and athletic ability in a mixed group of patients (some SGA) on GH therapy.[43] Further studies are thus needed to confirm these findings, although it is intuitive that an improved IQ would accompany an improvement in head circumference SDS.

SAFETY OF GROWTH HORMONE THERAPY

The pharmacological and metabolic safety of GH therapy in these children has been the subject of intensive study.

Safety: insulin–like growth factor I

Growth hormone stimulates the synthesis and secretion of IGF-I. In the Swedish SGA study IGF-I levels rose by 55 percent on day 10, 90 percent after 1 year and by 123 percent at the end of 2 years GH treatment ($0.033 \, mg \, kg^{-1} \, day^{-1}$).[10] This GH dose dependent increase is now well documented in other studies.[11,18,23] Correlation between rise in IGF-I and linear growth response has been reported suggesting that increasing the levels of IGF-I is probably the major mechanism of inducing catch-up growth in short SGA subjects.[11] IGF-I response predicts 42 percent of the variance of the 1 year growth response in the Swedish study.

IGF-I levels are typically lower in untreated short SGA subjects than in normal children, possibly linked to the influences of genetic variation and/or nutritional deficit on IGF-I production.[11] The data from long-term GH therapy studies in childhood into adult life are sparse. However, persistent elevation of serum IGF-I over a period beyond catch-up growth could theoretically increase the risk of cancer development and acromegalic symptoms and complications, including cardiomyopathy and bowel pathology.[44] The consensus statement therefore recommends measurement of serum IGF-I at least annually and reduction of the GH dose if IGF-I levels are more than two standard deviations above the mean of the age-adjusted normal range.[2]

Safety: Glucose homeostasis

Small birth size is associated with features of the metabolic syndrome (insulin resistance, type two diabetes, hypertension, hyperlipidemia, and cardiovascular disease).[45–47] Epidemiological studies initially reported this in adult life but more recently it has also been documented in children.

A reduction in insulin sensitivity (raised insulin levels following an oral glucose load compared to age matched controls) can be documented in childhood and early adulthood in subjects born SGA.[46,47] A study comparing SGA children with and without catch-up has reported higher fasting insulin levels and increased post-load insulin

secretion in those who had catch-up growth (weight and height) compared to non-catch-up SGA subjects and controls.[48] Thus short children who have not caught up may be at lower risk of this feature of the metabolic syndrome, but treatment with GH therapy may increase their risk while normalizing their linear growth.

Fasting glucose, insulin, and proinsulin levels rise and insulin sensitivity falls on GH therapy.[49,50] However, these studies have different findings 3 months after GH therapy has been discontinued with one showing significant improvement in insulin sensitivity and the other showing no improvement. Studies 6 months after stopping GH treatment show no differences in glucose and insulin levels on an oral glucose tolerance test between controls and SGA children (mean age 16 years).[51**] Thus the adverse effects on insulin sensitivity would appear to be reversible.

Safety: Blood pressure and lipids

The Dutch SGA study found that systolic blood pressure in untreated short children born SGA was elevated at baseline (0.7 SDS) but diastolic blood pressure was similar (-0.1 SDS).[36] The systolic and diastolic blood pressures fell compared with control data during 5 years of GH therapy. In the same group of patients, total cholesterol, LDL cholesterol, and the atherogenic index improved over 5 years although no change was noted in HDL cholesterol levels. On discontinuation of therapy this improvement in blood pressure and lipid profile was not lost over 6 months.[51]

In summary, the documented increased risk of hypertension, insulin resistance, hyperlipidemia, and cardiovascular disease in SGA subjects appears to be greatest for those subjects that show catch-up, particularly where this is rapid or exaggerated.[48] GH therapy in short SGA subjects is reported to improve blood pressure and lipid profiles but reversibly increase insulin resistance. The long-term impact of GH therapy is not known, so continued monitoring of variables of insulin sensitivity in these subjects is required into adulthood.

SELECTION OF PATIENTS

The varying designs of the GH therapy studies in short SGA patients give insights into potential patient and dose selection. The European license recommends therapy in children born SGA (birth weight or length < -2 SDS) with short stature (height < -2.5 SDS and more than 1 SDS below target height). Furthermore the child must be at least 4 years old with a height velocity below average (0 SDS). This excludes children who are experiencing spontaneous catch-up growth. Starting treatment before puberty is beneficial in terms of final height gain, suggesting that pre-pubertal height gain is the key to improved final height.[18,30**,34] The gains in height SDS during puberty are more modest.[31**] At the present time the recommended dose is standard

$(0.035\,\mu g\ kg^{-1}\ day^{-1})$, however variation of this dose depending on the height deficit at start or age of the patient may be beneficial.[23,31**,52***] Further studies are required to further define patient and dose selection recommendations. The response prediction model could be used as a tool to refine the recommended dose in individual cases in the future. Short SGA patients who are younger, shorter, and lighter at start of treatment and those with the GH receptor d3 allele respond best to conventional doses of GH.[24,25,30]

TREATMENT ENVIRONMENT

In order to optimally manage the SGA child short stature should be identified in the pre-pubertal years. This would require a chain of surveillance from birth to referral for specialist assessment. Although the majority of SGA infants will experience catch-up growth, the range of possible difficulties that such a patient may have, justifies an organized process of surveillance which co-ordinates maternity, community child health, secondary and tertiary services. A system of identification and appropriate assessment could significantly benefit the overall care of the SGA child.

When referred with short stature, SGA children should be clinically assessed and where indicated treated with GH by a pediatric endocrinologist.[53] Shared care with a general pediatrician or family doctor can follow similar shared care guidelines currently used for other GH indications. Ideally the pediatric endocrine clinic should offer neurodevelopmental and dysmorphology assessments in addition to auxological, endocrine, and metabolic investigation.

Detailed post licensing surveillance should include long-term follow-up and careful metabolic monitoring, as the implications of GH therapy on these subjects, at risk of the metabolic syndrome, will take many years to observe.

CONCLUSIONS

Short children born small for gestational age (SGA) account for approximately 20 percent of short children in a population and therefore contribute significantly to the workload of growth clinics.[5*] The licensed approval of recombinant human GH therapy offers a new therapeutic option in eligible children. Short children should first be investigated in order to identify causes of being born SGA and reasons for poor post-natal growth. Any specific cause found should be further investigated and treated appropriately. In the short child in whom no remediable cause has been identified, GH therapy may have a role to play in normalizing height and the earlier the child is identified the greater the potential response to treatment.

Studies of short SGA children, treated to final height, suggest that GH therapy is a safe and effective therapy in appropriate SGA subjects. However, long-term surveillance

is required to establish the effect therapy may have on the risk for developing features of the metabolic syndrome.

KEY LEARNING POINTS

- The etiology of small birth size for gestational age is complex involving both environmental and genetic factors.
- While around 85 percent of SGA children have post-natal catch-up growth, 21 percent of pre-pubertal short stature referrals were born SGA.
- GH therapy is licensed for treatment of short stature in children born SGA who have not had catch-up growth.
- Starting treatment at least 2 years before puberty can result in height gains of 1.7–1.9 SDS, whereas later initiation of treatment results in more modest height gains (0.7–0.9 SDS).
- Treatment should be monitored by a pediatric endocrinologist.
- IGF-I and glucose homeostasis, as a minimum review, should be assessed annually on treatment.
- Long-term surveillance is recommended to monitor the influence GH has on the development of the metabolic syndrome.

REFERENCES

● = Seminal primary article
◆ = Key review paper
＊ = First formal publication of a management guideline

1 Johnston LB, Clark AJ, Savage MO. Genetic factors contributing to birth weight. *Arch Dis Child Fetal Neonatal Ed* 2002; **86**: F2–3.

◆ 2 Yanney M, Marlow N. Paediatric consequences of fetal growth restriction. *Semin Fetal Neonatal Med* 2004; **9**: 411–8.

3 Strauss RS, Dietz WH. Growth and development of term children born with low birth weight: effects of genetic and environmental factors. *J Pediatr* 1998; **133**: 67–72.

4 Strauss RS. Adult functional outcome of those born small for gestational age: twenty-six-year follow-up of the 1970 British Birth Cohort. *JAMA* 2000; **283**: 625–32.

● 5 Karlberg J, Albertsson-Wikland K. Growth in full-term small-for-gestational-age infants: from birth to final height. *Pediatr Res* 1995; **38**: 733–9.

● 6 Hokken-Koelega AC, De Ridder MA, Lemmen RJ, *et al.* Children born small for gestational age: do they catch up? *Pediatr Res* 1995; **38**: 267–71.

7 Deiber M, Chatelain P, Naville D, *et al.* Functional hypersomatotropism in small for gestational age (SGA) newborn infants. *J Clin Endocrinol Metab* 1989; **68**: 232–4.

8 Ackland FM, Stanhope R, Eyre C, *et al.* Physiological growth hormone secretion in children with short stature and intrauterine growth retardation. *Horm Res* 1988; **30**: 241–5.

9 Boguszewski M, Rosberg S, Albertsson-Wikland K. Spontaneous 24-hour growth hormone profiles in prepubertal small for gestational age children. *J Clin Endocrinol Metab* 1995; **80**: 2599–606.

10 Giudice LC, de Zegher F, Gargosky SE, *et al*. Insulin-like growth factors and their binding proteins in the term and preterm human fetus and neonate with normal and extremes of intrauterine growth. *J Clin Endocrinol Metab* 1995; **80**: 1548–55.

11 Boguszewski M, Jansson C, Rosberg S, Albertsson-Wikland K. Changes in serum insulin-like growth factor I (IGF-I) and IGF-binding protein-3 levels during growth hormone treatment in prepubertal short children born small for gestational age. *J Clin Endocrinol Metab* 1996; **81**: 3902–8.

12 Cianfarani S, Maiorana A, Geremia C, *et al*. Blood glucose concentrations are reduced in children born small for gestational age (SGA), and thyroid-stimulating hormone levels are increased in SGA with blunted postnatal catch-up growth. *J Clin Endocrinol Metab* 2003; **88**: 2699–705.

13 Cianfarani S, Geremia C, Scott CD, Germani D. Growth, IGF system, and cortisol in children with intrauterine growth retardation: is catch-up growth affected by reprogramming of the hypothalamic–pituitary–adrenal axis? *Pediatr Res* 2002; **51**: 94–9.

14 Rochiccioli P, Tauber M, Moisan V, Pienkowski C. Investigation of growth hormone secretion in patients with intrauterine growth retardation. *Acta Paediatr Scand Suppl* 1989; **349**: 42–6.

* 15 Lee PA, Chernausek SD, Hokken-Koelega AC, Czernichow P. International Small for Gestational Age Advisory Board consensus development conference statement: management of short children born small for gestational age, April 24–October 1, 2001. *Pediatrics* 2003; **111(6 Pt 1)**: 1253–61.

16 Boguszewski M, Albertsson-Wikland K, Aronsson S, *et al*. Growth hormone treatment of short children born small-for-gestational-age: the Nordic Multicentre Trial. *Acta Paediatr* 1998; **87**: 257–63.

17 Butenandt O, Lang G. Recombinant human growth hormone in short children born small for gestational age. German Study Group. *J Pediatr Endocrinol Metab* 1997; **10**: 275–82.

18 Sas T, de Waal W, Mulder P, *et al*. Growth hormone treatment in children with short stature born small for gestational age: 5-year results of a randomized, double-blind, dose–response trial. *J Clin Endocrinol Metab* 1999; **84**: 3064–70.

● 19 Job JC, Chaussain JL, Job B, *et al*. Follow-up of three years of treatment with growth hormone and of one post-treatment year, in children with severe growth retardation of intrauterine onset. *Pediatr Res* 1996; **39**: 354–9.

20 de Zegher F, Du Caju MV, Heinrichs C, *et al*. Early, discontinuous, high dose growth hormone treatment to normalize height and weight of short children born small for gestational age: results over 6 years. *J Clin Endocrinol Metab* 1999; **84**: 1558–61.

21 Sas TC, Gerver WJ, De Bruin R, *et al*. Body proportions during 6 years of GH treatment in children with short stature born small for gestational age participating in a randomised, double-blind, dose-response trial. *Clin Endocrinol (Oxf)* 2000; **53**: 675–81.

22 Horikawa R, Tanaka T. Growth hormone treatment in short Japanese children born small for gestational age. *Horm Res* 2004; **62(Suppl 3)**: 128–36.

23 Czernichow P. Growth hormone treatment strategy for short children born small for gestational age. *Horm Res* 2004; **62(Suppl 3)**: 137–140.

● 24 Dos Santos C, Essioux L, Teinturier C, *et al*. A common polymorphism of the growth hormone receptor is associated with increased responsiveness to growth hormone. *Nat Genet* 2004; **36**: 720–4.

25 Binder G, Baur F, Schweizer R, Ranke MB. The d3-growth hormone receptor polymorphism is associated with increased responsiveness to GH in Turner syndrome and short SGA children. *J Clin Endocrinol Metab* 2006; **91**: 659–64.

26 Rosilio M, Carel JC, Ecosse E, Chaussainon JL. Adult height of prepubertal short children born small for gestational age treated with GH. *Eur J Endocrinol* 2005; **152**: 835–43.

27 Coutant R, Carel JC, Letrait M, *et al*. Short stature associated with intrauterine growth retardation: final height of untreated and growth hormone-treated children. *J Clin Endocrinol Metab* 1998; **83**: 1070–4.

28 Zucchini S, Cacciari E, Balsamo A, *et al*. Final height of short subjects of low birth weight with and without growth hormone treatment. *Arch Dis Child* 2001; **84**: 340–3.

● 29 Van Pareren Y, Mulder P, Houdijk M, *et al*. Adult height after long-term, continuous growth hormone (GH) treatment in short children born small for gestational age: results of a randomized, double-blind, dose-response GH trial. *J Clin Endocrinol Metab* 2003; **88**: 3584–90.

30 Dahlgren J, Wikland KA. Final height in short children born small for gestational age treated with growth hormone. *Pediatr Res* 2005; **57**: 216–22.

● 31 Carel JC, Chatelain P, Rochiccioli P, Chaussain JL. Improvement in adult height after growth hormone treatment in adolescents with short stature born small for gestational age: results of a randomized controlled study. *J Clin Endocrinol Metab* 2003; **88**: 1587–93.

32 Ranke MB, Lindberg A, Cowell CT, *et al*. Prediction of response to growth hormone treatment in short children born small for gestational age: analysis of data from KIGS (Pharmacia International Growth Database). *J Clin Endocrinol Metab* 2003; **88**: 125–31.

33 de Zegher F, Butenandt O, Chatelain P, *et al*. Growth hormone treatment of short children born small for gestational age: reappraisal of the rate of bone maturation over 2 years and metanalysis of height gain over 4 years. *Acta Paediatr Suppl* 1997; **423**: 207–12.

34 Boonstra V, Van Pareren Y, Mulder P, Hokken-Koelega A. Puberty in growth hormone-treated children born small for gestational age (SGA). *J Clin Endocrinol Metab* 2003; **88**: 5753–8.

35 Darendeliler F, Ranke MB, Bakker B, et al. Bone age progression during the first year of growth hormone therapy in pre-pubertal children with idiopathic growth hormone deficiency, Turner syndrome or idiopathic short stature, and in short children born small for gestational age: analysis of data from KIGS (Pfizer International Growth Database). Horm Res 2005; 63: 40–7.

36 Sas T, Mulder P, Hokken-Koelega A. Body composition, blood pressure, and lipid metabolism before and during long-term growth hormone (GH) treatment in children with short stature born small for gestational age either with or without GH deficiency. J Clin Endocrinol Metab 2000; 85: 3786–92.

37 Leger J, Garel C, Fjellestad-Paulsen A, et al. Human growth hormone treatment of short-stature children born small for gestational age: effect on muscle and adipose tissue mass during a 3-year treatment period and after 1 year's withdrawal. J Clin Endocrinol Metab 1998; 83: 3512–6.

38 O'Keeffe MJ, O'Callaghan M, Williams GM, et al. Learning, cognitive, and attentional problems in adolescents born small for gestational age. Pediatrics 2003; 112: 301–7.

39 Arends NJ, Boonstra VH, Hokken-Koelega AC. Head circumference and body proportions before and during growth hormone treatment in short children who were born small for gestational age. Pediatrics 2004; 114: 683–90.

40 van Pareren YK, Duivenvoorden HJ, Slijper FS, et al. Intelligence and psychosocial functioning during long-term growth hormone therapy in children born small for gestational age. J Clin Endocrinol Metab 2004; 89: 5295–302.

41 van der Reijden-Lakeman IE, de Sonneville LM, Swaab-Barneveld HJ, et al. Evaluation of attention before and after 2 years of growth hormone treatment in intrauterine growth retarded children. J Clin Exp Neuropsychol 1997; 19: 101–18.

42 van der Reijden-Lakeman I, Slijper FM, Dongen-Melman JE, et al. Self-concept before and after two years of growth hormone treatment in intrauterine growth-retarded children. Horm Res 1996; 46: 88–94.

43 Visser-van Balen H, Geenen R, Moerbeek M, et al. Psychosocial functioning of adolescents with idiopathic short stature or persistent short stature born small for gestational age during three years of combined growth hormone and gonadotropin-releasing hormone agonist treatment. Horm Res 2005; 64: 77–87.

44 Swerdlow AJ, Higgins CD, Adlard P, Preece MA. Risk of cancer in patients treated with human pituitary growth hormone in the UK, 1959–85: a cohort study. Lancet 2002; 360: 273–7.

● 45 Barker DJ, Gluckman PD, Godfrey KM, et al. Fetal nutrition and cardiovascular disease in adult life. Lancet 1993; 341: 938–41.

46 Leger J, Levy-Marchal C, Bloch J, et al. Reduced final height and indications for insulin resistance in 20 year olds born small for gestational age: regional cohort study. BMJ 1997; 315: 341–7.

47 Yajnik CS, Fall CH, Vaidya U, et al. Fetal growth and glucose and insulin metabolism in four-year-old Indian children. Diabet Med 1995; 12: 330–6.

48 Soto N, Bazaes RA, Pena V, et al. Insulin sensitivity and secretion are related to catch-up growth in small-for-gestational-age infants at age 1 year: results from a prospective cohort. J Clin Endocrinol Metab 2003; 88: 3645–50.

49 de Zegher F, Ong K, van Helvoirt M, et al. High-dose growth hormone (GH) treatment in non-GH-deficient children born small for gestational age induces growth responses related to pretreatment GH secretion and associated with a reversible decrease in insulin sensitivity. J Clin Endocrinol Metab 2002; 87: 148–51.

50 Cutfield WS, Jackson WE, Jefferies C, et al. Reduced insulin sensitivity during growth hormone therapy for short children born small for gestational age. J Pediatr 2003; 142: 113–6.

51 Van Pareren Y, Mulder P, Houdijk M, et al. Effect of discontinuation of growth hormone treatment on risk factors for cardiovascular disease in adolescents born small for gestational age. J Clin Endocrinol Metab 2003; 88: 347–53.

52 de Zegher F, Hokken-Koelega A. Growth hormone therapy for children born small for gestational age: height gain is less dose dependent over the long term than over the short term. Pediatrics 2005; 115: e458–62.

53 Johnston LB, Savage MO. Should recombinant human growth hormone therapy be used in short small for gestational age children? Arch Dis Child 2004; 89: 740–4.

54 Chatelain P, Job JC, Blanchard J, et al. Dose-dependent catch-up growth after 2 years of growth hormone treatment in intrauterine growth-retarded children. Belgian and French Pediatric Clinics and Sanofi-Choay (France). J Clin Endocrinol Metab 1994; 78: 1454–60.

55 Ranke MB, Lindberg A. Growth hormone treatment of short children born small for gestational age or with Silver–Russell syndrome: results from KIGS (Kabi International Growth Study), including the first report on final height. Acta Paediatr Suppl 1996; 417: 18–26.

40

The evaluation and treatment of the child with precocious puberty

JOAN DIMARTINO-NARDI, KATERINA HARWOOD

INTRODUCTION

The evaluation of children with early sexual development requires an understanding of the variable progression of normal puberty. The initial evaluation serves to identify the specific etiology of the sexual precocity. Further evaluation should then proceed to identify those children who might benefit from treatment with long-acting analogs of gonadotropin-releasing hormone (GnRHa) targeted to halt their pubertal progression and improve their final height.

NORMAL PUBERTY

Mechanisms of pubertal development

The physical changes during puberty are the result of two generally simultaneous processes: gonadarche, i.e., activation of the hypothalamic–pituitary–gonadal axis, and adrenarche, i.e., activation of the hypothalamic–pituitary–adrenal axis. The pulsatile release of gonadotropin-releasing hormone (GnRH) from the hypothalamus results in an increase in the amplitude and frequency of follicle-stimulating hormone (FSH) and an even greater increase in luteinizing hormone (LH) released from the pituitary gland.[1,2] In boys, LH stimulates increased testosterone production from the Leydig cells of the testes and FSH stimulates the maturation of the spermatogonia.[3] In girls, both FSH and LH are necessary for sex hormone production; FSH affects maturation of the ova.[1]

Adrenarche refers to the rise of adrenal androgen production from the zona reticularis of the adrenal gland.[4] It generally precedes gonadarche, and its control is poorly understood as the precise stimulating factor has not been identified. Adrenarche contributes to the development of sexual hair growth, body odor, as well as typical skin changes, including acne and oiliness.

The presence of gonadarche can be confirmed with a GnRH stimulation test.[5] After a bolus dose of exogenous GnRH, the gonadotropin response is diminished in the prepubertal child. As puberty progresses, there is an incremental rise of FSH, and an even greater rise of LH; the LH/FSH ratio becomes greater than 1. Thus LH response to an exogenous dose of GnRH is more indicative of pubertal maturation than the FSH response.

Clinical features

Puberty is the period in which sexual maturity is achieved. Pubertal onset occurs in 95 percent of girls between the ages of 8 and 13 years, with a mean age of 11 years.[6] In boys, the pubertal onset is between 9 and 14 years, with a mean of 11.5 years.[6] The pubertal changes have been staged by Marshall and Tanner.[7,8] For boys, Zachmann et al.[9] have introduced a set of elliptical models of known volume to assess testicular development.

In girls, the development of the breast bud (thelarche) and enlargement of the areola are the results of increased estradiol production from the ovary. Other estrogen effects include genital and uterine maturation and the development of the typical female fat distribution.[10] The duration of breast development spans about 3–3.5 years.[6] Sexual hair development (pubarche) results from androgens derived from the adrenals (adrenarche) and gonads (gonadarche). Other androgen-induced effects include the development of axillary hair and odor and acne. Generally, thelarche precedes pubarche, although it may occasionally be the other way around. Menarche, the first menstrual period, occurs at a mean age of 12.8 years in North America, but usually occurs 2.3 years after the onset of breast development.[11] Menarche generally occurs during Tanner stages IV–V. Frequently, girls have irregular menses with some anovulatory cycles for 1–2 years after menarche.

In boys, the first evidence of puberty is an increase in testicular volume to more than 3 mL using the models developed by Zachmann.[9] This generally begins at 11.5–12 years of age. Progressive genital enlargement spans 3–5 years and is the result of increasing testosterone production from the testes and androgens from the adrenals. Other androgen-induced effects include sexual hair development, increase in muscle mass, decrease in body fat and development of acne.[10] Gynecomastia (breast development) occurs in about two-thirds of boys during normal puberty.[3] Regression of breast tissue generally occurs when puberty is complete, usually by age 16 years.

In girls, the pubertal growth spurt occurs during the earlier Tanner stages. After menarche, growth is variable with an average increase in height of 4–6 cm. In boys, the pubertal growth spurt occurs during the later stages of puberty, Tanner stages III – IV. In both sexes, the pubertal growth spurt is the result of the combined effect of growth hormone and sex steroids.[12] Estrogen plays a major role in the maturation of the epiphyseal growth plate and the advancement of the bone age. The importance of estrogen in epiphyseal maturation has been supported by the delayed epiphyseal maturation in the estrogen-insensitive boy, and in aromatase-deficient boys and girls.[13–15] Furthermore, in either sex, estrogen is crucial for the accumulation of calcium in bones and the attainment of a normal bone mineral density.

PRECOCIOUS PUBERTY

Classically, a child is considered to have precocious sexual development when secondary sex characteristics appear before the age of 8 years in girls and 9 years in boys. The initial evaluation assesses whether the early pubertal development is the result of either the early activation of the hypothalamic–pituitary–gonadal axis (central precocious puberty) or increased sex steroid production from the gonads or adrenals independent of gonadotropin release (peripheral precocious puberty). The GnRH stimulation test is useful in distinguishing between the two subsets.

Recent surveys of large populations of children have suggested that the percentage of girls with breast development before the age of 8 years has increased from 2.5 percent in

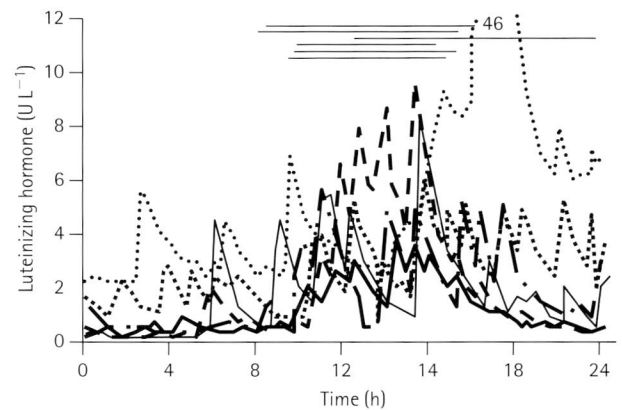

Figure 40.1 Twenty-four hour pulse patterns of luteinizing hormone (LH) in girls diagnosed to have idiopathic central precocious puberty (iCPP). Nighttime levels show a distinct pulsatile secretion pattern with increased levels compared to daytime values. Sleep periods are indicated with horizontal lines.

1969 to 10 percent in the 1990s.[16,17] In the 1997 study published by the Pediatric Research in Office Settings, 17 077 girls, 3–12 years of age, were evaluated for the age of onset of secondary sexual development. The authors of that study concluded that in girls 'across the United States, pubertal characteristics are developing at a younger age than currently used norms'.[16] On the basis of this study, the Drug and Therapeutics Committee of the Lawson Wilkins Pediatric Endocrine Society (LWPES) issued a statement lowering the normal age of puberty to 7 years in white girls and 6 years in black girls.[18]

Central precocious puberty

Central precocious puberty (CPP) refers to the early activation of the hypothalamic–pituitary–gonadal axis, which results in the development of sexual characteristics as well as the pubertal growth spurt. It accounts for >90 percent of cases of precocious puberty in published series.[19–22] Children have elevated basal levels of LH and FSH, which rise in response to a bolus dose of GnRH as seen in the normal pubertal child.[23] Furthermore, in girls with CPP, 24 h LH measurements at diagnosis reveal pulsatile secretion pattern with a distinct sleep–wake difference in LH amplitude (Fig. 40.1).[24] CPP is considered to be organic when it is associated with a lesion of the central nervous system (CNS), and as idiopathic when the computed tomography (CT) or magnetic resonance imaging (MRI) shows no such lesion. The incidence of idiopathic forms of CPP and its pattern of development vary according to gender.[11,25–29] Idiopathic CPP is rare in boys (fewer than 30 percent of CPP cases), while the opposite is true for girls (up to 80 percent of CPP cases). The pattern of development also varies according to gender and etiology. All boys with CPP and girls with organic CPP have rapidly progressive forms.

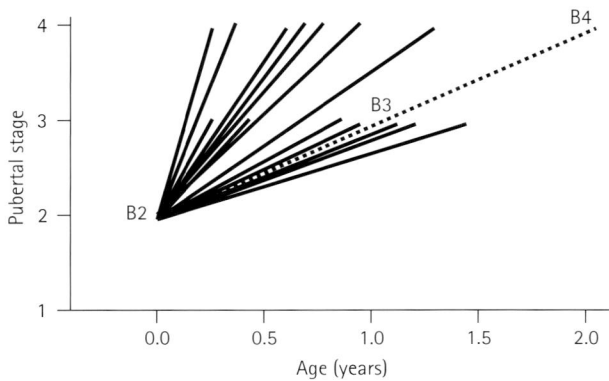

Figure 40.2 Progression of puberty from B2 to B3 or B4 in girls with idiopathic central precocious puberty. The broken line indicates approximate mean progression, calculated from transversal data in healthy Dutch girls.

In general, the rate of progression of puberty in idiopathic CPP in girls is faster than physiologic pubertal progression (Fig. 40.2). However, girls may also have a slowly progressive variant, in which predicted height is not altered after 2 years of spontaneous evolution.[30] For that reason, until recently (see below) all children with central precocious puberty underwent imaging of the pituitary using MRI with gadolinium.

The conditions known to be associated with CPP include:

- Idiopathic CPP
- CNS abnormalities: abscess, surgery, trauma, post-infection (meningitis, encephalitis), postchemotherapy, post-irradiation, granulomata, arachnoid cyst, suprasellar cyst, inflammatory disorders, septo-optic dysplasia, tumors (LH-secreting adenoma, astrocytoma, optic glioma, craniopharyngioma, dysgerminoma, ganglioneuroma, ependymoma, hypothalamic hamartoma, teratoma, pinealoma), hydrocephalus
- CPP secondary to chronic exposure to sex steroids (also referred to as combined precocious puberty): congenital adrenal hyperplasia, McCune–Albright syndrome, ovarian cysts, and familial gonadotropin-independent precocious puberty
- Miscellaneous conditions: Russell–Silver syndrome, hypothyroidism, von Recklinghausen's neurofibromatosis, tuberous sclerosis, epilepsy, and Prader–Willi syndrome

A hypothalamic hamartoma is an example of a CNS disorder associated with CPP. It is a benign congenital hyperplasia of nervous tissue with a normal histological appearance containing GnRH neurons and frequently presenting as a pedunculated mass at the base of the hypothalamus.[31] These tumors function as an ectopic GnRH pulse generator and function independently. Typically, patients with hamartomas present with CPP at an early age, more commonly among boys.

Transient central precocious puberty has also been described. Hence, for the early pubertal child, follow-up with confirmation of its progression should occur before therapy is initiated.[32]

Peripheral precocious puberty

Peripheral precocious puberty or pseudo-precocious puberty refers to the primary production of steroids from the adrenals or gonads without activation of the hypothalamic–pituitary–gonadal axis. Basal gonadotropins are suppressed, and there is a negligible gonadotropin response to GnRH testing. The conditions associated with pseudo-precocious puberty are:

- Congenital adrenal hyperplasia (CAH)
- McCune–Albright syndrome
- Familial gonadotropin-independent precocious puberty
- Adrenal lesion (adenoma, carcinoma)
- Ovarian lesion (granulosa cell tumor, granulosa–theca cell tumor, cystadenoma, gonadoblastoma, lipoid)
- Leydig cell tumor
- Human chorionic gonadotropin (hCG)-producing lesion: choriocarcinoma, chorioepithelioma, dysgerminoma, hepatoblastoma, teratoma, hepatoma
- Exogenous sex steroids
- Chronic primary hypothyroidism

Familial gonadotropin-independent precocious puberty refers to an autosomal dominant mutation in the LH receptor, resulting in a constitutively activated LH receptor and the resultant autonomous production of testosterone, which is independent of LH release.[33] Affected boys generally exhibit penile enlargement and bilateral testicular enlargement by the age of 4 years.[34] Gonadotropin levels are prepubertal. Boys with this condition can have secondary activation of the hypothalamic–pituitary–gonadal axis and concomitant true precocious puberty.

The McCune–Albright syndrome is another form of peripheral precocious puberty occurring most often in girls. They have an activating missence mutation in the gene for the alpha subunit of G_s, the G protein that stimulates cyclic adenosine monophosphate (cAMP) formation, which leads among others to an autonomous excessive hormone production.[35] Features of this syndrome include fibrous bone dysplasia, café-au-lait spots and multiple endocrinopathies including sexual precocity, hyperthyroidism, hyperadrenalism, pituitary gigantism or acromegaly, and hypophosphatemia. Patients may have autonomous ovarian estrogen production causing precocious puberty. As in boys with familial gonadotropin-independent precocious puberty, girls with this condition can eventually develop secondary true CPP as well.

Combined precocious puberty

Combined precocious puberty refers to the secondary activation of the hypothalamic–pituitary–gonadal axis that occurs after a long-standing sex steroid exposure associated with peripheral precocious puberty. As mentioned above, this can be seen for example with congenital adrenal hyperplasia, the McCune–Albright syndrome and familial gonadotropin-independent precocious puberty.

Contrasexual pubertal development

Contrasexual pubertal development is the development of secondary sexual characteristics inappropriate for the sex of the individual.

The conditions associated with contrasexual pubertal development are (1) virilization in girls, which includes:

- congenital adrenal hyperplasia
- virilizing adrenal neoplasm
- virilizing ovarian neoplasm

and (2) feminization in boys, which includes:

- adrenal neoplasm
- increased extraglandular conversion of circulating steroids to estrogen

Virilization of girls (sexual hair growth, oily skin, acne, clitoromegaly, and hirsutism) should prompt an adrenocorticotropic hormone (ACTH) stimulation test to identify a possible defect of adrenal steroidogenesis, because this is the most common cause. If hyperandrogenism occurs without identification of a specific enzymatic defect, adrenal suppression with dexamethasone and imaging of the adrenal glands and ovaries should be performed to exclude neoplasia.

Feminization (including gynecomastia) caused by abnormal estrogen production in a boy is unusual. Should it occur, gonadal and adrenal imaging should be performed to exclude neoplasia.

BENIGN CONDITIONS

Premature thelarche

Premature thelarche – isolated premature breast development – can be seen during two different stages of childhood; infancy/toddler-hood or after 6 years of age.

Quite commonly, small breasts (Tanner II–III) are seen in girls during the first 2 years of life caused by a persistence of infant gonadotropin secretion. There are no signs of estrogenization of the areola or vaginal mucosa and growth and bone-age maturation are normal as well. Ovarian ultrasound may detect small cysts. These breasts almost always resolve by 2–3 years of age.

In girls between the ages of 6–8 years breast development (Tanner II) may appear without any other evidence of puberty. Usually, normal puberty at the appropriate age ensues without an adult height compromise, but certain girls progress and develop central precocious puberty. For this reason, careful monitoring over time is needed.

Premature adrenarche

Premature adrenarche (PA) means early maturation of the zona reticularis of the adrenal glands. The modestly elevated androgens can bring about early changes associated with adrenarche (axillary and/or pubic hair, axillary odor, acne, oily skin). There should be no other associated findings such as virilization, advancement of growth, and bone-age maturation. Androgens levels (DHEA, DHEAS, androstenedione) are generally in the range of girls in the early (Tanner II–III) stages of puberty but need to be verified. Puberty is expected to start and progress normally.

In certain girls, premature adrenarche may be an early developmental phase of polycystic ovarian syndrome (PCOS) and insulin resistance.[36,37] In young minority girls with PA (Caribbean–Hispanic and African–American) ACTH-stimulated androgen levels were more than 2 standard deviations above the mean for normal girls in early puberty.[38] These girls were also found to have reduced insulin sensitivity when evaluated using the frequently sampled intravenous glucose tolerance test (FSIVGTT). The association of PA with PCOS has also been described in European Caucasian girls by Ibanez.

EVALUATION OF THE SEXUALLY PRECOCIOUS CHILD

The evaluation of a child with early sexual development needs to distinguish between true central precocious puberty, peripheral precocious puberty, and the benign conditions of premature thelarche or premature adrenarche. After the diagnosis of central precocious puberty has been established, the evaluation needs to identify those children with organic CNS pathology versus those without an identifiable etiology or idiopathic precocious puberty. Furthermore, among children with idiopathic PP, one must distinguish between those children with the slowly progressive form, from those with a more rapid course. The former more slowly progressive variant generally achieves a normal adult height, whereas the more rapidly progressive variant may result in early menarche, rapid epiphyseal maturation, and ultimately short stature.

Therefore, the evaluation of the child with early sexual development includes a complete history and physical examination, with particular attention to signs and symptoms suggestive of central nervous system (CNS) pathology. A family history should include the pubertal history and heights of family members. The physical examination should include blood pressure (elevated in adrenal hyperplasia–11 hydroxylase deficiency), height, weight, a careful evaluation of the skin for café-au-lait spots (McCune–Albright syndrome, neurofibromatosis), fibromas (neurofibromatosis), and hypopigmented lesions (tuberous sclerosis), and careful Tanner staging of pubertal development. In boys, testicular size should be measured using the Prader orchidometer. Bilateral or unilateral testicular enlargement can be seen with testicular tumors or adrenal rest tissue associated with adrenal hyperplasia. In girls, the presence of markedly hyperpigmented areola suggests the presence of an estrogen-secreting lesion (cyst of McCune–Albright, or estrogen-secreting tumor). Virilization (muscular habitus, clitoromegaly, penile enlargement) suggests the presence of an androgen-secreting lesion.

The laboratory evaluation involves direct measurement of basal sex steroids (testosterone and estradiol) and gonadotropins (FSH and LH). In boys, human chorionic gonadotropin should be measured. Thyroid function tests and adrenal androgen levels should also be obtained. In children with the early development of pubic hair, axillary hair or odor, measurement of early morning androgens (including 17-hydroxyprogesterone) or an ACTH stimulation test should be considered to evaluate for an enzymatic defect of adrenal steroidogenesis. A GnRH stimulation test is useful to confirm the activation of the hypothalamic–pituitary–gonadal axis. GnRH 100 µg is administered intravenously, with FSH and LH measured at 0, 20, 40 and 60 min after the administration of GnRH. Interpretation of the gonadotropin response requires a knowledge of the pre-pubertal and pubertal levels for the particular assay used. In CPP there is an exaggerated gonadotropin response to GnRH compared to physiologic puberty (Fig. 40.3), especially for LH, while basal gonadotropin and sex steroid levels

do not necessarily differ from children in a similar stage of puberty. The increased gonadotropin response may be explained by a more rapid development of the GnRH pulse generator and a retarded equilibrium between gonadal products and gonadotropin secretion.

Usually, an MRI of the pituitary gland with gadolinium is performed to rule out a CNS lesion in patients with CPP.[39] Adrenal and gonadal CT and/or ultrasonography should be performed if the GnRH test is consistent with peripheral precocious puberty to rule out tumor.

Traditionally, CPP evaluation – including MRI of the pituitary – has been performed if a child shows signs of sexual development before the age of 8 years in girls, and 9 years in boys. For girls this recommendation is based on a 5–10 percent incidence of intracranial lesions causing the CPP. However, in 90–95 percent of girls with CPP, brain imaging results are normal but the procedure is stressful, expensive and with potential side effects due to the need for sedation.[40] There is no dispute that all boys with precocious puberty should undergo neuro-imaging, as they have a much higher incidence of intracranial tumors.

On the basis of the previously mentioned surveys by Herman-Giddens, two American groups, Elders et al. and the LWPES, proposed different strategies for the selection of those young girls with evidence of early sexual development who should undergo full evaluation (including brain imaging) and treatment.[18,41] The recommendations suggest that the indications for an investigation of suspected precocious puberty in girls include:

- the presence of pubic hair or breast development in girls below the age of 6 years
- girls before the age of 8 years with any sign of puberty who appear to be developing more rapidly than is usual or who exhibit acceleration in linear growth or skeletal maturation
- girls with contrasexual PP[41]

In most cases, early breast and/or pubic hair development does not necessitate evaluation for pathologic etiology of precocious puberty in the case of white girls older than 7 years of age or African–American girls older than 6 years of age, unless there is evidence of one or more of the following factors:

- rapid progression (BA >2 years advanced and HP <2 SD below genetic target height (TH) or <150 cm),
- CNS-related signs and symptoms
- underlying neurological problems
- adversely affected emotional state of the patient or family[18]

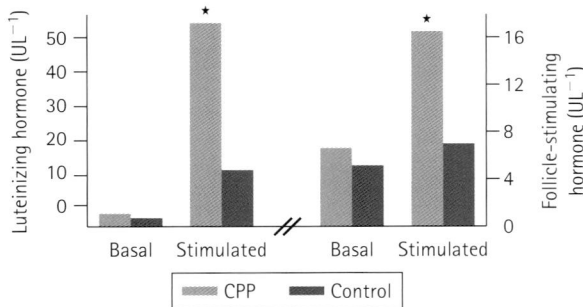

Figure 40.3 Basal and GnRH (100 µg, i.v.) stimulated levels of luteinizing hormone (LH) and follicle stimulating hormone (FSH) in 14 girls with idiopathic central precocious puberty (iCPP) and 21 controls in similar stages of puberty. Estradiol levels between iCPP and controls did not differ significantly (iCPP 92.7 ± 23 (SD), controls 65.4 ± 13 pmol L^{-1}, respectively). Basal levels of LH and FSH do not differ, while LH and FSH peak levels are significantly higher in the affected girls.

The report from Herman-Giddens[16] and the recommendation of the LWPES[18] that followed met with controversy and skepticism (e.g., references 42–44). Among the concerns is that use of the new guidelines will lead to significant underdiagnosis of endocrine conditions (such as

CAH, neurofibromatosis, hypothyroidism, and McCune–Albright syndrome), as well as delay in the diagnosis of intracranial lesions, which might initially become symptomatic only as CPP in 6- to 8-year-olds. Furthermore, a subset of girls with advanced bone age and reduced height potential may not be evaluated and not offered therapy to improve final adult height. It seems advisable, then, that all girls with secondary sexual development before 8 years of age have at least a bone-age assessment and close longitudinal follow-up, especially in view of the fact that breast and pubic hair development can be asynchronous in the early states of precocious puberty.[44]

Recent reports from Europe suggest a new set of criteria for selecting girls with PP for brain imaging.[45,46] The recommendations are that 'those girls with signs of sexual development before the age of 6 years or an estradiol level >45th percentile undergo imaging of the pituitary.' Using these guidelines, the sensitivity was 100 percent and the specificity was 39 percent. All patients with occult intracranial lesion were identified and more than 1/3 of the unnecessary brain MRIs were avoided. The caveats to directly applying the results of this study from Europe to practice in the US are that the European population is more homogenous and that different estradiol assays and value distributions were used in the European study. The need for validation for each specific patient population is obvious.

In a young child, difficulty coping with tall stature and advancing pubertal development may present with behavioral changes.[47–49] The discrepancy between physical appearance and chronological age may predispose certain children to stress, abuse, and early pregnancy. Psychological counseling may be helpful for the parents and child to decrease the fears that they may have regarding the early sexual development.

THERAPY

The premature exposure of the bones to sex steroids may cause rapid bone maturation with an adult height achieved at a younger age.[25,50,51] Short stature with a height below the 5th percentile can occur in 10–30 percent of girls with true precocious puberty.

The mean adult heights reported in untreated girls with idiopathic precocious puberty tend to be short (150.9–155.3 cm).[25,49,50,52,53] However, 29 of the 89 girls reported in these studies achieved an adult height greater than 5 feet (150 cm).[25,50,51,53,54] Hence, not all girls with precocious puberty are short as adults. The reported mean adult heights of untreated boys with precocious puberty also tend to be short and range from 149.8 to 159.6 cm.[25,51,53] However, not all boys in those studies were short as adults. The differences in adult height achieved by children with precocious puberty reflect genetic influences on height. In addition, mild, slowly progressive variants of precocious puberty have been reported. In these cases of idiopathic CPP with moderate estrogen activity and bone age advancement

less than 2 years above chronologic age, the height prediction was normal and did not deteriorate after 2 years of follow-up without therapy.[30,55,56] However, a careful clinical follow-up is necessary.[57]

The final heights and near final heights for 27 untreated children with precocious puberty were reported to be 161.4 ± 7.7 cm (32nd percentile) and 165 cm (59th percentile), respectively.[58] Ninety percent of the girls achieved a height of more than 153 cm (3rd percentile). Only 10 percent were shorter than 150 cm (1st percentile). Final height significantly correlated with the initial height prediction using the method of Bayley–Pinneau and with the degree of height age advancement. Furthermore, in a larger cohort of patients in many of whom adult height could not be obtained, there was no decrease in the height prediction after 3 years of follow-up. As this study did not include a large cohort of girls whose sexual precocity occurred before the age of 5 years, the Bayley–Pinneau method of height prediction for these younger girls should be interpreted with caution.

In true precocious puberty, the goal of therapy is to halt pubertal progression in order to avoid psychosocial problems, prevent early menarche and improve adult height in those children at risk for short stature.[59] The Bayley–Pinneau method of height prediction can be used to identify those patients at risk for short stature who might benefit from therapy.

Long-acting analogs of GnRH (GnRHa) cause reversible suppression of gonadotropins and a decline in gonadal sex steroid levels within 1 month of initiation.[60] GnRH testing may be used periodically to confirm suppression of the hypothalamic–pituitary–gonadal axis. GnRHa are not effective for the treatment of gonadotropin-independent precocious puberty as in McCune–Albright syndrome or familial gonadotropin-independent precocious puberty, unless secondary true precocious puberty occurs as well. Clinically, regression of breast development in girls and a decrease in testicular size in boys occur after several months of therapy. Sexual hair growth continues to progress because GnRHa do not suppress adrenarche.[61]

When treatment with GnRHa is discontinued, gonadotropin and sex steroid levels rise rapidly into the adult range.[62] One should take into account that the treatment with a GnRHa will not postpone central development of puberty. Since GnRHa activity is at the pituitary level, the hypothalamic GnRH release will not be affected and its maturation will continue. After discontinuation of the GnRHa, the characteristic pubertal day–night rhythm has disappeared.[24] Menses have been reported to occur in 65 percent of patients within 2 years after the discontinuation of GnRHa treatment. Fertility after GnRHa treatment has not been assessed as yet although pregnancies have been reported to occur in adolescents and young adults who had completed therapy with a GnRHa. A recent study published from Heger on long-term outcome after depot GnRHa treatment of CPP concludes 'long term depot GnRHa treatment of CPP girls preserved genetic height potential and improved final height (FH) significantly combined with normal body proportions. No negative effect on bone mineral density and reproductive function was seen. Treatment neither caused nor aggravated obesity'.[63]

GnRH therapy causes a decrease in growth velocity which results from a decrease in the amplitude of nocturnal growth hormone (GH) peaks without affecting GH pulse frequency.[64] The combined effect of the decrease in growth velocity, as well as a decrease in a rate of bone age maturation, results in an increase in the child's height prediction. The reported mean adult heights of treated girls with precocious puberty are very variable. Treated girls have been reported to achieve mean adult heights ranging from 154.7 cm to 164.9 cm with a height gain of about 2–5.2 cm when the final height is compared with the initial height prediction made at the time of diagnosis.[65–68] There is sparse information available regarding the adult height of boys treated with a GnRHa. Mean adult heights of treated boys range from 168 to 184 cm which constitute a 6.3–9.9 cm gain in adult height compared with the initial height prediction made at the time of diagnosis.[65,66] The tremendous variability of the impact of treatment on adult height reflects several factors, including genetic potential, the age of initiation of puberty, the degree of bone age advancement at the time of diagnosis, the speed of progression of puberty, and the timing of initiation of therapy. In the 1994 review by Kletter and Kelch, the adult height of GnRH-treated girls was assessed according to the age of the child when sexual precocity was diagnosed and evaluated.[69] In that review, the adult height of 17 treated children with precocious puberty, diagnosed before 6 years of age, was compared with the heights of 10 untreated children of the same age. The adult height of the treated children was 160.4 ± 1.8 cm in comparison to the untreated children who achieved an adult height of 153.9 ± 3.8 cm. The height of the 114 treated children, who were more than 6 years of age at the time of evaluation, was not significantly different from the height of the 54 untreated children (157.5 cm and 157 cm, respectively). The treatment of children who were diagnosed and treated before the age of 6 years resulted in a significant improvement in adult height.[70]

Brauner reserved GnRHa therapy for those girls with a poor height prediction that was less than 155 cm and did not treat those girls with a height prediction greater than 155 cm.[71] The group who received therapy achieved a mean adult height, which was 6.5 cm greater than their initial height prediction. In the untreated children, the adult height was similar to the predicted height at the initial evaluation.

In certain children with true precocious puberty, GnRHa therapy results in a marked decline in growth velocity below normal. In these children, standard provocative testing should be performed to evaluate for coexistent GH deficiency. Growth hormone therapy in these children can improve their growth velocity and height prediction.[72] This recommendation has also been extended to children with precocious puberty on GnRHa whose height prediction is impaired, even though they are not GH deficient by standard testing.[73] In these children, combination therapy (GnRHa + GH) can result in an improved growth velocity and predicted adult height.[74]

The therapy for pseudo-precocious puberty is dependent upon the etiology. Tumors are treated both surgically and with chemotherapy. In familial gonadotropin-independent precocious puberty, inhibitors of androgen biosynthesis (ketoconazole), antiandrogens (flutamide, spironolactone) and inhibitors of androgen-to-estrogen conversion (testolactone) are being investigated.[75] In the McCune–Albright syndrome, medroxyprogesterone acetate and testolactone have been used.[76] However, a recent study suggests a new and promising therapy with tamoxifen for girls with peripheral precocious puberty associated with the McCune–Albright syndrome.[77] During a 12 month trial the number of bleeding episodes significantly decreased along with reduction of growth velocity and rate of bone maturation.[77] Should true central sexual precocity develop, GnRHa can be added to the treatment regimen.

For congenital adrenal hyperplasia, replacement of deficient glucocorticoids and mineralocorticoids is used, although new forms of therapy are currently being investigated. Preliminary data suggest that a combination of antiandrogen (flutamide) and inhibitor of androgen to estrogen conversion (testolactone) allow for a reduction in the hydrocortisone dose in patients with adrenal hyperplasia.[78] This treatment regimen could lead to reduced risk of glucocorticoid excess and improved treatment outcome.[79] A long-term study of this new regimen is ongoing.

CONCLUSION

For the child who has early sexual development, the initial evaluation should be to identify the specific etiology so that appropriate treatment can be provided. For those children with true sexual precocity, therapy with long-acting analogs is effective in halting pubertal progression, improving adult height, and promoting the psychosocial adjustment of the child and family. There is a wide spectrum of clinical progression of early sexual development, ranging from the nonprogressive forms to the more rapidly progressive variants. Hence, not all children with sexual precocity will require GnRHa suppressive therapy. For those children whose families opt not to choose treatment because the height prediction is acceptable and the early development is not interfering with their psychosocial adjustment, careful follow-up of growth and development should continue.

Acknowledgment

Thank you to Henriette Delemarre for providing the figures for this chapter.

KEY LEARNING POINTS

- Evaluate girls <8 years old and boys <9 years old with early pubertal development.
- Distinguish central precocious puberty from peripheral precocious puberty.
- Rule out space occupying lesion in central precocious puberty.
- Obtain bone age and calculate height prediction.
- Assess the rate of progression of puberty.
- Offer treatment in those with poor height prediction, rapid progression and/or psychosocial issues.
- Consider growth hormone therapy for those with poor height prediction or poor growth velocity.

REFERENCES

● = Seminal primary article
◆ = Key review paper
✳ = First formal publication of a management guideline

1 Knobil E. The neuroendocrine control of the menstrual cycle. *Recent Prog Horm Res* 1980; **36**: 53–88.

2 Lee PA. Pubertal neuroendocrine maturation: early differentiation and stages of development. 1988.

● 3 Nielsen CT, Skakkebaek NE, Darling JA, *et al.* Longitudinal study of testosterone and luteinizing hormone (LH) in relation to spermarche, pubic hair, height and sitting height in normal boys. *Acta Endocrinol Suppl (Copenh)* 1986; **279**: 98–106.

4 Saenger P, Reiter EO. Premature adrenarche: a normal variant of puberty? *J Clin Endocrinol Metab* 1992; **74**: 236–8.

● 5 Reiter EO, Kaplan SL, Conte FA, Grumbach MM. Responsivity of pituitary gonadotropes to luteinizing hormone-releasing factor in idiopathic precocious puberty, precocious thelarche, precocious adrenarche, and in patients treated with medroxyprogesterone acetate. *Pediatr Res* 1975; **9**: 111–6.

6 Lee PA. Normal ages of pubertal events among American males and females. *J Adolesc Health Care* 1980; **1**: 26–9.

7 Marshall WA, Tanner JM. Variations in pattern of pubertal changes in girls. *Arch Dis Child* 1969; **44**: 291–303.

8 Marshall WA, Tanner JM. Variations in the pattern of pubertal changes in boys. *Arch Dis Child* 1970; **45**: 13–23.

9 Zachmann M, Prader A, Kind HP, *et al.* Testicular volume during adolescence. Cross-sectional and longitudinal studies. *Helv Paediatr Acta* 1974; **29**: 61–72.

● 10 de Ridder CM, Thijssen JH, Bruning PF, *et al.* Body fat mass, body fat distribution, and pubertal development: a longitudinal study of physical and hormonal sexual maturation of girls. *J Clin Endocrinol Metab* 1992; **75**: 442–6.

◆ 11 Kaplan SL, Grumbach MM. Clinical review 14: Pathophysiology and treatment of sexual precocity. *J Clin Endocrinol Metab* 1990; **71**: 785–9.

12 Attie KM, Ramirez NR, Conte FA, *et al.* The pubertal growth spurt in eight patients with true precocious puberty and growth hormone deficiency: evidence for a direct role of sex steroids. *J Clin Endocrinol Metab* 1990; **71**: 975–83.

✳ 13 Laue L, Kenigsberg D, Pescovitz OH, *et al.* Treatment of familial male precocious puberty with spironolactone and testolactone. *N Engl J Med* 1989; **320**: 496–502.

14 Federman DD. Life without estrogen. *N Engl J Med* 1994; **331**: 1088–9.

● 15 Smith EP, Boyd J, Frank GR, *et al.* Estrogen resistance caused by a mutation in the estrogen-receptor gene in a man. *N Engl J Med* 1994; **331**: 1056–61.

● 16 Herman-Giddens ME, Slora EJ, Wasserman RC, *et al.* Secondary sexual characteristics and menses in young girls seen in office practice: a study from the Pediatric Research in Office Settings network. *Pediatrics* 1997; **99**: 505–12.

17 Huen KF, Leung SS, Lau JT, *et al.* Secular trend in the sexual maturation of southern Chinese girls. *Acta Paediatr* 1997; **86**: 1121–4.

◆ 18 Kaplowitz PB, Oberfield SE. Reexamination of the age limit for defining when puberty is precocious in girls in the United States: implications for evaluation and treatment. Drug and Therapeutics and Executive Committees of the Lawson Wilkins Pediatric Endocrine Society. *Pediatrics* 1999; **104(4 Pt 1)**: 936–41.

19 Cisternino M, Arrigo T, Pasquino AM, *et al.* Etiology and age incidence of precocious puberty in girls: a multicentric study. *J Pediatr Endocrinol Metab* 2000; **13(Suppl 1)**: 695–701.

20 Garagorri JM, Chaussain JL, Job JC. Precocious puberty in girls. Study of 98 cases. *Arch Fr Pediatr* 1982; **39**: 605–11.

◆ 21 Pescovitz OH, Comite F, Hench K, *et al.* The NIH experience with precocious puberty: diagnostic subgroups and response to short-term luteinizing hormone releasing hormone analogue therapy. *J Pediatr* 1986; **108**: 47–54.

22 Bridges NA, Christopher JA, Hindmarsh PC, Brook CG. Sexual precocity: sex incidence and aetiology. *Arch Dis Child* 1994; **70**: 116–8.

● 23 Neely EK, Wilson DM, Lee PA, *et al.* Spontaneous serum gonadotropin concentrations in the evaluation of precocious puberty. *J Pediatr* 1995; **127**: 47–52.

● 24 Schroor EJ, Van Weissenbruch MM, Delemarre-van de Waal HA. Long-term GnRH-agonist treatment does not postpone central development of the GnRH pulse generator in girls with idiopathic precocious puberty. *J Clin Endocrinol Metab* 1995; **80**: 1696–701.

25 Sigurjonsdottir TJ, Hayles AB. Precocious puberty. A report of 96 cases. *Am J Dis Child* 1968; **115**: 309–21.

26 Chaussain JL, Savage MO, Nahoul K, *et al.* Hypothalamo-pituitary-gonadal function in male central precocious puberty. *Clin Endocrinol (Oxf)* 1978; **8**: 437–44.

27 Cacciari E, Frejaville E, Cicognani A, et al. How many cases of true precocious puberty in girls are idiopathic? J Pediatr 1983; **102**: 357–60.

28 Cutler GB Jr. Overview of premature sexual development. New York: Raven Press; 1990.

29 Oerter KE, Uriarte MM, Rose SR, et al. Gonadotropin secretory dynamics during puberty in normal girls and boys. J Clin Endocrinol Metab 1990; **71**: 1251–8.

30 Fontoura M, Brauner R, Prevot C, Rappaport R. Precocious puberty in girls: early diagnosis of a slowly progressing variant. Arch Dis Child 1989; **64**: 1170–6.

31 Judge DM, Kulin HE, Page R, et al. Hypothalamic hamartoma: a source of luteinizing-hormone-releasing factor in precocious puberty. N Engl J Med 1977; **296**: 7–10.

32 Schwarz HP, Tschaeppeler H, Zuppinger K. Unsustained central sexual precocity in four girls. Am J Med Sci 1990; **299**: 260–4.

● 33 Shenker A, Laue L, Kosugi S, et al. A constitutively activating mutation of the luteinizing hormone receptor in familial male precocious puberty. Nature 1993; **365**: 652–4.

34 Egli CA, Rosenthal SM, Grumbach MM, et al. Pituitary gonadotropin-independent male-limited autosomal dominant sexual precocity in nine generations: familial testotoxicosis. J Pediatr 1985; **106**: 33–40.

● 35 Weinstein LS, Shenker A, Gejman PV, et al. Activating mutations of the stimulatory G protein in the McCune-Albright syndrome. N Engl J Med 1991; **325**: 1688–95.

36 Dimartino-Nardi J. Premature adrenarche: findings in prepubertal African-American and Caribbean-Hispanic girls. Acta Paediatr Suppl 1999; **88**: 67–72.

◆ 37 Ibanez L, Dimartino-Nardi J, Potau N, Saenger P. Premature adrenarche–normal variant or forerunner of adult disease? Endocr Rev 2000; **21**: 671–96.

● 38 Vuguin P, Linder B, Rosenfeld RG, et al. The roles of insulin sensitivity, insulin-like growth factor I (IGF-I), and IGF-binding protein-1 and -3 in the hyperandrogenism of African-American and Caribbean Hispanic girls with premature adrenarche. J Clin Endocrinol Metab 1999; **84**: 2037–42.

39 Chemaitilly W, Trivin C, Adan L, et al. Central precocious puberty: clinical and laboratory features. Clin Endocrinol (Oxf) 2001; **54**: 289–94.

40 Kaplowitz P. Precocious puberty in girls and the risk of a central nervous system abnormality: the elusive search for diagnostic certainty. Pediatrics 2002; **109**: 139–41.

41 Elders MJ, Scott CR, Frindik JP, Kemp SF. Clinical workup for precocious puberty. Lancet 1997; **350**: 457–8.

42 Rosenfeld RL, Bachrach LK, Chernausek SD, et al. Current age of onset of puberty. Pediatrics 2000; **106**: 622–3.

43 Viner R. Splitting hairs. Arch Dis Child 2002; **86**: 8–10.

44 Midyett LK, Moore WV, Jacobson JD. Are pubertal changes in girls before age 8 benign? Pediatrics 2003; **111**: 47–51.

45 Chalumeau M, Chemaitilly W, Trivin C, et al. Central precocious puberty in girls: an evidence-based diagnosis tree to predict central nervous system abnormalities. Pediatrics 2002; **109**: 61–7.

46 Chalumeau M, Hadjiathanasiou CG, Ng SM, et al. Selecting girls with precocious puberty for brain imaging: validation of European evidence-based diagnosis rule. J Pediatr 2003; **143**: 445–50.

47 Money J, Clopper RR Jr. Psychosocial and psychosexual aspects of errors of pubertal onset and development. Hum Biol 1974; **46**: 173–81.

48 Ehrhardt AA, Meyer-Bahlburg HF, Bell JJ, et al. Idiopathic precocious puberty in girls: psychiatric follow-up in adolescence. J Am Acad Child Psychiatry 1984; **23**: 23–33.

49 Sonis WA, Comite F, Blue J, et al. Behavior problems and social competence in girls with true precocious puberty. J Pediatr 1985; **106**: 156–60.

50 Thamdrup E. Precocious sexual development: A clinical study of one hundred children. Dan Med Bull 1961; **8**: 140–2.

51 Werder EA, Murset G, Zachmann M, et al. Treatment of precocious puberty with cyproterone acetate. Pediatr Res 1974; **8**: 248–56.

52 Lee PA. Medroxyprogesterone therapy for sexual precocity in girls. Am J Dis Child 1981; **135**: 443–5.

53 Murram D, Dewhurst J, Grant DB. Precocious puberty: a follow up study. Arch Dis Child 1984; **59**: 77–8.

● 54 Paul D, Conte FA, Grumbach MM, Kaplan SL. Long-term effect of gonadotropin-releasing hormone agonist therapy on final and near-final height in 26 children with true precocious puberty treated at a median age of less than 5 years. J Clin Endocrinol Metab 1995; **80**: 546–51.

∗ 55 Leger J, Reynaud R, Czernichow P. Do all girls with apparent idiopathic precocious puberty require gonadotropin-releasing hormone agonist treatment? J Pediatr 2000; **137**: 819–25.

56 Kreiter M, Burstein S, Rosenfield RL, et al. Preserving adult height potential in girls with idiopathic true precocious puberty. J Pediatr 1990; **117**: 364–70.

● 57 Palmert MR, Malin HV, Boepple PA. Unsustained or slowly progressive puberty in young girls: initial presentation and long-term follow-up of 20 untreated patients. J Clin Endocrinol Metab 1999; **84**: 415–23.

● 58 Bar A, Linder B, Sobel EH, et al. Bayley-Pinneau method of height prediction in girls with central precocious puberty: correlation with adult height. J Pediatr 1995; **126**: 955–8.

59 Ritzen EM. Early puberty: what is normal and when is treatment indicated? Horm Res 2003; **60(Suppl 3)**: 31–4.

∗ 60 Crowley WF Jr, Comite F, Vale W, et al. Therapeutic use of pituitary desensitization with a long-acting lhrh agonist: a potential new treatment for idiopathic precocious puberty. J Clin Endocrinol Metab 1981; **52**: 370–2.

● 61 Wierman ME, Beardsworth DE, Crawford JD, et al. Adrenarche and skeletal maturation during luteinizing hormone releasing hormone analogue suppression of gonadarche. J Clin Invest 1986; **77**: 121–6.

● 62 Jay N, Mansfield MJ, Blizzard RM, et al. Ovulation and menstrual function of adolescent girls with central precocious puberty after therapy with gonadotropin-releasing hormone agonists. *J Clin Endocrinol Metab* 1992; **75**: 890–4.

● 63 Heger S, Partsch CJ, Sippell WG. Long-term outcome after depot gonadotropin-releasing hormone agonist treatment of central precocious puberty: final height, body proportions, body composition, bone mineral density, and reproductive function. *J Clin Endocrinol Metab* 1999; **84**: 4583–90.

● 64 DiMartino-Nardi J, Wu R, Varner R, *et al.* The effect of luteinizing hormone-releasing hormone analog for central precocious puberty on growth hormone (GH) and GH-binding protein. *J Clin Endocrinol Metab* 1994; **78**: 664–8.

65 Oerter KE, Manasco P, Barnes KM, *et al.* Adult height in precocious puberty after long-term treatment with deslorelin. *J Clin Endocrinol Metab* 1991; **73**: 1235–40.

66 Oostdijk W, Drop SL, Odink RJ, *et al.* Long-term results with a slow-release gonadotrophin-releasing hormone agonist in central precocious puberty. Dutch-German Precocious Puberty Study Group. *Acta Paediatr Scand Suppl* 1991; **372**: 39–46.

67 Boepple PA, Crowley WR Jr. Growth, final height and reproductive function following GnRH agonist-induced pituitary-gonadal suppression in central precocious puberty. In: *Proceedings of the 75th Annual Meeting of the Endocrine Society*; 1993: 10.

68 Cacciari E, Cassio A, Balsamo A, *et al.* Long-term follow-up and final height in girls with central precocious puberty treated with luteinizing hormone-releasing hormone analogue nasal spray. *Arch Pediatr Adolesc Med* 1994; **148**: 1194–9.

◆ 69 Kletter GB, Kelch RP. Clinical review 60: Effects of gonadotropin-releasing hormone analog therapy on adult stature in precocious puberty. *J Clin Endocrinol Metab* 1994; **79**: 331–4.

● 70 Klein KO, Barnes KM, Jones JV, *et al.* Increased final height in precocious puberty after long-term treatment with LHRH agonists: the National Institutes of Health experience. *J Clin Endocrinol Metab* 2001; **86**: 4711–6.

71 Brauner R, Adan L, Malandry F, Zantleifer D. Adult height in girls with idiopathic true precocious puberty. *J Clin Endocrinol Metab* 1994; **79**: 415–20.

● 72 Cara JF, Kreiter ML, Rosenfield RL. Height prognosis of children with true precocious puberty and growth hormone deficiency: effect of combination therapy with gonadotropin releasing hormone agonist and growth hormone. *J Pediatr* 1992; **120**: 709–15.

73 Saggese G, Pasquino AM, Bertelloni S, *et al.* Effect of combined treatment with gonadotropin releasing hormone analogue and growth hormone in patients with central precocious puberty who had subnormal growth velocity and impaired height prognosis. *Acta Paediatr* 1995; **84**: 299–304.

74 Pasquino AM, Pucarelli I, Segni M, *et al.* Adult height in girls with central precocious puberty treated with gonadotropin-releasing hormone analogues and growth hormone. *J Clin Endocrinol Metab* 1999; **84**: 449–52.

75 Holland FJ, Fishman L, Bailey JD, Fazekas AT. Ketoconazole in the management of precocious puberty not responsive to LHRH-analogue therapy. *N Engl J Med* 1985; **312**: 1023–8.

76 Foster CM, Pescovitz OH, Comite F, *et al.* Testolactone treatment of precocious puberty in McCune-Albright syndrome. *Acta Endocrinol (Copenh)* 1985; **109**: 254–7.

✳ 77 Eugster EA, Rubin SD, Reiter EO, *et al.* Tamoxifen treatment for precocious puberty in McCune-Albright syndrome: a multicenter trial. *J Pediatr* 2003; **143**: 60–6.

78 Laue L, Merke DP, Jones JV, *et al.* A preliminary study of flutamide, testolactone, and reduced hydrocortisone dose in the treatment of congenital adrenal hyperplasia. *J Clin Endocrinol Metab* 1996; **81**: 3535–9.

79 Merke DP, Keil MF, Jones JV, *et al.* Flutamide, testolactone, and reduced hydrocortisone dose maintain normal growth velocity and bone maturation despite elevated androgen levels in children with congenital adrenal hyperplasia. *J Clin Endocrinol Metab* 2000; **85**: 1114–20.

41

Delay of growth and puberty

HENRIETTE A DELEMARRE-VAN DE WAAL

INTRODUCTION

Puberty is the result of increasing gonadotropin releasing hormone (GnRH) release by the hypothalamus. This is followed by a complex sequence of endocrine changes with functioning of negative and positive feedback mechanisms, and is associated with the development of sex characteristics, a growth spurt and reproductive competence.

During fetal life the GnRH–gonadotropin axis is already functioning as can be observed by high levels of both luteinizing hormone (LH) and follicle stimulating hormone (FSH) at mid-gestation when the development of the vascular portal system is complete. This mid-gestational peak is followed by a decline of gonadotropin levels, due to a developing negative feedback system as well as central inhibiting influences on GnRH release.[1]

Low gonadotropin levels at birth are followed by a transient increase during the first months of life, the so-called post-natal peak. Thereafter levels return to a very low, often undetectable range during the pre-pubertal phase as a result of the intrinsic restraint.

The clinical signs of puberty are in boys an increase of testicular volume above 3 mL (G2), and in girls bud-shaped elevation of the areola and papilla (B2). In girls this early stage of puberty is associated with an immediate increase of height velocity, whereas in boys the pubertal growth spurt occurs in the second half of puberty. Girls experience menarche, a milestone of pubertal development, about 2.3 years after the start of breast development.

The secular trend includes an increase of adolescent height associated with an earlier start of pubertal development. In several European countries the trend to an earlier onset of pubertal maturation has come to a halt during the

last decades. In the Netherlands, breast development in girls started at mean ages of 10.5 and 10.7 years in 1980 and in 1997 respectively, whereas in boys testicular development started at the ages of 11.3 and 11.4 years.[2] The timing of puberty is the result of both a genetic constitution and the influence of environmental forces exerted on it.[3] For instance, delayed puberty is often familial, but will also occur in the case of systemic diseases associated with chronic malnutrition. Such conditions will not allow the body to expend energy on growth, puberty, and fertility. Many systems involved in the regulation of puberty have been elucidated; however, the genes regulating the timing of puberty are only partly known.[4,5]

Delayed puberty is defined when puberty starts at a chronological age older than +2SD of average maturers. From Dutch data, this is, for boys, when testicular growth (testes volume 4 mL or more) does not start before the age of 14 years and, in girls when breast development is not present at the age of 13 years or when menarche has not occurred by the age of 15 years (primary amenorrhea).[2] These age limits may vary only slightly in other European countries.

A delay of puberty may occur as an isolated condition, as in constitutional delay, or it may be the manifestation of a permanent condition recognized by lack of a pubertal onset or by a pubertal arrest.

The temporary form of delayed puberty is often associated with growth failure. When it is familial it is called constitutional delay of growth and puberty (CDGP).[6]

Delay of growth and puberty is the most common condition referred to the pediatrician. The adolescents present with growth failure, lack of pubertal characteristics, and psychosocial problems. Constitutional delay of growth and puberty will often be the diagnosis, but when in doubt,

Table 41.1 Causes of delayed puberty

Temporary form
> Isolated, constitutional or familiar
> Constitutional delay of growth and puberty (CDGP)
> Secondary to chronic diseases

Persistent form
Hypogonadotropic hypogonadism
> Idiopathic
> Mutations of LH β and FSH β subunits
> Kallmann syndrome
> GnRH receptor gene mutations
> *DAX1* gene mutation
> *GPR 54* gene mutation
> Transcription factor gene mutations: *PROP1*, *LHX3* and *HESX1*,
>   in combination with other pituitary hormone deficiencies
> Brain tumor
> Irradiation of the brain
> Hypothalamic dysfunction in combination with other
>   syndromes

Hypergonadotropic hypogonadism
> Gonadal dysgenesis in normal and abnormal karyotypes
> Anorchie (vanishing testes syndrome)
> LH and FSH receptor gene mutation
> Gonadal damage due to surgery, radiation and
>   chemotherapy

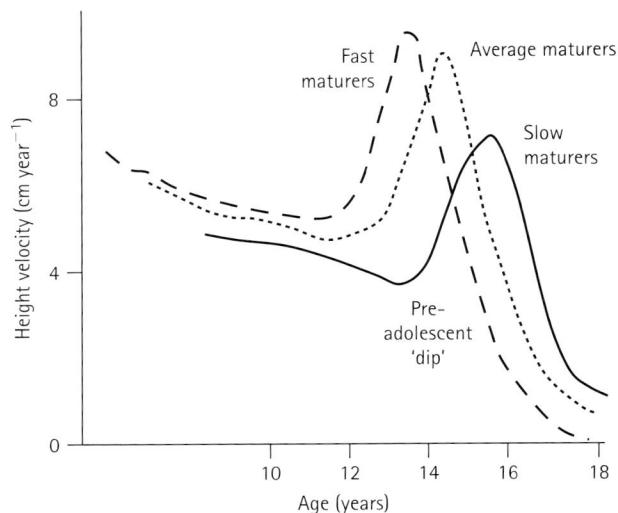

Figure 41.1 A physiologic phenomenon specifically seen in boys is the pre-adolescent dip, a lowering of height velocity, before the pubertal growth spurt. This dip can be very low, sometimes height velocities around 2 cm per year can be seen. The problem for these boys is that, during this period of slow growth, their classmates are in the full-blown spurt, and girls are at the end of puberty. At that moment, these boys are the shortest and most immature.

other causes of delayed puberty should be excluded. A summary of the causes of delayed puberty is given in Table 41.1.

PATHOPHYSIOLOGY: TEMPORARY DELAY OF PUBERTY

Delayed puberty presents with a wide individual variability. Late puberty is associated with a pre-pubertal dip of height velocity resulting in linear growth into a lower height SD as described by Hammer and Eddy in 1968[7,8] (Fig. 41.1). This decrease in height SDS is of particular concern in boys who are already short during pre-puberty. They are at risk of falling into an abnormally low SD range and well below their target range.

With respect to the diagnosis of constitutional delay of growth and puberty (CDGP), the delay of growth is defined as height for chronological age below -2 height SDs. Usually the child is born with a normal weight and length and his or her height curve decreases until the age of 3 years.[9] Thereafter height velocity remains reduced, below the 10th centile for chronological age and actual height is below the target height range. Bone maturation is often, but not invariably, retarded during pre-puberty. It can also suddenly slow down during late pre-puberty. Family history often includes a parent or sibling with delayed puberty, late menarche or late pubertal growth. Delayed puberty is

by definition associated with a late pubertal growth spurt. At the time of the pre-pubertal growth dip, bone age will be below 13 years. Final height will be attained in the target height range and comparable to the original, pre-pubertal height SD.

When pubertal development starts, bone age is comparable to the mean chronological age of onset of puberty. The progression of puberty, i.e., the time to complete the pubertal development, is normal compared to adolescents with a normally timed puberty. However, the impatient adolescent experiences his or her puberty as slowly progressive.[10]

It is unclear why more boys than girls present with delayed puberty. One explanation is that the distribution of timing of puberty is skewed with an increased number of male individuals in the late onset range. Another explanation is that boys experience more problems related to late development than girls. The latter option is most conceivable, since boys enter puberty at a later time than girls and sex characteristics such as increased height velocity, virilization and changing behavior do not occur until the second half of puberty.

In addition to the familial and idiopathic form, delayed puberty can be associated with chronic systemic diseases such as inflammatory bowel disease, asthma, and type 1 diabetes. These conditions often lead to growth failure and a delay of puberty. When the underlying condition is treated well, catch up growth will occur accompanied with pubertal onset.

Puberty is the result of reawakening of the GnRH pulse generator, which initiates the release of the gonadotropins LH and FSH. During the last decades several polymorphisms and mutations of the gonadotropins responsible for delayed and arrested puberty have been described.

Raivio et al.[11] reported a polymorphism of the LH β chain. Boys with this condition, either heterozygous or homozygous for the variant LH beta allele, have smaller testes, are shorter in height than the boys with the normal LH beta allele and have lower levels of insulin-like growth factor binding protein 3 (IGFBP-3). This LH variant resulting in constitutional delay of growth and puberty appears to affect testicular growth and puberty progression as well as the regulation of the IGF-I axis rather than affecting the reactivation of the GnRH release. This common polymorphism may contribute to a heterogenous phenotype of CDGP.

Mutations of the FSH β subunit gene may result in severe delayed puberty in girls and boys.[12,13] In both conditions hardly any sex steroid activity is present in the presence of increased LH and low FSH levels. In girls the pubertal arrest is the result of inappropriate follicular growth, while the two boys described with this mutation are azoospermic. These patients have a homozygous condition for the gene mutation, while their heterozygous family members are asymptomatic.

Except for the earlier described polymorphism of the LH β chain, all mutations and polymorphisms in gonadotropin genes and their receptors result in pubertal failure rather than in the phenotype of a simple delayed puberty.[14]

Delayed puberty in patients with chronic diseases may have consequences for their pubertal growth and final height as well as for the psychosocial dysfunction. In children with asthma, inhaled corticosteroids may have a systemic effect by absorption in circulation.[15] Growth failure will depend on the administered dose. However the individual sensitivity for the side effects of corticosteroids may be of importance as well. Suppression of adrenal function has also been described. It is important to appreciate that non-optimal treatment of asthma will also lead to growth failure. The pre-pubertal growth failure in asthmatic children is associated with a delayed bone maturation and delayed puberty. There is convincing evidence that final height will not be affected in these children. They reach their target height range, but at an older age.[16]

In children with chronic inflammatory bowel diseases (IBDs), Crohn's disease and ulcerative colitis, malnutrition seems to be the major factor interfering with normal growth and puberty. Especially in patients without complete remission and frequent relapses, puberty will be delayed.[17] In girls the mean age of the onset of puberty (stage B2) is 12.6 years versus 11.1 years in the reference group, whereas in boys testicular growth (testicular volume 4 mL) started at a mean age of 13.2 years versus 12.4 years in controls.[18] Since in girls with a pre-pubertal onset of Crohn's disease menarche occurred in 73 percent at age 16 or later, the progression of puberty seems to be retarded as well.[19] Girls with ulcerative colitis show less delay of puberty – in most of them menarche has occurred at the age of 14. Progression of puberty will depend on the activity of the disease. In addition to the nutritional status

of the patient, the inflammatory process will also interfere with linear growth. Surgical resection of the affected bowel may induce rapid onset of puberty, independent of the nutritional state.

Children with IBD, especially with Crohn's disease, are difficult to manage, since delay of puberty is not accompanied by a prolonged period of growth, as seen in asthmatic patients. One should consider treatment of these adolescents with the intent to improve final height.

PATHOPHYSIOLOGY: PERSISTENT PUBERTAL FAILURE

Pubertal failure may present by lack of onset of puberty, or a pubertal arrest. The defect can be localized either at the hypothalamus or pituitary resulting in hypogonadotropic hypogonadism. If the defect is localized at the gonadal level, then gonadotropins are increased – hypergonadotropic hypogonadism.

Hypogonadotropic hypogonadism

Hypogonadotropic hypogonadism (HH) can be primary, due to a developmental abnormality or secondary, due to an underlying disease such as a cerebral tumor.

The congenital form of hypogonadotropic hypogonadism is difficult to differentiate from simple delayed puberty (see under diagnosis). This is the reason that these patients are often referred at a late age, when they have developed many psychosocial problems. In general their height is not affected, since growth continues at a prepubertal rate. An eunuchoid disproportion with increased leg length resulting in a low upper-to-lower segment ratio is typical (in adult whites 0.9 or more is normal).[20] These patients have arm span exceeding their height as well.

In contrast to delayed puberty, when bone maturation remains retarded, bone age will eventually progress in hypogonadotropic patients (Fig. 41.2).

During pre-puberty both children with a delayed puberty and with hypogonadotropic hypogonadism have similarly low gonadotropin levels that do not increase in response to a GnRH test. A history of micropenis and undescended testes as well as cases of infertility in the family may suggest hypogonadism.

Mutations in gonadotropin genes are rare, as the natural selection of impaired fertility and reproduction will not be favored. Until now, several mutations for both the LH β subunit and FSH β subunit resulting in hypogonadotropic hypogonadism have been described.[14]

Defects in the GnRH gene would be a plausible cause for HH as well. However, although there is a naturally occurring hypogonadotropic mouse due to a mutated GnRH gene, no human mutations have yet been described.[21] Rather than to GnRH gene defects, hypogonadotropic hypogonadism often

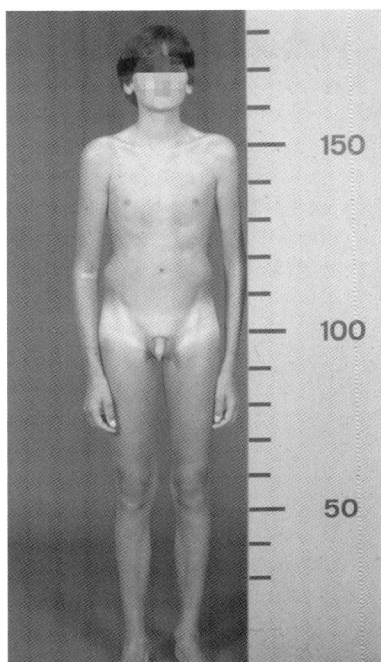

Figure 41.2 A boy with eunuchoidism due to hypogonadotropic hypogonadism. Please see Plate **23**.

relates to the development and function of the GnRH neuronal network, thus leading to GnRH deficiency.

A well known syndrome of hypogonadotropic hypogonadism due to GnRH deficiency is Kallmann syndrome, characterized by hypogonadism in combination with anosmia.[22] The prevalence is 1:10 000 to 1:86 000 births with a male to female ratio of about 3:1.[23] Many boys with Kallmann syndrome present with micropenis and cryptorchidism. One of the genes responsible for this syndrome is identified as the *KAL1* gene located in the Xp22.3 region encoding for a protein anosmia that shares homology with molecules involved in neuronal migration and axonal path finding.[24,25] Mutations of the *KAL1* gene will result in an arrest of migration of both the olfactory and GnRH neurons leading to the clinical picture of hypogonadotropic hypogonadism associated with anosmia. Recently, autosomal inheritance for Kallmann syndrome has been described as being due, amongst other factors, to a mutation of a gene encoding for the fibroblastic growth factor receptor1 located on the short arm of chromosome 8. This form is inherited in an autosomal dominant manner.[26] There is also an autosomal recessive form of Kallmann syndrome, for which the mutation has not yet been identified.

Dependent on inheritance, Kallmann syndrome is associated with other anomalies. In cases of the X-linked form the syndrome may present in combination with renal agenesis, often right-sided, neurological features such as mirror movements, ocular motor abnormalities, abnormal visual spatial attention, sensorineural deafness, cerebellar ataxia, epilepsia and mental retardation, pes cavus, cleft lip and

palate, café-au-lait macules and ichthyosis of the skin, ocular albinism, and ptosis.[27–29] The autosomal variant with heterozygous loss of function mutations of fibroblastic growth factor receptor1 (FGFR1) can be associated with midline and craniofacial defects such as cleft palate and dental agenesis.[26] Family members of the Kallmann patient are reported to have isolated anosmia with normal puberty or hypogonadotropic hypogonadism without smell dysfunction. In cases of anosmia, magnetic resonance imaging may demonstrate an absence of the olfactory bulbs and olfactory sulci.[30]

From genetic studies it appears that in familial cases of hypogonadotropic hypogonadism 11 percent have proved to have an X-linked form of Kallmann syndrome, in 64 percent the autosomal dominant form and in 25 percent the autosomal recessive form. In sporadic cases, a mutation of the *Kal1* gene is detected in less than 5 percent. This indicates that the majority of cases appear to be due to autosomal effects in genes not yet described.[23] The growth curve for a boy with Kallmann's syndrome is shown in Fig. 41.3.

Downstream of the GnRH neuron, in the human several inactivating mutations of the GnRH receptor are identified resulting in a wide spectrum of phenotypes varying from a complete condition of hypogonadotropic hypogonadism to a partial form.[31–34] In familial cases of HH about 40 percent of the patients lack the GnRH receptor function, whereas in sporadic cases this is 16 percent. Endocrinologically, there are absent to low pulsatile levels of gonadotropins associated with low sex steroid levels. These patients show an inadequate response to exogenous pulsatile GnRH administration, indicating that gonadotropin treatment is a more appropriate way to treat these patients to induce either spermatogenesis or ovulation.[35] Congenital adrenal hypoplasia caused by a mutation of the gene *DAX-1* can be associated with hypogonadotropic hypogonadism. The *DAX-1* gene is located at the X chromosome and encodes an orphan nuclear receptor that regulates the development and function of the adrenal gland as well as the hypothalamic-pituitary unit related to gonadotropin secretion via the gonadal axis.[36] Mutations of the *DAX-1* gene result in X-linked congenital adrenal hypoplasia, which will present in early childhood with adrenal insufficiency and lack of pubertal development in boys.[37] LH levels are particularly low, while FSH levels are in the low normal range. Testosterone levels are low. GnRH administration in a frequent pulsatile manner induces hardly any LH level increase, although free-alpha subunit may increase suggesting a pituitary defect in patients with *DAX-1* mutations. In young male infants a normal gonadotropin axis has been reported, suggesting that there is either a different control of gonadotropin secretion in the neonatal phase from that at puberty or that hypogonadotropic hypogonadism associated with congenital adrenal hypoplasia worsens in time.[37,38]

Heterozygous female carriers of the *DAX1*-gene mutation may present with delayed puberty.

Recently, the *GPR 54* gene has been described as a regulator of the control of puberty.[39] The *GRP 54* gene encodes

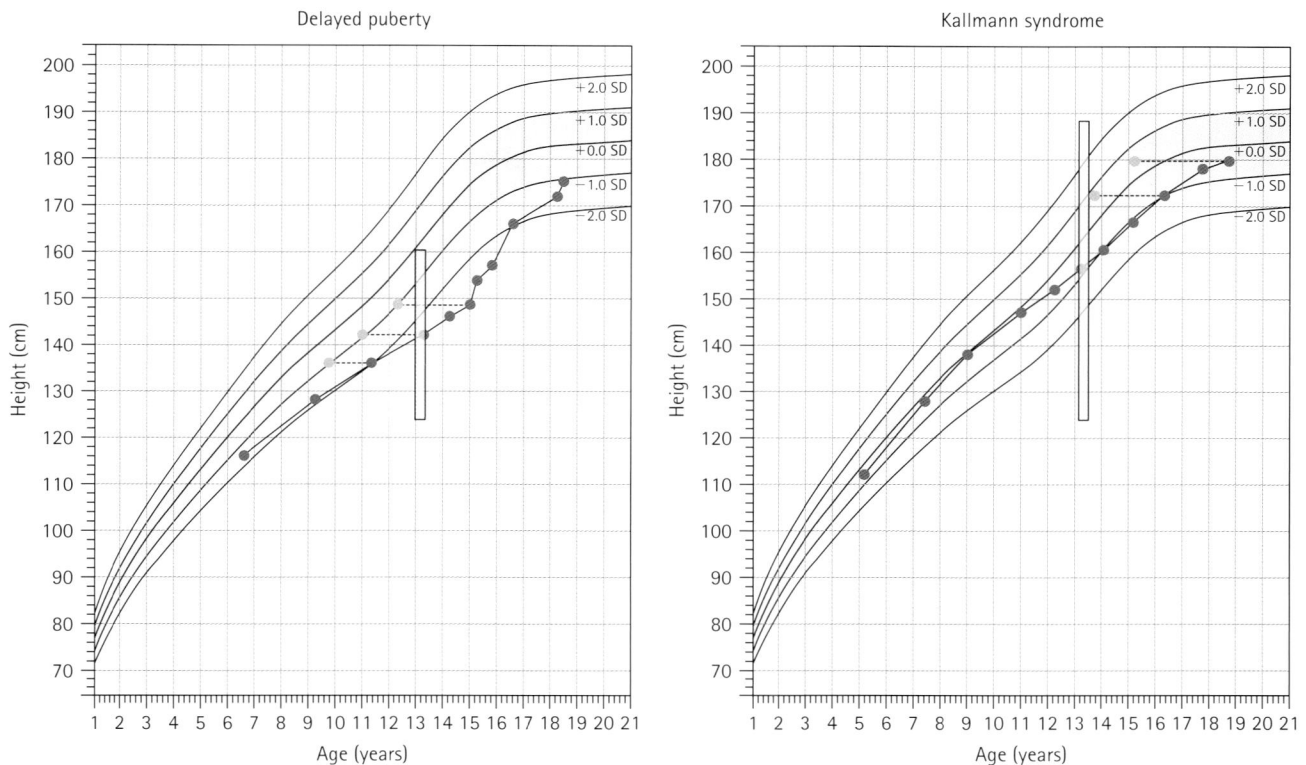

Figure 41.3 On the left side, the typical growth pattern of a boy with constitutional delay of growth and puberty. Bone maturation is delayed but will not cross a pubertal age without the appearance of pubertal characteristics. On the right side, the growth curve of a boy with Kallmann syndrome. Height velocity continues at a pre-pubertal rate, while the delayed bone age passes pubertal ages without the appearance of secondary sexual characteristics.

for a G protein-coupled receptor. Mutations of this gene result in hypogonadotropic hypogonadism in humans and mice. In humans the phenotype is lack of pubertal development in combination with low gonadotropin and sex steroid levels. In mice, mutations of the *GPR 54* gene result in infantile testes in the male and delayed vaginal opening due to lack of follicle maturation in the female. Both humans and mice respond to exogenous gonadotropin releasing hormone treatment. In affected mice, GnRH levels in the hypothalamic area are normal. Therefore it appears that the *GRP 54* gene plays a role in the release of GnRH rather than in its production.

In congenital hypopituitarism any combination of gonadotropin deficiency with another deficiency may occur as a result of a hypothalamic and/or pituitary developmental defect. Several developmental factors play a role in pituitary development. During the last decade several transcription factors have been identified. In the embryological phase these nuclear proteins have highly specific spatial and temporal expression patterns. They play a role in the proliferation and differentiation of the hormone precursor cells and form the pituitary anterior lobe.[40] PROP1 is one of these transcription factors and is involved in the early differentiation of gonadotrophic, somatotrophic, lactotrophic and thyrotrophic cells. *PROP1* gene defects are associated with hypogonadotropic hypogonadism, GH, TSH

and prolactin deficiency. The pituitary defect is inherited as an autosomal recessive trait. Heterozygous family members are not affected. Family studies show a variation in phenotypes depending on the gene defect. However, all *PROP1* mutations show multiple pituitary deficiencies. In general, affected children have severe short stature based on complete growth hormone deficiency, TSH deficiency and no spontaneous onset of puberty.[41] ACTH deficiency is described as presenting already at a young age, but can also present at a late age. The mechanisms underlying this late manifestation of one of the pituitary deficiencies are unknown. An enlarged anterior pituitary has been described in *PROP1* gene defects, which may precede later anterior pituitary hypoplasia.[42] Many patients with pituitary deficiencies have an ectopic posterior lobe on magnetic resonance imaging. However, patients with a *PROP1* gene defect have a normal posterior pituitary lobe.[43]

Until now two other transcription factors have been described as being involved with multiple pituitary hormone defects including gonadotropin deficiency. Mutations of the homeobox gene *HESX1* are associated with septo-optic dysplasia, a midline defect.[44] In addition to gonadotropins, these patients are deficient for growth hormone, prolactin, TSH and ACTH as well. Other features of the syndrome are optic dysplasia with impaired vision and subsequent pendular nystagmus and absence of the septum pellucidum.[45]

Patients with *LHX3* mutations have either an hypoplastic or an enlarged pituitary associated with a deficiency of all pituitary hormones except ACTH.[44,46]

Hypothalamic and pituitary tumors may affect gonadotropin and all other pituitary hormone secretion (see Chapter 38) . Clinical characteristics for a brain tumor are an abrupt failure of growth associated with an increase in weight and hormone deficiencies of both anterior and posterior pituitary lobes. Craniopharyngeoma is a common tumor in childhood, originating from Rathke's pouch. In addition to growth failure, children may complain of headache, polyuria, and polydipsia and other symptoms as a result of hormone deficiencies and increased intracranial pressure. Surgical treatment, with or without radiation, is the first treatment option for these tumors. Extirpation will lead to permanent damage of the hypothalamic area and therefore hypothalamic deficiencies, for which the patient needs lifelong replacement therapy. Hypothalamic dysfunction may be responsible for post-surgery adiposity. An increased 11 beta-HSD1 activity has been described in these patients, which correlates with the visceral to subcutaneous fat ratio. It is suggested that inhibition of 11 beta-HSD1 may help in order to prevent or in the case of post-surgery obesity to support the patient.[47]

Other brain tumors interfering with hypothalamic–pituitary function include germinomas, astrocytomas, gliomas, prolactinomas, and histiocytosis X.

Brain abnormalities such as a post-infectious state, vascular lesions and trauma may also result in delayed puberty. However, presumably as a result of pressure on the hypothalamic area, these central defects may also cause precocious puberty.

Irradiation and chemotherapy in the treatment of cancer in children may affect pubertal development by dysfunction at hypothalamic, pituitary and gonadal levels (see Chapter 38). An early puberty can occur, especially in girls, whereas hypogonadotropic hypogonadism is often observed at a later stage.[48]

Thalassemia is associated with iron deposition throughout the body. When the pituitary is affected, this will result in hypogonadotropic hypogonadism.[49] In addition to the pituitary, the gonads can also be involved, resulting in gonadal failure[50] (see Chapter 25).

Hypergonadotropic hypogonadism

Abnormalities at the gonadal level will result in hypergonadotropic hypogonadism associated with pubertal failure. Relatively frequently seen are girls with gonadal dysgenesis. They have streak ovaries containing stroma only. In the fetal period oogonia are present, but they involute before reaching maturation because they are unable to complete the meiotic prophase. Gonadal dysgenesis can be the result of X-chromosomal abnormalities such as 45 XO, a mosaicism, and in the presence of a normal 46 XX

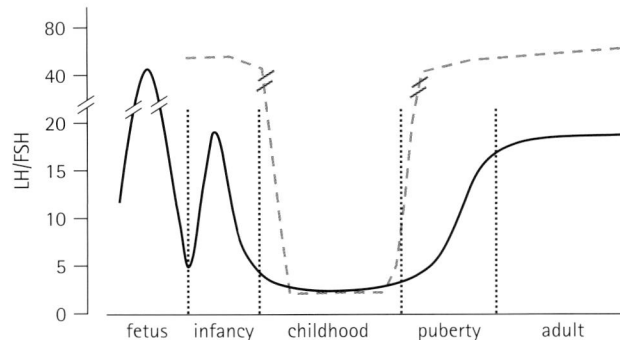

Figure 41.4 The gonadotropin pattern from the fetal period into adulthood in normal subjects (solid line) and subjects with gonadal failure (broken line).

karyotype. Autosomal gene abnormalities such as trisomies 13 and 18 are also associated with gonadal failure.[51]

During infancy and at late pre-puberty gonadotropin levels increase into very high or castrate ranges as a result of lack of feedback of gonadal steroids (Fig. 41.4). During childhood gonadotropin levels can be low and indistinguishable from physiological suppressed, pre-pubertal gonadotropin levels.[52]

Turner syndrome is characterized by an abnormal X chromosome pattern resulting in a phenotype including short stature and gonadal dysgenesis, first described by Turner in 1938[53] (see Chapter 35). Turner syndrome occurs in 1:2500 to 1:3000 live-born girls. The genotype may vary. Complete loss of a X or Y chromosome (45X), a mosaicism of this condition (45X/46XX and 45X/46XY), deletions of the short and long arm, ring conformation of the X-chromosome and other forms are possible. The phenotype of these X-chromosomal abnormalities has a wide spectrum.[54] Clinical features are in the neonatal period lymphedema of hands and feet and redundant neck tissue. Short stature is a major feature in combination with pubertal failure due to gonadal dysgenesis. Other developmental disorders are congenital heart disease with a prevalence of 17–45 percent, especially coarctation of the aorta and bicuspid aortic valve and renal malformations such as horseshoe kidney and duplication of the collecting system, which are found in 40 percent of patients with Turner syndrome.

Short stature is the result of haploinsufficiency of the short stature-homeobox (*SHOX*) gene, located in the pseudo autosomal region of Y and X short arm. Birth length is in the low normal range. The girls have a low height velocity with their height remaining in the low centiles. Because of their stable growth velocity on following a low centile the growth failure is often overlooked. Growth hormone treatment is a common treatment to increase final height in Turner syndrome patients (see Chapter 35).

Girls with Turner syndrome are often referred because of absence of puberty. Aneuploidy of the X chromosome will lead to a reduction of the number of developing oocytes. During the fetal period oogonia are present, but are not able to mature, and involute before completion of the meiotic phase. The streak gonads contain only stromal tissue. In the presence of a Y chromosome the girls are at risk of developing gonadoblastoma.[55] Gonadectomy is therefore advised. In a minority of Turner girls, puberty starts spontaneously, but in many pubertal arrest will occur. In about 90 percent primary sex steroid hormone replacement is necessary. Timing of starting estrogen treatment should be considered in relation to height. With growth hormone treatment the height of these girls is more appropriate, which makes it possible to start estrogens at an earlier, more physiological age.[56]

Spontaneous fertility has been described but, in general, girls with Turner syndrome are infertile. The infertility problems should be discussed with the parents, and with the girls at a pubertal age. In the future, possibilities may become available by preservation of ovarian tissue. Currently, the use of donor eggs and in vitro fertilization has been proven to be successful.

Another frequently encountered syndrome associated with gonadal failure is Klinefelter syndrome in boys. They usually have an XXY genotype. From cytogenetic surveys at birth prevalence of the XXY chromosomal pattern appeared to be 1.3 per 1000 male infants.[57] They have a birth weight and birth length in the low range. Between 5 and 8 years there is a notable increase of height velocity especially for leg growth with a slightly increased final height of about 186 cm. There is a tendency to central obesity.[57] Onset of puberty has a normal timing. At birth and pre-puberty the penis is relatively small. During puberty the testes start to grow but remain underdeveloped as a result of inappropriate growth of the seminiferous tubules. LH and FSH levels increase, for FSH into the elevated range already during early puberty, while LH and testosterone levels increase into the normal pubertal range. In late puberty, due to Leydig cell insufficiency LH becomes elevated as well. Because of gonadal failure a pubertal arrest will occur. Most of the adolescents with Klinefelter syndrome will have gynecomastia associated with increased estradiol levels. Since they are testosterone deficient, adolescents with Klinefelter syndrome need androgen replacement therapy as well as a personal guidance in order to achieve a proper puberty. In addition to the psychosocial aspects, these patients are at possible risk for other problems, such as an increased risk of malignancies. An increased risk for breast cancer has been suggested as well as for mediastinal germ cell tumors.[58]

Many cases remain undiagnosed during childhood and adolescence and even during adulthood because of insufficient awareness of the syndrome. Adults are diagnosed because of infertility. Small and firm testes are typical clinical findings. Most of the patients are azoospermic, but in half of them retrieval of spermatozoa from the testes is successful. In this situation procreation appears to be possible using intracytoplasmic sperm injection.[59] Gonadal failure can also be caused by surgery, irradiation and cytotoxic drugs (see Chapter 38).

Mutations of the gonadotropin receptors may be responsible for insufficient gonadal response to gonadotropin stimulation. Both inactivating as well as activating mutations are identified.

For the LH receptor inactivating mutation the phenotype will vary from complete lack of virilization to mild undervirilization. As for the clinical outcome, the endocrine status depends on the extent of the remaining activity of the LH receptor. In cases of complete inactivation the XY genotype will have a female phenotype associated with low testosterone levels, an increased LH, while the FSH level is within the normal range.[60] The internal sex organs are undeveloped because of the lack of testosterone. There is a gonadal unresponsiveness to LH and HCG.

The uterus is missing because of anti-Müllerian hormone production from the Sertoli cells. During puberty no development of sex characteristics, whether in a male or female direction will occur. The testes remain small and the testicular tissue contains immature Leydig cells and spermatogenesis is totally arrested.[60,61]

Only a few FSH receptor mutations have been described. Endocrinologically this is a hypergonadotropic state with increased FSH levels. In contrast to patients with hypogonadism due to ovarian dysgenesis with streak ovaries, women with a FSH receptor mutation have ovarian follicles. The ovaries contain follicles in the primordial phase, while a few will progress in their development. The patients have a variable development of secondary sex characteristics and primary or secondary amenorrhoea. As for the LH receptor mutation, there is a good correlation between the extent of FSH receptor inactivation and the phenotype.[14,62] Recently, a novel homozygous mutation of the FSH receptor has been reported in a female presenting with delayed puberty and primary amenorrhea.[63]

DIAGNOSTICS

Delayed puberty will be diagnosed from lack of pubertal development at two standard deviations above the mean age for the reference population. A growth curve, bone age, and family history may help to identify the underlying cause.

Micropenis at birth can be caused by gonadotropin deficiency. During the first months of life hypogonadotropic hypogonadism is easy to diagnose, since a post-natal increase of gonadotropins and testosterone is normally observed. Frequent blood sampling during this period will reveal a failure of this gonadotropin rise as a result of a GnRH or pituitary gonadotropin deficiency.[64]

Differentiation between hypogonadotropic hypogonadism and simple delayed puberty can be very difficult and sometimes impossible. Both conditions are associated with low spontaneous gonadotropin and gonadal steroid levels. In the absence of GnRH stimulation of the pituitary, either due to GnRH deficiency or late onset of puberty, the gonadotrophin response in a GnRH test will be blunted. In hypogonadotropic hypogonadism, pulsatile GnRH treatment may distinguish a hypothalamic from a pituitary defect, while in a pre-pubertal phase with normal low gonadotropin level, an increase into the elevated range may reveal gonadal failure.[65] It appears that pulsatile GnRH stimulation does not differentiate between a GnRH deficiency and simple delayed puberty. Over a period of 7 days of treatment the achieved increase of gonadotropin levels in both conditions is identical.[66]

Elevated spontaneous nocturnal pulsatile LH release, which can be present in a physically still pre-pubertal state, indicates that puberty is under way and that physical changes are imminent.[67] Therefore 24 h blood sampling for LH measurements and pulse analysis may provide a diagnostic tool.[68,69] In addition, as a result of increased nocturnal LH pulsatile release, an increased early morning plasma testosterone level can be a useful marker of the imminence of secondary sexual development in the investigation of cases of delayed puberty in boys.[70]

Similar diagnostics can be performed using long acting GnRH agonists. Boys with delayed puberty showing a night time LH increase, have a significantly higher response of LH to the GnRH agonist nafarelin.[71] Recently, reports describe that an hCG test appears to be more powerful in discriminating delayed puberty from hypogonadotropic hypogonadism than the GnRH agonist test.[72] During the hCG test the testosterone response is evaluated and in the GnRH agonist test the LH response. It is notable that in most studies the boys with the highest responses, either in GnRH agonist or in hCG test, have the highest testicular volumes.

It is clear that the combination of thorough history, physical examination and endocrine testing should provide the most useful diagnosistic information. If the diagnosis is not clear, temporary treatment to induce puberty is advised in order to prevent serious psychological side effects. This can be followed by subsequent re-evaluation.

In congenital hypergonadotropic hypogonadism, gonadotropin levels will be elevated during infancy. During pre-puberty, levels drop into the low normal range. During pre-puberty a GnRH test may be blunted as in physiological pre-puberty, but an increased response with higher levels for FSH than LH may occur as well. At the end of pre-puberty gonadotropin levels will rise into an elevated, castrate range.

In constitutional delay of growth and puberty, the pre-pubertal growth dip, when height SD progressively decreases, may suggest a growth hormone deficiency based on low IGF-I and IGFBP-3 levels. Growth hormone stimulation tests frequently confirm growth hormone deficiency. Short term priming with sex steroids will restore the growth hormone secretion pattern as well as IGF-I and IGFBP-3 levels.[73] Therefore priming with sex steroids should be considered in the evaluation of growth hormone secretion in patients with constitutional delay of growth and puberty. Boys can be treated with a testosterone depot 100 mg 2–8 days before testing and girls with 50–100 μg ethinylestradiol given over a period of 3 days prior to the test.[74]

When the diagnosis hypogonadotropic versus hypergonadotropic hypogonadism is confirmed one should perform additional tests related to the clinical symptoms. These investigations may include evaluation of other endocrine axes, chromosomal and DNA analysis, brain imaging, and genetic counseling.

MANAGEMENT OF DELAYED PUBERTY

In simple delayed puberty, the patient may have complaints with respect to short stature or to lack of virilization. Short stature is usually induced by the pre-pubertal growth deceleration. Patients can be treated with androgens or androgen derivatives. One should realize that in the case of simple delayed puberty, treatment intervention is not necessary, since puberty will start eventually and final height will be in the normal range. However, sometimes the doctor's goal is to improve the patient's well-being and temporarily optimize the growth pattern.[75]

In pre-pubertal boys and boys in early puberty with only a recent start of testicular growth, oxandrolone will increase height velocity without a progressive effect on bone maturation.[10] Unlike with testosterone, treatment with oxandrolone can be continued until the start of the pubertal growth spurt and will not suppress endogenous puberty. Follow-up of testicular volume makes it possible to discontinue oxandrolone at the time of an appropriate testicular volume of about 10–12 mL, when endogenous androgen secretion should be sufficient to induce the pubertal growth spurt. Oxandrolone thus only stimulates linear growth and does not promote virilization. Short term androgen treatment for periods of 3–6 months can be applied in boys with a start of pubertal development, who still have low androgen levels.[76] The treatment will induce an increase in height velocity and virilization. After discontinuation pubertal development will continue at a normal pace. If necessary the treatment can be repeated (Table 41.2). Experience with testosterone transdermal patches is limited.

Table 41.2 Treatment regimens in delayed puberty[76,80,96,97]

Boys
Oxandrolone 1.25–2.5 mg day^{-1} p.o. for 1–2 years
Testosterone 50–100 mg per 3–4 weeks for 3–6 months
Testosterone undecanoate 40 mg day^{-1} p.o. for 3–6 months
Testosterone transdermal patches
Aromatase inhibitor letrozole 2.5 mg day^{-1}; still experimental application

Girls
Ethinyl estradiol 0.05–0.1 μg kg^{-1} day^{-1} p.o. with increase to 5 μg day^{-1} for 3–6 months
17β-estradiol 5 μg kg^{-1} day^{-1} p.o. with increase to 10 μg kg^{-1} day^{-1} for 3–6 months
Transdermal 17β-estradiol 0.08–0.12 μg kg^{-1} day^{-1} for 3–6 months

In young boys these patches appear to deliver too high doses.[77]

In girls with simple delayed puberty there is hardly any experience with respect to intervention by exogenous estrogens. As for boys one may treat girls with short-term courses of estrogens. One should consider the growth inhibiting effect of estrogens, before starting this intervention. It is impossible to predict in individual cases whether and at which dose estrogen treatment will compromise height velocity. Estrogens can be administered orally as well as by transdermal patches (Table 41.2).

Recently, the use of an aromatase inhibitor in the management of delayed puberty in boys has been described. The aim of this treatment is to inhibit epiphyseal closure by estrogens, which may result in a longer period of growth with finally an increase of adult height.[78] During treatment with the aromatase inhibitor letrozole bone maturation is delayed, which confirms that estrogens are more potent with respect to bone maturation than androgens. No increase of IGF-I and IGFBP-3 is observed, while height velocity remains in a pubertal range. Treatment with an aromatase inhibitor resulted in a significantly increased adult height prediction. Until now these studies have been performed in boys with simple delayed puberty receiving either no treatment, or testosterone with placebo or testosterone with aromatase inhibitor. An effect of the aromatase inhibitor on endogenous estrogen synthesis was proven by decreased levels of estrogens in the aromatase inhibitor group compared to the untreated boys.[79] The high testosterone levels in the testosterone enanthate treated boys is associated with increased 17β-estradiol levels. The aromatase inhibitor group showed decreased estrogen levels compared to the placebo group, indicating that the conversion of androgens into estrogens is inhibited as well. The GnRH test showed increased gonadotropin responses in the aromatase inhibitor group, indicating that the negative feedback of sex steroid during puberty is mediated at least in part by estrogens and at the pituitary level.

The investigators consider treatment with aromatase inhibitors still as experimental and needing more extensive studies. The fact that the effect of endogenous estrogens can be diminished and adult height prediction improves, provides a rationale for studies of treatment to delay bone maturation in severe growth disorders as well.[80]

In persistent pubertal failure, a complete induction of puberty is necessary, followed by lifelong replacement therapy. Depending on the underlying cause, patients with hypogonadism can be treated with GnRH, gonadotropins or sex steroids. Sex steroid administration is the easiest and most feasible method of treatment. In girls, physiological development of sexual characteristics will occur with estrogens, while boys will undergo adequate virilization with testosterone, but the testes will remain undeveloped. In general, gonadotropins and GnRH in hypogonadotropic girls will be applied only to induce ovulation.[81,82] In pubertal and young adult boys gonadotropins can be applied to initiate testicular growth including androgen production

as well as spermatogenesis. However, in congenital hypogonadotropic hypogonadism gonadotropin replacement is not always successful.[83] In contrast, pulsatile GnRH results in a better development of the testes. Induction of puberty using pulsatile GnRH administration in hypogonadotropic boys will stimulate the pituitary to produce and secrete gonadotropins, which in turn initiate testicular growth.[66,82,84] After achieving spermatogenesis, treatment can be switched to one or two hCG injections per week. Local testicular testosterone levels will maintain sperm development and therefore fertility.

In congenital hypogonadism, boys may be born with a micropenis. Treatment with testosterone in the neonatal phase or during infancy is a feasible way to increase penile length without an effect on bone age.[85] In order to mimic the post-natal gonadotropin rise, which is assumed to be critical for late testicular development and fertility, one may treat infants with gonadotropins for several weeks.[8] This treatment is still experimental: follow-up of these patients is not available. Table 41.3 lists treatment regimens in persistent hypogonadism.

LONG-TERM FOLLOW-UP

Bone mineralization

Bone acquisition from birth through young adulthood leads to a gradual bone mass increase. During puberty the highest accumulation of bone mass occurs as a result of a complex sequence of hormones. We know that in both men and women estrogens play a major role in this process.[86] An appropriate peak bone mass is essential to prevent osteoporosis in later life.[87]

In 1992, Finkelstein and co-workers described osteopenia of the radius and spinal bone in adults with a history of delayed puberty, suggesting that pubertal timing plays a major role in achieving an appropriate peak bone mass during young adulthood.[88] This observation suggested that delayed puberty is associated with an increased risk for osteoporosis in later life.

Since this first report, normal bone mineralization in young adults with a history of constitutional delayed puberty has been reported as well.[89] The interpretation of bone measurements in children appears to be intricate and controversial, since it is dependent on the child's growth pattern, the techniques used to measure bone mass, its reference values as well as applied calculations. A recent study shows that the skeletal phenotype in delayed puberty has a normal bone mineral density at the lumbar spine and femoral neck and the trunk. A reduced total-body mass is the result of a reduced limb bone mass and reduced size of limbs and vertebrae.[90] This changed pattern of bone acquisition is presumably the result of a different growth pattern due to late exposure to sex steroids. However these data provide reassurance on the appropriate state of bone mineralization in delayed puberty.

Table 41.3   Treatment regimens in persistent hypogonadism

Boys

Treatment with testosterone esters in an increasing dose schedule every 6 months

25 mg m^{-2} per 2 weeks i.m.

50 mg m^{-2} per 2 weeks i.m.

75 mg m^{-2} per 2 weeks i.m.

100 mg m^{-2} per 2 weeks i.m.

Adult dose Sustanon 250® per 3–4 weeks

Induction of puberty with testosterone undecanoate is not very effective with respect to virilization

A very high and frequent dosed schedule is needed. In practice testosterone undecanoate is not applied frequently

Treatment with gonadotropins[83]

FSH 150 IU, 2–4 times per week i.m. in combination with hCG 2500 IU 2 times per week i.m.

Since, during early puberty FSH has increased more than LH, one may consider starting with only FSH for several weeks before the combination of both gonadotropins[98]

Doses should be adjusted on endocrine and clinical follow-up

Treatment with GnRH[66]

GnRH 2–20 μg per pulse s.c. of i.v. every 90–120 min using a portable pump

The GnRH dose should be adjusted based on testosterone levels and testicular growth

*In the above schedules, the doses are arbitrarily chosen based on the literature and own experience. No comparative studies are available

Girls

Treatment with 17-β-estradiol in an increasing dose schedule every 6 months

5 μg kg^{-1} day^{-1} p.o.

10 μg kg^{-1} day^{-1} p.o.

15 μg kg^{-1} day^{-1} p.o.

20 μg kg^{-1} day^{-1} p.o.

Treatment with ethinylestradiol in an increasing dose schedule every 6 months

0.1 μg kg^{-1} day^{-1} p.o.

0.2 μg kg^{-1} day^{-1} p.o.

0.4 μg kg^{-1} day^{-1} p.o.

0.6 μg kg^{-1} day^{-1} p.o.

Adult dose is about 30 μg day^{-1}. Then a contraceptive pill can be used

During both estrogen treatments, after 1–2 years a progesterone derivative should be added monthly to achieve menstrual bleeding and to prevent endometrium hyperplasia

* In the above schedules, the doses are arbitrarily chosen based on the literature and own experience. No comparative studies are available

---

In contrast to delayed puberty, it is well known that hypogonadism is associated with osteopenia when hormone replacement is not appropriate. Girls with gonadal dysgenesis and boys with Klinefelter syndrome are the most commonly seen patients with primary hypogonadism. Insufficient amounts of gonadal steroids will affect bone acquisition and consequently peak bone mass. In these conditions estrogens and androgens will normalize bone metabolism and bone mass gain.[91] In men with hypogonadotropic hypogonadism, hormone replacement at an early pubertal age as well as sex steroid levels in the high normal range are required in order to achieve a complete normalization of bone mineralization.[92]

Psychosocial aspects

Puberty is a period with great psychosocial changes which are related to the physical maturation. However, much about the relation between age of onset of biological puberty and psychosocial functioning remains unclear. It is known that delayed puberty forms a risk for social and psychological disturbances, whereas early maturation has been described as socially advantageous.[93,94] Hypogonadotropic hypogonadism is the most serious state of delayed puberty. In general the diagnosis will be made very late. It appears that adolescents with hypogonadotropic hypogonadism have problems in their identity development despite earlier treatment. This includes aspects of philosophy of life, friendships, school performance, and personal characteristics.[95] The problems in social interaction with peers and the strong dependency on their parents seem to be related primarily to the disorder and not to the burden of the treatment. These psychosocial aspects are an important issue in the treatment of delayed puberty and should receive more attention from a preventive point of view. The question arises whether treatment in young teenagers may diminish chances of personality and social problems in those with pubertal disorders.

KEY LEARNING POINTS

- Delayed puberty is defined as an absence of testicular growth at a chronological age of 14 years in boys and no thelarche at the age of 13 in girls. When familial and in combination with retarded growth it is known as constitutional delay of growth and puberty (CDGP).
- Chronic diseases are often associated with a delay of puberty.
- To distinguish hypogonadotropic hypogonadism from delayed puberty, the growth curve and skeletal maturation are important parameters.
- In cases of hypogonadism a genetic abnormality can be the underlying cause.
- Delayed puberty does not need medical intervention. However, short-term courses of sex steroid may support the patient with delayed puberty in a psychological manner.
- Sex steroid substitution in boys and girls with hypogonadism is an adequate treatment in order to induce development of the sex characteristics. In male patients, in the case of hypogonadotropic hypogonadism, pulsatile treatment with GnRH may initiate development of the testes including fertility.
- In contrast to hypogonadism, delayed puberty is not associated with an impaired peak bone mass.

REFERENCES

1 Kaplan SL, Grumbach MM. Pituitary and placental gonadotrophins and sex steroids in the human and sub-human primate fetus. *Clin Endocrinol Metab* 1978; **7**: 487–511.

2 Mul D, Fredriks AM, van Buuren S, *et al.* Pubertal development in The Netherlands 1965–1997. *Pediatr Res* 2001; **50**: 479–86.

3 Sedlmeyer IL, Hirschhorn JN, Palmert MR. Pedigree analysis of constitutional delay of growth and maturation: determination of familial aggregation and inheritance patterns. *J Clin Endocrinol Metab* 2002; **87**: 5581–6.

4 Delemarre-Van de Waal HA. Regulation of puberty. *Best Pract Res Clin Endocrinol Metab* 2002; **16**: 1–12.

5 Terasawa E, Fernandez DL. Neurobiological mechanisms of the onset of puberty in primates. *Endocr Rev* 2001; **22**: 111–51.

6 Traggiai C, Stanhope R. Delayed puberty. *Best Pract Res Clin Endocrinol Metab* 2002; **16**: 139–51.

7 Hammar SL, Eddy JA. The nurse and the hospitalized teenager. *RN* 1966; **29**: 68–71.

8 Main KM, Schmidt IM, Toppari J, Skakkebaek NE. Early postnatal treatment of hypogonadotropic hypogonadism with recombinant human FSH and LH. *Eur J Endocrinol* 2002; **146**: 75–9.

9 Horner JM, Thorsson AV, Hintz RL. Growth deceleration patterns in children with constitutional short stature: an aid to diagnosis. *Pediatrics* 1978; **62**: 529–34.

10 Schroor EJ, van Weissenbruch MM, Knibbe P, Delemarre-Van de Waal HA. The effect of prolonged administration of an anabolic steroid (oxandrolone) on growth in boys with constitutionally delayed growth and puberty. *Eur J Pediatr* 1995; **154**: 953–7.

11 Raivio T, Huhtaniemi I, Anttila R, *et al.* The role of luteinizing hormone-beta gene polymorphism in the onset and progression of puberty in healthy boys. *J Clin Endocrinol Metab* 1996; **81**: 3278–82.

12 Layman LC, Lee EJ, Peak DB, *et al.* Delayed puberty and hypogonadism caused by mutations in the follicle-stimulating hormone beta-subunit gene. *N Engl J Med* 1997; **337**: 607–11.

13 Phillip M, Arbelle JE, Segev Y, Parvari R. Male hypogonadism due to a mutation in the gene for the beta-subunit of follicle-stimulating hormone. *N Engl J Med* 1998; **338**: 1729–32.

14 Huhtaniemi IT. LH and FSH receptor mutations and their effects on puberty. *Horm Res* 2002; **57(Suppl 2)**: 35–8.

15 Rotteveel J, Potkamp J, Holl H, Delemarre-Van de Waal HA. Growth during early childhood in asthmatic children: relation to inhalation steroid dose and clinical severity score. *Horm Res* 2003; **59**: 234–8.

16 Shaw NJ, Fraser NC, Weller PH. Asthma treatment and growth. *Arch Dis Child* 1997; **77**: 284–6.

17 Ballinger AB, Savage MO, Sanderson IR. Delayed puberty associated with inflammatory bowel disease. *Pediatr Res* 2003; **53**: 205–10.

18 Brain CE, Savage MO. Growth and puberty in chronic inflammatory bowel disease. *Baillieres Clin Gastroenterol* 1994; **8**: 83–100.

19 Ferguson A, Sedgwick DM. Juvenile onset inflammatory bowel disease: height and body mass index in adult life. *BMJ* 1994; **308**: 1259–63.

20 McKusick VA. *Heritable Disorders of Connective Tissue.* St Louis: CV Mosby; 1972.

21 Cattanach BM, Iddon CA, Charlton HM, et al. Gonadotrophin-releasing hormone deficiency in a mutant mouse with hypogonadism. Nature 1977; 269: 338–40.

22 Kallmann FSW, Barrera SW. The genetic aspects of primary eunuchoidism. Am J Ment Defic 1944; 48: 203–36.

23 Seminara SB, Hayes FJ, Crowley WF Jr. Gonadotropin-releasing hormone deficiency in the human (idiopathic hypogonadotropic hypogonadism and Kallmann's syndrome): pathophysiological and genetic considerations. Endocr Rev 1998; 19: 521–39.

24 Franco B, Guioli S, Pragliola A, et al. A gene deleted in Kallmann's syndrome shares homology with neural cell adhesion and axonal path-finding molecules. Nature 1991; 353: 529–36.

25 Legouis R, Hardelin JP, Levilliers J, et al. The candidate gene for the X-linked Kallmann syndrome encodes a protein related to adhesion molecules. Cell 1991; 67: 423–35.

26 Dode C, Levilliers J, Dupont JM, et al. Loss-of-function mutations in FGFR1 cause autosomal dominant Kallmann syndrome. Nat Genet 2003; 33: 463–5.

27 Hardelin JP, Levilliers J, Blanchard S, et al. Heterogeneity in the mutations responsible for X chromosome-linked Kallmann syndrome. Hum Mol Genet 1993; 2: 373–7.

28 Sato N, Katsumata N, Kagami M, et al. Clinical assessment and mutation analysis of Kallmann syndrome 1 (KAL1) and fibroblast growth factor receptor 1 (FGFR1, or KAL2) in five families and 18 sporadic patients. J Clin Endocrinol Metab 2004; 89: 1079–88.

29 Prager O, Braunstein GD. X-chromosome-linked Kallmann's syndrome: pathology at the molecular level. J Clin Endocrinol Metab 1993; 76: 824–6.

30 Klingmuller D, Dewes W, Krahe T, et al. Magnetic resonance imaging of the brain in patients with anosmia and hypothalamic hypogonadism (Kallmann's syndrome). J Clin Endocrinol Metab 1987; 65: 581–4.

31 de Roux N, Young J, Misrahi M, et al. A family with hypogonadotropic hypogonadism and mutations in the gonadotropin-releasing hormone receptor. N Engl J Med 1997; 337: 1597–602.

32 de Roux N, Young J, Brailly-Tabard S, et al. The same molecular defects of the gonadotropin-releasing hormone receptor determine a variable degree of hypogonadism in affected kindred. J Clin Endocrinol Metab 1999; 84: 567–72.

33 Kottler ML, Chauvin S, Lahlou N, et al. A new compound heterozygous mutation of the gonadotropin-releasing hormone receptor (L314X, Q106R) in a woman with complete hypogonadotropic hypogonadism: chronic estrogen administration amplifies the gonadotropin defect. J Clin Endocrinol Metab 2000; 85: 3002–8.

34 Beranova M, Oliveira LM, Bedecarrats GY, et al. Prevalence, phenotypic spectrum, and modes of inheritance of gonadotropin-releasing hormone receptor mutations in idiopathic hypogonadotropic hypogonadism. J Clin Endocrinol Metab 2001; 86: 1580–8.

35 Caron P, Chauvin S, Christin-Maitre S, et al. Resistance of hypogonadic patients with mutated GnRH receptor genes to

pulsatile GnRH administration. J Clin Endocrinol Metab 1999; 84: 990–6.

36 Muscatelli F, Strom TM, Walker AP, et al. Mutations in the DAX-1 gene give rise to both X-linked adrenal hypoplasia congenita and hypogonadotropic hypogonadism. Nature 1994; 372: 672–6.

37 Seminara SB, Achermann JC, Genel M, et al. X-linked adrenal hypoplasia congenita: a mutation in DAX1 expands the phenotypic spectrum in males and females. J Clin Endocrinol Metab 1999; 84: 4501–9.

38 Peter M, Viemann M, Partsch CJ, Sippell WG. Congenital adrenal hypoplasia: clinical spectrum, experience with hormonal diagnosis, and report on new point mutations of the DAX-1 gene. J Clin Endocrinol Metab 1998; 83: 2666–74.

39 Seminara SB, Messager S, Chatzidaki EE, et al. The GPR54 gene as a regulator of puberty. N Engl J Med 2003; 349: 1614–27.

40 Cohen LE, Radovick S. Molecular basis of combined pituitary hormone deficiencies. Endocr Rev 2002; 23: 431–42.

41 Reynaud R, Chadli-Chaieb M, Vallette-Kasic S, et al. A familial form of congenital hypopituitarism due to a PROP1 mutation in a large kindred: phenotypic and in vitro functional studies. J Clin Endocrinol Metab 2004; 89: 5779–86.

42 Riepe FG, Partsch CJ, Blankenstein O, et al. Longitudinal imaging reveals pituitary enlargement preceding hypoplasia in two brothers with combined pituitary hormone deficiency attributable to PROP1 mutation. J Clin Endocrinol Metab 2001; 86: 4353–7.

43 Osorio MG, Marui S, Jorge AA, et al. Pituitary magnetic resonance imaging and function in patients with growth hormone deficiency with and without mutations in GHRH-R, GH-1, or PROP-1 genes. J Clin Endocrinol Metab 2002; 87: 5076–84.

44 Dattani MT, Martinez-Barbera JP, Thomas PQ, et al. Mutations in the homeobox gene HESX1/Hesx1 associated with septo-optic dysplasia in human and mouse. Nat Genet 1998; 19: 125–33.

45 Kaplan SL, Grumbach MM, Hoyt WF. A syndrome of hypopituitary dwarfism, hypoplasia of optic nerves and malformation of prosencephalon: report of 6 patients. Pediatr Res 1970; 4: 480.

46 Netchine I, Sobrier ML, Krude H, et al. Mutations in LHX3 result in a new syndrome revealed by combined pituitary hormone deficiency. Nat Genet 2000; 25: 182–6.

47 Hochberg Z, Friedberg M, Yaniv L, et al. Hypothalamic regulation of adiposity: the role of 11beta-hydroxysteroid dehydrogenase type 1. Horm Metab Res 2004; 36: 365–9.

48 Muller J. Disturbance of pubertal development after cancer treatment. Best Pract Res Clin Endocrinol Metab 2002; 16: 91–103.

49 De S V, Tangerini A, Testa MR, et al. Final height and endocrine function in thalassaemia intermedia. J Pediatr Endocrinol Metab 1998; 11(Suppl 3): 965–71.

50 Soliman AT, el Zalabany MM, Ragab M, et al. Spontaneous and GnRH-provoked gonadotropin secretion and testosterone response to human chorionic gonadotropin in adolescent

boys with thalassaemia major and delayed puberty. *J Trop Pediatr* 2000; **46**: 79-85.

51 Simpson JL, Rajkovic A. Ovarian differentiation and gonadal failure. *Am J Med Genet* 1999; **89**: 186-200.

52 Conte FA, Grumbach MM, Kaplan SL, Reiter EO. Correlation of luteinizing hormone-releasing factor-induced luteinizing hormone and follicle-stimulating hormone release from infancy to 19 years with the changing pattern of gonadotropin secretion in agonadal patients: relation to the restraint of puberty. *J Clin Endocrinol Metab* 1980; **50**: 163-8.

53 Turner HH. A syndrome of infantilism, congenital webbed neck, and cubitus valgus. *Endocrinology* 1938; **23**: 566-74.

54 Sybert VP, McCauley E. Turner's syndrome. *N Engl J Med* 2004; **351**: 1227-38.

55 Gravholt CH, Fedder J, Naeraa RW, Muller J. Occurrence of gonadoblastoma in females with Turner syndrome and Y chromosome material: a population study. *J Clin Endocrinol Metab* 2000; **85**: 3199-202.

56 Stephure DK. Impact of growth hormone supplementation on adult height in turner syndrome: results of the Canadian randomized controlled trial. *J Clin Endocrinol Metab* 2005; **90**: 3360-6.

57 Ratcliffe S. Long-term outcome in children of sex chromosome abnormalities. *Arch Dis Child* 1999; **80**: 192-5.

58 Manning MA, Hoyme HE. Diagnosis and management of the adolescent boy with Klinefelter syndrome. *Adolesc Med* 2002; **13**: 367-74, viii.

59 Lanfranco F, Kamischke A, Zitzmann M, Nieschlag E. Klinefelter's syndrome. *Lancet* 2004; **364**: 273-83.

60 Kremer H, Kraaij R, Toledo SP, *et al.* Male pseudohermaphroditism due to a homozygous missense mutation of the luteinizing hormone receptor gene. *Nat Genet* 1995; **9**: 160-4.

61 Latronico AC, Anasti J, Arnhold IJ, *et al.* Brief report: testicular and ovarian resistance to luteinizing hormone caused by inactivating mutations of the luteinizing hormone-receptor gene. *N Engl J Med* 1996; **334**: 507-12.

62 Aittomaki K, Herva R, Stenman UH, *et al.* Clinical features of primary ovarian failure caused by a point mutation in the follicle-stimulating hormone receptor gene. *J Clin Endocrinol Metab* 1996; **81**: 3722-6.

63 Meduri G, Touraine P, Beau I, *et al.* Delayed puberty and primary amenorrhea associated with a novel mutation of the human follicle-stimulating hormone receptor: clinical, histological, and molecular studies. *J Clin Endocrinol Metab* 2003; **88**: 3491-8.

64 Evain-Brion D, Gendrel D, Bozzola M, *et al.* Diagnosis of Kallmann's syndrome in early infancy. *Acta Paediatr Scand* 1982; **71**: 937-40.

65 Delemarre-Van de Waal HA, Van den Brande JL, Schoemaker J. Prolonged pulsatile administration of luteinizing hormone-releasing hormone in prepubertal children: diagnostic and physiologic aspects. *J Clin Endocrinol Metab* 1985; **61**: 859-67.

66 Delemarre-Van de Waal HA. Application of gonadotropin releasing hormone in hypogonadotropic hypogonadism –

diagnostic and therapeutic aspects. *Eur J Endocrinol* 2004; **151(Suppl 3)**: U89-94.

67 Wennink JM, Delemarre-Van de Waal HA, van Kessel H, *et al.* Luteinizing hormone secretion patterns in boys at the onset of puberty measured using a highly sensitive immunoradiometric assay. *J Clin Endocrinol Metab* 1988; **67**: 924-8.

68 Wu FC, Butler GE, Kelnar CJ, *et al.* Patterns of pulsatile luteinizing hormone and follicle-stimulating hormone secretion in prepubertal (midchildhood) boys and girls and patients with idiopathic hypogonadotropic hypogonadism (Kallmann's syndrome): a study using an ultrasensitive time-resolved immunofluorometric assay. *J Clin Endocrinol Metab* 1991; **72**: 1229-37.

69 Wu FC, Butler GE, Kelnar CJ, *et al.* Ontogeny of pulsatile gonadotropin releasing hormone secretion from midchildhood, through puberty, to adulthood in the human male: a study using deconvolution analysis and an ultrasensitive immunofluorometric assay. *J Clin Endocrinol Metab* 1996; **81**: 1798-805.

70 Wu FC, Brown DC, Butler GE, *et al.* Early morning plasma testosterone is an accurate predictor of imminent pubertal development in prepubertal boys. *J Clin Endocrinol Metab* 1993; **76**: 26-31.

71 Ghai K, Cara JF, Rosenfield RL. Gonadotropin releasing hormone agonist (nafarelin) test to differentiate gonadotropin deficiency from constitutionally delayed puberty in teenage boys – a clinical research center study. *J Clin Endocrinol Metab* 1995; **80**: 2980-6.

72 Degros V, Cortet-Rudelli C, Soudan B, Dewailly D. The human chorionic gonadotropin test is more powerful than the gonadotropin-releasing hormone agonist test to discriminate male isolated hypogonadotropic hypogonadism from constitutional delayed puberty. *Eur J Endocrinol* 2003; **149**: 23-9.

73 Marin G, Domene HM, Barnes KM, *et al.* The effects of estrogen priming and puberty on the growth hormone response to standardized treadmill exercise and arginine-insulin in normal girls and boys. *J Clin Endocrinol Metab* 1994; **79**: 537-41.

74 Ranke MB. Diagnosis of growth hormone deficiency an growth hormone stimulation tests. In: Ranke MB, ed. *Diagnostics of Endocrine Function in Children and Adolescents.* Basel: Karger, 2003: 107-28.

75 Kelnar CJ. Treatment of the short, sexually immature adolescent boy. *Arch Dis Child* 1994; **71**: 285-7.

76 De Luca F, Argente J, Cavallo L, *et al.* Management of puberty in constitutional delay of growth and puberty. *J Pediatr Endocrinol Metab* 2001; **14(Suppl 2)**: 953-7.

77 Houchin LD, Rogol AD. Androgen replacement in children with constitutional delay of puberty: the case for aggressive therapy. *Baillieres Clin Endocrinol Metab* 1998; **12**: 427-40.

78 Wickman S, Sipila I, Ankarberg-Lindgren C, *et al.* A specific aromatase inhibitor and potential increase in adult height in boys with delayed puberty: a randomised controlled trial. *Lancet* 2001; **357**: 1743-8.

79　Wickman S, Dunkel L. Inhibition of P450 aromatase enhances gonadotropin secretion in early and midpubertal boys: evidence for a pituitary site of action of endogenous E. *J Clin Endocrinol Metab* 2001; **86**: 4887–94.

80　Dunkel L, Wickman S. Novel treatment of delayed male puberty with aromatase inhibitors. *Horm Res* 2002; **57 (Suppl 2)**: 44–52.

81　Braat DD, Schoemaker J. Endocrinology of gonadotropin-releasing hormone induced cycles in hypothalamic amenorrhea: the role of the pulse dose. *Fertil Steril* 1991; **56**: 1054–9.

82　Schoemaker J, van Weissenbruch MM, Scheele F, van der MM. The FSH threshold concept in clinical ovulation induction. *Baillieres Clin Obstet Gynaecol* 1993; **7**: 297–308.

83　Schopohl J, Mehltretter G, von Zumbusch R, *et al.* Comparison of gonadotropin-releasing hormone and gonadotropin therapy in male patients with idiopathic hypothalamic hypogonadism. *Fertil Steril* 1991; **56**: 1143–50.

84　Delemarre-Van de Waal HA. Induction of testicular growth and spermatogenesis by pulsatile, intravenous administration of gonadotrophin-releasing hormone in patients with hypogonadotrophic hypogonadism. *Clin Endocrinol (Oxf)* 1993; **38**: 473–80.

85　Adan L, Couto-Silva AC, Trivin C, *et al.* Congenital gonadotropin deficiency in boys: management during childhood. *J Pediatr Endocrinol Metab* 2004; **17**: 149–55.

86　Smith EP, Boyd J, Frank GR, *et al.* Estrogen resistance caused by a mutation in the estrogen-receptor gene in a man. *N Engl J Med* 1994; **331**: 1056–61.

87　Genant HK, Cooper C, Poor G, *et al.* Interim report and recommendations of the World Health Organization Task-Force for Osteoporosis. *Osteoporos Int* 1999; **10**: 259–64.

88　Finkelstein JS, Neer RM, Biller BM, *et al.* Osteopenia in men with a history of delayed puberty. *N Engl J Med* 1992; **326**: 600–4.

89　Bertelloni S, Baroncelli GI, Ferdeghini M, *et al.* Normal volumetric bone mineral density and bone turnover in young men with histories of constitutional delay of puberty. *J Clin Endocrinol Metab* 1998; **83**: 4280–3.

90　Yap F, Hogler W, Briody J, *et al.* The skeletal phenotype of men with previous constitutional delay of puberty. *J Clin Endocrinol Metab* 2004; **89**: 4306–11.

91　Breuil V, Euller-Ziegler L. Gonadal dysgenesis and bone metabolism. *Joint Bone Spine* 2001; **68**: 26–33.

92　Guo CY, Jones TH, Eastell R. Treatment of isolated hypogonadotropic hypogonadism effect on bone mineral density and bone turnover. *J Clin Endocrinol Metab* 1997; **82**: 658–65.

93　Eichorn DH. Biological correlates of behavior. In: Stevenson HW, ed. *Child Psychology: Yearbook of the National Society for the Study of Education.* Chicago: University of Chicago Press, 1963: 4–61.

94　Reekers GA. Development of problems of puberty and sex roles in adolescence. In: Walker CE, Roberts MC, eds. *Handbook of Clinical Child Psychology.* New York: Wiley, 2005: 607–622.

95　Huisman J, Bosch JD, Roelofsen W, *et al.* The psychosocial development of boys treated with pulsatile LHRH administration for hypogonadotropic hypogonadism. *Ned Tijdschr Geneeskd* 1991; **135**: 2334–7.

96　Pozo J, Argente J. Ascertainment and treatment of delayed puberty. *Horm Res* 2003; **60(Suppl 3)**: 35–48.

97　Ankarberg-Lindgren C, Elfving M, Wikland KA, Norjavaara E. Nocturnal application of transdermal estradiol patches produces levels of estradiol that mimic those seen at the onset of spontaneous puberty in girls. *J Clin Endocrinol Metab* 2001; **86**: 3039–44.

98　Wennink JM, Delemarre-Van de Waal HA, Schoemaker R, *et al.* Luteinizing hormone and follicle stimulating hormone secretion patterns in boys throughout puberty measured using highly sensitive immunoradiometric assays. *Clin Endocrinol (Oxf)* 1989; **31**: 551–64.

42

Growth hormone insensitivity syndromes

CECILIA CAMACHO-HÜBNER, MARTIN O SAVAGE

PATHOGENESIS

The term growth hormone insensitivity syndrome (GHIS) describes a group of inherited disorders characterized by a reduction in the biological effects of GH in the presence of normal or elevated serum GH concentrations.

The first report of GHIS of genetic origin was published by Laron *et al.* in 1966.[1] Since then the description of this disorder has expanded, as has the spectrum of clinical and biochemical abnormalities. The clinical disorder known as Laron syndrome is associated with defects of the GHR gene usually defects in the extracellular domain.[2,3] Due to the large number of established GHR mutations it is impossible to describe them all in this chapter but this topic has been reviewed in detail.[4] The identification of several new genetic causes of GH deficiency or insensitivity has broadened the range of etiologies responsible for growth disorders as described in Table 42.1 and Fig. 42.1.[5]

Classical endocrine tests remain the most reliable for assessing the GH–IGF-I axis, analysis of appropriate candidate genes can contribute to the precise definition of the pathogenesis of the growth disorder.[5]

CLINICAL DIAGNOSIS OF GROWTH HORMONE INSENSITIVITY

The clinical characteristics of the affected patients are similar to those seen in GH deficiency secondary to mutations in the GH gene, namely hypoglycemic episodes presenting primarily in infancy and early childhood, severe post-natal growth

Table 42.1 Etiological classification of growth hormone insensitivity syndrome (GHIS)

Primary genetic defects of the GH–IGF-I axis	
GH receptor defects	Extracellular, transmembrane and intracellular mutations
Primary defects of IGF-I production or action	IGF-I gene mutations
	IGF-I receptor mutations
GH signal transduction defects	STAT 5b mutations
Acid labile subunit (ALS) defects	ALS gene mutations
Bioinactive GH molecule	

Secondary acquired dysfunction of the GH–IGF-I axis	
Malnutrition and nutritional disorders	Anorexia nervosa
Catabolic states	Severe burns
Chronic inflammatory disorders	Juvenile chronic arthritis
	Crohn's disease

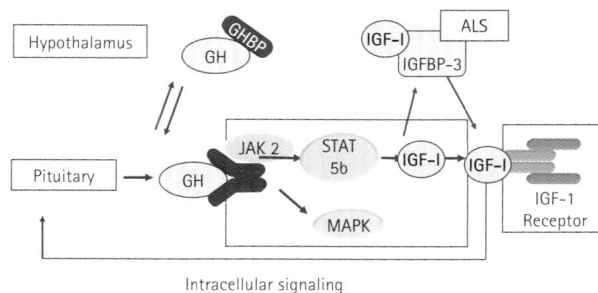

Intracellular signaling

Figure 42.1 Schematic representation of the growth hormone–insulin-like growth factor I (GH–IGF-I) axis.

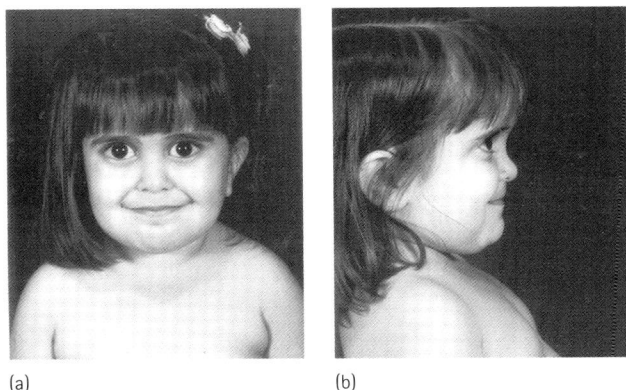

(a)   (b)

Figure 42.2 Photograph of a 5-year-old girl with classical growth hormone insensitivity syndrome (GHIS) or Laron syndrome. Her facial photographs show the protruding forehead and depressed nasal bridge.

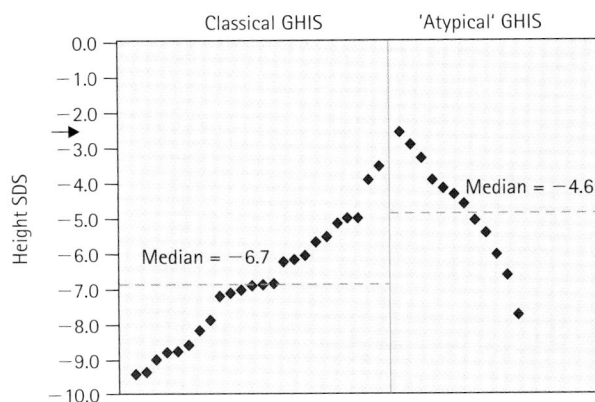

Figure 42.3 Height SDS (median) in a group of naive pre-pubertal patients with classical and non-classical or atypical growth hormone insensitivity syndrome (GHIS).

failure and typical craniofacial appearance specially associated with classical GHIS or Laron syndrome[1-6] (Fig. 42.2). In terms of linear growth, the most striking feature is the rapid decrease in height SDS during the early post-natal years. In the first 3 years of life there is a loss of approximately 3 SD below the mean per year as demonstrated in the Ecuadorian patients, the largest kindred with this disorder.[2,3] Final adult heights in a cohort of patients reported by Laron et al.[6] were only 119.5 ($\pm$8.5 SD) cm for girls and only 124.1 ($\pm$8.5 SD) cm for boys. Other clinical findings include the musculoskeletal system which can be underdeveloped and in older patients osteopenia that can be demonstrated by dual X-ray adsorptiometry (DEXA) scans.[7]

Intellectual retardation has been described in the original Israeli populations but is not a universal finding.

The heterogeneity of clinical and biochemical features has been demonstrated in a series of patients studied in Europe.[8] A recent analysis has been performed of 59 of the patients in this European series who were classified into 'classical' or atypical ('non-classical') based on their facial appearance. Fifty patients had classical facial features characterize by mid-facial hypoplasia due to an underdeveloped sphenoid and mandible, depressed nasal bridge and protruding forehead and the hair was usually sparse and thin with temporal and frontal recession. The seven patients classified as 'atypical' in this series had normal facies.[8] In addition, patients with atypical GHIS had less height deficit (height SDS -4.0 ± 1.4) compared with patients with classical GHIS (-8.6 ± 2.4). We have recently studied 36 naive GHI children with a median height SDS of -6.7 in classical patients and a median height SDS of -4.3 in children with non-classical or atypical GHI (Fig. 42.3).

Puberty is delayed in both males and females with GHIS and the pubertal growth spurt is generally absent. However, puberty starts spontaneously with normal progression to full sexual development, and adult patients have normal sexual and reproductive function.[6]

BIOCHEMICAL AND MOLECULAR INVESTIGATIONS

Severe short stature with or without classical features of Laron syndrome associated with normal to high serum GH concentrations and very low serum IGF-I, IGFBP-3, and ALS levels suggest impaired GH actions.[10] GH binding protein (GHBP), the circulating form of the extracellular domain of the GHR, was initially found to be absent but recent reports have found that some patients with GHIS may have normal or even elevated serum GHBP.[10] Usually, 'atypical' GHI patients have normal GHBP.

The molecular defect in GHIS originates in the GHR gene, which was cloned and characterized in 1987.[11] The GHR is encoded by a single gene located on the short arm of chromosome 5 (5 p13–p12). The gene expands $\approx$87 kb and is divided into 9 exons, starting in exon 2 through exon 10 and contains 8 introns.[12]

The mature GHR, a member of the cytokine receptor family, is a 620 amino acid, single-chain glycoprotein that is composed of a large extracellular domain involved in GH binding (exons 2–7), a transmembrane domain necessary for anchoring the GHR to the cell surface (exon 8) and an intracellular domain involved in GH signalling (exons 9–10).

In 1989 the first mutation in a patient with GHIS was described by Godowski et al. and their report led to genetic studies in a number of patients with GHIS.[12] Approximately 60 different mutations in the GHR have been identified to date.[2,3,8,10,13,14] These genes are almost all recessively inherited in either homozygous or compound heterozygous forms and range from exon deletions to more common point mutations which include nonsense (premature stop codon), missense (altered amino acid), splice site and frameshift mutations. The majority of the molecular defects in patients with GHIS have been identified as point mutations in exons 2–7 of the GHR gene.

Dusquenoy described the first patients with a D152H mutation and positive GHBP levels who presented with severe postnatal growth failure, no facial features of Laron syndrome and severe deficiencies of serum IGF-I and IGFBP-3.[15] In recent years other patients with GHBP positive levels and GHIS have been identified, including patients with heterozygous mutations with a dominant negative effect in which the mutant GHR formed heterodimers with the wild-type GHR and exerted a dominant negative effect on the normal protein.[16–18]

GROWTH HORMONE INSENSITIVITY DUE TO *STAT5b* MUTATION

A recent report describes a 16-year-old Argentinean girl from consanguineous parents, presenting with a clinical history of severe postnatal growth failure (Ht SDS −7.5), frequent upper respiratory infections, with immune dysfunction and marked IGF-I, IGFBP-3, and ALS deficiencies. She failed to respond to GH treatment and genetic studies were performed to elucidate the molecular defect associated with the clinical and biochemical diagnosis of GH insensitivity. Molecular studies showed that she has normal GH receptor gene but a novel GH post-receptor defect was identified. A homozygous missense mutation of the STAT5 gene was identified and the resulting protein proven to be incapable of phosphorylation in response to either GH or gamma interferon.[19] We have identified two siblings with clinical and biochemical features of GH insensitivity owing to a molecular defect in STAT5b (our unpublished data), and the frequency of abnormalities in STAT5b as a cause of GH insensitivity remains unknown.

TREATMENT

We have gained new insights into the growth-promoting and metabolic actions of IGF over the last few years primarily from studies of children with GHIS and studies of a single patient with IGF-I gene deletion.[20–23]

Treatment for IGF–I gene defects

In 1995, we were referred a 15.6-year-old male patient with extreme short stature (−6.9 SDS), markedly elevated GH levels and undetectable serum IGF-I with normal IGFBP-3 and elevated ALS concentrations. This patient had severe intra-uterine growth retardation (birth weight −3.9 SDS), post-natal growth failure, resistance to GH therapy, dysmorphic features of microcephaly, micrognathia, low hairline, and ptosis. A partial homozygous deletion of the IGF-I gene was identified as the molecular defect responsible for this clinical condition.[21] The ability of rhIGF-I to promote linear growth and normalize insulin sensitivity was clearly demonstrated during the 2 years of therapy[22,23] although many factors contributed to the final height achieved by the patient. This genetic defect is extremely rare and only one additional case in an adult has been reported.[24]

Treatment for growth hormone insensitivity syndromes

The possibility of rhIGF-I therapy improving childhood and adult height in patients with GHIS is an important advance for these previously untreatable patients.

Analysis of IGF-I pharmacokinetics using a single dose of rhIGF-I of $40\,\mu g\,kg^{-1}$ administered s.c. to adults with GHIS and normal subjects demonstrated the clearance and half-life in GHIS subjects to be $0.60\,mL\,min^{-1}\,kg^{-1}$ and 6 h, respectively, compared with $0.20\,mL\,min^{-1}\,kg^{-1}$ and 20 h in normal individuals.[25] The rapid clearance of rhIGF-I in GHIS patients, related to decreased serum levels of IGFBP-3 and ALS, and the reduced biological effect, was supported in a study of GH pulsatility in two children, where re-appearance of GH pulses occurred 4 and 7 h after administration of rhIGF-I given at $80\,\mu g\,kg^{-1}\,day^{-1}$ s.c.[26]

Clinical studies with rhIGF-I in GHIS started in the late 1980s. Most investigators administered rhIGF-I twice daily s.c., using doses from 40 to $120\,\mu g\,kg^{-1}$/dose.[20,27–29] Laron *et al.*[30] used a single daily dose of $150\,\mu g\,kg^{-1}$ s.c. All published reports demonstrated increases in growth rate during therapy[20,27–30] with a mean height velocity during the first year of treatment increased from <4 to 7.2–9.3 cm $year^{-1}$. During rhIGF-I therapy bone age did not advance more rapidly than chronological age (mean change in BA, 2.1 year; mean change in CA, 2.2 year) whereas, increased height velocity was accompanied by weight gain in most patients.

Prolonged therapy with rhIGF-I to children with GHIS and to those with GH gene deletion with neutralizing antibodies has proved to be safe and effective with side effects presenting mainly when high doses of rhIGF-I have been used.

In a sub-group of European patients treated with IGF-I at $80\,\mu g\,kg^{-1}$ twice daily, a negative relationship was demonstrated between height SDS and IGFBP-3 SDS, both reflecting the severity of the disorder and the response to IGF-I therapy.[28] These data suggest that the more severe is the biological defect the greater is the growth response to IGF-I therapy.

It is important to note that rhIGF-I treatment is associated with preferential tissue growth. The growth of the spleen determined by ultrasound was rapid in the first year of therapy and slowed down thereafter, whereas kidney growth remained relatively rapid but no structural abnormalities of the kidneys were observed by ultrasound.[27]

The adverse events reported during rhIGF-I therapy include: lipohypertrophy at injection sites, tonsillar hypertrophy, headaches and hypoglycemia. Transient increase of intracranial pressure with papilledema has also been reported.[20,27–30]

Most patients had an apparent increase in the size of nasopharyngeal lymphoid tissue and are frequently reported to develop snoring during sleep. IGF-I related hypoglycemia occurred mainly early in treatment or it was usually associated with an intercurrent illness, with concurrent loss of appetite. In these cases the symptoms improved after interrupting treatment and did not recur when IGF-I was restarted at a lower dose.[20]

Treatment of GHIS with rhIGF-I/rhIGFBP-3 complex

The majority of circulating IGF-I exists in the form of a ternary complex consisting of IGF-I, IGFBP-3, and ALS. IGFBP-3 and ALS regulate IGF-I bioavailability and bio-distribution. IGF-I carried within the ternary complex has a half-life of >12 h in healthy subjects. The development of rhIGF-I/rhIGFBP-3 as a therapeutic agent was driven by the need to enhance the biological effects of IGF-I and to eliminate the potential for acute insulin-like side effects. Efficacy of the complex has been demonstrated by diminished catabolism in severely burned children.[31]

We performed a pharmacokinetic study comparing the rhIGF-I/IGFBP-3 complex to rhIGF-I in four adolescents with GHIS. The complex induced an increase in serum concentrations of IGF-I within the normal range and was associated with an increased half-life (15–18 h) compared with rhIGF-I (8 h).[32] A trial of treatment with the rhIGF-I/IGFBP-3 complex in naive GHIS patients is currently in progress.

CONCLUSIONS

The integrity of the GH–IGF-I axis is essential for normal linear growth in childhood. Defects in either GH secretion or action will result in reducing serum IGF-I, the key growth promoting peptide. Genetic GH insensitivity may be viewed as a continuum ranging from classical GHIS to severe idiopathic short stature. This was evident from the European GHIS population, which consisted of patients with a broad range of clinical and endocrine defects. Investigation of children with severe idiopathic short stature may reveal molecular and endocrine features of partial GH insensitivity. The identification of several new genetic causes of GH deficiency or insensitivity has broadened the range of etiologies responsible for growth disorders. The availability of rhIGF-I alone or combined with rhIGFBP-3 is a positive development towards the treatment of this severe genetic growth disorder.

KEY LEARNING POINTS

- Growth hormone insensitivity syndrome (GHIS) describes a group of inherited disorders characterized by a reduction in the biological effects of GH in the presence of normal or elevated serum GH concentrations and low serum IGF-I, IGFBP-3 and ALS levels.

- Laron syndrome or classical GHIS is characterized by severe post-natal growth failure and typical craniofacial appearance. It is usually associated with a molecular defect in the extracellular domain of the GHR.
- Atypical or non-classical GHIS is characterized by severe post-natal growth failure but does not present the typical facies or any other dysmorphic features. It can be associated with a molecular defect in the GHR gene or a post-receptor defect.
- Treatment with rhIGF-I is efficacious and generally safe but careful monitoring is recommended.

REFERENCES

● = Seminal primary article
◆ = Key review paper

● 1   Laron Z, Pertezelan A, Mannheimer S. Genetic pituitary dwarfism with high serum concentration of growth hormone: a new inborn error of metabolism? *Isr J Med Sci* 1966; **2**: 152–5.

◆ 2   Rosenfeld RG, Rosenbloom AL, Guevara-Aguirre J. Growth hormone (GH) insensitivity due to primary GH receptor deficiency. *Endoc Rev* 1994; **15**: 369–90.

● 3   Rosenbloom AL, Guevara J, Rosenfeld RG, *et al*. The little women of Loja – growth hormone receptor deficiency in an inbred population of Southern Ecuador. *New Engl J Med* 1990; **323**: 1367–74.

◆ 4   Hull KL, Harvey S. Growth hormone resistance: clinical states and animal models. *J Endocrinol* 1999; **163**: 165–72.

◆ 5   Rosenfeld R, Hwa V. New molecular mechanisms of GH resistance. *Eur J Endocrinol* 2004; **151**: S11–5.

  6   Laron Z. Laron Syndrome (primary growth hormone resistance or insensitivity): the personal experience 1958–2003. *J Clin Endocrinol Metab* 2004; **89**: 1031–44.

  7   Benbassat CA, Esched V, Kamjin M, *et al*. Are adult patients with Laron syndrome osteopenic? A comparison between dual-energy X-ray absorptiometry and volumetric bone densities. *J Clin Endocrinol Metab* 2003; **88**: 4586–9.

  8   Woods KA, Dastot F, Preece MA, *et al*. Phenotype:genotype relationships in growth hormone insensitivity syndrome. *J Clin Endocrinol Metab* 1997; **82**: 3529–35.

● 9   Walker JL, Ginalska-Malinovska M, Romer TE, *et al*. Effects of the infusion of insulin-like growth factor I in a child with growth hormone insensitivity syndrome (Laron dwarfism). *N Engl J Med* 1991; **324**: 1483–8.

  10   Woods KA, Fraser NC, Postel-Vinay C, *et al*. A homozygous splice site mutation affecting the intracellular domain of the growth hormone receptor resulting in Laron syndrome with elevated GH binding protein. *J Clin Endocrinol Metab* 1996; **81**: 1686–90.

11 Leung DW, Spenser SA, Cachianes G, *et al.* Growth hormone receptor and growth hormone binding protein: purification, cloning and expression. *Nature* 1987; **330**: 537–43.

● 12 Godowski PJ, Leung DW, Meacham LR, *et al.* Characterization of the human growth hormone receptor gene and demonstration of a partial gene deletion in two patients with Laron-type dwarfism. *Proc Natl Acad Sci USA* 1989; **86**: 8083–7.

13 Amselem S, Dusquenoy P, Duriez B, *et al.* Spectrum of growth hormone receptor mutations and associated haplotypes in Laron syndrome. *Hum Mol Genet* 1993; **2**: 355–9.

14 David A, Metherell L, Clark AJ, *et al.* Diagnostic and therapeutic advances in growth hormone insensitivity. *Endocrinol Metab Clin North Am* 2005; **34**: 581–95.

● 15 Dusquenoy P, Sobrier ML, Duriez B, *et al.* A single amino acid substitution in the exoplasmic domain of the human growth hormone (GH) receptor confers familial GH resistance (Laron syndrome) with positive GH-binding activity by abolishing receptor homodimerization. *EMBO J* 1994; **13**: 1386–95.

16 Goddard AD, Covello R, Luoh SM, *et al.* Mutations of the growth hormone receptor in children with idiopathic short stature. *N Engl J Med* 1995; **333**: 1093–8.

17 Ayling RM, Ross R, Towner P, *et al.* A dominant-negative mutation of the growth hormone receptor causes familial short stature. *Nat Genet* 1997; **16**: 13–14.

18 Iida K, Takahashi Y, Kaji H, *et al.* Growth hormone (GH) insensitivity syndrome with high serum GH-binding protein levels caused by a heterozygous splice site mutation of the GH receptor gene producing a lack of intracellular domain. *J Clin Endocrinol Metab* 1998; **83**: 531–7.

● 19 Kofoed EM, Hwa V, Little B, *et al.* Growth hormone insensitivity associated with a STAT5b mutation. *N Engl J Med* 2003; **349**: 1110–2.

◆ 20 Savage MO, Camacho-Hübner C, Dunger DB. Therapeutic applications of the insulin-like growth factors. *Growth Horm IGF Res* 2004; **14**: 301–8.

● 21 Woods KA, Camacho-Hübner C, Savage MO, Clark AJL. Intrauterine growth retardation and post-natal growth failure associated with deletion of the insulin-like growth factor-I gene. *New Engl J Med* 1996; **355**: 1363–7.

22 Woods KA, Camacho-Hübner C, Bergman RN, *et al.* Effects of insulin-like growth factor I (IGF-I) therapy on body composition and insulin resistance in IGF-I gene deletion. *J Clin Endocrinol Metab* 2000; **85**: 1407–11.

23 Camacho-Hübner C, Woods KA, Miraki-Moud F, *et al.* Effects of recombinant human insulin-like growth factor-I (IGF-I) therapy on the growth hormone-IGF system of a patient with partial IGF-I gene deletion. *J Clin Endocrinol Metab* 1999; **84**: 1611–16.

24 Walenkamp MJE, Karperien M, Pereira MAM, *et al.* Homozygous and heterozygous expression of a novel insulin-like growth factor-I mutation. *J Clin Endocrinol Metab* 2005; **90**: 2855–64.

25 Grahnen, Kastrup K, Heinrich U, *et al.* Pharmacokinetics of recombinant human insulin-like growth factor I given subcutaneously to healthy volunteers and to patients with growth hormone receptor deficiency. *Acta Paediatr* 1993; **391(Suppl)**: 9–13.

26 Cotterill AM, Camacho-Hübner C, Holly JMP, Savage MO. The effect of recombinant human insulin-like growth factor-I treatment on growth hormone secretion in two subjects with growth hormone insensitivity (Laron syndrome). *Clin Endocrinol* 1993; **39**: 119–22.

27 Backeljauw PF, Underwood LE, and The GHIS Collaborative Group. Therapy for 6.5–7.5 years with recombinant insulin-like growth factor I in children with growth hormone insensitivity syndrome: a clinical research center study. *J Clin Endocrinol Metab* 2001; **86**: 1504–10.

28 Ranke MB, Savage MO, Chatelain PG, *et al.* Treatment of growth hormone insensitivity syndrome with insulin-like growth factor-I: long-term results of the European multicentre study. *Horm Res* 1999; **51**: 128–34.

29 Guevara-Aguirre J, Rosenbloom AL, Vasconez O, *et al.* Two year treatment of growth hormone receptor deficiency (GHRD) with recombinant insulin-like growth factor-I in 22 children: comparison of two dosage levels and to GH treated GH deficiency. *J Clin Endocrinol Metab* 1997; **82**: 629–33.

30 Laron Z, Anin S, Klipper-Aurbach Y, *et al.* Effects of insulin-like growth factor on linear growth, head circumference and body fat in patients with Laron-type dwarfism. *Lancet* 1992; **339**: 1258–61.

31 Herndon DN, Ramzy PI, DebRoy MA, *et al.* Muscle protein catabolism after severe burn: effects of IGF-I/IGFBP-3 treatment. *Ann Surg* 1999; **229**: 713–20.

● 32 Camacho-Hübner C, Rose S, Preece MA, *et al.* Pharmacokinetic studies of recombinant human insulin-like growth factor (rhIGF)-I/IGF binding protein-3 complex administered to patients with growth hormone insensitivity syndrome. *J Clin Endocrinol Metab* 2006; **91**: 1246–53.

43

Growth hormone releasing peptides/secretagogues

EZIO GHIGO, FABIO BROGLIO

INTRODUCTION

It is well known that the synthesis and secretion of insulin growth factor-I (IGF-I) mainly depend on growth hormone (GH) secretion which is, in turn, under the hypothalamic control exerted by growth hormone releasing hormone (GHRH) and somatostatin, integrated by the negative feedback action of IGF-I.[1,2] The role of neurotransmitters and neuropeptides as well as of peripheral hormones, metabolic fuels, GH and IGF-I binding proteins in controlling GH and IGF-I secretion has also been extensively studied.[1,2]

Recently, the complexity of the regulation of the somatotroph axis has been further enriched by the discovery of ghrelin.[3,4] Ghrelin is a 28 amino acid peptide endowed with a strong GH-releasing activity mediated by the activation of the GH secretagogues (GHS) receptors (GHS-R) that had been isolated because of their selective binding affinity with synthetic peptidyl and non-peptidyl GHS.[3,5,6]

GHS were invented more than 20 years ago and their strong GH-releasing activity even after oral administration suggested a potential clinical usefulness for the diagnosis and treatment of GH deficiency (GHD) in childhood and of somatopause in aging.[7,8]

GHS-R are expressed in the hypothalamus–pituitary unit but also in other central and peripheral tissues.[9–11] While the receptors in the hypothalamus and in the pituitary mediate the stimulatory effect of ghrelin on GH, prolactin (PRL) and adrenocorticotrophic hormone (ACTH) secretion, the identification of specific binding sites in other central and peripheral tissues explains other activities such as: (1) orexigenic

effect, (2) control of energy expenditure and influence on glucose and lipid metabolism, (3) influence on the endocrine pancreatic function, (4) influence on gastrointestinal motility and exocrine secretions, (5) influence on gonadal function, (6) cardiovascular actions, (7) anti-proliferative effects, (8) influence on behavior, and (9) influence on sleep.[3,4]

GHRELIN BIOCHEMISTRY: AN EXAMPLE OF REVERSE PHARMACOLOGY

Ghrelin is a 28 amino acid peptide predominantly produced by the stomach, with lower amounts also deriving from bowel, pancreas, kidney, lung, placenta, thyroid, pituitary, and hypothalamus.[3,4,10] Within the stomach ghrelin is produced by enteroendocrine cells, probably the X/A-like cells, a major endocrine population in the oxyntic mucosa, the hormonal product of which had not previously been clarified.[3,4,12] Ghrelin's discovery in 1999 was the result of lengthy research seeking an endogenous ligand of previously orphan receptors known as GHS-R.[5]

GHS is a term including several peptidyl and non-peptidyl molecules originally invented in the late 1970s as met-enkephalin derivatives devoid of any opioid activity[7,13] (Table 43.1).

GHRP-6 was the first peptidyl GHS able to release GH *in vivo* in humans even after oral administration though with low bioavailability and short-lasting effect.[7,13] In the following years, non-peptidyl molecules with higher and

Table 43.1 Growth hormone secretagogue/ghrelin milestones

1977 – to date	Synthesis and development of GH secretagogues; specifically	
	Synthetic peptidyl GHS	Synthetic non-peptidyl GHS
1977	(D-Trp2)-metENKH	
1984	GHRP-6	
1991	GHRP-1	
1992	Hexarelin	L-629,429
1993	GHRP-2	
1994		L-692,885
1995		MK-0677
1996	EP-51389	
1998	Ipamorelin	
1999		NN-703
2000		CP-424,391
1996	Identification and cloning of the GHS receptor type 1a	
1999	Isolation and cloning of ghrelin	

higher oral bioavailability and longer lasting effects were also synthesized.[7,13] Among them, MK-0677 was the most studied both in animals and in humans.[7,13]

In 1996, based on results coming from binding studies, an orphan receptor specific for GHS was isolated and its single gene cloned at chromosomal location 3q26.2.[14,15] Two types of GHS-R complementary DNA (cDNA) as the result of alternate processing of a pre-mRNA encode for two different receptors, the GHS-R type 1a, of 366 amino acids with seven-transmembrane regions, and the GHS-R type 1b, which consists of 289 amino acids and only five-transmembrane regions. Their sequences do not show significant homology with other known receptors, the closest relatives being the neurotensin receptor and the motilin receptor type 1A, with 59% and 52% similarity, respectively.[14,15] Both ghrelin as well as synthetic peptidyl and non-peptidyl GHS exhibit a high binding affinity to the GHS-R type 1a.[5,14] On the other hand, GHS-R type 1b does not bind GHS and therefore its functional role remains unknown.[7,14]

Ghrelin is the first circulating hormone in which the hydroxyl group of one of its residues is acylated, specifically by a n-octanoic acid on serine.[5,6] The acylation of the peptide has been supposed critical for crossing the blood–brain barrier and is essential for binding the GHS-R type 1a and for its GH-releasing activity and the other endocrine actions.[6,11,16,17] However, the non-acylated ghrelin form, which circulates in the bloodstream in amounts far higher than the acylated form, is not biologically inactive.[3,4] In fact, in vivo non-acylated ghrelin has been reported to promote adipogenesis and to counteract the effects of acylated ghrelin on insulin secretion and glucose levels.[18,19] Moreover non-acylated ghrelin is also able

to exert some non-endocrine actions including cardiovascular and anti-proliferative effects.[20,21] Since non-acylated ghrelin is unable to bind the GHS-R1a, it is likely that its biological effects are mediated by different GHS-R subtypes or receptor families, the existence of which is also suggested by binding studies.

The binding of ghrelin and synthetic GHS to the GHS-R type 1a activates the phospholipase C signaling pathway and inhibits K^+ channels, allowing the entry of Ca^{2+} through voltage-gated L- and T-type channels.[7] Expression of the GHS-R type 1a was shown in the hypothalamus and anterior pituitary gland[10,11] consistent with its role in regulating GH release. GHS-R type 1a is largely confined in somatotroph pituitary cells and in the arcuate nucleus, an hypothalamic area that is crucial for the neuroendocrine and the appetite-stimulating activities of ghrelin and synthetic GHS.[7,22]

Specifically, at the hypothalamic level, ghrelin has been shown to activate GHRH-containing neurons, but also cells expressing corticotropin-releasing hormone (CRH), arginine vasopressin (AVP), the appetite stimulating neuropeptide Y and the endogenous melanocortin receptor antagonist known as Agouti-related protein (AGRP).[23] Although with lower expression, GHS-R type 1a mRNA was also demonstrated in various extra-hypothalamic areas such as the hippocampus, substantia nigra, ventral tegmental area, and dorsal and medial raphe nuclei and Edinger–Westphal nucleus, pons, and medulla oblongata[7,24] possibly indicating an involvement in yet undefined physiological extra-neuroendocrine actions.

Recent studies have demonstrated the expression of GHS-R type 1a also in multiple peripheral organs as in the stomach and intestine, pancreas, kidney, heart and aorta, testis as well as in different endocrine neoplasms of lung, stomach, and pancreas.[3,10,25] Such a widespread distribution of GHS-R provided an explanation for the increasing amount of evidence showing various peripheral GH-independent actions of GHS such as cardiovascular and antiproliferative effects.[3,4]

Besides the 28 amino acid acylated ghrelin form, other endogenous ligands of the GHS-R type 1a have been described, among which several acylated ghrelin variants with different amino acid sequences or acyl chains,[4] adenosine, which acts as a weak agonist[26] and cortistatin, a neuropeptide homologous to somatostatin which, in turn, is unable to recognize this receptor.[27] It has been suggested that different molecules may bind different pockets of the GHS-R type 1a but not necessarily activate it. Further studies are required to clarify whether ghrelin is the sole ligand or just one of the ligands activating GHS-R and whether the GHS-R type 1a is the sole receptor or one of a group of receptors for one or more than one ligand.[3,7]

REGULATION OF GHRELIN SECRETION

Ghrelin secretion is pulsatile although, notably, its pulsatility does not correlate with that of GH and is related with food intake episodes.[28] Specifically, in humans, ghrelin levels show circadian variability with superimposed increases before meals and decreases after food intake.[29]

Pre-prandial increases have been found related to hunger score and, on this basis, suggested to play a role in meal initiation.[29,30] However, no correlation has been found between timing of request for food and increases in ghrelin levels and, moreover, 3 day fasting has been reported not to modify 24 h total ghrelin levels.[31,32]

Several factors have been implicated in the meal-induced decreases in total ghrelin levels in humans. Specifically, the reduction of circulating ghrelin levels after food ingestion has been reported to correlate well with the absolute meal caloric content[32] but not with gastric distension,[33] and among nutrients, carbohydrates, either given enterally and parenterally, show the most remarkable inhibitory effect on ghrelin secretion.[34,35]

The influence, if any, of amino acids and lipids is still a matter of debate. In humans, constant lipid infusion has been described not to influence plasma ghrelin levels[36] and oral fat administration has been reported to decrease, although to a lesser extent than after glucose ingestion,[33,37–39] or even to increase[40] circulating ghrelin levels. Protein intake has been reported either to increase[33,40–42] or not to affect[38] circulating ghrelin levels.

In agreement with the major influence of nutrition on ghrelin secretion, circulating ghrelin levels are increased in anorexia and cachexia while reduced in obesity and overfeeding, a notable exception being patients with Prader–Willi syndrome.[34,43–45] Both in anorexia and in obesity, ghrelin secretion is normalized by recovery of ideal body weight.[46,47] These changes are opposite to those of leptin suggesting that both ghrelin and leptin are hormones signaling the metabolic balance and managing the neuro-endocrine and metabolic response to starvation.[48]

Consistently with the negative association between ghrelin secretion and body mass index, a clear negative association between ghrelin and insulin secretion has been found in humans as well as in animals[49,50] suggesting an inhibitory influence of insulin on ghrelin secretion.[36,51–53] Indeed, during an euglycemic clamp, the steady state increase in insulin levels is associated with a clear reduction in circulating ghrelin levels[36,53] and insulin-induced hypoglycemia is followed by an increase of the classical counter-regulatory hormones (GH, PRL, ACTH, cortisol and catecholamine levels) which is coupled with a significant decrease of ghrelin secretion.[54]

Recently, it has been shown that post-prandial hyperinsulinemia is a decisive signal for meal-related ghrelin suppression.[55] In insulin-resistant states there is a lower decrement in post-prandial circulating ghrelin concentrations suggesting a negative cycle that augments nutrient intake in obese and type 2 diabetic subjects.[56]

However, at present, the most remarkable inhibitory input on ghrelin secretion has been shown to be somatostatin as well as its natural analogue cortistatin, with both also able to inhibit beta-cell secretion.[57–59]

Overall, evidence that insulin and somatostatin exert a critical inhibitory action on ghrelin secretion indicates that the latter is under major influence, mostly inhibitory, from the endocrine pancreas. A notable exception to the negative association between insulin and ghrelin secretion is represented by the Prader–Willi syndrome that is generally manifested by obesity but nevertheless associated with ghrelin hypersecretion.[45] In particular, in this condition ghrelin hypersecretion has been suggested to be responsible for hyperphagia and weight excess commonly present in this syndrome.[45,60]

In humans, ghrelin has been shown circulating in fetuses from 20 weeks of gestation to term and in neonatal blood at concentrations 1.5-fold to two-fold higher than those in normal weight adults.[61–63] The presence of ghrelin in fetal circulation is consistent with a real fetal production since neither significant umbilical veno-arterial difference of ghrelin levels nor correlation between maternal and fetal plasma levels were observed.[61] Interestingly, in contrast to post-natal life, during fetal life the stomach is not the major source of ghrelin secretion.[64] Specifically, in the fetal pancreas, ghrelin expression and release have been reported to precede and to be more marked than in the stomach.[62,64,65]

As in adulthood, plasma ghrelin levels in neonates have been reported to be negatively correlated with body weight[63,66,67] but, differently from adults, ghrelin secretion is refractory to the inhibitory effect of feeding.[68]

In post-natal life, plasma ghrelin levels have been reported to show a further increase in the first week of life probably as a function of increased nutritional needs in this period.[63] Some authors also reported further increases in circulating ghrelin levels during prepuberty followed by a decrease until the end of puberty.[69]

Interestingly, low ghrelin levels have been shown associated with slower weight gain from birth to 3 months of age[70] and, accordingly, among small for gestational age (SGA) infants, the degree of ghrelin suppression after glucose administration has been reported to be related to infancy weight gain.[71] The pathophysiological mechanisms underlying this relationship are at present unknown, and could theoretically be expression of either a direct influence of ghrelin status on the activity of the GH/IGF-I axis or related to ghrelin-induced variations in feeding behavior.

In elderly subjects, total ghrelin levels have been variably reported to be reduced[72] or increased[73] in comparison with middle-aged subjects. Notably, however, after multiple regression analysis including metabolic variables, no significant relationship between age and ghrelin levels persisted, thus suggesting that potential age related variations in ghrelin secretion are likely due to concomitant age related variations in energy metabolism rather than being a direct effect of age.[73]

Similarly evidence of higher ghrelin levels in women that in men have been reported to reflect differences either in body fat distribution and in body mass index rather being direct effect of gender on ghrelin secretion.[31,57]

BIOLOGICAL ACTIONS OF GHRELIN

As anticipated, the expression of GHS-R1a in several central and peripheral tissues explains the various endocrine actions of ghrelin[3,4] (Table 43.2). Among them, some have received particular attention due to their potential clinical implications.

Influence on endocrine hypothalamus–pituitary functions

GH-RELEASING ACTIVITY

Ghrelin and, long ago, synthetic GHS have been reported to possess strong and dose-related GH-releasing activity which is more marked in humans than in animals.[3,4,7] Specifically, in rats, differently from GHRH, the central administration of ghrelin stimulates GH release but does not augment its synthesis.[74]

Ghrelin/GHS and GHRH have a synergic effect indicating that they act, at least partially, via different mechanisms.[3,7,75–77] Nevertheless, GHS need GHRH activity to fully express their GH-releasing effect and it has been recently reported that in vitro ghrelin induces a significant stimulation of GHRH release from hypothalamic explants.[3,7,23,77]

Table 43.2 Endocrine and non-endocrine actions of acylated ghrelin versus synthetic GHS

Acylated ghrelin	Activities	Synthetic GHS
Endocrine activities		
Present	GH-releasing activity	Present
Present	PRL-releasing activity	Present
Present	ACTH-releasing activity	Present
Present	Influence on gonadal axis	Not studied
Central activities		
Present	Orexigenic activity	Present
Present	Influence on sleep and behavior	Discordant results according to the experimental models
Peripheral activities		
Present	Influence on gastric motility and acid secretion	Not studied
Present	Influence on exocrine pancreas secretion	Not studied
Present	Modulation of endocrine pancreas and glucose metabolism	Discordant results according to the experimental models
Present	Influence on lipid metabolism	Not studied
Present	Antiproliferative action	Present
Present	Cardiovascular activity	Present

On the other hand, the infusion of GHRH induces a significant increase in pituitary gene expression of both ghrelin and its receptors.[78,79] Moreover, to further underline the strict relationship between the GHRH and ghrelin systems, it has been recently demonstrated that the co-activation of GHS and GHRH receptors selectively potentiate the somatotroph responsiveness to GHRH.[79,80]

In humans the GH response to ghrelin/GHS is strongly inhibited, though not abolished, by a GHRH receptor antagonist as well as in patients with hypothalamus–pituitary disconnection or with GHRH-receptor deficiency, in agreement with the assumption that the most important action of GHS takes place at the hypothalamic level.[3,4,23,81]

Both ghrelin and synthetic GHS have been reported ineffective in modifying hypothalamic somatostatin release but there are data indicating that ghrelin and GHS might act as functional somatostatin antagonists at the pituitary and the hypothalamic level.[23,77,82,83] In humans the GH response to both natural and synthetic GHS is not modified by substances acting via somatostatin inhibition (such as acetylcholine receptor agonists and arginine) which, in turn, strongly potentiate the GH response to GHRH.[3] Moreover, the GH-releasing activity of ghrelin and synthetic GHS is partially refractory to the inhibitory effect of substances directly acting via stimulation of hypothalamic somatostatin (such as acetylcholine receptor antagonists, β-adrenoceptor agonists and glucose) which, in turn, almost abolish the somatotroph responsiveness to GHRH.[3] Indeed both ghrelin and GHS are partially refractory to the inhibition of substances acting on somatotroph cells such as free fatty acids, and even to exogenous somatostatin.[3] GHS are also partially refractory to the negative GH autofeedback but show peculiar sensitivity to the negative IGF-I feedback action.[3]

In vitro and in vivo ghrelin/GHS as well as GHRH induce homologous but not heterologous desensitization.[3,7,84,85] Despite a preserved pituitary GH releasable pool, desensitization to GHS activity has been demonstrated during continuous infusion of GHS as well as after frequent intermittent administration of these compounds.[3,7] Interestingly, this does not occur after less frequent daily intermittent GHS administration for up to 15 days.[3,7] Similarly to synthetic GHS, in dispersed pituitary cells in vitro, desensitization to serial ghrelin administration occurs at 1 h intervals, but not at 3 h intervals of stimulation.[86] In vivo, in humans, ghrelin has been reported insensitive to a previous administration of GHRH but undergoes partial desensitization during continuous infusion as well as after a previous administration of a synthetic GHS.[87]

The GH-releasing effect of ghrelin and synthetic GHS undergoes marked age-related variations decreasing in aging.[3,88] The mechanisms underlying the age-related variations in the GH-releasing activity of GHS differ by age. The enhanced GH-releasing effect of GHS at puberty reflects a positive influence of estrogen which could trigger an increase in GHS receptor expression.[3] However, estrogen insufficiency does not explain the reduced GH response to GHS in postmenopausal women.[3] In agreement with the reduction in hypothalamic GHS receptors in human aged brain, the GH response to hexarelin in elderly subjects is further increased but not restored by supramaximal doses.[3] The most important mechanism accounting for reduced GH-releasing activity of GHS in aging is probably represented by age-related variations in the neural control of somatotroph function including GHRH hypoactivity and somatostatinergic hyperactivity.[3,4]

PRL- AND ACTH-RELEASING ACTIVITY

The stimulatory effect of ghrelin on PRL secretion in humans is slight, independent of both gender and age and would reflect direct stimulation of somatomammotroph cells and/or central actions.[3,4]

The stimulatory effect of GHS on the activity of hypothalamic–pituitary–adrenal (HPA) axis in humans is similar to that of naloxone, AVP and even CRH.[3,4] The ACTH-releasing activity of ghrelin is independent of gender and does not show significant variations in aging (when the GH response is clearly reduced).[3,4]

In physiological conditions, the ACTH-releasing activity of ghrelin totally depends on CNS-mediated mechanisms via CRH-, AVP-, neuropeptide Y (NPY)- and gamma aminobutyric acid (GABA)-mediated actions and is generally sensitive to the negative feedback exerted by cortisol.[3,4]

INFLUENCE ON THE GONADAL AXIS

Intracerebroventricular injection of ghrelin decreases LH concentration in association with a decrease of the secretory LH pulse frequency. This effect likely reflects modulation of the activity of the GnRH pulse generator potentially via NPY/Y1 receptor mechanisms.[89]

A negative influence of ghrelin on the hypothalamus–pituitary–gonadal axis would explain the prompt turn-off of the axis during starvation. This turn-off would concomitantly reflect the starvation-induced decrease in leptin levels that, in turn, plays a facilitatory role on the same axis.[89]

GHS receptors are present in the testis as well as in the ovary.[9,10,90,91] Leydig cells have been reported able to synthesize ghrelin.[90] In vitro, ghrelin induces a significant inhibition of human CG- and cAMP-stimulated testosterone secretion coupled with a significant decrease in human CG-stimulated expression levels of the mRNAs encoding steroid acute regulatory protein.[90] More recently, strong ghrelin immunostaining was demonstrated in ovarian hilus interstitial cells and in young and mature corpora lutea but not in ovarian follicles.[91]

Influence on food intake and energy metabolism

OREXANT ACTIVITY

Among all the biological actions of ghrelin, particular attention has been focused on its role in the regulation of

appetite and energy balance. Long before ghrelin was discovered, different reports in rodents indicated that some GHS possess orexigenic activity.[3] Moreover, in the last decade, GHS have been shown able to activate neurons in hypothalamic areas strictly involved in the control of energy balance.[3,22,92,93] Accordingly, ghrelin turned out to be one of the most powerful orexigenic and adipogenic agents known so far.[92,94,95]

Ghrelin stimulates food intake in rodents, particularly after central administration.[96,97] Unlike other potent orexigenic agents that are active only when injected intracerebroventricularly (e.g., neuropeptide Y, AGRP, melanin-concentrating hormone), ghrelin has orexigenic and adipogenic effects even after systemic administration.[3,4,97] The efficacy of ghrelin as an orexigenic agent even after peripheral administration would be explained by its transport across the blood–brain barrier in the blood-to-brain direction. The hypothalamic areas playing a crucial role in the regulation of energy homeostasis, such as the ventromedial part of the arcuate nucleus, are not completely protected by the blood–brain barrier, contain neurons expressing GHS-R, and might therefore mediate ghrelin effects.[3,92,93,97]

It has also been demonstrated that ghrelin's influence on appetite and energy balance is, at least partially, mediated by hypothalamic leptin-responsive neurons.[3,92,98–100] Among the major hypothalamic pathways mediating ghrelin's influence on energy balance, one involves neuropeptide Y neurons, and the other involves melanocortin receptors.[101–104] Ghrelin increases AGRP and neuropeptide Y expression after both acute and chronic administration in rats.[101,105–107] Thus, NPY and AGRP likely co-mediate ghrelin's effects on energy balance, NPY might be more important for acute effects while AGRP might be involved in both chronic and acute ghrelin action in the hypothalamus.[3]

Accordingly, whereas deletion of either NPY or AGRP causes only a modest effect on the orexigenic effect of ghrelin, their simultaneous genetic ablation completely abolishes ghrelin's modulatory action on food intake.[107] However, other agents are likely involved in mediating the impact of ghrelin on appetite, food intake and energy balance; these include orexins, pro-opiomelanocortin (POMC), cocaine- and amphetamine-related transcript (CART), melanin-concentrating hormone (MCH), ciliary neurotropic factor (CNTF), GABA, galanin, CRH and somatostatin.[48,108,109] Besides the increase of appetite and food intake, reduced cellular fat oxidation and promotion of adipogenesis reportedly contributes to increased fat mass induced by ghrelin.[18,96]

It is noteworthy that ghrelin regulation of energy homeostasis seems mediated by efferent and afferent fibers of the vagal nerve.[110] Intravenously administered ghrelin decreases the afferent activity of the gastric vagal nerve at low doses.[110] Moreover, the blockade of the gastric vagal afferent fibers abolishes ghrelin-induced feeding, GH secretion, and activation of NPY-producing and GHRH-producing neurons in rats. Cholinergic influence on systemic ghrelin secretion has already been reported both in animals and humans.[39,111–115] Nevertheless, cholinergic agonists and antagonists do not influence the endocrine response to ghrelin administration in humans.[116]

Overall, as a result of central and peripheral actions, ghrelin administration in rodents causes weight gain.[96,101,117] This effect is not due to longitudinal growth or an increase in lean mass as one would expect to occur after stimulation of GH secretion.[3,96] Data in rodents clearly showed that ghrelin-induced weight gain is based on accretion of fat mass without changes in longitudinal skeletal growth and with a decrease of lean mass.[117]

Despite all these data, it has to be taken into account, however, that ghrelin-null mice do not differ from controls in terms of food intake, size, growth rate, and body composition[118] and even GHS-R-null mice show normal appetite and body composition while only a mild reduction of body weight compared with controls seems detectable.[119] Notably, however, a recent report indicated that transgenic mice over-expressing des-acyl ghrelin show small phenotype and alteration in the GH/IGF-I axis in the presence of normal nutritional behavior.[120]

INFLUENCE ON GLUCOSE METABOLISM AND ON ENDOCRINE PANCREATIC FUNCTIONS

Ghrelin expression has been reported to be variably localized in α-, β- and non-β non-α pancreatic cells.[65,121,122] Similarly, GHS-R1a and 1b have been found expressed in animal and human endocrine pancreas.[7,10,122]

Depending on the dose and experimental conditions, ghrelin has been reported to inhibit or stimulate insulin secretion in animals. Ghrelin stimulates insulin secretion from isolated rat pancreatic islets and in rats *in vivo*.[49,50] Conversely, ghrelin has been found able to blunt insulin secretion from the isolated rat pancreas after the stimulation with glucose, arginine, and carbachol.[49,50]

In humans, the administration of ghrelin is followed by an increase in plasma glucose levels coupled with a reduction in insulin levels without alterations in glucagon secretion.[3,49,50] The hyperglycemic effect of ghrelin is likely mediated by a glycogenolitic effect at hepatic level reflecting either a stimulation of catecholamine release and a direct action on hepatocytes.[3,49]

Notably, although unable to modify the insulin and glucose response to oral glucose load, ghrelin blunts the insulin response to arginine and enhances its hyperglycemic effect.[3,49] Ghrelin administration also increases circulating somatostatin and pancreatic polypeptide levels in humans, and the ghrelin-induced somatostatin increase could theoretically explain insulin decrease.[123] Independently of what the mechanisms mediating the impact of ghrelin on insulin secretion might be, it has to be emphasized that insulin and glucose negatively influence ghrelin secretion indicating the existence of feedback mechanisms linking ghrelin to the endocrine pancreas and glucose metabolism.[3,49,50] In this contest it is intriguing to speculate that the metabolic actions of ghrelin could well be coupled to its central actions playing a major role in the control of appetite, food intake and energy balance.

Influence on other non-endocrine functions

EFFECTS ON SLEEP AND BEHAVIOR

In rats, ghrelin has been reported to modify sleep–wake patterns by increasing wakefulness and decreasing the duration of rapid eye movement (REM) sleep periods. This might be caused either by a direct effect of ghrelin on sleep parameters or indirectly by the effects of the peptide on feeding behavior itself.[124] In humans, ghrelin administration has been reported to increase slow wave sleep, to enhance delta wave activity during the second half of the night and to reduce REM sleep during the second third of the night.[124]

Besides regulating eating behavior and sleep, ghrelin has been reported to increase anxiety-like behavior and memory retention in rats.[125] Similarly, in mice, both intracerebroventricular and intraperitoneal administration of ghrelin induce anxiogenic activities. Also, the administration of a CRH receptor antagonist significantly inhibits ghrelin-induced anxiogenic effects. Peripheral administration of ghrelin significantly increases CRH mRNA expression in the hypothalamus. These findings suggest that ghrelin may have a role in mediating neuroendocrine and behavioral responses to stressors and that the stomach could play an important role, not only in the regulation of appetite, but also in the regulation of anxiety.[114]

CARDIOVASCULAR ACTIONS

GHS-R1a expression has been shown in cardiac tissues as well as in endothelial cells.[10,126] Notably, specific binding sites able to recognize both acylated and non-acylated ghrelin as well as peptidyl GHS only have also been demonstrated by binding studies suggesting the existence of still uncloned GHS-R subtypes.[126]

In vitro, both ghrelin and synthetic GHS act as antiapoptotic factors at the cardiovascular level.[20] Notably, this action is exerted also by unacylated ghrelin indicating that the antiapoptotic effect of GHS might be mediated by a GHS-R non-type 1a.[20] *In vivo*, in animals, synthetic peptidyl GHS, but not ghrelin, exert a remarkable GH-independent protective action against cardiovascular damage while both ghrelin and GHS have been shown to improve cardiac performances in different pathophysiological conditions.[3,126] In humans, the acute administration of both synthetic GHS and ghrelin improve cardiac performances in different pathophysiological conditions, although with different hemodynamic profile, further supporting the hypothesis that not all the cardiovascular actions of ghrelin and synthetic GHS are mediated by the GHS-R1a.[3,126]

MODULATION OF NEOPLASTIC CELL PROLIFERATION

Most endocrine tumors at the pituitary level but also gastro-entero-pancreatic carcinoids, pulmonary carcinoids and thyroid tumors have been found to contain ghrelin, as detected by both immunohistochemistry or mRNA analysis.[3,25] In addition, non-endocrine lung, breast, colorectal, prostatic, and pancreatic carcinomas may produce ghrelin, as well.[3,25] The significance of ghrelin expression in human tumors is poorly understood, but it is of interest that concomitant expression of ghrelin binding sites also occurs in many of the above listed neoplasms.[3,25]

Interestingly, in some neoplastic tissues, results from binding studies indicate the existence of GHS-R subtypes also able to bind non-acylated ghrelin and this binding displaces radiolabelled acylated ghrelin from its binding sites.[3] Notably, in some human tumor cell lines, acylated ghrelin, unacylated ghrelin and synthetic GHS share similar anti-proliferative effects.[3] These findings open interesting perspectives in the control of tumor cell growth using synthetic ghrelin analogs. However, a complete mapping of the ghrelin receptor distribution in human tissues and – above all – tumors is necessary, together with the validation of *in vitro* data on *in vivo* models to better define the effects of different ghrelin analogs on human tumor growth.

GHRELIN AND SYNTHETIC GHS: WHAT CLINICAL PERSPECTIVES IN GROWTH DISORDERS?

Based on their strong and reproducible GH-releasing effect even after oral administration, the potential usefulness of ghrelin and its analogs in the diagnosis and treatment of diseases related to the GH/IGF-I axis has been widely investigated. When combined with GHRH, GHS represent one of the most potent and reliable tests to evaluate the pituitary GH releasable pool for the diagnosis of GH deficiency (GHD), at least in adulthood.[8,127–129] Testing with GHS is as sensitive and specific as insulin tolerance test (ITT) and GHRH + arginine, the two 'gold standard' tests for the diagnosis of adult GHD, provided that appropriate cut-off limits are assumed.[8,127,128] It is widely accepted that the diagnosis of GHD in childhood is not simply assessed by the GH response to either classical or maximal provocative tests.[130] A considerable number of short children with normal GH response to provocative tests show insufficient daily GH secretion reflecting neuro-secretory dysfunction and benefit from GH replacement.[130] Though a normal GH response to stimuli does not rule out GH insufficiency in childhood, potent and reproducible provocative tests of GH secretion such as GHS can provide definite information about the maximal secretory capacity of somatotroph cells in short children suspected for GHD.[127,130]

The possibility that GH-releasing substances, particularly if orally active, could represent a therapeutic approach alternative to rhGH in GHD patients received considerable attention. Clearly, GH-releasing substances have no place as alternatives to rhGH for treatment of severe GHD in patients with panhypopituitarism due to massive destruction of the pituitary gland. On the other hand, isolated GHD often reflects a hypothalamic pathogenesis, as shown by clear GH responses to GHRH in many short patients.[130]

The hypothesis was that patients with isolated GHD could benefit from treatment with GHRH and preferably with orally active GHS, which could have the advantage of restoring endogenous GH pulsatility, being, therefore, a more 'physiological' approach.

The potential usefulness of GHS for treatment of short stature with isolated GHD was suggested by some open studies reporting increase in height velocity in short children with idiopathic short stature or GHD after chronic treatment with intranasal or subcutaneous GHS.[131–135] When tested in double blind, placebo-controlled trials in short children with GHD, the efficacy of the most promising orally active GHS, MK-0677, was found to be lower than that of rhGH.[127] Treatment with MK-0677 transiently increased height velocity (approximately 3 cm year^{-1} increase) in a dose-independent manner in children with partial GHD but not in children with severe GHD who had no benefit from the treatment. Thus, it is unlikely that GHS can replace rhGH in the treatment of GHD in childhood. This evidence was also against the hypothesis that isolated GHD could reflect a defect in the activity of the endogenous GHS-like ligand, i.e., ghrelin. In any case, the failure of GHS as an alternative to rhGH for treatment of GHD, could have been predicted from the clear dependence of GHS's activity on the full integrity of the hypothalamic–pituitary axis and which is, by definition, compromised in most of the conditions leading to GHD in childhood.

On the other hand, GHS could provide anabolic treatment in frail elderly subjects after the somatopause based on the following evidence: (1) the age-related reduction in the activity of GH/IGF-I axis probably accounts for changes in body composition, structure functions and metabolism in normal elderly subjects which are remarkably similar to (but of lesser extent than) those in adult GHD, (2) the pituitary GH releasable pool is still significant in aged subjects, and (3) GH-releasing substances would represent a more physiological approach to increase endogenous GH pulsatility. GHRH needs to be administered parenterally while GHS are active even after oral administration. Among GHS, the non-peptidyl spiroindoline MK-0677 was the most promising candidate showing impressive bioavailability and long lasting effect after single oral daily administration.[127,136]

So far, the following results have been obtained by trials testing the effects of chronic treatment with MK-0677: (1) in elderly subjects it restores IGF-I levels in the normal young range indicating successful enhancement of somatotroph secretion, (2) in elderly subjects it increases REM sleep while decreasing REM latency, thus counteracting alterations in sleep pattern that are hallmarks of brain aging, (3) it reverses diet-induced catabolism in young volunteers indicating anabolic effect which increases fat-free mass and energy expenditure in obese patients, (4) in a large population of postmenopausal osteoporotic women, 1 year treatment with MK-0677 alone and in combination with alendronate, a bisphosphonate, attenuates the indirect suppressive effect of alendronate on bone formation but does not translate into significant increases in bone mass density at sites other than the femoral neck.[127,136] In all, at present, there is no definitive evidence showing the therapeutic efficacy of GHS as anabolic agents acting via rejuvenation of the GH/IGF-I axis in elderly subjects and further studies are needed to clarify this hypothesis.

CONCLUSION

GH secretagogues were introduced more than 20 years ago as synthetic molecules possessing strong GH-releasing activity. Based on this biologic activity, GHS have been reported to be a reliable provocative test for the diagnosis of GH deficiency but the tempting prospect of their clinical usefulness as orally active growth-promoting agents or anabolic anti-aging drugs has not been confirmed. In any case, synthetic GHS allowed the discovery of previously unknown specific receptors and, more recently, of their natural ligand, ghrelin.

Ghrelin, a 28 amino acid acylated peptide predominantly produced by the stomach, displays strong GH-releasing activity mediated by the hypothalamic–pituitary GH secretagogue (GHS) receptors which had been shown to be specific for a family of synthetic, orally active molecules known as GHS. However, despite the potent and reproducible GH-releasing activity, the tempting prospect of GHS as clinically useful tools as orally active growth-promoting agents or anabolic anti-aging drugs has not been confirmed. However, ghrelin and GHS, acting on central and peripheral receptors, also exert other actions including stimulation of ACTH and prolactin secretion, influence insulin secretion, glucose and lipid metabolism, orexigenic effect and modulatory activity on the neuroendocrine and metabolic response to starvation, influence on exocrine gastro-entero-pancreatic functions, cardiovascular activities and modulation of cell proliferation and apoptosis. The discovery of ghrelin and the characterization of these GH-independent biological activities has widened our knowledge of some critical aspects of neuroendocrinology and theoretically predicts these molecules as candidate drugs for treatment of pathophysiological conditions even unrelated to disorders in GH secretion.

KEY LEARNING POINTS

- GHS, when combined with GHRH, represent one of the most potent and reliable tests to evaluate the pituitary GH releasable pool for the diagnosis of GHD, at least in adulthood.
- Testing with GHS is as sensitive and specific as ITT and GHRH+arginine, the two 'gold standard' tests for the diagnosis of adult GHD, provided that appropriate cut-off limits are assumed.
- GH-releasing substances have no place as alternatives to rhGH for treatment of severe GHD in patients with panhypopituitarism due to massive destruction of the pituitary gland.
- The efficacy of chronic treatment with GHS to restore the function of the GH/IGF-I axis in idiopathic GHD has never been demonstrated.
- There is no definitive evidence, at present, showing the therapeutic efficacy of GHS as anabolic agents acting via rejuvenation of the GH/IGF-I axis in elderly subjects.

REFERENCES

● = Seminal primary article
◆ = Key review paper

1 Ghigo E, Arvat E, Gianotti L, et al. Hypothalamic growth hormone–insulin-like growth factor-I axis across the human life span. *J Pediatr Endocrinol Metab* 2000; **13(Suppl 6)**: 1493–502.

2 Giustina A, Veldhuis JD. Pathophysiology of the neuroregulation of growth hormone secretion in experimental animals and the human. *Endocr Rev* 1998; **19**: 717–97.

◆ 3 Van Der Lely AJ, Tschop M, Heiman ML, Ghigo E. Biological, physiological, pathophysiological, and pharmacological aspects of ghrelin. *Endocr Rev* 2004; **25**: 426–57.

◆ 4 Korbonits M, Goldstone AP, Gueorguiev M, Grossman AB. Ghrelin – a hormone with multiple functions. *Front Neuroendocrinol* 2004; **25**: 27–68.

◆ 5 Kojima M, Hosoda H, Matsuo H, Kangawa K. Ghrelin: discovery of the natural endogenous ligand for the growth hormone secretagogue receptor. *Trends Endocrinol Metab* 2001; **12**: 118–22.

● 6 Kojima M, Hosoda H, Date Y, et al. Ghrelin is a growth-hormone-releasing acylated peptide from stomach. *Nature* 1999; **402**: 656–60.

◆ 7 Smith RG, Van der Ploeg LH, Howard AD, et al. Peptidomimetic regulation of growth hormone secretion. *Endocr Rev* 1997; **18**: 621–45.

8 Baldelli R, Otero XL, Camina JP, et al. Growth hormone secretagogues as diagnostic tools in disease states. *Endocrine* 2001; **14**: 95–9.

● 9 Papotti M, Ghe C, Cassoni P, et al. Growth hormone secretagogue binding sites in peripheral human tissues. *J Clin Endocrinol Metab* 2000; **85**: 3803–7.

10 Gnanapavan S, Kola B, Bustin SA, et al. The tissue distribution of the mRNA of ghrelin and subtypes of its receptor, GHS-R, in humans. *J Clin Endocrinol Metab* 2002; **87**: 2988.

11 Muccioli G, Papotti M, Locatelli V, et al. Binding of 125I-labeled ghrelin to membranes from human hypothalamus and pituitary gland. *J Endocrinol Invest* 2001; **24**: RC7–9.

12 Date Y, Kojima M, Hosoda H, et al. Ghrelin, a novel growth hormone-releasing acylated peptide, is synthesized in a distinct endocrine cell type in the gastrointestinal tracts of rats and humans. *Endocrinology* 2000; **141**: 4255–61.

13 Fehrentz JA, Martinez J, Boeglin D, *et al*. Growth hormone secretagogues: past, present and future. *IDrugs* 2002; **5**: 804–14.

14 Smith RG, Leonard R, Bailey AR, *et al*. Growth hormone secretagogue receptor family members and ligands. *Endocrine* 2001; **14**: 9–14.

15 Howard AD, Feighner SD, Cully DF, *et al*. A receptor in pituitary and hypothalamus that functions in growth hormone release. *Science* 1996; **273**: 974–7.

16 Banks WA, Tschop M, Robinson SM, Heiman ML. Extent and direction of ghrelin transport across the blood–brain barrier is determined by its unique primary structure. *J Pharmacol Exp Ther* 2002; **302**: 822–7.

17 Broglio F, Benso A, Gottero C, *et al*. Non-acylated ghrelin does not possess the pituitaric and pancreatic endocrine activity of acylated ghrelin in humans. *J Endocrinol Invest* 2003; **26**: 192–6.

18 Thompson NM, Gill DA, Davies R, *et al*. Ghrelin and des-octanoyl ghrelin promote adipogenesis directly in vivo by a mechanism independent of the type 1a growth hormone secretagogue receptor. *Endocrinology* 2004; **145**: 234–42.

19 Broglio F, Gottero C, Prodam F, *et al*. Non-acylated ghrelin counteracts the metabolic but not the neuroendocrine response to acylated ghrelin in humans. *J Clin Endocrinol Metab* 2004; **89**: 3062–5.

20 Baldanzi G, Filigheddu N, Cutrupi S, *et al*. Ghrelin and des-acyl ghrelin inhibit cell death in cardiomyocytes and endothelial cells through ERK1/2 and PI 3-kinase/AKT. *J Cell Biol* 2002; **159**: 1029–37.

21 Cassoni P, Papotti M, Ghe C, *et al*. Identification, characterization, and biological activity of specific receptors for natural (ghrelin) and synthetic growth hormone secretagogues and analogs in human breast carcinomas and cell lines. *J Clin Endocrinol Metab* 2001; **86**: 1738–45.

22 Shuto Y, Shibasaki T, Otagiri A, *et al*. Hypothalamic growth hormone secretagogue receptor regulates growth hormone secretion, feeding, and adiposity. *J Clin Invest* 2002; **109**: 1429–36.

23 Wren AM, Small CJ, Fribbens CV, *et al*. The hypothalamic mechanisms of the hypophysiotropic action of ghrelin. *Neuroendocrinology* 2002; **76**: 316–24.

24 Katayama M, Nogami H, Nishiyama J, *et al*. Developmentally and regionally regulated expression of growth hormone secretagogue receptor mRNA in rat brain and pituitary gland. *Neuroendocrinology* 2000; **72**: 333–40.

25 Jeffery PL, Herington AC, Chopin LK. The potential autocrine/paracrine roles of ghrelin and its receptor in hormone-dependent cancer. *Cytokine Growth Factor Rev* 2003; **14**: 113–22.

26 Carreira MC, Camina JP, Smith RG, Casanueva FF. Agonist-specific coupling of growth hormone secretagogue receptor type 1a to different intracellular signaling systems. Role of adenosine. *Neuroendocrinology* 2004; **79**: 13–25.

27 Deghenghi R, Papotti M, Ghigo E, Muccioli G. Cortistatin, but not somatostatin, binds to growth hormone secretagogue (GHS) receptors of human pituitary gland. *J Endocrinol Invest* 2001; **24**: RC1–3.

28 Tolle V, Bassant MH, Zizzari P, *et al*. Ultradian rhythmicity of ghrelin secretion in relation with GH, feeding behavior, and sleep-wake patterns in rats. *Endocrinology* 2002; **143**: 1353–61.

29 Cummings DE, Purnell JQ, Frayo RS, *et al*. A preprandial rise in plasma ghrelin levels suggests a role in meal initiation in humans. *Diabetes* 2001; **50**: 1714–9.

30 Cummings DE, Frayo RS, Marmonier C, *et al*. Plasma ghrelin levels and hunger scores in humans initiating meals voluntarily without time- and food-related cues. *Am J Physiol Endocrinol Metab* 2004; **287**: E297–304.

31 Chan JL, Bullen J, Lee JH, *et al*. Ghrelin levels are not regulated by recombinant leptin administration and/or three days of fasting in healthy subjects. *J Clin Endocrinol Metab* 2004; **89**: 335–43.

32 Callahan HS, Cummings DE, Pepe MS, *et al*. Postprandial suppression of plasma ghrelin level is proportional to ingested caloric load but does not predict intermeal interval in humans. *J Clin Endocrinol Metab* 2004; **89**: 1319–24.

33 Erdmann J, Lippl F, Schusdziarra V. Differential effect of protein and fat on plasma ghrelin levels in man. *Regul Pept* 2003; **116**: 101–7.

34 Shiiya T, Nakazato M, Mizuta M, *et al*. Plasma ghrelin levels in lean and obese humans and the effect of glucose on ghrelin secretion. *J Clin Endocrinol Metab* 2002; **87**: 240–4.

35 Nakagawa E, Nagaya N, Okumura H, *et al*. Hyperglycaemia suppresses the secretion of ghrelin, a novel growth-hormone-releasing peptide: responses to the intravenous and oral administration of glucose. *Clin Sci (Lond)* 2002; **103**: 325–8.

36 Mohlig M, Spranger J, Otto B, *et al*. Euglycemic hyperinsulinemia, but not lipid infusion, decreases circulating ghrelin levels in humans. *J Endocrinol Invest* 2002; **25**: RC36–38.

37 Monteleone P, Bencivenga R, Longobardi N, *et al*. Differential responses of circulating ghrelin to high-fat or high-carbohydrate meal in healthy women. *J Clin Endocrinol Metab* 2003; **88**: 5510–4.

38 Greenman Y, Golani N, Gilad S, *et al*. Ghrelin secretion is modulated in a nutrient- and gender-specific manner. *Clin Endocrinol (Oxf)* 2004; **60**: 382–8.

39 Heath RB, Jones R, Frayn KN, Robertson MD. Vagal stimulation exaggerates the inhibitory ghrelin response to oral fat in humans. *J Endocrinol* 2004; **180**: 273–81.

40 Erdmann J, Topsch R, Lippl F, *et al*. Postprandial response of plasma ghrelin levels to various test meals in relation to food intake, plasma insulin, and glucose. *J Clin Endocrinol Metab* 2004; **89**: 3048–54.

41 Knerr I, Groschl M, Rascher W, Rauh M. Endocrine effects of food intake: insulin, ghrelin, and leptin responses to a single bolus of essential amino acids in humans. *Ann Nutr Metab* 2003; **47**: 312–8.

42 Groschl M, Knerr I, Topf HG, *et al*. Endocrine responses to the oral ingestion of a physiological dose of essential amino acids in humans. *J Endocrinol* 2003; **179**: 237–44.

43 Tschop M, Weyer C, Tataranni PA, *et al.* Circulating ghrelin levels are decreased in human obesity. *Diabetes* 2001; **50**: 707–9.

44 Ariyasu H, Takaya K, Tagami T, *et al.* Stomach is a major source of circulating ghrelin, and feeding state determines plasma ghrelin-like immunoreactivity levels in humans. *J Clin Endocrinol Metab* 2001; **86**: 4753–8.

45 Cummings DE, Clement K, Purnell JQ, *et al.* Elevated plasma ghrelin levels in Prader-Willi syndrome. *Nat Med* 2002; **8**: 643–4.

46 Otto B, Cuntz U, Fruehauf E, *et al.* Weight gain decreases elevated plasma ghrelin concentrations of patients with anorexia nervosa. *Eur J Endocrinol* 2001; **145**: 669–73.

47 Cummings DE, Weigle DS, Frayo RS, *et al.* Plasma ghrelin levels after diet-induced weight loss or gastric bypass surgery. *N Engl J Med* 2002; **346**: 1623–30.

48 Cummings DE, Foster KE. Ghrelin-leptin tango in body-weight regulation. *Gastroenterology* 2003; **124**: 1532–5.

49 Broglio F, Gottero C, Benso A, *et al.* Ghrelin and the endocrine pancreas. *Endocrine* 2003; **22**: 19–24.

50 Ukkola O. Ghrelin and insulin metabolism. *Eur J Clin Invest* 2003; **33**: 183–5.

51 Broglio F, Prodam F, Gottero C, *et al.* Ghrelin does not mediate the somatotroph and corticotroph responses to the stimulatory effect of glucagon or insulin-induced hypoglycaemia in humans. *Clin Endocrinol (Oxf)* 2004; **60**: 699–704.

52 Flanagan DE, Evans ML, Monsod TP, *et al.* The influence of insulin on circulating ghrelin. *Am J Physiol Endocrinol Metab* 2003; **284**: E313–6.

53 Saad MF, Bernaba B, Hwu CM, *et al.* Insulin regulates plasma ghrelin concentration. *J Clin Endocrinol Metab* 2002; **87**: 3997–4000.

54 Lucidi P, Murdolo G, Di LC, *et al.* Ghrelin is not necessary for adequate hormonal counterregulation of insulin-induced hypoglycemia. *Diabetes* 2002; **51**: 2911–4.

55 Murdolo G, Lucidi P, Di LC, *et al.* Insulin is required for prandial ghrelin suppression in humans. *Diabetes* 2003; **52**: 2923–7.

56 Anderwald C, Brabant G, Bernroider E, *et al.* Insulin-dependent modulation of plasma ghrelin and leptin concentrations is less pronounced in type 2 diabetic patients. *Diabetes* 2003; **52**: 1792–8.

57 Barkan AL, Dimaraki EV, Jessup SK, *et al.* Ghrelin secretion in humans is sexually dimorphic, suppressed by somatostatin, and not affected by the ambient growth hormone levels. *J Clin Endocrinol Metab* 2003; **88**: 2180–4.

58 Broglio F, Koetsveld PP, Benso A, *et al.* Ghrelin secretion is inhibited by either somatostatin or cortistatin in humans. *J Clin Endocrinol Metab* 2002; **87**: 4829–32.

59 Norrelund H, Hansen TK, Orskov H, *et al.* Ghrelin immunoreactivity in human plasma is suppressed by somatostatin. *Clin Endocrinol (Oxf)* 2002; **57**: 539–46.

60 DelParigi A, Tschop M, Heiman ML, *et al.* High circulating ghrelin: a potential cause for hyperphagia and obesity in Prader–Willi syndrome. *J Clin Endocrinol Metab* 2002; **87**: 5461–4.

61 Cortelazzi D, Cappiello V, Morpurgo PS, *et al.* Circulating levels of ghrelin in human fetuses. *Eur J Endocrinol* 2003; **149**: 111–6.

62 Wierup N, Sundler F. Circulating levels of ghrelin in human fetuses. *Eur J Endocrinol* 2004; **150**: 405.

63 Kitamura S, Yokota I, Hosoda H, *et al.* Ghrelin concentration in cord and neonatal blood: relation to fetal growth and energy balance. *J Clin Endocrinol Metab* 2003; **88**: 5473–7.

64 Chanoine JP, Wong AC. Ghrelin gene expression is markedly higher in fetal pancreas compared with fetal stomach: effect of maternal fasting. *Endocrinology* 2004; **145**: 3813–20.

65 Wierup N, Svensson H, Mulder H, Sundler F. The ghrelin cell: a novel developmentally regulated islet cell in the human pancreas. *Regul Pept* 2002; **107**: 63–9.

66 Farquhar J, Heiman M, Wong AC, *et al.* Elevated umbilical cord ghrelin concentrations in small for gestational age neonates. *J Clin Endocrinol Metab* 2003; **88**: 4324–7.

67 Onal EE, Cinaz P, Atalay Y, *et al.* Umbilical cord ghrelin concentrations in small- and appropriate-for-gestational age newborn infants: relationship to anthropometric markers. *J Endocrinol* 2004; **180**: 267–71.

68 Bellone S, Castellino N, Broglio F, *et al.* Ghrelin secretion in childhood is refractory to the inhibitory effect of feeding. *J Clin Endocrinol Metab* 2004; **89**: 1662–5.

69 Soriano-Guillen L, Barrios V, Chowen JA, *et al.* Ghrelin levels from fetal life through early adulthood: relationship with endocrine and metabolic and anthropometric measures. *J Pediatr* 2004; **144**: 30–5.

70 James RJ, Drewett RF, Cheetham TD. Low cord ghrelin levels in term infants are associated with slow weight gain over the first 3 months of life. *J Clin Endocrinol Metab* 2004; **89**: 3847–50.

71 Iniguez G, Ong K, Pena V, *et al.* Fasting and post-glucose ghrelin levels in SGA infants: relationships with size and weight gain at one year of age. *J Clin Endocrinol Metab* 2002; **87**: 5830–3.

72 Rigamonti AE, Pincelli AI, Corra B, *et al.* Plasma ghrelin concentrations in elderly subjects: comparison with anorexic and obese patients. *J Endocrinol* 2002; **175**: R1–5.

73 Purnell JQ, Weigle DS, Breen P, Cummings DE. Ghrelin levels correlate with insulin levels, insulin resistance, and high-density lipoprotein cholesterol, but not with gender, menopausal status, or cortisol levels in humans. *J Clin Endocrinol Metab* 2003; **88**: 5747–52.

74 Date Y, Murakami N, Kojima M, *et al.* Central effects of a novel acylated peptide, ghrelin, on growth hormone release in rats. *Biochem Biophys Res Commun* 2000; **275**: 477–80.

75 Hataya Y, Akamizu T, Takaya K, *et al.* A low dose of ghrelin stimulates growth hormone (GH) release synergistically with GH-releasing hormone in humans. *J Clin Endocrinol Metab* 2001; **86**: 4552.

76 Arvat E, Maccario M, Di VL, *et al.* Endocrine activities of ghrelin, a natural growth hormone secretagogue (GHS), in humans: comparison and interactions with hexarelin, a nonnatural peptidyl GHS, and GH-releasing hormone. *J Clin Endocrinol Metab* 2001; **86**: 1169–74.

77 Tannenbaum GS, Epelbaum J, Bowers CY. Interrelationship between the novel peptide ghrelin and somatostatin/growth hormone-releasing hormone in regulation of pulsatile growth hormone secretion. *Endocrinology* 2003; **144**: 967–74.

78 Kamegai J, Tamura H, Shimizu T, *et al.* Regulation of the ghrelin gene: growth hormone-releasing hormone upregulates ghrelin mRNA in the pituitary. *Endocrinology* 2001; **142**: 4154–7.

79 Kamegai J, Tamura H, Shimizu T, *et al.* The role of pituitary ghrelin in growth hormone (GH) secretion: GH-releasing hormone-dependent regulation of pituitary ghrelin gene expression and peptide content. *Endocrinology* 2004; **145**: 3731–8.

80 Cunha SR, Mayo KE. Ghrelin and growth hormone (GH) secretagogues potentiate GH-releasing hormone (GHRH)-induced cyclic adenosine 3′, 5′-monophosphate production in cells expressing transfected GHRH and GH secretagogue receptors. *Endocrinology* 2002; **143**: 4570–82.

81 Popovic V, Miljic D, Micic D, *et al.* Ghrelin main action on the regulation of growth hormone release is exerted at hypothalamic level. *J Clin Endocrinol Metab* 2003; **88**: 3450–3.

82 Kamegai J, Tamura H, Shimizu T, *et al.* Central effect of ghrelin, an endogenous growth hormone secretagogue, on hypothalamic peptide gene expression. *Endocrinology* 2000; **141**: 4797–800.

83 Tannenbaum GS, Bowers CY. Interactions of growth hormone secretagogues and growth hormone-releasing hormone/somatostatin. *Endocrine* 2001; **14**: 21–7.

84 Camina JP, Carreira MC, El MS, *et al.* Desensitization and endocytosis mechanisms of ghrelin-activated growth hormone secretagogue receptor 1a. *Endocrinology* 2004; **145**: 930–40.

85 Orkin RD, New DI, Norman D, *et al.* Rapid desensitisation of the GH secretagogue (ghrelin) receptor to hexarelin in vitro. *J Endocrinol Invest* 2003; **26**: 743–7.

86 Yamazaki M, Nakamura K, Kobayashi H, *et al.* Regulational effect of ghrelin on growth hormone secretion from perifused rat anterior pituitary cells. *J Neuroendocrinol* 2002; **14**: 156–62.

87 Micic D, Macut D, Sumarac-Dumanovic M, *et al.* Ghrelin-induced GH secretion in normal subjects is partially resistant to homologous desensitization by GH-releasing peptide-6. *Eur J Endocrinol* 2002; **147**: 761–6.

88 Broglio F, Benso A, Castiglioni C, *et al.* The endocrine response to ghrelin as a function of gender in humans in young and elderly subjects. *J Clin Endocrinol Metab* 2003; **88**: 1537–42.

89 Furuta M, Funabashi T, Kimura F. Intracerebroventricular administration of ghrelin rapidly suppresses pulsatile luteinizing hormone secretion in ovariectomized rats. *Biochem Biophys Res Commun* 2001; **288**: 780–5.

90 Tena-Sempere M, Barreiro ML, Gonzalez LC, *et al.* Novel expression and functional role of ghrelin in rat testis. *Endocrinology* 2002; **143**: 717–25.

91 Gaytan F, Barreiro ML, Chopin LK, *et al.* Immunolocalization of ghrelin and its functional receptor, the type 1a growth hormone secretagogue receptor, in the cyclic human ovary. *J Clin Endocrinol Metab* 2003; **88**: 879–87.

92 Zigman JM, Elmquist JK. Minireview: From anorexia to obesity–the yin and yang of body weight control. *Endocrinology* 2003; **144**: 3749–56.

93 Sainsbury A, Cooney GJ, Herzog H. Hypothalamic regulation of energy homeostasis. *Best Pract Res Clin Endocrinol Metab* 2002; **16**: 623–37.

94 Wren AM, Seal LJ, Cohen MA, *et al.* Ghrelin enhances appetite and increases food intake in humans. *J Clin Endocrinol Metab* 2001; **86**: 5992.

95 Lawrence CB, Snape AC, Baudoin FM, Luckman SM. Acute central ghrelin and GH secretagogues induce feeding and activate brain appetite centers. *Endocrinology* 2002; **143**: 155–62.

96 Tschop M, Smiley DL, Heiman ML. Ghrelin induces adiposity in rodents. *Nature* 2000; **407**: 908–13.

97 Wren AM, Small CJ, Ward HL, *et al.* The novel hypothalamic peptide ghrelin stimulates food intake and growth hormone secretion. *Endocrinology* 2000; **141**: 4325–8.

98 Shintani M, Ogawa Y, Ebihara K, *et al.* Ghrelin, an endogenous growth hormone secretagogue, is a novel orexigenic peptide that antagonizes leptin action through the activation of hypothalamic neuropeptide Y/Y1 receptor pathway. *Diabetes* 2001; **50**: 227–32.

99 Small CJ, Stanley SA, Bloom SR. Appetite control and reproduction: leptin and beyond. *Semin Reprod Med* 2002; **20**: 389–98.

100 Williams J, Mobarhan S. A critical interaction: leptin and ghrelin. *Nutr Rev* 2003; **61**: 391–3.

101 Kamegai J, Tamura H, Shimizu T, *et al.* Chronic central infusion of ghrelin increases hypothalamic neuropeptide Y and Agouti-related protein mRNA levels and body weight in rats. *Diabetes* 2001; **50**: 2438–43.

102 Wang L, Saint-Pierre DH, Tache Y. Peripheral ghrelin selectively increases Fos expression in neuropeptide Y-synthesizing neurons in mouse hypothalamic arcuate nucleus. *Neurosci Lett* 2002; **325**: 47–51.

103 Guan JL, Wang QP, Kageyama H, *et al.* Synaptic interactions between ghrelin- and neuropeptide Y-containing neurons in the rat arcuate nucleus. *Peptides* 2003; **24**: 1921–8.

104 Kalra SP, Kalra PS. Neuropeptide Y: a physiological orexigen modulated by the feedback action of ghrelin and leptin. *Endocrine* 2003; **22**: 49–56.

105 Tang-Christensen M, Vrang N, Ortmann S, *et al.* Central administration of ghrelin and agouti-related protein (AGRP (83–132)) increases food intake and decreases spontaneous locomotor activity in rats. *Endocrinology* 2004; Jul 1.

106 Tschop M, Statnick MA, Suter TM, Heiman ML. GH-releasing peptide-2 increases fat mass in mice lacking NPY: indication for a crucial mediating role of hypothalamic agouti-related protein. *Endocrinology* 2002; **143**: 558–68.

107 Chen HY, Trumbauer ME, Chen AS, *et al.* Orexigenic action of peripheral ghrelin is mediated by neuropeptide Y and agouti-related protein. *Endocrinology* 2004; **145**: 2607–12.

108 Ellacott KL, Cone RD. The central melanocortin system and the integration of short- and long-term regulators of energy homeostasis. *Recent Prog Horm Res* 2004, **59**: 395–408.

109 Seoane LM, Lopez M, Tovar S, *et al*. Agouti-related peptide, neuropeptide Y, and somatostatin-producing neurons are targets for ghrelin actions in the rat hypothalamus. *Endocrinology* 2003; **144**: 544–51.

110 Date Y, Murakami N, Toshinai K, *et al*. The role of the gastric afferent vagal nerve in ghrelin-induced feeding and growth hormone secretion in rats. *Gastroenterology* 2002; **123**: 1120–8.

111 Sugino T, Yamaura J, Yamagishi M, *et al*. Involvement of cholinergic neurons in the regulation of the ghrelin secretory response to feeding in sheep. *Biochem Biophys Res Commun* 2003; **304**: 308–12.

112 Williams DL, Grill HJ, Cummings DE, Kaplan JM. Vagotomy dissociates short- and long-term controls of circulating ghrelin. *Endocrinology* 2003; **144**: 5184–7.

113 Broglio F, Gottero C, Van KP, *et al*. Acetylcholine regulates ghrelin secretion in humans. *J Clin Endocrinol Metab* 2004; **89**: 2429–33.

114 Asakawa A, Inui A, Kaga T, *et al*. A role of ghrelin in neuroendocrine and behavioral responses to stress in mice. *Neuroendocrinology* 2001; **74**: 143–7.

115 Maier C, Schaller G, Buranyi B, *et al*. The cholinergic system controls ghrelin release and ghrelin-induced growth hormone release in humans. *J Clin Endocrinol Metab* 2004; **89**: 4729–33.

116 Broglio F, Gottero C, Benso A, *et al*. Acetylcholine does not play a major role in mediating the endocrine responses to ghrelin, a natural ligand of the GH secretagogue receptor, in humans. *Clin Endocrinol (Oxf)* 2003; **58**: 92–8.

117 Wren AM, Small CJ, Abbott CR, *et al*. Ghrelin causes hyperphagia and obesity in rats. *Diabetes* 2001; **50**: 2540–7.

118 Sun Y, Ahmed S, Smith RG. Deletion of ghrelin impairs neither growth nor appetite. *Mol Cell Biol* 2003; **23**: 7973–81.

119 Sun Y, Wang P, Zheng H, Smith RG. Ghrelin stimulation of growth hormone release and appetite is mediated through the growth hormone secretagogue receptor. *Proc Natl Acad Sci USA* 2004; **101**: 4679–84.

120 Ariyasu H, Takaya K, Iwakura H, *et al*. Transgenic mice overexpressing des-acyl ghrelin show small phenotype. *Endocrinology* 2004; Oct 7.

121 Date Y, Nakazato M, Hashiguchi S, *et al*. Ghrelin is present in pancreatic alpha-cells of humans and rats and stimulates insulin secretion. *Diabetes* 2002; **51**: 124–9.

122 Volante M, Allia E, Gugliotta P, *et al*. Expression of ghrelin and of the GH secretagogue receptor by pancreatic islet cells and related endocrine tumors. *J Clin Endocrinol Metab* 2002; **87**: 1300–8.

123 Arosio M, Ronchi CL, Gebbia C, *et al*. Stimulatory effects of ghrelin on circulating somatostatin and pancreatic polypeptide levels. *J Clin Endocrinol Metab* 2003; **88**: 701–4.

124 Steiger A. Sleep and endocrinology. *J Intern Med* 2003; **254**: 13–22.

125 Carlini VP, Monzon ME, Varas MM, *et al*. Ghrelin increases anxiety-like behavior and memory retention in rats. *Biochem Biophys Res Commun* 2002; **299**: 739–43.

126 Benso A, Broglio F, Marafetti L, *et al*. Ghrelin and synthetic growth hormone secretagogues are cardioactive molecules with identities and differences. *Semin Vasc Med* 2004; **4**: 107–14.

127 Broglio F, Arvat E, Gottero C, *et al*. Natural and synthetic growth hormone secretagogues. Do they have therapeutic potential? *Treat Endocrinol* 2003, **2**: 153–63.

128 Popovic V, Leal A, Micic D, *et al*. GH-releasing hormone and GH-releasing peptide-6 for diagnostic testing in GH-deficient adults. *Lancet* 2000; **356**: 1137–42.

129 Popovic V, Pekic S, Micic D, *et al*. Evaluation of the reproducibility of the GHRH plus GHRP-6 test of growth hormone reserve in adults. *Clin Endocrinol (Oxf)* 2004; **60**: 185–91.

130 Shalet SM, Toogood A, Rahim A, Brennan BM. The diagnosis of growth hormone deficiency in children and adults. *Endocr Rev* 1998; **19**: 203–23.

131 Klinger B, Silbergeld A, Deghenghi R, *et al*. Desensitization from long-term intranasal treatment with hexarelin does not interfere with the biological effects of this growth hormone-releasing peptide in short children. *Eur J Endocrinol* 1996; **134**: 716–9.

132 Laron Z, Frenkel J, Deghenghi R, *et al*. Intranasal administration of the GHRP hexarelin accelerates growth in short children. *Clin Endocrinol (Oxf)* 1995; **43**: 631–5.

133 Laron Z. Intranasally and orally active GH secretagogues are useful clinical tools: so why are they not on the market? *J Endocrinol Invest* 2003; **26**: 91–2.

134 Mericq V, Cassorla F, Garcia H, *et al*. Growth hormone (GH) responses to GH-releasing peptide and to GH-releasing hormone in GH-deficient children. *J Clin Endocrinol Metab* 1995; **80**: 1681–4.

135 Pihoker C, Badger TM, Reynolds GA, Bowers CY. Treatment effects of intranasal growth hormone releasing peptide-2 in children with short stature. *J Endocrinol* 1997; **155**: 79–86.

136 Smith RG, Sun Y, Betancourt L, Asnicar M. Growth hormone secretagogues: prospects and potential pitfalls. *Best Pract Res Clin Endocrinol Metab* 2004; **18**: 333–47.

44

Aromatase inhibitors

LEO DUNKEL

EVIDENCE SCORING OF THERAPY

   * Non-randomized controlled trials, cohort study, etc.
  ** One or more well-designed randomized controlled trials
*** Systematic review or meta-analysis

SUMMARY

The enzyme P450 aromatase, catalyzes the aromatization of C_{19} androgens (androstenedione and testosterone) to C_{18} estrogens (estrone and estradiol). In premenopausal women estrogen is predominantly synthesized in the ovary through P450 aromatase, but in males, testicular aromatization of androgens accounts only for about 15 percent of circulating estrogen. The estrogen synthesized within extragonadal tissues, particularly in bone and brain, is probably biologically active only locally in a paracrine or 'intracrine' fashion.

During puberty, in both sexes, the mechanism involved in the epiphyseal fusion is mediated by the action of estrogen through a cascade of events including proliferation, differentiation and apoptosis of chondrocytes. Inhibition of estrogen action by aromatase inhibitors (AIs) appears to decelerate this process, and therapeutically, AIs may increase adult height. The clinical experience with AIs in the pediatric setting is limited to testolactone, anastrozole, letrozole, and fadrozole. Testolactone, a non-selective steroidal AI, has been used successfully as adjunct to antiandrogen and GnRHa therapy for children with familial male limited precocious puberty and congenital adrenal hyperplasia, and with some success in girls with McCune–Albright syndrome. The limitations of testolactone include its relatively low potency, and the need for a frequent dosing. Letrozole, a selective non-steroidal AI, has been used in boys with delayed puberty in a randomized placebo controlled trial. In this study, delayed bone maturation simultaneously with good growth response resulted in the increase in predicted adult height in boys treated with testosterone and letrozole. In this study only minor differences in bone density were seen between the two treatment groups, both receiving concomitant testosterone therapy. No adverse effects on testis size or inhibin B concentration were noted. Anastrozole, a selective non-steroidal AI, did not cause any significant negative effects on body composition, protein synthesis, or kinetic measurements of bone calcium turnover in healthy young male volunteers in the short-term use. The therapeutic value of AIs in growth promotion now remains to be substantiated in controlled clinical trials.

SEX STEROIDS AND GROWTH

Increasing secretion of sex steroids in gonads during puberty induces acceleration of growth and development of secondary sexual characteristics. Androgens in boys and estrogens in girls have been generally assumed to be the primary sex steroids causing physical changes during puberty.

In 1994, the description of a man with inactivating mutation of the estrogen receptor (ER) revolutionized the traditional concept of the roles of sex steroids in males.[1] This 28-year-old man was 204 cm tall. He had a bone age of 15 years, open epiphyses of long bones, and consequently he was still growing. Moreover, he had no recollection of accelerated pubertal growth despite otherwise normal pubertal development. Soon thereafter, two males with similar phenotypes were described.[2,3] In these men, the effects of estrogens were suppressed due to mutations in the gene coding P450 aromatase enzyme, which converts androgens to

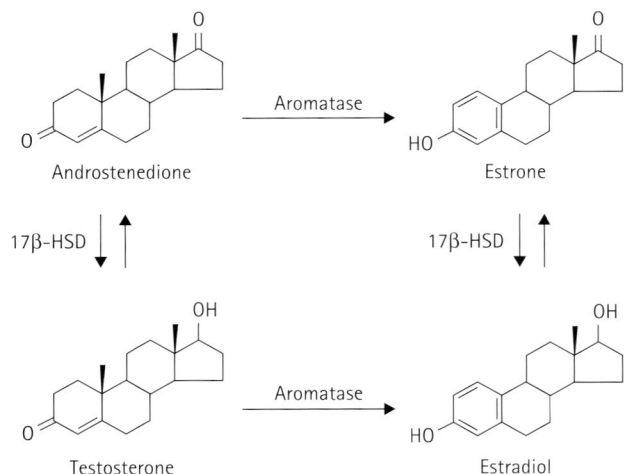

Figure 44.1 P450 aromatase catalyzes the aromatization of C_{19} androgens (androstenedione and testosterone) to C_{18} estrogens (estrone and estradiol). 17β-HSD = 17β-hydroxysteroid dehydrogenase.

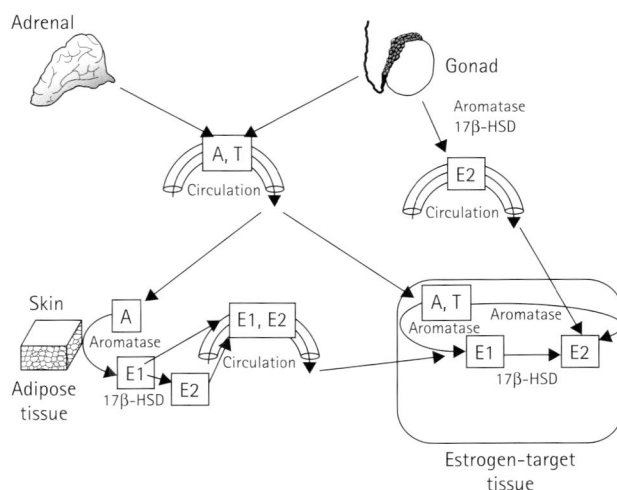

Figure 44.2 The concept of intracrine production of estrogen from adrenal and gonadal androgens by P450 aromatase in peripheral tissues.

estrogens. The administration of estrogen in these men closed the epiphyses and discontinued growth.[3,4] In all of these men, concentrations of androgens were normal or above normal. These case reports confirmed that estrogens are essential hormones for epiphyseal closure in males. Moreover, the reports suggest that estrogens probably do not participate in the regulation of linear growth, but induce growth acceleration during puberty. This newly discovered specific role for estrogen in growth regulation has significantly increased scientific interest for the use of specific aromatase inhibitors in treatment of short stature.

P450 AROMATASE

P450 aromatase is the enzyme that catalyzes the aromatization of C_{19} androgens (androstenedione and testosterone) to C_{18} estrogens (estrone and estradiol) (Fig. 44.1).

In premenopausal women the source of estrogens is predominantly of ovarian origin. After the menopause, estrogens are mainly synthesized in peripheral tissues (e.g., adipose tissue, skin, muscle, breast tissue, and bone) through local aromatization of circulating androgens, which are mostly produced by the adrenals, to estrogens.[5] In males, it has been estimated that the aromatase from testes can account for about 15 percent of circulating estrogens at best, and, hence, extragonadal production of estrogens is of physiological importance, like in postmenopausal women.[5] The same is probably also true for prepubertal children. Therefore, in the male the circulating levels of testosterone, produced by the testes, are converted efficiently by the P450 aromatase in extragonadal sites to give rise to local concentrations of estradiol sufficient to transactivate locally the estrogen receptor in the estrogen-dependent tissues.

These extragonadal sites of estrogen biosynthesis possess certain fundamental features which differ from ovarian estrogen biosynthesis, e.g., extragonadal estrogen biosynthesis is dependent on circulating precursor C_{19} steroids, and the estrogen synthesized within these compartments, particularly in the bone, breast and brain, is probably biologically active only at a local tissue level in a paracrine or 'intracrine' fashion (Fig. 44.2).[5,6]

AROMATASE INHIBITORS

The activity of P450 aromatase can be inhibited by several pharmaceutical compounds, which have been developed to block estrogen biosynthesis (for review, see Santen[7]). Clinical trials in 1960s with the first-generation aromatase inhibitor, aminoglutethimide, provided practical proof that aromatase inhibitors could be used for treatment of hormone-dependent breast cancer.[8] However, aminoglutethimide had substantial side effects, which diminished its usefulness. Over the last 30 years, several more potent and selective but less toxic aromatase inhibitors have been developed.[9,10] These new inhibitors can be divided into two categories with respect to mechanism of action: (1) the competitive inhibitors that bind to the active site of the aromatase enzyme and block estrogen formation, and (2) the inactivators that bind covalently to the active site of the enzyme and irreversibly destroy its enzymatic action. The latter are also called 'suicide' or mechanism-based inactivators. The current, third-generation compounds are nearly completely selective for the P450 aromatase enzyme, 1000-fold to 10 000-fold more potent than aminoglutethimide, and much better tolerated.

In several countries some of these third generation aromatase inhibitors have been approved for clinical use in hormone dependent breast cancer. Chemical structures for four competitive inhibitors, aminoglutethimide, anastrozole, fadrozole, and letrozole, and of an inactivator, exemestane are shown in Fig. 44.3.

AROMATASE INHIBITORS IN GROWTH INDICATIONS

Aromatase expression shown by immunohistochemistry, as well as aromatase mRNA detected by *in situ* hybridization

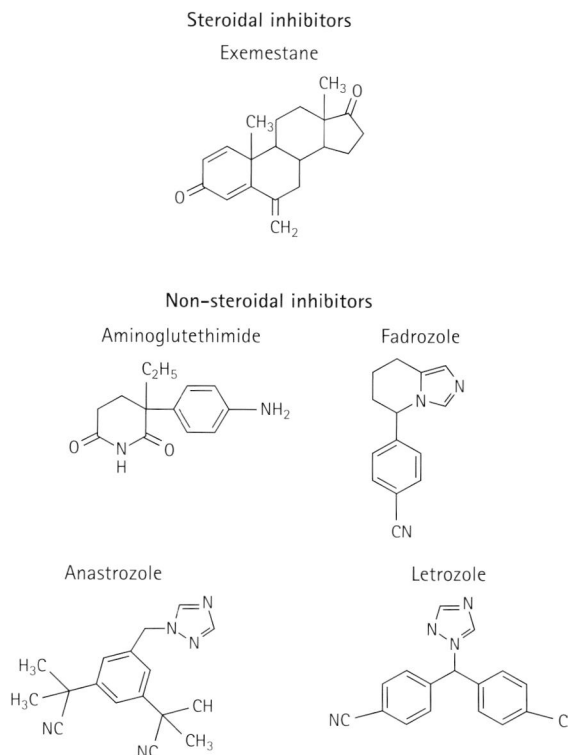

Figure 44.3 Chemical formulae of one steroidal and four non-steroidal aromatase inhibitors.

techniques, appear to be widely expressed in human bone tissue of male and female adults supporting the findings that the bone from both men and women have the capacity to form estrogen from androgen.[11] Evidence is also accumulating that estrogen is important for normal bone growth and mineralization not only of human females, but also of human males.[11,12]

These data together with the experience obtained from the clinical cases with inactivating mutations in estrogen receptor α and P450 aromatase genes,[1–3] provide a rationale for the use of aromatase inhibitors in growth indications. So far, the clinical experience with aromatase inhibitors in children is limited to four compounds, testolactone,[13*–16*] anastrozole,[17] fadrozole[18*] and letrozole[19**,20–22] (Table 44.1).

In general, aromatase inhibitors have been used in children at the same doses prescribed in adults, probably because adverse effects reported in the older patients are generally mild to moderate. Testolactone, a non-selective steroidal aromatase inhibitor, has been used as an effective adjunct to antiandrogen and GnRH therapy in children with familial male-limited pecocious puberty (FMPP) and congenital adrenal hyperplasia (CAH), and with partial results in reducing estrogen concentrations, frequency of menses and rate of bone maturation in girls with McCune–Albright syndrome (MAS). The limitations of testolactone include its relatively low potency, and the need for a frequent (every 6–8 h) dosing schedule.

Familial male precocious puberty

Familial male-limited precocious puberty (FMPP, also termed testotoxicosis) is a LH-releasing hormone (LHRH)-independent form of precocious puberty resulting from an activating mutation of the LH receptor. The mutation either occurs *de novo* or is inherited in an autosomal dominant fashion. Affected males usually begin pubertal development by 1–3 years of age, which leads to rapid growth and bone

Table 44.1 Aromatase Inhibitors in pediatric indications. Clinical experience with aromatase inhibitors in the pediatric setting is limited to four compounds, testolactone, anastrozole, letrozole, and fadrozole

Drug	Daily oral dosage	Indication (number of patients)	Reference
Testolactone	20–40 mg kg^{-1}	FMPP (9)	15
		MAS (12)	29,30
	3–4 divided doses	CAH (16)	16
Anastrozole	1 mg	MAS (NA)	Not published
		Pubertal gynecomastia (NA)	Not published
		Healthy young male volunteers	17
Letrozole	2.5 mg	Delayed puberty (10)	21
Fadrozole	240–480 µg kg^{-1}	MAS (16)	18

FMPP: familial male precocious puberty; MAS: McCune–Albright syndrome; NA: not available.

maturation, progressive virilization, and, ultimately, premature epiphyseal fusion and adult short stature.

In FMPP, in one trial, testolactone was combined with spironolactone (anti-androgen) and in those patients, who already had developed central precocious puberty also with GnRH analog.[13*–15*] During this combination treatment, after 1 year, growth rate decreased from 16.1 cm year^{-1} to 7.5 cm year^{-1}. During the subsequent 5 years of treatment, growth rate normalization was maintained (Fig. 44.4). Similarly, growth velocity SDS decreased from 6.9 to 1.1 after 1 year of treatment and continued to be significantly lower during the next 5 years of treatment. The rate of bone

maturation [change in the ratio of bone age to chronological age (BA/CA)] decreased from 2.5 to 1.7 after 1 year of treatment. After 2 years of treatment, BA/CA decreased to 0.8 and for the remainder of the 6 years of treatment, BA/CA remained normal or subnormal. Predicted height appeared to increase progressively after the first year of treatment. By the fourth, fifth, and sixth years, it had increased from 160.7 (pretreatment) to 173.6 cm (sixth year; $p < 0.005$ vs. pretreatment). Thus, long-term treatment with spironolactone, testolactone, and GnRH analog normalizes the rate of growth and bone maturation and improves predicted height in boys with FMPP. No adult height data are yet available in these patients.

Congenital adrenal hyperplasia

Worldwide the most common form of CAH is due to 21-hydroxylase (CYP21). This deficiency accounts for more than 90 percent of cases of adrenal hyperplasia. Classical CAH due to inactivating mutation in P450 *CYP21* gene occurs with an overall incidence of 1 per 13 000 to 1 per 16 000 births.[23]

The 21-hydroxylase deficiency results in increased production of adrenal androgens and decreased production of glucocorticoids and mineralocorticoids. The conventional medical treatment of CAH is to administer glucocorticoid and, if necessary, mineralocorticoid in order to substitute the missing hormones and in the attempt to suppress ACTH and adrenal androgen secretion to normal levels. However, suppression of ACTH secretion to normal levels may not normalize androgen production in patients with CAH because the intrinsic 21-hydroxylase defect shunts an excessive proportion of adrenal steroid intermediates into the androgen pathway. To overcome the intrinsic tendency of the adrenal gland to overproduce androgens, the level of adrenal steroid intermediates must be decreased to below normal levels, thereby preventing excessive shunting of these intermediates into the androgen pathway. This often requires supraphysiological glucocorticoid doses. Signs of glucocorticoid excess, such as obesity, poor growth velocity, are frequent among treated children. A common complication is central precocious puberty, which is most likely to develop when the diagnosis of CAH is delayed or when control of adrenal androgen secretion is poor. Excessive adrenal androgen production, excessive exposure to glucocorticoid, and precocious puberty, may cause short adult stature. However, short adult stature results even if good adrenal hormonal control is maintained throughout childhood and puberty.

In a recent meta-analysis of 561 patients, the average final height SD score of CAH patients was -1.37, and final height SD score was -1.21 SD below target height.[24***] Patients with early diagnosis had better outcomes, and good compliance was considered beneficial. Further, delay in the diagnosis of CAH has been found to result in more severely compromised adult height prognosis.[24–27] Conventional

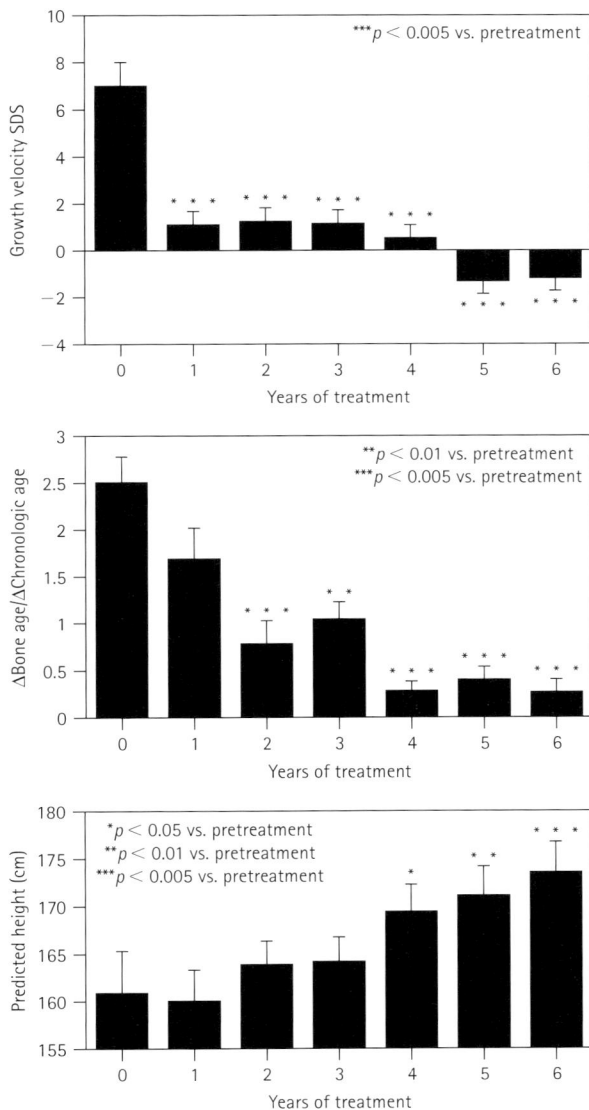

Figure 44.4 Six year results of treatment of boys with familial male-limited precocious puberty with an aromatase inhibitor (testolactone) and antiandrogen (spironolactone) with addition of deslorelin after central puberty onset. Asterisks denote the significant changes from the start: *$p < 0.05$; **$p < 0.01$; ***$p < 0.001$. From Leschek *et al.*[15] With permission from The Endocrine Society.

medical treatment still remains a challenging task, balancing between hypercortisolism and hyperandrogenism, which may lead to compromised adult height. Thus alternative treatment approaches are needed.[28***]

In one study, 28 children with CAH were randomised to receive 2 years treatment with either flutamide and testolactone, combined with reduced hydrocortisone dose (average of 8.7 ± 0.6 mg m^{-2} day^{-1}) and fludrocortisone ($n = 16$) or standard treatment with hydrocortisone (12.7 ± 2.9 mg m^{-2} day^{-1}) and fludrocortisone ($n = 12$). The investigators hypothesized that the clinical effects of excessive androgen and estrogen concentrations, which would result from decrease in hydrocortisone dose, could be blocked by the combination of an antiandrogen (flutamide) and an inhibitor of androgen to estrogen conversion (testolactone).[16*] In the flutamide and testolactone treated group, despite the reduction in hydrocortisone dose and rise in androgen levels, both of which were expected to increase the growth rate and bone maturation, growth rate and bone maturation rate declined significantly (for height velocity from 2.4 ± 0.5 to 0.1 ± 0.5 SDS; $p < 0.01$; for $\Delta BA/\Delta CA$ from 1.9 ± 0.3 to 0.7 ± 0.2). Children receiving the additional flutamide and testolactone regimen had some increase in predicted adult height (from -2.6 ± 0.5 at baseline to -2.0 ± 0.5 SD units at 2 years ($p < 0.30$)).

At 2 years of follow-up, four children in the experimental arm and two in the control arm were receiving GnRHa therapy. When these six children were omitted from the data analysis, children who remained prepubertal at the 2-year follow-up while on the standard treatment still had higher growth rate and bone age maturation (1.2 ± 0.7 $\Delta BA/\Delta CA$) as compared to the ones on the flutamide and testolactone regimen (0.7 ± 0.2 $\Delta BA/\Delta CA$). However the differences did not reach statistical significance. In both treatment arms there was no difference between the levels of estrogen, which was at or below the detection limit of the RIA method used in this study. Considerable vigilance was required in monitoring the safety of flutamide in these children due to its potential severe hepatotoxicity. No abnormalities in electrolytes, hematologic, hepatic and renal parameters were observed in both treatment arms. The only important adverse effects were mild cramping, nausea and diarrhea, which occurred early in treatment and resolved with a temporary reduction in dose. There were four cases of testicular adrenal rest tissue, two in each treatment arm. One boy receiving flutamide, testolactone, and reduced hydrocortisone developed significant bilateral testicular adrenal rest tissue, which decreased by increasing the doses of hydrocortisone.

McCune–Albright syndrome

The McCune–Albright syndrome is characterized (variably) by café-au-lait spots, fibrous dysplasia of bones, and sexual precocity. Girls with precocious puberty due to this syndrome have episodic increases in serum estrogen levels together with the formation of large ovarian cysts. The serum gonadotropin levels are typically suppressed, and the precocious puberty has not responded to treatment with long-acting analogs of luteinizing hormone-releasing hormone (LHRH).

In one study, aromatase inhibitor testolactone (40 mg kg^{-1} day^{-1}) was used to treat 12 girls with precocious puberty due to the McCune–Albright syndrome for periods of 0.5–5 years.[29*,30*,31] In the seven girls who received testolactone for at least 3 years, the mean $\pm$ SD serum estradiol level was 618 ± 268 pmol L^{-1} at the start of therapy and fell to 156 ± 84 pmol L^{-1} at 1 year, 116 ± 48 pmol L^{-1} at 2 years, and 241 ± 260 pmol L^{-1} at 3 years ($p < 0.05$ compared to the start of therapy), with recurrent ovarian cysts at 3 years in two patients. These seven girls averaged eight menses per year before therapy. The average frequency of menses decreased to two episodes per year during the first year of treatment, three per year during the second year, and four per year during the third year. The mean $\pm$ SD testosterone levels were slightly above the normal prepubertal range (0.51 ± 0.2 nmol L^{-1}) before treatment and did not change significantly during treatment. The mean $\pm$ SD androstenedione levels rose from 1.1 ± 0.6 nmol L^{-1} before treatment to 2.1 ± 0.1 nmol L^{-1} at 2 years and 2.8 ± 0.1 nmol L^{-1} after 3 years of treatment ($p < 0.05$ compared to before treatment) and were consistent with normal adrenarche.

In this group of patients, the mean predicted adult stature was 143.0 ± 7.8 cm before treatment and 147.3 ± 11.5 cm at 3 years ($p = $ NS). In three of 12 girls, all with bone age greater than 12 years, the gonadotropin responses to LHRH indicated early central precocious puberty after 1–4 years of treatment. The adverse effects of testolactone were transient abdominal pain, headache, and diarrhea in three girls and elevated hepatic enzymes in one girl who had abnormal liver function before treatment. Overall it appeared that testolactone was somewhat effective in the treatment of LHRH-independent precocious puberty in girls with McCune–Albright syndrome. However, in some patients the treatment becomes ineffective after 1–3 years.

In a more recent study an aromatase inhibitor fadrozole was given to 16 girls with gonadotropin-independent precocious puberty due to the McCune–Albright syndrome.[18*] The girls' ages ranged from 3.2 to 9.7 years, and their bone ages ranged from 5.75 to 14.25 years. After baseline evaluations, fadrozole was started at a dose of 240 µg kg^{-1} day^{-1} for 12–21 months and increased to 480 µg kg^{-1} day^{-1} for an additional 12 months in 10 girls. During treatment, seven girls had evidence of central precocious puberty; hence, the GnRH agonist deslorelin was added to their regimen. One girl was on a long-acting GnRH agonist from the start of treatment. After the first 6–12 months of treatment, fadrozole showed some benefits in 10 girls, including decrease in frequency of menses and/or rates of linear growth and bone maturation; however, fadrozole had no significant benefit in the group as a whole. The seven girls with evidence of central precocious puberty had no slowing in the progression of their puberty during the combined

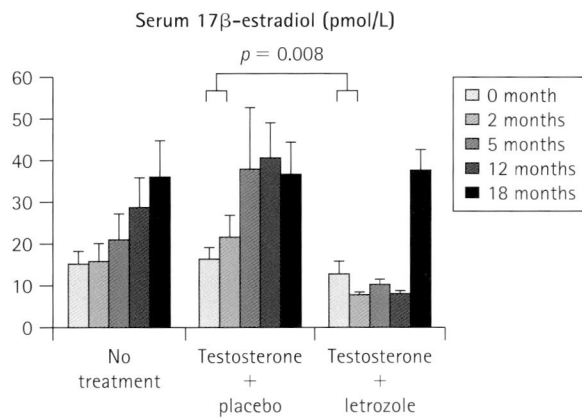

Figure 44.5   Mean ± SEM serum 17β-estradiol concentration. Asterisks denote the significant changes from the start within the group: *p < 0.05; **p < 0.01. From Wickman et al.[19]

fadrozole and GnRH analog treatment. Adverse effects of fadrozole included inhibition of cortisol and aldosterone biosynthesis at the dose of $480\,\mu g\,kg^{-1}\,day^{-1}$, without clinical evidence of adrenal insufficiency. In addition, three patients complained of nonspecific abdominal pain during fadrozole treatment.

Delayed puberty

One double blind placebo controlled study using testosterone enanthate combined either with letrozole inhibitor or placebo has been conducted in boys with constitutional delay of puberty.[19]** At entry, none of the boys had had any pubertal increase in growth velocity. Twenty-three boys with a mean age of 15.1 ± 0.2 years (range, 13.5–16.1) were randomly assigned to receive one or other of the two treatments.

In this study, letrozole inhibited estrogen synthesis effectively (Fig. 44.5). During the treatment with testosterone and placebo, the 17β-estradiol concentration increased, and an increase was also observed in the untreated group during the follow-up. In contrast, during the treatment with testosterone and letrozole, the concentration remained at the pretreatment level. After the discontinuation of letrozole treatment, the 17β-estradiol concentration increased in the testosterone-plus-letrozole-treated group also, and at 18 months, i.e., 6 months after discontinuation of the treatments, concentrations in all groups were similar.

The testosterone concentrations increased during the treatment with testosterone and letrozole five-fold higher than during the treatment with testosterone and placebo (Fig. 44.6). In the testosterone-plus-letrozole-treated group, the high concentration was sustained until discontinuation of the letrozole treatment, after which the concentration decreased to a level comparable with that of the testosterone-plus-placebo treated group.

In the testosterone-plus-letrozole-treated group, during treatment for 5 months, simultaneously with an increase of

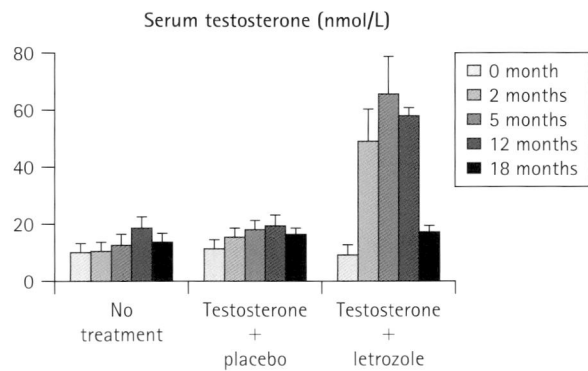

Figure 44.6   Mean ± SEM serum testosterone concentrations. Asterisks denote the significant changes from the start within the group: *p < 0.05; **p < 0.01; ***p < 0.001. From Wickman et al.[19]

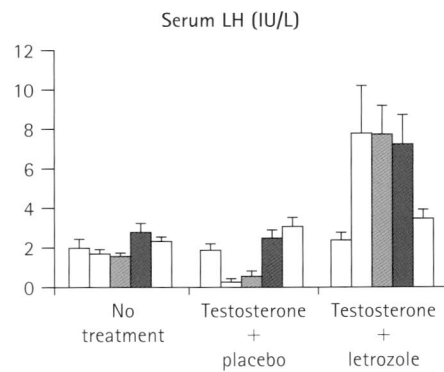

Figure 44.7   Mean ± SEM serum LH concentrations. Asterisks denote the significant changes from the start within the group: *p < 0.05; **p < 0.01; ***p < 0.001. From Wickman et al.[19]

and unchanged concentrations of 17β-estradiol, the basal LH concentration increased by 208 percent (p = 0.001) (Fig. 44.7), the basal FSH concentration by 167 percent (p = 0.0005), and the GnRH-induced LH response by 73 percent (p = 0.0005), but the GnRH-induced FSH response did not change significantly (p = 0.08). At 12 months, during the treatment with letrozole, the concentrations and GnRH-induced responses were at a similar level as at 5 months. These data show that when the action of endogenous estrogens is suppressed, LH and FSH concentrations increase despite very high androgen concentrations, indicating that the negative feedback between endogenous estrogens and gonadotropin secretion, established in adult men,[1–4,32] is already operative from early puberty onward. Furthermore, these observations suggest that androgens have a minor role compared with estrogens in regulating LH as well as FSH secretion in early- and midpubertal boys. When the action of endogenous estrogens was suppressed by the testosterone plus letrozole treatment in early and midpubertal boys, the LH pulse amplitude increased, but the LH pulse frequency, which is assumed to reflect the frequency of hypothalamic GnRH secretion,[33,34] did not change. These observations suggest that low concentrations of endogenous estrogens in early and midpubertal boys may

Table 44.2 Serum IGF-I and IGFBP-3 concentrations. From Wickman et al.[19]

	No treatment	Testosterone + placebo	Testosterone + letrozole	p value [a]
Inhibin B (ng L^{-1})				
0 month	153.7 ± 12.1	176.1 ± 12.5	161.2 ± 16.2	
5 months	186.4 ± 18.1	155.5 ± 21.8	200.5 ± 18.8	0.01
12 months	184.6 ± 10.3[c]	186.6 ± 19.0	219.8 ± 15.9[d]	0.1
18 months	180.6 ± 11.4[d]	216.8 ± 19.1	203.1 ± 16.6	0.8
IGF-I (nmol L^{-1})				
0 month	27.4 ± 3.8	28.3 ± 2.7	30.3 ± 3.4	
2 months	28.7 ± 2.9	34.0 ± 2.4[b]	25.6 ± 1.5	0.01
5 months	25.9 ± 2.0	34.5 ± 2.3[b]	25.2 ± 1.6	0.01
12 months	29.3 ± 3.3	34.3 ± 2.9[b]	27.4 ± 1.0	0.06
18 months	27.9 ± 2.6	31.9 ± 2.6	34.1 ± 1.2	0.9
IGFBP-3 (mg L^{-1})				
0 month	3.7 ± 0.2	3.8 ± 0.1	3.7 ± 0.2	
2 months	3.7 ± 0.3	4.1 ± 0.2[b]	3.6 ± 0.2	0.02
5 months	3.8 ± 0.2	4.3 ± 0.2[c]	3.4 ± 0.2	0.0004
12 months	3.9 ± 0.2	4.3 ± 0.1[d]	3.5 ± 0.2	0.008
18 months	4.5 ± 0.2[b]	4.7 ± 0.2[c]	4.4 ± 0.2[c]	0.8

Mean ± SEM. [a] p value refers to the difference between the treatment groups regarding changes in value from the start to the time-point indicated by p value. Change within group from the start to indicated time-point: [b] $p < 0.001$; [c] $p < 0.01$; [d] $p < 0.05$.

not influence the GnRH pulse generator, and that, in boys during early and midpuberty, the site of action of estrogens is the pituitary. The negative feedback regulation between FSH and endogenous estrogens has been reported in adult males.[33] The results of this study in adolescent boys suggest that this regulatory loop is already operative in early- and mid-pubertal boys. Although inhibin B participates in the regulation of FSH secretion from early and midpuberty onward,[35,36] the increase in FSH concentrations during letrozole treatment is probably not due to a diminished negative feedback signal from inhibin B, for inhibin B concentrations increased concomitantly with FSH concentrations.

In the testosterone-plus-placebo-treated group, the inhibin B concentration did not change (Table 44.2). In contrast, during the treatment with testosterone plus letrozole, the concentration was higher than at the start, but after discontinuation of the letrozole treatment, it did not differ from the pre-treatment concentration (Table 44.2). The changes in inhibin B concentration from the start to 5 months were different in the two treatment groups ($p = 0.01$) which is consistent with the difference in increases in testis volume and the divergent pattern of change in gonadotropin concentration.

The IGF-I and IGFBP-3 concentrations changed differently in the two treated groups during the treatments (Table 44.2). During the treatment with testosterone and

placebo, both concentrations increased immediately after the start of the treatment, but during the treatment with testosterone and letrozole, the concentrations remained at the pre-treatment level.

From the start to 5 months of treatment, the boys treated with testosterone and placebo grew slightly faster than the boys treated with testosterone and letrozole (9.9 ± 0.5 cm vs. 7.3 ± 0.9 cm, respectively, $p = 0.02$). After 5 months, no statistically significant differences in growth velocity was observed between the two treated groups, although a borderline higher growth velocity after the discontinuation of treatments was observed in the testosterone-plus-letrozole-treated than in the testosterone-plus-placebo-treated group ($p = 0.06$). Inhibition of estrogen synthesis by letrozole delayed bone maturation. Within the follow-up period of 18 months, the bone age increased 1.7 ± 0.3 years in the testosterone-plus-placebo-treated group, but only 0.9 ± 0.2 years in the testosterone-plus-letrozole-treated group (significance of the difference between the treatment groups, $p = 0.03$; Fig. 44.8). In the untreated group, the respective increment was 1.1 ± 0.3 years.

Delayed bone maturation simultaneously with good growth response resulted in the increase in predicted adult height in boys treated with testosterone and letrozole (Fig. 44.9). Letrozole treatment was associated with an increase in predicted adult height. In the testosterone-plus-placebo-treated group or in the untreated group, the

Bone age (yrs)

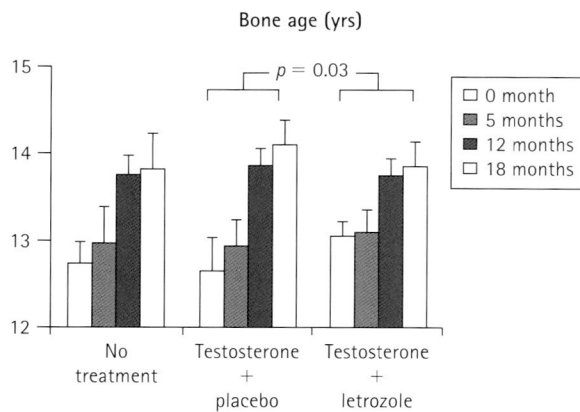

Figure 44.8 Mean ± SEM bone age. *p* value refers to the difference between the treatment groups regarding changes in bone age in 18 months. From Wickman *et al.*[19]

Change in predicted adult height in 18 months (cm)

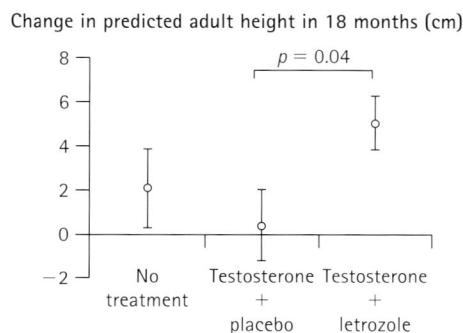

Figure 44.9 Mean ± SEM change in predicted adult height from the start to 18 months. From Wickman *et al.*[19]

predicted adult height did not change from the start to 18 months. In contrast, in the testosterone-plus-letrozole-treated group, an increase of 5.1 ± 1.2 cm (*p* = 0.004) in predicted adult height was seen; in one patient the predicted adult height decreased by 3.5 cm, the increases in the other boys ranged from 2.5 cm to 8.8 cm. The difference between the treatment groups regarding the change in predicted adult height was significant (*p* = 0.04). The mean near-adult-height was 6.9 cm higher in boys treated with letrozole than in boys treated with placebo (*p* = 0.04). In placebo-treated boys, the near-adult-height was 4.8 cm below target height (*p* = 0.006) whereas in letrozole-treated boys, there was no difference (*p* = 0.4). Also, the near-adult-height minus target height was 3.6 cm higher in boys treated with letrozole than in boys treated with placebo (*p* = 0.06).

The results of this study support the hypothesis that inhibition of estrogen synthesis in growing adolescents increases adult height. Since some boys with constitutional delay of puberty do not appear to exploit their genetic growth potential,[37–39] we can assume that these boys will achieve an adult height closer to their genetic growth potential if the estrogen action is inhibited. The observations that the predicted adult height did not change either

in the boys who received no treatment or in those who were treated with testosterone alone are consistent with previous studies, which have shown that androgen treatment does not increase adult height.[40–42]

Safety issues

For detecting possible side-effects of letrozole, bone mineral densities and the concentrations of total cholesterol, HDL-cholesterol, LDL-cholesterol, triglycerides, and transaminases, the leukocyte count, and the BMDs were determined during the follow-up of this study by Wickman *et al.*[20–22,43]

The increase in the BMD of lumbar spine from the start was observed in both treatment groups at 12 and 18 months. An increase from the start in the femoral neck BMD was observed in the testosterone-plus-placebo treated group at 12 and 18 months, but no change was seen in the testosterone-plus-letrozole-treated group. However, when the changes from the start in the lumbar spine and the femoral neck BMD were compared between the treated groups, no statistically significant differences were observed.[43] This indicates that a treatment for one year with a new, specific, and potent P450 aromatase inhibitor in pubertal boys is unlikely to have a significantly harmful effect on BMD. The cases with an inactive ERα[1] or defective aromatase enzymes[2,3] showed that an action of estrogen is needed for optimal development of peak bone mass in males. Patients with androgen insensitivity syndrome also have decreased BMD even before attainment of peak bone mass[44,45] indicating the importance of endogenous androgens in development of peak bone mass in males. The observation that no difference in the changes in BMD between the two treatment groups was found may be explained by the fact that during letrozole administration, high androgen concentrations have compensated for the disadvantageous effects of suppressed estrogen action.

However, minor disadvantageous effects on developing peak bone mass during the treatment with P450 aromatase inhibitors cannot be excluded on the basis of the study by Wickaman *et al.*[43.] They found no statistically significant increase in the femoral neck BMD during suppression of estrogen action by letrozole, while this parameter showed an increase in the testosterone-plus-placebo-treated group with intact P450 aromatase activity. For that reason, a close follow-up of bone metabolism during treatment with aromatase inhibitors is necessary.

In the study by Wickman *et al.* the HDL-cholesterol concentration decreased more during the treatment with testosterone and letrozole than during the treatment with testosterone and placebo.[22] In the testosterone-plus-placebo-treated group, no significant change in the HDL-cholesterol concentration was observed during the follow-up (*p* = 0.2; Table 44.3). In the testosterone-plus-letrozole-treated group, the concentration decreased from the start to the lowest level at 5 months (*p* = 0.002), but no subsequent decrease was observed thereafter (Table 44.3). In the untreated group, the concentration decreased to the lowest value at 18 months ($p = 0.047$). At 18 months, i.e., 6 months after discontinuation of all treatments, the concentrations were similar in all three groups. The concentrations of LDL-cholesterol or triglycerides did not change during the follow-up in any of the three groups (Table 44.3).

The difference in changes in HDL-cholesterol concentration between the boys treated with testosterone and letrozole and with testosterone and placebo indicates that the letrozole treatment may have minor disadvantageous effects on serum HDL-cholesterol concentrations. This is in accord with the finding of two aromatase deficient men who had subnormal HDL-cholesterol concentrations which increased during estrogen administration.[2-4] In the letrozole-treated group, the lowest level in the HDL-cholesterol concentration was observed at 5 months, and no subsequent decrease was observed thereafter despite the treatment with letrozole continued. Moreover, the HDL-cholesterol concentration in the letrozole treated boys was at a similar level to that in the boys in the other two groups after the discontinuation of all the treatments indicating that 1 year's treatment with letrozole in pubertal boys is unlikely to have a permanent harmful effect on HDL-cholesterol

concentration. However, these findings emphasize the importance of following-up HDL-cholesterol regularly during administration of P450 aromatase inhibitors.

The more profound decrease in the HDL-cholesterol concentrations during the treatment with testosterone and letrozole than during the treatment with testosterone and placebo may be due to the greater increase in androgen concentrations during the former than during the latter treatment. This is supported by the finding that decreasing HDL-cholesterol concentrations associated strongly with increasing testosterone concentrations. The important action of androgens in the regulation of HDL-cholesterol metabolism in adolescent boys was indicated by previous findings of inverse association between HDL-cholesterol and testosterone concentration even when factors affecting lipid metabolism had been taken into account,[46,47] and an association of testosterone[48,49] or DHT treatment[50,51] with the decrease in HDL-cholesterol concentration in boys with delayed puberty.

The concentrations of LDL-cholesterol and triglycerides did not change during either of the two treatments suggesting that treatment with P450-aromatase inhibitors do not contribute significantly in the regulation of concentrations of LDL-cholesterol or triglycerides in early and midpubertal boys. This finding of unchanged

Table 44.3   Serum concentrations of HDL-cholesterol, LDL-cholesterol, triglycerides, and insulin. From Wickman et al.[43]

	No treatment	Testosterone + placebo	Testosterone + letrozole	p value [a]
HDL-cholesterol (mmol L^{-1})				
0 month	1.8 ± 0.1	1.6 ± 0.09	1.6 ± 0.1	
5 months	1.6 ± 0.1	1.5 ± 0.1	1.2 ± 0.09[b]	0.005
12 months	1.5 ± 0.1	1.6 ± 0.1	1.4 ± 0.1[c]	0.06
18 months	1.4 ± 0.09[d]	1.4 ± 0.1	1.3 ± 0.09[c]	0.3
LDL-cholesterol (mmol L^{-1})				
0 month	2.2 ± 0.2	2.4 ± 0.2	2.5 ± 0.2	
5 months	2.7 ± 0.2	2.4 ± 0.2	2.5 ± 0.2	0.5
12 months	2.5 ± 0.2	2.4 ± 0.2	2.6 ± 0.2	0.4
18 months	2.3 ± 0.2	2.4 ± 0.2	2.3 ± 0.2	0.9
Triglycerides (mmol L^{-1})				
0 month	0.58 ± 0.06	0.91 ± 0.1	0.89 ± 0.1	
5 months	0.62 ± 0.08	0.86 ± 0.1	0.96 ± 0.1	0.6
12 months	0.70 ± 0.2	0.89 ± 0.1	0.85 ± 0.1	0.6
18 months	0.69 ± 0.1	0.85 ± 0.1	1.1 ± 0.2	0.3
Insulin (mU L^{-1})				
0 month	5.7 ± 0.8	7.1 ± 0.7	9.2 ± 1.3	
5 months	6.2 ± 1.2	6.8 ± 0.7	6.2 ± 0.9	0.2
12 months	6.6 ± 1.4	9.1 ± 1.2	6.5 ± 0.8[d]	0.02
18 months	7.6 ± 1.7	8.8 ± 1.2	9.4 ± 1.3	0.3

Mean ± SEM. [a] p value refers to the difference between the treatment groups regarding changes in value from the start to the time-point indicated by p value. Change within group from the start to indicated time-point: [b] $p < 0.01$; [c] $p < 0.02$; [d] $p < 0.05$.

concentrations of LDL-cholesterol and triglycerides in both treatment groups despite great difference in changes in sex steroid concentrations indicates that sex steroids may not have important regulatory roles in the metabolism of LDL-cholesterol and triglycerides in boys during early and midpuberty. However, previous studies have suggested that variation in lipoprotein concentrations in adolescent boys can be explained, to some extent, by the changes in body mass, testosterone, estrogen, and their interactions.[52,53]

Estradiol has been shown to act as a germ cell survival factor in the human testis *in vitro*.[54] The role of estrogen in human spermatogenesis can further be assessed by the findings in men with a mutation in a gene for ERα[1] and P450 aromatase enzyme.[3] The man with a mutation in the ERα gene, had a testis volume of 20–25 mL, a normal sperm density (25×10^6 mL^{-1}), but a decreased sperm viability of 18 percent (normal, >50 percent) α.[1] The aromatase deficient male had a subnormal volume of testis (8 mL), a decreased sperm count ($\leq 1 \times 10^6$ mL^{-1}; normal, >20 $\times$ 10^6 mL^{-1}) with 100 percent immotile spermatozoa.[3] However, abnormal findings in semen analysis in the aromatase deficient man may not be related to a suppression of estrogen action, since azoospermia and infertility were also reported in a brother of this man, who had a normal P450 aromatase gene.[3] Moreover, the results of semen analysis did not change during the treatment with transdermal estradiol[3] suggesting non-estrogen-dependent spermatogenic damage. In our study, neither the treatment with testosterone and placebo nor with testosterone and letrozole had an adverse effect on testis size or inhibin B concentration. These findings suggest that one year of treatment with P450 aromatase inhibitors in early and midpubertal boys did not interfere with spermatogenesis.

FUTURE PROSPECTS

The results of the studies currently published indicate that an increase in adult height may be attained in growing adolescent boys by inhibition of estrogen action.

Moreover, although our findings suggest that treatment for 1 year with a new P450 aromatase inhibitor in pubertal boys is unlikely to have a significantly harmful effect on developing peak bone mass, measuring BMD after the attainment of peak bone mass, at an age about 20–25 years, will resolve this issue.

Because bone maturation is delayed by suppressing the action of estrogens in growing children, the treatment with modern P450-aromatase inhibitors may prove to be an efficient treatment in various growth disorders. Further studies are needed to establish if treatment with these aromatase inhibitors can be used, e.g., in patients with precocious puberty or congenital adrenal hyperplasia with significantly advanced bone age. Moreover, they may be useful in some boys with delayed puberty and/or genetic short stature.

KEY LEARNING POINTS

- During puberty, in both sexes, epiphyseal fusion is mediated by the action of estrogen.
- Inhibition of estrogen action by aromatase inhibitors may decelerate this process.
- The clinical experience with aromatase inhibitors in the pediatric setting is limited to testolactone, anastrozole, letrozole, and fadrozole.
- Testolactone has been used successfully as adjunct to antiandrogen and GnRHa therapy for children with familial male limited precocious puberty and congenital adrenal hyperplasia, and with some success in girls with McCune–Albright syndrome.
- Letrozole treatment resulted in delayed bone maturation and increased predicted adult height in boys with delayed puberty in a randomized placebo controlled trial.
- Theoretically, aromatase inhibitors may have adverse effects on bone mineralization, serum lipid profiles, insulin sensitivity, spermatogenesis and cognitive functions. Short-term treatment has been found to be well tolerated.
- Further studies are needed to establish if treatment with aromatase inhibitors can be used, e.g., in patients with precocious puberty or congenital adrenal hyperplasia with significantly advanced bone age. They may be useful in some boys with delayed puberty and/or genetic short stature.

REFERENCES

● = Seminal primary article

◆ = Key review paper

1 Smith EP, Boyd J, Frank GR, *et al.* Estrogen resistance caused by a mutation in the estrogen-receptor gene in a man. *N Engl J Med* 1994; **331**: 1056–61.
2 Morishima A, Grumbach MM, Simpson ER, *et al.* Aromatase deficiency in male and female siblings caused by a novel mutation and the physiological role of estrogens. *J Clin Endocrinol Metab* 1995; **80**: 3689–98.
3 Carani C, Qin K, Simoni M, *et al.* Effect of testosterone and estradiol in a man with aromatase deficiency. *N Engl J Med* 1997; **337**: 91–5.
4 Bilezikian JP, Morishima A, Bell J, Grumbach MM. Increased bone mass as a result of estrogen therapy in a man with aromatase deficiency. *N Engl J Med* 1998; **339**: 599–603.
5 Labrie F, Belanger A, Cusan L, Candas B. Physiological changes in dehydroepiandrosterone are not reflected by serum levels of active androgens and estrogens but of their metabolites: intracrinology. *J Clin Endocrinol Metab* 1997; **82**: 2403–9.

6 Grumbach MM, Auchus RJ. Estrogen: consequences and implications of human mutations in synthesis and action. *J Clin Endocrinol Metab* 1999; **84**: 4677–94.

7 Santen RJ. Inhibition of aromatase: insights from recent studies. *Steroids* 2003; **68**: 559–67.

◆ 8 Santen RJ, Manni A, Harvey H, Redmond C. Endocrine treatment of breast cancer in women. *Endocr Rev* 1990; **11**: 221–65.

9 Sainsbury R. Aromatase inhibition in the treatment of advanced breast cancer: is there a relationship between potency and clinical efficacy? *Br J Cancer* 2004; **90**: 1733–9.

10 Miller WR. Biological rationale for endocrine therapy in breast cancer. *Best Pract Res Clin Endocrinol Metab* 2004; **18**: 1–32.

11 Sasano H, Uzuki M, Sawai T, *et al.* Aromatase in human bone tissue. *J Bone Miner Res* 1997; **12**: 1416–23.

12 Oz OK, Zerwekh JE, Fisher C, *et al.* Bone has a sexually dimorphic response to aromatase deficiency. *J Bone Miner Res* 2000; **15**: 507–14.

13 Laue L, Kenigsberg D, Pescovitz OH, *et al.* Treatment of familial male precocious puberty with spironolactone and testolactone. *N Engl J Med* 1989; **320**: 496–502.

14 Laue L, Jones J, Barnes KM, Cutler GB Jr. Treatment of familial male precocious puberty with spironolactone, testolactone, and deslorelin. *J Clin Endocrinol Metab* 1993; **76**: 151–5.

15 Leschek EW, Jones J, Barnes KM, *et al.* Six-year results of spironolactone and testolactone treatment of familial male-limited precocious puberty with addition of deslorelin after central puberty onset. *J Clin Endocrinol Metab* 1999; **84**: 175–8.

16 Merke DP, Keil MF, Jones JV, *et al.* Flutamide, testolactone, and reduced hydrocortisone dose maintain normal growth velocity and bone maturation despite elevated androgen levels in children with congenital adrenal hyperplasia. *J Clin Endocrinol Metab* 2000; **85**: 1114–20.

17 Mauras N, O'Brien KO, Klein KO, Hayes V. Estrogen suppression in males: metabolic effects. *J Clin Endocrinol Metab* 2000; **85**: 2370–7.

18 Nunez SB, Calis K, Cutler GB Jr, *et al.* Lack of efficacy of fadrozole in treating precocious puberty in girls with the McCune–Albright syndrome. *J Clin Endocrinol Metab* 2003; **88**: 5730–3.

19 Wickman S, Sipilä I, C. A-L, *et al.* A specific aromatase inhibitor and potential increase in adult height in boys with delayed puberty: a randomised controlled trial. *Lancet* 2001; **357**: 1743–8.

20 Wickman S, Dunkel L. Inhibition of P450 aromatase enhances gonadotropin secretion in early and midpubertal boys: evidence for a pituitary site of action of endogenous E. *J Clin Endocrinol Metab* 2001; **86**: 4887–94.

21 Wickman S, Sipila I, Ankarberg-Lindgren C, *et al.* A specific aromatase inhibitor and potential increase in adult height in boys with delayed puberty: a randomised controlled trial. *Lancet* 2001; **357**: 1743–8.

22 Wickman S, Saukkonen T, Dunkel L. The role of sex steroids in the regulation of insulin sensitivity and serum lipid

concentrations during male puberty: a prospective study with a P450-aromatase inhibitor. *Eur J Endocrinol* 2002; **146**: 339–46.

◆ 23 White PC, Speiser PW. Congenital adrenal hyperplasia due to 21-hydroxylase deficiency. *Endocr Rev* 2000; **21**: 245–91.

24 Eugster EA, Dimeglio LA, Wright JC, *et al.* Height outcome in congenital adrenal hyperplasia caused by 21-hydroxylase deficiency: a meta-analysis. *J Pediatr* 2001; **138**: 26–32.

25 Urban MD, Lee PA, Migeon CJ. Adult height and fertility in men with congenital virilizing adrenal hyperplasia. *N Engl J Med* 1978; **299**: 1392–6.

26 Brook CG, Zachmann M, Prader A, Murset G. Experience with long-term therapy in congenital adrenal hyperplasia. *J Pediatr* 1974; **85**: 12–9.

27 DiMartino-Nardi J, Stoner E, O'Connell A, New MI. The effect of treatment of final height in classical congenital adrenal hyperplasia (CAH). *Acta Endocrinol Suppl (Copenh)* 1986; **279**: 305–14.

28 Consensus statement on 21-hydroxylase deficiency from the Lawson Wilkins Pediatric Endocrine Society and the European Society for Paediatric Endocrinology. *J Clin Endocrinol Metab* 2002; **87**: 4048–53.

29 Feuillan PP, Foster CM, Pescovitz OH, *et al.* Treatment of precocious puberty in the McCune–Albright syndrome with the aromatase inhibitor testolactone. *N Engl J Med* 1986; **315**: 1115–9.

30 Feuillan PP, Jones J, Cutler GB Jr. Long-term testolactone therapy for precocious puberty in girls with the McCune–Albright syndrome. *J Clin Endocrinol Metab* 1993; **77**: 647–51.

31 Feuillan P, Merke D, Leschek EW, Cutler GB Jr. Use of aromatase inhibitors in precocious puberty. *Endocr Relat Cancer* 1999; **6**: 303–6.

32 Hayes FJ, Seminara SB, DeCruz S, *et al.* Aromatase inhibition in the human male reveals a hypothalamic site of estrogen feedback. *J Clin Endocrinol Metab* 2000; **85**: 3027–35.

33 Clarke IJ, Cummins JT. The temporal relationship between gonadotropin releasing hormone (GnRH) and luteinizing hormone (LH) secretion in ovariectomized ewes. *Endocrinology* 1982; **111**: 1737–9.

34 Levine JE, Pau KY, Ramirez VD, Jackson GL. Simultaneous measurement of luteinizing hormone-releasing hormone and luteinizing hormone release in unanesthetized, ovariectomized sheep. *Endocrinology* 1982; **111**: 1449–55.

35 Andersson AM, Juul A, Petersen JH, *et al.* Serum inhibin B in healthy pubertal and adolescent boys: relation to age, stage of puberty, and follicle-stimulating hormone, luteinizing hormone, testosterone, and estradiol levels. *J Clin Endocrinol Metab* 1997; **82**: 3976–81.

36 Raivio T, Saukkonen S, Jüüskelüinen J, *et al.* Signaling between the pituitary gland and the testes: inverse relationship between serum follicle-stimulating hormone and inhibin B concentrations in boys in early puberty. *Eur J Endocrinol* 2000; **142**: 150–6.

37 Crowne EC, Shalet SM, Wallace WHB, *et al.* Final height in boys with untreated constitutional delay in growth and puberty. *Arch Dis Child* 1990; **65**: 1109–12.

38 LaFranchi S, Hanna CE, Mandel SH. Constitutional delay of growth: expected versus final adult height. *Pediatrics* 1991; **87**: 82–7.

39 Albanese A, Stanhope R. Predictive factors in the determination of final height in boys with constitutional delay of growth and puberty. *J Pediatr* 1995; **126**: 545–50.

40 Albanese A, Stanhope R. Does constitutional delayed puberty cause segmental disproportion and short stature? *Eur J Pediatr* 1993; **152**: 293–6.

41 Martin MM, Martin ALA, Mossman KL. Testosterone treatment of constitutional delay in growth and development: effect of dose on predicted versus definitive height. *Acta Endocrinol Suppl* 1986; **279**: 147–52.

42 Blethen SL, Gaines S, Weldon V. Comparison of predicted and adult heights in short boys: effect of androgen therapy. *Pediatr Res* 1984; **18**: 467–9.

43 Wickman S, Kajantie E, Dunkel L. Effects of suppression of estrogen action by the p450 aromatase inhibitor letrozole on bone mineral density and bone turnover in pubertal boys. *J Clin Endocrinol Metab* 2003; **88**: 3785–93.

44 Bertelloni S, Baroncelli GI, Federico G, *et al.* Altered bone mineral density in patients with complete androgen insensitivity syndrome. *Horm Res* 1998; **50**: 309–14.

45 Marcus R, Leary D, Schneider DL, *et al.* The contribution of testosterone to skeletal development and maintenance: lessons from the androgen insensitivity syndrome. *J Clin Endocrinol Metab* 2000; **85**: 1032–7.

46 Morrison JA, Sprecher DL, Biro FM, *et al.* Sex hormones and lipoproteins in adolescent male offspring of parents with premature coronary heart disease and a control group. *J Pediatr* 1998; **133**: 526–32.

47 Morrison JA, Sprecher DL, Biro FM, *et al.* Estradiol and testosterone effects on lipids in black and white boys aged 10 to 15 years. *Metabolism* 2000; **49**: 1124–9.

48 Kirkland RT, Keenan BS, Probstfield JL, *et al.* Decrease in plasma high-density lipoprotein cholesterol levels at puberty in boys with delayed adolescence. Correlation with plasma testosterone levels. *JAMA* 1987; **257**: 502–7.

49 Arslanian S, Suprasongsin C. Testosterone treatment in adolescents with delayed puberty: changes in body composition, protein, fat, and glucose metabolism. *J Clin Endocrinol Metab* 1997; **82**: 3213–20.

50 Saad RJ, Keenan BS, Danadian K, *et al.* Dihydrotestosterone treatment in adolescents with delayed puberty: does it explain insulin resistance of puberty? *J Clin Endocrinol Metab* 2001; **86**: 4881–6.

51 Applebaum DM, Goldberg AP, Pykalisto OJ, *et al.* Effect of estrogen on post-heparin lipolytic activity. Selective decline in hepatic triglyceride lipase. *J Clin Invest* 1977; **59**: 601–8.

52 Laskarzewski PM, Morrison JA, Gutai J, *et al.* Longitudinal relationships among endogenous testosterone, estradiol, and Quetelet index with high and low density lipoprotein cholesterols in adolescent boys. *Pediatr Res* 1983; **17**: 689–98.

53 Laskarzewski PM, Morrison JA, Gutai J, *et al.* High and low density lipoprotein cholesterols in adolescent boys: relationships with endogenous testosterone, estradiol, and Quetelet index. *Metabolism* 1983; **32**: 262–71.

54 Pentikainen V, Erkkila K, Suomalainen L, *et al.* Estradiol acts as a germ cell survival factor in the human testis in vitro. *J Clin Endocrinol Metab* 2000; **85**: 2057–67.

45

Metabolic side effects and adverse effects of growth hormone therapy

SWATI BANERJEE, PAUL SAENGER

INTRODUCTION

The past decade has been remarkable for an increase in new indications for growth hormone (GH) treatment. As the use of GH becomes more widespread and the duration of treatment increases, new concerns have surfaced relating to the late onset of undesirable side effects. Fortunately, numerous studies and an excellent postmarketing surveillance have been instrumental in giving us a clear and ongoing understanding of possible effects from GH therapy. There appears to be no major problem yet with the use of recombinant GH. Having eliminated the risk of Creutzfeldt–Jakob disease, the indications have gradually extended beyond GH deficiency states in childhood and now include such diverse causes of short stature as Turner syndrome, chronic renal insufficiency (CRI), adult replacement therapy and more recently, Prader–Willi syndrome (PWS), short children born small for gestational age (SGA) and children with idiopathic short stature (ISS). Recombinant GH has been used in about 100 000 children so far, with an estimated 20 000 on active treatment in the USA. After more than 20 years of use in children with GH deficiency, growth hormone can be considered a safe drug with few serious side effects. However, with the widespread use of a product comes the inevitable reporting of various associations and effects, some of them serious and some relatively minor. For some an undeniable cause-and-effect relationship has been established; in others the role

of growth hormone is less convincing. The purpose of this chapter is to revisit and review the adverse effects of GH therapy and discuss the metabolic consequences in some detail. Additionally, some of the newer concerns will be addressed.

The limited knowledge of the long-term effects of recombinant growth hormone, together with the increasing number of patients being treated, led health authorities in Germany, Japan, the USA, and several other countries to organize long-term follow-up studies in a large cohort of patients. Two such ongoing studies document the use and reported adverse effects of therapy, in addition to other functions. The Kabi International Growth Study (KIGS) was based in Europe, Asia and Australia, and the National Cooperative Growth Study (NCGS) in the USA and Canada. Through these two agencies, thousands of children on growth hormone for an assortment of indications are being monitored for the assessment of their growth and in addition are being closely observed for any untoward event. As the product is being manufactured and distributed in ever increasing amounts, other databases have also been set up.

Growth hormone is a potent anabolic hormone with a multitude of biologic actions. It exerts its actions through the GH receptor which binds to growth hormone and causes intracellular signal cascading that results in a variety of subcellular events. The molecular basis of each individual effect has yet to be clearly elucidated. The mechanism of the various hormonal effects may be ascribed to growth hormone itself, or may be the result of production of growth factors such as insulin-like growth factor (IGF-I) and binding proteins such as IGFBP-3. This is of particular importance because of the increasing use of IGF-I as an independent therapeutic agent.

METABOLIC EFFECTS

Growth hormone therapy and carbohydrate metabolism (Figs 45.1 to 45.5)

Children have high turnover rates of substrates which provide most of the energy required for the oxidative needs of body tissues: glucose, free fatty acids and ketones. In the fasting state childhood glucose homeostasis is a balance between hepatic production and utilization (4–$6\,mg\,kg^{-1}min^{-1}$).

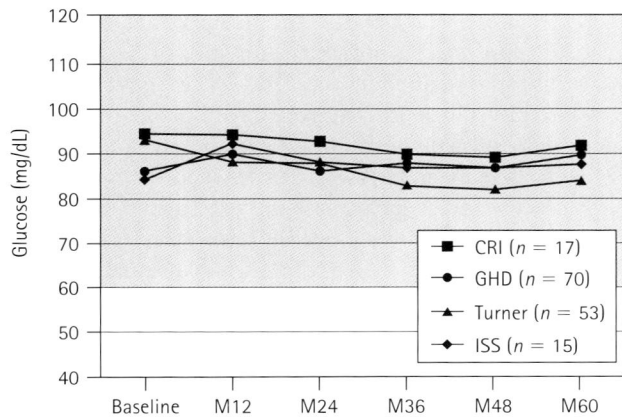

Figure 45.1 Fasting glucose (mean) throughout the 5 year study period in children with chronic renal insufficiency (CRI) and other growth disorders receiving GH treatment. (Reproduced with permission from Saenger et al.[10])

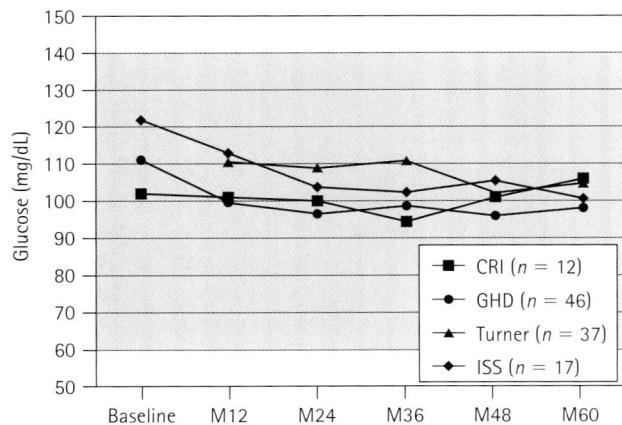

Figure 45.2 Postprandial glucose (mean) levels throughout the 5 year study period. Baseline postprandial glucose levels are not available for the Turner syndrome patients. (Reproduced with permission from Saenger et al.[10])

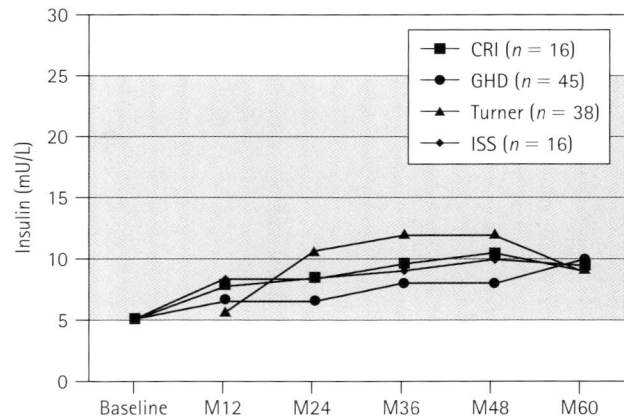

Figure 45.3 Fasting insulin (median) levels throughout the 5 year study period. Baseline postprandial insulin levels are not available for the Turner syndrome patients. (Reproduced with permission from Saenger et al.[10])

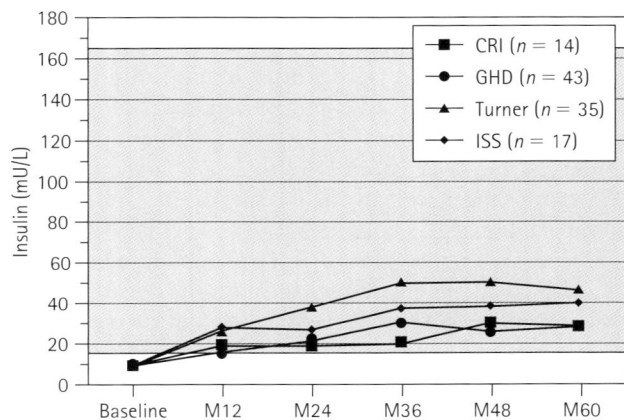

Figure 45.4 Fasting insulin (median) levels throughout the 5 year study period. Baseline postprandial insulin levels are not available for the Turner syndrome patients. (Reproduced with permission from Saenger et al.[10])

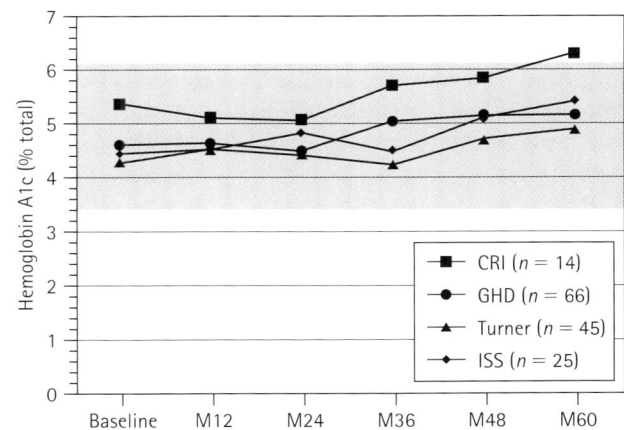

Figure 45.5 Hemoglobin A1c (mean) levels throughout the 5 year study period. Note assay changed 4/91. Reference range: 3.4–6.1 before; 4.4–6.1 after.

Gluconeogenesis and glycogenolysis contribute about 75 percent and 25 percent to glucose production in the fasting state, respectively. The utilization of glucose in children is remarkably different, because of the high non-insulin-mediated uptake by the brain, which contributes to 80 percent of the total glucose demand versus only 40 percent in adults. The regulation of glucose homeostasis in children is much the same as in adults, although the precise role of metabolic and hormonal factors has not been determined in children. Insulin suppresses hepatic glucose production and stimulates peripheral glucose use whereas glucagon, cortisol, growth hormone and catecholamines act as counter-regulatory influences. Although in adults with GH deficiency hypoglycemia is not a clinical problem, fasting hypoglycemia is seen in GH-deficient children. The cause of low plasma glucose is a diminished hepatic output through decreased gluconeogenesis and/or abnormal glycogen mobilization.[1] This may be the result of the lack of antagonism of growth hormone on insulin action. As a result of the relatively unopposed insulin action, there is also reduced secretion of insulin but this compensatory mechanism does not appear to be sufficient to prevent occasional hypoglycemia. Administration of growth hormone to deficient children restores glucose production to normal levels in these children.[2] In hypopituitarism, GH therapy has been associated with normalization of glucose turnover and insulin secretion, and has led to either unchanged or impaired responses to oral glucose administration.[2,3]

The clinical symptomatology of patients with acromegaly in which GH levels are elevated includes glucose intolerance and sometimes overt diabetes mellitus, and suggests that similar but more attenuated effects might be expected in individuals on pharmacological GH therapy. It has long been accepted that growth hormone exerts a 'diabetogenic' action in experimental animals.[4] Studies carried out with growth hormone led to the observation that there is an early insulin-like action lasting about 2 h, involving enhanced glucose use and antilipolysis (this effect is eliminated by prior GH administration), followed by a period of hyperglycemia despite elevated insulin levels.[5,6] Excess growth hormone appears to cause insulin resistance both in peripheral tissues and at the level of the liver with decreased peripheral glucose uptake and an increase in the hepatic glucose production.[6] Increased basal hepatic glucose production has been noted even in acromegalic individuals with normal glucose tolerance.[7]

In one study, ten pre-pubertal children with non-GH-deficient idiopathic short stature (ISS) had an almost two-fold rise in their insulin levels after 1 year of GH therapy, although none showed glucose intolerance. Interruption of treatment resulted in normalization of insulin secretion.[8] In a group of ten children with ISS, increased plasma insulin during oral glucose tolerance testing was found, but an almost complete reversal of hyperinsulinism within a year of discontinuation of GH therapy was observed.[9] The dose of growth hormone used in this group was almost two to three times the standard dose normally used. In a large

multicenter study, pubertal and pre-pubertal children with ISS displayed mean baseline glucose and 2 h postprandial glucose levels which remained unchanged throughout the 5 year treatment period. Although insulin levels showed a rise in the first 3 years of the study, they remained within the normal range and, after the third year, no further rise was observed. Hemoglobin A1c levels remained stable throughout the study.[10] It has been suggested that the effect of growth hormone on insulin sensitivity in pre-pubertal children with ISS appears to mirror the changes in carbohydrate tolerance seen in normal adolescence.[11] The long-term implication of the prolongation of this physiologic state of insulin resistance of normal puberty is unknown.

Mild insulin resistance is a feature of Turner's syndrome and this is exaggerated by GH therapy. A compensatory hyperinsulinemia appears to prevent the development of overt diabetes in most patients. After 6–12 months of GH treatment, both first- and second-phase insulin responses increased during a hyperglycemic clamp study. As the glucose infusion rates during the clamp did not change after growth hormone, the increased insulin response indicates decreased insulin sensitivity.[12] In a study evaluating treatment with growth hormone alone and in combination with oxandrolone in girls with Turner syndrome, there was an increased incidence of baseline pre-treatment glucose intolerance which is a well-known phenomenon in Turner syndrome, but there was no significant change in mean glucose, insulin or glucose tolerance in subjects treated with growth hormone alone during the first year of therapy.[13] On the contrary, therapy with oxandrolone, alone or in combination with growth hormone, resulted in significant glucose intolerance. In the same study, after the first week of GH therapy in a dose in excess of $0.375 \, mg \, kg^{-1}$ $week^{-1}$, a transient rise in the insulin levels was observed. In an Italian study, euglycemic hyperinsulinemic clamp studies were performed on six pre-pubertal girls with Turner syndrome before and 6 and 12 months after starting GH therapy. They demonstrated that although peripheral glucose use was not altered, there was a decrease in the hepatic insulin sensitivity.[14] After discontinuation of GH treatment, a group of Turner syndrome patients who had elevated insulin levels while on therapy showed a progressive normalization of insulin levels.[15]

Carbohydrate metabolism has been evaluated in children with CRI and compared with various other growth disorders treated with growth hormone. In one study, mean fasting and postprandial glucose remained unchanged throughout a 5 year period. Median fasting insulin levels rose from low normal levels into the normal range, with an average level of $10 \, mU \, L^{-1}$ at the end of 5 years. Mean HbA1c levels of the 16 children with CRI were slightly elevated compared with those of the others by the end of the study period.[10] Similarly, other studies have demonstrated that although no change in glucose tolerance was observed, an increase in insulin secretion occurred and persisted for the first 4 years in patients with

CRI on conservative treatment and in transplant recipients.[16,17] The increased insulin secretion remains a point of concern with regard to the possible development of glucose intolerance in the long term. This is particularly relevant in the transplant recipients, for whom GH treatment appears as a third risk factor for insulin resistance, in addition to chronic renal failure itself and the diabetogenic effects of glucocorticoid treatment.

Persistent poor growth in children who were born SGA is one of the newer indications for the use of GH treatment. There has been some concern that GH may worsen the pre-existing state of insulin resistance in these IUGR children. In a Dutch trial, researchers noted higher fasting and glucose stimulated insulin levels which however declined to normal after discontinuation of GH therapy, but clearly this cohort needs long term follow up to monitor their risk of developing the metabolic syndrome later on in life.[18]

Children with Prader–Willi syndrome (PWS) present an interesting combination of hyperphagia with obesity and growth hormone deficiency of hypothalamic origin, with GH treatment demonstrating multiple benefits.[19] Metabolic studies in children with PWS show that they have relatively normal insulin sensitivity as compared to other obese children, with a decrease and a delay of insulin secretion.[20] There is, however, a dose-dependent increase in insulin levels during GH treatment, along with some reports of type 2 diabetes mellitus.[21] Thus close surveillance of GH treatment in the PWS patient, especially in the very obese is recommended.

The NCGS in the USA has monitored the safety of recombinant growth hormone (rGH) since 1985 and after almost 20 years, data from over 47 000 patients representing 165 000 patient years have been collected. There are over 12 000 active subjects at 435 centers, providing extensive efficacy and safety data.[22] In 1996 they reported 22 children who developed diabetes mellitus during GH therapy. In nine children, it resolved when growth hormone was discontinued; four of them were on steroids and two had prior history of carbohydrate intolerance. In the remaining 13 subjects, all but three had pre-existing risk factors for developing diabetes.[23] In an update in 2000, 68 out of 33 161 enrolled patients in NCGS had diabetes mellitus or glucose intolerance.[24] Forty patients had diabetes, with 27 diagnosed as having type 1, consistent with the expected incidence for this condition.

KIGS is the worldwide counterpart to NCGS. Data from 1994 revealed 12 000 patients corresponding to more than 27 000 years of treatment. Their data suggest that there is a higher incidence of non-insulin-dependent diabetes mellitus (NIDDM) only in children who have predisposing risk factors and have subsequently received GH treatment. The incidence was 0.14 percent in the group treated for central nervous system (CNS) tumors, but the even larger figure of 0.55 percent in the group treated for leukemia, seems to be high. There are recent reports of T2DM in childhood leukemia survivors who received total body irradiation in preparation for bone marrow transplantation.

Thus, it is not possible to evaluate whether growth hormone, with its known effect of decreasing sensitivity to insulin, plays a role in the etiology of NIDDM or whether other factors, such as the initial very high dose of corticosteroids, are involved. The two cases of insulin-dependent diabetes mellitus (IDDM) in 2230 patient-years of GH treatment in Turner syndrome patients, where glucose intolerance occurs during the natural course of the condition, do not represent a statistically increased risk. An even lesser risk is represented by the one case in 11 972 patient-years of treatment comprising 4053 children with idiopathic GH deficiency, compared with the incidence of as many as 28 per 100 000 reported in normal children in various countries.[25]

A retrospective analysis of data from an international pharmacoepidemiological survey of children treated with GH was done to determine the incidence of impaired glucose tolerance and types 1 and 2 diabetes mellitus. Forty-three out of 23 333 children had confirmed glucose disorders (11 with type 1 diabetes, 18 with type 2 diabetes, and 14 with impaired glucose tolerance). The incidence and age at diagnosis of type 1 diabetes in children treated with GH did not differ from expected values. The incidence of type 2 diabetes was six-fold higher than reported in children not treated with GH. Type 2 diabetes did not resolve after GH therapy was stopped.[26]

Although there clearly appears to be some inherent risk of insulin resistance with pharmacological GH therapy, a recent consensus statement goes on to say that diabetes mellitus should not be considered as a contraindication to GH therapy, as long as standard clinical practice for routine diabetic care is followed.[27]

At this juncture it is prudent to monitor the HbA1c, glucose and insulin levels periodically while on GH therapy. Individuals known to be at risk of type 2 DM, such as girls with Turner syndrome, postchemotherapy patients, PWS, SGA, and children with CRI should be monitored closely.

Growth hormone and lipid metabolism

Adipose tissue is a well-known target for GH action. Growth hormone is known to have a dual effect on lipids. The acute, short-lived effect is insulin like, whereby lipolysis is acutely inhibited with a fall in the plasma free fatty acid (FFA) levels.[28,29] The second and more lasting effect is the anti-insulin and lipolytic effect and results in a rise in plasma FFAs and ketones.[30,31] The lipolytic effect results in a decrease of total body adipose tissue during long-term GH treatment. It decreases body fat by increasing the hydrolysis of triglycerides, releasing FFAs and glycerol while decreasing FFA re-esterification.[32,33] This lipolytic action of growth hormone allows lean body mass conservation at the expense of fat depots in obese individuals on a low-energy diet.[34] Lipoatrophy may occur at the site of GH injections, an adverse event only observed after repeated subcutaneous GH injections at the same site.

In adults with GH deficiency, high plasma cholesterol levels are accompanied by a rise in the concentrations of both low-density and very-low-density lipoproteins.[35] A raised plasma cholesterol (but not triglyceride) level was observed in children with GH deficiency, the cholesterol normalizing during long-term GH therapy.[36]

After receiving 3 months of GH therapy, seven GH-deficient children demonstrated a reduction in the lipid content of the abdominal subcutaneous adipocytes and a resultant redistribution of adipose tissue stores to a more peripheral pattern. This site-specific change in adipose distribution may be contributed by anatomically site-specific GH-mediated changes in insulin responsiveness of adipose tissue. The authors also demonstrated a decrease in de novo triglyceride synthesis with therapy.[37] Fifteen children, some with GH deficiency and some without, demonstrated an increase of their lean body mass with no change in their fat mass within 6 weeks of starting GH therapy.[38] In a study evaluating both carbohydrate and fat metabolism with GH treatment in non-GH-deficient children, despite relatively large doses of growth hormone $(0.3 \, \text{U} \, \text{kg}^{-1} \, \text{day}^{-1})$, FFA levels were unaffected and the relative contribution of carbohydrate and lipid oxidation to the energy expenditure, measured by indirect calorimetry methods, was unchanged by GH therapy.[9] In a large study comparing the effects of growth hormone on different groups of children, the modest changes that were observed in cholesterol and triglyceride levels were not statistically or clinically significant, and both levels remained in the normal range compared with age-appropriate standards.[10]

Growth hormone treatment in a group of Turner syndrome patients receiving higher GH doses than usual had no effect on lipid metabolism.[13,39] Whereas GH treatment did not affect the total plasma concentrations of triglyceride and cholesterol in children with CRI, recent evidence suggests that an increase in lipoprotein A may occur in some patients. An atherogenic plasma lipoprotein profile is characteristic of CRI, and these alterations are perpetuated after renal transplantation by cyclosporin A and glucocorticoid medication. Hence, growth hormone could theoretically contribute to early atherosclerosis in this group of patients, by both an increase in lipoprotein A and the observed increase in insulin secretion.[40]

At present, although the typical fat deposition pattern in GH-deficient children is well known, and the GH effect on fat mass in such subjects appears to be beneficial, very little can be concluded regarding its effects on lipid metabolism, especially in children with other underlying disorders.

The use of GH in Prader–Willi syndrome has presented some unique challenges in determining benefits versus risks in both carbohydrate and lipid metabolism. Studies have demonstrated sustained beneficial effects on body composition (decrease in fat mass and increase in lean body mass), after 4 years of GH therapy with doses of 1.0 and 1.5 mg m^{-2}, but not with lower doses.[19]

Water and salt retention in growth hormone therapy

In 1954, Ikkos et al. demonstrated that acromegalic individuals had an increase in total body water and sodium.[41] Increase in total body water, plasma volume, extracellular fluid, red cell volume, and exchangeable sodium are reported in acromegaly and reversed with normalization of the GH levels. Administration of growth hormone induces changes in electrolyte and fluid homeostasis, possibly as a result of a direct renal tubule action or mediated via the renin–angiotensin system.[42–45] Earlier studies demonstrated that both short-term and long-term administration of pituitary growth hormone to GH-deficient children resulted in an increase in total body water.[46,47] Edema appeared to be a common side effect of pituitary GH treatment in adults with or without GH deficiency.[48–50] Fluid retention continued to be observed in adults receiving recombinant growth hormone in both short-term and long-term trials.[51,52]

Symptoms such as increase in body weight, swollen ankles, and a sensation of tightness in the hands, were noted within a month of starting treatment. In adults the changes in sodium metabolism related to growth hormone, such as the expansion of the total body water compartment and weight gain, appear to be determined by the dose administered.[53] These effects and symptomatic edema appear to be much less common in children on recombinant growth hormone. Although adult subjects demonstrated an increase in extracellular volume and a significant suppression of atrial natriuretic peptide (ANP),[54] no changes in plasma renin activity (PRA) or ANP could be demonstrated in GH-deficient children on growth hormone, although their aldosterone levels, which were low initially, normalized with therapy.[55] A study of children with ISS treated with growth hormone demonstrated that there were no changes in PRA, aldosterone or ANP after a year of GH therapy.[56] Similar results were reported with no change in the fluid homeostasis in another study using both low and high doses of growth hormone.[57]

In healthy animals and humans, growth hormone induces glomerular hyperfiltration via an increased IGF-I production, and glomerular sclerosis is observed in transgenic, rGH-producing mice. Therefore concern was raised that GH treatment may accelerate the deterioration of renal function in patients with CRI. In uremic rats and in humans with a glomerular filtration rate (GFR) below 40 mL min^{-1} per 1.73 m^2, treatment with growth hormone did not affect the GFR, suggesting that its renotropic effect may be absent in CRI. Two published reports observed no significant difference in the average annual decline in GFR between children with CRI on conservative treatment receiving GH therapy and untreated control patients.[58,59] Nevertheless water retention is a known side effect during the first few weeks of GH therapy, and fluid overload is a concern especially in the children with CRI; therefore intensification of dialysis and/or antihypertensive treatment may be necessary.

Table 45.1   Patients with idiopathic intracranial hypertension (IIH) from the National Cooperative Growth Study (NCGS)

Diagnosis	Total no. of patients with IIH onset		Early IIH (cases/patient–year × 10^{-5})
	Early[a]	Late	
Growth hormone deficiency	5	4	158.5
Idiopathic short stature	0	0	0
Turner syndrome	2	0	369.7
Renal disease	3[b]	2	6218.9
Other diagnosis	1[c]	2[d]	313.4

[a] Onset in first 4 months of GH treatment.
[b] One child was also diagnosed as GH deficient.
[c] Prader–Willi syndrome with high doses of glucocorticoids.
[d] Osteopetrosis.
From Blethen et al.[23]

Eighteen cases of edema were reported by the NCGS group out of 19 000 children. In addition, eight girls with Turner syndrome and one boy with Noonan syndrome reported appearance or worsening of their lymphedema. It appears to affect those children with Turner syndrome who have a history of lymphedema during infancy. Three of 47 Turner syndrome patients treated with growth hormone developed lymphedema of the dorsum of their feet.[60]

In summary, growth hormone effects changes in the metabolism of water and sodium, probably via the renin–angiotensin system, leading to an expansion of the space occupied by total body water, including the intravascular volume. It is probable that the effect is dose dependent and transient. Finally, it is clearly age related, the effect being more pronounced in adults.

IDIOPATHIC INTRACRANIAL HYPERTENSION (Table 45.1)

The occurrence of pseudotumor cerebri or idiopathic intracranial hypertension (IIH), a benign condition with raised intracranial pressure and papilledema, has been attributed to fluid shifts; it is usually encountered, however, in patients who are also receiving glucocorticoids or who have other predisposing conditions. Although IIH is believed to be rare in children, it has been described in children with CRI and in association with replacement therapy in primary hypothyroidism. In children with GH deficiency, it is possible that rapid correction of long-standing hormone deficiency results in intracerebral fluid shifts and the development of IIH. In one of the earlier reports of cases with IIH, seven had GH deficiency and eight had CRI.[61,62] The others had Turner syndrome and Prader–Willi syndrome, but some had no underlying disorder. Obesity, CRI, and other metabolic and endocrine disorders such as hypothyroidism, apart from the use of higher doses of growth hormone, may by themselves increase the risk of mild IIH.

Of note has been the observation that intracranial hypertension can occur at any time during treatment, and not just during initiation of GH therapy.[24] Hence the patient

and parents should be instructed to report any untoward weight gain, feelings of tightness and especially headaches, photophobia, and visual changes, which may occur with raised intracranial pressure. Fundoscopy is recommended before treatment and at follow-up visits. Fortunately, almost all the reports of IIH have also shown that stopping treatment reverses the process and restarting it, especially with a lower dose, does not appear to cause a recurrence.

CARPAL TUNNEL SYNDROME

Carpal tunnel syndrome, felt to be secondary to soft tissue growth or edema, is less common in children compared with adults; only five children in the NCGS and two children in non-NCGS studies reported this syndrome.[23] This complication appears to be dose related.

NONMETABOLIC SIDE EFFECTS: GROWTH HORMONE TREATMENT AND THE RISK OF CANCER

Leukemia (Table 45.2)

A source of major concern has been the association of leukemia with GH therapy; this has received widespread publicity. Leukemia is one of the most common childhood malignancies, occurring in about one in 2000 children under the age of 15 years. Acute lymphoblastic leukemia (ALL) comprises 75–85 percent of these cases. Although most cases of childhood leukemia are idiopathic, known risk factors include a positive family history, underlying chromosomal disorders and prior treatment with radiation and chemotherapeutic agents. Children with ALL have a relapse rate of 10 percent/year in the first 2 years and 25–30 percent in the first 5 years. After 5 years of remission, the relapse rate is 1–2 percent/year. After one relapse the incidence of a second relapse is 80–90 percent. As there is a substantial risk of relapse in children who had leukemia, a study of these patients might be more sensitive in detecting an effect of GH treatment on the development of leukemia.

Table 45.2 Country-based reports of new onset leukemia in all patients treated with pituitary derived and recombinant GH (data up to 1996)

Country	No. of cases (no. without leukemia risk factors)
USA	18 (5)
Japan	15 (8)
France	4 (3)
Canada	2 (2)
Austria	1 (0)
Belgium	1 (0)
Finland	1 (0)
Germany	1 (1)
Italy	1 (1)
Netherlands	1 (1)
UK	1 (0)
Total	46 (21)
Total (non-Japanese)	31 (13)

From Allen.[98]

A specific questionnaire regarding these patients was sent to NCGS investigators.[23] More than 200 patients who had leukemia before GH therapy have been enrolled in the NCGS. As of June 1995, eight of these patients had recurrences reported. Four of them had at least one relapse before starting GH treatment, and three had received bone marrow transplants. Consequently, four of 200 (2 percent) patients relapsed for the first time while receiving growth hormone, with an average interval after initial diagnosis of 6 years. In each case, relapse occurred within 1 year of starting GH therapy. For patients with ALL in general, a relapse rate of 1–2 percent is expected 6 years after primary diagnosis.

Therefore, the reported relapse rate in the NCGS population was within the expected range. This is consistent with previous reports showing no effect of GH replacement therapy on the rate of ALL relapse.[63] However, occasional reports of ALL relapse several years after remission, but occurring within a year of GH replacement therapy, continue to caution the physician that the potential effect of growth hormone on ALL relapse should be assessed critically. By 1991 there had been about 10 cases of leukemia reported in patients undergoing GH treatment in the USA.[64] Eight of these children had previously diagnosed tumors of the CNS, seven having received radiotherapy or chemotherapy or both. Of significance was the fact that several patients with brain tumors and GH deficiency developed leukemia even before starting treatment with growth hormone.[65] Thus this group of patients may be more susceptible to the development of leukemias compared with others.

A worldwide review of children, who had been treated with growth hormone by 1989, revealed a total of 15 GH-deficient children who had leukemia after GH therapy.[66] Half of these children had other possible risk factors for the development of leukemia, such as cranial irradiation or various predisposing syndromes. A conservative analysis of the data suggested that the risk of leukemia in GH-deficient patients without other risk factors is roughly one case in 24 000 patient-years. The risk among normal (slightly younger) children is roughly one case in 42 000 subject-years. Growth hormone is known to be an immune modulator and GH deficiency itself, rather than GH therapy, may be the explanation for the possible increase in leukemia in GH-deficient patients. In an update in 1992 leukemia had occurred in 31 patients during and following GH therapy, with related malignancies in two other patients. Once again additional factors rather than GH increased the risk of leukemia.[67] In an extensive survey of 6284 patients treated with pituitary-derived growth hormone, no significant increase in the incidence of leukemia in patients treated for idiopathic GH deficiency was found.[68] Data collected since 1975 in Japan from more than 32 000 patients concluded that the incidence of leukemia in GH-treated patients without risk factors is not greater than that in the general population aged 0–15 years.[69]

Up to 1995, leukemia or preleukemic myelodysplastic syndromes have developed during or after GH therapy in 39 patients world wide.[70] In about half of these children, one or more risk factors for leukemia were present, including previous radiotherapy, chemotherapy, immunosuppressive therapy or other predisposing conditions. It was concluded that, with the currently available data, it is not possible to determine whether GH-deficient patients and other children with factors that predispose them to leukemia are being placed at a greater risk by exposure to growth hormone. A recent update by the same group concluded that based on current data,[69] the increased risk of leukemia is limited to children with underlying conditions that already predispose them to develop malignancies.[71] The demonstration of IGF-I and GH receptors on leukemia cells persuades one to be vigilant about the use of growth hormone in these patients.[72]

Hence, growth hormone should be offered to these individuals because their slow growth rate and short stature have a deleterious impact on their lives, although a full explanation of the potential risks should be imparted before starting treatment. There is no evidence at this time that GH therapy increases the incidence of leukemia in non-GH-deficient individuals with no other known risk factor.

Brain neoplasms

Brain tumors are the second most common childhood malignancy, the treatment of which usually includes cranial irradiation with adjuvant chemotherapy. With improved survival, the long-term management of the endocrine sequelae, including growth failure, is fundamental to the improved quality of life in these children. The use of growth hormone in children with radiation-induced GH deficiency is now widely accepted but questions still exist about the safety of this mitogenic hormone.

Several authors have studied the recurrence of brain tumors with growth hormone.[73–75] One study[74] compared the relapse rate of brain tumors in 47 children who were treated with growth hormone with that in another group of 170 children with brain tumors who did not receive it. Of the GH-treated children, 11 percent developed a recurrence of their tumor compared with 26 percent in the other group. An important observation made by these authors was that 16 of the children with previous brain tumors had abnormal findings on computed tomography at the start of GH treatment, two of whom later developed a recurrence. Thus, such abnormalities call for caution and frequent follow-ups but do not necessarily preclude GH treatment. Although the use of growth hormone does not increase the risk of tumor according to these studies, larger numbers need to be studied to resolve the issue fully. The NCGS group found no significant difference in the incidence of tumor recurrence compared with published (untreated) series, although with the data available a precise calculation of the tumor recurrence could not be made.[23] Current NCGS data are consistent with prior findings.[24] Recently the FDA added a class label warning stating that in childhood cancer survivors, an increased risk of a second neoplasm has been reported in patients treated with GH after their first neoplasm. Meningiomas were the most common of these second neoplasms. In adults it is unknown whether there is any relationship between GH replacement therapy and CNS tumour recurrence. Most recommend waiting at least a year after the completion of tumor therapy before starting GH treatment.

Other recently published studies include the UK series which followed 180 children with brain tumors who were treated with GH between 1965 and 1996, and 891 children with brain tumors who received radiotherapy but not GH. Thirty-five first recurrences occurred in the GH-treated children and 434 in the untreated children.[76] The relative risk of first recurrence in GH-treated compared with untreated patients, adjusted for confounding prognostic variables, was decreased as was the relative risk of mortality. There was no significant trend in relative risk of recurrence with cumulative time for which GH treatment had been given or with time elapsed since treatment was started.

Another group studied 361 GH-treated cancer survivors (including 172 brain tumor survivors). They were from among 13 539 survivors enrolled in the Childhood Cancer Survivor Study, a cohort of 5 year survivors of childhood cancer.[77] The relative risk of disease recurrence was 0.83 for GH-treated survivors. The relative risk of recurrence was not increased for any of the major cancer diagnoses. GH-treated subjects were diagnosed with 15 secondary neoplasms, all solid tumors and no secondary leukemias, for an overall relative risk of 3.21. This was mainly due to a small excess number of secondary neoplasms observed in GH-treated survivors of acute leukemia. Although this is of concern, the data need to be interpreted with caution given the small number of events.

Other neoplasms

Acromegaly, characterized by elevated levels of GH, IGF-I and IGFBP-3 has been linked with an increased incidence of colonic neoplasia. More recently, the association of IGF-I and IGFBP-3 levels and certain malignancies of adulthood such as breast, prostate and colorectal cancers has raised new concerns.[78–81] A report suggests that men with higher IGF-I levels are at a greater risk of developing prostatic cancer.[82] It has been reported that most cancer risk is increased in individuals in whom high IGF-I levels are accompanied with low IGFBP-3 levels. In subjects treated with GH, IGF-I and IGFBP-3 levels both rise together and are not within the elevated cancer-risk range, based on published studies. Until further research in the area dictates otherwise, ongoing surveillance and routine monitoring of IGF-I and IGFBP-3 levels in GH recipients must become standard of care.[83,84] Although there is no clear connection between GH use and increased incidence of these cancers, only very long term careful surveillance will be able to address these concerns satisfactorily.[85]

GROWTH–RELATED EVENTS

Unfavorable clinical events have occurred with GH treatment which appear to be related to the growth-promoting action of the hormone. Growth hormone produces its primary action, namely a growth-promoting effect on the body, by its action on bones, muscles and other tissues. The main effector appears to be IGF-I, but some of the actions are a direct result of growth hormone itself. The linear growth seen with GH therapy is a result of IGF-I as well as a direct effect of growth hormone on the cartilage resulting in differentiation and multiplication of cartilage precursor cells.[86]

Slipped capital femoral epiphysis (Table 45.3)

Obesity, male sex, rapid growth, and puberty are considered to be risk factors of slipped capital femoral epiphysis (SCFE) in the general population.[87] Twenty-one cases of SCFE were reported in 7719 GH-deficient patients. Twelve of them occurred during GH treatment, and six were before and three after the treatment.[88] In the NCGS, SCFE was reported in 27 children on GH therapy. There was no significant difference between boys and girls in the incidence of SCFE, unlike that seen in the normal adolescent population. Only one child with ISS developed SCFE.[89] GH deficiency, Turner syndrome and CRI appeared to be predisposing factors. SCFE occurs during normal adolescence and the growth spurt induced by growth hormone has been implicated in the pathogenesis of this entity. Animal models suggest that growth hormone can weaken the epiphyseal plate, thereby increasing the chances of slipped plates.[88] Although the precise mechanism is yet to be clarified, any knee, hip or thigh pain should be promptly investigated.

Table 45.3   Incidence of slipped capital femoral epiphysis (SCFE) in children treated with growth hormone (GH) and followed by the National Cooperative Growth Study (NCGS)

Diagnosis	Age at SCFE (years)	Time on growth hormone before SCFE (years)	Total patient–years years on growth hormone	SCFE cases per 10^5 patient–years
Idiopathic GH deficiency	15.9 ± 3.5	0.81 ± 0.47	15 829	69.5
Organic GH deficiency	14.9 ± 2.5	0.98 ± 1.07	5 055	158.3
Idiopathic short stature	14.5	0.75	10 562	9.5[a]
Turner syndrome	11.5 ± 2.3	1.4 ± 0.6	4 201	71.4
Other	13.8 ± 2.9	1.3 ± 0.8	2 579	116.3

[a]Significantly lower than risk in children with GH deficiency (<0.006)
From Blethen and Rundle.[89]

Facial features

There have been some reports of patients developing acromegaloid facial features with long-term GH treatment.[90] Levels of IGF-I ranging from 902 to 1241 ng mL^{-1} have been noted in these patients.

Scoliosis

Estimates of the prevalence of scoliosis vary widely, with girls being more commonly affected than boys. About three out of 1000 adolescent girls require treatment. The relationship between the pubertal growth spurt and scoliosis is well recognized, making the potential effects of growth hormone on this process very difficult to analyze. The frequency of scoliosis is increased by GH treatment, but it is not clear if it is the progression of already existing scoliosis that is influenced by the growth spurt after GH therapy.[91] Hence children with scoliosis who are treated with growth hormone should be carefully monitored for progression.

OTHER MISCELLANEOUS EFFECTS

Gynecomastia

Breast development appears to occur in about two-thirds of normal pubertal boys, whereas its appearance in pre-pubertal boys is rare.[92–94] Gynecomastia appears to be a common problem in adult men treated with growth hormone.[95] Twenty-two cases of gynecomastia have been reported in pre-pubertal children on GH therapy.[96] Breast development was noted between 4 and 84 months of treatment. The condition appears to be benign and self-limited and no intervention is warranted.

Pigmented nevi

The data currently available suggest that GH treatment may increase the number, size or degree of pigmentation of nevi.[97] The risk of malignant transformation of pigmented nevi does not appear to be increased with GH therapy. As there is a two-fold increase in the growth rate of the nevi in GH-deficient individuals and patients with Turner syndrome, long-term follow-up is required to identify delayed or unknown effects.

Acute pancreatitis

Acute pancreatitis during childhood is uncommon and is usually a feature of systemic disease such as uremia or valproate therapy. About 25 percent are idiopathic. Seven cases of pancreatitis were reported in children treated with growth hormone. Known risk factors were present in five of the seven cases.[98] A cause-and-effect relationship has not been clearly established except for one instance,[99] and symptoms usually resolve with continued GH treatment. Nevertheless, patients on GH treatment, especially in those with associated risk factors, should be carefully monitored.

Thyroid insufficiency

Administration of growth hormone to patients with GH deficiency has been reported to produce a variety of perturbations of thyroid function. An analysis of effects of recombinant growth hormone on thyroid function showed that after 4 days of growth hormone (0.125 mg m^{-2} per day), mean serum thyroxine (T_4) levels decreased by 8 percent and in contrast, mean serum triiodothyronine (T_3) levels increased by 21 percent. The increase in mean T_3 levels led to a 54 percent decrease in mean thyroid-stimulating hormone (TSH) level.[100] This is consistent with the suggestion that the predominant effect of GH therapy on thyroid function, in both GH-deficient and healthy subjects, with or without thyroid substitution is enhanced extrathyroidal conversion of T_4 to T_3.[100,101] It is suggested that the ensuing elevated T_3 levels would explain the blunted TSH response (via feedback inhibition) to thyrotropin-releasing hormone (TRH) stimulation. However, it still remains a possibility that GH therapy may accelerate the development of overt central hypothyroidism. As thyroid hormone is also required for normal growth, monitoring of thyroid hormone levels while on treatment with growth hormone appears to be a reasonable practice.

Adrenal insufficiency

The possibility of co-existing adrenal insufficiency should always be borne in mind in GH deficient states. GH replacement in such individuals can worsen the adrenal deficiency. All at-risk patients clearly need ongoing evaluation of the adrenal axis. A possible mechanism for the exacerbation of adrenal insufficiency with partial adrenocorticotropic hormone deficiency after commencing GH therapy is the inhibitory effect of GH on the conversion of cortisone to cortisol by 11 beta-HSD1.[102–104] Another reason for being aware of the possibility of later onset of adrenal insufficiency is the description of new genetic entities where there appears to be an evolving state of progressive hypopituitarism. For example, mutations in the PROP1 gene are one of the most frequent genetic defects in patients with combined pituitary hormone insufficiency. These patients apparently develop at least partial adrenal insufficiency, with a gradual decline of the function of the pituitary adrenal axis and eventually require substitution with hydrocortisone;[105] IMAGe syndrome (intrauterine growth restriction, metaphyseal dysplasia, adrenal hypoplasia congenita, genital abnormalities) is a multisystem disorder with a broad phenotype, which, if unrecognized, may result in major and possibly life-threatening complications with the development of late onset GH and adrenal insufficiency.[106]

Antibodies

Antibodies to growth hormone have appeared in patients treated with both pituitary and synthetic forms. Although the development of antibodies was observed in the earlier synthetic preparations with attenuation of growth,[107] the more recent products have been relatively free of this problem. In the rare case of antibody induced reduction in growth velocity, changing the product may be beneficial.[108]

Puberty

It had been suggested that the length of time of pubertal growth is shortened in GH-deficient children on GH treatment.[109] This observation has important implications in the management of children with growth failure being treated with growth hormone. An improvement in predicted adult height could easily be lost by shortening the period of pubertal growth. Subsequent studies have been able to refute this.[110] A confounding factor has been that patients with constitutional delay of growth and development have a shorter than normal puberty. This appears to

hold true especially in boys with this condition, with a relatively rapid progression from Tanner stages II–IV. This is independent of any GH effect but, if these children are treated as part of clinical protocols with GH therapy for ISS, erroneous conclusions of GH-mediated pubertal acceleration may be drawn. Kawai et al. recently reported suboptimal pubertal height gain in ISS.[111] In this light, it is interesting that the beneficial effects of growth hormone on adult height reported in patients with Turner syndrome may be attributable, in part, to the failure of most girls with gonadal dysfunction to enter puberty.[112] The recent use of high doses of GH during puberty to enhance growth results in higher levels of growth factors and will need long-term monitoring.[113]

Immune function

Although serum immunoglobulin levels do not appear to change significantly with GH therapy,[114] a decrease in the percentage of B-cell lymphocytes has been reported and in vitro studies have demonstrated a reduction in the expression of surface markers by B cells upon exposure to growth hormone.[115–117] Conflicting reports exist regarding the effects of GH administration on natural killer cell activity and mitogen response. With the demonstration of GH and IGF-I production by lymphocytes and the existence of GH and IGF-I receptors on lymphocytes, there clearly appears to be an active communication network between growth hormone and the immune system, although its significance has yet to be clearly defined.[118]

GROWTH HORMONE-STIMULATION TESTING

The discussion of adverse effects of growth hormone will not be complete without mention of the hazards associated with GH provocation testing using the insulin stimulation test, which is considered the gold standard of pharmacological GH testing. There have been reports of serious consequences secondary to hypoglycemia in children with hypopituitarism after these tests.[119] Hence great vigilance and expert management should be practiced while conducting provocation tests.

CREUTZFELDT–JAKOB DISEASE

Creutzfeldt–Jakob disease is a neurological disorder with progressive dementia associated with cerebellar dysfunction, myoclonus, and characteristic autopsy findings of astrocytosis and spongiosis with a diffuse neuronal loss. It is transmitted by a protein particle, or prion, which, in conjunction with PrPscrapie, a pathological isoform of a protein, prion protein, synthesized in healthy individuals and present on the neuronal surface, forms the characteristic amyloid plaques seen in Creutzfeldt–Jakob disease. There is a clear link between Creutzfeldt–Jakob disease and the use of pituitary growth hormone from contaminated human cadavers which may or may not be related to the genotype of the recipients. Although the risk does not apply any more with the use of recombinant growth hormone, in view of the prolonged incubation period, there is a theoretical risk that individuals treated with the pituitary growth hormone may yet develop the disease.[52]

CONCERNS RELATED TO CHRONIC RENAL INSUFFICIENCY AND GROWTH HORMONE THERAPY

The safety concerns for patients with CRI treated with growth hormone will continue to be an issue because of the wide variety of underlying renal conditions for which it can be used for its growth-promoting effect. In the narrowest context, effects can be categorized to those specific to renal disease, such as progression of chronic renal failure to end-stage renal disease, accentuation of carbohydrate intolerance, rejection episodes or loss of function post-transplantation, and adverse consequences of the combination of GH and immunosuppression therapy.

No current data support an acceleration of the progression of CRI to end-stage renal disease. However, small series, such as the three patients with cystinosis and chronic renal disease, in whom there was growth acceleration and an apparent increase in serum creatinine but not in creatinine clearance, raise the issue that somatic growth will exceed renal function and may hasten the need for transplantation.[120] Although the validity of the methods used in this study and the supporting data has been questioned, the net effects of the actions of growth hormone on kidney function need to be assessed prospectively. The issue of carbohydrate intolerance has already been addressed and to date it does not pose a serious problem.

In recipients post-transplantation, there are insufficient data available to determine whether there is an increase in rejection episodes or deterioration in renal function. Although efficacy is established, the safety of growth hormone continues to raise concerns. A large study showed a higher incidence of rejection in transplanted children on GH treatment, especially if they had pre-treatment rejection episodes.[121] In a group of 11 patients treated for 1 or more years with growth hormone, one patient had a precipitous drop in their creatinine clearance and two had biopsy-documented chronic rejection and loss of allograft function.[122] The authors point out that growth hormone *in vitro* has been shown to modulate the immune response and, although this has not yet been documented as clinically significant *in vivo*, growth hormone might interfere with the immunosuppressive effects of the drugs used to maintain successful graft tolerance. Further investigations of this potential interaction are warranted.

Of note is that focal segmental glomerulosclerosis (FSGS) has been described in association with acromegaly.[123] In a patient treated with GH for hypopituitarism, proteinuria was noted after many years of treatment and persisted despite cessation of GH. A renal biopsy specimen showed glomerular hypertrophy and limited glomerulosclerosis, compatible with FSGS.[124]

SUDDEN DEATHS WITH USE OF GROWTH HORMONES

Prader–Willi syndrome

The LWPES Drug and Therapeutics Committee was made aware by 2002 that seven patients with PWS died a median of 13 weeks after starting GH treatment.[71] These deaths were sudden and unexpected and sometimes associated with respiratory problems. Further analysis has clarified the risk to some extent. Irrespective of GH treatment, children with PWS are prone to upper airway obstruction related to insufficiency of respiratory muscles and pharyngeal narrowness which may be accentuated with intercurrent infections.[125] Obesity may play an important role by worsening the hypoventilation. A polysomnography and an otorhinolaryngologic examination are recommended in children with PWS before institution of GH therapy. Additionally, upper airway infections should be treated promptly and aggressively.

Adrenal insufficiency

Growth hormone deficiency is sometimes associated with other pituitary hormone deficiencies. Replacing GH can unmask the state of adrenal insufficiency. The possibility of co-existing adrenal insufficiency should always be borne in mind and may be the cause of sudden deaths. This possibility has been addressed in a cohort of 6107 patients who were known US pituitary-derived GH recipients from 1963 to 1985. There were 433 deaths and a quarter was sudden and unexpected. Hypoglycemia and adrenal insufficiency accounted for far more mortality than Creutzfeldt–Jakob disease.[126] Similar findings were noted earlier in a Canadian study.[127] All at risk patients clearly need ongoing evaluation of the adrenal axis.

GROWTH HORMONE TREATMENT IN ADULTS

The safety of GH use in adults is a subject of ongoing studies. It has been shown to be beneficial in adults with GH deficiency and in adults with AIDS. Conversely, we know now that in the intensive care setting in the critically ill adult, it causes increased mortality and hence has no

Table 45.4 Recommendations for management of possible side effects of growth hormone (GH)

Complaint	Concern	Evaluation	Management
Metabolic effects			
Polyuria, polydipsia	Diabetes mellitus	Urine glucose, serum glucose and insulin	Address risk factors, diet, insulin
Weight gain, swelling	Edema	On desmopressin	Alter desmopressin dose, stop growth hormone; if better, ?restart at lower dose
Headache	Pseudotumor cerebri	Fundoscopy and neurological evaluation, opening pressure of CSF	If papilledema, stop growth hormone, r/o space-occupying lesion, treat intracranial pressure
Paresthesiae	Carpel tunnel syndrome	Nerve conduction studies	Stop growth hormone and restart at lower dose if symptoms abate
Growth–related effects			
Limb, hip or knee pain	SCFE	Radiographs	Stop growth hormone till orthopedic evaluation
Poor growth	?Antibodies	Review dose, methods, compliance, bone age, nutrition, thyroid status, and then consider antibodies	If high titer of antibodies, change preparation after a washout period
Other effects			
Previous neoplasms	Recurrence or new neoplasm	Evaluate for recurrence before and during GH therapy	Stop growth hormone
Nevi	Rapid growth	Examine nevi as routine	Biopsy-suspicious lesions

Adapted from Blethen et al.[23]

role.[128] However, with the current approved indications, side effects are similar to those noted in children such as those effecting glucose metabolism, fluid retention, etc. In adults, abnormal carbohydrate metabolism occurs more in elderly people, in obesity, in postoperative states and in burns patients, on doses that are relatively smaller than GH doses in children.[129–132] Effects of fluid retention such as carpal tunnel syndrome appear to be more common too. There are increased levels of lipoprotein(a) with GH treatment but the clinical significance is unclear.[27] The occurrence of breast, colon and prostate cancers is a theoretical concern that needs to be monitored with long term surveillance.

CONCLUSION (Table 45.4)

A recent analysis of data collected from ≈60 000 patients (including 9000 with ISS) during long-term observational studies demonstrated the overall safety of recombinant human GH for the treatment of various pediatric growth disorders.[133] In general, the use of GH in children has been associated with remarkably few problems. However, it has to be kept in mind that GH is a potent anabolic agent and although this can be used to its advantage, as the therapeutic indications broaden and the dose increases, more unfavorable clinical consequences linked to the biologic actions of the hormone may emerge. Thus, constant surveillance

for rare but important associated events must continue, and pediatric and adult endocrinologists must be alert to the occurrence of adverse effects during and, maybe more importantly, after GH therapy.

KEY LEARNING POINTS

- Know the metabolic effects of growth hormone. They include:
  - carbohydrate metabolism, esp. insulin resistance
  - lipid metabolism
  - thyroid hormone metabolism
  - water, salt retention
  - increased intracranial hypertension
- Growth hormone and cancer: There is no clear connection between growth hormone use and cancer. Long-term surveillance is necessary, however.
- Growth-related events:
  - slipped capital femoral epiphysis
  - facial features
  - scoliosis
- New evidence implies that growth hormone might interfere with normal cortisol metabolism and may lead to clinically significant cortisol deficiency.
- Used appropriately, growth hormone is a remarkably safe drug.

REFERENCES

● = Seminal primary article
◆ = Key review paper
❋ = First formal publication of a management guideline

1   Haymond MW, Karl I, Weldon VV, Pagliara AS. The role of growth hormone and cortisone on glucose and gluconeogenic substrate regulation in fasted hypopituitary children. *J Clin Endocrinol Metab* 1976; **42**: 846–56.

● 2   Bougneres PF, Artavia-Loria E, Ferre P, *et al*. Effects of hypopituitarism and growth hormone replacement therapy on the production and utilization of glucose in childhood. *J Clin Endocrinol Metab* 1985; **61**: 1152–7.

3   Lippe BM, Kaplan SA, Golden MP, *et al*. Carbohydrate tolerance and insulin receptor binding in children with hypopituitarism: Responses after acute and chronic human growth hormone administration. *J Clin Endocrinol Metab* 1981; **53**: 507–13.

● 4   ]Houssay BA. The hypophysis and metabolism. *New Engl J Med* 1936; **241**: 961.

5   Rizza R, Miles J, Verdonk, C. Insulin sensitivity in man: A method for single day dose–response assessment using the euglycemic glucose insulin clamp technique. *Clin Res* 1980; **28**: 409–14.

◆ 6   Davidson MB. Effect of growth hormone on carbohydrate and lipid metabolism. *Endocr Rev* 1987; **8**: 115–31.

7   Karlander S, Vranic M, Efendic S. Increased glucose turnover and glucose cycling in acromegalic patients with normal glucose tolerance. *Diabetologia* 1986; **29**: 778–83.

8   Walker J, Chaussain JL, Bougneres PF. Growth hormone treatment of children with short stature increases insulin secretion but does not impair glucose disposal. *J Clin Endocrinol Metab* 1989; **69**: 253–8.

● 9   Lesage C, Walker J, Landier F, *et al*. Near normalization of adolescent height with growth hormone therapy in very short children without growth hormone deficiency. *J Pediatr* 1991; **119**: 29–34.

● 10 Saenger P, Attie KM, DiMartino-Nardi J, Fine RN, and the Genentech Collaborative Group. Carbohydrate metabolism in children receiving growth hormone for 5 years. Chronic renal insufficiency compared with growth hormone deficiency, Turner syndrome, and idiopathic short stature. *Pediatr Nephrol* 1996; **10**: 261–3.

11 Boulware SD, Caprio S, Jones TW, *et al*. Metabolic alterations induced by growth hormone treatment mirror changes during normal adolescence. *Pediatr Res* 1990; **27**: 72A.

● 12 Caprio S, Boulware SD, Press, M, *et al*. Effect of growth hormone treatment on hyperinsulinemia associated with Turner syndrome. *J Pediatr* 1992; **120**: 238–43.

13 Wilson DM, Frane JW, Sherman B, *et al*., and Genentech Turner Collaborative Group. Carbohydrate and lipid metabolism in Turner syndrome: Effect of therapy with growth hormone, oxandrolone, and a combination of both. *J Pediatr* 1988; **112**: 210–17.

14 Monti LD, Brambilla P, Caumo A, *et al*. Glucose turnover and insulin clearance after growth hormone treatment in girls with Turner's syndrome. *Metabolism* 1997; **46**: 1482–8.

15 Saenger P, Wesoly S, Wasserman EJ, *et al*. Safety aspects of GH therapy in Turner syndrome: no evidence for ventricular hypertrophy and normalization of insulin levels after discontinuation of GH. *Pediatr Res* 1996; **39**: 98A.

16 Tönshoff B, Haffner D, Mehls O, *et al*., and the German Study Group for GH Treatment in Children with Renal Allografts. Three year experience. *Kidney Int* 1993; **44**: 199–207.

17 Haffner D, Wuhl E, Tpnshoff B, Mehls O, and the German Study Group for Growth Hormone Treatment in Chronic Renal Failure. Growth hormone treatment in short children: 5 year experience. *Nephrol Dial Transplant* 1994; **9**: 960–1.

● 18 Hokken-Koelega AC, De Waal WJ, Sas TC, *et al*. Small for gestational age (SGA): endocrine and metabolic consequences and effects of growth hormone treatment. *J Pediatr Endocrinol Metab* 2004; **17(Suppl 3)**: 463–9.

◆ 19 Allen DB, Carrel AL. Growth hormone therapy for Prader–Willi syndrome: a critical appraisal. *J Pediatr Endocrinol Metab* 2004; **17(Suppl 4)**: 1297–306.

20 L'Allemand D, Eiholzer U, Schlumpf M, *et al*. Carbohydrate metabolism is not impaired after 3 years of growth hormone therapy in children with Prader–Willi syndrome. *Horm Res* 2003; **59**: 239–48.

21 Lindgren AC, Hagenas L, Ritzen EM. Growth hormone treatment of children with Prader–Willi syndrome: effects on glucose and insulin homeostasis. Swedish National Growth Hormone Advisory Group. *Horm Res* 1999; **51**: 157–61.

22 Wyatt D. Lessons from the national cooperative growth study. *Eur J Endocrinol* 2004; **151(Suppl 1)**: S55–9.

23 Blethen SL, Allen DB, Graves D, *et al*., on behalf of the National Cooperative Growth Study Safety of recombinant deoxyribonucleic acid derived growth hormone: the National Cooperative Growth Study experience. *J Clin Endocrinol Metab* 1996; **81**: 1704–10.

◆ 24 Maneatis T, Baptista J, Connelly K, Blethen S. Growth hormone safety update from the National Cooperative Growth Study. *J Pediatr Endocrinol Metab* 2000; **13(Suppl 2)**: 1035–44.

25 Taskinen M, Saarinen-Pihkala UM, Hovi L, Lipsanen-Nyman M. Impaired glucose tolerance and dyslipidaemia as late effects after bone-marrow transplantation in childhood. *Lancet* 2000; **356**: 993–7.

● 26 Oeffinger KC, *et al*. Chronic health conditions in adult survivors of childhood cancer. *New Engl J Med* 2006; **355**: 1572–82.

❋ 27 Consensus statement – the Growth Hormone Research Society. Critical evaluation of the safety of recombinant human growth hormone administration: statement from the Growth Hormone Research Society. *J Clin Endocrinol Metab* 2001; **86**: 1868–70.

28 Goodman HM. Antilipolytic effects of growth hormone. *Metabolism* 1970; **19**: 849–55.

29 Birnbaum RS, Goodman HS. Studies on the mechanism of the antilipolytic effects of growth hormone. *Endocrinology* 1976; **99**: 1336–45.

30 Swislocki NI, Szego CM. Acute reduction of plasma nonesterified fatty acids by growth hormone in hypophysectomized and Houssay rats. *Endocrinology* 1965; **76**: 665–72.

31 Chernick SS, Clark CM, Gardiner RJ, Scow RO. Role of lipolytic and glucocorticoid hormones in the development of diabetic ketosis. *Diabetes* 1972; **21**: 946–54.

32 Moskowitz J, Fain JN. Stimulation by growth hormone and dexamethasone of labeled cyclic adenosine 3′,5′ - monophosphate accumulation by white fat cells. *J Biol Chem* 1970; **245**: 1101–7.

33 van Vliet G, Bosson D, Craen M, *et al.* Comparative study of the lipolytic potencies of pituitary-derived and biosynthetic human growth hormone in hypopituitary children. *J Clin Endocrinol Metab* 1987; **65**: 876–9.

● 34 Clemmons DR, Snyder DK, Williams R, Underwood LE. Growth hormone administration conserves lean body mass during dietary restriction in obese subjects. *J Clin Endocrinol Metab* 1987; **64**: 878–83.

35 Merimee IJ, Hollander SE. Studies of hyperlipidemia in hGH-deficient state. *Metabolism* 1972; **11**: 1053–61.

36 Winter RJ, Thompson RG, Green OC. Serum cholesterol and triglycerides in children with growth hormone deficiency. *Metabolism* 1979; **28**: 1244–9.

37 Rosenbaum M, Gertner J, Leibe RL. Effects of systemic growth hormone administration on regional adipose tissue distribution and metabolism in GH deficient children. *J Clin Endocrinol Metab* 1989; **69**: 1274–81.

38 Gregory JW, Greene SA, Jung RT, *et al.* Changes in body composition and energy expenditure after six weeks growth hormone treatment. *Arch Dis Child* 1991; **66**: 598–602.

39 Stahnke N, Stubbe P, Keller E, Zeisel HJ, and the Serono Study Group, Hamburg. Effects and side effects of GH plus oxandrolone in Turner syndrome. In: Ranke MB, Rosenfeld RG, eds.*Turner Syndrome.* Amsterdam: Excerpta Medica, Elsevier, 1991: 241–7.

40 Querfeld U, Haffner D, Wuhl E, *et al.* Treatment with growth hormone increases lipoprotein (a) serum levels in children with chronic renal insufficiency. *Pediatr Nephrol* 1994; **8**: C54.

41 Ikkos D, Luft R, Sjögren B. Body water and sodium in patients with acromegaly. *Clin Invest* 1954; **33**: 989–94.

42 Ho KY, Weissberger AJ. The antinatriuretic action of biosynthetic human growth hormone in man involves activation of the renin–angiotensin system. *Metabolism* 1990; **39**: 133–7.

43 Cuneo RC, Salomon F, Wilmhurst P, *et al.* Cardiovascular effects of growth hormone treatment in growth hormone deficient adults: stimulation of the renin–aldosterone system. *Clin* Sci 1991; **81**: 587–92.

44 Herlitz H, Jonsson O, Bengtsson B-A. Effect of recombinant human growth hormone on cellular metabolism. *Clin Sci* 1994; **86**: 233–7.

45 Hoffman DM, Crampton L, Ho KKY. GH increases body sodium but not blood pressure in GH deficient adults. *Endocrinol Metab* 1994; **1(Suppl B)**: 29.

46 Parra A, Argote RM, Garcia G, *et al.* Body composition in hypopituitary dwarfs before and during human growth hormone therapy. *Metabolism* 1979; **28**: 851–7.

47 Rifkind AB, Saenger P, Levine LS, *et al.* Effects of growth hormone on antipyrine kinetics in children. *Clin Pharmacol Ther* 1981; **30**: 127–32.

48 Henneman PH, Forbes AP, Moldawer M, *et al.* Effects of human growth hormone in man. *J Clin Invest* 1960; **39**: L233–8.

49 Biglieri EJ, Wadlington CO, Forsham P. Sodium retention with growth hormone and its subfractions. *J Clin Endocrinol Metab* 1961; **21**: 361–70.

50 Rudman D, Chyatte SB, Patterson JH, *et al.* Observations on the responsiveness of human subjects to human growth hormone. *J Clinical Invest* 1971; **50**: 1941–9.

51 Manson JM, Wilmore DW. Positive nitrogen balance with human growth hormone and hypocaloric intravenous feeding. *Surgery* 1986; **100**: 188–96.

52 Hintz RL. Untoward events in patients treated with growth hormone in the USA. *Horm Res* 1992; **38(Suppl)**: 44–9.

53 Ranke MB. Effects of growth hormone on the metabolism of lipids and water and their potential in causing adverse events during growth hormone treatment. *Horm Res* 1993; **39**: 104–6.

54 Moller J, Jorgenson JO, Moller N, *et al.* Expansion of extracellular volume and suppression of atrial natriuretic peptide after growth hormone administration in normal man. *J Clin Endocrinol Metab* 1991; **72**: 768–72.

55 Carvalho D, Vinha E, Portocarrero MC, *et al.* Atrial natriuretic peptide and renin–aldosterone axis in pituitary dwarfism. In: Cavil L, Job JC, New MI, eds. *Growth Disorders: The State of the Art.* New York: Raven Press, 1991.

56 DiMartino J, Wesoly S, Schartz L, Saenger P. Lack of clinical evidence of sodium retention in children with idiopathic short stature treated with recombinant growth hormone. *Metabolism* 1992; **42**: 730–4.

57 Barton JS, Hindmarsh PC, Preece MA, Brook CGD. Blood pressure and the renin angiotensin aldosterone system in children receiving recombinant human growth hormone. *Clin Endocrinol* 1993; **38**: 245–51.

58 Tönshoff B, Dietz M, Haffner D. Effects of 2 years of growth hormone treatment in short children with renal disease. *Acta Paediatr Scand Suppl* 1991; **379**: 33–41.

● 59 Fine RN, Kohaut EC, Brown D, Perlman AJ, and the Genentech Cooperative Study Group. Growth after recombinant human growth hormone treatment in children with chronic renal failure. *J Pediatr* 1993; **124**: 374–82.

60 Price DA, Clayton PE, Crowne EH, Roberts CR. Safety and efficacy of human growth hormone treatment in girls with Turner syndrome. *Horm Res* 1993; **39(Suppl 2)**: 44–8.

61 Malozowski S, Tanner LA, Wysowski D, Fleming GA. Growth hormone, insulin-like growth factor 1, and benign

intracranial hypertension. *New Engl J Med* 1993; **329**: 665–6.

62   Malozowski S, Tanner LA, Wysowski DK, *et al.* Benign intracranial hypertension in children with growth hormone deficiency treated with growth hormone. *J Pediatr* 1995a; **126**: 996–9.

◆ 63   Ogilvy-Stuart AL, Ryder WDJ, Gattamaneni HR, *et al.* Growth hormone and tumor recurrence. *BMJ* 1992; **304**: 1601–5.

64   Lawson Wilkins Pediatric Endocrine Society. Addendum to the minutes of the Drug and Therapeutics Committee. Washington, May 1991.

65   Blatt J, Penchansky L, Phebus C, Horn M. Leukemia in a child with a history of medulloblastoma. *Pediatr Hematol Oncol* 1991; **8**: 77–82.

66   Stahnke N, Zeisel HJ. Growth hormone therapy and leukaemia. *Eur J Pediatr* 1989; **148**: 591–6.

67   Stahnke N. Leukemia in growth hormone treated patients: An update, 1992. *Horm Res* 1992; **38(Suppl 1)**: 56–62.

68   Fradkin JE, Mills JL, Schonberger LB, *et al.* Risk of leukemia after treatment with pituitary growth hormone. *JAMA* 1993; **270**: 2829–32.

69   Nishi Y, Tanaka T, Takano K, *et al.* Recent status in the occurrence of leukemia in growth hormone-treated patients in Japan. GH Treatment Study Committee of the Foundation for Growth Science, Japan. *J Clin Endocrinol Metab* 1999; **84**: 1961–5.

✳ 70   Furlanetto RW. Guidelines for the use of growth hormone in children with short stature A report by the Drug and Therapeutics Committee of the LWPES. *J Pediatr* 1995; **127**: 857–67.

✳ 71   Wilson TA, Rose SR, Cohen P, *et al.* The Lawson Wilkins Pediatric Endocrinology Society Drug and Therapeutics Committee. Update of guidelines for the use of growth hormone in children: the Lawson Wilkins Pediatric Endocrinology Society Drug and Therapeutics Committee. *J Pediatr* 2003; **143**: 415–21.

72   Lee PDK, Rosenfeld RG, Hintz RL, Smith SD. Characterization of insulin, insulin-like growth factor I and II, and growth hormone receptors on human leukemic lymphoblasts. *J Clin Endocrinol Metab* 1986; **62**: 28–35.

73   Clayton PE, Shalet SM, Gattamaneni HR, Price DA. Does growth hormone cause relapse of brain tumors? *Lancet* 1987; **i**: 711–13.

74   Ogilvy-Stuart AL, Shalet SM. Tumor occurrence and recurrence. *Horm Res* 1992; **38(Suppl 1)**: 50–5.

75   Moshang T Jr. Is brain tumor recurrence increased following growth hormone treatment? *Trends Endocrinol Metab* 1995; **10**: 205–9.

● 76   Swerdlow AJ, Reddingius RE, Higgins CD, *et al.* Growth hormone treatment of children with brain tumors and risk of tumor recurrence. *J Clin Endocrinol Metab* 2000; **85**: 4444–9.

● 77   Sklar CA, Mertens AC, Mitby P, *et al.* Risk of disease recurrence and second neoplasms in survivors of childhood cancer treated with growth hormone: a report from the Childhood Cancer Survivor Study. *J Clin Endocrinol Metab* 2002; **87**: 3136–41.

78   Renehan AG, Zwahlen M, Minder C, *et al.* Insulin-like growth factor (IGF)-I, IGF binding protein-3, and cancer risk: systematic review and meta-regression analysis. *Lancet* 2004; **363**: 1346–53.

79   Roberts CT Jr. IGF-I and prostate cancer. *Novartis Found Symp* 2004; **262**: 193–9.

80   Lonning PE, Helle SI. IGF-I and breast cancer. *Novartis Found Symp* 2004; **262**: 205–12.

81   Sandhu MS, Dunger DB, Giovannucci EL. Insulin, insulin-like growth factor-I (IGF-I), IGF binding proteins, their biologic interactions, and colorectal cancer. *Natl Cancer Inst* 2002; **94**: 972–80.

● 82   Chan JM, Stampfer MJ, Giovannucci E, *et al.* Plasma insulin-like growth factor-I and prostate cancer risk – a prospective study. *Science* 1998; **279**: 563–6.

◆ 83   Cohen P, Clemmons DR, Rosenfeld RG. Does the GH-IGF axis play a role in cancer pathogenesis? *Growth Horm IGF Res* 2000; **10**: 297–305.

84   Grimberg A, Cohen P. Growth hormone and prostate cancer: guilty by association? *J Endocrinol Invest* 1999; **22(5 Suppl)**: 64–73.

85   Ogilvy-Stuart AL, Gleeson H. Cancer risk following growth hormone use in childhood: implications for current practice. *Drug Saf* 2004; **27**: 369–82.

86   Isaksson OGP, Nilsson A, Isgaard J, Lindahl A. Cartilage as a target tissue for growth hormone and insulin like growth factor 1. *Acta Paediatr Scand Suppl* 1990; **367**: 137–41.

87   Kelsey JL, Keggi KJ, Southwick WO. The incidence and distribution of slipped capital femoral epiphysis in Connecticut and Southwestern United States. *J Bone Joint Surg Am* 1970; **52**: 1203–16.

88   Rappaport ED, Fife D. Slipped capital femoral epiphysis in growth-hormone deficient patients. *Am J Dis Child* 1985; **139**: 396–9.

89   Blethen S, Rundle AC. Slipped capital femoral epiphysis in children treated with growth hormone. A summary of the National Cooperative Growth Study Experience. *Horm Res* 1996; **46**: 113–6.

90   Bains-Bailon R, Foley TP, Hintz RL, Lee P. Excessive growth hormone dosing in growth hormone deficiency. *Pediatr Res* 1992; **31**: 73A.

91   Wang ED, Drummond DS, Dormans JP, *et al.* Scoliosis in patients treated with growth hormone. *J Pediatr Orthop* 1997; **17**: 708–11.

92   August GP, Chandra R, Hung W. Prepubertal male gynecomastia. *J Pediatr* 1972; **80**: 259–63.

93   Latore H, Kenny FM. Idiopathic gynecomastia in seven preadolescent boys. *Am J Dis Child* 1973; **126**: 771–3.

◆ 94   Braunstein GD. Gynecomastia. *New Engl J Med* 1993; **328**: 490–5.

95   Cohn L, Feller AG, Draper MW, *et al.* Carpal tunnel syndrome and gynecomastia during growth hormone treatment of elderly men with low circulating IGF-I concentrations. *Clin Endocrinol* 1993; **39**: 417–25.

96   Malozowski S, Stadel BV. Prepubertal gynecomastia during growth hormone therapy. *J Pediatr* 1995; **126**: 659–61.

97 Bourguignon J, Pierard GE, Ernould C, *et al.* Effects of growth hormone therapy on melanocytic naevi. *Lancet* 1993; **341**: 1505–6.

♦ 98 Allen DB. Safety of human growth hormone therapy: Current topics. *J Pediatr* 1996; **128**: S8–13.

99 Malozowski S, Hung W, Stadel BV. Acute pancreatitis associated with growth hormone therapy for short stature. *New Engl J Med* 1995; **332**: 401–2.

100 Grunfeld C, Sherman BM, Cavalieri RR. The acute effects of GH administration on thyroid function in normal men. *J Clin Endocrinol Metab* 1988; **67**: 1111–4.

101 Jorgensen JO, Molle J, Skakkaboek NE, *et al.* Thyroid function during growth hormone therapy. *Horm Res* 1992; **38(Suppl 1)**: 63–7.

102 Walker BR, Andrew R, MacLeod KM, Padfield PL. Growth hormone replacement inhibits renal and hepatic 11 beta-hydroxysteroid dehydrogenases in ACTH-deficient patients. *Clin Endocrinol (Oxf)* 1998; **49**: 257–63.

● 103 Stewart PM, Toogood AA, Tomlinson JW. Growth hormone, insulin-like growth factor-I and the cortisol-cortisone shuttle. *Horm Res* 2001; **56(Suppl 1)**: 1–6.

104 Giavoli C, Libe R, Corbetta S, *et al.* Effect of recombinant human growth hormone (GH) replacement on the hypothalamic–pituitary–adrenal axis in adult GH-deficient patients. *J Clin Endocrinol Metab* 2004; **89**: 5397–401.

● 105 Bottner A, Keller E, Kratzsch J, *et al.* PROP1 mutations cause progressive deterioration of anterior pituitary function including adrenal insufficiency: a longitudinal analysis. *J Clin Endocrinol Metab* 2004; **89**: 5256–65.

106 Pedreira CC, Savarirayan R, Zacharin MR. IMAGe syndrome: a complex disorder affecting growth, adrenal and gonadal function, and skeletal development. *J Pediatr* 2004; **144**: 274–7.

● 107 Kaplan SL, Underwood LE, August GP, *et al.* Clinical studies with recombinant-DNA derived methionyl hGH in GH deficient children. *Lancet* 1986; **i**: 697–700.

108 Pitukcheewanont P, Schwarzbach L, Kaufman FR. Resumption of growth after methionyl-free human growth hormone therapy in a patient with neutralizing antibodies to methionyl human growth hormone. *J Pediatr Endocrinol Metab* 2002; **15**: 653–7.

109 Darendeliler F, Hindmarsh PC, Preece MA, *et al.* Growth hormone increases rate of pubertal maturation. *Acta Endocrinol Scand* 1990; **122**: 414–6.

110 Hindmarsh PC, Brook CGD. Final height of short normal children treated with growth hormone. *Lancet* 1996; **348**: 13–6.

111 Kawai M, Momoi T, Yorifuji T, *et al.* Unfavorable effects of growth hormone therapy on the final height of boys with short stature not caused by growth hormone deficiency. *J Pediatr* 1997; **130**: 205–9.

112 Rosenfeld RG. Is growth hormone just a tall story? *J Pediatr* 1997; **130**: 172–3.

● 113 Mauras N, Attie KM, Reiter EO, *et al.* High dose recombinant human growth hormone (GH) treatment of GH-deficient patients in puberty increases near-final height: a randomized, multicenter trial. Genentech, Inc, Cooperative Study Group. *J Clin Endocrinol Metab* 2000; **85**: 3653–60.

114 Bozzola M, Maccario R, Cisternio M, *et al.* Immunological and endocrinological response to growth hormone therapy in short children. *Acta Paediatr Scand* 1988; **77**: 675.

115 Rapaport R, Oleske J, Ahdich H, *et al.* Effects of human growth hormone on immune functions: In vitro studies on cells of normal and growth hormone deficient children. *Life Sci* 1987; **41**: 2319–24.

116 Rapaport R, Peterson B, Skuza KA, *et al.* Immune functions during treatment of growth hormone deficient children with biosynthetic human growth hormone. *Clin Pediatr* 1991; **30**: 22–7.

117 Peterson BH, Rapaport R, Henry DP, *et al.* Effect of treatment with biosynthetic human growth hormone (GH) on peripheral blood lymphocyte populations and function in growth hormone deficient children. *J Clin Endocrinol Metab* 1990; **70**: 1756–60.

118 Rapaport R. Immunomodulation by GH in humans. In: Berczi I, Szelenyi J, eds. *Advances in Psychoneuroimmunology.* New York: Plenum Press, 1994: 83–98.

119 Shah A, Stanhope R, Matthew D. Hazards of pharmacological tests of growth hormone secretion in childhood. *BMJ* 1992; **304**: 173–4.

120 Andersson HC, Markello T, Schneider JA, Gahl WA. Effect of growth hormone treatment on serum creatinine concentration in patients with cystinosis and chronic renal disease. *J Pediatr* 1992; **120**: 716–20.

121 Guest G, Berard E, Crognier H, Broyer M. Effects of recombinant growth hormone on growth and renal function in short children after renal transplantation. Data of the French Society of Pediatric Nephrology. The 2nd International Congress on Pediatric Transplantation. *Pediatr Nephrol* 1996; **10**: C51.

122 Benfield MR, Parker KL, Waldo FB, *et al.* Treatment of growth failure in children after renal transplantation. *Transplantation* 1993; **55**: 305–8.

123 Takai M, Izumino K, Oda Y, *et al.* Focal segmental glomerulosclerosis associated with acromegaly. *Clin Nephrol* 2001; **56**: 75–7.

124 Fukasawa H, Kato A, Fujimoto T, *et al.* Focal segmental glomerulosclerosis in a case of panhypopituitarism: a possible role of growth hormone treatment. *Clin Nephrol* 2002; **58**: 317–20.

125 Eiholzer U. Deaths in children with Prader-Willi syndrome. *Horm Res* 2005; **63**: 33–9.

126 Mills JL, Schonberger LB, Wysowski DK, *et al.* Long-term mortality in the United States cohort of pituitary-derived growth hormone recipients. *J Pediatr* 2004; **144**: 430–6.

127 Taback SP, Dean HJ. Mortality in Canadian children with growth hormone (GH) deficiency receiving GH therapy 1967-1992. The Canadian Growth Hormone Advisory Committee. *J Clin Endocrinol Metab* 1996; **81**: 1693–6.

128   Takala J, Ruokonen E, Webster NR, *et al.* Increased mortality associated with growth hormone treatment in critically ill adults. *N Engl J Med* 1999; **341**: 785–92.

129   Belcher HJ, Mercer D, Judkins KC, *et al.* Biosynthetic growth hormone in burned patients: A pilot study. *Burns* 1989; **15**: 99–107.

130   Marcus R, Butterfield G, Holloway L, *et al.* Effects of short term administration of recombinant human growth hormone to elderly people. *J Clin Endocrinol Metab* 1990; **70**: 519–27.

131   Snyder DK, Underwood LE, Clemmons DR. Anabolic effects of growth hormone in obese diet restricted subjects are dose dependent. *Am J Clin Nutr* 1990; **52**: 431–7.

● 132   Ziegler TR, Young LS, Ferrari-Baliviera E, *et al.* Use of human growth hormone combined with nutritional support in a critical care unit. *J Parent Enter Nutr* 1990; **14**: 574–81.

133   Quigley CA, Gill AM, Crowe BJ, *et al.* Safety of growth hormone treatment in pediatric patients with idiopathic short stature. *J Clin Endocrinol Metab* 2005; **90**: 5188–96.

46

Medical management of tall stature

STENVERT L S DROP, SABINE M P F DE MUINCK KEIZER-SCHRAMA

EVIDENCE SCORING OF THERAPY

    * Non-randomized controlled trials, cohort study, etc.
  ** One or more well-designed randomized controlled trials
*** Systematic review or meta-analysis

INTRODUCTION

Whereas there are as many children growing above the 97th percentile (corresponding to +1.8 SDS) as below the 3rd percentile, tall stature is far less frequently a reason for seeking medical attention than short stature. Tall stature is more easily accepted in society and may be even, at some points, an advantage. This holds particularly true for boys and therefore girls are more often referred.

Growth is the result of complex processes. Multiple factors such as genetic constitution, nutrition, endocrine function and psychosocial well being are involved in the process of growth.[1,2] The genetic component of height has been estimated to be in the order of 0.75, i.e., 75 percent of the height variation is accounted for by genetic factors. Therefore, assessment of the parental height as an indicator of the genetic component of growth and development of the child is of critical importance.[3,4]

In addition socio-economic factors that are associated with growth are social class, family size, birth rank, housing, and crowding. Improved socio-economic conditions and more widespread health have led to the manifestation of a positive secular trend in growth and development over the past few centuries. As an example, in 1865 the mean adult height among Dutch recruits was 165 cm. One century later, in 1965, the mean adult height in boys was 178 cm. Fifteen years later, in 1980, the mean adult height had increased by another 4 cm to 182 cm and to 184 cm in 1997.[5] In the middle of the nineteenth century age of menarche in European girls was at about 16–17 years. Nowadays the mean age of menarche is 13 years or even younger.

Remarkably, studies of fossil remains of our hominid ancestors demonstrate that the stature of individuals living during the last hundreds to thousands of years reaches the range of heights seen today: the mean stature of early anatomically modern *Homo sapiens* in Europe was 184 cm in males and 167 cm in females.[6,7] Probably, phenomena responsible for positive and negative secular trends have affected height throughout all our history. Indeed, Maat found that the positive secular shift that has been occurring in the Netherlands since about 1850 was preceded by a negative secular shift. His observation is based on measurements of stature collected from deceased males, either *in situ* in the grave or from cadavers in the Low Countries during the years 50–2000 AD.[8]

In recent years knowledge with regard to the auxology and (neuro)endocrinology of tall stature has expanded. In addition long-term results of height reducing treatment modalities have become available. In this chapter the differential diagnosis and the therapeutic modalities available in the management of tall stature will be reviewed.

Studies of children with constitutional tall stature (CTS) indicate that tall stature may be due at least in part to increased growth hormone (GH) secretion. Studying children with various heights a significant positive correlation has been found between growth and GH secretion.[9–11]

More recent studies on the role of the system of the insulin-like growth factors, their receptors and binding proteins indicate that in CTS the most GH dependent component i.e., IGF-I levels are normal.[12] However, IGF-II levels may be increased, in agreement with the finding of high

IGF-II levels in some overgrowth syndromes.[13] Moreover, the IGF/IGFBP molar ratio may be increased and, therefore a greater availability of free IGF for target tissues may be responsible for overgrowth in CTS.[14]

Experiments of nature clearly illustrate the dominant role estrogens rather than androgens play in bone maturation and thus the attainment of adult height. In cases reported of men lacking estrogen activity as a result of aromatase deficiency or as a result of an inactivating mutation of the estrogen receptor,[15,16] bone maturation is severely retarded and growth continues far into adulthood as the epiphyses do not close. In contrast, XY females with the complete androgen insensitivity syndrome (AIS) have a pubertal growth spurt typical of normal females, both in magnitude and timing.[17]

Of particular interest are recent observations that overdosage of short stature homeobox containing (SHOX) genes located on the pseudo-autosomal region of the X-chromosome may be the mechanism explaining tall stature in 47,XXY, Klinefelter syndrome and the 47,XXX female syndrome.[18]

AUXOLOGY

Height prediction plays a key role in the management of children with growth disorders. In fact, possible intervention is based on the estimated height prognosis. Hence accurate techniques for reliable height prediction are essential. In clinical practice various methods have been developed of which the methods developed by Tanner, Bayley, and Pinneau are most commonly used.[19,20] They both share the use of bone age as an indicator of skeletal maturity in order to estimate final adult height. The first prediction method uses the bone age method developed by Tanner,[19] whereas the latter utilizes the method of Greulich and Pyle (1959). Many of the potential problems underlying bone age determination methods have to be considered. For instance both techniques make use of subjective processes and of discontinuous scales which result in considerable inter- and intravariability.[21-23]

An inventory among pediatricians has shown that up to 76 percent use the Greulich and Pyle technique to assess skeletal age.[24] The G and P technique is relatively easy to perform and can be incorporated easily into daily clinical practice. Although the radiographs for the atlas were collected between 1931 and 1942 in the Cleveland area of Ohio, USA, a recent study in the Netherlands has shown that the G and P atlas is still applicable in modern day Dutch Caucasian children and adolescents.[25]

Height prediction models are based on growth data derived from normal growing children of normal stature. This implies that these methods may not give accurate results when applied to children with growth disturbances. In a recent study the reliability of various prediction methods was evaluated in 55 healthy untreated boys and 88 girls with CTS.[26] In Table 46.1 the accuracy of the height prediction methods is expressed as predicted height minus actual adult

Table 46.1 Error of prediction of various final height prediction methods according to chronological age in 88 female and 55 male healthy tall individuals. Reproduced with permission from De Waal et al.[27]

Age (years)	No.	BP (cm)	TW (cm)	CASAS (cm)
Males				
12	7	4.2 (4.8)	0.3 (5.6)	−1.6 (6.8)
13	14	4.6 (4.3)	2.7 (4.7)	−0.6 (4.3)
14	16	2.7 (2.9)	0.2 (3.0)	−0.7 (2.6)
15	12	0.6 (1.3)	−5.8 (2.4)	−5.0 (2.0)
16	6	1.2 (3.4)	−4.2 (2.4)	−3.6 (1.9)
All	55	2.8 (3.6)	−0.9 (4.8)	−1.7 (4.2)
		[−6.0;11.5]	[−11.3;11.3]	[−15.6;6.4]
Females				
11	16	−0.1 (4.2)	−1.7 (4.7)	−2.5 (4.6)
12	21	1.4 (2.5)	−1.2 (2.5)	−1.0 (2.2)
13	26	0.5 (2.2)	−0.3 (1.9)	−0.1 (2.6)
14	13	0.5 (2.5)	0.5 (3.4)	−0.4 (3.5)
15	12	−0.2 (1.5)	−0.2 (3.0)	0.4 (2.4)
All	88	0.5 (2.7)	−0.8 (3.1)	−0.7 (3.2)
		[−6.8;7.6]	[−10.1;7.7]	[−13.3;9.6]

BP, Bayley and Pinneau; TW, Tanner and Whitehouse; CASAS, Computer-aided skeletal age scoring system.[27a]
Data are expressed as the mean (SD), with range in brackets.

height attained at a mean age of 25 years. Predictions are in general more accurate in girls than in boys, and, as expected, accuracy improves with advancement of (bone) age. From this study it is concluded that in boys and girls with CTS the most reliable prediction method is to extrapolate height SDS for BA (determined according to the method of Greulich and Pyle). In addition, in girls the prediction according to the method of Bailey and Pinneau is as reliable. Nevertheless the mean absolute errors of the single prediction methods were still considerable, varying from 2.3 to 5.3 cm in boys and from 1.9 to 3.7 cm in girls with individual errors up to 20 cm, reflecting the only relative reliability of the prediction in any one individual. Based on the above data, new prediction equations models were developed and additionally tested in untreated tall children.[27] The regression equations are given in Table 46.2. These equations showed satisfying accuracy in height prognosis: the mean (SD) error of prediction −1.4 (3.2) cm in boys and −0.5 (3.1) cm in girls.

DIFFERENTIAL DIAGNOSIS

Most children with tall stature are perfectly healthy. Nevertheless careful evaluation is indicated as tallness may be part of a disease or syndrome with far reaching consequences.

The possible etiology of tall stature is summarized in Table 46.3. A detailed description of the various syndromes is beyond the scope of this chapter and the reader is referred to excellent reviews.[28,29] Information specifically relevant

Table 46.2 Regression equations for prediction of final height in constitutional tall stature (Reproduced with permission from De Waal *et al.*[27])

	n	Equation to calculate the value of FH	RSD (cm)
Boys	71	$213.66 + 0.62 \times H + 0.29 \times TH - 10.49 \times CA - 12.98 \times BA_{GP} + 0.72 \times (CA \times BA_{GP})$	2.6
Girls	103	$129.42 + 0.74 \times H + 0.17 \times TH - 7.70 \times BA_{GP} - 5.90 \times CA + 0.41 \times (CA \times BA_{GP})$	2.7

FH, final height; H, height; TH, target height; CA, chronological age; BA_{GP}, bone age by Greulich and Pyle method; RSD, residual standard deviation.

Table 46.3 The differential diagnosis of tall stature

A   Variants of normal growth: Constitutional (familial) tall stature
B   Primary growth disorders
1   Sex-chromosome related disorders
  • Klinefelter syndrome and variants
  • XXY syndrome
  • XYY syndrome
2   Overgrowth syndromes with advanced bone maturation
  • Sotos syndrome
  • Weaver syndrome
  • Marshall-Smith syndrome
3   Additional syndromes with overgrowth and advanced bone maturation
  • Beckwith Wiedemann syndrome
  • Hyperinsulinism
4   Syndromes with tall stature as outstanding feature
  • Marfan syndrome
  • Marfanoid phenotype
  • MEN IIB
  • Homocysteinuria
  • Estrogen inactivity/resistance
C   Secondary growth disorders
  • GH excess
  • Precocious (pseudo) puberty

from the history and physical examination is given in the table. Whenever available, use should be made of population based or disorder specific growth charts (www. Growth analyzer.org). A diagnostic algorithm is presented in Fig. 46.1.

Constitutional tall stature

Constitutional tall stature (CTS) is a variant of the normal pattern of childhood growth and constitutes 3–10 percent of the normal population, depending on the definition used. Usually, one or both parents are also tall reflecting the importance of genetic and familial factors in etiology and pathogenesis. Mean birth length is at or above the 75th percentile (0.7 SDS) and tall stature becomes evident at the age of 3–4 years. Growth velocity is accelerated in early childhood but slows down after 4–5 years of age when the growth curve starts to parallel the normal curve.[30] The diagnosis is generally made from the family history, a record of growth and physical examination. No apparent abnormalities are present on physical examination which makes it possible to distinguish CTS from primary or secondary excessive growth syndromes (see Tables 46.3 and 46.4).

Primary growth disorders

SEX-CHROMOSOME RELATED DISORDERS

Klinefelter syndrome (and variants)

This syndrome was first described by Klinefelter in 1942 and results from the presence of one or more additional X-chromosomes (47,XXY, 48,XXXY, 49,XXXXY). Aneuploidy of the X chromosome is the result of non-dysjunction during first or second meiotic partition during gemeogenesis, or during one of the first mitotic partitions following fertilization. The additional X-chromosome in the 47,XXY karyotype is as frequently of maternal or paternal origin. The phenotype is similar. A correlation between parental age and the occurrence of this syndrome has been claimed. In addition an increased incidence following *in vitro* fertilization (ICSI) has been suggested.[31] The prevalence is 1:1000/1500 boys.

The clinical features include excessively long legs, poor school performance, and small testes already present at a pre-pubertal age. Tall stature is not only the result of additional chromosomal material but also from inadequate sexual development, allowing growth to continue at a normal rate beyond the usual age of cessation. This explains the eunuchoidal body proportions. The testes are small because of hyelinization and fibrosis of the seminiferous tubules. However, most often puberty develops normally although testosterone levels may be low to low normal. Gonadotrophin levels, specifically FSH levels are increased after the age of 12 years. The increased estrogen/testosterone ratio explains the occurrence of gynecomastia during adolescence. Whereas the height is frequently in the upper percentiles it is seldom far above the 97th percentile and for that reason height reducing therapy is most often not indicated. Mental retardation is not an obligatory feature. There may, however, be behavioral problems at home or at school and it is for that reason that an early diagnosis is recommended to enable proper psychosocial counseling.

XXX syndrome

Girls with a 47,XXX karyotype are frequently tall, albeit not excessively.[32,33] Their phenotype is completely female, pubertal development is normal and the body proportions are not eunuchoidal. The prevalence is 1:1000 girls and a

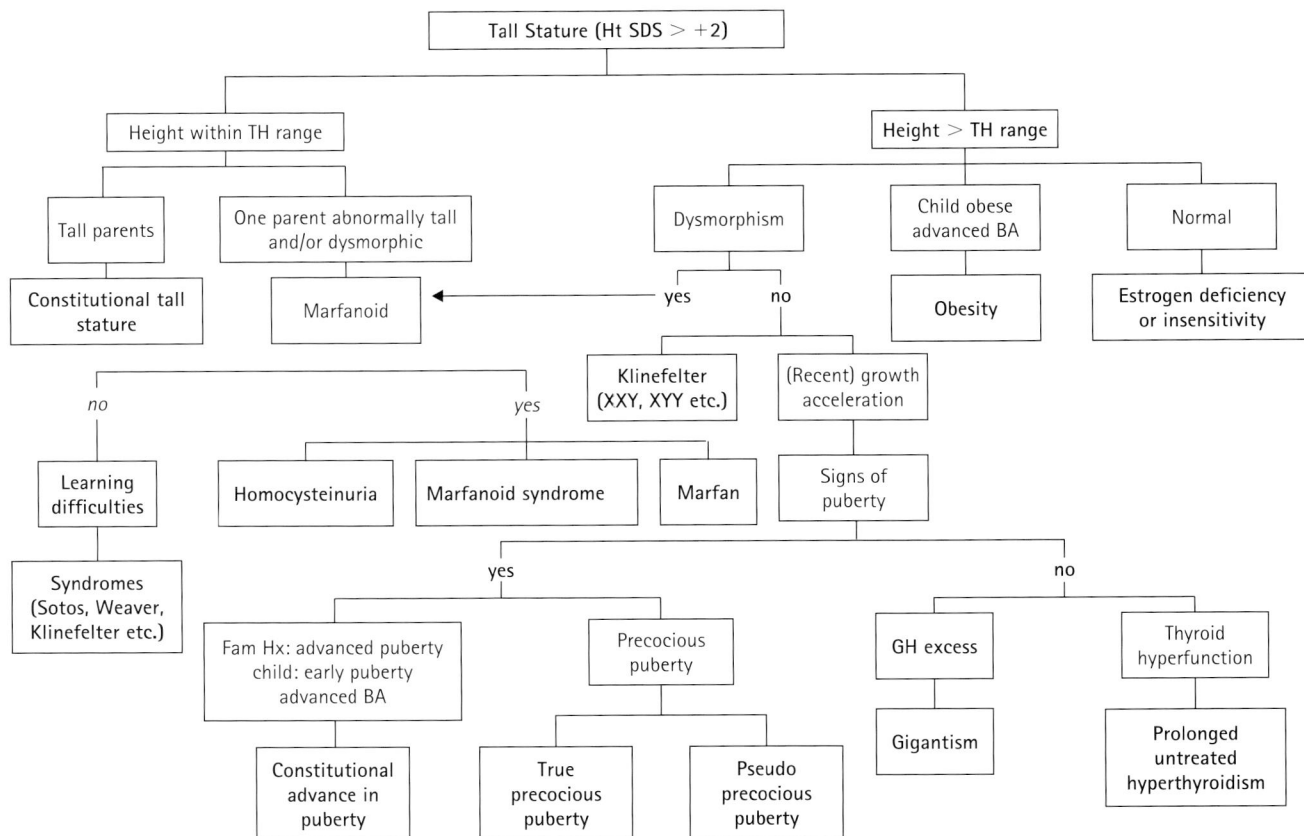

Figure 46.1 Diagnostic flow chart to aid the differential diagnosis in individuals with conditions causing overgrowth.

Table 46.4 History and physical examination in a tall child

History
Pregnancy and birth details
Birth weight, length, head circumference
Parents and sibling heights[a] and pubertal timing
Developmental milestones
Family history of ocular or cardiovascular disease
Neurological abnormalities
Nutrition
System review, e.g. hypoglycemia

Physical examination
Height, weight, head circumference
Growth chart: growth velocity
Body proportions: sitting height; lower segment; arm span
Dysmorphic features
Pubertal status
Thyroid status
Musculoskeletal status: joint laxity, contractures, arachnodactyly, acral enlargement, spinal deformity
Gynecomastia
Neurological examination
Cardiovascular examination

[a]Obtain actual measurements.

relation with increased parental age has been suggested. Because of lack of specific symptoms it is estimated that many girls with this syndrome remain undiagnosed. In girls with a final height prognosis above the target height range,

specifically if there is evidence of dysmorphism and psychomotor retardation, the possibility of triple X syndrome should be considered.[34,35] Even after onset of puberty pubertal development may slow down or even arrest, leading to an increment of final height prognosis.

XYY syndrome

With a prevalence of 1:1000 in the normal population, most boys with the 47,XYY syndrome remain undiagnosed. They may be rather but not excessively tall.[32,36] They may suffer from severe acne during puberty and sometimes radio-ulnar synostosis is found. Other features include psychomotor delay.

OVERGROWTH SYNDROMES WITH ADVANCED BONE MATURATION

These overgrowth syndromes are not always sharply defined and comprise a group of disorders with the following common characteristics: increased birth length and weight, advanced growth and bone maturation during the first years of life, but retarded mental development.

Sotos syndrome

Sotos syndrome is characterized by pre- and post-natal overgrowth, macrocephaly, advanced bone age and typical facial features. Haploinsufficiency of the *NSD1* gene has been identified as the major cause, with intragenic mutations or submicroscopic micro-deletions found in about 50–75 percent of clinically diagnosed patients.[37,38]

Most often final height remains within the normal range and height reducing therapy is not indicated. These children have the physical appearance of being older accentuating their developmental retardation.

Weaver syndrome

Weaver syndrome is a condition closely linked to Sotos syndrome. However, there are distinctive craniofacial features. Final height might be beyond the normal range, which is remarkable in view of the advanced bone maturation. *NSD1* mutations have been found in a significant percentage of patients.[39,40]

Marshall–Smith syndrome

Children with the Marshall–Smith syndrome may have some clinical similarities with the Weaver syndrome. Phenotypically there are heavy eyebrows, proptosis, and megalocornea with blue sclerae. X-ray of the hand reveals not only a markedly advanced bone age but also abnormalities of the metacarpal bones and the phalanges.[41]

ADDITIONAL SYNDROMES WITH OVERGROWTH AND ADVANCED BONE MATURATION

Beckwith–Wiedemann syndrome

Characteristic features of the Beckwith–Wiedemann syndrome are macroglossia, abdominal wall defects, visceromegaly, embryonal tumors, hemihyperplasia, ear and renal abnormalities, and neonatal hypoglycemia. Dysregulation of imprinted growth-regulating genes within chromosome 15 is considered the major cause.[42] During the first 4–6 years of life there is an advanced growth rate but thereafter height and weight normalize because of an advanced bone maturation and final height remains most often within the normal range.

Perinatal macrosomia

Hyperinsulinism, as in persistent hyperinsulinemic hypoglycemia of infancy (PHHI, nesidioblastosis) or in infants of diabetic mothers, will result in overgrowth. Following proper treatment and resolution of hypoglycemia normal growth will resume.

SYNDROMES WITH TALL STATURE AS OUTSTANDING FEATURE

Marfan syndrome

Marfan syndrome is an autosomal dominant inherited disorder with complete penetrance but highly variable expression even within families. The prevalence is 1:10 000. In the early 1990s mutations were discovered in the fibrillin gene (*FBN1*) located on the long arm of chromosome 15 and a large gene mutation data base is now available.[43] The syndrome involves many systems and diagnostic criteria have been proposed and recently revised.[44,45] In young children the diagnosis may be

difficult. Later on, symptoms such as tall extremities, hyperlaxicity of joints, and visual problems resulting from myopia or lens subluxation may become more prominent. Cardiac anomalies may be found on echocardiography. A dissecting aneurysm is a life-threatening condition.

Height limiting therapy may be considered because of the excessively tall stature[46] and it may also arrest kyphosis and scoliosis. A multidisciplinary approach involving pediatric cardiologist, orthopedic surgeon, ophthalmologist, and endocrinologist is highly recommended.

Marfanoid phenotype

The marfanoide habitus has been described in several syndromes of which the MENIIB syndrome and homocysteinuria are the most prominent.

MEN IIB syndrome

The multiple endocrine neoplasia syndrome II B is an autosomal dominant inherited disorder caused by an activating mutation (*M918T*) in the tyrosine kinase domain of the *RET* proto-oncogene localized on chromosome 10. The syndrome is characterized by the almost obligatory occurrence of medullar thyroid carcinoma, pheochromocytoma, and hyperparathyroidism. The type IIB form has additionally typical phenotypical characteristics such as diffuse ganglioneuromatosis of the digestive tract and Marfanoid body proportions.[47]

Homocysteinuria

Homocysteinuria is an autosomal-recessive disorder caused by a deficiency of the enzyme cysthionine L-synthetase. The gene is located on chromosome 21q22.3 and many mutations have been identified. Clinically, this disorder is characterized by a marfanoid habitus, arachnodactyly, pectus excavatum or carinatum, and subluxation of the lens of the eye, mental retardation, and juvenile osteoporosis. The diagnosis is confirmed by increased serum levels of methionine and homocysteine or increased homocysteine excretion in the urine. Optimizing metabolic control may help to reduce excessive growth.[48]

Estrogen deficiency/resistance

Cases have been reported of men lacking estrogen activity as a result of aromatase deficiency or secondary to an inactivating mutation of the estrogen receptor. Bone maturation is severly retarded and long bones continue to grow far into adulthood as the epiphyses do not close.[15,16,49,50]

Secondary growth disorders

GROWTH HORMONE EXCESS

Pituitary gigantism is caused by excessive GH secretion before fusion of the epiphyses, while acromegaly occurs after their fusion. The possibility of pathologic growth should be considered in all individuals who exceed mean normal height by 3 SD. Probably a more rigorous criterion would be to consider growth abnormal in those individuals whose growth exceeds that predicted by midparental height by 2 SD.[51] The syndromes of childhood gigantism and adult acromegaly are most often due to excess pituitary GH production. In most patients this is caused by well-defined pituitary adenomas, but somatotroph or mammosomatotroph hyperplasia with detectable or undetectable circulating GH-releasing hormone (GHRH) levels has also been reported.[52,53] Very rarely excessive growth may be secondary to an optic glioma.[54] About 30–50 percent of pituitary adenomas of patients with gigantism have mutations of the alpha-subunit of stimulatory GTP binding proteins.[55,56] The mutation leads to constitutive activation of the G_s protein, causing increased adenylate cyclase activity. The oncogene that is generated by these mutations is termed *gsp*. This increased second messenger activation is thought to induce tumor growth.[57] In about 20 percent of patients with gigantism excessive pituitary GH secretion from an adenoma and/or somatotroph hyperplasia is associated with the McCune–Albright syndrome.[58,59] Polyostotic fibrous dysplasia, café-au-lait pigmentation of the skin and a number of other endocrine syndromes like sexual precocity, hyperthyroidism, and adrenal hyperplasia can complicate the signs and symptoms of gigantism in such patients. Affected tissues from patients with McCune–Albright syndrome have also been reported to contain activating mutations of the G_s alpha gene.[60–62] This suggest that a single point mutation of the G_s alpha gene might in some individuals lead to both the development of McCune–Albright syndrome and pituitary adenomas causing gigantism.

Ectopic secretion of GHRH from peripheral neuroendocrine tumors such as carcinoids located in the lung, thymus and gut, or islet cell tumors, very seldomly cause the clinical picture of childhood gigantism.[63–65] Even rarer are cases of eutopic GHRH hypersecretion from hypothalamic hamartomas or gangliocytomas.[63,66]

The clinical picture of gigantism during childhood is best characterized by excessive growth (see above), while the classical signs and symptoms of acromegaly as they occur in adults (soft tissue swelling, paraesthesia, carpal tunnel syndrome, headaches, excessive perspiration) are less impressive in children. Stigmata of McCune–Albright syndrome can help early diagnosis.

The diagnosis of pituitary gigantism is established by demonstration of the clinical features, the result of laboratory testing, and radiological investigation.

Although randomly sampled levels of GH in children with pituitary gigantism are typically high, normal children and adolescents may also have episodically high GH levels, that are not suppressed by oral glucose loading,[67] or respond with a paradoxical increase in response to the intravenous administration of thyrotropin releasing hormone.[68] Excessive secretion of GH is in most individuals confirmed by clearly elevated circulating IGF-I levels above the age standards, but interpretation can be misleading during pubertal years.[51] Most patients with gigantism and

pituitary adenomas have macroadenomas at the time of diagnosis. These tumors with a diameter above 1 cm often cause hypopituitarism, and in the case of supra-sellar extension headaches and/or visual field impairments. Apart from secondary hypothyroidism, hypoadrenalism and hypogonadism ('reversal of puberty'), increased circulating prolactin (PRL) levels often indicates the presence of a (mixed GH/PRL) secreting pituitary macroadenoma.

In children with excessive, potential pathologic, growth, and biochemical evidence of high GH release, an early differential diagnosis between physiologic and pathologic growth remains difficult, while the results of laboratory tests can be ambiguous. Most practising pediatricians tend to wait for 3–6 months in order to document the growth rate. However, radiological and nuclear medical techniques can be helpful to visualize pituitary abnormalities. Magnetic resonance imaging (MRI) investigation reveals pituitary adenomas with very small sizes (below 3 mm in diameter), while somatostatin receptor imaging (Octreoscan) visualizes virtually all peripheral carcinoids and islet cell tumors secreting GHRH ectopically.

PRECOCIOUS PUBERTY

For the sake of completeness, precocious puberty, either central or pseudo-precocious puberty, is mentioned here as it results in relative tall stature at a pre-pubertal age. However, final height may be seriously compromised as a result of advanced progression of bone maturation and early closure of the epiphyses. A detailed description of the pathophysiology of precocious puberty is beyond the scope of this chapter and the reader is referred to Chapter 40.

TREATMENT OF CONSTITUTIONAL TALL STATURE

Psychosocial problems in tall adolescents have been recognized by pediatricians and endocrinologists and treatment of constitutional tall stature is generally on psychological grounds. Although psychosocial factors form the main reason for treatment, extensive psychological investigations before or during height reductive therapy has never been performed.[69] However, many clinicians share their experiences that some children with excessive growth may suffer considerably from being much taller than others. Many tall adolescents feel different from their peers and may develop coping mechanisms such as kyphotic posture and social withdrawal. In addition, practical problems such as clothing and shoe sizes, fear about future compatible partnering and career-planning are also frequently reported problems faced by tall adolescents. On the other hand, there is no doubt that many tall adolescents have no concern at all about their height. In fact in our culture tallness is generally valued positively. An association between physical stature and achievement has been documented; tall individuals score higher on intelligence tests than short individuals and persons who achieved higher social status tend to be taller than those of lower status.[70–72] Various studies in adolescent boys and girls have shown an association between physical status and self-esteem or body-satisfaction.[73–76] Studies relating height and self-esteem showed conflicting results.

In a retrospective survey among young adults with CTS no major psychological maladjustment was found in previously treated tall children compared to tall controls.[69]

As discussed above the indication for treatment is practically limited to CTS perhaps with the exception of individual cases of children with Marfan syndrome.[46]

Sex steroids (***)

The basis for the use of sex steroids to limit adult height stems from observations in children with precocious puberty. Early closure of the epiphyses due to premature secretion of gonadal steroids limits their eventual final height.

Since the original description of Goldzieher in 1956[77] treating adolescent tall girls with high doses of sex steroids, many reports have appeared describing the height reducing effects of administration of high doses of estrogens in girls and androgens in boys.[78–84] There is general agreement that a favorable effect on ultimate height results from such pharmacological therapy, the height reduction being greater when the treatment has begun at a younger age and/or bone age.

In a large scale retrospective study investigating the reliability and accuracy of the various prediction methods in children with CTS the effect of sex-steroid treatment was evaluated in 60 boys and 159 girls.[26] At the end of the treatment period an average height reduction was obtained of 4.1–6.9 cm in girls and 2.7–6.9 cm in boys. At a mean age of 25.1 years final height measurements were obtained. A post-treatment growth had occurred averaging from 2.4 in boys and 2.7 cm in girls. This post-treatment growth was clearly negatively correlated with the bone age at the time of discontinuation of sex-steroid therapy.

As shown in Fig. 46.2 the ultimate height reduction corrected for differences between treated and non-treated controls and for inaccuracy of the prediction methods is strongly related to the bone age at the time of start of treatment.

A remarkable finding is that in boys in whom treatment was initiated at or beyond a bone age of 14 years and in girls at or beyond a bone age of 15 years[85] no improvement or even additional growth was observed.

It is of specific interest to note that in boys the addition of estrogens to androgen treatment for the first 6 weeks of treatment had no effect on height reduction.[86]

Side effects of sex–steroid treatment (***)

In girls supraphysiological doses of ethinyl estradiol have been advocated ranging from 100 to 300 μg day⁻¹ orally in combination with progestagens (medroxy-progesterone

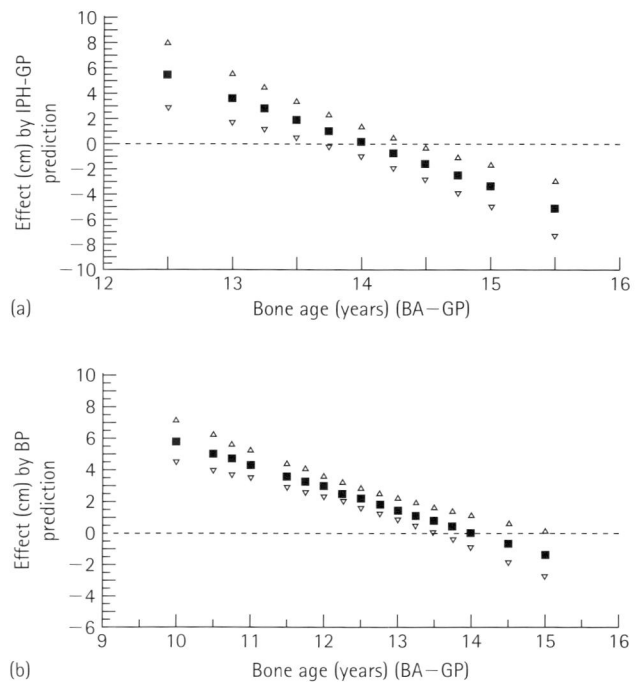

(a)

(b)

Figure 46.2 Adjusted effect of (a) androgen or (b) estrogen therapy and 95 percent confidence intervals by bone age (BA) in (a) constitutionally tall boys and (b) constitutionally tall girls. IPH, index of potential height; BP, Bayley and Pinneau; GP, Greulich and Pyle (final height was predicted on the assumption that the height SDS for bone age, determined according to BP, remains constant. (Reproduced with permission from De Waal et al.[26])

5–10 mg day⁻¹ orally every 5–12 days of the month). Boys have been given testosterone in the form of intermuscularly administered testosterone-ester depot preparations at a dosage of 250–1000 mg per month.[69]

It is well-known that treatment with sex steroids may have effects on hemostasis, lipid metabolism, and functioning of the hypothalamo-gonadal axis. In addition, there is an impressive body of data available on the association between the long-term use of oral contraceptives (OCs) and possible health risks reflecting prospective risks in estrogen-treated girls. Nevertheless, so far, most unwanted side effects reported during or shortly after discontinuation of therapy were found to be mild and, specifically, suppression of the hypothalamo-gonadal axis was found to be reversible.[87–90]

Long-term effects were evaluated in a retrospective study pertaining to 64 tall adult men and 180 adult women who received supra-physiological doses of sex-steroids during puberty. Sixty-one untreated tall men and 94 untreated tall women served as controls. They were interviewed in a standardized way at a mean follow-up period of 10 years after cessation of treatment.[91] Most reported side effects were mild: in girls menstrual cycle characteristics of previously treated women were comparable with controls. Post-treatment amenorhea of longer than 6 months was found in 5 percent of the women. Information about

127 pregnancies was gathered and revealed no significant differences. Malignancy was not reported. In a recent large retrospective survey in Australia pertaining to 371 estrogen-treated women and 409 untreated tall women, treated women were more likely to have difficulty in becoming pregnant.[92]

In boys aggravation of acne was most often reported during treatment (39 percent) followed by gynecomastia (13 percent). In a subset of 43 treated and 30 untreated tall men a detailed evaluation of gonadal function was performed. Sperm quality and testis volumes were comparable between treated and non-treated men. Serum values of testosterone, SHBG and gonadotrophins were in the normal range although FSH levels were higher in treated men. Varicocele (left-sided) was present in the combined group of treated and untreated men in 42 percent.[93]

In a retrospective study, psychosocial information was obtained via various questionnaires in 424 adult men and women with constitutional tall stature of whom 243 had been treated for their tallness during childhood with high doses of sex hormones. In retrospect, previously treated tall men and women indicated that they experienced more problems related to their height than tall controls: they were teased more frequently and experienced more remarks and jokes about their stature. Tall subjects did very well in terms of education and employment. In conclusion, no major psychological maladjustment was found in previously treated compared to untreated tall controls.[91]

A similar study[89] did not reveal any major psychological maladjustment in previously treated tall children compared to untreated children. No distinct differences were found in psychological well-being, social anxiety self-esteem, and body perception. Compared to the normal population tall subjects did very well in terms of education and employment confirming the idea that tallness is linked to occupational success.

Surgery (*)

Limb shortening, for instance by bilateral epiphysiodesis above and below the knee, has been suggested for the treatment of excessive tall stature. The risk of major complications does not outweigh the potential benefits in otherwise healthy children.[94] Epiphysiodesis is discussed in detail in Chapter 47.

Treatment of secondary tall stature (*)

Most patients with gigantism have pituitary macroadenomas with extrasellar extension. Trans-sphenoidal surgery is indicated in order to debulk or totally remove the tumor. In some patients 'cure' is accomplished by this surgical procedure,[95,96] but persistent excessive GH release from tumor remnants is often observed. Apart from re-operation, resulting in near total hypophysectomy[51] alternatives include

external pituitary irradiation and medical therapy. The effects of external irradiation are slow, involving several years during which excessive growth is not controlled. Also in long-term follow-up anterior pituitary insufficiency is observed in more than 50 percent of acromegalic patients.[97] Medical therapy with dopamine agonists such as bromocriptine only seldomly normalizes GH and IGF-I levels.[58,97] A long-acting somatostatin analog such as octreotide suppresses GH release from pituitary tumor remnants or somatotroph hyperplasia in most patients with gigantism with achievement of satisfactory GH and IGF-I levels in about 60 percent of the patients.[52,53,98–100] However, insufficient data are currently available concerning the question whether octreotide therapy controls GH and IGF-I levels to such an extent that excessive body growth is also suppressed.

Most recently growth hormone receptor antagonists have become available. GH inhibiting activity is based on the fact that it prevents proper dimerization of the GH receptor and therefore inhibits GH action. In adults it has been proven to be the most effective drug to normalize IGF-I levels (in over 90 percent of the patients).[101] Clinical follow-up in these patients is further complicated by the simultaneous presence of partial or total hypopituitarism.[102]

In conclusion, the primary treatment of childhood gigantism involves trans-sphenoidal surgery or the surgical removal of peripheral neuroendocrine tumors secreting GHRH ectopically.

KEY LEARNING POINTS

- It is recommended that tall children are referred in the late pre-pubertal period to secure proper pre-treatment evaluation of growth and bone maturation. Treatment is restricted to excessive tallness (i.e., $< +2.5$ SDS) or when there is a very outspoken professional desire where height forms a clear limitation (such as ballet dancer, pilot).
- Careful attention should be paid to the individual psychosocial problems related to tallness, especially in relation to the socio-cultural environment, when considering treatment. The family need a full explanation of possible risks and benefits of treatment and to be aware of limitations of height prediction methods. In girls a thorough family history is taken for thrombo-embolic disorders and breast cancer.
- Treatment may be initiated at an early bone age (bone age <13 years (boys); <11 years (girls)), psychosocial constraints permitting, i.e., not before an age corresponding to the 10th percentile of the first stage of pubertal development.
- With respect to follow-up of patients previously treated, while no hard evidence of testicular damage has been established after androgen treatment in tall boys, the finding in one study of marginally

elevated FSH levels along with normal sperm counts, testicular volumes and endocrinological parameters including inhibin B levels, warrants further study. In view of an association between use of oral contraceptives (OCs) at a young age and duration of OC use with increased risk of breast cancer (but reduced risk of ovarian cancer) there is a need for long-term follow-up of individuals treated with pharmacological doses of estrogens.

- Meta-analysis of follow-up studies in many countries, as well as combining disease registries for cancer and cardiovascular disorders, may give important information of relevance to concerns of patient support groups.

REFERENCES

● = Seminal primary article
◆ = Key review paper
✳ = First formal publication of a management guideline

◆   1   Tanner JM. *Growth at adolescence*, 2nd ed. Oxford: Blackwell, 1962.

◆   2   Mascie-Taylor CGN. Biosocial influences on stature: a review. *J Bio Soc Sci* 1991; **23**: 113–28.

3   Sorva R, Tolppanen EM, Lankinen S, Perheentupa J. Growth evaluation: parent and child specific height standards. *Arch Dis Child* 1989; **64**: 1483–7.

4   Luo ZC, Albertsson-Wikland K, Karlberg J. Target height as predicted by parental heights in a population-based study. *Pediatr Res* 1998; **44**: 563–71.

●   5   Fredriks AM, Van Buuren S, Burgmeijer RJ, *et al.* Continuing positive secular growth change in The Netherlands 1955–1997. *Pediatr Res* 2000; **47**: 316–23.

6   Garralda MD. Evolution of human height. In: Hernandez M, Argente J, eds. *Human Growth: Basic and Clinical Aspects.* Amsterdam: Elsevier Science Publishers, 1998: 135–42.

7   Styne DM, McHenry H. The evolution of stature in humans. *Horm Res* 1993; **39(suppl)**: 3–6.

●   8   Maat GJR. Male stature; a parameter of health and wealth in the low countries 1950–1977 AD. In: Metz WH ed. *Wealth, Health and Human Remains in Archeology.* Symposium Nederlands Museum Anthrop. Praehist. Amsterdam 2003.

9   Albertsson-Wikland, Rosberg S. Analyses of 24-hour growth hormone profiles in children: relation to growth. *J Clin Endocrinol Metab* 1988; **67**: 493–500.

10   Rochiccioli P, Messina A, Tauber MT, Enjaume C. Correlation of parameters of 24-hour growth hormone secretion with growth velocity in 93 children of varying height. *Horm Res* 1989; **31**: 115–8.

11   Tauber M, Pienkowski C, Rochiccioli P. Growth hormone secretion in children and adolescents with familial tall stature. *Eur J Pediatr* 1994; **153**: 311–6.

12   Gourmelen M, Le Bouc Y, Girard F, Binoux M. Serum levels of insulin-like growth factor (IGF) and IGF binding protein in constitutionally tall children and adolescents. *J Clin Endocrinol Metab* 1984; **59**: 1197–203.

13   Bentov I, Werner H. IGF, IGF receptor and overgrowth syndromes. *Pediatr Endocrinol Rev* 2004; **1**: 352–60.

14   Garrone S, Radetti G, Sidoti M, *et al.* Increased insulin-like growth factor (IGF)-II and IGF/IGF-binding protein ratio in prepubertal constitutionally tall children. *J Clin Endocrinol Metab* 2002; **87**: 5455–60.

●   15   Conte FA, Grumbach MM, Ito Y, *et al.* A syndrome of female pseudohermaphrodism, hypergonadotropic hypogonadism, and multicystic ovaries associated with missense mutations in the gene oncoding aromatase (P450arom). *J Clin Endocrinol Metab* 1994; **78**: 1287–92.

●   16   Smith EP, Boyd J, Frank GR, *et al.* Estrogen resistance caused by a mutation in the estrogen-receptor gene in a man. *N Engl J Med* 1994; **331**: 1056–61.

●   17   Zachmann M, Prader A, Sobel EH, *et al.* Pubertal growth in patients with androgen insensitivity: indirect evidence for the importance of estrogens in pubertal growth of girls. *J Pediatr* 1986; **108**: 694–7.

●   18   Ogata T, Matsuo M, Muroya K, *et al.* 47,XXX male: A clinical and molecular study. *Am J Med Genet* 2001; **1**: 98: 353–6.

19   Tanner JM, Whitehouse RH, Cameron N, *et al. Assessment of Skeletal Maturity and Prediction of Adult Height (TW2-method).* London: Academic Press; 1983.

20   Bayley N, Pinneau S. Tables for predicting adult height from skeletal age. *J Pediatr* 1952; **40**: 423–41.

21   Roche AF, Davila GH, Eyman SL. A comparison between Greulich–Pyle and Tanner–Whitehouse assessments of skeletal maturity. *Radiology* 1971; **98**: 272–80.

22   Kemperdick HF. Skelettalter-Bestimmung bei Kindern mit normalen und abweichendem Wachtumsverlauf. *Fortschr Med* 1981; **99**: 152–6.

23   Wenzel A, Melsen B. Replicability of assessing radiographs by the Tanner Whitehouse-2 method. *Hum Biol* 1982; **54**: 575–81.

●   24   Buckler JM. How to make most of bone ages? *Arch Dis Child* 1983; **58**: 761–7.

25   Van Rijn RR, Lequin MH, Robben SGF, *et al.* Is the Greulich and Pyle atlas still valid for Dutch caucasian children today? *Pediatr Radiol* 2001; **31**: 748–52.

●   26   Waal de WJ, Greyn-Fokker MH, Toolens AMP, *et al.* Accuracy of final height prediction and effect of growth reductive therapy in 362 constitutionally tall children. *J Clin Endocrinol Metab* 1996; **81**: 1206–16.

27   Waal de WJ, Stijnen Th, Lucas IS, *et al.* A new model to predict final height in constitutionally tall children. *Acta Pediatr* 1996; **85**: 889–93.

27a   Van Teunenbroek A, De Waal WJ, Roks A, *et al.* Computer aided skeletal age scores in healthy children, girls with Turner syndrome and children with constitutional tall statue. *Pediatr Res* 1996; **39**: 360–7.

28   Sotos JF. Overgrowth disorders. *Clin Pediatr (Phila)* 1996; **35**: 517–29.

29   Cohen MM Jr, Neri G, Weksberg R. *Chromosomal Disorders with Overgrowth. Overgrowth Syndromes.* Oxford: Oxford University Press, 2002: 161–5.

30   Dickerman Z, Loewinger J, Laron Z. The pattern of growth in children with constitutionally tall stature from birth to age 9 years. A longitudinal study. *Acta Paediatr Scand* 1984; **73**: 530–6.

31   In 't Veld P, Brandenburg H, Verhoeff A, *et al.* Sex chromosomal abnormalities and intracytoplasmic sperm injection. *Lancet* 1995; **346**: 773.

32   Ratcliffe SG, Pan H, McKie M. Growth during puberty in the XYY boy. *Ann Hum Biol* 1992; **19**: 579–87.

33   Linden MG, Bender BG, Harmon RJ, *et al.* 47,XXX: what is the prognosis? *Pediatrics* 1988; **82**: 619–30.

34   Kanaka-Gantenbein C, Kitsiou S, Mavrou A, *et al.* Tall stature, insulin resistance, and disturbed behavior in a girl with the triple X syndrome harboring three SHOX genes: offspring of a father with mosaic Klinefelter syndrome but with two maternal X chromosomes. *Horm Res* 2004; **61**: 205–10.

35   Rooman RP, Van Driessche K, Du Caju MV. Growth and ovarian function in girls with 48,XXXX karyotype – patient report and review of the literature. *J Pediatr Endocrinol Metab* 2002; **15**: 1051–5.

36   Borgaonkar DS, Shah SA. The XYY chromosome male – or syndrome? *Prog Med Genet* 1974; **10**: 135–222.

● 37   Kurotaki N, Imaizumi K, Harada N, *et al.* Haploinsufficiency of NSD1 causes Sotos syndrome. *Nat Genet* 2002; **30**: 365–6.

38   Visser R, Matsumoto N. Genetics of Sotos syndrome. *Curr Opin Pediatr* 2003; **15**: 598–606.

● 39   Douglas J, Hanks S, Temple IK, *et al.* NSD1 mutations are the major cause of Sotos syndrome and occur in some cases of Weaver syndrome but are rare in other overgrowth phenotypes. *Am J Hum Genet* 2003; **72**: 132–43.

40   Rio M, Clech L, Amiel J, *et al.* Spectrum of NSD1 mutations in Sotos and Weaver syndromes. *J Med Genet* 2003; **40**: 436–40.

● 41   Williams DK, Carlton DR, Green SH, *et al.* Marshall–Smith Syndrome: the expanding phenotype. *J Med Genet* 1997; **34**: 842–5.

42   Baujat G, Rio M, Rossignol S, *et al.* Paradoxical NSD1 mutations in Beckwith–Wiedemann syndrome and 11p15 anomalies in Sotos syndrome. *Am J Hum Genet* 2004; **74**: 715–20.

43   Collod-Beroud G, Le Bourdelles S, Ades L, *et al.* Update of the UMD-FBN1 mutation database and creation of an FBN1 polymorphism database. *Hum Mutat* 2003; **22**: 199–208.

44   Beighton P, de Paepe A, Danks D, *et al.* International Nosology of Heritable Disorders of Connective Tissue, Berlin, 1986. *Am J Med Genet* 1988; **29**: 581–94.

45   De Paepe A, Devereux RB, Dietz HC, *et al.* Revised diagnostic criteria for the Marfan syndrome. *Am J Med Genet* 1996; **62**: 417–26.

∗ 46   Knudtzon J, Aarskog D. Estrogen treatment of excessively tall girls with Marfan syndrome. *Acta Paediatr Scand* 1988; **77**: 537–41.

47   Bongarzone I, Vigano E, Alberti L, *et al.* Full activation of MEN2B mutant RET by an additional MEN2A mutation or by ligand GDNF stimulation. *Oncogene* 1998; **16**: 2295–301.

48   Topaloglu AK, Sansaricq C, Snyderman SE. Influence of metabolic control on growth in homocystinuria due to cystathionine B-synthase deficiency. *Pediatr Res* 2001; **49**: 796–8.

● 49   Morishima A, Grumbach MM, Simpson ER, *et al.* Aromatase deficiency in male and female siblings caused by a novel mutation and the physiological role of estrogens. *J Clin Endocrinol Metab* 1995; **80**: 3689–98.

∗ 50   Carani C, Qin K, Simoni M. Effect of testosterone and estradiol in a man with aromatase deficiency. *N Engl J Med* 1997; **337**: 91–5.

51   Daughaday W. Pituitary gigantism. *Endocrinol Metab Clin North Am* 1992; **21**: 633–47.

52   Moran A, Asa SL, Kovacs K, *et al.* Gigantism due to pituitary mammosomatotroph hyperplasia. *N Engl J Med* 1990; **323**: 322–7.

53   Zimmerman D, Young WF, Ebersold MJ, *et al.* Congenital gigantism due to growth hormone-releasing hormone excess and pituitary hyperplasia with adenomatous transformation. *J Clin Endocrinol Metab* 1993; **76**: 216–22.

54   Drimmie FM, MacLennan AC, Nicoll JA, *et al.* Gigantism due to growth hormone excess in a boy with optic glioma. *Clin Endocrinol* 2000; **53**: 535–8.

55   Lyons J, Landis CA, Harsh G, *et al.* Two G protein oncogenes in human endocrine tumors. *Science* 1990; **249**: 655–9.

56   Landis CA, Harsh G, Lyons J, *et al.* Clinical characteristics of acromegalic patients who's pituitary tumors contain mutant Gs protein. *J Clin Endocrinol Metab* 1990; **71**: 1416–20.

● 57   Landis CA, Masters SB, Spada A, *et al.* GTPase inhibiting mutations of the stimulatory G protein activate the alpha chain of Gs and stimulate adenylyl cyclase in human pituitary tumours. *Nature* 1989; **340**: 692–6.

58   Cuttler L, Jackson JA, Saeed-us Zafar, *et al.* Hypersecretion of growth hormone and prolactin in McCune–Albright syndrome. *J Clin Endocrinol Metab* 1989; **68**: 1148–54.

59   Dötsch J, Kiess W, Hanze J, *et al.* G$_s$ alpha mutation at codon 201 in pituitary adenoma causing gigantism in a 6-year-old boy with McCune Albright syndrome. Clinical Case Seminar. *J Clin Endocrinol Metab* 1996; **81**: 3839–42.

● 60   Weinstein LS, Shenker A, Gejman PV, *et al.* Activating mutations of the stimulatory G protein in the McCune Albright syndrome. *N Engl J Med* 1991; **325**: 1688–95.

61   Shenker A, Weinstein LS, Sweet DE, Spiegel AM. An activating Gs alpha mutation is present in fibrous dysplasia of bone in the McCune Albright syndrome. *J Clin Endocrinol Metab* 1994; **79**: 750–5.

62   Shenker A, Weinstein LS, Moran A, *et al.* Severe endocrine and non-endocrine manifestations of the McCune Albright

syndrome associated with activating mutations of stimulatory G protein Gs. *J Pediatr* 1993; **123**: 509–18.

63 Scheithauer BW, Kovacs K, Randall RV, *et al.* Hypothalamic neuronal hamartoma and adenohypophysis choristoma: their association with growth hormone adenoma of the pituitary gland. *J Neuropath Exp Neurol* 1983; **42**: 648–63.

64 Garcia-Luna PP, Leal-Cerro A, Montero C, *et al.* A rare cause of acromegaly: ectopic production of growth hormone-releasing factor by a bronchial carcinoid tumor. *Surg Neurol* 1987; **27**: 563–8.

65 Sano T, Asa SL, Kovacs K. Growth hormone-releasing hormone producing tumors: clinical, biochemical, and morphological manifestations. *Endocr Rev* 1988; **9**: 357–73.

66 Asa SL, Scheithauer BW, Bilbao JM, *et al.* A case for hypothalamic acromegaly: a clinicopathological study of six patients with hypothalamic gangliocytomas producing growth hormone-releasing factor. *J Clin Endocrinol Metab* 1984; **58**: 796–803.

67 Pieters GFFM, Smals AGH, Kloppenborg PWC. Defective suppression of growth hormone after oral glucose loading in adolescence. *J Clin Endocrinol Metab* 1980; **51**: 265–70.

68 Evain-Brion D, Garnier P, Schimpff RM, *et al.* Growth hormone response to thyrotropin-releasing hormone and oral glucose. Loading tests in tall children and adolescents. *J Clin Endocrinol Metab* 1983; **56**: 429–32.

◆ 69 Drop SL, De Waal WJ, De Muinck Keizer-Schrama SM. Sex steroid treatment of constitutionally tall stature. *Endocr Rev* 1998; **19**: 540–58.

70 Humpreys LG, Davey TC, Park RK. Longitudinal correlation analysis of standing height and intelligence. *Child Dev* 1985; **56**: 1465–78.

71 Taesdale TW, Owen DR, Sornssen TIA. Intelligence and educational level in adult males at the extremes of stature. *Hum Biol* 1991; **63**: 19–30.

72 Hensley WE, Cooper R. Height and occupational success: a review and critique. *Psychol Rep* 1987; **60**: 843–9.

73 Brooks-Gunn J, Warren MP. The psychological significance of secondary sexual characteristics in nine-to eleven-year-old girls. *Child Dev* 1988; **59**: 1061–9.

74 Blyth DA, Simmons RG, Bulcroft R, *et al.* The effect of physical development on self-image and satisfaction with body-image for early adolescent males. *Res Comm Health* 1982; **2**: 43–73.

75 Davies E, Furnham A. Body satisfaction in adolescent girls. *Br J Med Psychol* 1986; **59**: 279–87.

76 Martin S, Housley K, McCoy H, *et al.* Self-esteem of adolescent girls as related to weight. *Percept Mot Skills* 1988; **67**: 879–84.

∗ 77 Goldzieher M. Treatment of excessive growth in the adolescent female. *J Clin Endocrinol* 1956; **16**: 249–52.

78 Zachmann M, Ferrandez A, Mürset G, Prader A. Estrogen treatment of excessively tall girls. *Helv Paediat Acta* 1975; **30**: 11–30.

∗ 79 Zachmann M, Ferrandez A, Mürset G, *et al.* Testosterone treatment of excessively tall boys. *J Pediatr* 1976; **88**: 116–23.

● 80 Wettenhall HNB, Cahill C, Roche AF. Tall girls: A survey of 15 years of management and treatment. *J Pediatr* 1975; **86**: 602–10.

81 Bierich JR. Estrogen treatment of girls with constitutional tall stature. *Pediatrics* 1978; **62**: 1196–201.

82 Sorgo W, Scholler K, Heinze F, *et al.* Critical analysis of height reduction in oestrogen-treated tall girls. *Eur J Pediat* 1984; **142**: 206–65.

● 83 Grüters A, Heidemann P, Schlüter H, *et al.* Effect of different oestrogen doses on final height reduction in girls with constitutional tall stature. *Eur J Ped* 1989; **49**: 11–3.

84 Brämswig JH, Schellong G, Borger HJ, Breu H. Testosteron-Therapie hochwüchsiger Jungen. Ergebnisse bei 25 Jungen. *Dtsch Med Wschr* 1981; **106**: 1656–61.

85 Greulich WW, Pyle SI. *Radiographic Atlas of Skeletal Development of the Hand and Wrist,* 2nd ed. Stanford: Stanford University Press; 1959.

● 86 Decker R, Partsch CJ, Sippell WG. Combined treatment with testosterone (T) and ethinylestradiol (EE2) in constitutionally tall boys: is treatment with T plus EE2 more effective in reducing final height in tall boys than T alone? *J Clin Endocrinol Metab* 2002; **87**: 1634–9.

87 Hanker JP, Schellong G, Schneider HPG. The functional state of the hypothlamo-pituitary axis after high dose oestrogen therapy in excessively tall girls. *Acta Endocrinol* 1979; **91**: 19–29.

88 Bramswig JH, Nieschlag E, Schellong G. Pituitary–gonadal function in boys after high dose testosterone treatment for excessively tall stature. *Acta Endocrinol* 1984; **107**: 97–103.

89 Binder G, Grauer ML, Wehner AV, *et al.* Outcome in tall stature. Final height and psychological aspects in 220 patients with and without treatment. *Eur J Pediatr* 1997; **156**: 905–10.

90 Weimann E, Bergmann S, Bohles HJ. Oestrogen treatment of constitutional tall stature: a risk–benefit ratio. *Arch Dis Child* 1998; **78**: 148–51.

91 Waal de WJ, Torn M, Muinck Keizer-Schrama de SMPF, *et al.* Long term sequelae of sex steroid treatment in the management of constitutionally tall stature. *Arch Dis Child* 1995; **73**: 311–5.

● 92 Venn A, Bruinsma F, Werther G, *et al.* Oestrogen treatment to reduce the adult height of tall girls: long-term effects on fertility. *Lancet* 2004; **364**: 1513–8.

93 Waal de WJ, Vreeburg JTM, Bekkering F, *et al.* High dose testosterone therapy for reduction of final height in constitutionally tall boys: does it influence testicular function in adulthood? *Clin Endocrinol* 1995; **43**: 87–95.

∗ 94 Plaschaert VF, van der Eijken JW, Odink RJ, *et al.* Bilateral epiphysiodesis around the knee as treatment for excessive height in boys. *J Pediatr Orthop B* 1997; 6: 212–4.

∗ 95 Arafah BM, Brodkey JS, Kaufman B, *et al.* Transsphenoidal microsurgery in the treatment of acromegaly and gigantism. *J Clin Endocrinol Metab* 1980; **50**: 578–85.

∗ 96 Lüdeke DK, Herrmann HD, Schulte FJ. Special problems with neurosurgical treatments of hormone-secretion pituitary adenomas in children. *Prog Exp Tumor Res* 1987; **30**: 362–70.

∗ 97   Ritzen EM, Wettrell G, Davies G, *et al*. Management of pituitary gigantism. The role of bromocriptine and radiotherapy. *Acta Paediatr Scand* 1985; **74**: 807–14.

98   Gelber SJ, Heffez DS, Donohoue A. Pituitary gigantism caused by growth hormone excess from infancy. *J Pediatr* 1992; **120**: 931–4.

99   Schoof E, Dorr HG, Kiess W, *et al*. Five-year follow-up of a 13-year-old boy with a pituitary adenoma causing gigantism – effect of octreotide therapy. *Horm Res* 2004; **61**: 184–9.

● 100   Consensus statement. Biochemical assessment and long-term monitoring in patients with acromegaly: statement from a joint consensus conference of the GH research society and the pituitary society. *J Clin Endocrinol Metab* 2004; **89**: 3099–102.

101   Muller AF, Van Der Lely AJ. Pharmacological therapy for acromegaly: a critical review. *Drugs* 2004; **64**: 1817–38.

102   Shalet SM. Pituitary adenomas in childhood. *Acta Endocrinol (Copenh)* 1986; **79**: 750–5.

47

Surgical management of tall stature

M F MACNICOL

INTRODUCTION

The etiology of tall stature has already been discussed in Chapters 18 and 46, including its medical management. The surgical approach to the problem is constrained by the risks of surgery, particularly those attendant upon shortening the femur or tibia by excision of a segment of bone. Thus, the only absolute indication for reducing the length of a limb, whether by growth arrest or shortening, is in significant hemihypertrophy. Overgrowth (gigantism) of a limb produces disproportionate enlargement of part or all of the extremity. Only the skeletal elements may be involved, with apparently normal soft tissue, or there may be additional enlargement with fat, lymphedema or angioma formation. By definition, the affected limb is larger than the normal side, although in rare instances both legs may be enlarged. The correct height of the child or adult can be gauged from the span of the outstretched arms, and thence the decision made to label the leg hypertrophic if its contribution causes the estimated height to be exceeded. In the absence of neurological deficit or systemic disease, which may produce atrophy, any discrepancy in length can be ascribed to the oversized limb, which is therefore labelled as hemihypertrophy.

INDICATIONS

A relative indication for correcting tall stature surgically arises when the child (and parents) is distressed by the prospect of increased height. Arbitrarily, a projected height at maturity of 185 cm (6 feet 1 inch) in women and over 213 cm (7 feet) in men would make a reduction in height appropriate. Obviously, athleticism and good coordination mitigate the concern, particularly if competitive sport is possible to a high standard. But if muscle weakness, angulatory deformity of the limb and poor posture are associated with tall stature, the condition may be poorly tolerated, making surgical intervention justified. In certain skeletal dysplasias, particularly Marfan syndrome with its associated ligament laxity, bilateral epiphysiodeses are relatively simple to perform. Similarly, acquired forms of gigantism, including those secondary to vascular stimulus (for example, arteriovenous shunts and hemangiomas), may be reduced by surgical techniques.

The operations described for slowing growth or shortening a limb properly apply to discrepancies in length of one or both segments. Yet in the management of tall stature there may occasionally be a place for epiphysiodesis above and below both knees[1] if there is sufficient growth remaining (Fig. 47.1) [2,3] to produce a reduction in height of 5 cm or more. The decision is not an easy one to make, and no reduction in spinal growth can be effected. In addition, the arms may appear disproportionately long if the legs are shortened significantly.

This chapter deals with the relatively atraumatic procedure of percutaneous epiphysiodesis (growth plate arrest) as it may be applied to tall stature. The operation is preferred to stapling of the growth plate[4] which does not guarantee predictable tethering of the physis, so that angular deformity or inadequate shortening may result. Surgical shortening techniques are also outlined.

EPIPHYSIODESIS

The relative contributions of the growth plates to lower limb elongation in normal children indicate that 65 percent

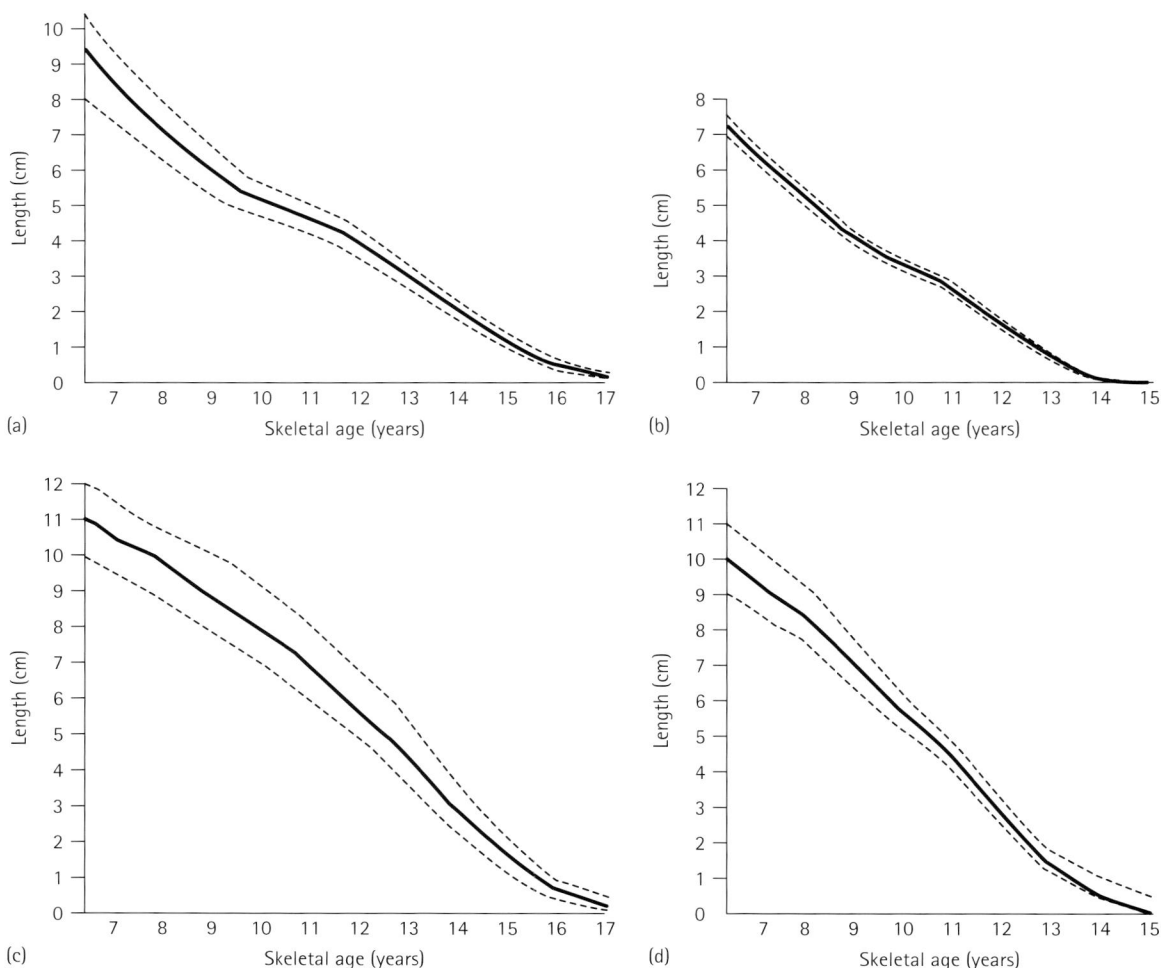

Figure 47.1 'Growth remaining' curves for the (c, d) distal femur and (a, b) proximal tibia in (a, c) boys and (b, d) girls.

of growth occurs around the knee with the distal femur providing 37 percent and the proximal tibia 28 percent. Westh and Menelaus[5] have pointed out that epiphysiodesis will produce about a 1 cm (3/8 inch) reduction of growth annually at the lower femur, from the ages of 10 to 14 years in girls and 12 to 16 in boys, and in the upper tibia the retardation per annum is 0.7 cm (1/4 inch). Combined and bilateral epiphysiodeses at the age of 10 years would therefore reduce height by some 7 cm in a girl, although rather more than if she was very tall for her age. Epiphysiodesis before the age of 10 years is rarely indicated, but is theoretically appropriate if height is likely to be excessive.

The first description of permanent growth arrest is credited to Phemister[6] who termed it 'epiphysiodiaphysial fusion'. The operation required incisions on either side of the limb, and over each growth plate. A block of bone was excised with an osteotome, and through these medial and lateral windows the growth plate was excised and curetted out, before reinserting the bone blocks (turned through 90° to augment the arrest) and closing the wound. Morbidity

after the operation was considerable, and stiffness of the knee, although temporary, was increased by the need to splint the limb with a plaster cylinder for 6 weeks.

A percutaneous epiphysiodesis was pioneered by Bowen and Johnson,[7] using curettage through cortical holes under image intensifier control. The procedure still requires medial and lateral incisions and newer modifications, using powered reamers and burrs, are hazardous. A newly developed tubesaw[8,9] makes it possible to approach the growth plate from the lateral side only, providing an aperture in the bone large enough to permit further curettage of the growth plate without resorting to the potentially risky use of a dental burr or other powered instrumentation.

TECHNIQUE

The operation is performed with the patient anesthetized on a radiolucent table and the image intensifier positioned over the knee. The limbs are prepared and draped after

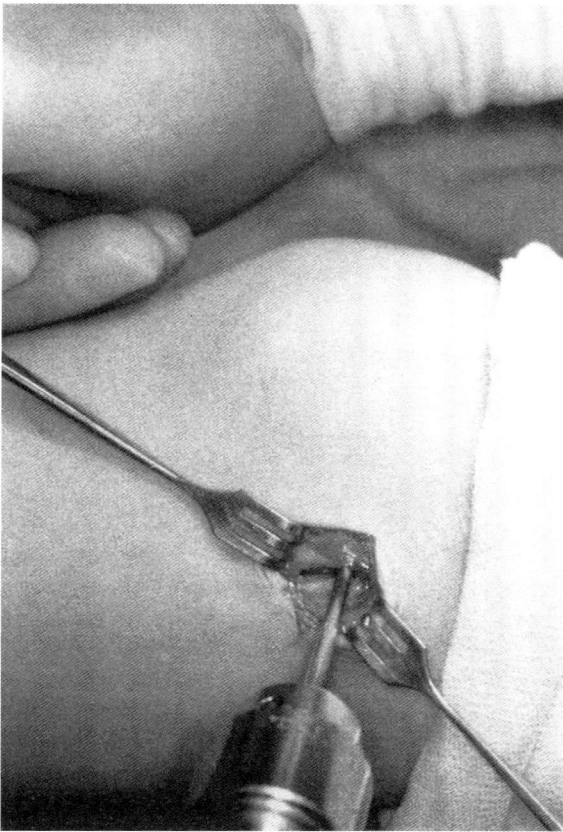

Figure 47.2   The guidewire is inserted across the growth plate by hand, using a Jacob's chuck. The illustration shows the lateral side of the distal femur.

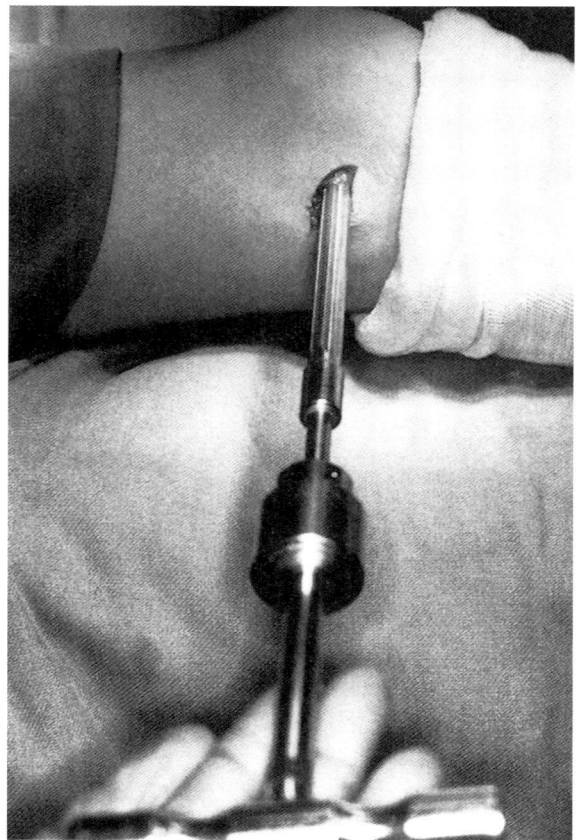

Figure 47.3   The tubesaw is driven across the femur, again by hand.

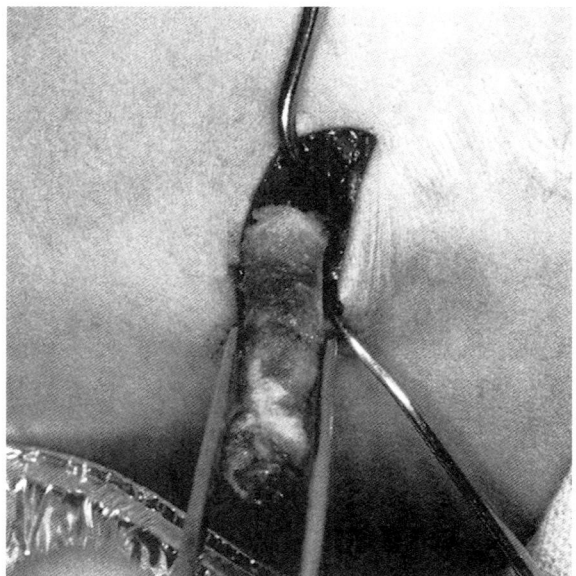

Figure 47.4   The core of cancellous bone contains the spiralling white line of the growth plate cartilage (seen between the teeth of the forceps).

exsanguination, and inflation of the upper thigh tourniquet. As the procedure takes about 15 min per epiphysiodesis, the tourniquets can be inflated together for those cases where bilateral operations are planned for tall stature because the procedure is completed in 1 h.

A 2 cm incision is placed longitudinally over the growth plate, and the periosteum exposed by gentle spreading with dissecting scissors. The growth plate is revealed by dividing the periosteal sleeve, midway between the anterior and posterior surfaces of the bone.

Using a guidewire and centralizing cylinder (Fig. 47.2) short tubes of cancellous bone are cored out across the crescent of the growth plate (Fig. 47.3).

The removed core of bone should demonstrate a spiral 'white line' of growth cartilage contained within the cancellous bone (Fig. 47.4). A small curette is used to clear away further accessible portions of the growth plate, thus ensuring sufficient ablation of the physis. The bone plug is replaced within the tunnel. The proximal fibular growth plate should be excised with a scalpel through the same lateral wound, which offers access to the tibia. Immobilization of the knees is unnecessary, but elbow crutches should be provided until the patient is walking comfortably, usually 2–3 weeks after the operation.

The ablation of the growth plate becomes apparent in 3–6 months and can be demonstrated more readily with magnetic resonance imaging or computed tomography scanning than with conventional radiography. It is customary to monitor the correction of leg length discrepancy with leg length films (scanograms) postoperatively (Fig. 47.5), but in the case of tall stature the only measurement is that of height. Leg lengths should remain the same if epiphysiodesis has been successful at the four sites, but it is as well to check periodically that the pelvis is level when the patient is standing.

SEGMENTAL SHORTENING

If the patient is reaching maturity or has ceased to grow, physeal arrest will be ineffective. Shortening of the femur or tibia, or of both bones, may then be appropriate for limb length discrepancy. It would be very unusual to recommend shortening for tall stature, and the operative risks merit thorough discussion. In purely surgical terms, excision of segments of up to 4.0 cm from the tibia and 5.0 cm from the femur can be safely achieved. However, shortening carries with it the risks of vascular compromise, including compartment syndrome, and muscle weakness.[10,11] These complications, and a cosmetically ugly postoperative thickening of the limb at the operative site, are unlikely if the shortening is constrained to the limits mentioned above.

A four-segment shortening would therefore produce a decrease in height of almost 10 cm (4 inches) in an adult. The

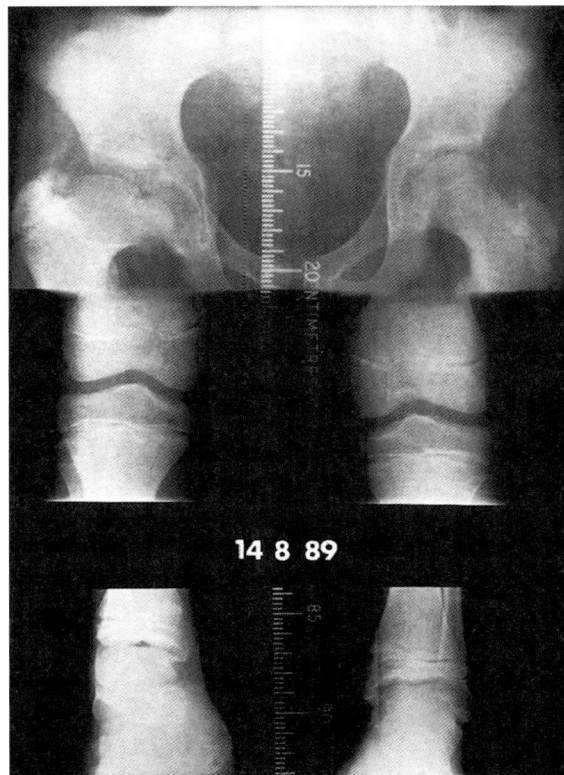

(a)

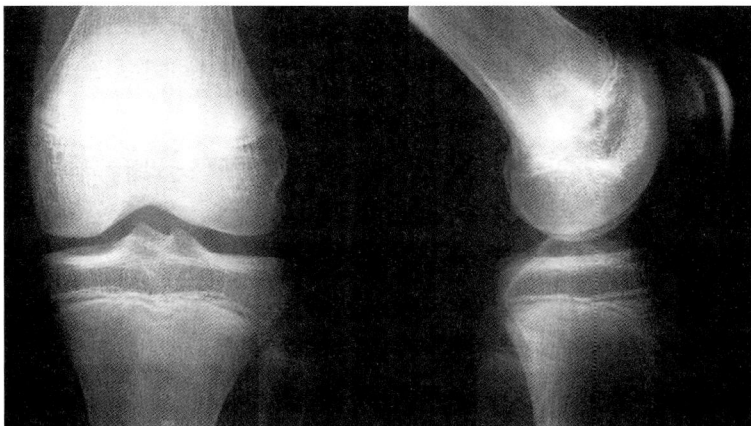

(b)

Figure 47.5 (a) Perthe's disease resulted in shortening of 2.5 cm, shown by the grid of the leg length film. (b) The radiographs, particularly the lateral projection, reveal that the growth plate is closing after a contralateral distal femoral epiphysiodesis. Note the reinserted bone plug, acting as a central physeal tether.

method would only be justifiable if tall stature was associated with leg length discrepancy or major disproportion between femoral and tibial lengths. A step-cut osteotomy (Fig. 47.6) is preferred to excision of a diametrical segment of bone if the procedure is being carried out by direct exposure of the bone to be shortened. Menelaus[12] uses an anteromedial incision and a sufficient step-cut osteotomy to provide 5–7.5 cm of bone overlap after the shortening (2.5–5.0 cm in his series). The shaft of the fibula is shortened by excising a segment from the middle of the shaft, and the tibial fragments fixed by two screws, rather than a plate. Compression plating may be used after excision of a measured length of the middle to upper tibial shaft, but the bulk of the implant leads to a greater risk of vascular compromise. Skin closure may also prove difficult.

The proximal femur is a safer site for shortening, even if the contralateral overgrowth is principally tibial. Likewise, it would be the elective site for the rare case of bilateral shortening. Wagner[11] has described the open technique which should not be placed too distal in the isthmus of the femoral shaft. The lesser trochanter with its attached iliopsoas tendon

should not be removed and hence the proximal osteotomy is made as shown in Fig. 47.7. If the distal osteotomy is carried out first, the proximal fragment can then be abducted to facilitate the step-cut osteotomy. An AO compression blade plate (Fig. 47.8) is preferred to a Richard's screw and plate device as the latter may lead on to delayed union.[13] Liposuction has been suggested if the thigh looks too squat postoperatively, but the bulk is principally muscle. The osteotomy should unite within 3 months and the implant is

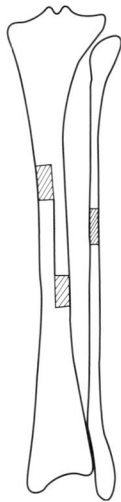

Figure 47.6 A step-cut tibial osteotomy with excision of a similar length of the fibular shaft.

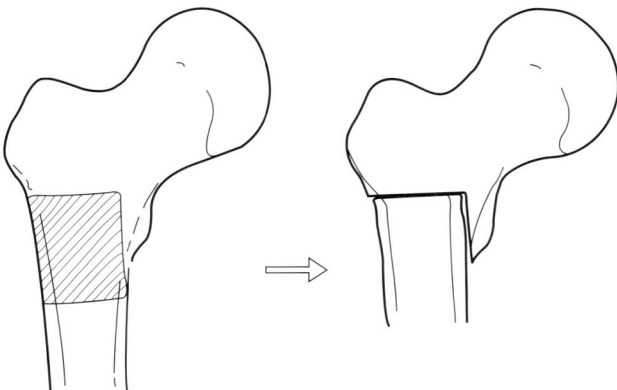

Figure 47.7 Step-cut osteotomy of the proximal femur preserving the attachment of the iliopsoas tendon.

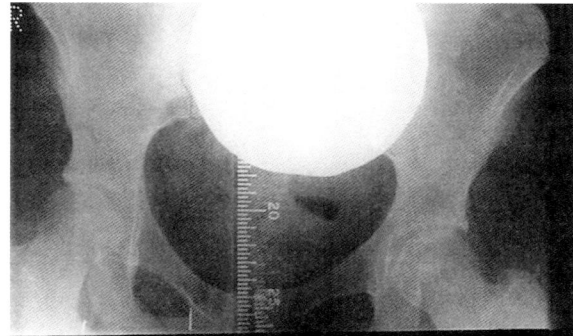

(a)

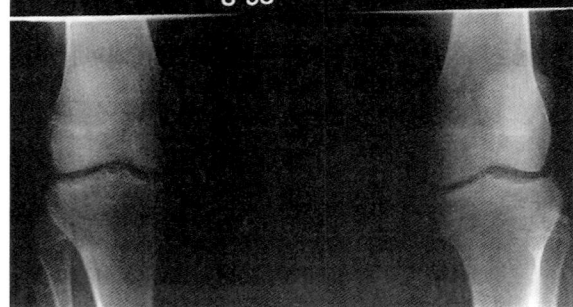

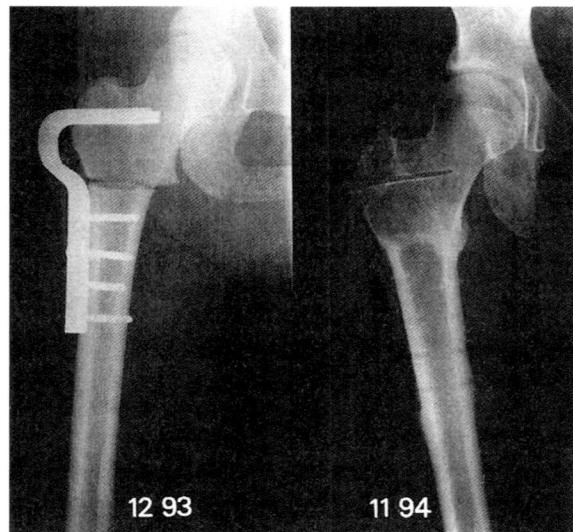

(b)

Figure 47.8 (a) Overgrowth of the right femur after a diaphyseal fracture 3 years previously, at the age of 12 years. The patient has reached maturity so that epiphysiodesis is impossible. (b) A subtrochanteric shortening of 2.5 cm was carried out using a blade plate for internal fixation.

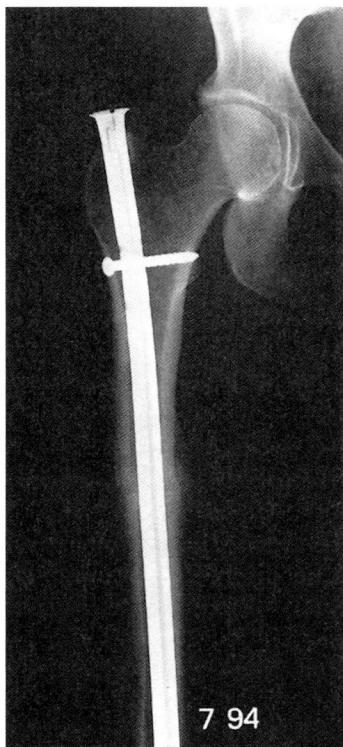

Figure 47.9 Interlocking nail fixation after femoral shortening.

removed after 1 year, once the proximal femoral shaft has remodelled.

Kuntscher[10] stimulated interest in closed femoral shortening using a specially developed intramedullary cam saw. The technique is reported for leg length discrepancy, and calls for a precise and careful use of the image intensification, guidewire, reamers, saw and intramedullary rod. Blair *et al.*[14] preferred to carry out the distal osteoclasis (breakage of the osteotomy by external, manual pressure) first, whereas Oppenheim and Namba[15] devised a series of cannulated splines that fit over the intramedullary rod, making it possible to complete the proximal osteotomy initially. The instrumentation is introduced via the piriform fossa through a 5 cm incision over the buttock, and a second incision may be required so that a small osteotome can be inserted to complete the proximal osteotomy.[16] On completing the two osteotomies the intercalary segment of bone is split longitudinally and the rod driven down to hold the two major femoral segments, once the measured, shortening segment has been displaced on either side. There must be no distraction of the residual osteotomy site and if the rod is a proper fit the patient can weight bear with crutches once the quadriceps muscle is functioning again. An interlocking nail allows greater stability after the osteotomy (Fig. 47.9). Kenwright[17] and Menelaus *et al.*[18] have suggested that femoral shortening of up to 8 cm is now safe and so the general view is that tibial shortening should be avoided whenever possible.

REFERENCES

1 Plaschaert VFP, van der Eijken JW, Odink RJH, *et al.* Bilateral epiphysiodesis around the knee as treatment for excessive height in boys. *J Pediatric Orthop B* 1997; **6**: 212–4.

2 Anderson M, Green WT, Messner MB. Growth and prediction of growth in lower extremities. *J Bone Joint Surg Am* 1963; **45**: 1–14.

3 Menelaus MB. Correction of leg length discrepancy by epiphyseal arrest. *J Bone Joint Surg Br* 1966; **48**: 336–9.

4 Blount WP, Clarke GR. Control of bone growth by epiphysial stapling. *J Bone Joint Surg Am* 1949; **31**: 464–78.

5 Westh RN, Menelaus MB. A simple calculation for the timing of epiphyseal arrest – further report. *J Bone Joint Surg Br* 1981; **63**; 117–9.

6 Phemister DB. Operative arrest of longitudinal growth of bones in the treatment of deformities, *J Bone Joint Surg Am* 1933; **15**: 1–15.

7 Bowen JR, Johnson WJ. Percutaneous epiphysiodesis. *Clin Orthop* 1984; **190**: 170–6.

8 Macnicol MF, Krishnan J, Draper ERC. Epiphysiodesis using a cannulated tubesaw: comparison with the Phemister technique. *J Paediatr Orthop B* 1993; **2**: 70–4.

9 Alexeeff M, Macnicol MF. Epiphysiodesis in the management of limb length inequality. *Curr Orthop* 1995; **9**: 178–84.

10 Kuntscher G. Intramedullary surgical technique and its place in orthopaedic surgery: My present concept. *J Bone Joint Surg Am* 1965; **47**: 809–18.

11 Wagner H. Surgical lengthening or shortening of femur and tibia; techniques and indications. In: Hungerford DS, ed. *Progress in Orthopic Surgery. Leg Length Discrepancy: the Injured Knee.* Berlin: Springer-Verlag, 1977: 71–94.

12 Broughton NS, Olney BW, Menelaus MB. Tibial shortening for leg length discrepancy. *J Bone Joint Surg Br* 1989; **71**: 242–5.

13 Jackson AM. Leg length discrepancy. In: Benson MKD, Fixsen JA, Macnicol MF, eds. *Children's Orthopaedics and Fractures,* 1st ed. Edinburgh: Churchill Livingstone, 1994: 487–502.

14 Blair VP, Schoenecker PL, Sheridan JJ, Capelli AM. Closed shortening of the femur. *J Bone Joint Surg Am* 1989; **71**: 1440–5.

15 Oppenheim WL, Namba R. Closed femoral shortening. Modification using an internal splint. *J Paediatr Orthop* 1988; **8**: 609–12.

16 Winquist RA, Hansen ST Jr, Pearson RE. Closed intramedullary shortening of the femur. *Clin Orthop* 1978; **136**: 54–61.

17 Kenwright J. Shortening by bone resection. *Semin Orthop* 1992; i: 194–200.

18 Menelaus MB, Doig WA, Oppenheim WL. Shortening procedures. Femoral shortening, tibial shortening and intra-pelvic limb shortening. In: Menelaus MB, ed. *The Management of Limb Inequality*. Edinburgh: Churchill Livingstone, 1991: 95–107.

Appendix to Chapter 12

Example of calculation of midparental height and target range (for Buckler-Tanner charts):

Parental heights: Mother 164 cm   Father 180 cm

FOR DAUGHTERS

1. Plot mother's height: 164 cm
2. Plot father's height **minus** 13 cm to give corrected height:

$$180 - 13 = 167\,\text{cm}$$

3. Plot the mid-parental height (MPH) i.e. the mean of these two measurements:

$$\text{MPH} = \frac{164 + 167}{2} = 165.5\,\text{cm}$$

4. Plot the target range (MPH $\pm$ 9 cm):

$$165.5 \pm 9 = 156.5 \text{ to } 174.5\,\text{cm}$$

FOR SONS

1. Plot father's height: 180 cm
2. Plot mother's height **plus** 13 cm to give corrected height:

$$164 + 13 = 177\,\text{cm}$$

3. Plot the mid-parental height (MPH) i.e. the mean of these two measurements:

$$\text{MPH} = \frac{180 + 177}{2} = 178.5\,\text{cm}$$

4. Plot the target range (MPH $\pm$ 10 cm):

$$178.5 \pm 10 = 168.5 \text{ to } 188.5\,\text{cm}$$

Index

Note: 'vs' indicates the differential diagnosis of conditions. Abbreviations: SGA, small-for-gestational age.

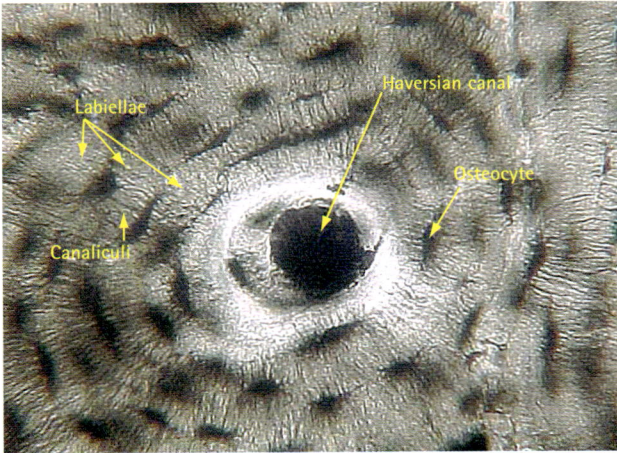

Plate 1 The osteon, or the Haversian system. A central haversian canal is surrounded by layers of lamellae and canaliculi. (This figure appears in balck and white on page 43.)

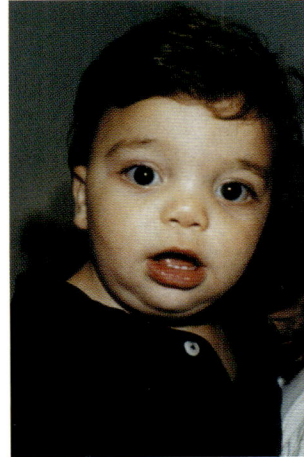

Plate 3 Boy with Aarskog syndrome. Typical facial features include hypertelorism, short nose with anteverted nares and long philtrum. (The figure appears in black and white on page 263.)

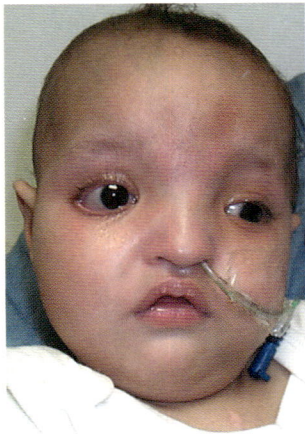

Plate 2 Infant with Wolf–Hirschhorn syndrome. Note the high forehead, prominent glabella, broad nasal root and hypertelorism (Greek helmet). (The figure appears in black and white on page 261.)

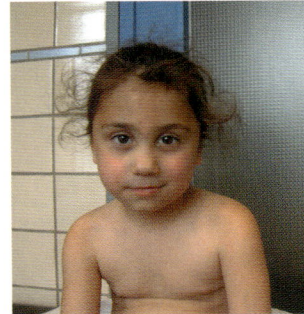

Plate 4 Girl with Albright hereditary osteodystrophy due to a mutation in the GNAS1 gene. (The figure appears in black and white on page 264.)

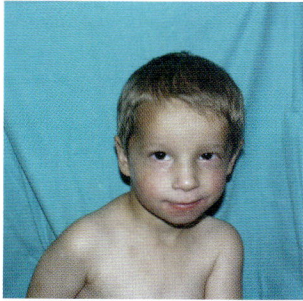

(a)

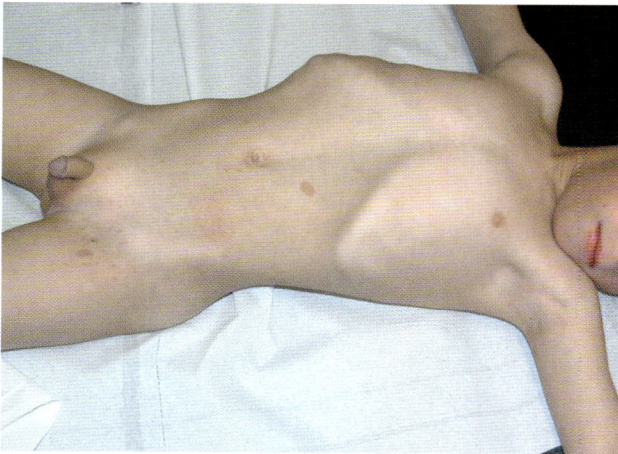

(b)

Plate 5 Boy with Bloom syndrome showing (a) the telangiectatic rash on the cheeks and (b) hyperpigmented spots on the abdomen and in the left groin. (The figure appears in black and white on page 265.)

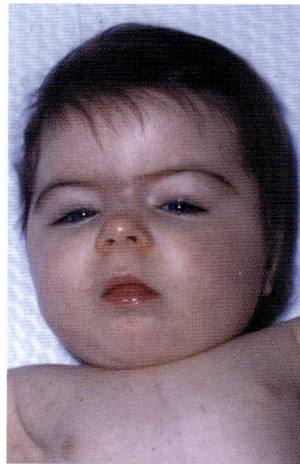

(a)

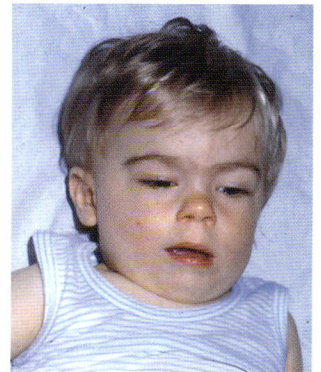

(b)

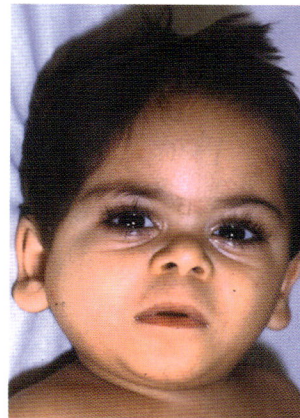

(c)

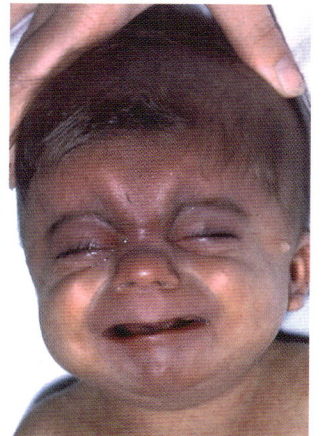

(d)

Plate 6 Typical facial features of the Brachmann–de Lange syndrome in four unrelated children. (Courtesy of J. Leroy) (The figure appears in black and white on page 267.)

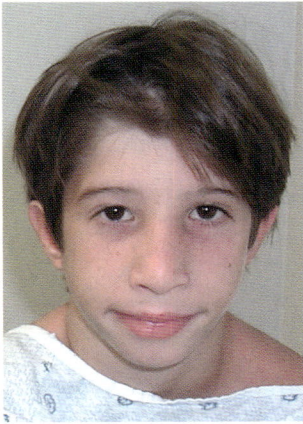

Plate 7 Patient with Dubowitz syndrome. A mild ptosis of the right upper eyelid is present. (The figure appears in black and white on page 268.)

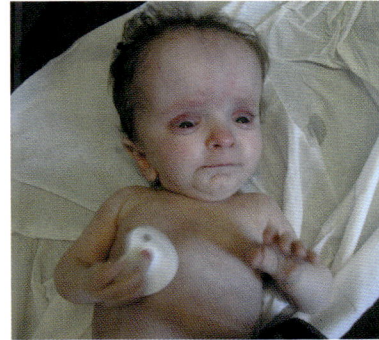

Plate 9 Infant with Wiedemann–Rautenstrauch syndrome. The skull is relatively large with high and prominent forehead, sparse hair and prominent veins. (The figure appears in black and white on page 270.)

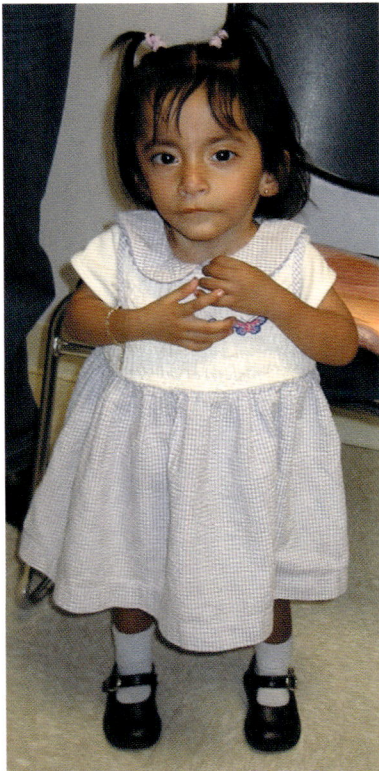

Plate 8 Girl with the Russell–Silver syndrome. (The figure appears in black and white on page 269.)

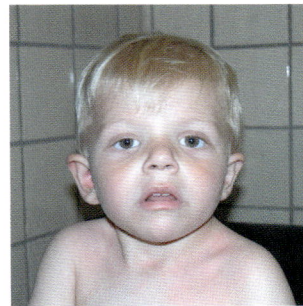

Plate 10 Typical facial features in a boy with Noonan syndrome: hypertelorism with downslanting palpebral fissures, low-set ears with thickened helix and clearly outlined philtrum. (The figure appears in black and white on page 271.)

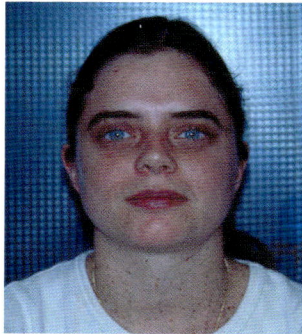

Plate 11   Woman with LEOPARD syndrome showing light-colored irides and multiple lentigines in face and neck. (The figure appears in black and white on page 271.)

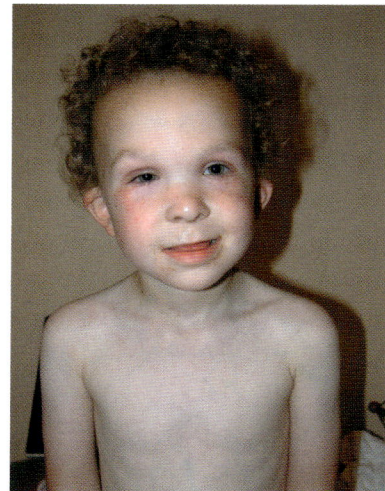

(a)

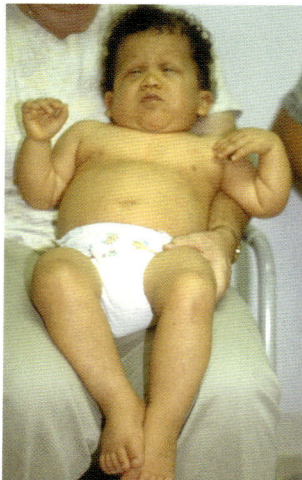

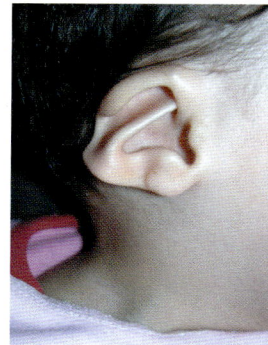

(b)

Plate 13   (a) Girl with CHARGE syndrome. Note the facial asymmetry due to paresis of the right facial nerve. (b) Typical shape of the external ear in CHARGE syndrome. (The figure appears in black and white on page 272.)

Plate 12   Coarse facial features in a child with the cardiofaciocutaneous syndrome. (The figure appears in black and white on page 272.)

(a)

(b)

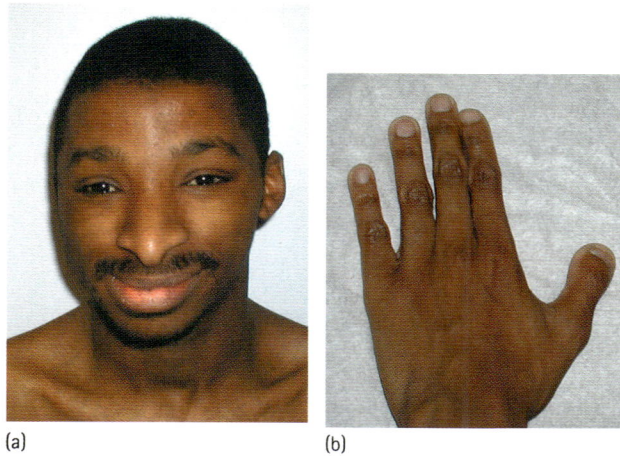

Plate 14 Boy with Rubinstein–Taybi syndrome. Note (a) the typical nose with the columella extending below the alae and (b) broad thumb. (The figure appears in black and white on page 274.)

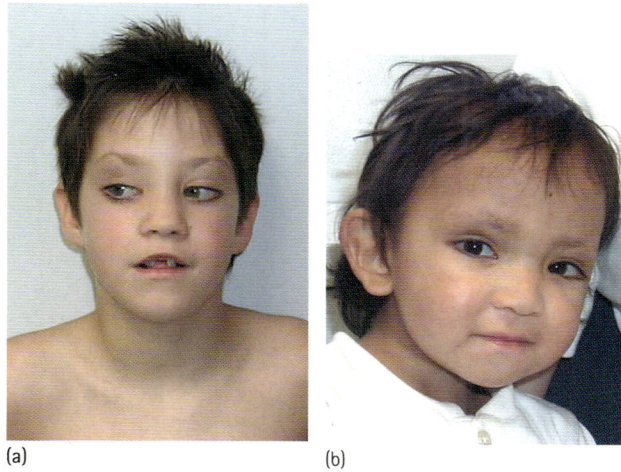

(a)

(b)

Plate 15 Two unrelated patients with Kabuki syndrome. Typical are the arched eyebrows, long palpebral fissures and eyelashes, and eversion of the lateral part of the lower eyelids. (The figure appears in black and white on page 274.)

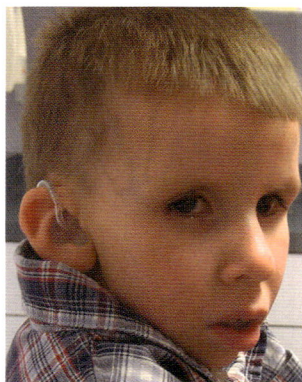

Plate 16 Characteristic facial features in a boy with Cockayne syndrome. (The figure appears in black and white on page 275.)

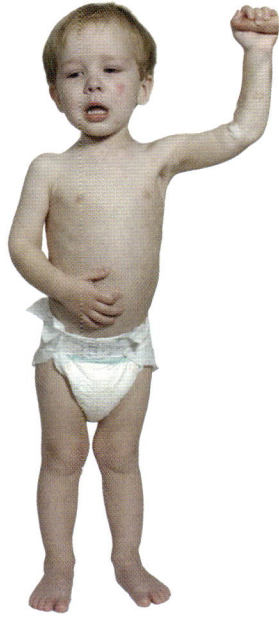

Plate 17 Child with celiac disease at presentation age 2 years. Note the misery, pallor, wasting and abdominal distension. (The figure appears in black and white on page 331.)

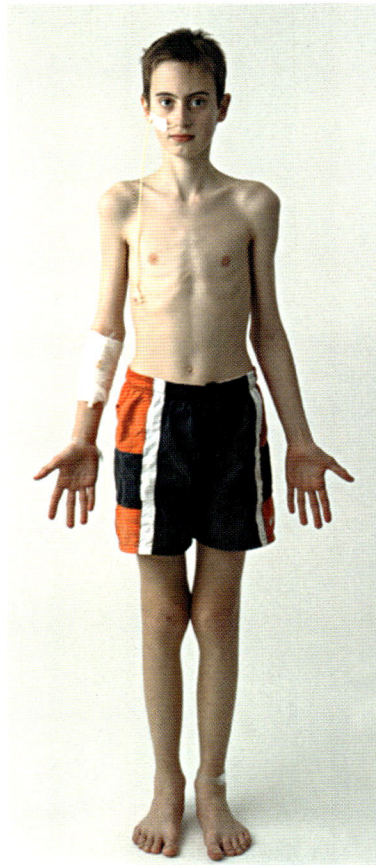

Plate 18 A 14-year-old boy with Crohn's disease at presentation. Note the pre-pubertal fascies, pallor, reduced subcutaneous fat and poor muscle bulk. (The figure appears in black and white on page 334.)

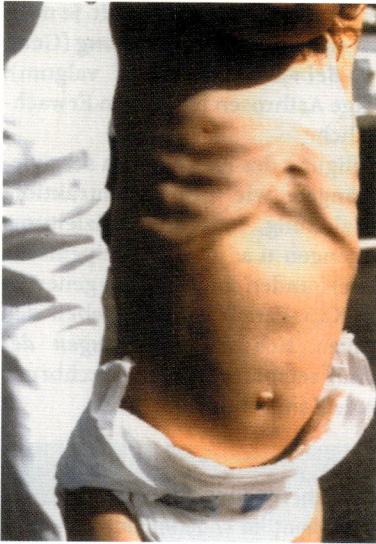

Plate 19   An 18-month-old girl with vitamin D deficiency. Costochondral enlargement of ribs from the rachitic rosary. (The figure appears in black and white on page 361.)

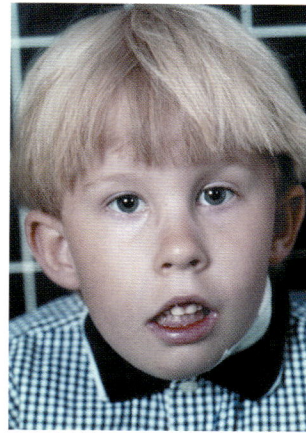

Plate 21   A boy with Prader–Willi syndrome. (The figure appears in black and white on page 527.)

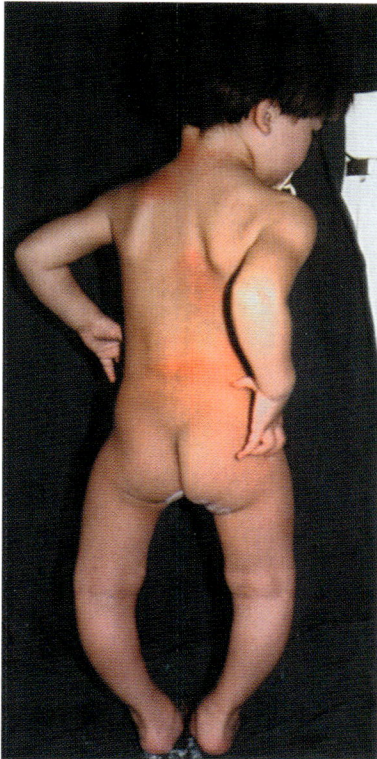

Plate 20   Extreme bowing of the femur and tibias in a 2.5-year-old girl with hypophosphatemic rickets. (The figure appears in black and white on page 365.)

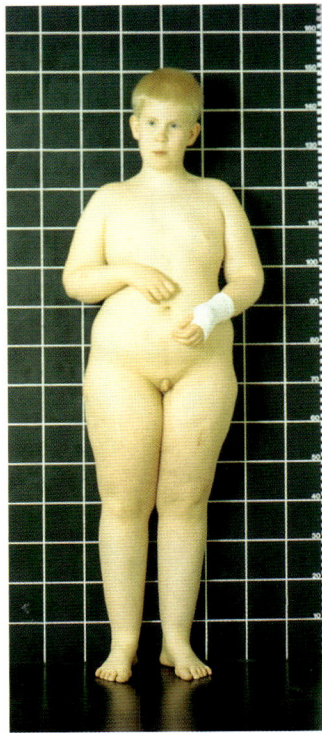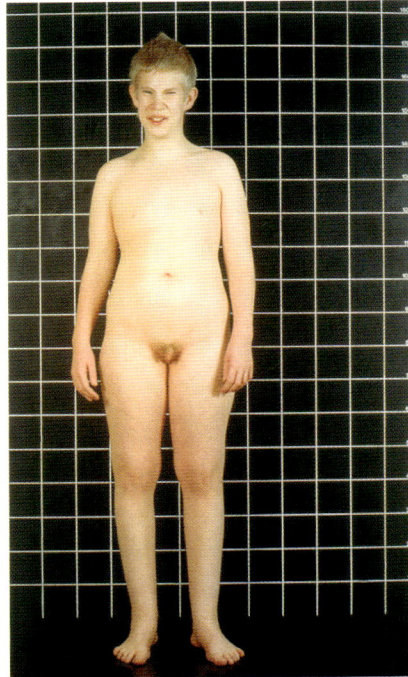

(a)   (b)

Plate 22   A boy before the start of growth hormone treatment and 1 year after commencing treatment. (The figure appears in black and white on page 532.)

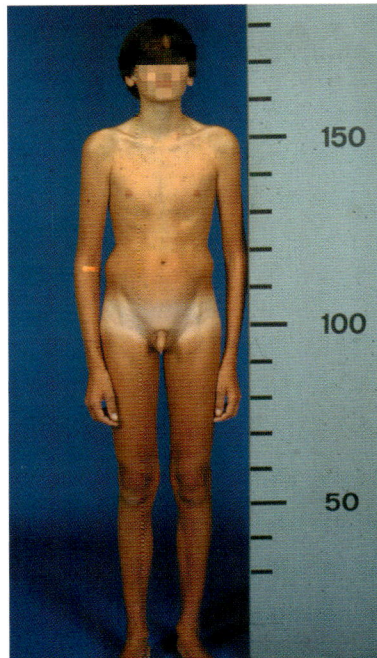

Plate 23   A boy with eunuchoidism due to hypogonadotropic hypogonadism. (The figure appears in black and white on page 598.)